VETERINARY GASTROENTEROLOGY

VETERINARY GASTROENTEROLOGY

Edited by

NEIL V. ANDERSON, D.V.M., Ph.D.

Professor
Department of Surgery and Medicine
College of Veterinary Medicine
Kansas State University
Manhattan, Kansas

Lea & Febiger   1980   Philadelphia

Library of Congress Cataloging in Publication Data
Main entry under title:

Veterinary gastroenterology.

   Includes bibliographical references and
index.
   1. Veterinary gastroenterology.
I. Anderson, Neil V. [DNLM: Gastrointestinal
diseases—Veterinary.   SF851 V586]
SF851.V45   636.089'63   79-20234
ISBN 0-8121-0632-6

Published in Great Britain by Bailliere Tindall, London

PRINTED IN THE UNITED STATES OF AMERICA

Print No.:   4   3   2   1

*Dedicated by the authors
to their spouses and families,
and to all students of veterinary medicine*

PREFACE

Veterinary gastroenterology has existed as a body of knowledge since man's earliest observations of animal disease. Early man could readily perceive the gastrointestinal system as being open-ended, with its conveyor-belt movement and clearly defined input and output. Dietary indiscretions and excesses were recognized, in both man and animals, by their cause-and-effect relationship to vomiting, diarrhea, and abdominal pain. General knowledge of gastrointestinal function preceded by centuries man's comprehension of body systems that were less accessible to observation and examination.

The recent knowledge explosion in medicine has provided impetus for the defining of a number of specialties within veterinary internal medicine. Yet veterinary gastroenterology has remained until recently an unidentified subdiscipline, without a unifying perspective. This book is written to define veterinary gastroenterology as a first approximation. Through reiteration by ourselves and others, that definition will come into clearer focus, for the benefit of society, the animals we serve, our students, and our colleagues.

It is the thesis of this book that veterinary gastroenterology is, in fact, an identifiable and understandable body of knowledge, and that the common features of gastrointestinal disease of herbivore, omnivore, and carnivore outweigh the variations and differences that seem so striking at first impression. Thus, gastroenterology is presented as the general case except where distinct species differences require separate discussion. Where that occurs, the species are usually presented in this sequence: (1) equine, (2) bovine, and (3) canine. The chapters are organized into four sections, each with its own emphasis.

The first ten chapters describe the animal patient as presented in clinical practice. History, signs of disease, and physical and laboratory examinations are described. Technique and indications for special physical examinations are discussed. Symptomatic therapy is then detailed, indicating those treatments that can be given on a rational basis even though the diagnosis has not yet been made. This first section is broad and general, emphasizing the sick animal and the ways in which veterinarians might react to that animal in the case workup. It may be most useful to the beginning student of clinical veterinary medicine, since it introduces definitions and concepts in a linear fashion and at a measured pace.

The second section consists of general topics from both preclinical and clinical sciences. Form and function of the gastrointestinal system are followed by discussions of gut microflora, pathophysiology of diarrhea, and gut function testing procedures. Strategies for parasite control, the influence of feeding practices, gastrointestinal pharmacology, and antimicrobial drugs conclude the section. These chapters provide depth of background for the didactic presentation of gastrointestinal diseases that follows.

A regional presentation of gastrointestinal diseases is made in Section Three, beginning at the mouth and proceeding aborally. Specific diseases of the several domestic species are discussed in detail, including both the similarities and differences in clinical expression. Sections Two and Three may be of interest to both practitioners and students desiring a comprehensive discussion of diseases of the digestive tract, with a discussion of basic mechanisms by which agents cause those diseases.

The fourth section explores the real and apparent relationships between the gastrointestinal and other systems. The signs of gastrointestinal disease do not arise exclusively from within the digestive tract. Section Four illustrates, again primarily for the beginning student of clinical veterinary medicine, that gastroenterology is inextricably interwoven with the state of the whole animal.

Manhattan, Kansas   Neil V. Anderson

ACKNOWLEDGMENTS

The authors are indebted to observers and investigators in many disciplines who patiently gathered the information and formulated the principles presented here. While each author has properly acknowledged sources pertinent to that chapter, a historic overview brings into perspective certain persons whose work has been critical to the advancement of veterinary gastroenterology. While no listing could be complete, to omit mention of those who have worked at the cutting edge of new knowledge would be to ignore and thus diminish their stature as veterinary gastroenterologists. Thus, the following stand unranked as our North American colleagues deserving of special mention: Alvin F. Sellers, Charles E. Stevens, Harley W. Moon, Charles E. Cornelius, D. L. Harris, Robert D. Glock, Donald L. Ross, Charles A. Mebus, Herbert J. Van Kruiningen, Robert W. Dougherty, Donald R. Strombeck, and Otto M. Radostits. The work of D. E. Kidder and F. W. G. Hill and their colleagues at Bristol has had great impact on this side of the Atlantic. To the late S. Hoflund of Stockholm, G. Esperson of Copenhagen, and G. Dirksen of Munich and their colleagues, we express our sincere appreciation.

While this textbook's contributors, with appropriate modesty, would exclude themselves from the preceding list, the editor is unburdened by such constraints. Many of the authors of *Veterinary Gastroenterology* have pioneered in the area in which they write and deserve to stand with those listed above. All of them have brought to bear on their chapter(s) the seasoned experience necessary to convey understanding to the reader. I hold them in high regard for their willingness to participate.

In offering *Veterinary Gastroenterology* to the reader, I invite comment and criticism. For whatever help you may receive from it, appreciation is due to the authors. For error or poor judgment, the responsibility is mine.

The authors join me in acknowledging the support of family and friends throughout the writing of manuscripts. Special thanks are due to those colleagues who relieved us of clinical and teaching duties so that the writing and rewriting could proceed. To those patient and talented persons who converted our pencilled manuscripts to typescript, only to be rewarded with the opportunity to type yet another smooth draft, we extend our thanks. In that regard, warm thanks to Alice M. Davidson.

This undertaking was neither begun nor advanced by the editor alone. Eric I. Williams graciously agreed to meld his "manuscript aborning" into this volume, and he joined Ralph C. Buckner and Alfred M. Merritt II in encouraging me by being the first to accept authorship. Carl A. Osborne, Robert M. Kirk, and H. Fred Troutt gave helpful suggestions about concepts and organization. Each author participated in developing the chapter outline, thus bringing forward the concepts pertinent to the topic in a more readable way. The reader will recognize that a standard format for all chapters, even those within Section Three, would have yielded a tedious, cramped literary effort.

Christian C. F. Spahr, Jr. graciously provided the opportunity for *Veterinary Gastroenterology* to become a reality. His warm friendship, wise counsel, and constant encouragement are greatly appreciated. Mary E. Mansor brought about a sense of organization at the outset and throughout the editorial process. Thomas J. Colaiezzi orchestrated the production of the book and the cross-country flow of galley and page proof, so that there always seemed to be another large manila envelope in the mailbox just when I was beginning to get a bit restive. To Kit, Mary, and Tom, and to their colleagues at Lea and Febiger, I express my deep appreciation.

Special acknowledgment is made to those who helped shape my understanding of gastroenterology: Donald G. Low, Alan P. Thal, and James C. Rhodes. Their counsel was sound; the imperfections of my understanding are of my own doing. Personal and professional counsel came from George C. Mather, B. Franklin Hoerlein, and Jacob E. Mosier. During more than a decade, three colleagues at Kansas State University stand out as having been unfailingly helpful in advancing my understanding of gastroenterology: John L. Noordsy, Mark M. Guffy, and David A. Schoneweis.

My wife Betty is a constant source of strength and encouragement and I thank God for our life together. Our children developed an unabashed pride in the project, but were very careful never to allow the master of the House with the Orange Door to think that he was indispensable to the process.

Manhattan, Kansas   NEIL V. ANDERSON

CONTRIBUTORS

Bettina G. Anderson, Ph.D.
Associate Professor
Department of Veterinary Anatomy
College of Veterinary Medicine
The Ohio State University
Columbus, Ohio

Neil V. Anderson, D.V.M., Ph.D.
Professor
Department of Surgery and Medicine
College of Veterinary Medicine
Kansas State University
Manhattan, Kansas

Wesley D. Anderson, D.V.M., Ph.D.
Professor and Chairman
Department of Veterinary Anatomy
College of Veterinary Medicine
The Ohio State University
Columbus, Ohio

Robert A. Argenzio, Ph.D.
Physiologist
National Animal Disease Center
Ames, Iowa

J. Desmond Baggot, Ph.D.
Associate Professor of Pharmacology and
   Chemotherapy
School of Veterinary Studies
Murdoch University
Western Australia

Robert S. Brodey, D.V.M.†
Professor of Surgery
University of Pennsylvania School of Veterinary
   Medicine
Head, Small Animal Tumor Clinic
University of Pennsylvania Small Animal Hospital
Philadelphia, Pennsylvania

†Deceased.

Ralph G. Buckner, D.V.M.
Professor of Medicine and Surgery
Department of Medicine and Surgery
Chief, Small Animal Section
College of Veterinary Medicine
Oklahoma State University
Stillwater, Oklahoma

Colin F. Burrows, B. Vet. Med.
Assistant Professor of Medicine
University of Pennsylvania School of Veterinary
   Medicine
Philadelphia, Pennsylvania

James R. Coffman, D.V.M.
Professor
Department of Medicine and Surgery
College of Veterinary Medicine
University of Missouri
Columbia, Missouri

Lloyd E. Davis, D.V.M., Ph.D.
Professor of Clinical Pharmacology
Departments of Veterinary Clinical Medicine and
   Veterinary Biosciences
College of Veterinary Medicine
University of Illinois
Urbana, Illinois

Albert S. Dorn, D.V.M.
Associate Professor of Surgery
Department of Urban Practice
College of Veterinary Medicine
University of Tennessee
Knoxville, Tennessee

Sidney A. Ewing, D.V.M., Ph.D.
Professor and Head
Department of Veterinary Parasitology,
   Microbiology, and Public Health
College of Veterinary Medicine
Oklahoma State University
Stillwater, Oklahoma

Robert M. Hardy, D.V.M.
Associate Professor
Department of Veterinary Clinical Sciences
College of Veterinary Medicine
C 339 Veterinary Hospitals
St. Paul, Minnesota

Stanley G. Harris, D.V.M., Ph.D.
Associate Professor
Department of Medicine
Veterinarian, Department of Laboratory Animal
  Resources
University of Texas Health Science Center
San Antonio, Texas

Colin E. Harvey, B.V.Sc., M.R.C.V.S.
Associate Professor of Surgery
University of Pennsylvania School of Veterinary
  Medicine
Diplomate, American College of Veterinary Surgeons
Chief, Section of Small Animal Surgery
University of Pennsylvania Small Animal Hospital
Philadelphia, Pennsylvania

Dwight C. Hirsh, D.V.M., Ph.D.
Associate Professor of Microbiology
Department of Veterinary Microbiology
School of Veterinary Medicine
Chief, Microbiology Service
Veterinary Medical Teaching Hospital
University of California
Davis, California

William E. Hornbuckle, D.V.M.
Assistant Professor
Department of Clinical Sciences
New York State College of Veterinary Medicine
Cornell University
Ithaca, New York

Bruce L. Hull, D.V.M.
Associate Professor
Department of Large Animal Surgery
College of Veterinary Medicine
The Ohio State University
Columbus, Ohio

Gerald F. Johnson, D.V.M.
The Animal Medical Center
New York, New York

Jerry H. Johnson, D.V.M.
Equine Practitioner
Lexington, Kentucky
Formerly Professor and Head of Equine Surgery
College of Veterinary Medicine
University of Missouri
Columbia, Missouri

Helen E. Jordan, D.V.M., Ph.D.
Professor
Department of Veterinary Parasitology,
  Microbiology, and Public Health
College of Veterinary Medicine
Oklahoma State University
Stillwater, Oklahoma

David S. Kronfeld, Ph.D.
Professor of Nutrition
Department of Clinical Studies
University of Pennsylvania School of Veterinary
  Medicine
Kennett Square, Pennsylvania

Robert E. Lewis, D.V.M.
Professor and Chairman
Department of Anatomy and Radiology
College of Veterinary Medicine
University of Georgia
Athens, Georgia

H. Dwight Mercer, D.V.M., Ph.D.
Professor of Veterinary Pharmacology/Toxicology
Center for Sciences Basic to Medicine
College of Veterinary Medicine
Mississippi State University
Starkville, Mississippi

Alfred M. Merritt, D.V.M.
Professor of Medicine
Department of Medical Sciences
College of Veterinary Medicine
University of Florida
Gainesville, Florida

William E. Moore, D.V.M., Ph.D.
Professor of Clinical Pathology
Department of Laboratory Medicine
College of Veterinary Medicine
Kansas State University
Manhattan, Kansas

John A. Mulnix, D.V.M.
Practitioner
Anderson Animal Hospital and Moore Animal
  Hospital
Denver, Colorado

Joan A. O'Brien, V.M.D.
Professor of Medicine
University of Pennsylvania School of Veterinary
  Medicine
Chief, Section of Small Animal Medicine
University of Pennsylvania Small Animal Hospital
Philadelphia, Pennsylvania

Carl A. Osborne, D.V.M., Ph.D.
Professor and Chairman
Department of Small Animal Clinical Sciences
College of Veterinary Medicine
Professor
Department of Pediatrics
University of Minnesota
St. Paul, Minnesota

David J. Polzin, D.V.M.
Veterinary Medical Associate
Department of Small Animal Clinical Sciences
College of Veterinary Medicine
University of Minnesota
St. Paul, Minnesota

Thomas E. Powers, D.V.M., Ph.D.
Professor and Chairman
Department of Veterinary Physiology and
  Pharmacology
College of Veterinary Medicine
The Ohio State University
Columbus, Ohio

J. Harold Reed, D.V.M., Ph.D.
Professor of Medicine
Department of Clinical Studies
Coordinator, The Small Animal Clinic
Ontario Veterinary College
The University of Guelph
Guelph, Ontario

William D. Schall, D.V.M.
Associate Professor
Department of Small Animal Medicine and Surgery
School of Veterinary Medicine
Michigan State University
East Lansing, Michigan

Jerry B. Stevens, D.V.M., Ph.D.
Professor
Department of Veterinary Pathobiology
College of Veterinary Medicine
University of Minnesota
St. Paul, Minnesota

Bud C. Tennant, D.V.M.
Professor of Comparative Gastroenterology
Chief of Medicine
Department of Clinical Sciences
New York State College of Veterinary Medicine
Cornell University
Ithaca, New York

Donald E. Thrall, D.V.M., Ph.D.
Assistant Professor
Section of Radiology
School of Veterinary Medicine
University of Pennsylvania
Philadelphia, Pennsylvania

H. Fred Troutt, V.M.D.
Head
Department of Veterinary Sciences
Virginia Polytechnic Institute and State University
Blacksburg, Virginia

J. Thomas Vaughan, D.V.M.
Dean
Professor of Large Animal Surgery and Medicine
School of Veterinary Medicine
Auburn University
Auburn, Alabama

Shannon C. Whipp, D.V.M., Ph.D.
Laboratory Chief
National Animal Disease Center
Ames, Iowa

Robert H. Whitlock, D.V.M., Ph.D.
Associate Professor of Medicine
Department of Clinical Studies
Chief, Section of Large Animal Medicine
University of Pennsylvania School of Veterinary
  Medicine
Kennett Square, Pennsylvania

Eric I. Williams, D.V.M.
Professor of Medicine and Surgery
Department of Medicine and Surgery
College of Veterinary Medicine
Oklahoma State University
Stillwater, Oklahoma

Wayne E. Wingfield, D.V.M.
Associate Professor
Department of Clinical Sciences
College of Veterinary Medicine
Colorado State University
Fort Collins, Colorado

CONTENTS

_____

SECTION FOUR: SYSTEMIC DISEASES AND THE GASTROINTESTINAL SYSTEM

Section One

VETERINARY GASTROENTEROLOGY

Chapter 1

THE HISTORY

NEIL V. ANDERSON

The history of gastrointestinal disease is obtained as part of the history of the animal, the herd, or the flock. It is always obtained against the background of, and is usually confluent with, the complete history of the case. Illness affects the whole animal, even though the lesion may be limited to a system. "If one organ suffers, they all suffer together."[1] Therefore the history should always be taken in a broad perspective, even though the clinical evidence seems to point to the gastrointestinal system as the site of disease.

All histories have one of two characteristics. They are either too extensive or too brief! In reality, all histories have more potential information than is pertinent to the case. The goal of the veterinarian is to acquire enough history to guide the workup and treatment of the patient. By standardizing the method of obtaining the history, the veterinarian will, with experience, encounter fewer indeterminate histories and will be able to expand the verbal output of even the most taciturn client.

When the veterinarian agrees to accept the case, the interview begins. From the client's viewpoint, many aspects of a veterinary practice that are interpreted as representing skill and competence are found in the interview and in subsequent communications. The initial opportunity to see the patient may in large degree be a matter of random selection by the client or of geographic proximity, especially in a metropolitan area. But the opportunity to continue serving the needs of the patient and client will depend to a considerable degree on the effectiveness of communication, even if the outcome of the initial case is less than satisfactory. Conversely, the best of professional skill and patient care may go for naught if the felt needs of the client are not also met in the process.

The client (owner, herdsman, agent) is an integral part of the health-care delivery system, and should be recognized as such by the veterinarian. It may even be said that the client is the continuous member of the system and the veterinarian the discontinuous member. Signs of illness are noticed by the client before the veterinarian enters the case, and nursing care of the patient continues after the veterinarian departs. It is only during hospitalization that the client assumes a rather passive role in the system. The wise veterinarian will ensure that the client recognizes and accepts the concept of the health-care team, and his shared part in it. This recognition and acceptance process begins with the interview.

THE INTERVIEW AND ITS SETTING

All of the communications that occur in the initial encounter, whether verbal or nonverbal, are part of the interview. While the most valuable portion of the interview is the history, certain preliminaries are in order before the history-taking can proceed.

The initial verbal and nonverbal contact with the client influences every element of the relationship thereafter. One should face the client squarely, establish eye-contact, and give undivided attention during the brief seconds that introductions are made. The client must feel assured of both our personal and professional attention before the interview can be expected to proceed smoothly. In short, the client must sense an attitude of acceptance and helpfulness on our part. This impression is particularly important when veterinarian and client have not previously met, but that same impression should be formed in any interview. A first-interview format is assumed in this discussion.

When introductions have been completed, the veterinarian should take control of the interview by choosing the setting. Creature comfort and freedom from distraction—for the client primarily and for the veterinarian secondarily—are important considerations. The simple act of moving to the leeward side of a self-feeder may be all that is needed if the interview is to be held in a feed-yard on a windy day. Seeking out a shaded area to avoid intense heat or providing a chair for an elderly client are other examples. The principle to adopt in choosing the setting is to elicit passive or active cooperation by the client, all the while making the client the real

3

center of attention. Even though it may be the veterinarian's total effort in the case that ultimately produces a favorable outcome, the client must be made to feel needed, both during the interview and thereafter.

The client should begin to feel more at ease once the interview setting has been established. Achieving this initial goal is the responsibility of the veterinarian. A cold, nonsmiling countenance, a brusque, impatient attitude, or inadvertent upstaging by the veterinarian are potential causes of difficulty. Since the interview cannot effectively begin until the client can give full attention, he should be encouraged to deal with actual or potential distractions at the outset. This type of participation usually produces greater subsequent cooperation, especially when the interview is held at the farm, ranch, or kennel. In the hospital setting, the veterinarian should limit intrusions by staff personnel during the interview.

It is extremely helpful to conduct the interview with the patient or herd in view. The client will then be able to recall previous observations more correctly, and the veterinarian will be stimulated to ask questions in a more precise manner.

THE PRIMARY COMPLAINT

Asking the client for the primary complaint is a time-honored part of obtaining the history, because it permits the client to express the concern that prompted the call to the veterinarian.[2] Whether the information proves accurate and helpful or, as in some instances, misleading is of secondary importance. The mere act of helping the client to bring this concern to the fore minimizes confusion, outright misunderstanding, and time-loss. "What have you observed (noticed, seen) and when did you first observe (notice, see) it?" is a positive request for information that invites an objective answer. Variations on this type of opener—"How may I help you this morning?"—will be devised to suit the almost infinite variety of circumstances in which interviews are held. One should never ask, "What's wrong?" This question often produces a feeling of consternation and resentment in the client, and is an open invitation for a negative, even sarcastic reply.

Shifting visual attention from the client to the patient as the opening question is asked is a very useful technique. It tends to reduce the tension which many persons experience when they feel inadequately prepared to answer the veterinarian's questions. Many clients feel uncomfortable, lose their objectivity, and become defensive in a direct face-to-face interview, but will be able to cope if the object of the interview (the patient) is kept in view. Frequent reestablishment of eye-contact when responding to the client is usually adequate to provide assurance that the veterinarian continues to respect the primacy of the client in the interview.

When the primary complaint has been stated and defined, the narrative history should proceed. Other complaints may surface later on, but the client's immediate need has been met and the initial goal of the interview has been achieved. However, the primary complaint is sometimes stated in terms of the veterinarian's expectations rather than in terms of the client's concerns. Failure to recognize what the client really wants is a common cause of difficulty in the remainder of the interview.

THE NARRATIVE HISTORY

The early part of the history will be, or should be, narrated by the client. Later dividends will accrue to the veterinarian who can assess the client's communication abilities during the narrative. The type of question that can be asked with reasonable expectation of an objective answer must be graded according to the client's communication abilities, state of knowledge, and state of calmness or agitation. The veterinarian is responsible for adjusting to the client's communication level, as a true measure of professional ability. Properly phrased questions go far to forestall the client from gaining the impression that he is regarded as ignorant, unobservant, or deliberately untruthful.

When the client's initial narrative is finished, and, unfortunately, sometimes long before that point, it will be apparent how much effort the veterinarian must expend in organizing the remainder of the interview. The observant client, particularly the one who expects large financial benefit to be gained from the patient's recovery, usually presents the more organized and objective history. Those clients whose interest in the patient is largely emotional may have difficulty in being either organized or objective. The care with which questions are formulated and the order in which they are asked will be helpful to the disorganized client. Questions designed to clarify points in the history should usually be kept to a minimum until the client has finished the narrative. Even though one may occasionally be subjected to a seemingly unending narrative by allowing the client this freedom, most clients give brief narratives and need to be encouraged to remember and describe events relating to the patient. Direct questions by the veterinarian, made in the light of the client's complaint and expectation, will help make the use of time more efficient.

DIRECT QUESTIONS

Four categories of historic information pertain to every case, whether a single animal or a herd, drove, or flock is involved: (1) the patient(s), (2) the environment, (3) management factors, and (4) client factors.

By segregating the direct question into these categories, the veterinarian can help the client organize the narrative. Informing the client about the categories before beginning the direct questions will simplify the interview by permitting the client to concentrate on each item in turn.

Questions should be asked about the order in which abnormal events have occurred (e.g., dietary change and vomiting), and the time-lapse between events (e.g., eating and vomiting). The client's observations should be identified, and the client's interpretations of events should be clarified. Many clients cannot distinguish between events which have some common features; e.g., vomiting, regurgitation, and expectoration. Additionally, it is tempting for the client to agree (or disagree) with a leading question rather than admit ignorance of the definition of a term. Thus, it is better to ask, "Has there been any change in the bowel movement?" than to say, "Has there been diarrhea?" Many clients have never acquired even a layman's medical vocabulary, and can describe the excretions from the animal body only by their common or vulgar names. The variant terms for "bowel movement" will have to be chosen with regard to the situation, the species in question, and one's assessment of what terms the client will relate to most easily. Finally, each client should be assured that "I don't know" is a perfectly acceptable answer.

The patient(s) should be clearly identified as to intended use, such as food production, reproduction, work, or pleasure. The presumed reproductive status of intact females should be ascertained. If a single animal is being presented, how many other animals (and of what species) are at the household, farm, ranch, or kennel? What is the animal's immediate environment, what shelter is provided, what surface does it stand on, what are the limits of its range, and what other animals come in contact with it? The current feeding practice should be described, and the source of feed identified, at an appropriate point in the interview. What feed supplier serves the ranch? Are hay bales wire-tired? When was the last bag of dog food purchased? When was it opened? The status of vaccinations should be determined, including what products and what vaccination schedules are used.

The greatest put-down that can be given to a salesperson is to accuse him of "not knowing the territory," in this case, the environment. To avoid that fate, the veterinarian should be aware of regional geography and soil type, the characteristics of the local water-bearing rock strata, the water supply, and standards of husbandry and pet-care in the area. If a public utility water system is not used, one should determine whether the well is shallow or deep, and where it is located with respect to drainfields and feed-yards. Ponds filled from run-off water should be identified for possible inspection. Recent changes in environmental temperature and humidity, as well as current climatic conditions, should be known when the interview is conducted.

Management factors may be the key to understanding the onset of disease. Changes in care of animals frequently occurs during holiday and vacation seasons, during periods of maximum effort in other areas of farming and ranching, and during periods of altered use of the animals (exhibitions and shows, trail rides, long-distance transport). Direct questions should be made about recent movements of the patient that might have increased the opportunity for exposure to infection or environmental hazards. However, the most important management factor that influences the gastrointestinal system is abrupt change in quality, constituents, or quantity of the ration. All species are susceptible to indigestion due to ration changes, and manifest signs of anorexia, discomfort, abdominal distention, vomiting, and/or diarrhea. Immature animals and particularly neonates are more susceptible to changes in ration than are adults.

Client factors are those events (interactions) in which the client as a person impinges on the patient, whether for good or ill. Emotional bonds between client and patient, dominance by patient or client, hostility or resentment, and rivalries for attention and affection within the household setting are examples of interactions that may initiate or influence disease processes. While it is true that companion animals are more likely to be influenced by client factors, it is sometimes difficult to separate management factors from client factors for any species of patient. Thus, it is useful to identify client factors even for commercial production units.

Direct questioning should be done in a non-threatening way that is designed to clarify rather than complicate the issue. ("Then you did ___?" rather than "Why didn't you do ___?"). The client who is made to feel on trial for some supposed sin of omission or commission can be relied upon to retreat into silence or into an uncooperative attitude rather than risk further offense. It is well to learn early on whether the animal has been treated for the current problems, by whom, and with what. The direct questioning should always conclude with "Is there anything that I haven't asked that you think I should know about?" This question provides yet another opportunity for the client to present a more accurate impression of the case.

The history should then be reviewed and the important items identified, both by asking the client's opinion and by making one's own judgment. This process will give rise to direct questions which will expand the historic part of the data base. Few clients come to the interview with a strong sense of organization; rather, fact, observations, and opinions are usually freely admixed. Two direct questions that should always be asked are, "Has this problem (sign, disease) ever occurred before?" and "Have any disease problems occurred before?" These questions may help the client recall one or more similar occurrences, which in turn may help greatly in ultimately defining the patient's problems.

PAST PERTINENT HISTORY

A review of the past pertinent history should follow the current history. It should include both the history of the individual animal of the present herd or flock, and the past history of the ranch, farm, stable, or kennel, as appropriate. Have similar signs of illness been observed in the past? Are other animals on the premises presently affected with these or other signs of disease? When was the animal, herd, or flock acquired? Have any animals been brought to the premises recently for any purpose? As one continues to provide veterinary service to a client, the past pertinent history becomes more and more a part of the knowledge set of the veterinarian. Once the past pertinent history is recorded for an animal or herd, it is relatively easy to update it.

REVIEW OF THE SYSTEMS

A review of systems function should be included in the summation of the current history. Questions should be phrased in terms of the commonly recognized functions of a system rather than in terms that would require the client to know what the signs of systemic disease are. "Is the cow ruminating normally" (or, "Is she chewing her cud")? "Is the dog eating and drinking as usual?" "Have you noticed coughing, sneezing, or other breathing difficulty?" is an appropriate question about the respiratory system. "Does he hear and see well?" will elicit the client's impressions about the organs of special

sense. "Has there ever been lameness, pain, or difficulty in walking?" aids in evaluating musculoskeletal function. A more direct mode of questioning than that used in obtaining the current history seems appropriate, since the client may need reminders to begin thinking beyond the scope of a patient's current major problems. Questions should extend back in time if the client presents information suggesting that one or more systems may have been diseased in the past.

The historic data is recorded as soon as it is received, as a general rule. However, many narrative histories contain superfluous or inaccurate information, so a word-for-word transcription of the history quickly becomes unwieldy and counterproductive. It is better to identify the salient features of the history as they are related, and then record as much as is needed to help the clinician in diagnosis and to constitute a legal record.

The experienced veterinarian is often able to complete the general physical examination of a dog or cat in 3 to 5 minutes while the history is being related. The entries for history and physical examination can then be made simultaneously. One accepts some risk of overlooking an important detail by combining these events, but the efficient use of time commends it. One principal advantage of combining history-taking and physical examination is that the client can be asked to comment on findings as they are made.[2] This is especially true regarding externally visible findings which are evident to the owner. The method of recording historic data is a matter of personal choice by the veterinarian. Systems that vary from total prose to elaborate checklists are used, although many records systems are too brief to be useful in the future. Well-constructed records that are organized on the basis of the patients' (and clients') problems (Problem-Oriented Veterinary Medical Records) are most helpful in improving total patient care.

TERMINATION OF THE INTERVIEW

When the veterinarian senses that enough pertinent information has been gained, he should terminate the interview and give undivided attention to the physical examination. In the instance where the loquacious client persists in providing information beyond that needed by the veterinarian, one can simply begin the physical examination and expect that the torrent of words will subside. The interview that is proceeding unsatisfactorily from the standpoint of either client or veterinarian is probably best adjourned immediately and tactfully. After the general examination has been completed, enough information may have come to light to resume a more fruitful line of questioning. Calling attention to a physical finding, particularly one that the client can see, will often permit resumption of the interview in a more positive vein. Many clients can begin to build the history more accurately on the sense of organization provided by the veterinarian.

At some point in every interview, the veterinarian must make the decision that the history is complete. In doing so, one accepts the risk of losing some potentially valuable information. If questions have been carefully worded, the risk is small. Histories are seldom truly completed in one interview, and a further review of the history occurs with most cases.

REFERENCES

1. New English Bible, I Cor. 12:26. New York, Oxford University Press, 1970.
2. Low, D. C., Osborne, C. A., and Finco, D. R.: The pillars of diagnosis: history and physical examination. *In* Textbook of Veterinary Internal Medicine, Vol. 1. Edited by S. J. Ettinger. Philadelphia, W. B. Saunders Co., 1975.

Chapter 2

SIGNS OF GASTROINTESTINAL DISEASE

NEIL V. ANDERSON

Signs of disease in animals are externally discernible events which differ in one or more respects from normal behavior or function. The client has a concept of what is normal for that animal, herd, or flock, based on previous observations and experience. The narrative history includes a description of those abnormal or unusual events that the client perceives as being associated with disease.

Veterinarians find that signs of gastrointestinal disease tend to cluster around one or more of seven major themes, as described by clients: (1) anorexia, (2) dysphagia, (3) vomiting, (4) diarrhea, (5) abdominal distention, (6) abdominal and pelvic pain, and (7) dullness, personality disturbance, and seizures. None of these signs excludes the possibility of disease of another system or of the body as a whole. However, with the exception of the sign mentioned last, all these signs are so commonly associated with the gastrointestinal tract as to constitute the primary signs of gastrointestinal disease in animals.

The client's description may not include the exact terms listed. In reviewing the history and before concluding the interview, one will want to understand not only what the client said but what he meant. This is particularly true of the common signs of gastrointestinal disease, namely, vomiting and diarrhea.

When the client has finished the initial narrative and has cited a sign of disease, the veterinarian can ask several direct questions in an attempt to characterize the client's observations further. Questions are phrased in such a way that the client can answer briefly with "yes" or "no" whenever possible and with greater specificity than could be inferred from the narrative history. In this way, the client may be able to segregate and isolate events so as to help identify probable, plausible reasons for the presence of those signs.

Many of these questions are never verbalized. Some answers are available at a glance if the interview is taking place at the stable, feed-yard, or kennel. However, if the animal is brought to a hospital or clinic, it is often necessary to ask a greater number of questions in order to form the mental images so necessary for correct interpretation of the client's observations.

ANOREXIA

This condition exists when an animal refuses to ingest readily available, palatable food in its usual feeding pattern. Anorexia may be complete or partial. Some of the following questions may be asked. "When was the horse last observed to be normal? When did the horse last eat? Was the onset of anorexia abrupt or gradual? Did other horses eat the food? Has there been a change in ration in association with onset of anorexia? Has an adequate amount of fresh water been continuously available? Does the bull move toward the feed bunk as if to eat? Does the bull make attempts to prehend food? Does the cow ruminate? Have any changes been made in management recently? Has this animal, herd, or flock been recently moved into a new environment? Have any pigs been introduced onto the premises in the past 7 to 10 days? What treatments have been given? Have any chemicals or sprays been applied on or near this animal, herd, or flock? Does the dog drink water? Can the dog open and close its mouth in a normal manner? Is its mouth held open or closed when the dog is not eating? Does the tongue protrude from the dog's mouth? Does the dog have access to trash or garbage?" These and other questions can be used to add perspective to the client's observations.

The anorectic patient should be regarded as having a lesion within or near the mouth or pharynx, or as having a centrally mediated inhibition of the normal desire to eat and drink. That the latter is often the case is easily understood when one considers that fever or hypothermia, acute or chronic pain in many parts of the body, localized abscess and/or generalized infection, metabolic or endocrine disturbances, and primary diseases of the central nervous system are all frequently accompanied by anorexia. Thus, it is the least specific sign of gastrointestinal disease unless an additional localizing sign is observed that directs one's attention to the mouth.

DYSPHAGIA

Difficulty in swallowing or an inability to swallow, a condition called dysphagia, is strongly suggestive of an oropharyngeal lesion or of disease of the central nervous system. Dysphagia may be perceived as difficult or painful swallowing, in that there is extension and lowering of the head and neck as the bolus is swallowed. Mild lesions may simply elicit hesitation in swallowing. Alternatively, severely painful or difficult swallowing may be associated with ventral flexion of the head and arching of the neck, so that the chin is held close to the chest, followed by extension of the head and neck. Noticeable contraction of the muscles of the pharyngeal wall may be seen with parting and retraction of the lips at the commissures even though the mouth is held closed as the act of swallowing is completed. Grunting or crying may occur in conjunction with difficult or painful swallowing.

Dysphagia may be characterized by persistent swallowing efforts accompanied by repeated bobbing or shaking of the head and neck at each swallowing attempt. This motion may continue to occur even after the pharynx is cleared of ingesta. Cyclic protrusion and retraction of the tongue may be observed between the repeated swallowing attempts, particularly in the horse, cow, cat, and dog, which have a rather mobile tongue. When dysphagia is accompanied by such flicking movements of the tongue, one should search carefully for ulcers, foreign bodies, broken or loosened teeth, or evidence of oropharyngeal trauma or inflammation.

Questions are asked in a manner similar to those described for anorexia, but the questions may not be readily answered with "yes" or "no." Rather, it may be useful to ask the client to pantomime the observed events. If the client is shy or unable to act out what he has observed, the veterinarian may pantomime and thus get a better indication from the client as to the nature of the observed sign.

Dysphagia is frequently confused with anorexia, and reported as such by the client. If the animal prehends and chews food, however reluctantly, one can be assured that complete anorexia is not a consideration in the case, and the mouth and pharynx should be carefully examined. When the dysphagic animal has become fully aware that repeated attempts to swallow are unproductive, fatiguing, or painful, eating usually ceases or greatly decreases in frequency. In this instance, the client may correctly report that the animal is anorectic but may not be aware that it is also dyphagic.

Ptyalism. This increased flow of saliva frequently accompanies dysphagia. Other common causes include oropharyngeal or generalized infection, mechanical or chemical irritation of the buccal or pharyngeal mucous membranes, or central nervous system stimulation or depression from ingested chemicals and drugs. Certain plants seem to cause ptyalism when chewed or ingested. Ptyalism may exist even if most of the saliva is swallowed. Thus, the client may describe frequent swallowing without mentioning saliva directly. However, escape of excessive salivary secretion from the mouth is almost inevitable, and the visible overflow of fluid or foam from the lips or its presence on the ground reveals that ptyalism exists.

Pseudoptyalism. This condition occurs when the animal is unable or unwilling to swallow, and allows the normal flow of saliva to overflow from the lips. It is frequently difficult to distinguish between ptyalism and pseudoptyalism at the time of examination, since buccal, oral, and pharyngeal lesions may both stimulate salivary flow and cause pain sufficient to inhibit swallowing.

Ptyalism and pseudoptyalism are helpful in localizing the site of disease to the mouth and pharynx. However, either sign may be a clue to central nervous system stimulation or depression. The veterinarian should observe the whole animal within the context of the history and the results of the general physical examination before concluding that the cause of ptyalism is indeed localized to the mouth or pharynx.

Spillage of food, fluid, or foam from the mouth during swallowing attempts suggests that pharyngeal paralysis exists. One should evaluate the patient for a possible central nervous disorder, e.g., medullary paralysis in the dog or rabies in any mammal, to avoid having an incorrect interpretation of oropharyngeal signs mislead the handling of the case.

VOMITING SYNDROMES

These conditions share the common feature of expulsion or ejection of food and fluid through the mouth and nasopharynx, although *regurgitation* and *expectoration* differ from vomiting in a number of particulars.

Vomiting. A coordinated, centrally mediated act, vomiting is initially characterized by a sense of apprehension on the part of the patient, with uneasiness, restlessness, and pacing, licking of the lips, ptyalism, and repeated swallowing efforts. These initial events, which are probably evidence of a sense of nausea, are followed by retching with the mouth held either open or closed. The head is lowered, the patient ignores nearby persons, animals, or events, the abdominal muscles contract rhythmically and repeatedly, and sloshing, fluid sounds emanate from the patient's body. The sense of premonition may exist for several seconds to several minutes, while active retching may wax and wane for seconds to a minute or more before vomiting occurs. Gastric content is ejected from the mouth one or more times, with head lowered, accompanied by gurgling sounds, during which time respiration is delayed and the thorax is expanded. Contraction of the abdominal musculature is particularly strenuous and, along with the negative pressure in the expanded thorax, is largely responsible for expulsion of gastric content. Relaxation of the body and a brief episode of deep, rapid respirations are observed after vomiting is completed. The sequence of events may be repeated at intervals of minutes or hours if the cause persists.

Vomiting is common in dogs, but less so in cats and pigs. It is uncommon in horses, cattle, sheep, and goats. Vomitus passes through the nasopharynx and external nares of the horse because of the length and position of the soft palate. In other species, vomitus is expelled through the mouth, for the most part. The volume of vomitus is quite variable and reflects the volume of gastric content prior to onset. Successive episodes of vomiting yield smaller volumes, especially if the interval between episodes is short. If the stomach is essentially emptied, subsequent episodes of vomiting may culminate with intense retching but without expulsion of gastric content. The affected animal usually does not consume the vomitus if a sense of illness persists. Cats seldom do so under any circumstances, but dogs and pigs will consume their own and the vomitus of others. When puppies or gluttonous adult dogs vomit after engorging with food, they will frequently consume the vomitus later.

The components of vomitus should be identified by questioning the client and/or by personal inspection. Food, clear fluid, and mucus are usually present. The state of maceration ("digestion") of food is an indication of the duration of time that the food was retained within the stomach, and of the motor and secretory activity of the stomach. The time-lapse after eating is a crude indication of the

severity of the problem; the sooner after eating that vomiting occurs, the more severe the lesion may be. But vomiting may also be a sign of extragastric disease; it is stimulated as often as not by something other than an organic lesion of the stomach. Vomiting is not the equivalent of gastritis in any sense of the word. In fact, vomiting is so frequently a sign of other systemic or generalized diseases that extragastric causes of vomiting must always be ruled out before confirming a diagnosis of gastric disease. Bile vomitus is evidence of duodenal reflux, and therefore of duodenal or periduodenal irritation, or peritonitis.

When the clinician identifies hematemesis, there should be a search for the source of hemorrhage in the stomach, duodenum, esophagus, pharynx, oral cavity, or sinuses. Blood that originates in or enters the stomach from elsewhere and is retained therein for more than a few minutes will coagulate and become dark in color if gastric acid is present. Blood is irritating to the gastric mucosa, and vomiting often occurs after it enters the stomach. The dark flecks of coagulated blood impart the appearance of "coffee grounds" to the vomitus, while hemorrhage from the oral cavity, sinuses, or pharynx is bright red and often frothy if expelled immediately.

Macroparasites, notably ascarids and cestodes, are often identified in vomitus. Fecal vomitus occurs in bowel obstruction while tissue shreds, rarely found, strongly suggest an ulcer and/or neoplasia of the stomach.

Projectile vomiting occurs in that particular instance where premonitory signs are absent or brief. In contrast to the much more usual non-projectile vomiting described previously, the stomach provides much of the motive force in projectile vomiting. Injury to the base of the skull or hypothalamus, acute panencephalitis, and pylorospasm initiate an abrupt expulsion of gastric content, so forceful that the vomitus is "projected" some distance from the mouth. Since premonitory signs are brief or absent, the head is not lowered and the projectile nature of the vomiting act is evident. Projectile vomiting occurs as a "normal" event in certain brachycephalic breeds of dogs. Boxers and Boston Terriers in particular are easily stimulated to vomit. They are uncommonly cheerful throughout the episode, and will frequently consume and retain the vomitus shortly after projectile vomiting has occurred.

Clients frequently refer to the vomiting patient as having been "sick," regardless of the type of vomiting. The visual and auditory aspects of vomiting are readily identified by the client, but rather than identify the event by name, many clients refer to it as being "sick to the stomach." Direct questioning may permit identification of projectile vomiting, which may not be characterized by "sickness" either before the act or after it is completed. Fortunately, trauma or fever is evident as the cause of projectile vomiting in such patients.

Regurgitation. In contrast to vomiting, regurgitation is the act of expelling esophageal food and fluid through the mouth or nasopharynx, without the extreme premonitory signs that precede gastric vomiting. It is readily observed as part of the physiologic events of rumination, except that in the ruminant the cud is retained in the mouth, masticated, and swallowed. Persistent regurgitation is distinctly pathologic in non-ruminants and occurs most commonly in dogs. It is the most common sign of esophageal disease. The act is abrupt and brief, physically much more passive than vomiting, and does not seemingly engender a sense of severe distress on the part of the animal. Food and fluid are most often regurgitated through the mouth in carnivores, but through the external nares in horses. Abnormal esophageal motility, or overflow from a filled, dilated, or obstructed esophagus are the usual causes. The horse with esophageal obstruction ("choke") may have a persistent nasal discharge because of nasal regurgitation, and the client may describe this condition by saying that the horse has a "cold." Close inspection may reveal food particles at the external nares.

The animal that regurgitates will cast its head ventrally, cough or retch briefly, and expel esophageal content. The animal usually remains alert afterward, will usually swallow several times to clear the pharynx, may cough once or twice, and then seems outwardly unchanged. Esophageal content varies from firm to fluid, lacks the acid odor of gastric content, and usually has a pH of 6 or higher. Repeated consumption of regurgitated material occurs in those animals with congenital or acquired dilatation of the esophagus, while those with organic obstruction are more likely to exhibit signs of depression, and, perhaps because of dull pain associated with obstruction, to refrain from eating and will thus be regarded as anorectic. Regurgitation accompanied by explosive sneezing or coughing, in conjunction with swallowing of food or water, suggests that the lesion is at the level of the hypopharynx and that the patient has both dysphagia and regurgitation. Cricopharyngeal achalasia in the dog is classically accompanied by dysphagia and regurgitation, and one should assess that possibility carefully if food or fluid is also expelled from the mouth or nares as part of the dysphagic act.

Expectoration. By this act fluid, mucus, food, or exudate is ejected from the pharynx and nasopharynx. This sign of nasopharyngeal or upper respiratory disease is common to all species. It occurs at least as commonly as vomiting in dogs and cats and much more often than regurgitation. Expectoration is frequently confused with vomiting by both clients and veterinarians.

Expectoration is often preceded by stertorous inhalation through the nares in dogs and cats, which represents an attempt to dislodge and withdraw mucus from the nasopharynx into the pharynx. Even though domestic animals are not able to keep their lips closed during this maneuver, it resembles in most other respects the manner in which man clears mucus from the nasopharynx and soft palate. The subsequent act of expectoration differs from that of man only in the particulars that small animals utilize gravity and flicking movements of the tongue to expel mucus from the mouth, instead of the lip and tongue movements with forceful expulsion of air that characterize "spitting" or expectoration in man. Cows clear the pharynx by extending the head and neck while blowing air forcefully through the pharynx and mouth, while horses expectorate through the nasopharynx and nares. Both species cough in conjunction with expectoration.

To many clients, expectoration resembles and is frequently confused with vomiting, because it is frequently preceded by brief retching and lowering of the head. However, it differs greatly in volume, since expectoration in dogs and cats seldom yields more than a few milliliters. In fact, expectoration may be completed without the ejection of pharyngeal content if the mucus or exudate is quite viscous. The animal simply swallows and then expectorates again later. It is noteworthy that clients who describe vomiting as "getting sick to the stomach" or "spitting up" may in another instance describe expectoration as "vomiting." It may be necessary to describe or pantomime the act of expectoration before the client can give a clear indication of what he observed.

Dysphagia and expectoration may exist concurrently because pharyngeal lesions give rise to both signs. The importance of the history is magnified when one becomes aware that pharyngitis is not always accompanied by intense reddening. Knowing that these signs coexist may help the veterinarian avoid the mistake of treating a dog for an unspecified gastric disease ("vomiting") when the lesion is actually in the pharynx.

DIARRHEA

This condition is characterized by the passage of feces of increased water content, and with greater frequency than normal. Tenesmus may be present. The magnitude of increase is an important clue to the site of disease in the digestive tract. Volume and frequency of defecation are two characteristics that should always be determined from the history or by personal observation. Failure to do so greatly impedes diagnostic effort and may hinder effective treatment. The presence or absence of tenesmus and pain at defecation should be noted, as well as their intensity.

The volume of diarrheal feces is directly related to the proportional increase of water content. Each species has a characteristic form to normal feces, a reflection in part of the degree of colonic reabsorption of water. Horses, sheep, goats, rabbits, guinea pigs, and humans have typical rounded or ovoid fecal masses. The normal feces of cattle vary from segmented and firm to soft and unformed, depending on age, diet, and availability of water, while that of dogs, cats, and pigs is normally firm and segmented to soft and formed. In each instance, the pediatric age-group of the domestic species has softer feces during the initial suckling period than after adjustment to a growth ration. It is from these considerations that the client and the veterinarian share their understanding of what is normal volume for the species; i.e., normal from each fecal passage and normal for a 24-hour period.

When fecal volume is increased 5 to 10 times above that which is usual in the monogastric animal, the small bowel is implicated as the probable site of disease. The large volume of diarrhea is a direct reflection of incomplete water reabsorption by the small intestine of monogastric animals, regardless of the cause. Conversely, small-volume diarrhea, defined as a several-fold increase in the volume of feces passed in a 24-hour period, is an indication of colonic disease. Herbivores absorb a considerable proportion of their total nutrients from the cecum and colon and have a considerably greater absorption of total gastrointestinal water from the large, long cecocolic segment than does the monogastric animal from its short colon. Thus, diarrhea in adult herbivores, particularly in horses, is a large bowel phenomenon. In all species, the total 24-hour fecal volume is an important consideration and should be part of the history.

Increased frequency of defecation is an almost invariable feature of diarrhea. Local irritation of the rectum and anus produces a considerable increase in frequency of defecation, while colonic irritation produces a lesser increase. Small bowel disease in monogastric animals is likely to result in the least increase in frequency of defecation. For example, 2 to 6 large volume bowel evacuations per day by a dog that usually defecates once or twice daily would be a typical sign of small bowel disease. Colon disease, on the other hand, frequently causes an affected dog to defecate as often as 12 to 15 or more times daily.

An inverse relationship tends to exist between fecal volume and frequency in dogs and cats. Disease of the small intestine tends to produce a large increase in total 24-hour fecal volume, while causing a modest increase in the frequency of defecation. Colon and rectal disease may cause little increase in total 24-hour fecal volume, while the frequency with which small quantities of soft or formed feces or mucus are passed is greatly increased.

When diarrhea exists, the feces are more fluid because of increased water content. The fecal material may be well-mixed, so that a pool of fluid feces results after defecation. In some instances, there has not been thorough mixing of the fluid and particulate components, so that fluid separates and flows away from the solid particles. In severe small bowel disease, the feces may contain more than 90% water. Color may vary from the normal brown or dark green, to light green or yellow or an even lighter color. Bilirubin, in its several stages of bacterial-mediated change, accounts for brown, green, and yellow color; the more rapid the intestinal transit time, the lighter the bilirubin-related color of feces. Fresh or well-preserved forage, when eaten by herbivores, may yield a green fecal color. Fecal lipid imparts a light greyish hue to the fecal mass as it cools and dries.

The fluidity of diarrhea yields some information about probable etiology and the depth of the lesion in the intestinal wall, and considerable information about the severity of the disease. Voluminous, fluid diarrhea suggests that net water flux across the intestinal mucosa has been altered, and perhaps reversed. Clarity of the diarrheal fluid suggests that the mucosal cells are primarily affected and that blood vascular integrity is largely intact. In diarrheas of abrupt onset, large volume suggests that the lesion is diffuse. Viruses, bacteria and bacterial toxins, and ingested irritants are known to cause this type of diarrhea and may be assessed in the light of known causes of diarrhea in the species of animal thus affected. Salmonellosis in stressed horses, panleukopenia in young kittens, transmissible gastroenteritis in suckling piglets, and canine distemper in young puppies are examples of this type of fluid diarrhea. The fluid diarrhea of Johne's disease in cattle usually has a bubbly appearance.

Gas is passed per rectum by all animals throughout life. A large and variable proportion of flatus in monogastric animals is atmospheric air that has been swallowed, while in herbivores de novo synthesis by intestinal bacteria is the source of much of the gas. Oligosaccharides and proteins, particularly soy protein, are substrates that yield gas as a by-product of bacterial action. The gas may be free or admixed with feces. This is normal in herbivores that have recently gained free access to lush forage. Chronic giardiasis in adult dogs is frequently characterized by such a frothy diarrhea.

Undigested food may be passed in normal or diarrheal feces. The cuticle of many whole cereal grains largely resists the digestive action of certain species. Whole corn and oats are passed in the feces of cattle since they do not crush grains efficiently by mastication. Horses, pigs, sheep, and goats chew grains much more thoroughly, and fecal passage of disproportionate amounts of whole grains in these species is a clue to abnormal dentition. Dogs may eat dry grains but do not digest them well, while they digest cooked grains more completely. Cooked, undigested corn and barley may be observed in the feces of normal dogs, the above notwithstanding. Cats eat and digest cooked cereals in both canned and dry foods and as part of the digestive tract of their prey.

Other undigested foods that may appear in feces include fats and oils, meats and cartilage, and bones. Normal dogs and cats digest and absorb dietary fats and oils very well, so their presence in feces indicates great dietary excess, or digestive or absorptive failure. The same applies to meats, while cartilage is not quite as well digested under any circumstance. Green or uncooked bone is digested quite well if ground or finely chewed, while cooked bone seems not to be as well digested by dogs.

Certain indigestible materials are frequently found in dog feces, including hair, grass, cellulose, and synthetic materials. Small amounts may cause no clinical problem; large amounts may cause diarrhea or constipation, depending on whether the material is locally irritating.

When blood is extravasated into the digestive tract, the resultant fecal color varies from black to bright red, depending on the site of blood loss. Assuming that transit time is not altered, duodenal and jejunal blood loss, e.g., due to blood-sucking endoparasites, results in a uniformly dark, almost black ("tarry") appearance to the feces. Breakdown of hemoglobin by bacterial action accounts for the black color, also known as melena.

Hemorrhage into the ileum and proximal colon is less altered and less admixed, and is therefore less dark in color. The terms "plum-pudding," "raspberry jam," or "currant jelly" can hardly be improved upon, however much one tries to avoid speaking in terms of "food pathology." Formed, blood-coated feces may be interspersed with blood clots and blood-stained mucus to yield the appearance of bowel hemorrhage described previously. Dysentery, defined as diarrhea with bloody mucus, rectal tenesmus, and abdominal pain, is probably the best term to apply to this type of diarrhea.

Hemorrhage from the distal colon and rectum is usually evacuated quickly, thus the bright, easily recognizable character of the blood. The term hematochezia is reserved for the bloody coating observed on, but not admixed with feces.

Coagulative necrosis of gut epithelium may result in the passage of a gray, tenacious pseudomembrane. Diarrhea may not accompany this type of lesion, particularly in the cow. Shreds of mucosa may be shed from ulcer margins, intussuscepted bowel or epithelial neoplasms of the bowel. Blood loss is almost invariably noted when shreds of mucosa are found.

Transit time is seldom normal in intestinal disease, and changes in motility may greatly modify the appearance of blood in feces. Very rapid motility in a diffusely irritated, bleeding small bowel may result in the passage of voluminous, bright bloody bowel movements, even though the site of blood loss is the duodenum or jejunum. Conversely, blood lost into the distal small bowel, if retained for many hours, may be quite dark when passed. Blood lost into the distal colon or rectum is usually passed rather quickly because the associated inflammation results in tenesmus and increased frequency of defecation. Finally, it is common in many instances of intestinal blood loss to observe fecal blood in several color variations, particularly if increased mucous secretion accompanies blood loss.

ABDOMINAL DISTENTION

Distention of the abdomen due to problems associated with the gastrointestinal tract can be classified clinically as follows:

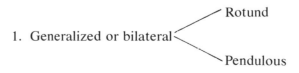

1. Generalized or bilateral — Rotund / Pendulous

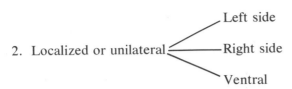

2. Localized or unilateral — Left side
— Right side
— Ventral

Gastrointestinal distention may be caused by food, fluid, gas, feces or neoplasm.[1] An additional cause of abdominal distention is the presence of fat, or of a fetus in the gravid female.

Rotund distentions are often caused by gas, and pendulous distentions by fluid or tissue masses. Rapid consumption of feed or water produces transient generalized abdominal distention in all species. Experienced clients may be able to help define the problem of abdominal distention from their previous experiences; e.g., bloat in cattle and gastric dilatation in dogs. Abdominal distentions will be discussed further in Chapter 4.

ABDOMINAL AND PELVIC PAIN

Signs of abdominal pain, often referred to as colic, include restless movements with alternate pacing and recumbency, occasional turning of the head and neck towards the abdomen, sweating, and in some species, grinding of the teeth (bruxism) and grunting, groaning, or whining.

If pain is very severe, the patient may collapse suddenly, only to rise quickly and move about again. This pattern is particularly true in horses. Whether standing or recumbent, the patient may stretch out as if to minimize pressure on the abdomen. Geldings are known to develop a penile erection and even masturbate during an episode of severe abdominal pain. Horses may void small volumes of urine repeatedly when abdominal pain is present.

Kicking at the abdomen is characteristic of abdominal pain in cattle, although it also occurs in cows with sore teats. The iatrogenic pain of cardiac catheterization may cause a horse to kick at the xiphoid cartilage. Bruxism may occur due to acute or chronic abdominal pain in cattle and sometimes in pigs. Puppies and kittens may whine due to the discomfort of abdominal distention.

In cattle, the manifestation of abdominal pain may be in the form of a grunt or a groan. Groaning is more characteristic of severe abdominal distention, especially if the patient is recumbent. A grunt may be related to contraction of a digestive organ; e.g., in the early stage of traumatic reticuloperitonitis in a cow, a grunt can be detected during reticular contraction.

Arching of the back is associated with abdominal pain in horses, cattle, and dogs. Sweating (hyperhidrosis) may accompany abdominal pain in horses and less frequently in cattle. Dogs with acute abdominal pain may recline with the abdomen on a cool surface, or assume a prayer position, with forequarters and head lowered and extended. The abdomen may decrease in size because of anorexia. Fatigue and depression are later manifestations of abdominal pain in all species.

Tenesmus, the most common sign of pain or discomfort within the pelvis, is vigorous straining to evacuate the rectum, uterus, or urinary bladder, usually without passage of content. It is characterized by an arched back, elevated tail, and intermittent abrupt contractions of the abdominal muscles. It is mild or absent in small bowel disease but is commonly associated with colonic disease; indeed, it is one of the hallmarks of distal colonic and rectal disease in all species. Clients usually infer correctly that the patient is in pain or is quite uncomfortable. Tenesmus frequently continues after fecal passage, with resumption of the posture typically associated with defecation but without further passage of feces. Small amounts of mucus and blood will frequently be passed per rectum after persistent, prolonged tenesmus. In severe cases there may be protrusion of the anus or vagina, and prolapse of the rectum or uterus. The patient may remain standing or assume recumbency, or alternate from one position to the other. Until physical examination is performed, one cannot be certain whether the rectum has been emptied, or whether the animal is unable to pass a rectal fecalith and is thus constipated, or whether the patient is attempting unsuccessfully to micturate. The lesion may be adjacent to, rather than within, one of the pelvic organs. Signs of rectal tenesmus are more pronounced in cattle than in other species. The cause of tenesmus may be remote from the pelvic area, notably in cattle afflicted with rabies or seneciosis.

The subjective impression of pain accompanying tenesmus is often gained by the client or veterinarian observing an animal in the act of defecation. It may be manifested as crying, panting, or other visible signs of discomfort. Tenesmus alone usually localizes the lesion; evidence of pain provides a subjective estimation of the intensity of physical distress that the affected animal is experiencing.

DULLNESS, PERSONALITY DISTURBANCE, AND SEIZURES

Although primary signs of disease of the central nervous system, dullness, personality disturbance, and seizures are often secondary to disease of other systems. Occasionally, they may be signs of liver failure in all species. Excessively high concentration of ammonia in the body fluids due to inadequacy of the liver in converting ammonia to urea is a postulated cause for the central nervous system signs. Other parameters may be detectably abnormal and should be tested in the diagnostic workup, in order to rule out liver disease as a cause. The observant client may notice icterus or bilirubinuria.

The degree of dullness may vary from mild depression to stupor and recumbency. Afflicted animals may perform certain actions repetitively, such as walking compulsively or pressing the head against a fixed object. The personality may change from being normal to being distant and withdrawn or sluggish in responsiveness, followed by an apparent return to normal. Since the seizures, should they occur, are centrally mediated, they are indistinguishable from those of primary central nervous system disease. Finally, liver disease may be manifested by anorexia, ptyalism, vomiting, or diarrhea.

REFERENCE

1. Blood, D. C., Henderson, J. A., and Radostits, O. M.: Veterinary Medicine, 5th ed. Philadelphia, Lea & Febiger, 1979.

Chapter 3

GENERAL PHYSICAL EXAMINATION OF THE GASTROINTESTINAL SYSTEM

ERIC I. WILLIAMS
RALPH G. BUCKNER

The enduring base for the general physical examination is an understanding of the physical characteristics of the normal animal. To acquire and improve basic skills in physical examination, one must observe and examine normal animals regularly. Normal animals far outnumber abnormals in most populations and represent a built-in opportunity to improve one's skill in differentiating them. Vaccination and health maintenance programs provide a continually available source of normal animals. The veterinarian must gain the ability to create a mental image of what would be normal for each animal, given the variables of species, age, sex, breed, reproductive status, feeding program, and environment. Failure to refine and upgrade the concept of normal hinders improvement in one's ability to diagnose disease and treat patients.

The general physical examination of the gastrointestinal system, as described in this chapter, is made as part of the standardized examination of regions of the body. "Examine by regions, and record findings by systems"[1] is a sound way to begin understanding the sick animal's problems. The standardized physical examination begins at the head and continues along the neck, thorax, and abdomen to the rear quarters. Inspection (both at a distance and at arm's length), palpation, auscultation, and percussion each have a place in every examination. The trend toward greater use of instrumentation in physical examination has added greater specificity to the physical findings (see Chapters 7 and 8). However, instruments are useful adjuncts for diagnosis only when the general physical examination has been well done. Transistors, tubes, and fiber bundles are additive to, not a substitute for, the hands-on examination.

An effective way of making the transition from taking the history to beginning the examination is to address one's actions to the primary complaint. It assures clients that first priority has been assigned to their concern. A limited examination directed at the primary complaint may confirm that the client's concern is justified, that "abdominal pain is indeed present" or "that diarrhea is severe." The reassured client will usually relax at this point, and the veterinarian can proceed with the examination.

Inspection of the patient, begun at some distance, can yield a sense of perspective about the patient's digestive tract. It should include observation of the patient both at rest and in motion whenever possible. The sequence of events is variable; one may have been able to observe the patient as it mingled with other animals in the feed-yard, pasture, or kennel-exercise area while the history was being narrated. Valuable impressions can be gained while the client and the dog are escorted to the examination room, or while the client unloads the horse and leads it into the hospital. For example, the state of nutrition can be assessed from the sleekness of the coat, the flesh cover of ribs, and the thickness of muscling.

The mouth, abdomen, and perineum are the principal regions in which visual findings can be related to the gastrointestinal system. One may observe an abnormal head posture related to an oropharyngeal lesion, the influence of abdominal pain in reducing the length and ease of stride, and the abnormal tail carriage (twitching, tightly held to the body, or held somewhat raised) associated with anorectal lesions. When the patient is examined at the paddock, pen, or kennel, one should observe type and quality of feed, evidence of food intake, and characteristics and components of the feces.

Clients appreciate humane and gentle handling of their animals. The use of a chute is essential in handling range cattle for the physical safety of all persons in the area. Yet one can use that framework of steel in a humane manner. The same is true for the use of lip and ear restraint of horses; head, neck, and tail restraint of cattle; and hand or muzzle restraint of dogs and cats. The client's feelings and attitudes toward, and knowledge of, restraint should be assessed. His need to know the method of and the necessity for physical restraint should be dealt with before initiating it. A calm demeanor, gentle voice, and the use of minimal restraint consistent with personal safety reassure both patient and client.

During the examination, the clinician should be aware of and routinely practice techniques that demonstrate concern for the patient's well-being, such as stroking the hair in its natural pattern except when examining the skin directly. Animals to be shown at exhibitions may be placed at a disadvantage if the hair has been clipped. When clipping is necessary, hair must be removed in a neat, well-defined pattern. Regrowth of clipped hair may be of different color or texture, notably in Arabian horses, Poodle dogs, and Siamese cats, and the client should be so informed beforehand. It is advisable to elevate extremities toward the trunk for inspection rather than extending them away from the trunk. The clinician should not support his own weight on any animal except as necessary for restraint.

THE MOUTH

The muzzle, face, and submandibular area should be examined by visual inspection and palpation before opening the mouth. Special attention should be given to crusting or peeling of the muzzle, an abnormal nasal discharge, foaming at the mouth, or drooling of food and/or saliva. One should palpate for swelling of the submandibular area, for enlargement of submandibular or retropharyngeal lymph nodes, and for the presence of firm or soft, diffuse or localized swellings of the face.

Examination of the mouth can be performed in young animals of all domestic species by manually elevating and extending the head and depressing the mandible. Insertion of a thumb or finger between the maxilla and mandible in the premolar region usually elicits opening of the mouth, especially if the digit is gently pressed against the hard palate. Foals and calves are usually restrained with the head held against one's side and with the tongue drawn rostrally and to the side. Tilting one's head forward permits a downward view into the patient's mouth. Puppies and kittens are set at table height or higher and the mouth is examined from a direct frontal position. Hand restraint alone is usually adequate because the patient is quite small. In all instances, the patient is positioned so that the mouth is brought in line with the brightest available light. A penlight or headlamp may be used; natural

light is preferred for viewing mucous membranes. Pallor, cyanosis, and icterus are more readily seen by natural light.

When the mouth of the puppy or kitten is to be opened, a restraining hand is placed transversely across the crown of the head, with the thumb below the mandible. Then, the thumb is shifted onto the hard palate, as described, or is lodged against the upper premolars or the canine tooth if the mouth is small. Next, the mouth is gently levered open by downward pressure on the lower incisors with the index finger of the opposite hand. As the mouth opens, the index finger may be quickly directed caudally over the base of the tongue to expose the soft palate, tonsils, and proximal pharynx. This latter maneuver may be done in rather leisurely fashion in many puppies, but should be done quickly in kittens because they resent having a finger in their mouth. The caudally directed papillae of the feline tongue can be used to advantage in further exposing the pharynx, by simply maintaining sufficient digital pressure on the tongue so that it "adheres" to the finger momentarily as the finger is withdrawn from the oral cavity.

The mouth can be examined repeatedly by this method without injury or undue excitement of the patient. Several quick inspections are better tolerated by the patient than one prolonged inspection under vigorous restraint. The ventral surface of the tongue and the floor of the mouth are exposed by dorsal pressure in the intermandibular region with the second finger as the mandible is depressed by the thumb on the lower incisors. The lips of puppies and kittens should never be compressed during any of these hand manipulations.

The foal and calf require more vigorous restraint. The upper lip and the tongue may be used as levers to hold the mouth open. Digital pressure on the upper lip is applied by inserting the fingertips into the dorsal aspect of the buccal space near the commissure and pressing the lip into the palm of the hand. The tongue is grasped and withdrawn laterally at the opposite commissure of the lips. Draping a dry towel over the hand before grasping the tongue greatly facilitates the maneuver in horses and cattle of all ages.

GLOVES MUST ALWAYS BE WORN IF MANUAL EXPLORATION OF THE MOUTH IS CONTEMPLATED IN A PATIENT SHOWING EXCESSIVE SALIVATION OR SIGNS OF CHOKING, LEST THE UNDERLYING CAUSE BE RABIES!

Mature horses should be restrained in stocks, and growing and mature cattle in a chute. The clinician should avoid standing squarely in front of the patient, to protect against being struck by the forelimb of a horse, or to prevent being covered with saliva or sputum if the steer coughs! A suitable mouth speculum should be inserted in horses and cattle if a prolonged examination is to be undertaken. Mature dogs are examined in the same manner as puppies except that giant breeds of dogs may be restrained in a standing position on the floor and examined without recourse to a table.

Examination of the mouth is begun by everting the lips and observing the gums for the pallor of anemia and for petechial hemorrhages, icterus, vesicles or ulcers, swelling, and wounds. The lips and tongue are checked for vesicles, ulcers, injury, or swelling and are palpated for evidence of induration. The dental pad of cattle is always closely examined, because coarse roughage and virus infections may cause inflammation and erosion at this site. The incisor teeth are examined for signs of discoloration and/or loss of enamel. It is important to know that the incisor teeth of normal cattle are relatively loose, as compared to the incisors of the horse.

In order to examine the premolar and molar cheek teeth, the tongue should be held against the commissure of the lip opposite the teeth to be examined. Bovine patients between 12 and 18 months old should be carefully checked for premolars which are being shed and which thus interfere with chewing. Old cattle or horses may have a molar tooth that is overgrown due to the absence of the apposed tooth.

The buccal surfaces should be examined for areas of necrosis, as in calf diphtheria, and for a food bolus or foreign body lodged between the teeth or in the pharynx. The palate is observed for congenital deformity in the young animal and for ulcers, petechial hemorrhages, swellings, or areas of necrosis in animals of all ages.

THE PHARYNX

Direct examination of the pharynx can be performed by visual inspection with the aid of artificial light. Special attention should be paid to the tonsils in the dog and cat and to the possibility of an embedded foreign body in all species. Other pathologic lesions are as described for mouth, lips, and tongue. The pharyngeal region can be examined externally by inspection and palpation, with special attention to the regional lymph nodes.

In order to conduct a more complete examination of the mouth and pharynx, sedation or light general anesthesia may be necessary, especially if the patient is fractious. Restraint of the head and use of a mouth speculum facilitate the examination.

THE ESOPHAGUS

The cervical esophagus lies in a sheltered location between the cervical vertebrae and the left lateral aspect of the trachea. Thus, the normal esophagus is not readily delineated in domestic animals by palpation unless it is distended or thickened. Passing a stomach tube into the esophagus and palpating its course along the neck is an aid in becoming better acquainted with its location. Observing the unimpeded passage of a food bolus along the course of the cervical esophagus assures normal function of that segment. Special methods of physical examination are used to examine the thoracic esophagus, i.e., passing a tube or sound, radiography, esophagoscopy, and thoracotomy.

THE STOMACH

The physical examination of the stomach is described separately for monogastric and ruminant animals because of the differences of structure and function of the stomach in these two groups.

Monogastric Animals. The emptied monogastric stomach is contained within the rib cage in all species and is essentially impalpable. When food-filled, the corpus of the stomach enlarges so that a firm, doughy mass protrudes caudally from the hypochondrium along the left lateral body wall. If the body wall is thin and supple, as in cats and dogs, the food-filled stomach is palpable. An enlarged gas-filled stomach, usually palpable in dogs and cats, may be detected by auscultation along with percussion in a horse.

Cradling the anterior abdomen of the dog or cat in the palm of the hand and gently palpating across the abdomen with thumb and fingers, then moving posteriorly as digital pressure is alternately applied and released, will entrap and outline intra-abdominal organs. Digital pressure should be used to define the margins, to determine the degree of firmness, and to sense the presence or absence of fluid in organs or in masses. Although this method suffices for small cats and dogs, it is usually necessary to place a hand on either side of the abdomen when palpating the abdomen of larger cats and dogs. Experienced clinicians find that two-handed abdominal palpation is probably superior to the one-handed method.

Palpation of the anterior abdomen in a dog or cat is made easier by raising the forequarters and thorax. The sternum should be pressed upward to elevate the animal, with the forelimbs relaxed in partial flexion. The abdominal muscles become more tense if the forelimbs are extended. Anterior abdominal organs or masses tend to move slightly caudally during this maneuver, improving one's chances of palpating them well. Placing the dog or cat in lateral or dorsal recumbency may facilitate palpation of liver, kidneys, or masses, especially in the obese patient.

The normal resistance of the abdominal wall, and the heightened resistance induced by fear or by an inexperienced examiner's hands, should be differentiated from the resistance to abdominal palpation induced by localized or generalized abdominal pain. In this regard, a physically relaxed hand and arm are essential; even gentle palpation elicits a response when the animal is in pain. Remember that the severely depressed animal may not yield a pain response in some instances.

Auscultation of the abdomen permits one to distinguish normal peristalsis, aperistalsis, hypermotility, and gaseous distention of hollow viscera. Percussion may reveal an enlarged organ or mass, and a combination of percussion and auscultation may reveal ascites.

Ruminants. The clinician must be thoroughly acquainted with the anatomic structure and motility pattern of the ruminant forestomachs and stomach if he is to conduct a thorough physical examination. The bovine will serve as the ruminant type in this discussion.

The rumen is the largest forestomach, occupying the left half of the abdomen and lying immediately adjacent to the left abdominal wall and left flank. It lies caudal and ventral to a slightly convex, curved line drawn from the left elbow to the top of the last rib, thence caudal to the tuber coxae. This imaginary line approximates the anterior border of the diaphragm and delineates the anterior boundary of the abdominal cavity.

The anatomic size and location of the rumen enable the clinician to examine this organ by auscultation, percussion, and palpation over a wide area of the left lateral abdominal wall. In addition, the motility of the dorsal sac of the rumen can be observed and the texture of rumen content can be palpated at the left paralumbar fossa. One can palpate the contraction wave of the dorsal sac by placing the palm or fist at the left paralumbar fossa. About two waves per minute is usual in the dairy cow, whereas feedlot cattle on high-concentrate rations often have only one ruminal contraction wave per minute. Auscultation along the left flank will reveal normal borborygmus and the characteristic crunching, mixing sounds during ruminal

contractions. Gurgling sounds that occur during eructation of rumen gases can also be auscultated. The rumen can be evaluated for pain by deep palpation with the fist in the lower left flank immediately caudal to the rib cage.

The reticulum is a relatively small organ encased within the rib cage (sixth to eighth interspaces on the left side) between the rumen and the diaphragm to the left of the midline. With the animal standing in a normal position, the position of the reticulum can be located by placing the hand on the left lateral body wall immediately caudal to the left elbow. Auscultation over the lower third of the seventh intercostal space on the left side reveals the soft but crunching sounds that occur during normal contraction of the reticulum. The reticulum is inaccessible for percussion or direct palpation. Examination for pain may be done by applying pressure dorsally with the fist or knee, or with a rigid bar directed transversely under the xiphoid. An assistant is needed for the latter maneuver. The animal may flinch or grunt as upward pressure is applied, or when pressure is abruptly released. By auscultation of the reticulum and concurrent palpation at the left paralumbar fossa, motility of the rumen and reticulum can be correlated.

Clinical Interpretation of Reticuloruminal Motility. The clinical interpretation for forestomach motility has been described.[2] An examination of the normal, adult bovine will reveal the following cycle of events:

1. A biphasic contraction of the reticulum, recognized on auscultation as a mild "swishing" sound, is followed by a contraction wave proceeding caudally over the dorsal sac of the rumen. The contraction of the dorsal rumen can be seen and/or palpated at the left paralumbar fossa. (When the hand is placed on the flank, the rumen can be felt pressing against the lateral body wall as it contracts.) This phase is not accompanied by the eructation of ruminal gases because the cardia is covered with ruminal ingesta.

2. Following the relaxation of the reticulum and the rumen, there is a contraction of the rumen only, again recognizable at the left flank. The reticulum remains relaxed, the cardia is cleared of ingesta, and ruminal gases that collect in the dorsal sac are expelled by eructation. The act of eructation can be heard quite easily in the normal adult bovine. The wave of eructated gas can also be observed in the left ventral neck region as it ascends the

esophagus. Immediately before eructation begins, the animal holds its breath. By observing the left costal arch during a ruminal contraction, the clinician can follow this sequence of events.

The two phases of forestomach contractions can thus be recognized by observing the left flank and identifying the noneructating and the eructating contractions. In most normal animals they alternate. However, variations occur, depending on the diet and the degree of fullness of the rumen; e.g., two noneructating contractions may follow an eructating contraction or vice versa. Contractions occur at the rate of 1 to 3 per minute in cattle on forage, being more frequent after food intake.

The ability to recognize these contractions is invaluable to the clinician in the diagnosis of traumatic reticuloperitonitis in the early stages, because the animal may grunt or hold its breath as the reticulum contracts (Williams reticular grunt test). The clinician is also well-advised to become familiar with the normal "crunching" sounds that occur within the rumen during normal contractions.

A final point should be made about the reticulorumen. The region where the esophagus enters the reticuloruminal atrium (cardia) is located by drawing a horizontal line from the submandibular region to the diaphragmatic plane previously described. Assuming that the animal is standing with the head in the normal position, the bisection will occur at the junction of the upper and middle third of the eighth intercostal space. The clinician will find this information invaluable in estimating the location of an esophageal obstruction. By first placing a stomach tube along this imaginary line and marking the distance to the cardia on the tube, the obstructing mass can be rather accurately located with respect to the cardia.

The omasum lies medial to the lower third of the eighth to the eleventh ribs on the right side, within the rib cage. In the normal adult animal it is approximately the size of a basketball. Direct examination of this organ is quite limited. Auscultation may permit one to hear gurgling sounds as ingesta passes through the omasum. Disorders of the omasum may be detected by the animal's grunting response to pain when deep digital pressure or percussion is applied to the intercostal spaces adjacent to it.

The abomasum is much more developed than the forestomachs in the young calf, occupying most of the hypochondrial region. The fundus or anterior blind sac of the abomasum is located in the xiphoid region in close proximity to the reticulum. The pylorus joins the duodenum at the ventral aspect of the right ninth or tenth ribs. Direct physical examination of the abomasum in the adult bovine is limited by the thick tense ventral abdominal muscles. As with the reticulum, forceful pressure dorsally in the right hypochondrium may elicit abomasal pain. A combination of ballottement and auscultation in the ventral aspect of the right anterior quadrant of the abdomen is helpful in detecting large quantities of gas or fluid in the abomasum. Tympany of the abomasum in the calf can be recognized visually as an asymmetric right-sided abdominal distention, and by auscultation, percussion, and ballottement.

The pylorus is impalpable in the normal adult bovine. It may be palpable in a thin animal at the ventral aspect of the eleventh rib when the pylorus is greatly enlarged and projecting caudally as in lymphosarcoma.

Exploration of the Reticuloruminal Sac. In many instances a thorough surgical exploration of the abdomen and the reticuloruminal sac is indicated in order to make a positive diagnosis of a digestive disorder.

The laparotomy is done with the animal in the standing position if possible. Under regional or local anesthesia of the left paralumbar area, the dorsal rumen is exposed following incision of the skin, muscles, and peritoneum. A sterile long-sleeved glove is worn. A manual exploration of the abdominal viscera is done before the rumen is incised. The hand should pass freely along the dorsal and left lateral aspects of, and caudal to, the rumen. Similarly, the hand should pass freely toward the right side as it is moved ventral to the anterior dorsal blind sac and reticulum. Movement of the hand between the diaphragm and normal reticulum should be unimpeded and cause no discomfort to the patient. The terminal esophagus is palpated as a tubular structure that traverses the diaphragm and attaches to the rumen dorsal and to the right of the reticulum. The iliac lymph nodes, reproductive tract, urinary bladder, kidneys, spleen, and liver are palpated for abnormalities of form and position. Intestine, omasum, pylorus, abomasum, and mesenteric lymph nodes may be palpable, depending on the size of the rumen.

When exploration of the abdomen has been completed, the rumen is sutured to the margins of the incision to prevent contamination of the peritoneal cavity with rumen content, and a vertical incision is made in the dorsal sac. The right arm is introduced through the rumen incision. In the normal animal, one feels a gas pocket in the dorsal rumen, with the ventral sac containing fluid ingesta. Solid ingesta floats on the fluid layer. A thorough exploration of the rumen can be made without removing any solid ingesta, although ingesta may be removed if desired.

The rumen, a large storage vat lined by papillae, is partially divided into dorsal and ventral sacs by two pillars which are infoldings of the wall, with corresponding grooves on the serosal surface. The pillars project into the anterior and posterior regions, forming blind sacs at each extremity. The anterior pillar projects obliquely dorsal and caudal, with a thick concave free-edge which lies medial to the eleventh and twelfth ribs. The pillar is covered with papillae on both sides but there are none on the concave surface. The posterior pillar lies almost horizontally and separates the dorsal and ventral posterior blind sacs.

Following a thorough exploration of the rumen, it is advisable to proceed toward the reticulum along the inside of the dorsal wall of the rumen and follow its contour until the reticulum, with its characteristic honeycomb lining, is reached. The reticulum contains semi-liquid ingesta and there is usually a considerable amount of foreign material such as sand or gravel on its floor. This organ is separated from the rumen by a rather slender structure, the reticuloruminal fold. This structure is almost perpendicular at rest and is lined by honeycomb epithelium on the anterior surface and by ruminal papillae posteriorly. It is important for the clinician to be familiar with the differences between the anterior pillar and this fold, for an inexperienced person with a short arm may easily "get lost" in the anterior ruminal sac of one of the larger cattle breeds when trying to locate the reticulum!

By placing the fingertips against the anterior wall of the reticulum, the veterinarian will readily feel the heartbeats and thus appreciate the close proximity of these organs. It is vitally important that a thorough exploration of the total inner surface of the reticulum be conducted, especially when one suspects the presence of a penetrating foreign body such as a nail or wire. In most adult cattle, part of the reticulum extends to the right beyond the midline and curves slightly around the anterior border of the omasum in the form of an ill-defined blind sac. A penetrating foreign object located in this area may remain undetected unless a thorough exploration of the entire reticulum is made.

The cardia is easily located at the dorsal aspect of the anterior reticular wall. A stomach tube passed via the mouth or nostril until it protrudes through the cardiac opening will greatly assist in the identification of this structure. At the cardia, the fingertips can be diverted ventrally into the reticular groove, whose spiral-shaped course can then be followed to the omasal orifice.

THE LIVER

Palpation of the normal liver is most readily done in the cat. Pressing the fingers anteromedially at the hypochondrium, while holding the thumb lateral to the opposite rib cage, one is able to locate the liver and evaluate its size and firmness. Reversing the position of the hand brings the opposite side of the liver against the fingers. Elevating the thorax tends to allow the liver to move caudally. Normal lobar margins are sharply angled in cats and dogs. The normal dog liver can best be palpated by pressing anterodorsally at the hypochondrium with both hands, recurving the fingers with palms held flattened on the ventrolateral thorax on either side. Standing by the shoulder of the animal with an arm directed caudoventrally past each shoulder of the dog toward the ventrum expedites the maneuver. In deep-chested dogs, the normal liver may be impalpable.

The normal liver of horses and cattle is not felt by transabdominal palpation. Percussion of an enlarged liver may be possible in cattle by deep palpation immediately posterior to the right rib cage.

THE PANCREAS

The normal pancreas is impalpable in all species.

THE INTESTINE

The scope of the physical examination of the intestine varies with the species. For example, more extensive examination of the colon is possible in the horse, because of the size and proximity of its segments. Conversely, in the dog and cat, the small intestine is readily examined because the abdominal wall is relatively thin and supple. Auscultation along the right and left posterior flanks of the horse will detect normal intestinal sounds (borborygmus) or the classic "tinkling" sounds of intestinal obstruction, which is a valuable physical finding in the sick horse. Abdominal distention may be due to intestinal obstruction in all species, and may be detected visually.

In the cat and the dog, the intestine can be asucultated, palpated, and percussed across the abdominal wall. If the abdominal muscles are tense owing to severe pain, it may be advisable to defer abdominal palpation until after radiographs have been obtained and interpreted. Only the imprudent clinician persists in palpating an exquisitely tender abdomen.

Manual examination of the small and large intestine, and of adjacent intra-abdominal organs is done in both horse and cow by the rectal approach. The patient should be suitably restrained for the protection of the clinician. Shoulder-length, well-lubricated rubber or polyethylene gloves should be worn. Evacuation of feces and introduction of the arm past the elbow, coupled with relaxation of the arm, will elicit greater relaxation of the rectum. Abdominal structures are outlined with the fingertips and are evaluated for thickness, degree of firmness or turgidity, and for content, i.e., solid, liquid, or gas. In the dog, rectal palpation is done with a gloved finger, combined with deep abdominal palpation by the other hand to bring intra-abdominal structures toward the pelvis.

THE RECTUM AND ANUS

The anorectal examination is begun by visual inspection of the perineum, perianal region, and anus for inflammation, erosion, ulcer, swelling, and hemorrhage. Rectal examination should include evaluation of the musosa for tenderness, mucosal defects, mucosal or mural mass, prolapse, or stricture. The anal sacs are palpated in dogs and cats for swelling or tenderness. The content of the anal sacs is noted.

Fecal material should be inspected visually and examined digitally for abnormal components at the time of rectal examination. Form, degree of firmness or estimation of fluid content, color, presence or absence of food particles, mucus, foreign material, blood, and tissue should be noted. Specimens for laboratory examination may be collected as the rectal examination is done.

REFERENCES

1. Low, D. G.: Personal communication, 1959.
2. Williams, E. I.: A study of reticulo-ruminal motility in adult cattle in relation to bloat and traumatic reticulitis with an account of the latter condition as seen in a general practice. Vet. Rec. 67:907, 922, 1955.

Chapter 4

PHYSICAL FINDINGS IN GASTROINTESTINAL DISEASES

RALPH G. BUCKNER
ERIC I. WILLIAMS

Physical findings in gastrointestinal diseases are abnormalities of form and function perceived by seeing, hearing, feeling, and smelling. When findings are assessed accurately, the veterinarian is able to develop a more complete data base, establish the diagnosis and prognosis, and administer rational therapy.

The findings in the digestive tract are detected principally in the mouth and on mucous membranes, in vomitus and diarrhea, in the abdomen, and in the rectum and anus. Some findings are so characteristic as to be virtually pathognomonic, e.g., the "sausage-loop" of an intussusception in a cat. Other findings may lack an immediately recognizable relationship to a diagnosis. As one learns that "clusters" or groups of signs and findings are characteristic of certain gastrointestinal diseases, definition of the problem begins to take form.

EXTERNAL FINDINGS

A visual survey of the patient frequently yields findings that not only guide the subsequent examination but are valuable as direct diagnostic clues as well. Ptyalism is common in digestive diseases, but is also found in other diseases. It is often associated with lesions of the oropharynx, and its presence calls for careful examination of those structures. Local infections (glossitis, stomatitis, tonsillitis, or pharyngitis), injuries such as fractured teeth and lacerations of the tongue, and foreign bodies embedded in the palate, buccal space, tongue, tonsillar crypt, or pharynx are examples. Foreign objects may be impacted between or over the teeth. Linear foreign objects such as sticks and bones may become impaled between the last premolar or molar teeth in either arcade, causing ptyalism as well as bizarre behavior, including rage. The visual image can easily be associated with rabies, to such an extent that the patient may experience an untimely demise at the request of the client.

Self-protection should be prominent in the veteri-narian's mind when examining the patient with ptyalism. Gloves should always be worn whenever examining the mouth that spills saliva. Because oral lesions seem to induce rage in some patients, there is a greater than usual danger of being bitten.

Alopecia or abrasion of the muzzle, associated with scratching with a foot or with rubbing of the muzzle on fixed objects or on the ground, is a clue to painful oropharyngeal lesions and particularly to foreign bodies. The outflowing saliva is likely to be cloudy if inflammation has developed from infection or trauma. Bloody saliva is a clue to oral wounds, deep ulcers, or fractured teeth or bones, including injury to the sinuses. However, sinus lesions drain primarily through the external nares or into the pharynx, where the exudate stimulates coughing and expectoration.

The patient that holds its mouth agape as it spills saliva may be experiencing pain, or may be prevented from closing the mouth because of an oral foreign body or fracture. This must be differentiated from the slackly drooping mandible of medullary paralysis in the dog. Animals with brain abscess or other central nervous system lesions may masticate compulsively without swallowing, and may exhibit pseudoptyalism.

Continuous protrusion of the tongue occurs if motor function of the hypoglossal nerve is lost. It also occurs in actinobacillosis of cattle. Repetitious protrusion and withdrawal of the tongue is a clue to an oropharyngeal lesion, and calls for careful examination of mouth and pharynx.

When the observer's attention is drawn to the oropharynx by one of the externally visible findings, he should observe for swallowing before approaching the patient more closely. Pharyngeal paralysis with inability to swallow occurs in a relatively few specific diseases, including rabies. Unwillingness to swallow is much more common than pharyngeal paralysis and accompanies many of the lesions causing ptyalism. Pharyngeal inflammation, mass,

23

or tonsillitis are likely to cause intensification of pain when swallowing occurs; thus, the patient refrains from swallowing or has exaggerated extension and flexion of the head and neck when it does swallow.

A distended cervical esophagus may be observed, particularly in the short-coated patient. The dilated esophagus frequently fills with gas (air). During the expiratory phase of respiration, the column of gas may shift anteriorly and further distend the cervical esophagus. This visual finding is made most commonly in dogs.

Abdominal distention may be visually assessed by comparing the abdomen with other parts of the body. Obese animals often have a large, seemingly distended abdomen. An obese patient that is able to move about freely and with no apparent discomfort may not have true abdominal distention. On the other hand, a thin nonpregnant patient with a large abdomen is likely to have a pathologic lesion within the digestive tract.

Gaseous distentions tend to be symmetric and rotund because of the plasticity of abdominal viscera. Prompt rebound to external palpation and high-pitched resonance, heard when the abdomen is percussed and auscultated, are characteristic of gaseous distentions. Fluid distentions, on the other hand, tend to be pendulous. Sharp percussion with the hand generates a fluid wave that can be sensed with the other hand at the opposite abdominal wall. Percussion of fluid elicits a lower-pitched sound than does percussion of a gas-filled viscus. Severe gaseous and fluid distentions of the abdomen cause anterior displacement of the diaphragm and produce respiratory embarrassment even at rest.

Gaseous distentions tend to be contained within the digestive tract; rupture of a gas-filled viscus is usually followed by peritonitis and death unless recognized and treated quickly. Fluid distentions, although commonly occurring within the obstructed digestive tract, may occur in any hollow viscus. Accumulation of fluid within the peritoneal cavity has many causes, some of which are compatible with minimal discomfort and long survival.

When the abdominal distention has been tentatively classified as primarily gaseous or fluid in nature, several special techniques are used to localize the site and extent of the distention. Gaseous distentions of the stomach and rumen are confirmed and may be temporarily relieved by stomach tube. Fluid within stomach or rumen may also be detected and removed by siphoning with a tube. Peritoneal fluid can usually be detected by paracentesis abdominis. Ascites, exudate from peritonitis,

spilled gastrointestinal content, bile, hemorrhage, urine, and fluids from neoplastic tissue may be detected. Other special techniques of physical examination, including radiography and endoscopy, are described in Chapters 7 through 9.

Reduced size of the abdomen (contracted abdomen) is not necessarily a finding of disease, nor does it imply that the abdomen is painful. It is not necessarily associated with abnormal function of the digestive tract. Simple lack of food and water may be the cause. Any lesion proximal to the esophagogastric junction that inhibits or prevents ingestion of food and water is another consideration. Severe diarrhea may result in dehydration through repeated evacuation of the small intestine and colon, with visible reduction of normal abdominal girth.

Abdominal pain may be suspected in the patient if the following are observed: kyphosis, unwillingness to move about, stilted gait, kicking at the abdomen, turning of the head toward the abdomen (pleurothotonos), restlessness, and repeated lying down and arising to a standing position.

Diarrhea is usually evident on the tail, anus, perineum, and hocks. When examining the patient in its usual environment, one can often find an abundance of evidence for further characterizing the diarrhea: mucus, blood, macroparasites, undigested food, steatorrhea, and foreign material.

Pelvic pain is observed as tenesmus, with an abrupt abdominal press coinciding with bulging of the perineum and elevation of the tail. Close inspection and rectal examination usually localize the problem to rectum and anus or to the vagina and uterus.

DENTITION

Physical findings involving the teeth include retained deciduous teeth, discoloration or loss of enamel, absence of teeth, overgrown, uneven, or fractured teeth, periodontal disease, and, occasionally, dental caries.

Since dental abnormalities can interfere with the prehension and mastication of food, there are likely to be signs of ptyalism and foaming at the mouth, dropping of food from the mouth (quidding), shaking of the head, or other obvious interference with chewing. In horses and cattle, impaired mastication results in an abnormal amount of whole grain in the feces. However, intact oat hulls are passed in the feces of horses and cattle with normal teeth. Unmacerated grain on the ground or floor adjacent to the feed box or bunk is a clue to abnormal dentition in herbivores. A localized swelling on the side of the face may be a clue to an abscessed tooth in any species.

Discolored teeth with loss of enamel are seen in cases of fluorosis and in dogs that survive severe viral infection, e.g., distemper in the early months of life. Yellow to brown discoloration of a puppy's or kitten's deciduous teeth may be observed after tetracycline has been administered during the early weeks of life. A brownish-purple discoloration of the incisors occurs in cattle and cats with porphyria. The absence of incisor teeth, usually the central incisors, is referred to as "broken mouth," a common syndrome in sheep that graze rough forage. Affected sheep have difficulty in grazing and in the prehension of root crops. Reduced numbers of permanent teeth, usually caused by failure of eruption of incisors or premolars, are sometimes observed.

Abnormalities of the cheek teeth (premolars and molars) commonly occur in horses and cattle. These include the incomplete shedding of the shells of one or more deciduous (premolar) teeth in adolescent cattle, an overgrown molar tooth with absence of the opposite tooth in older animals, or irregular occlusal surfaces of the cheek teeth in aged horses. In all instances, there is visible evidence of interference with mastication. Fractures of the upper fourth premolar tooth due to trauma are fairly common in dogs.

MUCOUS MEMBRANES

Pallor of the mucous membranes results from reduced tissue perfusion. The normal pink mucous membrane may be so pale that it fails to blanch, or blanches only slightly, upon digital pressure. Evaluation of perfusion should be done with caution in animals that have submucous pigment deposition, i.e., black Cocker Spaniels, Chow Chows, and some Holstein and Angus cattle. The color of the mucous membrane of the oral cavity of the cat must be judged carefully, since the normal pink color is less ruddy than in dogs. The vaginal mucosa may be a more reliable area for judging the color of the mucous membrane in some domestic animals; however, in dogs and cats the conjunctiva is preferred.

Pallor of mucous membranes accompanied by tachypnea after exercise should lead one to search for acute hemorrhage, perhaps into the bowel, peritoneal space, or thorax. Lethargy, depression, faltering gait, weakness, and polydipsia frequently occur after acute blood loss. Pallor is a hallmark of the shock syndrome, with cyanosis in endotoxic shock. The mucous membrane may be cool to the touch. A site of gram-negative infection should be sought if endotoxic shock is suspected. As an example, rupture of a digestive viscus releases gram-negative bacteria into the adjacent body space, thus providing the source of endotoxin.

Congestion of mucous membranes may occur in gastrointestinal disease, usually as a manifestation of dehydration. The visible mucous membranes are ruddy to dusky blue in proportion to the severity of hemoconcentration. Vomiting, diarrhea, and prolonged failure to ingest water are the usual gut-associated causes. The congested mucous membrane blanches only slightly with digital pressure. A somewhat adhesive or "tacky" sensation is sensed when the fingertip is touched to the congested buccal mucous membranes. Whether acute or chronic, it accompanies passive venous overfilling from any cause.

Hyperemia, reddening of mucous membranes due to increase in oxygenated blood, occurs in any part of the digestive tract but is immediately visible only at the mouth or anus. While it may be evidence of local irritation or infection, hyperemia may also be a clue to more deep-seated disease elsewhere in the body. Severe azotemia, septicemia, acute hepatic disease, or acute pancreatitis are but a few of the disorders in which hyperemia of oral mucous membranes occurs.

Edema and *inflammation* of oral mucous membranes tend to occur together. When deep gingival and labial infections occur, the sites are particularly likely to appear both swollen and red. Edematous tissues of the oral cavity are smooth, glistening, and turgid; the red hue of the tissues is a clue to the presence of inflammation. Infection is by far the most common cause; trauma or other predisposing cause should be sought.

Exudation into the gastrointestinal tract is serous to mucous in character, but is not commonly purulent except in the buccal and oral cavities. The exudate contains large quantities of protein and leukocytes, and is most readily visible at the mouth or anus. It accompanies vesicle formation in the mouth and ulceration of the oral or rectal mucosa. The exudate may be tenacious and fetid when tissue necrosis has occurred. It can be associated with viral and bacterial agents, e.g., bovine virus diarrhea of cattle, feline viral rhinotracheitis, and leptospirosis in dogs. Exudation from the mucosa of the small intestine is cloudy to bloody, depending on severity. It may be detected in vomitus containing refluxed intestinal content, but if gastric and intestinal exudate is passed per rectum, it may be admixed with feces and thus be obscured. Hematemesis, the vomiting of blood, is an inconstant sign observed when the gastric mucosal capillary bed is breached, as in ulceration, neoplasia, or uremia. Inflammation of the colon is characterized by the passage of viscous, adhesive, cloudy to yellowish mucus or exudate per rectum.

Icterus or jaundice is a yellow discoloration of the mucous membranes, also observable in the skin, subcutaneous fat, plasma, and urine. It should not be confused with the normal yellow color of the mucous membranes of Jersey and Guernsey cattle and of some horses.

Conjugated bilirubin usually stains the tissue visibly at 2.0 mg/dl of serum. It has a tendency to localize in tissues with a high concentration of elastic fibers, e.g., skin and sclera. Equivalent intensity of staining of the mucous membranes by unconjugated bilirubin occurs at a higher plasma concentration than that of conjugated bilirubin, because unconjugated bilirubin is not as readily bound to tissue.

The oral cavity is not a reliable location for the detection of icterus, because of the abundant capillary blood supply and submucous pigment deposition. The sclera, vaginal mucosa, or skin of the posterior abdomen and groin are preferred locations. Natural light is superior to artificial light for the visual detection of icterus; fluorescent lighting is likely to obscure it.

Erosion is the loss of mucosa resulting in exposure of the underlying tissue. It is characterized by erythema, transudation, and exudation. Microbial invasion of eroded epithelia usually occurs before exudation is observed. Erosion is observed on the lips or in the oral cavity as a denuded, slightly depressed, irregularly circumscribed area of mucous membrane. Causes include viral or bacterial infection, azotemia, trauma, the abrasive action of food substances or foreign bodies, congenital dental deformities, or exposure to caustic chemicals. Epithelial necrosis may precede erosion, e.g., in acute bovine viral diarrhea, infectious bovine rhinotracheitis, and feline rhinotracheitis.

Ulceration may accompany or follow erosion and is characterized by local excavation of submucous tissue, exudation, and variable hemorrhage. Severe ulceration may be observed on the lateral borders of the tongue and buccal mucosa of the horse. Ulceration is frequently observed in the oral cavity of cattle due to bacterial and viral diseases. The azotemic dog frequently displays ulceration of the lateral margins and the tip of the tongue. It is commonly observed in the cat on the upper lips, and on the lateral borders and dorsal surface of the tongue.

Erosion and ulceration of the mucosa and submucosa of the lips, tongue, palate, gingiva, and pharynx may be observed directly in all animals. The signs are: ptyalism, which is often hemorrhagic and fetid, anorexia, and/or dysphagia. Pseudoptyalism and dysphagia may be observed if erosion and ulceration of the oropharynx inhibit swallowing.

Denuding of the mucosa of the esophagus and stomach may stimulate regurgitation or vomiting, the latter usually in monogastric animals. The horse does not vomit unless gastric rupture is imminent or has already occurred, and the ruminant seldom vomits. Both species can and do regurgitate, however. Anorexia often follows due to pain associated with the act of swallowing.

Erosion and ulceration of the small intestine in monogastric animals may result in vomiting of bile- or blood-tinged (dark brown to black) mucus, if intestinal content refluxes into the stomach.

Erosion and ulceration of the colon and rectal mucosa in all species are characterized by tenesmus and the frequent passage of small quantities of feces containing fresh blood and mucus. These signs are observed in colitis in the horse, salmonellosis in calves, and ulcerative colitis in the dog. Erosion, ulceration, and the response to chronic inflammation of the deep structures of the wall of the colon result in cicatrix formation, stenosis, stricture, and obstruction. The frequent passage of small quantities of soft to fluid feces, tenesmus, and anorexia are observed.

Further evaluation of the gastrointestinal tract can be made by radiographic and endoscopic methods.

Hemorrhage from the alimentary tract can be observed in the saliva, vomitus, or feces. Blood in saliva is bright red to pink and may also be indirectly observed as a similar discoloration of the water in the drinking bowl.

When the source of hemorrhage is the ulcerated mucosal surfaces of the oral cavity or oropharynx, the color is bright red. Blood originating in the esophagus, stomach, or small intestine causes the vomitus to be brown-to-black-flecked if gastric acid has altered hemoglobin to hematin. The collection of dark, bloody, fetid, tenacious saliva on the teeth and gingiva in the dog is found in acute leptospirosis and other diseases characterized by azotemia. Melena is the passage of black, tarry feces, while hematochezia is the passage of fresh blood in or on the feces. The former is characteristic of hookworm infection in the dog, for example. Melena with dark red mucus occurs in intussusception in the horse, cow, dog, and other species. Hematochezia may be observed in any acute inflammatory, chronic granulomatous, neoplastic, or parasitic disease of the large intestine, i.e., histoplasma colitis in the dog.

Fresh blood from the anus unaccompanied by the passage of feces can be due to parasites in the terminal colon or to a fecalith, foreign body, or tumor in the rectum.

A *tumor* may be defined generally as a space-occupying mass of tissue, or specifically as an uncontrolled proliferation of cells. Tumors may be found within an organ or protruding through the mucosal surface. They may be soft or firm, when observed on the mucosal surface of the alimentary tract, and produce a variety of signs, depending upon location, size, and number.

The epulides of the Boxer dog are nodular, proliferating masses of gingival tissue that may be erythematous, ulcerated, and necrotic. Oral papillomas in dogs and cattle are discrete or coalescent pedunculated tufts of tissue with papillary surfaces, occurring on any mucous surface. Involvement of the oral cavity, palate, or pharynx by papillomas is characterized by ptyalism or pseudoptyalism that is serous to mucoid, occurs with or without blood, and has a strong odor of necrotic tissue. Dysphagia and subsequent anorexia accompany tumors in the palate and oropharynx. Melanomas of the oral cavity are often ulcerated deeply, and may have caused loosening or actual loss of teeth before examination is made.

Tumors involving the esophagus are relatively rare in all domestic animals. Esophageal tumors cause obstruction, anterior dilatation, pseudoptyalism, and regurgitation. Extension of malignancies from the cardiac portion of the stomach into the thoracic esophagus results in regurgitation of bright red and/or hemolyzed (dark) blood. Polydipsia frequently accompanies gastritis caused by tumor, resulting in further vomiting. Carcinoma of the stomach, although uncommon, occurs in all domestic animals, and is suspected in the face of persistent vomiting in dogs and cats. Hematemesis, polydipsia, anorexia, and weight loss are frequently part of the cluster of signs associated with gastric carcinoma in these species.

The small intestine responds to the presence of a tumor as it would to the presence of an obstructing foreign body. Depending upon the location and degree of blockage, vomitus tinted with blood or greenish yellow bile will be observed. The latter signifies reflux of duodenal contents into the stomach. Partial to complete obstruction with ces-

sation of peristalsis may occur if the intestinal wall is deeply invaded, e.g., lymphosarcoma in the bovine.

Tumors of the large intestine tend to cause obstruction, with dilatation anterior to the tumor. Hemorrhages, either bright or dark, are passed with mucus in the feces. Tumors of the distal colon are characterized by repeated tenesmus, hematochezia, and passage of quantities of mucus. Transabdominal or rectal palpation of the tumor frequently elicits pain and tenesmus.

Tumors of the rectum or anus with ulcerated mucosal surfaces often yield fresh hemorrhage preceding the passage of feces, or blood may drip intermittently from the anus following defecation. Tenesmus often occurs in such cases and pain is elicited by manual exploration of the rectum.

ABDOMINAL DISTENTION

A rotund abdomen is usually associated with excessive gas production and/or accumulation in the digestive tract. Abdominal distention in the horse may be detected at the paralumbar fossae, although the small size of the fossae and the thick abdominal wall of the horse limit the degree of visible distention. In cattle and sheep, however, tympany of the rumen (bloat) first causes unilateral distention at the left paralumbar fossa, progressing toward rotund bilateral distention in more severe cases. In the dog, gastric tympany results in a flaring of the posterior rib cage and the hypochondrium. As gastric distention increases, the posterior abdomen also becomes visibly distended.

The effect of excess fluid on abdominal contour depends on the location of such fluid. Voluminous ascites will give rise to a bilaterally pendulous abdomen in most species, because the distending fluid has much greater mass per unit volume than does gas. Muscle weakness accentuates the pendulous appearance of the fluid-filled abdomen. Great accumulation of abdominal fluid may noticeably alter the stance and gait of the animal, tending to produce a flat-footed posture and causing veering and staggering during locomotion. The latter is visible evidence of the inertial effect of a large fluid mass. When fluid accumulates within a digestive viscus, the site and degree of the resulting abdominal distention depend on the organ involved. There will tend to be an asymmetric left-sided distention if the rumen is fluid-filled.

The accumulation of fluid within the small intestine due to an intestinal obstruction (torsion, intussusception) eventually results in rotund bilateral abdominal distention in all species. In cattle, it will also cause stasis of fluid in the rumen, which becomes distended and as a characteristic "slushy" feel on palpation at the left paralumbar fossa.

Unilateral abdominal distention of gastrointestinal origin may occur on either side. In cattle, reference has already been made to unilateral (left side) bloat. A tympanitic swelling immediately caudal to the left costal arch is seen in an advanced case of left-sided abomasal displacement. Likewise, with the same disorder, observation of the animal from the rear may reveal a localized distention of the abdomen at the lower left flank. However, medial displacement of the rumen from the left body wall by the intruded abomasum may result in a "slab-sided" appearance of the left abdominal wall.

Abdominal distention involving the right flank is characteristic of abomasal or cecal problems in cattle. A tympanitic swelling immediately caudal to the right costal arch occurs in a case of advanced displacement of the abomasum to the right. The tympany is more obvious if abomasal torsion develops. A localized tympanitic swelling in the right paralumbar fossa, immediately cranial to the tuber coxae, is characteristic of cecal torsion in cattle. A localized distention in the lower right flank below the costal arch is observed with advanced abomasal impaction.

Weakness or a tear in the abdominal musculature results in a change in the contour of the abdomen. Unilateral distention arises from a ventral abdominal rupture and may occur to the left or right of the midline. Rupture of the prepubic tendon, whether in mares or in cows, will produce a bilateral ventral distention of the caudal abdomen. In cases of ventral midline abdominal distention, such as umbilical hernia, part of the gastrointestinal tract is likely to be involved.

An inguinal hernia may cause a localized distention of the caudal abdomen in bulls, which may extend to the hypochondrium in severe cases. More often, the hernia extends only into the scrotum, as a unilateral swelling. The clinician must always check for scrotal hernia in a male animal showing signs of colic and, if hernia is present, for possible strangulation of the incarcerated segment of intestine. The examination should include external palpation of the scrotum and rectal palpation of the inguinal rings.

ABDOMINAL PAIN

The manifestation of abdominal pain in cattle may be in the form of a grunt or a groan at intervals. Groaning is more characteristic of severe abdominal distention especially if the patient is recumbent. This must not be confused with pain arising from other areas, such as from thoracolumbar disc protrusion in the dog. A grunt may be related to a contraction of a digestive organ; e.g., in the early stage of traumatic reticuloperitonitis, a grunt can be detected during reticular contractions. Kyphosis, associated with abdominal pain, is most commonly seen in cattle and dogs. Sweating (hyperhidrosis) may accompany abdominal pain in horses and less frequently in cattle. Dogs with acute abdominal pain may recline with the abdomen on a cool surface, or may assume a prayer posture with the forequarters and thorax lowered to the floor, or may pace restlessly about the area, alternatively seeking recumbency only to arise and pace about again. Horses with severe abdominal pain are likely to be active, especially in the early hours after onset. Some of their characteristic actions include lying down abruptly, rolling over, getting up, circling, and pawing at the earth.

Fatigue, depression, and inactivity are later manifestations of abdominal pain in all species.

ABDOMINAL MASS

Rectal palpation is used to detect abdominal masses in horses and cattle. Less commonly, one may detect an abdominal mass in a thin pig or a sheep by transabdominal palpation. Goats have a fairly thin abdominal wall and one can palpate reasonably well by hand pressure across the abdominal wall.

Abdominal organs with fixed position give rise to masses that are relatively fixed, e.g., liver, kidney, and stomach. Mobile, pendulous organs give rise to masses that have a noticeable degree of mobility, e.g., small intestine, mesenteric lymph nodes, and spleen. Including a routine of palpation (transabdominal, rectal) in the general physical examination and repeatedly using that technique will prepare one to distinguish the mass or abnormal organ from normal structures.

RECTUM AND PELVIS

Rectal palpation usually differentiates normal from abnormal structures. Solid masses, with or without tenderness, and fluid- or gas-filled viscera are the abnormalities usually found. The abnormal finding is then related to digestive, reproductive, urinary, or blood or lymph vascular systems, based on anatomic relationships. Detailed descriptions of rectally palpable abnormalities of the digestive system are presented with discussions of specific disease entities in Section Three.

ANUS AND PERINEUM

The findings at the anus and perineum are often painful, giving rise to tenesmus. Barring the presence of inspissated feces occluding the anus, most anal lesions are either inflammatory or neoplastic. These pathologic processes are not always readily differentiable at physical examination, since either inflammation or neoplasia may cause similar signs of swelling, hemorrhage, ulceration or erosion, and exudation. The diagnostic procedure of incisional biopsy is probably superior to impression (smear)

biopsy, since most lesions in this heavily contaminated region have exudate on the surface.

The anus of the dog may become eroded and ulcerated in association with neoplasia of the circumanal glands, while the perianal region of the grey horse may be eroded by melanoma. The anus and perineum of German Shepherd dogs are often affected with numerous tortuous fistulous tracts. Erosion and ulceration of the perianal region precede the appearance of the problem, one seen almost exclusively in this breed and in Irish Setters. Rectal lesions often accompany perianal fistulae and may be detected by rectal digital examination and by colonoscopy.

Chapter 5

DEFINING GASTROINTESTINAL PROBLEMS

Part I. Problem-Oriented Veterinary Medical Record

WILLIAM D. SCHALL

Solving gastrointestinal problems is a challenging task for the veterinarian, because the problems are often ill-defined. Many patients recover without precise definition of the problem, i.e., without an etiologic diagnosis. The difficulty in plodding through a complex case with a maze of poorly defined and partially resolved problems can be lessened if a logical and systematic approach is taken. Use of the Problem Oriented Veterinary Medical Record (POVMR) well-nigh forces the clinician to be more logical and systematic in case workups.

OUTLINE OF POVMR

The first premise of the POVMR is that the patient's problems should be identified at a defensible level of understanding, titled in standard terms, and numbered. Diagnostic and therapeutic efforts can then be directed to each problem in turn. This concept is especially important when the patient has multiple problems, even though the individual problems are really of common origin and are ultimately resolved to a single diagnosis. In the POVMR, a problem is defined as a client's complaint or as a sign of disease (dysphagia), an abnormal laboratory test result (hypoalbuminemia), a pathophysiologic syndrome (hepatic failure), or an etiologic diagnosis (enteric colibacillosis). A problem, then, is something that requires veterinary medical management,[1] whether by diagnostic effort (Dx), treatment (Rx), or client education (CE) so that the client understands the problem better.

It is essential that the clinician entitle problems honestly as he presently understands them. For instance, diarrhea may be due to uremia and not to a primary enteritis. Until sufficient objective data are gathered to redefine the problem at a higher level of understanding, it should remain titled as honestly understood, i.e., diarrhea, a clinical sign, rather than enteritis, which implies that one has proven that intestinal inflammation exists.

After problems are identified, titled, and numbered, initial diagnostic plans should be formulated for each problem. Each procedure in the diagnostic plan should be included with the specific intent of ruling out some disease or category of disease. When these new objective data are obtained, the problem may be redefined at a higher level of understanding. After initial diagnostic plans are formulated, the plan for therapy (Rx) is made. In many instances therapeutic actions are undertaken hastily and obscure proper definition of the problem. Not infrequently, therapy is inappropriate and may contribute to the patient's problems. It is important that diagnostic and therapeutic plans for one problem be considered in the context of all of the patient's problems.

After initial diagnostic and therapeutic plans are carried out, analysis of data and observations are done and further plans for action are recorded in the progress notes in the following manner. First, new subjective and objective data are recorded under the headings cited at the end of the paragraph. Next, assessments of these data are made and recorded, which leads to follow-up diagnostic and therapeutic plans. Client education is also documented so that subsequent client communication by any member of the veterinary medical care team is always made in the light of what was said previously. Entries to the progress notes made in this standard fashion have led to the acronym, SOAP:

S	= Subjective data	= Clinical observations
O	= Objective data	= Laboratory data
A	= Assessment	= "What decisions can be made based on what I have learned since the previous entry," and "what likely diagnoses must be tested for (rule-outs)" and "what must I do to rule-out that diagnosis with reasonable assurance."
P	= Plans	
Dx	= Diagnostic plans	
Rx	= Therapeutic plans	
CE	= Client education	

PROBLEM-SPECIFIC DATA BASE

The set of data that must be obtained for a given problem is the problem-specific data base. By implication, assessment of those data will, in a high percentage of instances, permit resolution of the problem, i.e., yield a diagnosis. The concept is a familiar one in veterinary medicine, except that formerly the data were related specifically to an etiologic diagnosis rather than to a clinical problem. The large number of possible diagnoses tended to discourage the clinician, because the gap between the sick patient and the diagnosis was wide and a logical plan was often lacking. Using the POVMR, the problem-specific data base is related to the disease as it exists rather than to the hypothetic diagnosis.

Just as one could not readily utilize etiology-related data bases because of the very large number of possibilities, one cannot even define a specific data base for all problems that might be encountered. What the clinician can and should do, however, is design problem-specific data bases for those problems regularly encountered in his practice. Geographic location, animal species, and cost-yield ratios are factors that must be considered in the establishment of problem-specific data bases. While defining problem-specific data bases is to a degree arbitrary, it is far less so than attempting to manage frequently encountered problems without the same amount of objective data each time. Moreover, only the concept, not the content, remains intact. If it is learned after 6 months of experience that a specific item of a problem-specific data base has a low yield, the procedure (e.g., lab test, radiograph, EKG) can be deleted from the list. Rarely encountered or extremely simple problems may not deserve a problem-specific data base, but many problems often associated with gastrointestinal disease are best approached with such a defined data base. Suggested problem-specific data bases are included for most of the problems in this chapter as part of the initial diagnostic plan.

The remainder of this chapter is devoted to the presentation of common gastrointestinal problems in a POVMR format. The cases are not resolved in ultimate terms but are developed to the initial level of definition. The intent is to provide some exercise in defining problems; the remaining chapters of Section One expand on the initial workup of the case.

Part II. Clinical Cases

JAMES R. COFFMAN

Initial synthesis and orderly evolution of a data base are intuitive in some clinicians and not in others. The methodology described here is intended to aid the veterinarian in developing an orderly and, more important, an open-ended approach to data gathering. A traditional, finite cause-and-effect approach limits one to knowledge in use at a given point in time. However, the problem-oriented approach allows the clinician to assimilate new and changing information without altering the approach to problem-solving.

WEIGHT LOSS

Loss of body weight is not a problem specific to the digestive system, but it is a common clinical manifestation of gastrointestinal disease. When loss of weight is due to decreased fat and muscle mass rather than to loss of gastrointestinal content and total body water, it could also be an expression of other chronic disease or starvation.

Inadequate Total Digestible Nutrients (TDN). Regardless of the species involved, inadequate caloric intake is probably the most common cause of weight loss. Thus, one must be familiar with feedstuffs commonly fed to the various species within the geographic area. One must know the approximate TDN content of different feedstuffs and be able to recognize feed quality. This capability and knowledge are particularly valuable in large animal practice where labels with minimum nutritional analysis are often not readily available. When dealing with two or more animals, the veterinarian must also establish whether the feed provided by the client is actually accessible to the animals, or whether the social structure of the herd or flock might prevent one or more individuals from consuming a full share.

Endoparasitism. Next to TDN deficiency, endoparasitism is the most important cause of weight loss. Many veterinarians, particularly those lacking experience, tend to limit their scrutiny of endoparasitism to a fecal examination and a history of the medication program (if any), while forgetting the most important feature, i.e., management. The fallibility of quantitative egg counts is well established. No medical control program for endoparasitism can compensate for bad management; it can only complement good management. Thus, when the history and an examination of the facilities suggest endoparasitism, the suspicion should not be too hastily set aside on the basis of recent deworming, or by a low or negative fecal flotation result.

Specific Nutrient Deficiency. While deficiencies of specific nutrients are common, they are not frequently associated with loss of body weight. In other words, when an adequate amount of TDN is present, specific nutrient deficiency is not likely if weight loss is the only presenting problem. A prominent exception to this is protein deficiency. Animals receiving adequate calories may lose weight on a protein deficient diet if extra metabolic demands exist, such as growth, hard performance, reproduction, or lactation.

Chronic Liver Disease. All species of domestic animals affected with chronic liver disease may exhibit weight loss, frequently as the only presenting problem. However, the liver is seldom the only organ damaged, and therefore further investigation may reveal chronic liver disease to be only one of several disease processes.

One must remain cognizant that chronic liver disease is frequently a subtle, indolent pathologic process, much less clinically apparent than acute necrotizing liver disease. Abdominal palpation and radiographic examination are helpful when the animal is small enough to render them feasible. An extensive panel of hepatic tests, as well as biopsy, may be used to rule-out chronic liver disease, as described in Chapters 6 and 25.

Neoplasia. Development of the data base in the non-parasitized, weight-losing patient receiving an adequate diet will occasionally reveal evidence suggestive of neoplasia. Suspicion may be raised by detection of a mass by transabdominal or rectal palpation, visualization of a mass by radiography, laparoscopy, a finding of malabsorption (as from intestinal lymphoma), detection of changes in peritoneal fluid, or paradoxic increase of serum enzyme activities.

Malabsorption. Failure to absorb nutrients adequately, even though they are present in adequate amounts, is not common. When the syndrome is due to disease processes such as intestinal lymphoma or villous atrophy, many nutrients will be malabsorbed. However, it is not uncommon for a specific nutrient to be poorly absorbed. Fat malabsorption in intestinal lymphangiectasia and lactose malabsorption in congenital or acquired lactase deficiency are examples.

Obviously, weight loss is not specific for digestive disease. A broad range of causes exists, potentially involving most systems. However, the most common causes of weight loss are related to the digestive system, and the probable digestive abnormalities should be ruled out early in the medical workup.

Suggested Problem-Specific Data Base for Weight Loss:

1. Review of ration for energy content   ☑
2. Review protein content of ration   ☑
3. Fecal examination: direct/flotation   ☑
4. Total serum protein   ☑

This data base is a beginning point in the workup, applicable to any species. It is intended to identify common probable causes, if they exist, or to begin to rule them out of consideration. Furthermore, one cannot abandon the data-collecting process simply because a positive (abnormal) result is obtained for any given item (e.g., 1 and 2 on the preceding list may be interrelated). It must be emphasized that all of these data are collected for all animals that have a problem of weight loss. Similarly, a negative (normal) result for item 4 does not rule out liver disease by any means. Rather, it is an economically useful though crude estimate of liver function and protein-losing diseases. As with many tests that provide a limited view of organ function/status, a negative value does not prove the organ or system to be free of disease.

Case History

A 9-year-old castrated male Thoroughbred Hunter, 16.2 hands tall, has become a matter of concern to his owner and trainer because of progressive weight loss. The normal weight of the horse is 600 kg (1320 lb); he presently weighs 500 kg. Upon visiting the stable to examine the horse, the veterinarian obtained the following history.

Narrative History

The horse was purchased and moved to this stable a year ago and was in good condition at that time. He has been ridden for 30 minutes to an hour, 5 days a week since that time and has been shown 2 to 3 times a month for the past 4 months. During the past 2 months, weight loss has been noted, becoming rapid during the past 2 weeks. He is fed equal parts of oats and sweet feed (a mixture of corn, oats, bran, and molasses), and grass hay. The horse has been dewormed twice via stomach tube during the past year. He always cleans up his feed and does not "slobber grain." The horse has had "all his shots."

Direct Questions

Question: "Are any other horses in the stable affected with a similar disorder?"

Answer: "None."

Q: "What vaccinations are current?"

A: "Tetanus toxoid, bivalent encephalomyelitis, influenza, and rhinopneumonitis."

Q: "With what medication was the horse dewormed, and when was it given?"

A: "He was dewormed about 8 months ago and again about 4 months ago. I don't know what with; the vet said it was supposed to get everything."

Q: "Now regarding the ration, how much of the grain mix is fed daily?"

A: "We feed about 2 gallons of total grain morning and night, about 16 pounds."

Q: "I see you are feeding good quality timothy hay. How much does the horse eat per day?"

A: "About a third of a bale, so that would be about 20 pounds."

Q: "Has colic been observed?"

A: "No, although we have found the horse cast against the wall two or three times during the past few weeks, so he may have been rolling a little from colic and we just didn't see it."

Q: "How much water does the horse consume?"

A: "Most days about 7 or 8 gallons unless it is quite hot; then he may drink 12 to 15 gallons."

Q: "Does the horse urinate normally?"

A: "As far as we know. He urinates without difficulty and his bedding is not unusually wet."

Physical Examination

The mucous membrane color is normal, as is heart rate and pulse quality. Body temperature is normal. The eyes are normal, the facial features are symmetric, and respiratory movements are normal. The haircoat is somewhat harsh and lacks lustre. Auscultation of the thorax reveals no abnormalities. Placement of a mouth speculum allows the identification of normal dentition.

At this point, two problems are identified and an initial plan for diagnosis can be established.

1. Weight loss
2. Occasional abdominal pain

The occasional abdominal pain is probably associated with the cause of the weight loss. Certain possible causative factors worthy of consideration do not apply directly to the digestive system. Equine infectious anemia would be one, requiring a Coggins immunodiffusion test. Adrenal dysfunction could be a factor, but is well down on the list of probabilities, largely because a long haircoat and polyuria/polydipsia are not present. Having auscultated a normal thorax and having established the preceding list of problems, the initial diagnostic plan is related primarily to the digestive system and may be organized as follows: Notice that the problem-specific data base is expanded for this case because of the identification of the second problem.

1. Weight Loss
   Dx: A. Review energy content of ration ☑
   B. Review protein content of ration ☑
   C. Fecal flotation and fecal occult blood ☑
   D. Total serum protein ☑
2. Occasional Abdominal Pain
   Dx: A. Rectal palpation ☑
   B. Complete blood count ☑

Discussion

The diet is adequate in energy and protein. Good quality timothy hay has about 40% TDN, and 20 × 0.40 = 8 lb TDN in this example. This type of grain mix has about 80% TDN, and 16 × 0.80 = 12.8 lb TDN. At his present level of work, the horse would require approximately 55 cal per kg (500 kg × 55 cal = 27,500 cal). Since a pound of TDN contains about 2000 cal, it is obvious that the horse is obtaining more than enough energy to maintain his weight, since 20 lb TDN = 40,000 cal. In 20°C weather (70°F), the daily water requirement for most domestic animals is around 50 ml/kg/24 hours (30,000 ml for this horse). Since a gallon of water approximates 4000 ml, this horse's average consumption (about 30,000 ml) is within normal limits.

Rectal examination is of key importance, primarily related to palpation of the cranial mesenteric artery and its immediate right branch, which is feasible in about 80% of full-size horses. It is also possible that a neoplastic mass or abdominal abscess may be palpated. Fecal flotation is indicated as an estimate of the severity of internal parasitism, although a single flotation is an extremely unreliable parameter when only one horse is tested. A fecal occult blood test is indicated because gastric ulcer, gastric habronemiasis, and neoplasia are potential causes of both recurrent colic and weight loss. A complete blood count is indicated since internal parasitism commonly causes anemia and leukocytosis involving all classes of mature white cells, while active chronic infections such as salmonellosis frequently induce a neutrophilic leukocytosis.

The problem may be resolved and treatment begun on the basis of the results of the initial workup. However, experience suggests that additional diagnostic effort will be necessary in many cases with these two problems. Chronic liver disease may be present as either a primary, concurrent, or intercurrent disease process. Thus, a liver profile is indicated (see Chapters 6 and 25). The total protein and serum protein electrophoresis can provide additional insight regarding protein-losing gastroenteropathy, as well as chronic infection and parasite migration. Performance of an abdominal paracentesis speaks directly to the possibility of strongyle larval migration, chronic septic peritonitis, or neoplasia.

ABNORMAL PREHENSION AND/OR MASTICATION

Inability to prehend or chew food in a normal manner is not uncommon and suggests a primary disease process in the head. The problem may relate to a mechanical inability to move the lips, tongue, and mandible, or to a pharyngeal or retrobulbar mass, or to a neurologic deficit affecting the musculature of the tongue and mandibles, or to some painful affectation of the oral mucosa.

Stomatitis/glossitis. Inflammatory and degenerative alterations in the oral mucosa may occur for a variety of reasons. Among the more common causes are trauma and infection. However, niacin deficiency is also a cause of glossitis. Probably the most common cause is ingestion of irritating or caustic compounds, including certain plants.

Dental Disease. Dental abnormalities can contribute to difficult mastication through infliction of pain or through mechanical obstruction. For example an abscessed, loose, or broken tooth will induce a pain response and discourage prehension, mastication, or both, whereas an elongated tooth may prevent complete closure of the jaws. Uneven wear of dental arcades produces sharp points on the teeth, which can cause numerous small abrasions and lacerations of the tongue and cheeks.

Foreign Body. Occasionally a foreign body will become lodged between two teeth or even across the roof of the mouth between upper premolars or molars. Sticks, wire, glass, and bone fragments are commonly involved. Initially, the animal may exhibit active attempts to remove the object by rubbing the head and by intermittent frustrated attempts to eat. Later, because previous attempts to eat have proven painful, the animal may simply appear anorectic and depressed. Rage may occur when the head is examined.

Fracture and Arthritis. Fracture of one or more bones surrounding the buccal cavity is virtually always preceded by a traumatic episode. However, the traumatic event may not be observed by the owner. Thus if the fractured part is not located in such a manner as to manifest visible swelling, careful palpation will be necessary to identify the affected area. Occasionally radiography is necessary as a screening procedure even though fracture is not specifically suspected. Fracture of the hyoid bone can be an example of an occult lesion producing pain in this area. Luxation, abscess, or arthritis of the temporomandibular articulation can be suspected when pain is produced by opening the jaws and is confirmed by radiography unless the arthritis is confined to the joint capsule.

Masseter Myopathy. On occasion masseter muscle dysfunction may occur. Trauma is probably the most common cause. Primary disease processes do affect these muscle groups, an example being eosinophilic myositis in dogs.[2]

Neurogenic. Neurologic disorders cause difficult prehension or mastication of food through damage to the cranial nerves. Trauma, tumor, intoxications, and infections are common causes. One should attempt to differentiate the animal that has given up trying to overcome difficulties in prehension or mastication from the animal that is depressed and anorectic. Furthermore, careful, repeated examinations are necessary to differentiate the animal that cannot identify food (as in encephalitis) from the animal that cannot swallow (as in rabies).

Case History

A crossbred Hereford-Angus cow weighing 400 kg (880 lb) has been observed by the owner to be gaunt and losing weight. She has been on grass for 2 months, as it is now late June. The grass is very lush. The rest of the cows are fat. The owner moved the cow into a small lot and gave her one-half bale of hay and some water. Upon arriving at the ranch to examine the cow, the following history was obtained.

Narrative History

"The cow was wintered with the rest of the cow herd on corn ensilage and brome hay and turned onto bluestem pasture the first of May. She was doing well then and no weight loss was observed until 4 or 5 days ago when she seemed to be a little "gaunt-up." The last few days she has lost weight at a terrific rate and yesterday was standing off by herself. All these cows were dewormed this spring and vaccinated for leptospirosis. This cow nosed around in her hay last night but didn't really eat. She slobbers some."

Direct Questions

Question: "What type of water source is available and how accessible is it?"

Answer: "These cows water from a free-flowing stream; they can wade right out in it."

Q: "Is the stream flowing now?"

A: "Yes. It always flows except for a few weeks some dry years."

Q: "Are any other cows similarly affected?"

A: "None."

Q: "Did the cow seem to have normal locomotion when you moved her to this lot?"

A: "Oh, yes, she could trot right along."

Q: "Is leptospirosis the only disease against which the cow is vaccinated?"

A: "Yes."

Q: "Was she depressed?"

A: "No."

While taking the history, the veterinarian observes the cow walk to the water tank and drink a small amount, then put her muzzle in the hay. She nudges the hay back and forth, paws at it, attempts to prehend some hay, but stops and walks away.

Client: "I get the impression this cow can drink and would like to eat, but can't."

D.V.M.: "I would say that's true."

Physical Examination

Having run the cow down an alley into a chute, the initial physical examination is conducted. The cow is 8% dehydrated. Heart rate and pulse quality are normal. Respiratory rate is somewhat increased, but not abnormally so considering the midday heat. Rectal temperature is normal. Ruminal contractions are depressed. Auscultation of the thorax reveals no abnormality. Pain or swelling is not detected when the head and neck are examined externally. Examination of the muzzle reveals a broad ulcer on the upper lip and when the lips are drawn apart, several small ulcers are visualized on the dental pad and gingival mucosa. Saliva drips from the mouth in small amounts.

At this point, four problems are identified and an initial plan for diagnosis can be established. It is logical to assume that the weight loss is related to the inability to eat and drink normally. Given other problems that tend to localize the true cause of the problem to the head region, the prudent clinician is content to limit the initial diagnostic workup of weight loss to simple visual observation. Since it is an important problem to the client, it is desirable that the client education process include an explanation that the primary lesion in the mouth region probably caused the weight loss. It is not to be assumed that all clients are able to see that relationship intuitively.

The initial plan for diagnosis is to elucidate the cause of the ulcers and to rule out a possible foreign body in the mouth.

1. Rapid Weight loss
   Dx: A. Observe ☑
   CE: A. Explain probable relationship to other problems in head region; in the pharynx. ☑
2. Abnormal Prehension
   Dx: A. Insert mouth speculum ☑
       Visual
       Manual (rubber gloves)
3. Ulcers of Lips and Oral Mucous Membranes
   Dx: A. Impression smear of lesions ☑
       B. Inspect pasture and perimeter fence for corrosive agent ☑

4. Ptyalism
   Dx: A. Observe   ☑
5. Dehydration, 8%
   Dx: A. None   ☑

Discussion

Only one animal in the herd is affected and the disease process has apparently been present for 5 to 7 days. These facts suggest that a herd problem is not present.

While buccal ulceration may occur with infectious diseases, it is also commonly due to ingestion of a caustic compound. In this instance, thorough examination of the mouth is necessary both to determine the extent and severity of the lesions and to rule out the presence of a foreign body in the mouth or pharynx. Impression smears may give a clue as to the causative agent.

The lush grass tends to rule out some of the irritant weeds (such as bull nettles), but a search should be made for some caustic agent that the cow may have been licking or chewing.

This type of case calls for careful physical examination, since the signs appear to localize the lesion to the mouth and head. Vesicular diseases and bovine virus diarrhea are less likely causes in circumstances such as this, but one should consider them if the first line of inquiry does not yield a diagnosis.

DYSPHAGIA

Difficulty in swallowing is an abnormality common to a number of disease processes involving the head and neck. One of the more common clinical signs of dysphagia is pseudoptyalism, since the animal continues to secrete saliva but cannot or will not swallow it.

Pharyngitis and/or Para-pharyngeal Infection. Pain due to mucosal inflammation may cause difficult or painful swallowing. Displacement of the pharyngeal wall by a para-pharyngeal lesion (e.g., abscess) may cause mechanical interference in swallowing. Dysphagia would be more severe in the latter instance.

Tonsillitis. Enlargement and pain associated with tonsillitis may cause dysphagia as well as vomiting.

Foreign Body or Tumor. Foreign bodies such as fragments of bone or wood may become lodged in the pharynx or esophagus as well as the mouth. Tumors may also cause dysphagia by obstruction. Obviously, one would expect a short term acute history with a foreign body and a more insidious history with a tumor.

Esophageal Disease. Insufficient innervation, obstruction (by tumor or foreign body), or dilatation of the esophagus can all result in dysphagia. In most instances food and saliva will be regurgitated through the mouth and/or nasal passages, depending upon the species involved.

Neurogenic. One of the classic infectious neurologic diseases, rabies, causes pseudoptyalism due to neurogenic inability to swallow. While other afflictions of the brain stem (e.g., tumor, trauma, abscess) may cause similar signs, rabies is and should be the foremost consideration in the workup of dysphagia.

Case History

A 4-year-old intact male Bassett weighing 22 kg (48 lb) is presented because of difficulty in eating and drinking.

Narrative History

"My dog has had all of his vaccinations and has not been ill since he was a little puppy. For the past 3 or 4 days he hasn't been feeling at all well. I didn't think too much of it when he refused food, but when his water dish remained filled, I became very concerned. Yet he seems to want to eat and drink because he goes to his water dish rather frequently. He seems to cough when he tries to drink. Several times he has picked up food as if to eat. When he tries to swallow, he vomits or something because the food comes out of his mouth along with some clear fluid. He seems to swallow a lot, even though he isn't eating or drinking.

Today I noticed that he was very depressed, and when I petted his back, the skin seemed stiff."

Direct Questions

Question: "What food do you usually feed your Bassett?"

Answer: "Meat-type canned food."

Q: "Does he go outdoors very often?"

A: "Seldom, and then only in the fenced yard."

Q: "Do you feed table foods?"

A: "Occasionally."

Q: "Does he ever get into the trash?"

A: "No."

Q: "Has he had any difficulty in breathing?"

A: "No."

Physical Examination

The dog is somewhat depressed. The rectal temperature is 101.6°F. The eyes are noticeably sunken; the mucous membranes are ruddy and tacky. The skin lacks normal turgor. Dehydration is estimated at 10%. The heart and lungs are normal to auscultation. The abdomen is contracted but non-tender.

Although the dog is docile, he very strongly resists attempts to open his mouth. There is a dark viscous film of saliva on the lips, and saliva exudes from the lips after attempts to open the mouth are abandoned. A fetid odor emanates from the mouth.

The problems are identified:

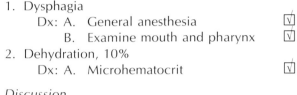

1. Dysphagia
   Dx: A. General anesthesia   ☑
       B. Examine mouth and pharynx   ☑
2. Dehydration, 10%
   Dx: A. Microhematocrit   ☑

Discussion

The physical examination is incomplete until the mouth and pharynx are properly visualized. The narrative history strongly suggests that the dog desires to eat and drink but is unable to do so, perhaps because of pain. His distinct unwillingness to allow his mouth to be opened raises the index of suspicion that a lesion exists in or adjacent to the mouth or pharynx. Pseudoptyalism is present. The fetid odor suggests that an open lesion, perhaps with local tissue destruction, exists in the mouth or pharynx. Finally, the repeated attempts to swallow also suggest that there is a lesion, perhaps a foreign body, in the oropharynx.

The clinician must consider a number of alternatives before inducing anesthesia, including but not limited to the following: Is even ultra-short general anesthesia necessary or would narcosis or tranquilization provide proper restraint? Should survey radiographs be taken before anesthesia is induced? Am I prepared to perform endotracheal intubation quickly? What will be the course of action if a foreign object interferes with intubation? Are grasping forceps immediately at hand? How will hemorrhage be controlled? Is cautery available? What postoperative care may be needed, aside from fluid therapy? Should fluid therapy precede anesthesia, so that the plasma volume, cardiac output, and renal perfusion are more nearly normal? These and other questions must be answered in the affirmative before proceeding with the examination.

VOMITING

Vomiting is a common, nonspecific clinical sign. Among the principal domestic animals, the dog, cat, pig, and occasionally the cow, vomit. The horse vomits only when the stomach is severely dilated or ruptured and then the vomitus is discharged primarily through the nostrils. Of particular clinical importance is the differentiation between regurgitation and vomiting. Vomiting also functions as a protective mechanism in instances of intestinal obstruction. This is exemplified by the cataclysmic effect of gastric dilatation in the horse with small bowel obstruction, as compared to species which readily vomit. Dogs affected with gastric torsion are unable to vomit effectively and react much as do horses to gastric dilatation. The more commonly encountered causes of vomiting with gastrointestinal tropisms are briefly dicussed.

Gastric Causes. Inflammatory alterations in the gastric mucosa may result from a variety of insults, such as ingestion of spoiled food, dirt, pesticides, fertilizer, and foreign bodies. Viral infections such as canine distemper, infectious canine hepatitis, feline panleukopenia, and porcine transmissible gastroenteritis (TGE), as well as bacterial infections such as salmonellosis and leptospirosis also cause vomiting. Internal parasites such as ascarids and tapeworms are common causes of vomiting in dogs and cats. Except for internal parasitism, most of the factors listed result in acute gastritis. Chronic gastritis is less common and is apt to be due to chronic or intermittent exposure to an irritant. A pathologic process apart from the digestive tract may also result in chronic gastritis, e.g., azotemia. In a young dog, pyloric stenosis causes projectile vomiting.

Ulcers. Ulceration of the stomach may be a cause of vomiting. Swine and cattle in confinement feeding programs are probably the most frequently encountered ulcer victims. Peptic ulcers are occasionally observed in dogs and are most frequently associated with liver disease.[3]

Intestinal Obstruction. Obstruction of the bowel exists as a continuum from partial to complete. Outright occlusion of the intestinal lumen, as with torsion, may produce vomiting, whereas partial obstruction is less likely to cause vomiting. However, ileus due to circulatory or neurogenic deficit may also result in vomiting. Peritonitis could cause vomiting by direct inflammation of the peritoneum or by secondary ileus with pooling of fluid in the bowel. Electrolyte imbalances resulting in ileus can also produce vomiting secondary to physiologic obstruction of bowel. When intestinal obstruction is associated with vomiting, abdominal pain is characteristically a concurrent finding.

Pancreatitis. Acute, necrotizing pancreatitis, most common in middle-aged, obese, female dogs frequently causes vomiting.[4] Food may be vomited initially, but after the stomach is emptied, gastric or upper intestinal content is vomited. As with intestinal obstruction, abdominal pain is characteristic and therefore pancreatitis may be confused with intestinal displacement as well as acute renal diseases and ruptured bladder.

A problem-specific data base for vomiting may comprise the following:

1. Abdominal Palpation   ☑
2. Total Serum Protein   ☑
3. CBC   ☑
4. BUN   ☑
5. Fecal Examination   ☑

The parameters may be expanded upon as other problems appear and as the clinician's level of understanding of the problem increases.

Case History

A 6-year-old, obese, spayed female Cocker Spaniel weighing 20 kg (44 lbs) is examined because she has vomited several times during the past week and is now somewhat depressed.

Narrative History

"The dog is current on all her immunizations. She is fed a commercial canned dog food and occasionally some table scraps. She is particularly fond of bread and gravy. She has never been sick.

At first I thought it might have just been something she ate, but she kept vomiting so I thought I had better get her examined. She seemed to feel real good until last night, when she started feeling a little droopy. The first two or three times she vomited food soon after eating. The last few times I have found foamy mucus on the carpet. She seems to drink a lot of water and yesterday I saw her vomit water right after drinking. There was a little greenish tinge to that. She hasn't eaten for about a day."

Direct Questions

Question: "Is this the only pet you have?"
Answer: "Yes, it is."
Q: "Is the dog kept in the house most of the time?"
A: "The only time she is outdoors is when I take her out. Usually early in the morning, around noon, late afternoon, and before I go to bed."
Q: "Do you know of any instance where the dog might have been chewing on indigestible things?"
A: "Well, no, but my grandchildren were here for a few days last week. They had their little toys scattered all over the house."
Q: "About how much volume has the dog vomited?"

A: "Well, at first about half of a cup full, but more recently less than that."
Q: "Was there a characteristic color to the vomitus?"
A: "After the first two or three times, it was foamy mucus, but it always had a greenish tinge to it."
Q: "Has the dog ever had diarrhea during this time or during the preceding week or two?
A: "No, at least not that I have observed."
Q: "Has anything been changed regarding the way or the place in which the dog is fed and watered?"
A: "No."
Q: "Have you or any of your neighbors been using any sprays or insecticide powders of any kind where the dog could possibly be exposed?"
A: "No, I think I would know about that. Anyway, it's too early in the year for any kind of yard work."

Physical Examination

Body temperature is 102°F. The heart rate is somewhat elevated. Mucous membrane color is normal. The skin is somewhat inelastic suggesting dehydration of 8%. Auscultation of the thorax reveals no abnormality, but intestinal borborygmi are reduced. The abdomen is tensed when palpated. Because of tenseness, obesity, and the heavy haircoat, the abdomen cannot be adequately palpated.

At this point, the following list of problems is made and an initial plan for diagnosis established:

1. Vomiting
   Dx: A. Fecal examination
         Flotation   ☑
         Direct microscopic   ☑
       B. Serum Na^+, K^+, Cl^-, and plasma HCO_3^- ☑
2. Abdominal Pain
   Dx: A. CBC   ☑
       B. Total plasma protein   ☑
       C. BUN and urinalysis   ☑
       D. Liver profile   ☑
       E. Abdominal survey radiographs   ☑
       F. Serum amylase and lipase   ☑
   CE: Discuss rule-outs described below and give prognosis to client   ☑
3. Dehydration: 8%
   Dx: A. Compare total protein and microhematocrit   ☑
       B. Evaluate electrolyte values   ☑

Discussion

Since the vomitus originally contained food and later was bile stained, esophageal obstruction may be tentatively ruled out. Fecal examinations will yield positive or negative evidence for parasitism and digestion of foodstuffs. A CBC would give an indication whether viral or bacterial infection or allergy is involved. A total protein determination compared with the microhematocrit would provide a crude estimate of fluid deficit. Blood urea nitrogen is important from 2 points of view: (1) the vomiting could be due to azotemia, or (2) dehydration resulting from a primary gastrointestinal problems could be causing pre-renal uremia. Performance of a urinalysis would bring greater resolution to this question. Since pancreatitis can cause both vomiting and abdominal pain, amylase and lipase determinations are indicated. Liver disease occurs not only as a primary problem, but as a concurrent or intercurrent problem accompanying intestinal disorders, thus the liver profile. Because the history suggested the possibility of foreign body, and because the abdomen is tender, abdominal radiographs are indicated.

That this dog is seriously ill is evident from the history and physical findings. Although the problem of dehydration is not studied directly in a diagnostic way, the specificity of fluid therapy is greatly enhanced by using data gathered for other problems, i.e., the state of hemoconcentration and the electrolyte values. Blood pH and pCO_2 determinations would be helpful, particularly if the dog's condition deteriorated. Positive findings from the amylase and lipase or from the abdominal radiographs would indicate the need for an abdominal paracentesis.

DIARRHEA

The clinical sign of diarrhea may be considered as representing more water in the feces than is normal, for purposes of this dicussion. Many etiologic agents are involved in these alterations. Pathophysiology of diarrhea is discussed in detail in Chapter 14.

Enteritis. Inflammatory changes in the bowel wall may induce alterations in secretion, absorption, and motility. Causes include infections, irritant dietary constituents, and preformed toxins. One must also be cognizant of the high level of oxygen dependency of intestinal mucosa and therefore the adverse influence of circulatory insufficiency on the intestine.

Malabsorption Syndrome. Basically, chronic failure to absorb nutrients from the bowel is due to decreased exocrine secretion by the pancreas or changes in the bowel mucosa or wall, e.g., villous atrophy or neoplasm.[5] Loss or congenital absence of disaccharidase enzymes at the microvillus border of the intestinal epithelial cells is also a cause, particularly in the young. Osmotic diarrhea due to malabsorption may be mimicked by osmotic diarrhea due to excess dietary starch.

Drug-Induced. Intentional or inadvertent drug administration is a common cause of diarrhea. Notable examples are broad-spectrum antibiotic treatment and organophosphate intoxication.

Peritonitis. Irritation of the serosal surface of the bowel may induce alterations in motility resulting in diarrhea. Peritonitis is a secondary disease; thus when peritonitis is diagnosed, one must search for a primary disease process.

Suggested Problem-Specific Data Base for Diarrhea:

1. Review Ration   √
2. Fecal Examination (include culture)   √
3. CBC   √
4. Total Serum Protein   √

Case History

A 3-year-old Quarterhorse filly weighing 450 kg (990 lb) was housed in a stall in a training stable. She had several "cow-consistency" bowel movements last evening. This morning she had fluid diarrhea. Since 6:00 a.m. (it is now 10:30 a.m.) she has had four voluminous bowel movements varying from very soft "cow consistency" to "watery."

Narrative History

"This filly was brought here to be trained 60 days ago. At that time she was 'poor' and has probably gained 150 pounds since her arrival. I do not know if she had ever been dewormed before, but we have dewormed her twice; once the first week and again a week or so ago. She has not been vaccinated for anything. We received a new load of hay 4 or 5 days ago; I do not know if that could have anything to do with it or not. We feed all the horses oats, a mixed grain and molasses combination, and grass hay."

Direct Questions

Question: "Are any of the other horses affected?"
Answer: "No."
Q: "Have any of the horses in the stable been sick recently?"
A: "Last week three or four were coughing but we gave them antibiotic and they straightened right out."
Q: "Was this filly treated?"
A: "I believe she was. Yes, I'm sure she was—two or three times."

Q: "Do you recall what antibiotic was used?"

A: "The vet that prescribed it said it was a tetracycline."

Q: "How much grain are you actually feeding this filly?"

A: "About 2 to 2½ gallons morning and night, so that's about 18 or 20 pounds."

Q: "Do you know what drugs were used when the filly was dewormed?"

A: "The first time she had TBZ (Thiabendazole) in her grain. The last time she was tubed and the other vet said he used an 'organic phosphate'."

Physical Examination

The filly is depressed, but shows no evidence of abdominal pain. Heart rate is 45 beats per minute and respiratory rate is normal. Haircoat is normal. Mucous membranes are pink. There is no evidence of dehydration. Body temperature is high normal (101.5°F). The water bucket is empty.

At this point the following problems can be identified and an initial diagnostic plan organized:

1. Diarrhea
   Dx: A. Fecal Examination
   - Flotation ☑
   - Direct microscopic ☑
   - Culture and antibiotic sensitivity ☑
   - B. CBC ☑
   - C. Total Serum Protein ☑
   - D. Review Ration ☑
2. Depression
   Dx: A. Observe ☑

Discussion

The potential involvement of a bacterial or parasitic agent must be considered; thus the fecal examinations and culture may yield diagnostic clues. The total serum protein gives an additional clue as to water balance. Also, a low total protein would suggest a protein-losing syndrome, such as would occur with disease of the mucosa or lamina propria of the bowel. One should quantitate albumin and globulin for further elucidation of that probability. In addition, an occult blood test would indicate denudation of the gut mucosa.

The history of 18 to 20 pounds of grain daily strongly suggests grain overload resulting in osmotic diarrhea. However, it is doubtful that grain overload would explain the weight loss prior to arrival at the stable.

A clue is found in the history for predisposition to diarrhea by disturbance of intestinal microflora through antibiotic administration. Cholinergic effects of the organophosphate dewormer could be contributory. If such was the case here, signs of diarrhea would ameliorate with time.

ABDOMINAL PAIN

Signs of abdominal pain are similar in all species, but are much more profoundly expressed in some, particularly the horse. Specific clinical manifestations have been discussed in Chapter 4. Causes may be manifold and do not always involve the digestive system.

Peritonitis. Peritoneal pain may arise from any inflammatory lesion within the abdominal cavity which involves, either primarily or by extension, the visceral or parietal peritoneum. Unfortunately the most common cause of peritonitis is infection, frequently due to rupture of a hollow viscus or to intentional or accidental invasion of the abdomen. Primary gastrointestinal disease processes such as pancreatitis and gastric or duodenal ulceration may lead to secondary peritonitis which persists or recurs.

Ileus. Ileus in itself does not cause pain. However, gut stasis inevitably leads to gas and/or fluid accumulation resulting in distention and pressure on the gut wall. The resultant combination of ischemia and pressure causes pain.

Pancreatitis. Acute inflammatory and degenerative changes involving the pancreas are described in all the domestic species but are most important in the dog. In addition to being a primary cause of pain, pancreatitis can lead to localized or generalized peritonitis.

Ischemia of the Intestine. Decreased blood flow may occur in several ways. Pressure on the bowel wall inhibits capillary filling. This is usually secondary to ileus, which can have many causes. Also, the presence of a hard mass within the lumen of the gut can lead to focal pressure necrosis in a few days. The most drastic type of ischemic damage to the bowel is interruption of mesenteric circulation as with primary thrombus formation, incarceration, or directional displacement of the gut.

Case History

A 2-year-old Quarterhorse stallion weighing 500 kg (1100 lb) was exhibiting moderately severe signs of abdominal pain when the owner went to feed him at 7:30 a.m. The horse had been observed at 10:00 p.m. the previous evening and seemed normal at that time.

Narrative History

"This horse seemed all right last night but when I came in this morning, he was getting up and down and pawing. He stretched out a time or two like he had to urinate but then he would start circling again and lie down. Last night, he ate a good deal of the hay I gave him and cleaned up his grain. He drank a gallon or so of water."

Direct Questions

Initial questioning reveals that there are 10 horses in the stable and this is the only one affected. All the horses have been dewormed at 8-week intervals for the past year, the last time 3 weeks ago. The horses have been vaccinated for encephalomyelitis, tetanus, influenza, and rhinopneumonitis.

Question: "How much grain is the horse being fed, and how often?"

Answer: "He gets 1 gallon of mixed grain morning and night. We also feed mixed alfalfa and grass hay free choice. I would guess he eats about a third of a bale a day."

Q: "Do you have any way of knowing how much water he drinks?"

A: "Well, he'll average about 4 to 5 gallons a day."

Physical Examination

The horse is in excellent physical condition. The haircoat is glossy. Body temperature is normal. The heart rate is 70 beats per minute, which is about 80% greater than normal. Although the pulse is normal in amplitude, the mucous membranes are somewhat congested and the capillary refill time is prolonged (4 to 5 seconds). The abdomen is tense and auscultation reveals decreased borborygmi on both sides.

At this juncture two problems are identified and an initial plan for diagnosis is made.

Problem list:
1. Abdominal pain

    Dx: A. Pass stomach tube ☑

        B. Give 5 g dipyrone IV ☑

        C. Rectal examination ☑

2. Altered circulation

    Dx: A. Packed cell volume (PCV) and total plasma protein ☑

        B. Abdominal paracentesis ☑

Discussion

Introduction of a stomach tube will usually determine whether the stomach is under fluid or gas pressure. If the stomach contains fluid under pressure, gastric dilatation (either primary or secondary to small bowel displacement) may be identified. Rectal examination is helpful in identifying gas-distended loops of bowel, turgid, incarcerated, or otherwise displaced segments of bowel, impactions, and verminous arteritis. Since the possibility of iatrogenic rupture of the rectum is always present, this must be done with great care. Increase in PCV and total plasma protein values represents loss of plasma water, suggesting significant circulatory compromise and an increased likelihood of irreversible morphologic change. Abdominal paracentesis gives immediate and direct evidence of a compromised segment of bowel, verminous migration, or primary idiopathic peritonitis. Administration of dipyrone, an analgesic with little or no effect on the circulatory system, is a helpful diagnostic maneuver because good response to such a compound decreases the likelihood of an irreversible morphologic alteration.

ABDOMINAL DISTENTION

Conceptually, distention of the abdomen may result from:

1. Gas in the intestinal lumen.
2. Fluid in the intestinal lumen.
3. Fluid in the peritoneal cavity.
4. Pregnancy.
5. A space-occupying mass other than pregnancy, e.g., tumor or abscess.

Enlargement or apparent enlargement of the abdomen may also be due to:

1. Depot fat in the body wall, with increased mesenteric and omental fat.
2. Accumulation of dietary fiber in the gut lumen.
3. Loss of muscle mass or muscle tone in the abdominal wall leading to a dependent configuration of the abdomen.

More than one of the factors may be present at one time.

Obesity. Deposition of fat within the abdominal cavity or within the abdominal wall occurs in animals that are receiving excess dietary energy or are comparatively low on the thyroactive scale. Examination of the animal and the observation of fat deposition in other areas usually makes this apparent.

Bulky Ration. Frequently an animal will be forced to consume large volumes of a ration high in fiber and low in energy. If adequate energy is ultimately obtained, the animal may have normal subcutaneous depot fat. However, it is possible for animals to be thin and have a large abdomen due to dietary bulk. One should keep in mind that this type of ration is frequently low in protein, so ascites may also be contributing to the size of the abdomen. Internal parasitism frequently accompanies a poorly balanced ration, further compounding the problem.

Pregnancy. This straightforward cause of abdominal distention is occasionally overlooked. When the patient is a female of appropriate age, this should always be investigated since mating frequently occurs in any species without the client's knowledge.

Ileus. Decreased intestinal motility is apt to be associated with accumulation of gas within the lumen. When small bowel is involved, there is a greater tendency for fluid accumulation within the gut lumen as well. Distention of the abdominal wall will occur rapidly and the resultant configuration will vary depending upon the species involved.

Fluid in the Peritoneal Cavity. Accumulation of fluid within the peritoneal cavity may have many causes. Any inflammatory alterative lesion which causes capillary wall damage results in plasmapheresis into the peritoneal cavity resulting in accumulation of an exudate. Congestive heart failure, hepatic cirrhosis, and chronic kidney disease may result in accumulation of a transudate within the abdomen. Urine may accumulate and distend the abdomen; marked distention with urine is usually not apparent unless the urinary bladder is ruptured.

Muscle Weakness. Loss of muscle tone or mass frequently results in a pendulous abdomen. This is usually the result of mobilization of muscle protein for gluconeogenesis. Starvation and Cushing's disease are common causes.

Neoplasm/Abscess. The presence of a space-occupying lesion other than pregnancy will also distend the abdomen. Most commonly the lesion is a neoplasm or an abscess. Palpation across the abdominal wall or via rectal examination may reveal the firm, localized nature of such a mass.

Case History

A 400-kg (880-lb) feedlot steer has been on feed for 60 days. The steer is anorectic and has a distended abdomen, with low-grade abdominal pain.

Narrative History

"This pen of steers was brought off wheat pasture and put on feed about 2 months ago. They were vaccinated for IBR, PI3, and blackleg. They have been on corn silage and 2 pounds of 40% protein supplement per day. They are now getting about 10 pounds of ground milo in addition.

This steer was off by himself last night but came up and ate. This morning he was laying down and we had to urge him to get him up. He looked about like he does now, and we brought him on down here to the sick pen."

Direct Questions

Question: "Have you had any other cattle affected this way in the past few weeks?"

Answer: "Well, we've had a couple bloaters and a water belly or two. No more than usual."

Q: "Are all the rest of the steers in this pen normal?"

A: "Yes."

Q: "Have you seen this steer urinate?"

A: "I haven't seen him. He dribbled a little when I got him up."

Physical Examination

The steer has somewhat labored, rapid respirations. The abdomen is best described as rotund. As he is pushed into a chute, one can feel a heavy cover of fat. The heart rate is increased. The lung field sounds normal but tidal volume is decreased. Both flanks are somewhat distended. Auscultation and palpation in the left paralumbar fossa suggest atony of the rumen. Body temperature is 103°F. The steer passes normal feces and urine while in the chute.

One can now identify several problems and establish an initial plan for diagnosis:

1. Abdominal distention
   Dx: A. Rectal examination   ☑
         B. Pass stomach tube   ☑
         C. Check rumen pH   ☑
         D. Paracentesis abdominis   ☑
2. Depression
   Dx: A. Observe   ☑
3. Anorexia
   Dx: A. Observe   ☑

Discussion

Rectal examination will go a long way toward explaining the cause of the abdominal distention. The rumen may have become large enough to cause displacement of the right flank as well as the left. A fluid line might be detected by percussion and auscultation. An empty or nondetectable bladder would raise the index of suspicion for a ruptured bladder secondary to urethral calculus. Pulsations of the pelvic urethra would direct attention to a urethral calculus. Passage of a stomach tube would rule out choke and test for excessive gas in the forestomachs. Determining rumen pH would assist in the rule-out process for rumen acidosis. Abdominal paracentesis would reveal the presence of peritonitis, sanguinous changes due to a compromised segment of bowel, or the presence of free urine. Uremia, lactic acidosis, and endotoxemia or a combination of these are all plausible causes of depression and anorexia in this patient.

REFERENCES

1. Welser, J. R.: Problem oriented veterinary medical record. *In* Textbook of Veterinary Internal Medicine, Vol. 1. Edited by S. J. Ettinger. Philadelphia, W. B. Saunders Co., 1975.
2. Whitney, J. C.: Eosinophilic myositis in dogs. Vet. Rec. *67*:1140, 1955.
3. Cornelius, L. M., and Wingfield, W. E.: Diseases of the stomach. *In* Textbook of Veterinary Internal Medicine, Vol. 2. Edited by S. J. Ettinger. Philadelphia, W. B. Saunders Co., 1975.
4. Anderson, N. V., and Strafuss, A. L.: Pancreatic disease in dogs and cats. J.A.V.M.A. *159*:885, 1971.
5. Roberts, M. C., and Hill, F. W. G.: The oral glucose tolerance test in the horse. Equine Vet. J. *5*:171, 1973.

Chapter 6

LABORATORY EXAMINATIONS

WILLIAM E. MOORE

Clinical pathology consists of a variety of special examinations aimed at expansion of the patient's diagnostic data base. Proper usage of these and other special examinations requires selection by the clinician after evaluating clinical history and physical signs of disease. As with other examinations, abnormal and normal results observed in the laboratory are rarely pathognomonic for a specific disease, but when pathogenetic mechanisms of abnormalities are considered from a problem-oriented approach, the diagnostic specificity of the data base is greatly enhanced. It is from this viewpoint that the clinical pathology of the gastroenteric system has been considered. Preferred specific laboratory methods and detailed tabulations of normal values for each test are available in textbooks of clinical pathology.[1-4] Rather, pathogenetic mechanisms for abnormal gastroenteric organ function will be described, including the indications for laboratory determinations most likely to define the abnormality and discussion of the various lesions that may create such abnormalities. Since hematologic, fluid, electrolyte, and acid-base balance and microbiologic abnormalities are seen with many gastroenteric disorders, a general description of these is provided; the more specific clinical pathology of the organs is discussed with the same aboral organization found in the remainder of the text.

SCREENING PROFILE

Screening profiles are indicated in veterinary medicine to detect problems in apparently healthy animals prior to elective stressful procedures (e.g., surgery) or in aged animals, to help define and localize problems in animals in which signs of disease are ill-defined, and to detect secondary or concurrent problems hidden by an obvious disease condition. In addition, economics may dictate profiling when the expense is less than performing the several desired tests individually.

The survey profile procedure has been altered so much by technologic advances of the past decade

Table 6–1. Tests available in screening profiles

Typical Survey Profile	Additional Profile Tests
*Glucose	†SGPT
Urea nitrogen	Iron
Uric acid	Triglycerides
Cholesterol	Creatine phosphokinase
Total protein	Creatinine
*Albumin	Sodium
*Alkaline phosphatase	Potassium
SGOT	Total CO_2
LDH	Chloride
Phosphorus	*Amylase
Calcium	*γ-glutamyl transpeptidase
*Total bilirubin	

*Tests for which abnormal results suggest gastroenteric disease.
†Increased activity suggests hepatic disease only in dogs, cats, and some laboratory animals.

that it is now difficult to define a "typical" screening profile. While the original 10 to 12 test survey profiles consisted of sensitive but often nonspecific indicators of disease, many newer profiles are larger and contain some specific indicators for organ dysfunction. Tests that are frequently included in profiles are listed in Table 6–1. Abnormalities of tests marked by asterisks indicate the likelihood of gastroenteric disease, although none are entirely specific.

In brief, elevated glucose and amylase results suggest, respectively, endocrine and acinar pancreatic disease, while decreased glucose values may be due to islet hyperfunction or neoplasia or hepatic dysfunction. Abnormally low albumin values suggest malnutrition, maldigestion, malabsorption, hepatic dysfunction, or excessive albumin loss. Elevated bilirubin concentration and elevated alkaline phosphatase, serum glutamic-pyruvic transaminase (SGPT), more properly called alanine amino transferase, and γ-glutamyl transpeptidase activities suggest hepatic dysfunction. Of the other tests, normal results of serum glutamic oxalacetic transaminase (SGOT), more properly called aspartate amino transferase, and lactic dehydrogenase (LDH) indicate that active hepatocellular damage is unlikely; however, elevated values for these enzyme are too nonspecific to serve as diagnostic indicators. Many of the other profile tests may yield abnormal results in gastroenteric disease but all are nonspecific and are rarely helpful in delineating the nature or cause of the disease except in combination with more specific indicators. The diagnostic value and limitations of each potentially useful indicator of gastroenteric disease will be discussed in greater detail in relationship to specific clinical problems.

FLUID, ELECTROLYTE AND ACID-BASE PROBLEMS

Correction of serious fluid, electrolyte, and hydrogen ion imbalance in gastrointestinal diseases is often life-sustaining during the time required to establish a specific diagnosis and begin proper specific therapy. Indeed, in some cases with severe imbalance, proper and adequate fluid therapy may be the major determinant for success. Depleted electrolytes and water must be replaced in the amounts and proportions necessary to restore and maintain the approximate homeostatic concentration of each. The underlying cause for the imbalance must then be corrected if therapy is to be successful. While the type of imbalance is usually predictable from history and clinical signs, the magnitude of the change is not. In severe cases of imbalance, therapy should be initiated on the basis of clinical judgment but laboratory evaluation of a pre-therapy sample will indicate the therapeutic adjustments necessary to correct the imbalance. Since the electrolyte, fluid, and acid-base balance of the animal patient may be continuously altered by the course of the disease, response to therapy, and normal homeostatic control mechanisms, it is important that the clinician anticipate these changes in order to modify the therapy schedule for maximum response-effectiveness. Reassessment of clinical and laboratory evaluations will aid in making therapeutic adjustments and recognizing seemingly inappropriate responses that may warn of undetected disorders.

Pre-gastric disorders that severely reduce the oral intake of fluids result in dehydration from obligatory water and electrolyte losses, but changes in electrolyte and hydrogen ion concentrations are rarely serious until renal failure occurs. Since such animals are in a fasting state, a mild progressive metabolic acidosis generally results. Ruminants continually secrete large volumes of saliva containing sodium and bicarbonate in concentrations similar to plasma, to the extent that cattle and sheep with experimental total salivary fistulae may become seriously depleted of these ions. Salivary losses alone are rarely of primary clinical significance but are often associated with insufficient water consumption and dehydration.

Bloat and carbohydrate intoxication represent special forms of "pregastric" problems occurring in the ruminant. In bloat due to overeating of lush young grasses, a moderate metabolic acidosis becomes progressively more severe when ruminal distention reduces normal thoracic volume and lung compliance. Intra-abdominal pressure upon the posterior vena caval and portal venous return causes splanchnic pooling of blood and arterial hypotension. Among animals with carbohydrate intoxication, the highly fermentable starchy grain results in a marked increase in ruminal organic acid content, particularly in D- and L-lactic acid. As the pH of the rumen approaches the pK (3.1) of these organic acids, the concentration of undissociated acid molecules increases and diffuses directly across ruminal mucosa. (Undissociated acid equals 1/100 and 1/10 of total concentration at pH 5.1 and 4.1, respectively.) The H^+ of both acids immediately dissociates upon entering the extracellular fluid resulting in metabolic lactic acidosis. Unless hepatic circulation is depressed by increasing intraruminal pressure, much of the L-lactate is oxidized to restore buffer bicarbonate. D-lactate is non-metabolizable and is excreted. When L-lactic acid influx exceeds the metabolic capacity of the liver, metabolic acidosis and associated hyperkalemia become progressively more severe. Hyperammonemia and associated central nervous system damage may also play a role in some cases of carbohydrate intoxication.[5]

Vomiting of consumed fluids, saliva, and secretions from the unstimulated gastric mucosae result in fluid imbalances similar to those due to pregastric fluid loss. Basal gastric secretions are small in volume, have an electrolyte content similar to plasma, and are only moderately acidic in nature. However, vomiting of acid gastric juices secreted in response to food, histamine or catecholamine stimulus, or *sequestration* of gastric fluid (e.g., abomasal dilatation or displacement) leads to metabolic alkalosis in direct proportion to the net hydrogen ion loss. Once initiated, metabolic alkalosis is frequently potentiated by renal mechanisms that result in inappropriate secretion of an acid urine. This seemingly paradoxical renal response is related to hypokalemia and hypochloremia caused by (1) decreased dietary intake, or loss in vomitus, (2) the alkalosis-induced shift of extracellular potassium into intracellular fluid, (3) decreased proximal tubular reabsorption of sodium due to low chloride content of glomerular filtrate, and (4) the aldosterone-mediated distal nephron mechanisms for conservation of sodium ions at the expense of potassium and hydrogen ion excretion. As the distal nephron cell becomes relatively depleted of intracellular potassium, hydrogen ion excretion increases perpetuating the alkalotic imbalance. Unless potassium therapy is administered, the renal loss of acid may continue even after loss of significant quantities of gastric acid has ceased.

Although vomiting is a frequent clinical sign of systemic or metabolic disease in many dogs and cats, the small volume of the vomitus and/or partial neutralization of the gastric acid by *reflux* of alkaline intestinal secretions prevents significant gastric acid loss. Characteristically, these animals show signs of mild to severe acidosis related not to the fluids lost by vomiting but rather to concurrent disease processes.

Observation of the composition, color, and pH of vomitus may help to differentiate among pregastric, gastric, and gastrointestinal fluids. Pregastric fluids and resting gastric secretions are seromucoid in nature, unstained by bile and have a pH of 6.0 to 7.5. Food particles in these fluids appear undigested. Stimulated gastric secretions will have a pH less than 4.0 and may or may not be bile stained depending upon the extent of intestinal reflux. Food particles that have been in contact with gastric secretions may appear partially digested, the extent depending upon the time in contact. If substantial intestinal reflux has occurred, the pH of the vomitus may range from 4 to 7 with definite bile staining.

While vomiting is rarely a clinical problem among cattle, sequestration of gastric secretions in the abomasum due to obstruction by torsion, displacement, intraluminal objects, or neurogenic flaccidity results in metabolic alkalosis. As in the vomiting dog, the alkalosis is often potentiated by hypokalemia and inappropriate aciduria. Since an excess of potassium is present in the sequestered fluid and the rumen content, correction of the abomasal obstruction usually results in prompt recovery from hypokalemia and alkalosis without extensive intravascular fluid therapy. However, if the alkalosis is particularly severe or prolonged, fluids containing potassium and sodium chloride may be required to correct the fluid and electrolyte deficiencies.

Although gastric dilatation and volvulus as seen in large dogs and horses results in sequestration of fluids, the quantity of acid sequestered is usually too small to create significant metabolic alkalosis. In fact, at the time of initial examination, these animals may have a rapidly developing severe metabolic acidosis. Although lactic acidosis might be expected to result from the severe arterial hypotension and splanchnic pooling of blood, this has not been confirmed in clinical or experimental studies[6,7] and the mechanism of the acidosis is not yet known.

Diarrhea of any cause increases fecal loss of water and electrolytes, especially of sodium and bicarbonate and in some cases potassium as well. The resultant hypovolemia stimulates aldosterone-mediated renal conservation of sodium in exchange for potassium and hydrogen ions. When diarrhea is not severe, renal mechanisms and respiratory compensation by hyperventilation may maintain essentially normal blood pH and Na^+ and K^+ concentrations. However, in severe diarrhea the loss of bicarbonate is so great that renal acid secretion is unable to maintain body pH and metabolic acidosis results. As excess H^+ is buffered by intracellular proteins, potassium ions diffuse from cells into extracellular fluid resulting in hyperkalemia. Fortunately, in hyperkalemia, potassium excretion takes precedence over hydrogen ion excretion by the distal nephron and as long as adequate glomerular filtration is maintained, distal nephron function usually maintains plasma potassium concentrations below the critical level for adverse cardiac effects. However, if glomerular filtration decreases due to hypovolemia, the efficiency of potassium excretion also decreases. Since most of the sodium ion is reabsorbed in the proximal tubule at low GFR, little remains for aldosterone-mediated K^+ or H^+ exchange in the distal nephron. In extreme cases of *hypovolemia*, glomerular filtration pressure may drop so low that anuria occurs, totally eliminating this potential mechanism for homeostatic correction of acidosis and hyperkalemia.

Although the mechanisms stated above apply to all animal species, horses usually do not develop hyperkalemia even with extreme diarrhea; in fact, horses are often hypokalemic. The mechanism by which horses maintain normo- or hypokalemic values is not entirely known; however, it is known that animals exchange potassium for sodium in the colon by methods analogous to the aldosterone-mediated mechanisms of the distal nephron, and that the horse appears to be extremely efficient in this mechanism.[8] Perhaps the effectiveness of this mechanism is sufficient to provide the horse with an extra margin of safety in severe diarrhea.

The net result of severe diarrhea is severe contraction of both intracellular and extracellular fluid compartments, severe metabolic acidosis, and sodium and potassium depletion, although both of these ions may be present in normal or excess concentration in the plasma. As metabolic acidosis is corrected during therapy, serious intracellular potassium deficits may develop unless this ion is included in the replacement fluids. Periodic reevaluation of electrolytes during replacement therapy may be useful in detecting hypokalemia. Interpretation of such results depends in part upon recognizing the inverse relationship between blood pH and potassium concentration; e.g., plasma potassium increases approximately 0.6 mEq/L for each 0.1 pH unit of fall in blood pH.[9]

Urine pH is helpful in indicating an abnormal state of fluid balance only when considered in conjunction with other clinical signs. When severe dehydration exists, urine volume will be low and the pH of preformed urine may not be a true indicator of current acid-base status. A freshly collected alkaline urine specimen implies that plasma bicarbonate is probably in excess of 27 to 30 mEq/L, but acid urine may be excreted in states of metabolic acidosis or hypokalemic metabolic alkalosis. Since animals with metabolic acidosis will usually attempt respiratory compensation (hyperventilation), this sign together with other findings and history often help in clinical differentiation between acidotic and alkalotic states.

GENERAL HEMATOLOGIC CHANGES

Hematologic changes associated with gastroenteropathy are general in nature and usually give no indication of the specific type or location of the lesion.

Increased packed cell volume (PCV) and hemoglobin values are expected in states of hemoconcentration due to simple fluid loss. Normal or low PCV values in a clinically dehydrated animal suggest a pre-existing anemia.

Mild to moderate decreases in PCV and hemoglobin are expected with chronic anorexia, debilitation, chronic inflammation of any cause, or neoplasia. Such anemias are usually non-regenerative normocytic-normochromic in nature. Mild to moderate anemia is also a common finding among dogs with maldigestion or malabsorption and in the chronic state the erythrocytes are often moderately hypochromic.

Hemorrhage into the gastrointestinal tract may occur with intestinal parasitism, ulcerative lesions, thrombocytopenia, or inherited or acquired coagulopathies. These anemias are usually regenerative as indicated by polychromasia (reticulocytosis) and are generally associated with macrocytes and leptocytes within 24 to 48 hours after initial occurrence of the hemorrhage. Occasional cases of very chronic hemorrhage (e.g., intestinal parasites) cause an apparent marrow-exhaustive, "non-regenerative" change characterized by hypochromic anisocytosis with macrocytic and normocytic leptocytes. If iron deficiency has occurred due to blood loss, hypochromic microcytes are seen as well.

Changes in numbers of circulating leukocytes associated with gastroenteric disease are general and appropriate to the nature of the lesion. As in other diseases, the changes reflect the balance among production and release, distribution among body pools, and rate of exodus from the blood stream at normal and abnormal sites of destruction.

In the general gastroenteric disease model, clinically significant hormonal effects upon leukocyte response are those induced by catecholamines and glucocorticoids. Epinephrine-like hormones (catecholamines) induce increased peripheral capillary blood flow and cause a shift of marginated leukocytes into the circulating pool; this results in a mature neutrophilia. Less predictably, extreme and prolonged muscular activity, particularly in young animals, may cause peripheral lymphocytosis as well. These changes are unlikely to distort the problem list for seriously ill animals but must be considered as possible causes of mature neutrophilia and/or lymphocytosis among excitable animals with signs of mild to moderate gastroenteric disease.

Increased *circulating glucocorticoid* concentrations occur in states of severe stress, overproduction (Cushing-like syndromes), decreased clearance (occasionally seen in liver disease) and with therapeutic administration of natural or synthetic glucocorticoids. This group of hormones tends to decrease margination and egress of leukocytes from the circulating pool and causes release of the bone marrow storage pool. Both of these effects increase circulating mature neutrophils with minor to moderate increase in "old" (hypersegmented) forms.

The acute effect of glucocorticoids upon *circulating lymphocytes* is redistribution from the circulating pool to tissue pools. Persistently elevated cortisol concentration results in reduced production of lymphocytes due to inhibition of mitosis and to lympholysis of germinal centers. These effects both contribute to lymphopenia. Eosinophil release from marrow is decreased by excess circulating corticosteroids resulting in an eosinopenia although the reduction is often incomplete if the peripheral blood itself is a site of eosinotaxis. In the dog, circulating monocytes are generally increased in response to excess circulating glucocorticoids; a similar response may occur in other animal species but is less predictable than in dogs. In summary, the general effect of increased glucocorticoids alone is a mature neutrophilia, lymphopenia, and eosinopenia with or without monocytosis. In stressful disease conditions these changes are superimposed with the changes due to disease, and the combined effects must be considered in interpreting the data.

Inflammatory or necrotic lesions of the gastroenteric organs generally result in a regenerative neutrophilia of a degree and time-course typical for the species. In dogs, this response is generally rapid, reaching a peak that may be extreme (e.g., 50,000+ leukocytes/μl) within 3 to 4 days while cattle make a relatively moderate (17 to 20,000+) and slow response requiring 5 to 7 days to reach a peak. Among the other domestic species, the response of the cat and pig is similar to that of the dog but less extreme; in the horse both the rapidity and the degree of response are intermediate, and the response of the other ruminants is similar to that of the cow.

Acute gram-negative *bacterial infections* of the intestinal tract which progress to generalized septicemia or endotoxemia (e.g., salmonellosis) result in a sequence of peripheral leukocyte changes. Very small amounts of circulating endotoxin cause increased margination of peripheral neutrophils, which results in neutropenia, followed within 2 to 6 hours by release of the large marrow storage pool of band and mature neutrophils (with neutrophilia). However, pinocytotic uptake of endotoxin by neutrophils leads to release of enzymes with subsequent cytoplasmic autolysis (mature toxic neutrophils) and cellular destruction, and larger amounts of endotoxin cause a neutropenia due to destruction of the mature cells. Thus, depending upon the stage of disease at the time of sampling, infections may result in either a neutropenia or a mature toxic neutrophilia. Later in the disease, the regenerative response of the marrow becomes apparent, but continued endotoxemia may cause dysphasic development of the maturing neutrophils with decreased numbers of segmented neutrophils and relatively large numbers of toxic neutrophilic bands, metamyelocytes and even myelocytes in the circulation.

Nearly all of the *viral diseases* that frequently occur with predominantly gastroenteric signs cause destruction of mature neutrophils and thus a tran-

sient neutropenia. If the disease is stressful, lymphopenia and eosinopenia also occur. The epitheliotropic viruses damage or destroy surface epithelium allowing entry of bacteria which stimulate a regenerative neutrophilia. Several of the more severe viral diseases (e.g., feline panleukopenia, rinderpest) are caused by viruses that are pantropic but have their worst pathogenic effects upon rapidly dividing cells. These viruses seriously damage both the marrow and lymphoid mitotic pools and the intestinal mucosae. In these diseases severe leukopenia without evidence of marrow response is the rule in spite of intercurrent bacterial infection.

Cats with the panleukopenia-like syndrome caused by feline leukemia virus may present a leukogram similar to that caused by panleukopenia virus. The FeLV virus leukogram in these cases usually remains unchanged for some time; whereas in feline panleukopenia, if natural defenses of the animal and therapy are adequate, regeneration of marrow will be signalled by increased numbers of neutrophilic myelocytes and metamyelocytes in the peripheral blood approximately 4 to 6 days after the onset of the disease. As convalescence progresses over the next 1 to 2 days, the peripheral blood count of immature and mature neutrophils will continue to increase with a shift to a more normal ratio of mature:immature forms. The large numbers of immature neutrophils seen during the convalescent phase of feline panleukopenia will be quite similar to leukograms seen in FeLV-induced granulocytic forms of myeloproliferative disease, except that the leukogram of the convalescent panleukopenia case will return to normal within a few days while the myeloproliferative disease case generally remains leukemic in nature.

Eosinophilia is a common response to gastrointestinal parasitic nematode infection, either to adults within the intestinal lumen or to migrating or encysted larval forms in tissues. Other causes of eosinophilia which may present with signs referrable to gastroenteric disease include such conditions in dogs as severe dirofilarial infestation with secondary liver disease; eosinophilic gastroenteritis, and hypoadrenocorticism (addisonian-like syndrome). The addisonian dog often has a lymphocytosis in addition to eosinophilia.

In man, eosinophilia is commonly associated with many chronic gastrointestinal inflammations, and perhaps a similar conclusion will be reached for some animal species when the data base for nonparasitic gastrointestinal diseases is closely analyzed. Furthermore, eosinophilia is commonly associated with chronic exposure to ectoparasites, airborne and "contact allergens," and may be present but unrelated to the cause of concurrent mild to moderate gastroenteric signs.

The young of all domestic animal species have much higher normal lymphocyte values than do aged animals of the same species; thus, interpretation of lymphocytosis and lymphopenia must always be age-related. As indicated previously, lymphocytosis may occur in some cases of "physiologic" leukocytosis and in hypofunction of the adrenal. Lymphocytosis also may be present at various stages of lymphocytic neoplasia in any of the domestic animal species. While gastroenteric signs are not the most common signs of lymphocytic neoplasia, the disease is of frequent occurrence in cats, cattle, and dogs, and the signs may mimic diseases of gastroenteric origin. Other causes of lymphocytosis likely to exist concurrently with problems of gastroenteric origin are uncommon although several viruses capable of inducing lymphocytosis in cattle have been isolated during the search for the etiology of lymphocytic neoplasia. It is possible that these are more common infections than is generally known.

Lymphopenia is a common sign of increased plasma glucocorticoid concentration and occurs in many viral diseases. *Lymphopenia* also occurs occasionally in lymphocytic neoplasia. In man, intestinal lymphangiectasia results in a persistent lymphopenia due to constant lymphocytic loss into the lumen of the intestine. Reported cases of lymphangiectasia in domestic animals are few; some have been characterized by extreme lymphopenia without concurrent eosinopenia and monocytosis. However, all of these dogs were seriously ill and no data on cortisol concentrations or lymphocyte turnover are available to clearly establish a causal relationship between lymphopenia and lymphangiectasia.

CLINICAL PATHOLOGY OF INDIVIDUAL ENTERIC ORGANS

Laboratory examination of the mouth, pharynx, and salivary glands has been of limited clinical usefulness except for cytologic and bacteriologic findings. Hematologic findings are usually those expected for each species in inflammatory disorders. Chemistry determinations are rarely useful although conditions that result in prolonged anorexia may lead to hypoproteinemia and those that prevent water intake will lead to the various abnormalities associated with dehydration. In horses, anorexia from any cause for longer than 48 to 72 hours' duration will cause moderate to severe

hyperbilirubinemia. Less than 20% is direct reacting bilirubin, apparently due to decreased hepatic uptake of the albumin-bound unconjugated bilirubin. Such icteric horses may cause a diagnostic enigma unless proper history is available or unless specific liver function tests are performed.

Salivary Glands. The simple, qualitative mucin clot test has been useful in conjunction with cytologic examination to allow differentiation of salivary cysts and abscesses from other subcutaneous accumulations of fluid in the salivary gland area. This test consists of mixing a small amount of aspirated fluid with 2.5% acetic acid, and observing for the tightly condensed "clot" that occurs when hyaluronic acid or certain other glycoproteins (mucin) polymerize in acid media.[10] Serum (from hematomas) and lymph accumulations (due to local lymphatic blockage) form clear solutions while viscous inflammatory exudates from sources that do not secrete mucin form a turbid suspension of coarse flakes. Since some salivary glands do not contain high mucin content, the test is not useful in detecting abscessation of these glands. Infection due to bacteria which elaborate necrotoxins may diminish the mucin secretory ability of infected glands and these fluids also yield a negative mucin clot test. Exudates containing heavily encapsulated microorganisms (e.g., *Cryptococcus spp.*) will give a strongly positive mucin clot test but the cytologic examination should be diagnostic.

Amylase activity is sometimes used in man to determine whether fluid accumulations contain salivary secretions and this has been erroneously reported to be of value in animals. None of the domestic animals except the pig have significant salivary amylase. This test should not be used in veterinary medicine.

Cytologic examination of aspirated fluids, fine needle biopsy of firm enlargements in the mouth, and scrapings from oral lesions may allow classification of these lesions as non-inflammatory, inflammatory, or neoplastic. When many neutrophils, monocytes, and macrophages are present, the inflammatory lesion may be classified as toxic or nontoxic on the basis of neutrophil appearance even if the etiologic agent is not evident. Sialocele fluid contains a non-toxic neutrophil accumulation with many cells showing old age changes such as hypersegmentation and karyorrhectic or pyknotic degeneration. Bacterial abscesses usually result in karyolytic degeneration and vacuolation of neutrophils. Pasteurella and pathogenic staphylococci are especially toxic and cause marked karyolytic changes in neutrophils. Actinomyces organisms often are found in typical clusters of coccobacillary rods with or without slender branching filamentous forms. The neutrophils that make up the granule surrounding this colony are usually highly toxic; neutrophils elsewhere in the fluid exudate may only show hypersegmentation and pyknotic degeneration. If organisms of one type are seen, a presumptive diagnosis is frequently possible on the basis of history, type of lesion, and the morphologic characteristics of the bacteria. Such findings are always helpful in assisting the laboratory to identify the predominant or most likely causative agent.

Among the neoplasms likely to be found, some may be identified readily by exfoliative cytology while others require histopathologic examination of punch, wedge, or excision biopsies. Neoplasms such as melanomas usually are easily recognized by the characteristic appearance of the melanin granules in young melanocytes. Occasional amelanotic forms may be impossible to diagnose by exfoliative means. Biopsy of enlarged tonsils or submandibular nodes usually allows differentiation between reactive lymphoid hyperplasia, lymphadenitis, and lymphosarcoma or recognition of metastases from neoplasms such as squamous cell carcinoma. If generalized lymphadenopathy exists, nodes other than those in the submandibular area should be examined since these are often reactive because of frequent entry of inflammatory agents through abrasions of the oral mucosae.

Mouth and Tongue. Squamous cell carcinomas of the mouth or tongue in cats often appear as a raised ulcerative lesion. Cytology of these lesions has been disappointing in diagnostic efficiency because epithelial cells at the margin of an inflammatory lesion often are highly anaplastic in appearance and because invasiveness and architectural abnormalities of tissue cannot be detected by exfoliative cytology. Such lesions are more accurately diagnosed by punch or incision biopsy of the margin of the lesion. Scrapings of ulcerative lesions of the tongue of dogs or cats may be helpful in diagnosing eosinophilic granulomas and granulomas due to foreign bodies, such as plant awns or similar agents.

Esophagus and Stomach. The clinical pathology of the esophagus, stomach and ruminant forestomachs and abomasum also are rather limited in scope. Acute traumatic reticuloperitonitis in cattle commonly results in emergence into circulation of band and metamyelocyte neutrophils but without mature neutrophilia until the fifth to seventh day of abscess development. Hematologic changes are not common with other diseases of these organs.

Acid-base, electrolyte, and organic anion changes are commonly associated with abnormal loss or sequestration of fluids from the stomach or abomasum. These changes have been described in detail earlier. Examination for parasite eggs in feces may be helpful in the diagnosis of parasitic disease of these organs although such examinations are of no value in detecting infestation of the esophagus or stomach by arthropod larvae. Cytologic examination of esophageal and stomach washings have been useful to detect cancer cells among human patients but have been totally unrewarding in my experience with animal samples. This difference probably is a reflection of the much lower incidence of esophageal and gastric exfoliating neoplasms among animals and may reflect the relative inexperience of veterinary clinical pathologists in dealing with such specimens.

Small Intestine. Laboratory evaluation of the duodenum, jejunum, and ileum is generally performed to determine possible causes for diarrhea or to evaluate the health of an animal with suspected intestinal obstruction. The minimum data base for animals with diarrhea must include at least one evaluation of a fecal specimen for evidence of parasitic infection; if results are negative, especially in a high volume diarrhea, at least two additional specimens should be checked to increase the sensitivity for detecting certain parasites. Negative results, especially in young animals, must always be assessed with consideration for the parasite life cycle since severe signs of intestinal disease may occur prior to sexual maturation and egg production by intestinal parasites.

Bacterial enteritis is a common cause for diarrhea among all animal species. Although specific identification of the bacterial etiologic agent for diarrhea may be useful to determine therapy for an individual animal, the epidemiologic value is often of far greater importance. Many different aerobic and anaerobic bacteria inhabit the digestive tracts of animals and identification of the "one" etiologic agent requires careful sampling, appropriate primary and secondary cultures, and in some cases serotyping, phage typing, or identification of specific toxin production. At present the greatest clinical application for fecal culturing is to identify or "rule out" the presence of specific known enteric pathogens such as the *Salmonella spp.*, or enterotoxin-producing strains of *Escherichia coli*.

Aside from identification of bacterial causes for diarrheas, laboratory determinations are useful to detect and differentiate abnormalities related to bacterial enteritis and other causes of malabsorption, maldigestion, or protein-losing enteropathies.

Acute bacterial enteritis may result in significant hemorrhage and/or protein exudation into the digestive tract, but the extent is often not reflected in PCV or plasma protein values until the concurrent hemoconcentration is corrected. Maldigestion and malabsorption produce a moderate anemia with poor regenerative response which may be slightly hypochromic in nature and accompanied by moderate hypoproteinemia.

Except for specific intestinal disaccharidase deficiency, most causes of maldigestion are a result of pancreatic exocrine deficiency (rarely bile salt deficiency), and laboratory tests to detect this are discussed under that heading. A specific disaccharidase deficiency usually results in diarrhea when that disaccharide is fed. A presumptive diagnosis may be proven by challenge feeding of a disaccharide (e.g., lactose) and evaluating plasma for evidence of digestion and absorption of the monosaccharide components (e.g., glucose). Alternatively, intestinal biopsy specimens may be incubated in vitro with specific disaccharides to detect these deficiencies.

Malabsorption may be detected by challenge testing with simple compounds that require no digestion prior to active or passive absorption and measurement of plasma or urine levels at timed intervals after oral administration of the compound. A crude but commonly used test for this purpose in dogs has been the feeding of corn oil with and without added pancreatic lipase. If lipemia occurs at 2 to 3 hours following either feeding, intestinal absorption is considered to be normal. Determination of xylose absorption following oral dosage provides more quantitative and reliable results and is the test now generally recommended to confirm malabsorptive conditions. A detailed discussion of methods and interpretation of challenge testing to evaluate intestinal function may be found in Chapter 16.

When evidence exists for intestinal malabsorption, presumptive evidence for the type of lesion involved may sometimes be gained by reviewing the hematologic findings of the case. Persistent eosinophilia in a dog with no evidence for intestinal parasites strongly suggests a diagnosis of eosinophilic gastroenteritis. Similarly, evidence in peripheral blood for lymphosarcoma or histoplasmosis provides a presumptive etiologic diagnosis for these causes of malabsorption.

Although cytologic examination of fecal smears may demonstrate large numbers of eosinophils in dogs with eosinophilic gastroenteritis, intestinal biopsy is often required to detect or confirm the lesion causing malabsorption. Cytologic imprints of the biopsies, examined after staining with new methylene blue or Romanowsky's stains, will provide a rapid assessment of inflammatory, invasive, or neoplastic lesions, but histopathologic examination of the biopsy sections is recommended to establish the final diagnosis.

Protein-losing enteropathies have many clinical similarities to malabsorption and maldigestion and have many laboratory similarities as well. Albumin concentration is generally decreased as are plasma total lipid, cholesterol, and triglyceride concentrations. Such findings together with a marked decrease in peripheral blood lymphocytes without simultaneous reduction in eosinophils or increase in monocytes indicate that intestinal biopsy and/or studies to detect intestinal loss of albumin should be performed. Large numbers of neutrophils may be detected by cytologic examination of feces in exudative protein-losing enteropathies due to inflammatory lesions of intestinal mucosae. Definite confirmation of these lesions may also require biopsy.

Other lesions of the small intestine cause only general changes in hematologic and chemistry values. Fluid loss or sequestration resulting from intestinal obstruction generally produces a mild to moderate metabolic acidosis except when the obstruction is very high in the duodenum causing marked loss or sequestration of gastric fluids.

Ulcerative lesions of the duodenum result in chronic hemorrhage usually associated with a regenerative anemia, although the anemia may be nonregenerative in very chronic cases. Occult blood in feces may confirm gastric or intestinal hemorrhage provided the diet is not high in heme-containing compounds. Chronic blood loss also results in a hypoproteinemia of both albumin and globulin fractions and may cause a moderate prerenal uremia due to digestion of the blood. If the ulcer perforates the intestinal wall, reabsorption of intestinal fluids from the peritoneal cavity may cause marked elevation of plasma bilirubin (mainly direct reacting), alkaline phosphatase, amylase, lipase, and other normal constituents of biliary or pancreatic secretions.

Large Intestine. Cecal, colonic, rectal, and anal disorders cause few specific changes in the laboratory data base. The general acid-base, electrolyte, and hematologic changes resulting from dysfunction of the large intestine have been discussed earlier in this chapter. Parasite infestation, when present, can usually be detected by examination of concentrated fecal preparations. Tape impressions of the anus and perineum may be useful in horses and other species which may be infested with "pinworms" (e.g., *Oxyuris equi*). Bacterial pathogens may be identified by appropriate culture techniques of fecal or rectal biopsy specimens. Cytologic examination of the feces will reveal numerous neutrophils in exudative forms of colitis, but the colonic source of the leukocytes must be distinguished from small bowel exudation on the basis of other signs. As with gastric or small intestinal hemorrhage, bleeding from the cecum, colon, or rectum will produce a positive fecal occult blood test, but the feces are characterized by frankly red blood or "currant-jelly" clots rather than a dark homogeneous color. Erythrocytes may be identified in cytologic preparations from such feces.

Cytology of abnormal masses found in the rectum, anal or perianal regions may be very helpful in establishing a diagnosis. In dogs, one of the more common neoplasms is the perianal gland or hepatoid adenoma characterized by cells which are similar to hepatic parenchymal cells in appearance. These neoplasms are easily diagnosed by imprint or aspiration biopsy. Rectal adenocarcinomas and other neoplasia of the anal area are relatively accessible to biopsy and diagnosis by imprint cytology or histopathologic means.

The Pancreas. Acute inflammatory or traumatic lesions of the pancreas in dogs usually result in a characteristic regenerative neutrophilia with stress-associated changes (lymphopenia, eosinopenia, and monocytosis), lipemia, and increased serum amylase and lipase activity. Alkaline phosphatase and glutamic-pyruvic transaminase are often moderately elevated (two to three times normal). These changes in enzyme activity are nondiagnostic and often remain elevated for several days after amylase and lipase return to normal. Other signs of hepatic disease are rarely observed. Hyperglycemia is common, and in some cases transient overtly diabetic glucose concentrations (>200 mg/dl) occur. Extremely severe hemorrhagic pancreatitis occasionally results in only moderate increases in amylase and lipase activity, presumably due to decreased capillary reabsorption and obstructed lymphatic circulation of the pancreas.

In typical cases of pancreatitis, plasma glucose values usually return to normal within 24 to 48 hours, and amylase and lipase values within 48 to 96 hours as inflammation subsides. Chronic foci of inflammation may progressively destroy pancreatic tissue and lead to recurrent acute pancreatitis with only slight to moderate elevations of amylase and lipase. In fact, in some cases the activity of these enzymes may not reach the diagnostic range. For maximum diagnostic sensitivity, both amylase and lipase should be determined as there is much individual variation in the degree of elevation of these enzymes in response to pancreatitis. A high normal or slightly elevated value of either amylase or lipase in conjunction with a significantly elevated value of the other is common in dogs with chronic or recurrent pancreatitis. When history suggests pancreatitis but neither amylase nor lipase values are increased to the diagnostic range, a prediabetic response (K = 1 to 2) to a high-dose IV glucose tolerance test (H-IVGTT) may be taken as additional evidence for pancreatic destruction since prediabetic curves are unusual among dogs without concurrent or previous pancreatic disease. Glucose tolerance testing should not be performed on clinically ill animals. In some cases exploratory laparotomy and biopsy may be necessary to confirm the diagnosis of chronic pancreatitis.

Two techniques commonly used to aid in diagnosing acute pancreatitis in human patients have been of little value for dogs, in our experience. Urinary amylase values are generally greatly increased among human patients with pancreatitis, and increased activity often remains after serum values have returned to normal. Peritoneal fluid amylase and lipase values are also often elevated in these patients. Dogs with clinical or experimental pancreatitis often have little peritoneal fluid accessible for analysis, and urine amylase activity is extremely variable even among dogs with very high serum amylase activity.[11]

Amylase activity during acute pancreatitis in cats rarely exceeds two to three times normal values. Glucose tolerance testing is generally of no diagnostic value for pancreatitis among cats since the prediabetic state may occur in apparently normal cats with no other laboratory or histologic evidence of pancreatitis. Amylase activities in pancreatitis in sheep and cattle are unlikely to reach values as high as those for dogs because pancreatic tissue activities are much less.

Laboratory determinations useful in detecting acinar pancreatic hypofunction due to fibrosis or juvenile atrophy include those which will differentiate maldigestion from malabsorption. In pancreatic insufficiency decreased secretion of proteases such as trypsin may be detected by determination of fecal tryptic activity. This is best determined by the test-tube gelatin digestion method and should be performed at fecal dilutions of 1:10 and 1:100. Dogs with digestive hypofunction may have adequate fecal protease activity at the 1:10 dilution, but the origin of this enzyme may be bacterial rather than pancreatic; normal pancreatic acinar function nearly always results in gelatin digestion even at the 1:100 dilution.

Failure of the animal to develop lipemia within 2 to 3 hours after consuming 3 ml corn oil/kg indicates malabsorption, maldigestion, delayed gastric emptying or, rarely, deficiency of bile salt secretion. If lipemia develops within 2 to 3 hours following oral administration of the oil plus exogenous pancreatic enzymes, pancreatic exocrine insufficiency can be assumed. Other challenge tests (e.g., xylose absorption) also may be used to differentiate maldigestion and malabsorption. Unfortunately, the fecal trypsin and fat absorption tests are semiquantitative at best and occasionally the results may appear equivocal or contradictory (e.g., slight fat absorption with negative 1:100 fecal trypsin or negative fat absorption even with supplemental enzymes, positive fecal trypsin, and positive xylose absorption). In such cases additional evidence of reduced pancreatic mass may be obtained by H-IVGTT with results in the prediabetic range.

Other simple tests that may prove maldigestion include microscopic examination of a thin film of feces stained with a propylene glycol solution of Sudan III or with Lugol's iodine solution. In severe cases of maldigestion many orange-staining neutral fat droplets will be observed in the Sudan III stained slide. Large numbers of purple to black starch granules and reddish-brown stained undigested muscle fibers with visible cross-striations may be visible in the iodine-stained smear. The most reliable of the microscopic examinations is that for fecal fat and this may be equivocal in some malabsorption problems.

A 24-hour quantitative fecal fat determination usually provides a definitive diagnosis of maldigestion or malabsorption of fats since most animals with these diseases excrete far more than the maximum normal 7 g of fat in their feces/day. If digested and undigested fractions of the fecal fat are quantitated, maldigestion may be differentiated from malabsorption since neutral fats will predominate in pancreatic exocrine insufficiency.

Since polyuria is a common sign of diabetes mellitus, glucosuria, ketonuria, and low urine pH are often the first laboratory signs of the disease. Since glucosuria often occurs among animals following parenteral administration of glucose solutions and among those with pathologic urinary stasis, urinary hemorrhage or rarely those with specific renal tubular defects, plasma glucose values should be determined to confirm the diagnosis of diabetes mellitus. Conversely, hyperglycemia may

not be detected in some cases by measurement of urinary glucose. The glucose oxidase reaction is inhibited in the presence of ascorbate concentrations normally found in the urine of some dogs, and some animals with severe glomerular filtration defects may reabsorb all glucose filtered. In cases such as these, diabetes mellitus can be diagnosed only by plasma glucose determination.

Fasting glucose concentrations in excess of 200 mg/dl are generally considered evidence for overt diabetes mellitus while hyperglycemia of a lesser degree may indicate insufficient insulin secretion or excessive glucocorticoid or catecholamine secretion. When persistent unexplained fasting hyperglycemia of less than 200 mg/dl is found, the H-IVGTT should be done. In this test,[12] K values of less than 1.0 are usual in overt diabetes mellitus; K values of 1.0 to 2.0 are evidence for the relative insulin-deficient prediabetic state. Alternatively or additionally, fasting insulin or glucagon levels may be determined by radioimmunoassay and, if necessary, insulin response to intravenous glucose challenge may be measured. In the prediabetic dog fasting insulin concentrations are generally normal but secretion in response to induced hyperglycemia is subnormal. Overtly diabetic dogs usually have subnormal fasting insulin and increased plasma glucagon concentrations; even when the insulin value is within normal range, it is always less than it should be for the hyperglycemic state of the animal.

Hypoglycemia when not due to improper sample handling may be a sign of pancreatic neoplasia, functional hypoglycemia ("puppy" or "hunting-dog" hypoglycemia), hepatic disease, or rarely glycogen storage disease. In ruminants, hypoglycemia is a common finding in metabolic diseases such as pregnancy toxemia of sheep and ketosis of cattle. Generalized hepatic disease can cause hypoglycemia, but other clinical and laboratory signs would be expected in hepatic disease of this severity.

The Liver. Destructive *hepatic* diseases cause appropriate leukocyte response although often less extreme than would be expected for similar lesions in organs with greater epithelial surface. Diffuse bacterial microabscesses (dogs) and large hepatic abscesses (cows) generally result in regenerative neutrophilia but often of a relatively modest degree. As in the case with other chronic infections, hepatic bacterial abscesses may cause a moderate nonregenerative anemia. Other chronic liver lesions also may result in anemia due to erythrocyte membrane changes, especially when hepatic lipid metabolism is abnormal.

A consumption thrombocytopenia may occur in patients with acute destructive, or neoplastic hepatic lesions as a result of disseminated intravascular coagulation. Patients with severe chronic liver disease may have deficient production of coagulation factors which may result in severe hemorrhage.

Biochemical tests for functional hepatocellular integrity may be divided into several general categories including: (1) quantitation of serum constituents normally metabolized or excreted by the liver, (2) the quantitation of hepatic enzyme activity in serum, and (3) quantitation of serum constituents normally produced by the liver. Biochemical evaluation of the liver should include at least one test from each group plus other determinations indicated by clinical signs or results of preliminary laboratory evaluation.

Bilirubin is formed mainly by degradation of hemoglobin from senescent erythrocytes and in lesser amounts from other heme sources and is excreted almost entirely by the liver. Increased plasma bilirubin concentration in the absence of evidence for hemolytic disease represents an important indicator of hepatic excretory dysfunction, although correlation between the degree of hyperbilirubinemia and the extent of hepatic lesions is not always apparent.

Among cattle hyperbilirubinemia is an insensitive indicator of hepatic dysfunction, and many cattle with extensive hepatic cholestasis show little increase in plasma bilirubin concentration. In contrast, moderate hyperbilirubinemia is easily induced by fasting of horses that have no other apparent hepatic dysfunction. In other domestic animals, general hepatic cholestasis usually results in hyperbilirubinemia but focal cholestasis even as severe as the obstruction of the biliary tree of an entire hepatic lobe may cause no significant increase in plasma bilirubin.

Total bilirubin determination is usually of little diagnostic value unless the proportion of conjugated (direct-reacting) bilirubin is also determined. In domestic animals other than horses, intrahepatic and posthepatic cholestasis usually results in hyperbilirubinemia with a predominance of the conjugated form. The hyperbilirubinemia of horses with cholestasis due to hepatic disease is predominantly due to unconjugated bilirubin, but conjugated values in excess of 30% of the total are indicative of hepatocellular dysfunction.[13] Acute hemolytic disease in all species results in hyperbilirubinemia with a majority of non-conjugated bilirubin, although among dogs the conjugated (direct-reacting) portion may become predominant after 2 to 3 days of continuing hemolysis. Conjugated hyperbilirubinemia in dogs during a progressive hemolytic disease is generally associated with other evidence of hepatocellular damage such as elevated serum GPT enzyme activity.

Enzymes for which increased serum activity usually indicates damage to hepatocellular membranes are sorbitol dehydrogenase (SDH), arginase, ornithine carbamyl transferase (OCT), each in all species, glutamic dehydrogenase (GD; ruminants), and glutamic-pyruvic transaminase (GPT; dogs, cats and some laboratory animals). When there is no evidence for skeletal or cardiac muscle damage or recent exceptional muscular activity, increased serum activity of glutamic oxalacetic transaminase (GOT), and of lactic dehydrogenase (LDH), or more specifically LDH isoenzyme 5, also indicates probable hepatocellular membrane damage.

All of these enzymes except OCT and GD are normally present in the cytosol of the hepatic cell and readily escape into the serum when exterior cell membranes are damaged. The degree and duration of increased serum activity are directly related to the intracellular concentration and the serum half-life of the enzyme and indirectly related to the molecular size of the enzyme molecule. However, it is impossible to differentiate between severe damage to moderate numbers of cells and moderate damage to many cells on the basis of serum enzyme activities alone. Theoretically, serum elevation of membrane bound (e.g., OCT) and mitochondrial enzymes (e.g., GD and one isoenzyme of GOT) will occur only with disruption of intracellular organelles and serve as a more specific indicator of severe hepatocellular disease than elevation of cytosol enzymes. In practice, however, the interpretation of ''biochemical biopsies'' is difficult, and correlation with specific hepatocellular lesions is often disappointing. At this time, the only justifiable assumption is that the elevation of serum enzyme activity generally parallels the severity of the lesion.

Alkaline phosphatase (AP), leucine amino peptidase (LAP), 5'nucleotidase (5'N) and γ-glutamyl transpeptidase (γ-GT or GGTP) are enzymes with relatively low intracellular concentration, and cellular destruction alone will not cause substantial elevation of serum activity. Alkaline phosphatase, the most commonly measured among this group, is present in two forms (isoenzymes) in the hepatic cell, one originating in cytosol and the other from nuclear and microsomal membranes. Determination of AP activity has been most helpful diagnostically in dogs, useful in cats, but of less obvious value in other species. The apparent species variation is often attributed to wide "normal" ranges among horses and ruminants but may represent misinterpretation of an inadequate data base. Focal or general intrahepatic cholestasis and extrahepatic biliary obstruction induce excess synthesis of the membrane-bound isoenzyme and may result in extreme elevations of AP activity in dogs with values ranging from 2 to 50 times normal. Elevations of cat enzyme activity in similar conditions is generally less extreme (2 to 5 times normal).[14] Hyperbilirubinemia will always be present when cholestasis is general, but focal cholestasis often results in marked elevation of AP activity without concurrent signs of icterus.

Cortisol and its synthetic analogs also induce excessive formation of either a new or an altered AP isoenzyme of hepatic origin in dogs.[15] Extreme elevation of serum AP activity may occur as a result of chronic excess glucocorticoid stimulation of either endogenous (Cushing's syndrome) or exogenous (iatrogenic) origin.

Extreme elevations of AP activity, apparently due to this same isoenzyme, are often found in dogs with diabetes mellitus when severe fatty infiltration of the liver is present. Neither cortisol excess nor diabetes mellitus commonly results in hyperbilirubinemia.

Leucine amino peptidase, 5'nucleotidase, and γ-glutamyl transpeptidase have had little usage in veterinary medicine. LAP in cats appears to parallel changes seen for alkaline phosphatase. Although the data base for GGTP cannot fully describe its indications or interpretation, this enzyme is mainly associated with the biliary tree. Increased serum GGTP activities are generally observed in acute hepatic disease and in general and focal cholestasis. In man increases are also seen with biliary neoplasia, pancreatitis, drug stimulation of the microsomal biotransformation system, and occasionally in renal disease. Advantages for GGTP over alkaline phosphatase include the greater specificity of GGTP for biliary origin and the tendency for GGTP to remain elevated after transaminases and alkaline phosphatase have returned to normal.

Among the various serum constituents produced or controlled by hepatic function are total serum proteins, albumin, several coagulation factors, glucose, and urea nitrogen. Serum albumin and the majority of serum globulins other than the immunoglobulins are formed by the liver, but abnormal rates of synthesis are often masked by changes in fluid balance unless the deficient production is chronic.

Acute hepatitis rarely results in a detectable albumin decrease because the half-life of albumin is approximately 6 to 10 days, minor decreases are masked by hemoconcentration, and only a small amount of hepatic tissue is required to maintain adequate protein synthesis. Chronic fibrosis or atrophy of the liver due to vascular anomalies (portal shunts) may result in severe depletion of albumin to concentrations of less than 1 g/dl resulting in ascites and/or peripheral edema. However, many young dogs with vascular anomalies may show no evidence of hypoalbuminemia until the signs of disease are advanced.

Coagulation proteins synthesized by the liver usually are only slightly decreased during viral hepatitis. This results in a slightly prolonged prothrombin time but severe hemorrhage occurs only with hepatitis-induced disseminated intravascular coagulation. Coagulation factor analysis is an insensitive means of detecting hepatic disease and usually is not performed for this purpose. When clinical signs or history suggests that coagulation factors are deficient, the analyses are of value to ascertain the etiology of the disease.

Glucose production and release during glycolysis and gluconeogenesis are especially important features of hepatic metabolism. Although an inconstant sign of hepatic disease, hypoglycemia associated with signs of degenerative liver lesions indicates general hepatocellular dysfunction.

The amino nitrogen released by deamination reactions in gluconeogenesis must be detoxified by hepatic synthesis of urea. In severe acute or chronic hepatic failure with decreased gluconeogenic ability, urea synthesis is decreased and, in the presence of normal glomerular filtration rates, plasma urea nitrogen levels will be decreased. As in the case with hypoglycemia, this is an inconstant but important indicator of serious hepatic dysfunction.

Special tests for hepatic function include bromosulfophthalein (BSP) and other anion dye excretion tests, plasma bile acid and blood ammonia concentrations. BSP is bound to plasma albumin after injection and is cleared from the plasma by active hepatocellular uptake, conjugation, and excretion into the bile. When injected intravenously, BSP dye is removed from plasma in exponential fashion among horses, cattle, and sheep. Prolongation of the time required to halve the plasma concentration ($t_{1/2}$) is one of the most sensitive indicators for hepatic dysfunction, including acute destructive hepatocellular lesions, general cholestasis, decreased hepatocellular mass, and decreased hepatic arterial blood flow. Decreased portal blood flow, fatty infiltration of hepatocytes, and hyperbilirubinemia without general cholestasis also result in minor but significant increases in BSP $t_{1/2}$. In addition to its value as a sensitive detector of hepatic dysfunction, repeated determinations of BSP clearance at 3- to 7-day intervals may serve as a prognostic indicator of hepatic recovery or progressive disease.

Among normal dogs, a semilogarithmic plot of plasma BSP clearance reveals at least two overlapping exponential excretory components; a rapid initial phase and a slower second phase. The biphasic curve complicates interpretation of the $t_{1/2}$ and renders it insensitive as a detector of acute hepatocellular damage in dogs. The percent of the initial BSP concentration that remains in the plasma 30 minutes after injection (BSP_{30} retention) is generally a more sensitive indicator for canine hepatic function than is BSP $t_{1/2}$. In spite of these difficulties, BSP_{30} retention has been more consistently abnormal among dogs with anomalous hepatic vascular lesions than any other common laboratory measurement of hepatic function.[16,17,18]

Other anion dyes, including indocyanine green (ICG) and rose bengal, have been used in a manner similar to BSP excretion as a measure of hepatic function but have not gained equal popularity in veterinary medicine. ICG excretion in the dog appears more nearly exponential than that of BSP and may be a more sensitive indicator of minor hepatic dysfunction. However, the greater cost of ICG and inability to determine ICG concentration with inexpensive laboratory instruments have resulted in less frequency of usage and, at this point, an inadequate development of a data base for interpretation of clinical results.

Ammonia (NH_3) is produced within the digestive tract of all domestic animals by microbial metabolism and absorbed in amounts that would be extremely toxic or lethal if allowed to reach peripheral circulation. Hepatocytes normally remove nearly all of this NH_3, metabolizing it to urea. When hepatic function is severely decreased by acute hepatocellular damage or by acquired or anomalous vascular shunts that allow a portion of portal blood to enter the peripheral circulation without passing through functional hepatic sinusoids, peripheral blood ammonia concentrations increase to toxic levels. Increased peripheral blood ammonia levels also may be caused by congenital urea cycle enzyme deficiencies. Among animals with acute hepatocellular damage or those with cirrhosis severe enough to result in acquired portal-caval shunting, other signs of hepatic disease will clearly identify the diseased organ and indirectly suggest the likely cause for abnormal central nervous system signs. However, among animals with congenital anomalies of the hepatic vascular system and those with hepatic urea-cycle enzyme deficiencies, other indicators of hepatic function are often normal. Such cases often have postprandial exacerbations of abnormal central nervous system signs because peak microbial production of NH_3 occurs at that time. In either case ammonia concentration should be determined in a freshly collected blood sample. If blood NH_3 is increased, the type of lesion must be confirmed by other evidence of hepatic dysfunction, by specific urea cycle enzyme analysis of a hepatic tissue biopsy sample, or by radiographic means.

Bile acids are produced by the liver in all species, excreted in the bile, largely reabsorbed by the intestine, transported to the liver by the portal system, and re-excreted by the hepatocytes into the bile.

When hepatic efficiency in removal of the bile acids is reduced by severe hepatocellular damage, chronic cirrhosis, or shunting of peripheral blood, bile acid concentrations increase and in some cases cause severe cutaneous pruritus. Until recently, determination of plasma bile acid concentration has been difficult and our data base for interpretation is inadequate. However, some reports[19,20] have suggested that determination of plasma bile acid concentration may provide a very sensitive indicator of hepatic dysfunction.

Biopsy allows visual examination of hepatic tissue, and when lesions are general or diffusely scattered, a definite diagnosis often may be obtained. Techniques for percutaneous hepatic needle biopsy are well described for the dog,[21,22] and the procedure has had relatively few complications and contraindications. Similar satisfactory results should be expected from other animal species, although practical experience may be inadequate to select the best techniques. Indications for biopsy include hepatomegaly, hyperbilirubinemia, or evidence for progressive hepatic disease, which cannot be satisfactorily explained on the basis of other clinical and laboratory determinations. Obvious contraindications would include severe hemorrhagic tendencies, shock, and severe acute onset of disease conditions. Procedures requiring anesthetic agents that must be metabolized by the liver should be avoided in patients with evidence for severe hepatic disease. Specimens obtained by percutaneous needle biopsy may be unsatisfactory for diagnosis of hepatic lesions that are only focally distributed, are limited to one hepatic lobe, or involve extensive cirrhosis. In these cases the clinician must determine the relative indications and contraindications for exploratory surgery and surgical biopsy.

Percutaneous hepatic needle biopsies of the core type are generally more satisfactory for diagnosis of hepatic disease than are aspiration biopsies, but material from either should be examined immediately by cytologic means to detect evidence for inflammatory or suppurative lesions and allow appropriate cultures of the specimen when indicated. When examined with new methylene blue or Wright's stain, slide films of aspiration biopsies or imprints of core biopsies may allow presumptive identification of some diseases including infectious canine hepatitis, histoplasmosis, toxoplasmosis, lymphosarcoma, reticulum cell sarcoma, and some metastatic neoplasms. Although fatty infiltration of hepatocytes and focal cholestasis may sometimes be recognized by examination of imprints, examination of sections of the core biopsy are more likely to result in a definitive diagnosis.

The Peritoneum. Peritoneal fluid assay may be very helpful in diagnosis or prognosis of certain disorders involving the gastroenteric tract. Normal fluid is small in quantity and contains few cells, mainly lymphocytes and mononuclear cells.[23] Any obstruction to the normal return of this fluid to circulation via the lymphatics of the peritoneal surface of the diaphragm or any transudation or exudation of fluid exceeding the capacity of lymphatic flow will result in peritoneal fluid accumulation.

Classic transudative peritoneal effusions are clear, low specific gravity (<1.018) fluids of low cellularity and low protein concentration. Fibrinogen is absent and the fluid will not clot. These effusions are associated with hypoproteinemia. Common causes of severe hypoproteinemia and associated hypoalbuminemia are intestinal malabsorption, protein-losing enteropathies, severe hepatic atrophy or cirrhosis, and glomerulonephritis or nephrosis with associated urinary protein loss.

Congestive heart failure and other causes of hepatic congestion due to inadequate hepatic venous return often result in effusion of a higher specific gravity (>1.018) and protein concentration (>3.0 g/dl) than that found in classic transudates. These fluids may contain small amounts of fibrinogen resulting in soft clots or wisps of fibrin in the fluid.

With chronicity, transudates, especially those due to hepatic congestion, are modified cellularly by moderate influx of neutrophils, erythrocytes, monocytes, and macrophages but generally remain less cellular than exudative fluids. The mesothelial cells of the peritoneal lining are stimulated to exfoliate and proliferate in clusters of young basophilic staining cells easily mistaken for cancer cells by inexperienced cytologists.[24]

Peritoneal exudates are generally cloudy and often bloody in appearance due to high leukocyte and erythrocyte cellularity and are generally more viscous than transudates due to higher protein content. Examination of the peritoneal fluid that accumulates during colic in horses is very helpful in diagnosis and prognosis. These fluids are generally low in specific gravity and are not highly cellular prior to infarction of the intestinal wall. Early in intestinal ischemia the major cellular content of the fluid changes from lymphocytes to neutrophils with some monocytes, macrophages, and mesothelial cells present. The cellular population (especially neutrophils) and protein content of peritoneal fluid increase abruptly as intestinal wall viability decreases and becomes unmistakably an inflammatory exudate. Less severe ischemia of the intestine due to recurrent embolic episodes often results in modified transudate formation with increased numbers of individual and clustered monocytes.[25]

Traumatic reticuloperitonitis in cattle may lead to peritoneal exudative effusion while torsion of the abomasum or intestine and intestinal intussusception result in a modified transudative effusion which becomes exudative as the viability of the affected organ decreases.

Among dogs and cats, peritoneal exudates may be associated with bacterial infections such as Actinomyces species or systemic fungi such as *Histoplasma capsulatum.* The cellular content of the fluid is mainly neutrophils with a mixture of cells showing hypersegmentation and karyolysis. A presumptive diagnosis can be made when typical organisms are observed.

Mixed bacterial species are often observed following traumatic rupture of the intestine or dehiscence of an intestinal surgical incision. Such lesions cause severe peritonitis and are generally associated with severe karyolysis of the many neutrophils present. If the lesion is relatively large, particles of intestinal content may be observed in the fluid.

The viscous slightly cloudy straw-colored exudate of feline infectious peritonitis is atypical by classic standards and generally of low cellularity, but it has high protein content (specific gravity >1.018) and contains fibrinogen which will form a fibrin clot.

Neoplastic effusions are extremely variable in characteristics, depending upon the mechanism by which the effusion is formed and upon its tendency to exfoliate cells. Lymphosarcoma may obstruct lymph flow in mesenteric nodes and may result in a relatively low volume transudative fluid containing variable numbers of lymphocytes, many of which may appear neoplastic.

Exfoliating neoplasms that cause partial obstruction of diaphragmatic lymphatics result in accumulation of fluid containing large numbers of neutrophils and macrophages, as the exfoliated cells become degenerate. Neoplastic exudates can be specifically identified only by observation of the exfoliated neoplastic cells in the fluid.

Frank hemorrhage may result from traumatic injury to abdominal organs or rupture of a vascular neoplasm such as splenic hemangioma. When hemorrhage is fresh, the protein content is similar to that of plasma and the sample will usually clot unless an anticoagulant is added. Leukocyte numbers and distribution will be similar to those of peripheral blood. The presence of platelets always indicates fresh hemorrhage except when a portion of the sample is aspirated directly from a blood vessel. In the 48 to 72 hours following hemorrhage, much fluid and many erythrocytes will be returned to the peripheral circulation via the diaphragmatic lymphatics and the thoracic duct. This autotransfusion often causes a sudden, partial correction of the acute anemia and in retrospect is an important diagnostic feature of abdominal hemorrhage. As the erythrocytes and protein return to the circulation, the peritoneal fluid progressively changes in appearance to that of a modified transudate except that erythrocytes and macrophages showing active erythrophagia will remain for several days.

REFERENCES

1. Coles, E. H.: Veterinary Clinical Pathology, 3rd ed., Philadelphia, W. B. Saunders Co., 1974.
2. Henry, R. J., Cannon, D. C., and Winkelman, J. W.: Clinical Chemistry. Principles and Techniques. 2nd ed., Hagerstown, MD, Harper & Row Publishers, 1974.
3. Kaneko, J. J., and Cornelius, C. E.: Clinical Biochemistry of Domestic Animals, 2nd ed., Vols. 1 and 2. New York, Academic Press, 1971.
4. Schalm, O. W., Jain, N. C., and Carroll, E. J.: Veterinary Hematology, 3rd ed. Philadelphia, Lea & Febiger, 1975.
5. Cho, D. Y., and Leipold, H. W.: Experimental spongy degeneration in the brain. Acta Neuropathol. 39:115, 1977.
6. Merkley, D. F., Howard, D. R., Eyster, G. E., Krahwinkel, D. J., Sawyer, D. C., and Krehbeil, J. D.: Experimentally induced acute gastric dilatation in the dog: cardiopulmonary effects. J.A.A.H.A. 12:143, 1976.
7. Datt, S. C., and Usenik, E. A.: Intestinal obstruction in the horse. Physical signs and blood chemistry. Cornell Vet. 65:152, 1975.
8. Tasker, J. B.: Fluid and electrolyte studies in the horse. V. The effects of diarrhea. Cornell Vet. 57:668, 1967.
9. Weisberg, H. F.: Water, electrolytes, acid-base and oxygen. In Todd-Sanford Clinical Diagnosis by Laboratory Methods, 15th ed. Edited by I. Davidsohn and J. B. Henry. Philadelphia, W. B. Saunders Co., 1974, p. 775.
10. Van Pelt, R. W.: Interpretation of synovial fluid findings in the horse. J.A.V.M.A. 164:91, 1974.
11. Moore, W. E., and Anderson, N. V.: Unpublished data.
12. Greve, T., Dayton, A. D., and Anderson, N. V.: Acute pancreatitis with co-existent diabetes mellitus: an experimental study in the dog. Am. J. Vet. Res. 34:939, 1973.
13. Tennant, B., Baldwin, B. H., Silverman, S. L., and Makowski, C.: Clinical significance of hyperbilirubinemia in the horse. In Proc. 1st Int. Symp. Equine Hematol. Edited by H. Kitchen and J. D. Krehbeil. Golden, CO, Am. Assoc. Equine Pract., 1975, p. 246.
14. Everett, R. M.: Personal communication.
15. Dorner, J. L., Hoffman, W. E., and Long, G.: Corticosteroid induction of an isoenzyme of alkaline phosphatase in the dog. Am. J. Vet. Res. 35:1457, 1974.
16. Cornelius, L. M., Thrall, D. E., Halliwell, W. H., Frank, G. M., Kern, A. J., and Woods, C. B.: Anomalous portosystemic anastomoses associated with chronic hepatic insufficiency in six young dogs. J.A.V.M.A. 167:220, 1975.
17. Ewing, G. O., Suter, P. F., and Bailey, C. S.: Hepatic insufficiency with congenital anomalies of the portal vein in dogs. J.A.A.H.A. 10:463, 1974.
18. Strombeck, D. R., Weiser, M. G., and Kaneko, J. J.: Hyperammonemia and hepatic encephalopathy in the dog. J.A.V.M.A. 166:1105, 1975.
19. Gronwall, R.: Plasma bile acids. In Proc. 1st Int. Symp. Equine Hematol. Edited by H. Kitchen and J. D. Krehbiel. Golden, CO, Am. Assoc. Equine Pract., 1975, p. 255.
20. Gronwall, R.: Personal communication.
21. Osborne, C. A., Hardy, R. M., Stevens, J. B., and Perman, V.: Liver biopsy. Vet. Clin. North Am. 4:333, 1974.
22. Feldman, E. C., and Ettinger, S. J.: Percutaneous transthoracic liver biopsy in the dog. J.A.V.M.A. 169:805, 1976.
23. Perman, V.: Transudates and exudates. In Clinical Biochemistry of Domestic Animals, 2nd ed., Vol. 2. Edited by J. J. Kaneko and C. E. Cornelius. New York, Academic Press, 1971.
24. Perman, V., Osborne, C. A., and Stevens, J. B.: Laboratory evaluation of abnormal body fluids. Vet. Clin. North Am. 4:255, 1974.
25. McGrath, J. P.: Exfoliative cytology of equine peritoneal fluid—an adjunct to hematologic examination. In Proc. 1st Int. Symp. Equine Hematol. Edited by H. Kitchen and J. D. Krehbiel. Golden, CO, Am. Assoc. Equine Pract., 1975, p. 408.

Chapter 7

GASTROINTESTINAL RADIOGRAPHY

Part I. Indications for Radiography

ROBERT E. LEWIS

Evaluation of the clinical signs observed provides the indications for radiography. Since radiography will increase the cost of the diagnostic workup of the case, the veterinarian must always judge the cost versus the expected return in diagnostic information. Any procedure performed should have an acceptable probability of changing and upgrading the management of the case. It has never been shown what percent of positive findings are necessary to justify the cost of a procedure. However, it is often thought that the higher the cost, the higher the percent of positive findings that must be obtained. Potentially lethal acute disorders may justify more procedures early in the workup of the case. It should be kept in mind, however, that negative results may help rule out one or more diseases that had been considered as probable causes of the clinical signs. Although negative films may not have proven the definitive diagnoses, they will have assisted greatly in the management of the case and are probably well worth the cost to the client. Radiography is expensive, particularly the special procedures, so there should be a strong expectation that diagnosis or treatment will be advanced before the procedure is done.

REGIONAL APPROACH FOR SURVEY RADIOGRAPHY

Survey radiographs may be made of three regions of the body when clinical signs of alimentary disease are present: (1) head and/or neck, (2) neck and/or thorax, and (3) abdomen. The clinical signs of gastrointestinal disease tend to localize the probable site of the lesion to one of these regions. Anorexia is such a general clinical sign that it alone does not justify a radiographic study.

Survey radiographs are always the first step in a radiographic evaluation of the patient. Many times the diagnoses can be determined from the survey radiographs and the time-loss, added trauma to the patient, and expense associated with special procedures can be avoided. It is advisable to decide what diseases are to be ruled out before radiography is done. The specific diseases in the rule-out list will influence the choice of which part to study radiographically and whether any special procedures are necessary.

When the clinical signs are primarily related to the head (dysphagia, ptyalism, and expectoration), the major contribution of survey radiography is to identify radiopaque foreign bodies and to evaluate the teeth. Proper evaluation of the teeth in horse, cow, or dog requires oblique radiographs, so that the arcades of teeth are not superimposed upon each other. In most cases, the roots of the teeth are the focus of attention and two radiographs must be made to evaluate them adequately in both arcades.

Radiographs of the neck and/or thorax are indicated by the clinical sign related to the esophagus, i.e., regurgitation. The size, location, and margination of the esophagus can be studied on survey radiographs if the esophagus contains air. If no air is present within the esophagus, a contrast esophagram is required to evaluate the esophagus properly. When the thorax has been radiographed, evaluation of the heart and lungs is possible and may often assist in diagnosing complications of alimentary tract disease or other intercurrent diseases.

Radiography of the abdomen in both the horse and cow is difficult to accomplish because of technical limitations. Radiography of the abdomen in the dog and cat is within the capability of a wide range of machines and can provide much useful information. Vomiting, diarrhea, abdominal distention, and abdominal pain are indications for abdominal radiography. The roentgen signs of density, size, shape, location, and margination are useful in delineating the segments of the alimentary tract and also the other abdominal organs.

SPECIAL PROCEDURES

If the specific diagnosis cannot be determined from the survey radiographs, special contrast procedures must be considered. Each of the special procedures will be discussed relative to the indications for doing that particular procedure.

Esophagram. An esophagram is indicated when clinical signs of dysphagia and/or regurgitation exist and the physical examination and survey radiographs have not provided the diagnosis. The type of esophagram will be indicated by the age of the animal and by evaluation of the survey radiographs.

If the animal is less than 5 months of age and has been regurgitating since being placed on solid food, the most important evaluations to make are:

1. What portions of the lumen of the esophagus are enlarged?

2. Can the esophagus propel solid food into the stomach?

To accomplish this, a $BaSO_4$-food mixture is the best medium. This combination should never be used if a foreign body is suspected, as the foreign body will often be camouflaged by the heterogeneous appearance of the medium.

The *barium-paste esophagram* should be used in those cases where dysphagia and/or regurgitation are present and where the esophagus cannot be visualized on survey radiographs by air contrast within the lumen. The paste will outline the location of intraluminal objects and mucosal marginations.

The *aqueous organic iodide esophagram* should be used when there is suspicion of a foreign body and/or perforation. If perforation has occurred, there may be pleural effusion and/or severe lung disease that has been caused by ingesta leaking from the esophagus into either the pleural cavity or lung. Barium paste is preferred for demonstration of small perforations, because visualization of small quantities of aqueous media outside of the esophageal lumen is very difficult.

Upper Gastrointestinal Tract Study. The primary clinical indications for an upper gastrointestinal examination (upper GI study) are vomiting and abdominal pain. If the vomiting is acute and persistent (duration of more than 3 days with high frequency), the possibility of making a specific diagnosis is greater. The number of diagnoses made from upper gastrointestinal studies in dogs and cats with clinical signs referable to the gastrointestinal system is quite low. It has been stated that the reason for the popularity of this study is the tremendous therapeutic effects of the barium suspension, not the diagnostic accuracy.[1] Similarly, an upper gastrointestinal study in cases where diarrhea is the only clinical sign is almost always a waste of time, money, and effort. Other laboratory tests and procedures are much more likely to lead to a definitive diagnosis.

Barium Enema. Diarrhea and tenesmus are the clinical signs that usually indicate the need for a barium enema, but it frequently does not provide a diagnosis because few colonic diseases cause radiographically demonstrable changes in the colon. In animals with abdominal masses, the barium enema will identify the colon and aid in determining whether the colon or an adjacent structure is associated with the mass. If the diarrhea contains red blood and mucus, the diagnostic return for the barium enema would likely be higher because of the stronger possibility of ulcerative colitis, intussusception, or a colonic neoplasm. Tenesmus alone may be an indication for a barium enema, since there is a strong likelihood that the lesion would be in the descending colon or rectum. Depending upon the method used, the rectum may not be visualized well on a barium enema.

Cholecystography. Cholecystography may be indicated whenever disease of the gallbladder is suspected. The clinical sign of icterus might indicate obstructive gallbladder disease. With gallbladder obstruction the gallbladder is not filled normally; therefore the contrast media may not accumulate as completely as in the normally functioning gallbladder. The test is likely to be falsely positive if total serum bilirubin exceeds 3 mg/dl. Gallstones are quite rare in the dog and cat and have usually been reported to be radiopaque and should be visualized on survey films. Radiolucent gallstones also occur and can be diagnosed only by cholecystography or at surgery.

Portography. Portography is necessary to diagnose portacaval shunts, which have been described in the dog. Indications for portography are the presence of neurologic signs, a low BUN, or a distended abdomen caused by ascites, in addition to other signs of liver disease.

Horizontal Beam Radiography. This technique allows gravity to displace certain organs so that other abdominal structures can be better visualized. The position in which the animal is placed depends upon which abdominal organs are to be visualized. Horizontal beam radiography can also be useful in detecting very small quantities of gas within the peritoneal cavity. Free gas is usually associated with perforation of the gut or ruptured urinary bladder in the female and may be suspected following trauma and/or gunshot wounds. The animal should be in right lateral recumbency to allow the air to become trapped in the dome of the abdominal cavity just caudal to the rib cage. In left lateral recumbency, the liver can usually be separated from the lateral abdominal wall, and visualization of as little as 10 to 20 ml of gas is often possible. In dorsoventral recumbency, as little as 2 to 3 ml of free gas can be visualized. Horizontal beam radiography can also be utilized in conjunction with an upper gastrointestinal examination, by allowing the contrast media to shift to different portions of the stomach as the position of the dog is varied. Radiography of the head and neck of the horse and cow is usually done with a horizontal beam and with the animal standing. Metallic objects and boluses embedded in soft tissue, e.g., in the parapharyngeal tissues, may be visualized particularly if gas is present adjacent to the object.

Part II. Technique for Radiographic Examination of the Canine and Feline

DONALD E. THRALL

SURVEY FILMS

When making survey films of the neck or chest to examine the esophagus, no special patient preparation is required. However, any patient scheduled for abdominal radiography should be prepared. Critical evaluation of survey films of the abdomen is difficult unless the stomach is free of ingesta and the colon free of fecal material. In the acutely ill patient, preparative procedures may be detrimental to the patient.

Ideally, proper patient preparation involves withholding all solid food per os for 24 hours prior to the examination and administering a warm water enema 2 or 3 hours prior to the examination. If the enema is given immediately prior to radiography, one usually finds that a large volume of gas has been introduced into the bowel, which detracts from the diagnostic quality of the radiograph. Some commercial enema preparations also tend to result in substantial gas accumulation, thus the specification of a warm water enema. While not every patient requiring abdominal radiography can be subjected to the rigors of ideal preparation, it is the rare patient indeed that cannot tolerate a gently administered warm water enema. Time invested in this procedure is time well spent.

Visualization of various soft tissue structures in the abdomen is enhanced by surrounding fat. Fat is slightly less capable of absorbing diagnostic x-rays than are other soft tissues. Therefore, areas of fat will appear darker on a radiograph than other surrounding soft tissues and fat will also outline the soft tissues. This difference in radiographic density between fat and other soft tissues is referred to as subject contrast. Subject contrast can be either minimized or enhanced by altering certain technical factors associated with the radiographic equipment. In the case of abdominal survey radiography, one should attempt to enhance subject contrast so that a greater distinction between abdominal organs can be achieved. The two most practical means of enhancing subject contrast are: (1) utilization of a grid and (2) utilization of a high mas-low kVp technique.

A grid absorbs radiation scattered by the patient before it reaches the film. It is therefore placed between the patient and the film. Since thin patients do not scatter a significant amount of radiation, a grid is not necessary if the patient measures less than 10 cm in thickness.

The description of the physical phenomena leading to enhancement of subject contrast through the use of a high mas-low kVp technique is beyond the scope of this book. This principle can be practiced, however, by using at least 10 mas, with an appropriate kVp, when survey radiographs are made.

Survey films of a patient suspected of having esophageal disease should include ventrodorsal and lateral radiographs of the neck and chest. The anatomic landmarks of the neck are easy to identify, and no particular problems are associated with radiography of this area. On the other hand, several problems exist when radiography of the chest is undertaken. The first problem is that of identifying the anatomic limits of the chest so that the entire part is included on the film. The cranial limit of the chest is the thoracic inlet and the caudal limit is the last rib. When one properly positions a patient for chest radiography, the center of the x-ray beam usually intersects the heart. When the patient is positioned for the lateral or ventrodorsal radiograph, the front legs should be pulled cranially to remove as much of the tissue mass of the shoulders from the cranial thorax as possible. In the ventrodorsal position, the sternum should be superimposed over the spine. One should routinely attempt to make the exposure at the height of inspiration.

The survey radiographic examination of the abdomen consists of ventrodorsal and lateral radiographs. The cranial anatomic limit of the abdomen is the tenth rib; the caudal limit is at the coxofemoral joints. Extreme caudal tension should not be placed on the rear legs as this will result in the formation of tension bands of skin tissue which will be visible radiographically. The exposure can be made at the height of either inspiration or expiration.

SPECIAL PROCEDURES

Esophagraphy. No patient preparation is necessary prior to the conduction of an esophagram.

The contrast medium used for esophagraphy depends upon the reason the examination is being conducted. If the clinician is primarily interested in the character of the esophageal mucosa, a thick barium sulfate ($BaSO_4$) paste (Esophatrast or Microtrast) should be used. Such pastes are available commercially or they can be prepared by mixing $BaSO_4$ powder U.S.P. with water until a thick paste is formed. The inconvenience of formulating one's own $BaSO_4$ paste points out the advantage of purchasing the commercially prepared product. To begin the procedure, a quantity of paste, ranging in volume from 5 to 20 ml, is placed upon a tongue depressor and then transferred to the mouth of the patient. The region of the junction between the hard palate and soft palate is a suitable landmark. Care

must be taken not to overwhelm the swallowing capability of the patient, so as not to cause tracheal aspiration. Also, one must avoid staining the skin with contrast medium, which causes radiographic artifacts. Once the paste has been administered, the patient's mouth should be restrained in the closed position in order to thwart an attempt to expectorate the paste rather than to swallow it. Once the majority of the paste has been swallowed, ventrodorsal and lateral neck radiographs and ventrodorsal-oblique and lateral chest radiographs should be made as quickly as possible. The ventrodorsal-oblique is utilized rather than the standard ventrodorsal so that the esophagus will not be superimposed on the spine and cardiac silhouette. If delay between administration of the paste and radiography is avoided, an excellent delineation of the esophageal mucosa is usually obtained.

If the clinician is primarily interested in the integrity of the esophagus, an aqueous organic iodine contrast medium intended for oral administration (Oral Hypaque or Gastrografin) should be used. These media are absorbed from body tissues and their use obviates the deposition of insoluble $BaSO_4$ contrast medium in structures such as the lung or mediastinum, if a perforation or fistula of the esophagus does exist. Five to 10 ml of contrast medium placed into the patient's mouth via a syringe should be sufficient. Care should be taken not to inject the medium too rapidly or the patient may aspirate rather than swallow. Staining the skin of the patient with contrast medium should be avoided. Radiographs of the neck (ventrodorsal and lateral) and chest (ventrodorsal and lateral) made immediately after administration of the contrast medium will not delineate the esophageal mucosal pattern as the aqueous media is transported rapidly to the stomach without coating the mucosa. If a perforation or fistula is present, however, identification of contrast medium outside the esophagus will usually be possible.

If the clinician is primarily interested in alterations of the diameter of the lumen of the esophagus, as may occur in esophageal dilatation, vascular ring disease, or an esophageal stricture, $BaSO_4$-impregnated food should be used. This contrast medium is easily prepared by mixing either a commercial $BaSO_4$ suspension (redi-Flow) or $BaSO_4$ powder U.S.P. with commercially available moist or semimoist food. The $BaSO_4$-impregnated food mixture will usually be eaten readily by the patient. Following ingestion of the contrast medium, ventrodorsal and lateral radiographs of neck and chest should be made. If no abnormalities of the esophagus are present, the contrast medium will have been moved rapidly to the stomach and the esophageal mucosa will not have become coated. If a stricture exists or peristalsis of the esophagus is depressed, the contrast medium will remain in the esophagus and the extent of associated esophageal dilatation can be evaluated.

Upper Gastrointestinal Examination. Before an upper gastrointestinal examination (upper GI) is conducted, the patient must be properly prepared by withholding all solid food and medication per os for a period of 24 hours prior to the procedure and administration of a warm water enema 2 or 3 hours prior to the procedure. All drugs affecting gastrointestinal motility should be withheld prior to the examination for a period of time long enough to assure that gastrointestinal motility is normal. Failure to prepare the patient properly will compromise the diagnostic quality of the study. In critically ill patients, the urgent need for diagnostic information may supersede the requirement for strict patient preparation.

One has a choice of two basic types of contrast media: (1) BaSO$_4$ suspensions and (2) oral aqueous organic iodine contrast media. The oral aqueous organic iodine contrast media are undesirable for a number of reasons:

1. They have a tendency to induce vomiting.

2. They are hyperosmolar and tend to become diluted as they draw fluid into the bowel lumen.

3. By drawing fluid into the bowel, an already disturbed fluid and electrolyte balance may be worsened. They are useful, however, in cases of suspected gastrointestinal perforation.

When using BaSO$_4$ for an upper gastrointestinal examination or for an esophagram, one has the choice of using a commercially available BaSO$_4$ suspension or formulating a suspension out of BaSO$_4$ powder U.S.P. and water. To prepare a suspension, BaSO$_4$ powder U.S.P. should be mixed with water in a blender at a 30% w/w concentration. This mixture has the undesirable characteristics of sedimenting in vitro and both sedimenting and flocculating in vivo when mixed with normal gastrointestinal secretions. Sedimentation and flocculation are not routinely encountered when commercially available BaSO$_4$ suspensions which contain suspending agents are used. The mechanics of preparing a BaSO$_4$ U.S.P.-water suspension as well as the problems of sedimentation and flocculation make the choice of using redi-Flow an easy one.

Most clinicians have the tendency to underestimate the amount of contrast medium necessary for an upper gastrointestinal study. An adequate dose is 13 ml per kilogram of body weight given via gastric intubation. Gastric intubation is favored over oral administration because of the tendency of the patient to swallow large quantities of air when the latter method is used.

Ventrodorsal and lateral abdominal radiographs should be made at the following times after administration of the contrast medium: immediately, 15 minutes, 30 minutes, 60 minutes, and then hourly until all contrast medium is in the colon or until a definitive diagnosis is made. Radiographs made late in the series are useful in detecting barium adherence to a gastric foreign body or mucosal lesion. If fluoroscopy is available, the peristaltic activity of the stomach as well as the status of pyloric function should be evaluated immediately after administration of the contrast medium.

The rate of transit of barium through the gastrointestinal tract is a function of the rate of peristalsis of the stomach and small intestine, the functional status of the pylorus, and the viscosity of the contrast medium. Considering these variables, it is difficult to define the normal gastrointestinal transit time. The schedule in Table 7–1 is approximately correct for a commercially available 30% w/w BaSO$_4$ suspension administered via gastric intubation to a healthy dog.

Pneumogastrography. A pneumogastrogram can be easily performed by instilling air into the stomach through a gastric tube. A rigid dose schedule has not been worked out for the dog, but 30–35 ml of air per kg of body weight should provide adequate gastric distention without endangering the patient's life. The air should be removed following completion of the procedure. It may be necessary to decrease the mas by a factor of 0.5 to avoid overexposing the radiograph.

Barium Enema. The colon must be thoroughly cleansed prior to the conduction of a barium enema. If not removed, residual fecal material may be mistaken for a lesion, or at the very least, the

Table 7–1. Radiographic appearance of the upper gastrointestinal study as a function of time after administration of the contrast medium

Time After Administration of BaSO$_4$ (min)	Radiographic Appearance of Upper Gastrointestinal Tract
15	Duodenum well filled
30	Jejunum well filled
120	Stomach completely empty
360	Jejunum and ileum empty

diagnostic quality of the study is compromised. Proper patient preparation includes denying solid food per os for a period of 24 hours prior to the examination as well as giving at least one enema 2 or 3 hours prior to the examination. The procedure may be done on conscious patients that are under tranquilization or general anesthesia. Narcotic drugs, such as morphine or fetanyl-droperidol must be avoided owing to their spasmogenic effect on the large bowel.[1]

The contrast medium of choice is a commercially available 30% w/w $BaSO_4$ suspension diluted to approximately 10% w/w with water. Aqueous organic iodine contrast media should be reserved for cases of suspected large bowel perforation. The exact dose required to distend the colon properly has not been established for the dog or the cat. Twenty to 30 ml/kg of body weight is recommended for the dog and 10 to 20 ml/kg of body weight for the cat.[1] The contrast medium can be infused with a dose syringe. However, gravity flow from a suspended enema bag through an inflated balloon tip catheter inserted in the rectum is recommended. The catheter should be attached to the enema bag and filled with contrast medium prior to insertion so that air will not be injected into the colon. A clamp must be available to regulate the flow of contrast medium as desired. Pressure, other than gravity, must not be applied to the colon. Gravity flow of contrast medium from the enema bag will usually cease when the colon is distended. In a small percentage of cases, retrograde flow through the ileocolic valve will fill the distal small bowel with contrast medium, making the study more difficult to interpret. Ventrodorsal and lateral radiographs of the abdomen should be made when one half of the calculated dose has been given. These radiographs will allow one to assess the degree of distention of the colon and whether ileocolic reflux has occurred. If ileocolic reflux has not occurred, another set of radiographs, possibly including oblique projections, should be made when the entire calculated dose has been given. These radiographs allow one to evaluate the fully distended colon.

A more critical evaluation of the colon mucosa can be made with the double contrast barium enema, made by injecting air (22 to 23 ml/kg) into the colon after the contrast medium from a conventional barium enema has been allowed to flow out of the colon through the balloon catheter. A double contrast barium enema can also be performed by injecting a small amount (2.2 ml/kg) of $BaSO_4$ suspension into the colon of a dog thoroughly prepared for abdominal radiography and then filling the colon with air (22 to 23 ml/kg). Several patient positions may be necessary to allow the entire colon to be visualized, as the air will not fill the entire colon simultaneously.

Cholecystography. Prior to conduction of a cholecystogram, the patient's abdomen must be prepared for radiography as described previously. Various contrast media are available for cholecystography, some of which are designed for oral administration while others are for intravenous administration. The obvious advantage of the intravenous agents is the rapidity with which the gallbladder becomes opacified. Iodipamide (Cholografin Meglumine), an intravenous agent, given at a dose of 0.5 mg/kg produces gallbladder visualization consistently at 30 minutes after administration.[2] Gallbladder opacity should be further improved by 120 minutes. Ipodate calcium (Oragrafin calcium granules), an oral agent, at a dose of 450 mg/kg, should produce gallbladder opacification at 12 hours following administration of the medium.[2]

Generally speaking, gallbladder opacification and visualization of intra- and extrahepatic bile ducts will be enhanced when an intravenous agent is used.

Gallbladder opacification failure may occur even in healthy dogs due to physiologic cholestasis. Other causes of opacification failure include pathologic cholestasis, acute pancreatitis, and acute cholecystitis.[2]

Portography. The following five techniques are available for radiographic examination of the portal venous system:

1. Operative splenic vein portography.
2. Operative mesenteric vein portography.
3. Transabdominal splenoportography.
4. Celiac arterial portography.
5. Cranial mesenteric arterial portography.

Operative splenic vein and mesenteric vein portography are probably the techniques of choice for the conduction of portography by the practicing veterinarian. In these techniques, the splenic vein or jejunal vein, or both, are cannulated through a laparotomy incision. Polyethylene catheter-needle combinations are strongly recommended. Once the desired vein(s) are cannulated, organic iodine contrast media of the triiodinated benzoic acid derivative type (Conray-400) are injected by hand at a dose of 0.50 to 1.0 ml/kg body weight. Lateral abdominal radiographs are then made over the 3- to 10-second period after injection at the rate of one exposure per second. If rapid filming is not available, a single exposure made at 5 to 7 seconds after injection may suffice. Operative portography is the most practical of all methods of portography for the practicing veterinarian, but requires careful attention to surgical technique.

Transabdominal splenoportography involves placing an intravenous catheter through the abdominal wall into the spleen, with the tip situated near the hilus. General anesthesia is required. With the animal in right lateral recumbency, the spleen is palpated and the catheter is inserted into the intraperitoneal space through a small skin incision. The catheter is passed into the spleen and an attempt is made to position the tip at the hilus. Backflow of venous blood indicates proper catheter position. Once the catheter is positioned properly, organic iodine contrast medium is hand injected at a dose of 0.50 to 1.0 ml/kg of body weight. Serial radiographs are then made with the x-ray beam centered over the cranial abdomen and caudal thorax. Radiographs are made over the 3- to 10-second period after injection at the rate of one exposure per second. If rapid filming is not available, a single exposure made 5 to 7 seconds after injection may suffice. Transabdominal portography is technically difficult, and potentially hazardous complications, such as splenic lacerations, do occur.

Celiac and cranial mesenteric arterial portography require the use of image-intensified fluoroscopy in order to position the angiographic catheter properly.[3] Since fluoroscopy is not available to most practitioners, these techniques will not be discussed here.

Horizontal Beam Radiography. In this easy and useful technique, the beam is horizontal, the cassette must be fixed in a vertical position, and the animal is supported in the desired position against the cassette. The cassette can be held with gloved hands if the primary beam is restricted. A better method is to use a commercially available, wall-mounted cassette holder so that the radiographer's entire attention can be devoted to positioning the patient. If the measurement of the animal indicates the need for a grid, it can be taped to the front of the cassette or a special cassette containing a grid may be used. The use of horizontal beam radiography obviously requires that the tube head of the x-ray machine rotate and be movable in a vertical plane.

Part III. Normal Radiographic Presentations

DONALD E. THRALL

SURVEY FILMS

The description of the normal abdominal radiograph will be limited to the gastrointestinal tract. Other guides are available for those desiring a comprehensive presentation of other organs and systems within the abdomen.[4,5]

The esophagus is routinely not visualized on survey radiographs of the thorax. Occasionally, it will contain a small volume of gas, particularly in anesthetized patients.

The stomach is routinely visualized on survey abdominal radiographs as a result of gas present within the lumen. The stomach is divided into five anatomic regions: the cardia, fundus, body, pyloric antrum, and pylorus (pyloric canal or pyloroduodenal junction) (Fig. 7–1). The portion of the stomach visualized on the survey radiograph depends upon the position of the patient and therefore the location of intragastric gas at the time the exposure is made[6] (Table 7–2 and Fig. 7–2).

The thickness of the stomach wall, which is a function of the degree of gastric distention, is extremely difficult to evaluate from survey films. The mucosal surface frequently appears very irregular owing to visualization of the rugal folds (Fig. 7–1). The less distended the stomach, the more prominent the rugal folds will be. Occasionally, varying degrees of gastric contractions will be evident on survey films (Fig. 7–3).

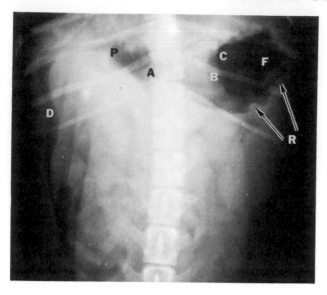

Figure 7–1. Ventrodorsal radiograph of the cranial abdomen (canine) showing the relative position of the gastric fundus (F), cardia (C), body (B), pyloric antrum (A), and pylorus (P). Gas is present in the descending duodenum (D). Rugal mucosal folds (R) are visible.

Table 7–2. Location of gas within the canine stomach as seen on survey abdominal radiographs as a function of the position of the patient during radiography

Patient Position During Radiography	Location of Gas Within Stomach
Dorsal recumbency	Body
	Pyloric antrum
Ventral recumbency	Fundus
Right lateral recumbency	Greater curvature
Left lateral recumbency	Lesser curvature
	Pyloric antrum

The duodenum is infrequently visualized on survey films. When seen, usually only the descending portion is noted (Fig. 7–1). Gas in the descending duodenum has been implicated as resulting from pancreatitis. However, far more instances of duodenal gas are seen in normal patients than in patients with pancreatitis.

The jejunum and ileum are located in the mid-ventral abdomen and are freely movable. The normal range of diameter of the jejunum and ileum has not been determined in the dog or the cat. As a general rule, all normal segments of small bowel should have a diameter less than three times the diameter of a caudal thoracic rib. The amount of gas present within the small bowel varies tremendously (Figs. 7–4 through 7–6). Essentially all gas present within the small bowel is air that has been swallowed. Dyspneic and nauseated patients have a tendency to swallow large quantities of air (Fig. 7–5).

The cecum, which is a diverticulum of the ascending colon, can be identified on survey abdominal radiographs (canine only) owing to the presence of gas within it. The cecum has a characteristic "comma" shape and is located in the midportion of the right hemi-abdomen (Fig. 7–6). The diameter of the cecum is larger than that of the small bowel.

The colon is divided into three areas: (1) the ascending colon, (2) transverse colon, and (3) descending colon (Fig. 7–7). The ascending and transverse colons are relatively fixed. The ascending colon begins at the cecum and extends cranially. At the level of T12 or T13, the colon turns at the right colic (hepatic) flexure and crosses to the left as the transverse colon. In the cranial left hemi-abdomen, the transverse colon turns caudally at the left colic (splenic) flexure and becomes the descending colon. The descending colon usually lies along the left lateral portion of the abdomen, but is relatively loosely attached because of the long mesocolon, and may deviate into the right hemi-abdomen. Visualization of the colon depends on the amount of fecal material and/or gas within the lumen (Figs. 7–4, 7–5, and 7–7).

SPECIAL PROCEDURES

Esophagraphy. The esophagus begins at the cricopharyngeal sphincter, which separates the laryngeal portion of the pharynx from the cervical esophagus (Fig. 7–8). The diameter may vary owing to the presence of peristaltic waves. At the thoracic inlet, the esophagus may abruptly course ventrally for a short distance (Fig. 7–9). This has been reported as an esophageal diverticulum, but represents only a normal anatomic variant. A slight dorsal deviation of the esophagus may be present as it passes over the base of the heart (Fig. 7–9). The mucosal pattern of the entire canine esophagus is linear (Fig. 7–9). In the feline thoracic esophagus, only the cranial one-half is characterized by a linear mucosal pattern. The caudal one-half of the feline esophagus has a "herringbone" mucosal pattern

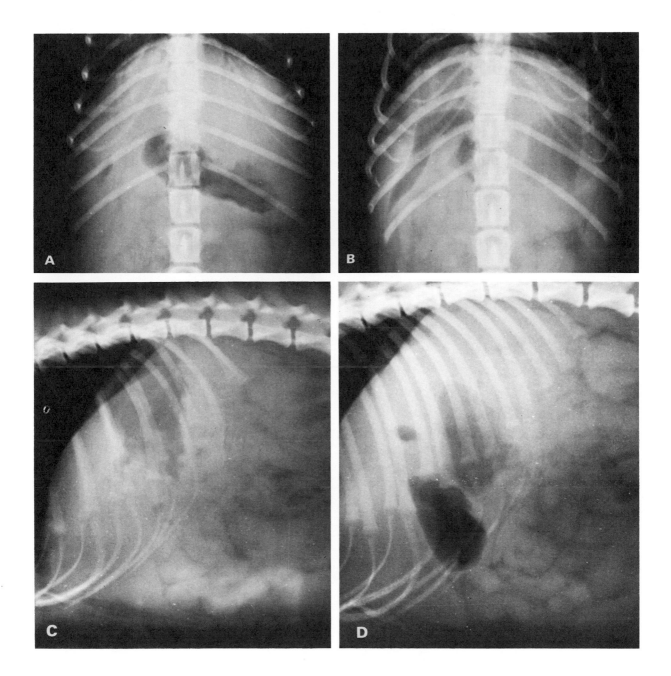

Figure 7–2. Radiographs of the cranial abdomen (canine) made with the patient positioned in the dorsal (**A**), ventral (**B**), right lateral (**C**), and left lateral (**D**) recumbent positions demonstrating the effect of patient positioning on the radiographic presentation of stomach gas. Gas is present in the duodenum in **B**. See text and Table 7–2.

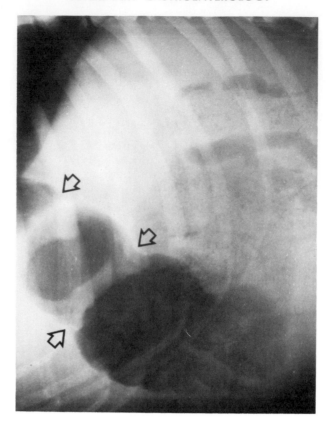

Figure 7–3. Lateral radiograph of the cranial abdomen (canine) made with the patient in left lateral recumbency showing two antral peristaltic waves (arrows). Rugal folds are also visible.

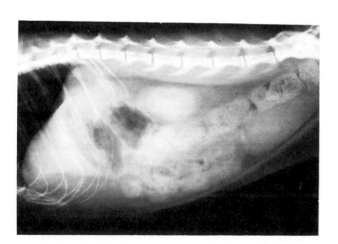

Figure 7–4. Lateral abdominal radiograph (feline) showing only minimal small bowel gas. The cranial colon contains gas while the caudal colon contains fecal material.

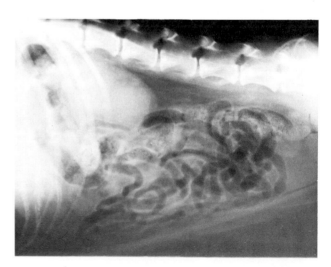

Figure 7–5. Lateral abdominal radiograph (canine) of a patient with dyspnea. Note the large amount of small bowel gas. Without knowing that dyspneic patients tend to swallow a large volume of air, this radiograph may be incorrectly interpreted as inhibition ileus.

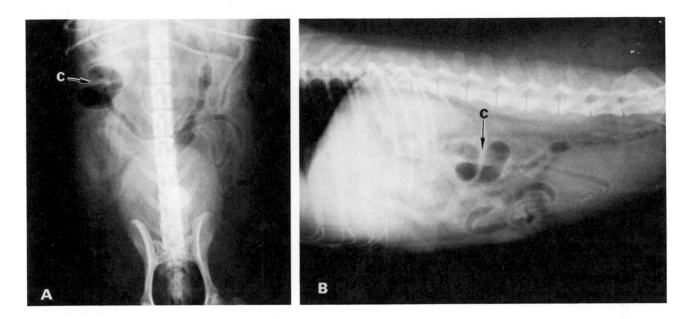

Figure 7–6. Ventrodorsal **(A)** and lateral **(B)** abdominal radiographs (canine) showing an intermediate amount of small bowel gas. The cecum (C) is distended with gas.

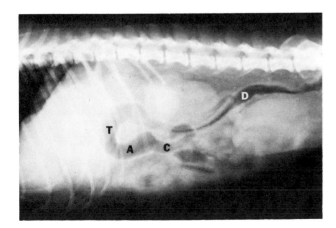

Figure 7–7. Lateral abdominal radiograph (canine) showing a moderate amount of colon gas. The cecum (C) as well as the ascending (A), transverse (T), and descending (D) portions of the colon are visible.

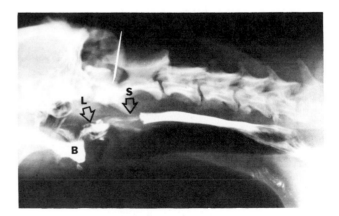

Figure 7–8. Lateral radiograph of a cervical esophagram (canine) showing the base of the tongue (B), laryngeal pharynx (L), and the cricopharyngeal sphincter (S) as well as the cervical esophagus. Note the linear mucosal pattern in the cervical esophagus.

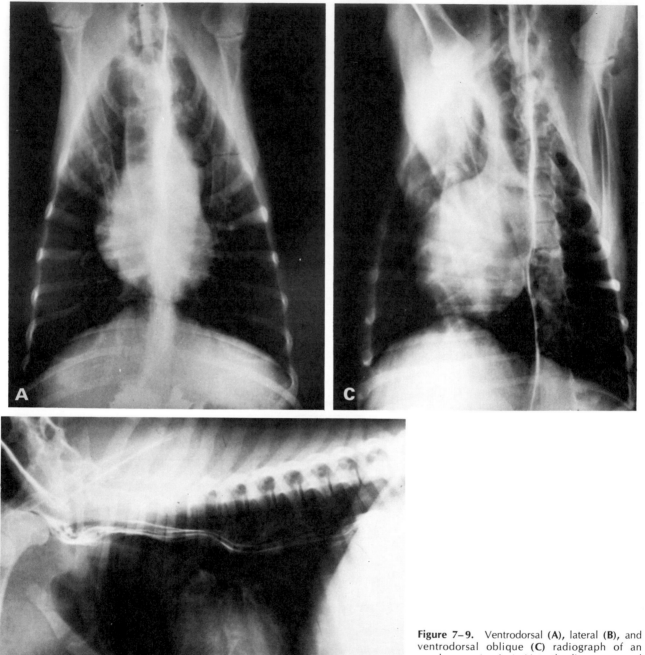

Figure 7–9. Ventrodorsal **(A)**, lateral **(B)**, and ventrodorsal oblique **(C)** radiograph of an esophagram (canine). Note the linear mucosal pattern in the esophagus. Note, also, the superior quality of the ventrodorsal oblique in comparison to the ventrodorsal projection. In the lateral projection, note the esophageal depression at the thoracic inlet and the esophageal elevation over the tracheal bifurcation.

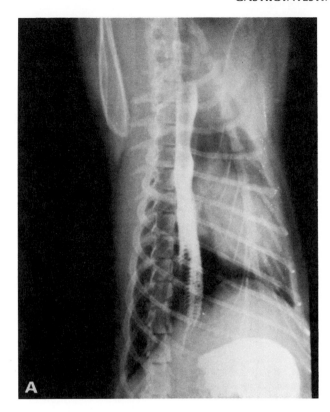

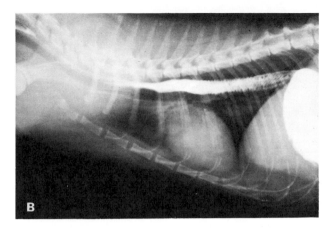

Figure 7–10. Ventrodorsal oblique (A) and lateral (B) radiograph of an esophagram (feline). Note the linear mucosal pattern in the cranial thoracic esophagus and the normal "herringbone" mucosal pattern in the caudal thoracic esophagus.

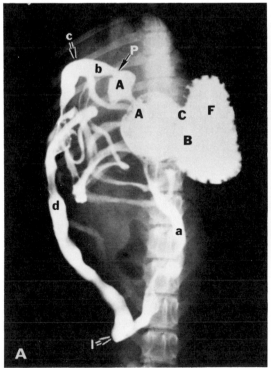

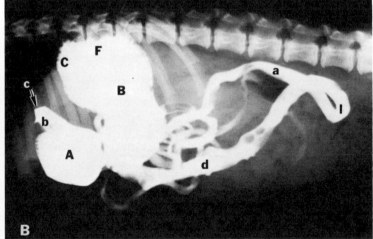

Figure 7–11. Ventrodorsal (A) and lateral (B) abdominal radiographs after administration of a $BaSO_4$ suspension via gastric intubation. The following components of the upper gastrointestinal tract are visible: cardia (C), fundus (F), body (B), pyloric antrum (A), pylorus (P), duodenal bulb (b), descending duodenum (d), ascending duodenum (a), cranial duodenal loop (c), caudal duodenal loop (l). Notice the antral peristaltic contractions visible on both radiographs. Pseudoulcers are visible in the descending duodenum in the lateral radiograph.

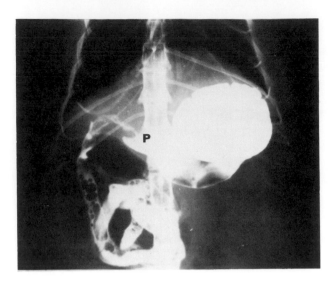

Figure 7–12. Ventrodorsal abdominal radiograph from an upper gastrointestinal study (feline). Notice the midline position of the pylorus (P).

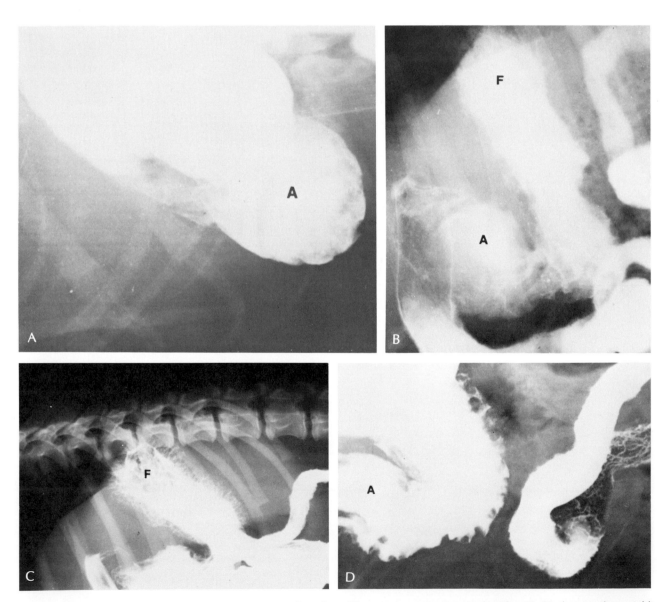

Figure 7–13. Close-up view of the gastric region (canine) from four different upper gastrointestinal studies **(A–D)** showing the variable appearance of the normal gastric mucosa that may be encountered. The location of the fundus (F) or pyloric antrum (A) is indicated.

72

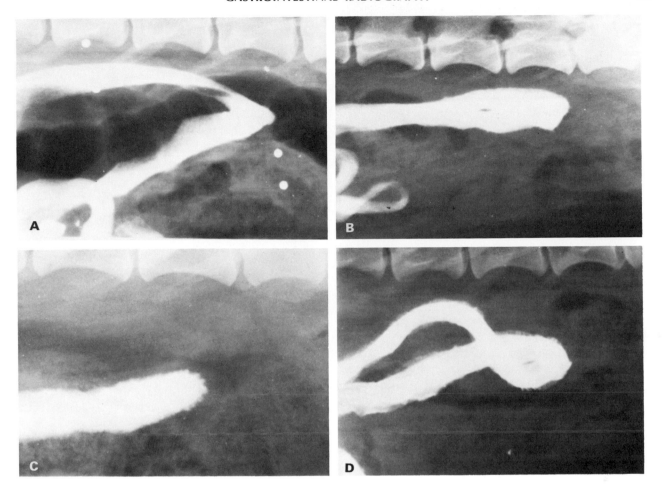

Figure 7–14. Close-up view of the caudal duodenal loop from four different upper gastrointestinal studies **(A–D)** showing the variable appearance of the mucosa that may be encountered. (Reprinted with permission of Dr. D. E. Thrall and The Journal of Small Animal Practice.)

(Fig. 7–10), which must not be mistaken for inflammatory mucosal change. The ventrodorsal oblique view of the thoracic esophagus is more valuable than the straight ventrodorsal radiograph (Fig. 7–9).

Upper Gastrointestinal Study. The anatomic areas of the stomach are much easier to identify during an upper gastrointestinal study than on survey radiographs (Fig. 7–11). The radiographic architecture of the feline stomach is the same as that of the canine, except that the pylorus of the cat is located much nearer the midline (Fig. 7–12). The appearance of the gastric mucosa varies considerably from patient to patient and is somewhat related to the degree of distention of the stomach (Fig. 7–13).

The duodenum is divided into bulbar, descending, and ascending portions by the cranial and caudal duodenal flexures respectively. These areas are usually identifiable on early films made during an upper gastrointestinal study (Fig. 7–11).

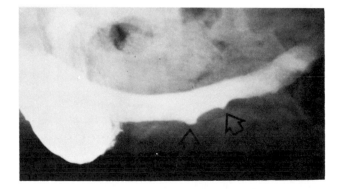

Figure 7–15. Close-up view of the descending duodenum from an upper gastrointestinal study showing two pseudoulcers (arrows).

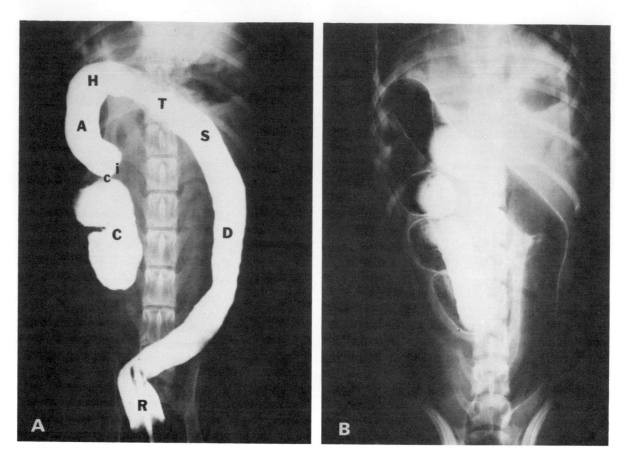

Figure 7–16. Routine **(A)** and double contrast **(B)** barium enema. The following structures and/or regions can be identified: cecum (C), cecocolic valve (c), ileocolic valve (i), ascending colon (A), hepatic flexure (H), transverse colon (T), splenic flexure (S), descending colon (D), and rectum (R). Notice the smooth margination of the colonic mucosa. The double contrast barium enema allows a more critical evaluation of the mucosa.

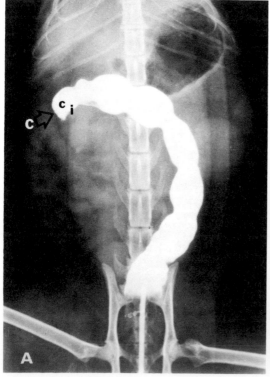

Figure 7–17. Ventrodorsal **(A)** and lateral **(B)** abdominal radiographs (feline) from a barium enema. Note the comparatively small feline cecum (C). The regions of the ileocolic (i) and cecocolic (c) valves are indicated.

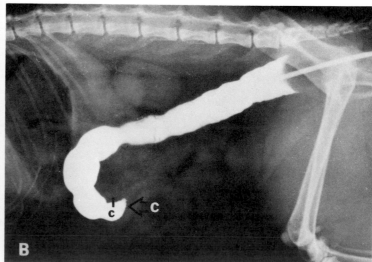

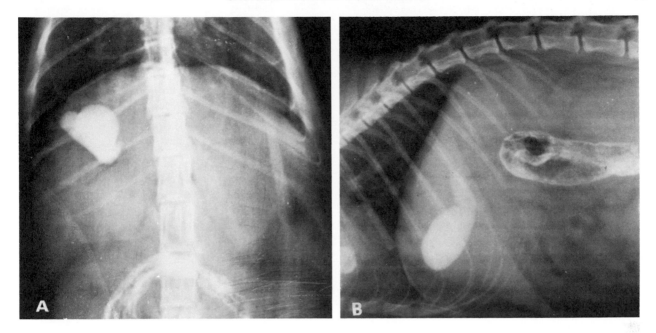

Figure 7–18. Ventrodorsal (**A**) and lateral (**B**) radiographs of an abdomen from a cholecystogram (feline). No bile ducts are visible. The contrast medium that was not absorbed from the intestine is present in the colon.

The mucosal pattern of the small intestine varies widely from smooth to noticeably fimbriated (Fig. 7–14). In the past, it has been suggested that the coarsely fimbriated mucosal pattern might represent a mucosal inflammatory change. Of late, however, it has been shown that this pattern is normal and is most likely due to intervillar penetration of the contrast medium.[7] The mucosa of the canine duodenum is occasionally characterized by "crater-like" depressions into the mucosa (Fig. 7–15). These depressions represent mucosal thinning over submucosal lymphoid follicles and are called pseudoulcers.[8] They are seen only in the canine duodenum.

Barium Enema. The anatomic portions of the colon are easily identified on a radiograph of a barium enema (Figs. 7–16 and 7–17). The mucosal pattern should be very smooth and essentially featureless in a normal patient properly prepared for the examination. In both the dog and the cat the cecum is a diverticulum of the proximal portion of the ascending colon; however, the canine cecum is proportionally larger than the feline cecum (Figs. 7–16 and 7–17). The mucosa can be much more critically evaluated from a double contrast barium enema than from a standard barium enema (Fig. 7–16).

Cholecystography. The gallbladder is located in the right cranial abdomen nestled between the quadrate

and right medial lobes of the liver in the dog and is embedded in the visceral surface of the right medial lobe in the cat. Normal limits for the size of the gallbladder have not been determined for the dog or the cat. Cholecystographically, the gallbladder should be of uniform density and not greatly distended (Fig. 7–18). Extrahepatic and intrahepatic bile ducts may or may not be visible.

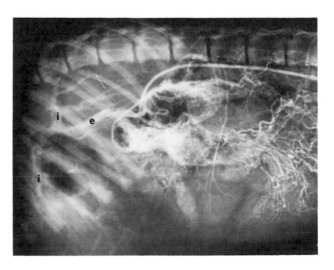

Figure 7–19. Normal portal venogram obtained via cranial mesenteric arterial injection of contrast medium. Both the extrahepatic (e) and intrahepatic (i) portions of the portal vein are visible.

Portography. Any of the five previously mentioned means of conducting a portogram should result in satisfactory visualization of the portal vein in the normal patient. Both the extrahepatic and intrahepatic portions of the portal system should be discernible (Fig. 7–19). No contrast medium should be present in the vena cava if the study has been conducted properly. The hepatic vein is frequently not visualized.

REFERENCES

1. Gomez, J. A.: The gastrointestinal contrast study: methods and interpretation. Vet. Clin. North Am. *4*:805, 1974.

2. Allan, G. S., and Dixon, R. T.: Cholecystography in the dog: the choice of contrast media and optimum dose rates. J. Am. Vet. Radiol. Soc. *16*:98, 1975.

3. Suter, P. F.: Portal vein anomalies in the dog: their angiographic diagnosis. J. Am. Vet. Radiol. Soc. *16*:84, 1975.

4. Root, C. R.: Interpretation of abdominal survey radiographs. Vet. Clin. North Am. *4*:763, 1974.

5. Thrall, D. E.: The abdomen. *In* Carlson's Veterinary Radiology, 3rd ed. Philadelphia, Lea & Febiger, 1977.

6. Grandage, J.: The radiological appearance of stomach gas in the dog. Aust. Vet. J. *50*:529, 1974.

7. Thrall, D. E., and Leininger, J. R.: Irregular intestinal mucosal margination in the dog: normal or abnormal? J. Small Anim. Pract. *17*:305, 1976.

8. O'Brien, T. R., Morgan, J. P., and Lebel, J. L.: Pseudoulcers in the duodenum of the dog. J.A.V.M.A. *155*:713, 1969.

Chapter 8

ENDOSCOPIC EXAMINATIONS

Part I. Endoscopes

JERRY H. JOHNSON

Instrumentation should be used as an aid to diagnosis—a part of but never a substitute for logical diagnostic effort. The mystique of instrumentation should be replaced by a sound knowledge of its strengths and limitations. In order to be responsible professionally, the veterinarian must gain expertise in proper use of endoscopes and in interpretation of findings. Such expertise should be gained under the instruction of an experienced endoscopist. When both skill and confidence have been acquired, the clinical patient may be examined.

Many of the indications for gastrointestinal endoscopy in veterinary practice are found at the orifices of the tract. For this reason, pharyngoscopy, proctoscopy, and distal colonoscopy are done more frequently in veterinary practice than are esophagoscopy, gastroscopy, and duodenoscopy.

Rigid endoscopes have been available to the medical profession for many years but the development of flexible, long-shaft fiberoptic endoscopes allows visual examinations of areas that previously could not be examined. Endoscopy is becoming a viable, even routine, alternative to exploratory laparotomy for visualization and biopsy of the stomach and colon. More uses of flexible fiberoptic endoscopes will probably emerge in future years as instrument technology improves further. Photographic equipment that attaches to the endoscope eyepiece has helped to develop uniform nomenclature by enabling endoscopists to compare the pathologic processes observed and by providing a definite advantage in teaching.

Selection of the Endoscope. For the veterinarian, selection of the endoscope depends primarily on the types of examinations to be performed in the practice. Versatility of application is an important consideration. The skills that the veterinarian wishes to acquire should be another guide in selecting the most useful instrument. Sophisticated endoscopes are of little value if the veterinarian does not be-

come proficient in their use; instruments of limited utility or of poor quality may prevent the most proficient endoscopist from making the correct diagnosis. Finally, purchase cost and maintenance costs must be evaluated in the light of probable frequency of usage. If endoscopy is to be partly subsidized by other practice activities, as many surgical procedures are, it is possible to justify obtaining one or more endoscopes of a quality that would not be justified on an economic basis alone.

Most of the endoscopes used in veterinary practice are designed for use in humans. Adult or pediatric models are selected, depending on the size of the animal patient.

There are many types of endoscopes, but each usually has four characteristics: hollow or solid, rigid or flexible, proximally or distally lighted, and "hot" or "cold" light. Some rigid endoscopes, both hollow and solid, have the light bulb in the distal tip of the instrument. These instruments are usually battery-powered and portable. Light is lost through the optics in these instruments but the optics have been improved in recent years. Rigid endoscopes may also be equipped with a "cold" fiberoptic light source, with illumination being delivered through a bundle of flexible glass fibers from the power source to the endoscope. This lighting system does not produce heat as does the instrument with the light bulb on the distal tip, but it has a disadvantage common to all fiberoptic systems in that a nearby electrical outlet is necessary. The endoscope can be moved only the length of the "umbilical cord" from the power source.

Endoscopes are available in varying lengths (50 to 187 cm) and diameters (3.7 to 15.8 mm). The viewing window may be anterior or lateral. Of the solid rigid scopes, the type with a forward-viewing right angle head is used most frequently in examining the pharynx and larynx of the horse. A forward-viewing flexible scope is more useful for visualization of the digestive tract of the dog, although it can also be used for pharyngoscopy of the horse and for esophagoscopy and bronchoscopy in any species. Rigid hollow endoscopes of 3.5 mm and larger diameter, and of several lengths may be selected. The size of animal dictates the size of instrument needed; therefore, pediatric models are used for cats and small dogs.

Rigid, battery-powered solid endoscopes are the most economical, but their use is largely limited to examination of the pharyngeal and laryngeal area of the horse. Rigid fiberoptic endoscopes have an advantage over the battery-powered instrument in that the light intensity is greater.

Flexible fiberoptic endoscopy is possible in virtually all patients. The instruments are fully flexible and possess distal tip manipulation whereby the distal 5 to 6 cm of the endoscope can be deviated by remote control. Instruments of advanced design allow either a four-way controlled angling to 120° in two planes at right angles, or polydirectional control up to 200°. A controlled biopsy taken under direct vision is possible as a result of the controlled angulation of flexible biopsy forceps. Also, brush cytology under direct vision is possible and is much preferred to gastric lavage. Aspiration controlled by a hand-operated valve is available on all modern instruments that offer biopsy capability. The biopsy channel doubles as an aspiration channel. Catheters and other devices of suitable diameter and construction may be passed down the biopsy channel. Air insufflation by an electric pump controlled by a hand- or foot-operated valve is helpful in maintaining a clear field of view and in distending a hollow viscus such as an equine uterus or canine stomach. Distal lens washing "in situ" is also possible in the modern endoscope either by using a hand- or power-operated water spray or by injecting water down the lens-washing channel with a syringe.

An insulated electrosurgery probe may be passed down the biopsy channel to snare and excise pedunculated masses or to cauterize a biopsy site, and thus spare the patient a major surgical procedure.

Failure of fiberoptic illumination is quite infrequent compared to that of incandescent distal illumination. The lamp in the fiberoptic scope can be changed without removal of the endoscope from the patient. Some fiberoptic light sources have a built-in alternate bulb that can be used at the flip of a switch. Also, since heat is not a problem in fiberoptic illumination, quartz halogen and xenon arc lamps can be employed for increased light intensity.

Photography through the fiberoptic endoscope is done with a single lens reflex camera using automatic exposure control or through-the-lens metering. Whole or half frame 35-mm color photographs can be made to document the lesion. Distal cameras (intragastric cameras) producing 5- or 6-mm color pictures are also available. Camera adapters and light sources are available for motion photography and for closed-circuit color television viewing.

A second eyepiece (teaching head) is available for some endoscopes, allowing two persons to examine the patient at once. Such an attachment is valuable for instructional purposes.

In selecting an endoscope, one should not overlook used equipment, which is often available at reduced cost. The buyer should check for excessive wear or damage before purchase. Obviously, new instruments should also be checked in the same manner and should be free of defects, although quality control is generally quite good. Rigid solid scopes should be checked to ensure that they have not been bent and that the viewing window glass and eyepiece glass have not been scratched. The rheostat in the battery-powered source should move smoothly. Few things are more discouraging than to position a rigid endoscope correctly in a nervous horse, only to have the procedure fail because the rheostat is inoperable owing to corrosion.

A fiberoptic endoscope is more complex and requires checking more systems. The power supply with some instruments contains a water and air pump that flushes the viewing window; it should be functional.

The polyvinyl covering over the distal end of the instrument should be checked carefully for holes or roughened areas or cracks that might leak. Fluid leakage in the instrument could result in considerable expense, such as replacement of a fiber bundle. By looking through the eyepiece at a nearby light source, one can estimate the number of black dots that are seen. These dots indicate broken fibers that transmit a small amount of light or no light within the image-transmission bundle. If black dots are excessive in number, the image may not be clear enough for proper endoscopic viewing. Connect the instrument to the power supply and check the light transmission bundle for intensity of light. Some endoscopes have two transmission bundles; both should be checked. Check the eyepiece for scratches and for fluid condensation on the inside of both the eyepiece and distal-tip viewing window.

Care and Maintenance. Care and maintenance of equipment are vital to the conduct of an efficient endoscopic procedure. Misuse, whether from ignorance or neglect, will soon result in damage to the endoscopic equipment, requiring costly repairs or replacement. Careful maintenance and knowledge of inherent limitations will prolong the life of the equipment.

Rigid endoscopes, whether hollow or solid, are not as fragile as flexible instruments, but care should be taken in handling and storage of these instruments. The battery-operated instruments frequently have electrical short circuits resulting from multiple connections between the battery box and the light bulb on the tip. Therefore, care should be taken to keep these connections clean and protected. A fiberoptic rigid endoscope has a flexible cord that is usually permanently attached to the instrument. This component should be handled gently and not bent acutely because bending could damage the light-transmitting fiber bundle.

Cleaning these rigid instruments is best done with mild soap, taking care not to submerge the proximal tip. Sterilization is limited to ethylene oxide treatment, because the glass and synthetic materials used in construction of the instrument are not tolerant of such high temperatures as in autoclaving. Rigid hollow endoscopes should be cleaned thoroughly on all surfaces after use, rinsed free of cleansing agents, and set in a vertical position to drain and dry. The light carrier should be replaced after the drying process is complete.

Flexible fiberoptic endoscopes should be handled carefully since these instruments are fragile. When picking up the instrument, take hold at each end. If the instrument is held only by the proximal end, the distal tip should not contact anything that would damage the tip nor should one allow it to swing violently. This motion could damage the head or the flexible glass fibers. Do not demonstrate the flexibility by tying the instrument into a knot as this practice causes undue stress to the fiber bundles. In general, do not form a circle of less than 8-cm radius when bending the endoscope.

Fiber bundles should be used at 20°C, even though it may require extra effort to warm the instrument, particularly in large animal practice. Fibers subjected to extreme cold, as in a veterinarian's vehicle, are more brittle and may fracture. Warming the instrument before use should be done carefully because continued submersion of the proximal end in warm fluid may cause leakage into the instrument with resultant corrosion.

The protective polyvinyl chloride sheath of the endoscope has several important functions. This covering forms a smooth outer coat that reduces friction on tissues and encloses the flexible metal mesh that sheaths the bending tube containing the fiber bundles, channels, and cables. The outer coat also forms a watertight and hermetically sealed case preserving a greater than atmospheric pressure within the endoscope shaft. Even a small hole into this outer sheath will allow water to seep into the tube. If water enters a fiber bundle, the bundle ceases to function normally.

The endoscope should be cleaned immediately after an examination so that fluids will not dry on or in the endoscope. The biopsy channel, suction, and water flush should be cleaned thoroughly. The outer coating of the flexible shaft should be washed with a suitable antiseptic solution such as an organic iodine soap and rinsed with water. Some manufacturers suggest that 30 to 70% alcohol be wiped over the flexible shaft after rinsing. Also, the proximal end and eyepieces could be wiped with alcohol. It is best to check the manual of the specific endoscope for the proper cleaning solutions and technique.

Sterilization of fiberoptic endoscopes can be accomplished with gas (ethylene oxide) sterilization. Steam sterilization (autoclaving) will destroy the instrument. Cold sterilization using a 0.1% solution of benzalkonium chloride to swab the outer sheath twice, rinsing with sterile water, and flushing the biopsy channel with 10 ml of the benzalkonium chloride twice followed by a sterile water rinse is as effective as gas sterilization and is much less time consuming.[1]

Part II. Pharyngoscopy

JERRY H. JOHNSON

Pharyngoscopy is done to differentiate naso-pharyngeal disease from tracheobronchial problems. Nasal discharge is a prime indication for pharyngoscopy in the horse, while gastrointestinal-related indications are dysphagia and nasal expectoration of food. Choke must be ruled out in the latter instance in all species. Primary pharyngeal problems affecting gastrointestinal function are rare in the horse, but are common in cattle, dogs, and cats, in which infections and foreign bodies predominate.

The pharynx of the horse and pig cannot be examined under direct vision through the mouth. While a surgical approach through the cricothyroidean space will allow partial direct examination in the horse, endoscopy has eliminated the need for this surgery as a diagnostic procedure. Pharyngoscopy is far less traumatic and eliminates in most cases the need for anesthesia and postoperative care.

Instrumentation. The endoscopic equipment should be assembled and checked to make certain that it is operable before approaching the patient. The rigid endoscope (V-902-A) should be warmed to prevent fogging after passage by placing the tip in warm water, blowing on the viewing window, or briskly rubbing it with a gauze sponge. A surfactant solution (Nolvasan) should be applied to the viewing window immediately before passage.

A flexible fiberoptic endoscope (see sources of instruments, p. 107) should be used at room temperature, to prevent damage to the fiber bundle. All systems should be checked before passage, including a look through the eyepiece to check for cleanliness of the optics.

Radiographic Studies. Pharyngoscopy in horses often precedes radiography because of economic considerations and the predominance of soft-tissue lesions. Radiography is utilized more commonly in the workup of pharyngeal disease of dogs and cats.

Preparation and Restraint of the Patient. Restraint for pharyngoscopy in a quiet, well-mannered horse may be as little as a firm hold on the halter. Restraint and limited movement are essential when using a rigid endoscope, to prevent damage to the

nasal turbinates. The preferred place is a quiet stall with subdued lighting, with two assistants plus the examiner present. A twitch is used in all cases unless the horse struggles against the twitch. In those cases, a chain lead shank is passed under the upper or lower lip and may work just as well. If the examination is to be made via the right nostril, the twitch should be applied by the assistant positioned on the left side of the horse. The twitch handle should be rotated clockwise to prevent excessive distortion of the nostrils. A second assistant positioned on the right side of the horse puts the left shoulder under the mandible with the left hand over the bridge of the horse's nose. The right hand is on the halter. If stocks are available, they may be used to prevent lateral movement of the horse. All assistants should be instructed in their duties and about the type of examination that is to take place before the horse is twitched. Once the twitch is applied, noise and rapid movement should be kept to a minimum so that the horse does not try to strike and/or rear. The twitch should be left on no longer than needed. When using a flexible endoscope, a twitch may be needed to pass the instrument, but it may be removed after passage in a cooperative horse.[2,3,4]

In horses that have been handled very little, sedation in the form of a phenothiazine tranquilizer and/or a small dose of xylazine (Rompun) may be needed. Sedation may inhibit laryngeal movement, and the examiner should be aware of that problem. If the horse violently objects to the nose twitch even with a sedative, and if, in the veterinarian's opinion, there is insufficient air passage through both nostrils, a tracheostomy should be considered.

If it is determined that the horse is fractious when handled or examined about the nose, the twitch may be applied to the lower lip or an assistant can twist an ear. A stomach tube coated with an anesthetic jelly passed into the nostril several times will anesthetize the mucosa and will usually allow endoscopy without additional restraint or sedation.

If the horse cannot be controlled by proper sedation or restraint, general anesthesia may be necessary. An endotracheal tube should be available before the anesthetic is administered, in case of respiratory difficulty.

Technique and Normal Findings. Depth of passage can be measured by placing the instrument lateral to the horse's head and parallel to the intended course. Either nostril may be used for endoscopy. With the horse restrained and assuming the right nostril is to be used, the endoscope is cradled in the left hand, between the thumb and index finger, as a writer holds a pen. The external nare is flared and the tip of the endoscope is inserted into the ventral meatus. As soon as the endoscope has been introduced 8 to 10 cm past the nostril, the left hand is used to hold the endoscope against the septum in case the horse shakes its head. If the veterinarian holds the endoscope with the left hand, the instrument moves with the horse's head and minimizes damage to the turbinates. Should the tip of the endoscope strike a firm obstruction, most probably the ethmoid turbinate, the instrument should be withdrawn slightly, the distal tip directed ventrally, and the instrument advanced gently. The same technique applies to the flexible scope but instead of redirection, the distal tip can be deviated ventrally using the control knob.

The pharynx of the horse is somewhat funnel shaped, the larger anterior part joining the mouth and nasal cavity, while the small end is continued by the esophagus. The pharynx of the horse has several openings: posterior nares, pharyngeal orifices of the guttural pouches, the oral cavity, larynx, and esophagus.

Pathologic Findings. Infectious and inflammatory changes in the pharynx should not be confused with normalcy. The age of the horse and the history are essential to distinguish a normal from a pathologic pharynx. In the young horse the submucosal tissue contains numerous glands. The lymph follicles form a chain dorsally between the eustachian openings and are referred to as the pharyngeal tonsil. If this area has a cobblestone appearance, a follicular pharyngitis may be present. Any exudate in this area should be considered to be pathologic.

The pharyngeal recess, which is the most dorsal aspect, may appear to be an ulcerated area to the untrained eye. Pathologic changes include an exudate at the recess, swelling and inflammation, and polyps that are composed of swollen lymphoid nodules.

Primary tumors, although rare in this area, may be observed as causing a partial blockage.

Complications. The most frequent complication of pharyngoscopy in the horse is epistaxis. This generally subsides without treatment after the horse has succeeded in blowing blood all over the veterinarian and the assistants. Other complications depend on the horse and the experience of the assistants. The objective of pharyngoscopy is to get a clear view of the pharynx without injury to the patient, the veterinarian, the assistants, or the equipment. An improperly restrained horse can shake its head vigorously enough to dislodge the endoscope from the nostril, resulting in injury to the turbinates, the nostril, or the endoscope.

Part III. Esophagoscopy

JOAN A. O'BRIEN

Endoscopic examination of the esophagus is indicated whenever there is evidence of esophageal disease.[5] This evidence may be historic; i.e., the owner observes the patient swallow an object, or it may be based on signs of esophageal disease, e.g., dysphagia or regurgitation, or on a radiographic finding.

Dysphagia is a cardinal sign of many diseases of the esophagus. It may vary from mild, repeated attempts to swallow while eating or drinking to severe straining and gagging with reluctance to eat. The clinician should attempt to evaluate the owner's report of dysphagia by watching the animal eat and drink. It is sometimes possible to observe whether the dysphagia is pharyngeal or esophageal in origin, or both. The consistency of the food should be varied so that it can be noted whether the animal has difficulty swallowing liquids, solids, or all forms of food and water.

Regurgitation is very common in esophageal disease. It is important to distinguish regurgitation from vomiting, although the later may rarely occur in esophageal disease. The time after eating, and the volume, character, and consistency of regurgitated material should be noted. Immediate regurgitation is more common with cricopharyngeal achalasia and strictures, whereas it may be more delayed in functional disorders. The character may vary from undigested food to mucus mixed with food or it may be mucus alone. An alkaline pH of regurgitated mucus is fairly reliable evidence of an esophageal source. The regurgitation of "sausage"-shaped undigested food is evidence of esophageal disease but is not diagnostic of any single entity. Regurgitation in association with an overfilled, dilated esophagus is quite passive. If the lesion is localized and especially if it is near the pharynx, the animal may exhibit more evidence of distress.

Hematemesis is a rarer sign of esophageal disease but should be investigated endoscopically since it can signal esophagitis, which can be malignant, inflammatory, or mechanical in origin. It is important to rule out oral, pharyngeal, gastric, or pulmonary sources of blood. Hematemesis in esophageal disease is rarely frank hemorrhage but more often blood-streaked or pink-stained mucus.

Instrumentation. A flexible fiberoptic endoscope designed as a gastroduodenoscope (see sources of instruments, p. 107) for use in humans has been adapted for esophagoscopy in veterinary medicine. The great length of both the pediatric and adult gastroduodenoscopes offers versatility for patients of differing sizes and permits examination of distal parts of the upper gastrointestinal tract in small animals. All endoscopes of this type permit excellent visualization, are flexible, and have been designed to obtain small punch and brush biopsies as well as washings for culture and cytology.[6] They are primarily diagnostic instruments and are rarely used to retrieve foreign bodies or to dilate strictures.

The most useful endoscope for both diagnostic and therapeutic procedures in small animals is the standard, rigid, distally lighted hollow esophagoscope. These instruments are available with either bulbs or rigid fiberoptic light carriers. The latter, while more expensive, are cooler, more reliable, and provide better illumination. It is necessary to have several sizes of the rigid esophagoscopes in order to examine animals of differing sizes. It is possible to use the same instruments for bronchoscopy and esophagoscopy. For very large dogs a minimum length of 75 to 80 cm is suggested. In addition to the esophagoscopes, lumen finders (soft probes to locate the lumen of the esophagus) and aspirators of compatible diameters and lengths are needed. For removal of foreign bodies, at least one alligator grasping forceps long enough for use through each esophagoscope is required. Many other kinds of forceps are available for more specialized work. Several types and sizes of bougies are useful for dilatation of esophageal strictures.

Esophagrams. Radiographic examination of the normal esophagus has been described previously. It is important to emphasize that normal survey thoracic or cervical films do not rule out esophageal disease. Swallowing-function esophagrams in the awake animal are necessary to evaluate certain types of esophageal disease. Evaluation of esophageal function may involve swallowing of liquid, paste, or food mixed with contrast material. In the presence of stricture, the passage of a No. 5 French soft catheter to the distal esophagus permits filling the esophagus in a retrograde fashion, in order to evaluate the diameter of the lumen along the entire length of the esophagus.

Esophagrams should be performed prior to esophagoscopy in an effort to delineate the type and site of esophageal disorder, ideally at least 24 hours prior to esophagoscopy so that the contrast material will not interfere with endoscopic visualization. If this is not possible, saline lavage may be utilized to wash out the contrast medium. A normal esophagram does not negate the necessity for esophagoscopy in the face of definite signs of esophageal disease. Radiographic abnormalities characteristic of specific disease states are discussed in Chapter 21.

Preparation and Restraint of the Patient. In the dog, cat, foal, and calf, where general anesthesia is required, fasting for 12 hours is recommended. Preanesthetic and general anesthesia are utilized and an endotracheal tube is placed and tied to the mandible. The endotracheal tube is particularly important in preventing collapse of the cervical trachea from the pressure of a rigid esophagoscope.[7] In most horses and cattle, sedation and restraint with a twitch will permit passage of the flexible fiberoptic esophagoscope to the area of the cricopharyngeal sphincter, where swallowing will be stimulated. The esophagoscope can then be advanced gently to examine the lumen to the full length of the instrument.

Technique and Normal Findings. Esophagoscopy is performed in the small animal under general anesthesia; sedation and restraint are used in the horse and cow. The small animal is placed in left lateral recumbency with the head extended, while the large animal may be examined standing or in the left lateral position. A lubricated esophagoscope is directed through the mouth toward the recess bounded by the right lateral surface of the larynx and the wall of the pharynx. In the mature horse and cow the endoscope is passed nasally. As the mucosa of the right arytenoid cartilage comes into view, the instrument is directed dorsally into the esophagus. In an anesthetized animal there is generally very little resistance to the passage of an esophagoscope. If resistance occurs at any point, a lumen finder should be inserted through the esophagoscope and gently manipulated until the lumen of the esophagus becomes visible.

The cervical part of the esophagus is normally collapsed and will appear as pliant longitudinal folds which part readily as the esophagoscope is inserted. The normal esophageal mucosa is clear, glistening, and pink to pink-gray. The folds are more prominent in the horse and cow than in the dog and cat. In the large animal it is usually only possible to examine the cranial half of the cervical esophagus owing to the limitations of instrument length. The lumen of the thoracic part of the esophagus can be seen to expand with inspiration and collapse with expiration, because of changes in intrapleural pressure. If the animal's neck is not fully extended, there may be some resistance to the passage of the esophagoscope at the thoracic inlet. At the base of the heart, there is an area normally narrowed by the impingement of the great vessels. This point can be overcome by elevating the bevel of the esophagoscope dorsally and advancing it when the lumen is seen. Pulsations of the heart and aorta are transmitted through the esophageal wall at this point. At the gastroesophageal junction, the esophagus normally forms a small closed rosette. There is often a rush of fluid into the esophagus as the stomach is entered. The gastric mucosa is bright red and is sharply demarcated from the pale esophageal mucosa. Normally a small amount of mucous secretion is present in the esophagus and must be aspirated as examination of the mucosa is performed.

Pathologic lesions of the esophagus are described in Chapter 21.

Complications. Esophagoscopy when performed gently by an experienced endoscopist with proper instrumentation and patient control results in few complications.

The most dreaded complication is perforation of the esophagus. It is important to realize that perforation may occur and not be immediately recognized by the endoscopist. In one study in people, perforation was recognized immediately in only half of the cases. Perforation can occur through the hypopharynx, cervical or thoracic esophagus. Hypopharyngeal perforations with infection usually become localized by fascial planes and result in a retropharyngeal abscess. Cervical perforations may become localized or can dissect along fascial spaces to the mediastinum to cause mediastinitis. Most perforations of the thoracic esophagus lead to mediastinitis.

Treatment of localized infection after perforation is regional surgical drainage and broad-spectrum antibiotic, since the infection is usually due to the mixed aerobic and anaerobic flora of the pharyngeal region. Treatment for mediastinitis due to esophageal perforation is thoracotomy and drainage. Medical therapy alone has not been effective.

Signs of perforation are subcutaneous cervical or mediastinal emphysema, usually rapid in onset; fever, tachycardia, dysphagia, and occasionally hydropneumothorax and pyothorax. Chest and lateral neck films should be taken if there is any suspicion of perforation. A Gastrografin swallow may be helpful in delineating the site if given early after perforation.

Impaction of the flexible fiberoptic scope which has turned on itself has been reported as a rare occurrence in people, but has not been reported in veterinary medicine.

Part IV. Gastroscopy

GERALD F. JOHNSON

Indications for gastroscopy include signs referable to gastric disease such as vomiting, hematemesis, and melena. Valuable information regarding the nature of the lesion is obtained in differentiating types of inflammation and mucosal defects, and in detecting and differentiating neoplasms. Occasionally an etiologic agent such as occurs in mycotic gastritis can be discerned. Gastroscopy is useful in evaluating the extent of disease, both inflammatory and neoplastic, thus permitting the clinician to make better judgments regarding future management, including the need for surgical intervention.

Another indication for gastroscopy is to monitor therapy. The response to medical treatment and the healing of lesions can be followed, as can the progress of surgically reconstructed stomachs.

In animals, the restraint involved limits the procedure more than the gastroscopy procedure itself. Gastroscopy is very safe and has only one absolute contraindication, cardiopulmonary decompensation. Relative contraindications include a perforated viscus and varying degrees of esophageal obstruction. As in other clinical judgments, the risk involved must be balanced against the anticipated benefits.

Although disease conditions in veterinary medicine for which gastroscopy should be used are still being defined, gastroscopy is no longer a supplementary tool but is being established as a procedure of major clinical value. Gastroscopy has advantages over other methods of studying gastric disease. Compared to radiology, gastroscopy affords visualization and photographic documentation and enables samples to be taken for laboratory analysis. Gastroscopy involves no radiation exposure. Compared to surgery, gastroscopy is noninvasive, and has a lower morbidity and mortality, but it has limited therapeutic capability and biopsy specimens are not as rewarding as those taken surgically. Yet gastroscopy permits excellent scrutinization of both normal and abnormal stomach and often permits the clinician to establish the need for surgery. Gastroscopy can often detect the presence of neoplasia and determine type.

The value of gastroscopy is enhanced greatly when the endoscopist has knowledge of gastric physiology and pathophysiology. One should be familiar with gross gastric pathology and have an understanding of the type, incidence, and species variation of gastric disease. In the same sense, gastroscopy can be used as a tool to enhance one's understanding of physiology and pathophysiology.

Through the use of teaching attachments, still- and cine-photography, and even television, gastroscopy is valuable in training endoscopists as well as teaching students of gastroenterology. The use of gastroscopy as an experimental tool in studying physiology and pathophysiology has also proven to be of value.

Results of gastroscopic procedures should be recorded as are results of other procedures such as radiography, surgery, and laboratory data. This recording assists in the future management of the case and is useful for data retrieval. A form documenting the pertinent patient information and a description of the endoscopic findings along with endoscopic photographs can serve as a permanent record.

Instrumentation. Gastroscopy in small animals is done with a multipurpose endoscope (Fig. 8–1) with several important features (see sources of instruments, p. 107). The flexible portion of the endoscope has a diameter of 6.8 mm and a diameter of 7.2 mm at the distal tip. The controllable distal 6 cm has a bending angle of 150° up and 150° down. It has a two-way, one-plane bending system and a working length of 110 cm with a viewing angle of 65°. This endoscope has a channel that serves the dual purpose of suction channel and biopsy channel. Through this channel, fluid and air can be aspirated to improve visualization, and endoscopic biopsy forceps, biopsy brush, snares, and grasping instruments can be passed (Fig. 8–2). Photographic documentation is obtained using the camera which attaches to the eyepiece. It is easy to use and requires no focusing; the exposure is automatically set at the light source.

This endoscope has proven to be durable and has maintained its excellent optics; over 500 procedures have been performed with no need for major repairs. Details as minute as individually ingested hairs can be well visualized and easily grasped with

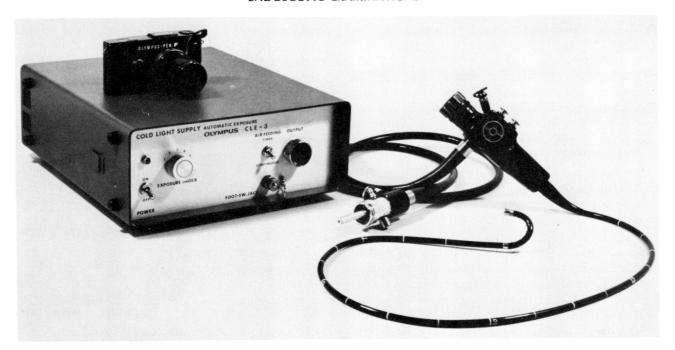

Figure 8–1. The Olympus CLE-3 light source with the Pen-F camera for use with the Olympus endoscopes. The GIF-P pediatric endoscope is to the right of the light source.

the biopsy forceps, yet large areas can be equally well examined.

This endoscope, designed for use in pediatrics, is particularly well suited for endoscopy in small animals because its length of 110 cm makes it desirable

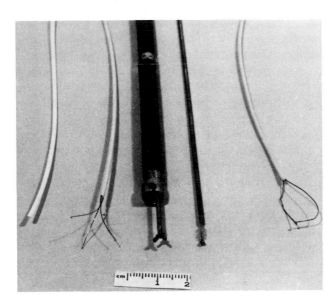

Figure 8–2. Various instruments for use through the endoscope. From left to right: catheter, four-pronged grasping forceps, endoscope tip with biopsy forceps positioned through the biopsy channel, cytology brush, and snare.

for larger breeds of dogs that may have an esophagus as long as 80 cm. Its small diameter, light weight, and increased flexibility make it more practical in examining small dogs and cats than the standard-sized bulkier instruments. Although the angle of vision and photographic capabilities are somewhat restricted by the smaller imaging and light transmitting bundles (compared to the more standard sized endoscopes), the versatility and advantages of this endoscope outweigh the disadvantages encountered in its use. Its two-way, one-plane (up and down) controllable tip, as compared to the four-way controllable tips available with other endoscopes, has not been a major disadvantage. Torque is applied to the flexible portion of the tube to permit visualization to the left or right.

The greatest disadvantage of this smaller diameter endoscope compared to other larger diameter endoscopes is the small size of the biopsy/suction channel, which technically limits the biopsy specimens to 1.5 mm in diameter and 2.0 mm in length. In addition, this size limits the use of instrumentation such as snares and grasping forceps.

Gastrograms. Radiographic examination of the normal stomach has been described earlier. Gastroscopy is used to elucidate radiographic findings further and is indicated when signs are not explained by the absence of radiographic findings.

The limits of radiology should be appreciated. Gastroscopy can add a further dimension to the study of gastric disease.

Gastrograms are not always indicated prior to gastroscopy, as in the case of gastric foreign bodies that are to be removed endoscopically, or prior to repeat gastroscopy used to monitor therapy or follow the course of disease. Gastrograms are not always indicated when gastric lesions are expected to involve mainly the mucosa, as in gastritis associated with mast cell neoplasia or ingested agents such as aspirin. Gastrograms, in general, however, contribute valuable information to gastroscopy whether findings are negative or positive.

Several techniques used to obtain a gastrogram can enhance its value. Fluoroscopy used with changes in patient positioning and spot film exposures increases the accuracy of diagnosis, but its availability is limited. Double contrast gastrograms using air and positive contrast media are valuable in examining the mucosal pattern. Triple contrast with gas introduced into the peritoneum as well as air and positive contrast medium in the stomach aids in detecting increased thickness of the stomach wall and extrinsic lesion. Using four positions (dorsoventral, ventrodorsal, and right and left lateral), different areas of the stomach can be scrutinized. Using a sufficient quantity of contrast medium to fill and distend the stomach is important. When air is used, this can be removed after several exposures and additional positive contrast material added for further study. Exposures should be taken at recommended intervals to evaluate early emptying, how long contrast media is retained, and how completely the stomach empties. Gastroscopy can be performed when contrast medium is out of the stomach.

Preparation and Restraint of the Patient. For gastroscopy in the dog and cat, general anesthesia is usually required although oxymorphone and atropine have been used successfully as the sole agents in dogs. A mouth gag is always used to protect the instrument, and the endotracheal tube is tied to the mandible.

Left lateral recumbency is preferred so that the antrum and pylorus are away from the tabletop and are thus more free to move and less distorted. Using the same patient position with each procedure affords proper orientation and recognition of landmarks.

Technique and Normal Findings. After the instrument is checked for proper working order, the instrument panel is grasped in one hand and the tip gently inserted through the cranial esophageal sphincter with the other. Traversing the cranial esophageal sphincter is done blindly as if passing a stomach tube. Whether one uses the right or left hand on the instrument panel and the opposite hand on the flexible portion depends on the individual preferences of the endoscopist and the type of endoscope being used. A general rule for use in all endoscopy is not to advance the tip unless the lumen is in focus. Following this rule prevents perforation when obstruction, diverticula, mass, or areas of diseased organ walls are encountered. The instrument should not be advanced against resistance.

After the cranial esophageal sphincter has been traversed and the cranial two-thirds of the esophagus has been examined with the forward viewing endoscope, a tunnel view of the distal third of the esophagus is obtained. The slit-like gastroesophageal orifice is generally closed (Plate I, Fig. 1). At the normal gastroesophageal junction, a distinct circumferential margin can be identified where the light-colored esophageal mucosa joins the darker red gastric mucosa (Plate I, Fig. 2). The normal gastric mucosa is pink to bright red in the dog and somewhat lighter in the cat. While maintaining the orifice in the field of vision, the tip is advanced. Because the orifice is usually eccentrically located, deviation of the tip to one side and slightly downward often is necessary. Doing these maneuvers as the endoscope is advanced will permit the tip to enter the gastric lumen. The most common error made at this time is not having the tip centered at the gastroesophageal orifice. If this occurs, the instrument should be retracted, the orifice revisualized, orientation again established, and the maneuvers repeated.

A second common error at this junction is to advance the tip too far, so that the objective contacts the mucosa of the collapsed stomach or the posterior gastric wall and obscures the visual field. Retracting the tip and insufflating air to distend the stomach moderately permit visualization within the gastric lumen. It is important to realize when the tip has entered the gastric lumen. This area is identified by the darker red mucosa compared to the lighter esophageal mucosa and by the presence of rugae. Rugae can be seen to flatten as the stomach is distended. The endoscope tip should be positioned just through the gastroesophageal lumen so that an overview and orientation within the lumen of the stomach are obtained. Most of the body of the stomach can be examined by moving the tip up and down and by using left and right torque in the two-way controllable tip or, in a four-way endo-

Plate I

Plate I

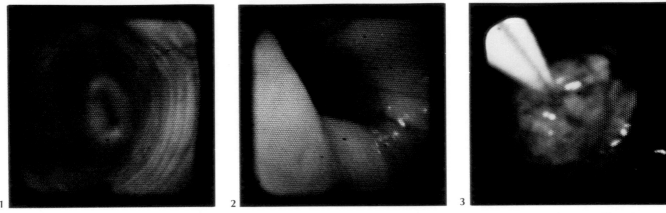

Figure 1. In this tunnel view of the normal feline esophagus, the slit-like esophagogastric junction (A) can be seen. Note the circumferential folds of the distal feline esophagus and normal superficial blood vessels (B). (The letters A and B in the legends are shown in the line drawings that match each color photo. Small black dots are artifacts.)

Figure 2. A closer view of the normal canine esophagogastric junction partially open reveals the light-colored esophageal mucosa (A) in the forefield demarcated from the normal darker red gastric mucosa (B).

Figure 3. The endoscopic biopsy forceps (A) are apparent in the visual field grasping a gastric lymphoma tumor in a dog.

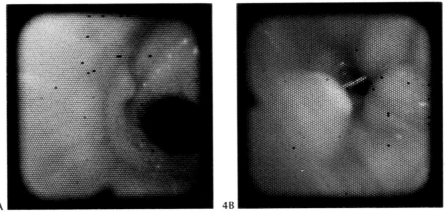

Figure 4. **(A)** A distal view of the pancreatic papilla (A) is obtained in the descending duodenum of a dog. **(B)** A stream of pancreatic juice (A) emanates from the pancreatic duct at its opening on the papilla, (B).

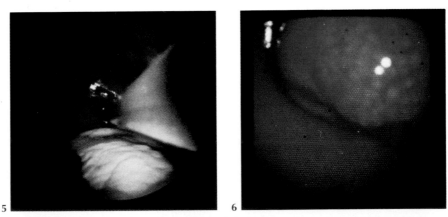

Figure 5. This more distant view obtained during laparoscopy performed through the right side with an operating scope shows the biopsy forceps (A) in the field of vision about to grasp the liver. The duodenal limb of the pancreas (B) can also be seen in the forefield. The diaphragm (C) is seen in the background.

Figure 6. Lymphoma of the ileocolic area was a consideration when this dog's upper gastrointestinal series was interpreted. At colonoscopy the ileum (A) is intussuscepted into the descending colon (B).

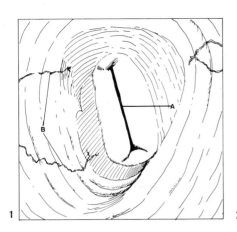

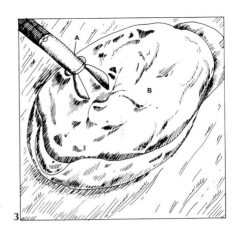

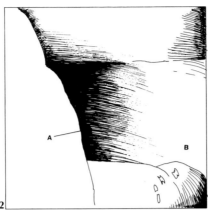

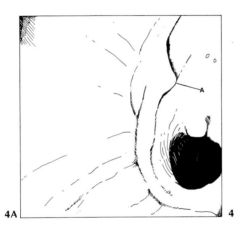

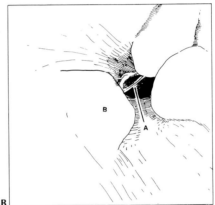

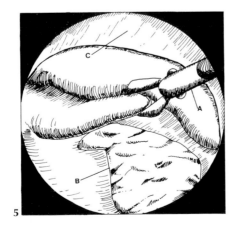

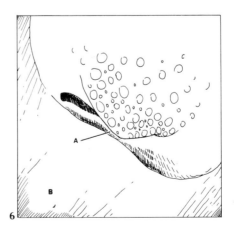

scope, by using the four-way control knob. The instillation of fluid containing defoaming agents or the aspiration of accumulated fluid and secretions through the suction channel provides adequate visualization.

By insufflating or aspirating air, the degree of gastric distention is varied, enabling folds and rugae to be flattened which enhances the detection of lesions. Moving the tip nearer to and farther from lesions and looking at them from different angles provides an appreciation for size, protuberance, and depth. Lesions should be carefully studied. Performing gastroscopy in a darkened room with a quiet comfortable ambience facilitates concentration.

Next it is important to identify a large fold, the incisura, on the lesser curvature as a landmark which separates the body of the stomach from the antrum. The antrum extends distally from this fold. With the animal in left lateral recumbency, the antrum will be directed up or away from the tabletop and somewhat cranially. To visualize the pylorus, the tip of the endoscope must be advanced into the antrum by giving the tip an upward bend and advancing it along the greater curvature (Fig. 8–3A). During distention of the body of the stomach,

the antrum distends very little but is displaced to the right of the abdominal cavity. When this occurs, the incisura and the entrance to the antrum as viewed from the stomach appear as a crescent-shaped orifice, smaller in size than the distended body of the stomach. This makes the antrum difficult to enter, and overdistention causes cardiopulmonary embarrassment.

Because the area along the lesser curvature of the antrum is more difficult to examine and because it is a frequent site for neoplasia as well as a site for other lesions, special care must be taken to visualize it. A second area that is difficult to examine at gastroscopy is the cardiac portion of the stomach. In order to examine this area, the endoscope must be retroflexed or placed in a J-position so that the portion of the endoscope entering through the cardia as well as the surrounding area is seen (Fig. 8–3B).

As the gastroscopist looks through the eyepiece, a notch in the field of vision indicates the upward direction of the distal end. In addition to this, an appreciation of normal anatomic sites relative to the patient's position enables the gastroscopist to maintain orientation with the field of vision and movements of the remote tip. For instance, in left lateral

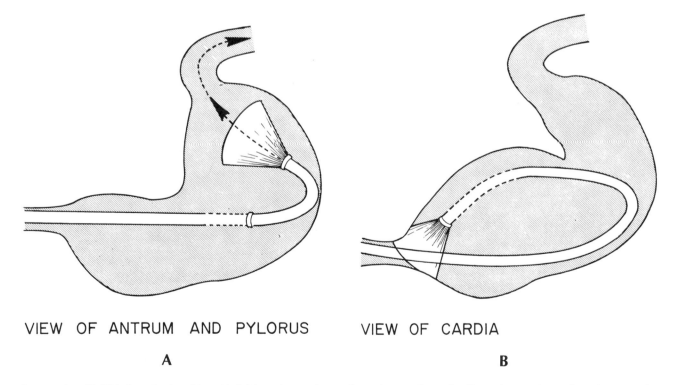

VIEW OF ANTRUM AND PYLORUS   VIEW OF CARDIA

A   B

Figure 8–3. **(A)** With the animal positioned in left lateral recumbency, the endoscope tip can be directed upward away from the supporting surfaces and toward the uppermost pyloric antrum. As the endoscope is advanced in this curved position, it slides along the caudal fundus of the stomach directing the tip into the antrum. **(B)** The tip of the endoscope is shown in a retroflexed position. The endoscopist can visualize the scope traversing the cardia, and is then able to examine that portion of the stomach immediately surrounding the cardia.

recumbency, the gastroscopist will gain a view such that the antrum is superior and the body of the stomach is inferior in position or closest to the tabletop. A mobile foreign body would most likely fall out of the antrum and be found in the body of the stomach, closest to the left or "down" side of the patient. This is also where fluid accumulates. The instrument tip must, therefore, be straight ahead or directed slightly downward to visualize the foreign body lying along the greater curvature.

The primary goal in gastroscopy is to examine the entire luminal surface of the stomach. Once an abnormality is found, care must be taken to ensure that others are not overlooked. The reasons for not examining portions of the stomach should be recorded. Unsuccessful gastroscopy occurs because of faulty equipment, inexperienced endoscopists, poor preparation or restraint, esophageal obstruction, or the presence of foreign material (e.g., ingested hair, cage paper), viscous secretions, excessive blood, and intrinsic and extrinsic deformities.

The time for gastroscopy varies considerably and depends on the location of the lesion, the presence of fluid or foreign material, the use of photography, specimen collection, the number of individuals observing, and the skill of the endoscopist. A thorough gastroscopy can take as little as 10 minutes from insertion of the endoscope to its removal.

An adequate number of biopsy specimens must be taken to establish a diagnosis. Endoscopes having biopsy capabilities are a distinct advantage. With these instruments, the biopsy forceps are passed through the biopsy channel and guided precisely to the biopsy site in the field of vision (Plate I, Fig. 3). Due to the small size of the specimens obtained and because they are taken from the surface, numerous biopsies should be taken from carefully selected sites. For instance, biopsies should be taken from the margin of ulcerating lesions. Unless the mucosal integrity is compromised, obtaining specimens from submucosal lesions is difficult. To obtain specimens for cytologic examination, impression smears can be made from tissue taken with the biopsy forceps or cytology brush. An endoscopically directed pulsating stream of water can also be used to obtain cells for cytology.[8] The success of obtaining a pathologic diagnosis depends on adequate specimen collection in addition to the skill of the pathologist or cytologist. If a tissue diagnosis is necessary and cannot be established endoscopically, full thickness biopsies should be taken surgically.

Pathologic Findings. Gastritis is a diagnosis based on the histologic examination of the stomach tissue. In general, endoscopic impressions of gastritis correlate poorly with biopsy material in humans[9] and in the dog.[10] If, however, obvious mucosal defects such as erosions and active bleeding are seen, a gastroscopic diagnosis of gastritis becomes more reliable. Even then, biopsies should be taken to elucidate the type of gastritis present. With likely etiologies such as aspirin ingestion, a histologic diagnosis may be unnecessary.

Gastroscopy can detect gastritis not detectable with radiography and greatly contribute to an understanding of the pathogenesis, incidence, and management of gastritis in small animals.

Gastroscopy has proved to be beneficial in detecting and managing gastric cancer. It often establishes a histologic diagnosis and aids in determining the extent of disease, thus providing valuable information for the management of the case.[11]

Gastroscopy is valuable in detecting sources of gastric bleeding and providing information as to the nature of the lesion. It is a valuable adjunct in the workup of an animal with melena and/or hematemesis and in animals suspected of having blood loss anemia. It is valuable in detecting the rare peptic ulcer of dogs.[12]

Therapeutic gastroscopy with the aid of biopsy forceps, grasping forceps, and snares is used to extract gastric foreign bodies. Objects such as coins, wires, lead foreign bodies, and malleable foreign bodies such as cloth can often be removed, thus obviating the need for a gastrotomy. This procedure sometimes requires considerable endoscopic skill and patience; at other times, foreign bodies can be removed in as little as 10 minutes.

Complications. Complications are rare when gastroscopy is performed by a capable endoscopist. While perforation of the stomach is a serious complication, it has not occurred during 350 consecutive gastroscopy procedures for evaluation of naturally occurring disease, as performed by four of my colleagues and by me. Impaction of the endoscope in J-shaped position in the esophagus has been reported in human endoscopy, but it is rare.[13]

Hypotension and bradycardia are sometimes seen in association with gaseous distention of the stomach, due to the interference with venous return to the right heart, vagovagal stimulation, and compromise of respiratory muscles. This problem is managed by removing the intragastric air, withdrawing the endoscope, and discontinuing administration of an anesthetic agent.

Part V. Duodenoscopy

GERALD F. JOHNSON

Few indications now exist for duodenoscopy in small animal veterinary medicine. However, it can be useful in elucidation of abnormal radiographic findings, in evaluation of inflammatory disease, and in biopsy of the occasional neoplastic lesion. As endoscopy is more widely practiced and instruments with improved capabilities are developed, it is likely that further indications for endoscopy of the small intestine will be established and a better insight will be gained into the physiology and pathophysiology of this inaccessible area.

Instrumentation. For veterinary duodenoscopy, a versatile endoscope is needed. Features of the controllable tip should include a short bending section with four-way control that can be moved through the acute angle formed by the cranially directed antrum and the caudally directed descending duodenum. For examination of the intestine of animals weighing as little as 3 kg, a very flexible endoscope with a small diameter is needed to pass through the pylorus and into the intestine. Compared to endoscopes designed for duodenoscopy in humans, an increased working length is needed for the larger breeds of dogs. Primarily due to the longer esophagus in these animals, the distance from the incisor teeth to the pylorus is greater than the corresponding distance in humans.

The endoscope described under Gastroscopy (Part IV) is suitable for duodenoscopy in dogs and cats. Although its features of forward viewing, small diameter, flexibility, and a tip that can be moved through angles of 300° are advantageous, its two-way, one-plane bending and long-bending section of 6 cm are less desirable. However, newer instruments have shorter bending sections and four-way tip control among other advantages. A working length of 110 cm is long enough to reach the duodenum of most dogs.

Radiographic Studies. Survey films and an upper gastrointestinal tract study may be done prior to duodenoscopy. Negative findings on radiography do not preclude duodenoscopy. Rather, they can be used by the veterinarian as part of the data base on which to plan the procedure.

Technique. Greater expertise is required to pass the tip of the endoscope into the duodenum of the dog and cat than into the stomach because of the position of the pylorus and because the pylorus does not open as readily as the esophagogastric junction. Animals are prepared, restrained, and positioned in the same manner as for gastroscopy. The stomach should be examined after duodenoscopy since distention and manipulation within the stomach seem to increase the tone of the pyloric sphincter, thus making insertion of the endoscope into the duodenum more difficult.

With the tip of the endoscope positioned in the antrum and with minimal manipulation and distention, the pylorus is kept in the center of the visual field as it is approached. Sometimes the pylorus is open and the tip is advanced directly through it. Usually the pylorus is closed and the tip is advanced up to the orifice. The field of vision is obscured by a red hue as the mucosa contacts the objective and, with continued gentle advancement, the tip may pass through. If three to five attempts are unsuccessful, glucagon is given intravenously at 0.05 mg/kg body weight (not to exceed a total dose of 1 mg). Because glucagon has a hypotonic effect on the gastrointestinal tract, the pylorus relaxes and the passage of the tip is facilitated. When the pyloric sphincter is passed, the control knob should be free to move or be gently directed downward as the tip is advanced into the descending duodenum. A moderate amount of air is then insufflated to reestablish the field of vision and to provide spatial orientation.

In attempting to advance the tip of the endoscope through the pylorus, a redundancy may be created in the flexible portion of the tube proximal to the tip, along the greater curvature. Withdrawing the endoscope to eliminate the redundancy and to bring the flexible tube closer to the lesser curvature may bring the controllable tip into better alignment with the pylorus and facilitate its entry into the duodenum. When the pyloric sphincter is passed, the tip of the endoscope often advances quickly to the flexure joining the descending and ascending duodenum. It may be retracted slightly for orientation. Only the descending duodenum is usually examined, for the following reasons:

1. The flexure joining the descending and ascending duodenum is difficult to negotiate.

2. The length of the scope limits further insertion in larger animals.

3. There are fewer indications for examining the ascending duodenum once the descending duodenum is examined.

The descending duodenum is best examined while the tip is being retracted. Good visualization with tunnel-like views can be obtained, and procedures such as duodenal aspirations and biopsies should be performed at this point.

When duodenoscopy is completed, excessive air is removed and the endoscope is withdrawn, bringing the tip back into the gastric lumen. Endoscopy is terminated at this point or the stomach and esophagus can be examined as the instrument is removed.

Seven cats and 40 dogs have undergone duodenoscopy in my practice.* With administration of glucagon and increased expertise in performing the procedure, the success rate has increased to approximately 70%. Simply put, the greatest reason for failure to complete the procedure is the inability to advance the tip of the endoscope through the pylorus. Other reasons are poor patient preparation, overdistention of the stomach, neoplastic obstruction of the pylorus, and, in larger dogs, the fact that the distance from the oral cavity to the pylorus is greater than the working length of the endoscope.

Normal Findings. The normal duodenal mucosa appears velvety or shaggy due to the presence of villi that can be individually discerned when observed at close range through the endoscope. As the tip of the endoscope is retracted caudally to cranially through the canine duodenum, two papillae can be identified, although this varies.[14] The first to come into view, and the easier to identify, is the more distally located pancreatic papilla, which is white compared to the reddish pink of the surrounding mucosa. This papilla appears round to oval (1.5 to 2 mm in diameter) and can be observed to change

in shape from flat to conical. Rarely a pancreatic papilla can be observed to actively discharge secretion (Plate 1, Fig. 4A). With further withdrawal of the endoscope, the biliary papilla comes into view (Plate 1, Fig. 4B).

In the cat, only one papilla exists for the pancreatic and biliary ducts. This papilla and the biliary papilla in the dog are more difficult to identify because of their location just a short distance past the pyloric sphincter, near the convex curve formed by the junction of the antrum and the descending duodenum. This papilla resembles the pancreatic papilla but its more cranial position and the fact that bile can sometimes be seen coming from it aid in identifying it.

Pathologic Findings. Duodenoscopy coupled with duodenal aspiration via an endoscopically placed catheter has been used to diagnose giardiasis in several dogs when other methods of diagnosis failed. *Stronglyloides stercoralis* larvae have been aspirated while performing duodenoscopy on a dog to evaluate a suspected inflammatory enteropathy. Though numerous fecal flotations and direct smears were negative for *S. stercoralis* larvae previously, it is likely that examination of a fecal sediment preparation would have yielded a diagnosis as well.

A duodenal ulcer not detected on barium radiography has been detected endoscopically.[15] Diffuse involvement of intestinal mucosa with lymphosarcoma has also been diagnosed in endoscopic biopsies in a cat. Because of the difficulty in passing blind mucosal capsules into the intestine of animals to evaluate diffuse enteropathies, duodenoscopy may offer a valuable alternative especially if improved biopsy capabilities provide more adequate mucosal sampling that can be better oriented for histologic examination.

Complications. Complications of duodenoscopy have included cyanosis, poor peripheral perfusion, and alterations in heart rate of several animals, particularly smaller animals. These were presumably due to (1) vagovagal reflexes associated with distention of the intestine and stretching of the mesentery and its vessels, despite atropine premedication or (2) poor venous return to the right heart. Other complications may occur as duodenoscopy is more widely used in veterinary medicine.

---

*Animal Medical Center, 510 E. 62nd Street, New York, NY 10021.

Part VI. Endoscopic Cannulation of Duodenal Papillae

GERALD F. JOHNSON

In veterinary medicine, cannulation of the pancreatic ducts would be of value since few direct methods exist for evaluating pancreatic diseases—other than laparoscopy[16] and laparotomy. Endoscopic cannulation of the pancreatic duct may provide information regarding pancreatic function, inflammation, and neoplasia.

Cannulation of the biliary and pancreatic ducts is performed under direct vision by passing a cannula through a specially designed endoscope. Radiographic contrast media is then injected to facilitate cholangiography or pancreatography studies. This procedure was first performed on humans in 1968[17] and on the dog in 1974.[18] Its practical use in human medicine was reported by Japanese workers[19,20,21] and later by others in the United States and Europe. Recent reviews are available[22,23] and its value has been emphasized.[24] Endoscopic techniques have also been employed for the peroral removal of choleliths[25] and recently, peroral cholangiopancreatoscopy has been performed providing a view of the major bile ducts and pancreatic ducts.[26] Cannulation has also been used to evaluate organ function and to obtain specimens for cytology.

Though indications for endoscopic cannulation of the biliary and pancreatic ducts are few and its cost-benefit ratio presently prohibitive, the procedure may be at the ready disposal of veterinarians as veterinary medicine becomes more sophisticated and as technology improves. Like so many other techniques, its value will be appreciated as indications are defined and experience is gained.

Instrumentation. The most popular endoscope used in human endoscopic cholangiopancreatography (ECP) is a side-viewing endoscope, which is suitable for dogs weighing 15 to 30 kg (see sources of instruments, p. 107). The catheter, serving as a cannula, is passed through a channel and exits at a right angle to the long axis of the endoscope in the field of vision. This angle can be varied by a lever at the control panel. Under endoscopic guidance, the papilla is identified and the cannula inserted into the duct.

Preparation and Restraint of the Patient. Preparation, premedication, and position of the dog are the same as for gastroscopy and duodenoscopy.

Technique and Normal Findings. The side-viewing instrument is manipulated through the stomach and into the duodenum. The duodenal papillae are located on the medial aspect of the duodenal wall a few centimeters distal to the pylorus. In the dog, two separate papillae usually exist.[27] Because the biliary papilla is close to the pylorus and because the duct and its papillae are directed caudad, this duct is difficult to cannulate. The pancreatic papilla is located 1 to 2 cm more caudad than the biliary papilla and its duct enters nearly perpendicular to the gut lumen, making it easier to cannulate than the biliary duct. To prevent duodenal motility during cannulation, glucagon or other hypotonic agents can be administered intravenously or intramuscularly. Hypaque 50% or another suitable water-soluble radiographic contrast substance is injected by hand when the duct is cannulated. Approximately 35 ml is injected into the biliary system and 2 to 5 ml into the pancreatic duct system. Fluoroscopy with image intensification is needed to determine filling of the duct systems. The normal canine pancreatic duct system empties within minutes of removal of the cannula. If the pancreatic duct is injected with excessive pressure on the plunger, individual acini can be uniformly seen throughout the gland and an acinargraph is obtained. In one dog this was associated with a dramatic rise in pancreatic enzymes though no overt signs of pancreatitis and no loss of appetite were observed after the study.

The disadvantages of endoscopic cannulation of the papillae are that the equipment is expensive and the procedure requires considerable endoscopic skill and training. In addition, fewer indications exist in veterinary medicine since cholelithiasis, which has been a major incentive for developing the technique in humans, seldom occurs in animals, and endoscopes designed for ECP in people can be adapted to only a limited size of animal. For giant breeds of dogs, they are too short, and miniaturization of the instruments will be necessary for smaller breeds and species, but this is not economically feasible at present.

The major advantages of ECP are that the procedure is noninvasive, and good pancreatograms and cholangiograms can be obtained.

Pathologic Findings. Cholangiograms can be an aid in evaluating jaundiced animals that are suspected of having mechanical obstruction due to cholelithiasis, scarring from pancreatitis or peritonitis, or neoplasia. However, cholangiography performed with laparoscopy is likely to give more information and requires less cost, time, and expertise than ECP. The gallbladder, major bile ducts, duodenum, and pancreas are usually directly seen at laparoscopy, which may make the localization of and reason for obstructive biliary tract disease apparent.

Cholangiography performed at laparoscopy opacifies the biliary tree proximal to the obstruction, which provides more valuable information than opacifying the biliary tree distal to the obstruction, as occurs with ECP. If no obstruction is present, however, retrograde cholangiography is more likely to opacify the biliary tree than cholangiography performed at laparoscopy which, in the unobstructed biliary tree of the dog, opacifies the gallbladder, cystic ducts, and common bile duct. The contrast material then exits into the duodenum without opacifying the more proximal segments of the biliary tree.

Complications. Excessive force used in injecting the contrast material for pancreatography is likely to produce pancreatitis. Pancreatitis has been infrequently encountered in humans after ECP.[28] Complications of retrograde cholangiography are also infrequent in man. The most frequent is cholangitis, usually occurring in patients with previously infected biliary tract secondary to cholelithiasis.

Part VII. Laparoscopy

GERALD F. JOHNSON

Laparoscopy is an endoscopic technique that provides a view of the abdominal contents and peritoneal surface. Known also as peritoneoscopy, the procedure has long been used as a diagnostic and therapeutic tool in humans. The procedure was used as early as 1910 to study peristalsis in animals.[29] This discussion will deal primarily with the use of laparoscopy to evaluate liver disease in small animals.

Liver diseases in small animal veterinary medicine are not well defined. The clinician is seldom able to fit them into classifications that provide a rationale for specific treatment or prognosis. Sophisticated techniques such as radioisotope scanning, endoscopic retrograde cannulation of the biliary tract, transhepatic cholangiography, sonography, and computed tomography are not at the ready disposal of veterinarians. Limited methods used to evaluate liver disease antemortem in veterinary medicine include history, physical examination, clinical pathologic evaluation, radiography, blind liver biopsy,[30,31,32] and laparotomy. Though liver biopsy in veterinary medicine can be valuable for the diagnosis, prognosis, and treatment of liver disease, a simple, safe, high-yield method of obtaining liver biopsies has not attained general acceptance.

Laparoscopy in animals has seldom been used in North America, but has been used in Europe.[16,33] Because of its ease, safety, and accuracy of diagnosis, laparoscopy is an important but underused method for evaluating liver disease in animals. Blind liver biopsy has limited value when compared to laparoscopy. Laparoscopy's advantages over blind liver biopsy include a direct view of the liver and surrounding structures, while its choice over guided biopsy is that it may be taken under direct visual control. Laparoscopy, therefore, greatly enhances the diagnostic accuracy and has been demonstrated to have a lower morbidity and mortality than one method of blind liver biopsy.[33] Inadvertent puncture of vascular masses, the major hepatic ducts, gallbladder, and other abdominal viscera is minimized. The amount of bleeding after biopsy can be assessed during laparoscopy and measures taken to stop the bleeding whenever necessary. The disadvantages of laparoscopy are the cost of the equipment and the additional time required compared to that required for blind liver biopsy. These disadvantages, however, are outweighed by the added safety and additional information obtained.

Due to the morbidity, mortality, and unsatisfactory yield of blind liver biopsy I abandoned this procedure soon after the values of laparoscopy were established. Laparoscopy is now my preferred method for obtaining liver biopsies other than those taken at laparotomy when surgically treatable disease is suspected.

Compared to laparotomy, laparoscopy is safer in animals with liver disease complicated by hypoproteinemia, ascites, or portal systemic encephalopathy. In addition, few hepatopathies of the dog and cat can be treated surgically. Laparoscopy can often provide the same information that can be had from exploratory laparotomy. Less time, less surgical trauma, and less chemical restraint are required for laparoscopy. Indeed, major surgery for diagnostic purposes may be contraindicated. Laparoscopy is also accompanied by faster recovery rate and shorter hospitalization. When the proper indications and contraindications are observed, laparoscopy can be valuable in animals that are unable to tolerate major surgery.

In addition to being used whenever liver biopsy is indicated, laparoscopy is also used to perform splenoportography and cholangiography by puncture of the spleen and biliary system under direct vision. This is helpful in selected cases to establish the need for surgery, and it gives the surgeon valuable information regarding the localization and type of surgical treatment to be performed.

Contraindications for laparoscopy are few. Absolute contraindications for laparoscopy include cardiopulmonary decompensation, abnormal blood coagulation, surgically treatable disease within the abdomen, and extensive intra-abdominal adhesions. When adhesions between abdominal viscera and parietal peritoneum are present, puncture of abdominal viscera can occur when the trocar or peritoneum needle is introduced through the abdominal wall. Obviously, laparoscopy should not be performed on any animal if the risks outweigh the benefits to be gained.

In animals with extensive ascites, some of the fluid should be removed either medically or by abdominocentesis and the patient stabilized prior to laparoscopy.

Laparoscopy performed with laparoscopes 5 mm in diameter and larger should not be used in smaller breeds of dogs and in cats because entry of the trocar and sleeve is more likely to result in complications. More important, the pneumoperitoneum needed to provide adequate space for visualization and maneuvering the larger telescope and sleeve is greater, and it cannot be well tolerated in these smaller animals. However, a 1.7-mm laparoscope has been used with good success in cats, in smaller breeds of dogs, as well as in the larger breeds of dogs.[34]

Thus, with recent technical advances, laparoscopy coupled with ancillary procedures for biopsy and splenoportography offers the veterinarian a needed, safe, easy, and accurate method of evaluating liver disease in animals.

Instrumentation. The development of laparoscopes incorporating high-resolution optical lens systems and glass fiber light-carrying bundles along with the development of high-intensity cold light sources has provided excellent visualization of the abdominal cavity. The instruments are available from several manufacturers.

Endoscopes used for laparoscopy are rigid and of variable diameter and length. Some laparoscopes have a channel for passing various operating instruments, in addition to being designed for use with electrocoagulation. Miniaturized telescopes having an outside diameter as small as 1.7 mm to be used with a cannula having an outside diameter of 2.2 mm (the size of a 14-gauge needle) are available. Somewhat larger telescopes of 2.5 mm with sleeves of 4 mm should also prove valuable in these smaller animals.

The equipment for laparoscopy consists of a trocar, sleeve, and telescope. The sleeve is fitted with a Luer-Lok adapter to permit insufflation of gas for maintaining pneumoperitoneum. A trumpet valve prevents the escape of gas from the peritoneal cavity when the trocar is removed, and the telescope is introduced into the abdominal cavity through the sleeve. A suitable light source and light transmitting cables that attach to the telescope are used to illuminate the peritoneal cavity.

A Wolf fiber-light laparoscope with Lumina optics has been used by my colleagues and me in over 100 laparoscopies on dogs. The telescope is 10 mm in diameter with a field of vision of 170°. It has an operating channel of 5 mm (Fig. 8–4) in diameter that accommodates biopsy forceps of 45 cm in

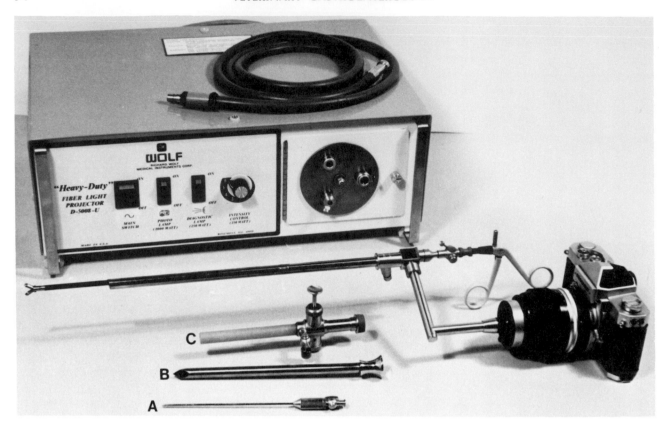

Figure 8–4. An operating laparoscope with the camera attached and forceps through the operating channel. In the foreground is the Verres pneumoperitoneum needle (A), trocar (B), and sleeve (C). The light source is shown with the light transmitting cable lying on top.

length. The spring-operated pneumoperitoneum needle, a Verres needle, has an inner blunt-tipped cannula with a side hole. This aids in preventing the puncture of abdominal viscera when establishing pneumoperitoneum.

For establishing pneumoperitoneum, normal air can be insufflated manually with a rubber bulb insufflator or carbon dioxide can be gently introduced from a small hand dispenser which has been adapted for this purpose. Nitrous oxide can also be introduced from tanks having a suitable regulator.

Devices available from laparoscope manufacturers can measure the quantity of gas insufflated and monitor the intra-abdominal pressure achieved. This contributes a further measure of safety to laparoscopy. For longer instrument life, a sterilizing tray for use with ethylene oxide ampules can be used to sterilize the telescope and other items that could be damaged by heat sterilization, though newer laparoscopes and light cables can be autoclaved.

A simple surgery pack containing towels, towel clamps, hemostats, sponges, scalpel, thumb forceps, scissors, Verres needle, and the laparoscope trocar and sleeve is used. Tru-Cut needles are used for liver biopsy. Spinal needles (18 to 20 gauge) are used for splenoportography, and 20-gauge spinal needles or Chiba needles are used for cholangiography. The Chiba needle is a flexible 22-gauge needle with a stylet, available in 6-, 8-, or 10-inch lengths.

Radiographic Studies. A radiographic finding of hepatomegaly, reduced liver size, or localized hepatic mass are indications for laparoscopy. Preoperative radiocontrast studies, particularly pneumoperitoneum, may be helpful in supporting the indications for laparoscopy. However, if there is persuasive evidence from the history, physical examination, and survey films that liver disease exists, it may be wise to forego further radiographic studies in favor of laparoscopy.

Preparation and Restraint of the Patient. Preparation of the animal for laparoscopy should include a period of fasting for 12 to 24 hours, with fresh water available except during the 3-hour period immediately prior to the procedure. The urinary bladder, colon, and stomach should be empty. Before laparoscopy is performed, plain films of the abdomen should be studied, and the cardiopulmonary and blood coagulation status should be assessed.

Chemical restraint varies depending on the species, patient manageability and ability to tolerate the chemical restraint. Drugs primarily metabolized by the liver, such as short-acting barbiturates, are avoided in dogs with disorders such as cirrhosis and portal vein anomalies. Oxymorphone (Numorphan) is preferred for most laparoscopies performed on dogs because of its favorable analgesic properties and because it can be rapidly reversed with specific antagonists such as naloxone hydrochloride (Narcan). Oxymorphone is used with local anesthesia, or it can be used for endotracheal intubation with the animal being maintained on inhalation anesthesia. Atropine is also used as a premedication.

Technique and Normal Findings. For laparoscopy, the animal is placed on a table that can be raised to a comfortable level. A table that can be tilted to shift abdominal viscera if needed affords slightly better visualization. It is not necessary to perform laparoscopy in an operating room since the peritoneal cavity is exposed for only a few seconds while inserting or removing the telescope from the sleeve and then a positive intra-abdominal pressure exists relative to outside atmospheric pressure.

Selection of the right or left side for insertion of the trocar and sleeve is based on the procedures to be performed and the area to be examined. If just visualization of the liver and liver biopsy are to be done, the right side is selected. The left side is selected only if the spleen or a left-sided liver lesion is to be visualized. Other sites of entry have not been adequately evaluated, although fat within the falciform ligament obscures vision when a ventral midline site is used.

To perform laparoscopy through the right abdominal wall, the animal is placed in left lateral recumbency and an area of skin at the laparoscopy site is clipped, surgically scrubbed, and draped. Sterile technique is adhered to with the laparoscopist wearing surgical gloves, gown, cap, and mask. The pneumoperitoneum needle is inserted into the peritoneal cavity away from the site selected for insertion of the trocar and sleeve. The underlying area should be palpated to avoid placing the needle into an abdominal organ or abdominal mass. A moderate pneumoperitoneum is established, based on observable distention and ballottement. Respiration is not compromised, but the body wall is lifted away from the viscera. Attention must be given to respiration and vascular perfusion while the pneumoperitoneum is maintained.

A ventrolateral site on the right abdominal wall and a variable distance caudal to the ribs is selected (Fig. 8–5). The exact site varies depending on the preference of the laparoscopist and on the size and body condition of the animal. In a large dog with microhepatica, a site close to the ribs and more ventral is chosen, whereas in animals with hepatomegaly, a site more caudal is selected.

After the pneumoperitoneum is established, a skin incision is made, the length of which should equal the diameter of the trocar. Blunt dissection using curved scissors with rounded tips should be performed, paralleling the muscle fibers down to the peritoneum. The skin incision and blunt dissection should not be excessive, since the sleeve must fit snugly to prevent the leakage of gas from the pneumoperitoneum. The tissue planes should not overlap during dissection, so that a safe, clean insertion of the trocar and sleeve can be made without excessive trauma to the body wall and abdominal viscera. The trocar is then withdrawn, leaving the sleeve in place. The trumpet valve on the sleeve prevents escape of gas from the pneumoperitoneum. Warming the telescope prior to its insertion prevents moisture from condensing on the objective. This can be accomplished by holding the tip in the closed hand for a short time or by using a warmed saline bath. Preheaters are available through the manufacturer. The objective can be easily cleared by gently touching it against an abdominal organ.

The laparoscopist should begin looking through the telescope as soon as it is inserted in the sleeve and the trumpet valve is depressed. This aids in making certain the sleeve has been introduced into the peritoneal cavity and not between the muscle layers or adipose tissue. This also helps determine whether the pneumoperitoneum is adequate and helps detect adhesions of abdominal viscera to parietal peritoneum. The laparoscopist should next examine the viscera underlying the entry site to be certain no trauma has occurred due to insertion of the trocar and sleeve. The telescope tip is then advanced a varying distance past the end of the sleeve depending on the size of the animal and the space afforded by the pneumoperitoneum. If the sleeve is inserted too far, it should be retracted somewhat, taking care to maintain the tip of the sleeve in the peritoneal cavity. To detect any abnormalities that may not have been previously suspected, the cranial and caudal portions of the abdomen are examined first from a distance and then at closer range, if necessary.

The liver and surrounding structures should then be examined. The telescope, which provides an

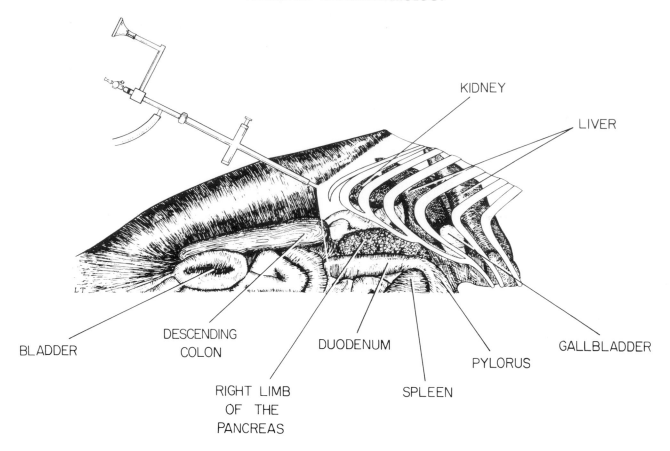

KIDNEY

LIVER

BLADDER

DESCENDING
COLON

DUODENUM

GALLBLADDER

PYLORUS

RIGHT LIMB
OF THE
PANCREAS

SPLEEN

Figure 8–5. The laparoscope is inserted through the right ventral abdominal wall. The right hepatic lobes, pancreas, and gallbladder are in the field of vision.

excellent macroscopic view of the liver parenchyma or lesions, can be introduced further to examine lesions at close range. To perform a needle biopsy of the liver, a small skin incision is made for insertion of the biopsy needle. A site is selected on the abdominal wall close to the area of the liver to be biopsied. The telescope should be retracted so that the biopsy needle will be seen just after it enters the peritoneal cavity. The needle is inserted into the peritoneal cavity and observed through the laparoscope as the needle is directed to the biopsy site. One or more biopsies are then taken under direct vision. Most laparoscopies are performed by one individual but having an assistant scrubbed in is helpful. The laparoscopist should direct the biopsy needle to, and insert it into, the biopsy site with one hand while holding the laparoscope with the other. Assistance is needed when using the Tru-Cut needle, since it requires manipulation with both hands.

In larger breeds of dogs, particularly if the liver is small, a biopsy instrument longer than the 15-cm Tru-Cut needle is needed to reach the liver, which

may be located more than 15 cm cranial to the caudal rib margin. In these instances, an operating laparoscope is advantageous because biopsy forceps 45 cm in length (Plate I, Fig. 5) can be passed through the operating channel, providing the length needed to obtain the biopsy specimen. A second smaller trocar or sleeve can be used with laparoscopes not having biopsy channels. This second puncture with the smaller trocar and sleeve can be used to accommodate biopsy forceps, probes, and other instruments. After the biopsy or biopsies are performed, the sites should be observed for excessive bleeding, which rarely occurs. Pressure can be applied to the bleeding site with the closed forceps or a probe and hemostatic agents can be injected at the site if needed. Electrocoagulation can also be used for hemostasis with those laparoscopes designed for its use.

When the laparoscopy is completed, the telescope is withdrawn and the pneumoperitoneum is relieved by depressing the trumpet valve on the sleeve. The sleeve is then withdrawn and the incision closed. The animal should be observed for a period of time after the procedure for any untoward effects.

When *splenoportography* is indicated, laparoscopy is performed through the left side with the animal placed in right lateral recumbency on an x-ray table. Plain films should be taken, with exposure factors and kVp determined before laparoscopy is performed. The site of entry is close to the spleen and its selection is based on plain films and palpation. Though not usually a problem, care should be taken that the spleen is not punctured when the trocar and sleeve are inserted, especially if splenomegaly is present. Chlorothiazide tranquilizers are avoided because they are often not metabolized properly in most animals in whom splenoportography is indicated and because they produce engorgement, which may interfere with splenic pulp pressure recordings. When liver biopsy is performed, it is done before the splenoportography and pressure measurements. An 18- to 20-gauge, 10-cm spinal needle with stylet is inserted at a point usually on the ventrolateral abdominal wall close to the spleen. Under direct vision, the needle bevel is inserted under the splenic capsule and firmly seated 1 to 2 cm into the parenchyma. The telescope is removed and the intraperitoneal gas is permitted to escape through the sleeve before pressure recordings and splenoportography are performed. Fluoroscopy and image amplification are advantageous but not necessary.

For *cholangiography*, laparoscopy is performed through the right abdominal wall as for liver biopsy, with the animal on an x-ray table. First the liver and biliary structures are examined and liver biopsies performed. A 20-gauge spinal needle or Chiba needle with stylet is inserted through the abdominal wall at a site close to the gallbladder or major ducts and, under direct vision, the needle tip is placed into the biliary tree. Cholecystocholangiography has been performed in people[35,36] and in dogs.[37] Most of the bile is aspirated and can be submitted for laboratory analysis. A syringe is fitted with venous extension tubing which is attached to the needle positioned in the biliary tract, and 35 ml of 50% Hypaque are drawn up. This system should be free of bubbles, which would ordinarily interfere with radiographic interpretation.

Fluoroscopic control and image amplification are again helpful in determining the degree of filling of the biliary tree and the amount of dye to be injected. If the biliary tree is patent, dye should be seen entering the duodenum. When the radiographs are completed, the dye can be removed. If the needle is to be withdrawn and laparoscopy completed with the contrast material remaining in the biliary system, excessive biliary pressure due to the injected dye should be relieved prior to withdrawing the needle to prevent leakage of dye or bile. This enables radiographs to be taken in different positions.

In humans, the gallbladder is approached with a needle at laparoscopy via a transhepatic route, enabling the liver parenchyma to tamponade the gallbladder puncture, thus preventing bile or dye from leaking.[38] This approach is difficult in the dog because the gallbladder adheres to the liver surface at its dorsal aspect and the gall bag is approached from the ventral aspect. The transhepatic approach to the major bile ducts using the Chiba needle[39] coupled with laparoscopy in the dog would prevent leakage but would require more expertise than direct gallbladder puncture.

In general, training, experience, and a thorough familiarity with gross pathology of the liver, gallbladder, pancreas, and spleen as well as other intra-abdominal organs contribute greatly to the value and safety of laparoscopy. Adequate records and photographic documentation are helpful in organizing data, training, and teaching. A form can be used which includes patient description, data from ancillary procedures such as splenic pulp pressure and cholangiographic findings, in addition to follow-up results such as biopsy interpretation and necropsy findings.

Pathologic Findings. Guided liver biopsies are more easily obtained and the chances of detecting focal lesions are increased when laparoscopy is performed through the right abdominal wall. This provides a view of much more liver surface than when laparoscopy is performed through the left abdominal wall. This approach is recommended if only liver biopsy is to be done. The caudate process of the caudate lobe can be seen in the more distal portion of the abdomen and the right lateral lobe ventral to it. The right medial lobe, along with the quadrate lobe, is seen in the cranial ventral aspect of the abdominal cavity. Much of the visceral and parietal surfaces of the liver can be seen and, for more careful inspection, a probe can be used through an operating laparoscope or through a second puncture site for gently lifting or moving various lobes. Laparoscopy performed through the right abdominal wall also provides a view of structures related to the liver and biliary tract, which is valuable in assessing liver disease. The gallbladder and often the major biliary ducts, the right limb of the pancreas,[40] the descending duodenum, and the pylorus can be seen. Other structures that can be visualized are the tendinous and muscular portions of the diaphragm, portions of the spleen, the right kidney, the loops of the small intestines, the colon, and the parietal peritoneum.

Laparoscopy performed through the right abdominal wall coupled with guided liver biopsy has proven valuable in detecting diffuse as well as focal liver disease. The severity and extent of disease are often apparent merely by the view provided at laparoscopy. The macroscopic appearance contributes valuable information to the diagnosis of such diseases as cirrhosis and focal neoplasia, when coupled with the biopsy interpretation. I used this procedure to evaluate a series of 23 dogs with diffuse, non-neoplastic hepatocellular disease. Seven of these were believed to have cirrhosis based on the macroscopic appearance and histopathologic diagnosis.

Laparoscopy has proven useful in the detection and management of animals with cancer.[11] Neoplasia of the liver was detected in 11 dogs; four had lymphoreticular tumors, three had primary hepatic neoplasms, two had mast cell tumors, and one had fibrosarcoma. Only one of these 11 dogs was felt to be surgically treatable. A benign primary liver tumor was resected, and the dog was doing well when lost to follow-up 9 months after surgery.

Mechanical obstruction of the biliary tree is a relatively infrequent cause for jaundice in the dog, compared to intrahepatic cholestasis. However, cholecystocholangiography performed by the author under direct vision at laparoscopy has provided valuable information in three icteric dogs. Mechanical obstruction of the biliary system was excluded in two dogs. The detection of an obstruction at the intramural portion of the common bile duct at the duodenum provided valuable information for the surgical treatment of the third dog (Fig. 8–6). No complications occurred in these few cases, but further evaluations and variations in technique are necessary before risk-data can be compiled. Cholecystocholangiography or cholangiography performed by puncture of the gallbladder or major bile duct under direct vision could prove to be a valuable procedure to evaluate the canine and feline biliary tract.

I have used laparoscopy to perform splenoportography in 30 dogs. Seventeen of these dogs had cirrhosis and had splenic pulp pressures recorded. In one dog with cirrhosis, unsuspected lymphosarcoma in the spleen was documented by guided fine needle aspiration of that organ. Splenoportography at laparoscopy has been used to document anomalies of the portal vein associated with portal-systemic encephalopathy in 13 dogs.[41] This technique was unsuccessful in two very small dogs, and an alternate method of obtaining angiography of the portal vasculature should be considered in these cases. Biopsies of the liver were obtained in all cases except one in which a laparoscope without a biopsy channel had to be used. This was a large breed dog with microhepatica and a portal vein anomaly. The biopsy needle was not long enough to obtain tissue. Further information was obtained in some cases by simultaneously measuring right atrial, caudal vena caval, hepatic vein, and hepatic wedge pressures via a catheter placed through the jugular vein.

Laparoscopy and its ancillary procedures have also proven valuable in studying the course of disease and in evaluating treatment. I have used it to study 25 Bedlington Terriers for a copper metabolism defect. It has been used to detect the recurrence, metastasis, or remission of cancer in animals treated with surgery or chemotherapy. Seven of eight dogs that had surgery and were on treatment for their cancers were demonstrated by laparoscopy to have cancer still present. Of the seven, two had lymphoreticular tumors, four had hemangiosarcoma, and one had ovarian cancer. One of these dogs was treated for systemic mast cell neoplasia and was believed to be in remission, based on a normal-appearing liver and spleen with a negative liver biopsy and a negative fine needle aspirate of the spleen.

Complications. These complications can be categorized according to the steps involved. When pneumoperitoneum is established, puncture of a hollow viscus such as the urinary bladder or gut can result in distention of that viscus. If the pneumoperitoneum needle is inserted in a vessel, in the spleen, or in a vascular mass, gas emboli may result. Subcutaneous emphysema and emphysema within the body wall can also occur if the needle is not introduced all the way through the peritoneum.

By using carbon dioxide and nitrous oxide, these risks are minimized because the gases rapidly diffuse through tissue, as opposed to air, which diffuses less readily. In contrast to air and nitrous oxide, carbon dioxide is irritating to the peritoneum and is therefore tolerated less well by the animal when laparoscopy is performed with local anesthesia. Respiratory embarrassment can occur with any gas if the volume is excessive.

Introduction of the trocar and sleeve is the most critical step in performing laparoscopy and if done improperly can result in trauma to the abdominal

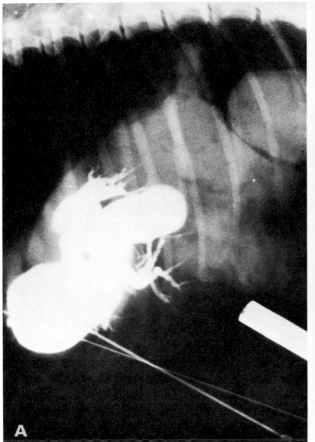

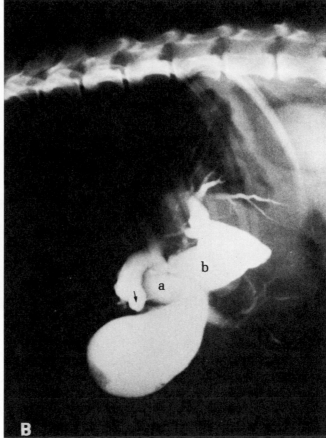

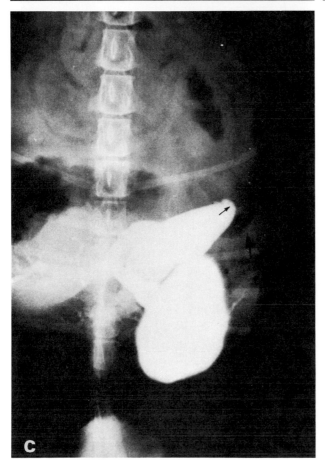

Figure 8–6. A cholecystocholangiogram performed during laparoscopy on a dog.

(A) Two needles are inserted into the gallbladder (a second needle of larger diameter was placed to enable aspiration of the abnormally viscous bile). The trocar sleeve can also be seen. (The telescope was removed to prevent radiation damage to the fiberoptic bundles.)

(B) After the needles were removed, a slight variation in patient position demonstrates an obstruction at the very distal end of the common bile duct (arrow). Note the tremendous dilation of the cystic duct (a) and the intrahepatic ducts (b).

(C) On the ventrodorsal view, gas fortuitously outlines the descending duodenum (large arrow). Note that no radiographic contrast medium enters it. A greatly dilated biliary tree is again shown. The obstruction (small arrow) was produced by a scirrhous reaction from a carcinoid tumor located along the mesenteric border of the duodenum.

wall and abdominal viscera. These complications can be minimized by taking the following precautions. Adequately prepare the patient, study plain films, avoid using excessively large laparoscopes, palpate the underlying area, dissect through the abdominal wall properly so that excessive force is not needed to insert the trocar and sleeve, and establish an adequate pneumoperitoneum.

In obese animals, adipose tissue is stored on the dorsum and therefore the abdominal cavity is located relatively more ventral. With this ventral "shift" of the abdominal cavity, care should be taken to select a site more ventral than usual to avoid entering the retroperitoneal space or to avoid trauma to the kidney.

Complications can also occur at the time of liver biopsy. Obtaining guided forceps biopsy is safer than obtaining guided needle biopsy in smaller breeds, in larger breeds with microhepatica, and in laparoscopy performed through the left abdominal wall where only a small portion of the liver may be seen. In obtaining needle biopsies in these instances, the needle may traverse the liver parenchyma and puncture underlying structures. However, the biopsy forceps allow specimens to be taken from the surface or edge of the liver lobe, thus avoiding this complication. If the diaphragm is punctured, a pneumothorax develops because a positive intra-abdominal gas pressure exists relative to the intrathoracic pressure when the pneumo-peritoneum is established. Other potential complications of the biopsy include bile peritonitis and bleeding. Infection within the peritoneal cavity, although a potential hazard, has not occurred in my cases. Minor infection within the body wall and subcutaneous tissues has occurred rarely and, in one animal, was believed to be due to contamination of the wound with hypertonic radiographic contrast material.

In my first 105 consecutive laparoscopies using the 10-mm Wolf laparoscope, three deaths occurred related to the procedure. One dog with jaundice and hepatosplenomegaly died an hour after the procedure. The liver biopsy revealed malignant mast cells, and it was believed that the procedure stimulated mast cell degranulation that resulted in death. A second dog evaluated for ascites bled from the liver biopsy and had to be transfused. A severe coagulopathy was demonstrated, and the dog died the following day. Adequate evaluation of this animal's coagulation status prior to laparoscopy would have revealed this problem to be a contraindication. This case also represents one of the few missed diagnoses. Improper respiratory monitoring while the pneumoperitoneum was established resulted in death of the third dog, a 3.5-kg Yorkshire Terrier with a portal vein anomaly, on which splenoportography was attempted during the laparoscopic procedure.

Part VIII. Colonoscopy

GERALD F. JOHNSON

Indications for colonoscopy in animals are: (1) suspicion of colonic disease, owing to signs of tenesmus or blood and mucus in the feces, (2) suspicion of diffuse bowel disease, such as lymphoma, inflammatory or infectious diseases, (3) abnormal radiographic findings, (4) evaluation of surgical or medical treatment, and (5) unexplained diarrhea.

Indications for colonoscopy are fewer in the dog and cat than in man for the following reasons:

1. The incidence of colon cancer is not as high as in man.[42,43]

2. Colon carcinomas in the dog are usually within reach of the standard rigid colonoscopes.

3. Polyps rarely occur in the dog and cat.

Colonic polyps in man prompted the development

of operative colonoscopy utilizing specialized double lumen colonoscopes that accommodate grasping forceps and an electrocautery snare for polypectomy.[44] Operative colonoscopy is rarely indicated in veterinary medicine.

Localization of gastrointestinal lesions in dogs and cats is often difficult. Upper and lower gastrointestinal endoscopy, in conjunction with biopsy, can be valuable in defining the problem, and exploratory surgery and full thickness biopsies of the bowel are sometimes avoided in the process.

Reasons for not performing colonoscopy are few but include lack of proper indications, an incompletely prepared bowel, and inability of the patient to tolerate the necessary restraint. Discretion must be used in the biopsy of animals with coagulopathies.

Focal lesions suspected of being limited to the rectum or being within reach of the standard rigid colonoscope can be examined with that instrument. The greatest use for colonoscopy has been in detecting and evaluating naturally occurring colitides in the dog. Colonoscopy also has potential value as an investigative and experimental tool. Improved skill and improved instrumentation should permit routine evaluation of the ascending colon, cecum, ileocolic valve, and even the ileum.

Flexible fiberoptic endoscopy provides a meticulous and thorough inspection of the luminal surface of the entire colon in the dog and cat that no other method of examination can provide. This offers the veterinarian an invaluable technique with which to study the colon in animals. The value of colonoscopy in human medicine has been reviewed.[45] The veterinarian is at an advantage in examining the colon of the carnivore since its anatomy is relatively simple, lacking haustrations and complex flexures. The rectum is short and straight, with the remaining colon shaped like a question mark, permitting rather easy passage of fiberoptic colonoscopes in these animals.

Instrumentation. The same endoscopes used for upper gastrointestinal endoscopy are suitable for colonoscopy as well; this circumvents the expense of an additional endoscope. Using the same instrument for both orifices of the digestive tract of humans is undesirable from the aesthetic viewpoint, but is acceptable in veterinary medicine. Contamination of the upper gastrointestinal tract with microorganisms from the lower gut has not been a problem and, from a practical standpoint, is unlikely to become a major deterrent to using the same endoscope for upper and lower gastrointestinal endoscopy in animals if proper instrument care and cleaning are provided.

Several endoscopes have been used successfully for colonoscopy in the dog and cat. Once again, the varying size of animals presents problems in designing endoscopes strictly for veterinary use. A working length of 110 cm is preferred over shorter lengths. Those with greater diameter (12.5 mm) and decreased flexibility are more difficult instruments to use for colonoscopy on cats and small dogs. However, the latter instrument has better biopsy capabilities because of its larger biopsy channel and forceps. Features of an endoscope designed for small animal veterinary gastrointestinal endoscopy should include: (1) biopsy and photographic capabilities, (2) small outside diameter, (3) a working length of approximately 150 cm, (4) increased flexibility, and (5) a short bending section with four-way tip control that can be deflected greater than 150° from the long axis.

Radiographic Studies. Although abnormal radiographic findings detected on a colonogram are indications for colonoscopy, colonograms are not necessary prior to performing colonoscopy in the dog and cat. A thorough colonoscopy procedure provides more information than a colonogram primarily because it provides direct visualization of the mucosal surface, which is involved in the majority of diseases affecting the colon of the dog and cat. The two procedures can be complementary. Colonoscopy provides information directly to the colonoscopist and a colonogram can then be performed after endoscopy to evaluate the thickness of the colon wall or to examine areas above a stricture.

Preparation and Restraint of the Patient. Since incomplete preparation of the intestinal tract is the major reason for failure to complete colonoscopy, this step must be emphasized. Even the small bowel should be emptied if the ascending colon, cecum, and ileocolic valve are to be examined. Whenever possible, a 24-hour liquid diet is followed by a 24-hour fast. Laxatives may also be used. Enemas with large volumes of water or dioctyl sodium sulfosuccinate solution are administered with a long soft enema tube, at least 1 hour prior to colonoscopy. Visual artifacts may be produced by an enema, and it should not be given immediately prior to examination. The administration of phosphate enema solutions can be hazardous[46] because of fluid and electrolyte imbalances that may follow.

Restraint is similar to that suggested for use in upper gastrointestinal endoscopy. The left lateral recumbent position is preferred since this position keeps the right colon and cecum area away from the supporting table, thus facilitating examination of this area.

Technique and Normal Findings. A digital examination should always be performed prior to colonoscopy to detect sites of potential complications such as diverticula associated with perineal hernias or rectal strictures. Plain or contrast radiographs should be studied when available, to alert the veterinarian to the presence of diseased bowel and to emphasize specific areas to be examined.

In the anesthetized dog, particularly, but also in the cat, a vestibule of a few centimeters in length is often present between the anus and the rectum. This area is not described in anatomy texts but probably corresponds to the area between the medial coccygeal muscle and the external sphincter where rectal diverticula occur with perineal hernias. When the tip of the endoscope is inserted through the anal canal and air is insufflated, this vestibule is entered and the endoscopist must then find the orifice leading to the rectum and the colon. This should be done while viewing through the endoscope, so that the tip is not advanced through a cul-de-sac in the vestibule, causing perforation. Again, as for upper gastrointestinal endoscopy, the tip of the endoscope should not be advanced unless the lumen is in focus.

Once the rectum has been entered, air is insufflated, and a tunnel view of the descending colon is obtained. With the lumen of the splenic flexure in view, the scope is advanced, giving the tip a slight upward deflection. In this way, the tip of the endoscope is directed caudally and ultimately advanced into the ascending colon. A slide-by technique is sometimes used in negotiating curves, whereby mucosa can be visualized passing by the field of vision as the tip is advanced through flexures, but the lumen itself is not in full view. The examiner must feel resistance to the passage of the endoscope, thus avoiding bowel perforation resulting from excessive force when advancing the tip. The ascending colon, ileocolic valve, and cecum are important areas to examine, since they are frequent sites of such diseases as parasitism, lymphoma, intussusception, and inverted cecum.

Using the GIF-P endoscope, good visualization of the ileum has been obtained only rarely since the ileocolic valve is difficult to negotiate and offers significant resistance to passage of the endoscope tip. The cecum, however, appearing simply as a gaping cul-de-sac marked by a definite rim, can more frequently be entered with the tip of the endoscope either intentionally or inadvertently. To avoid perforation, the colonoscopist must be aware that the cecum is a blind pouch. Instruments designed for veterinary use may, in the future, provide routine examination of the distal small bowel.

Colonic biopsies are diagnostically valuable and safe to perform. They are usually obtained in conjunction with colonoscopy. Target biopsies are taken with the endoscopic forceps, and, if diffuse disease is suspected, a suction mucosal biopsy instrument with a capsule designed for use in animals is used.

The contribution of biopsy in evaluating diseases of the colon cannot be overemphasized. Seldom is colonoscopy or proctoscopy performed without biopsies being taken, and the taking of multiple biopsy specimens is strongly urged. It does no good simply to look at an inflammatory, ulcerative, or mass lesion and then guess what it is and how to treat it. Histologic examination may establish a diagnosis in cases of neoplasia or reveal an etiologic agent that would not be apparent without biopsy. The type of inflammatory response detected in histopathologic preparations, such as an eosinophilic inflammation, often leads to more specific treatment and more accurate prognosis.

The pathologist who has attempted to interpret endoscopic forceps biopsies will attest to the fact that they leave something to be desired because of their small size, distortion, and inconsistent orientation on the slide. The endoscopist should reserve these for target sites. On the other hand, biopsies taken with suction mucosal biopsy capsules when diffuse disease is suspected yield much more information. Less distortion occurs when this type of biopsy is taken, the sample is larger and easier for the histology technician to orient properly on a slide. Obtaining tissue with the biopsy capsule, when done properly, is extremely safe. Usually three to five biopsies are taken during an examination, and no complications have occurred in my series of more than 300 colonic biopsies taken with a mucosal biopsy capsule. A colonogram should not be performed until 2 weeks after a suction mucosal biopsy has been taken because the pressure required to distend the colon with contrast may cause perforation at the biopsy site.

Pathologic Findings. In a series of 70 colonoscopies, 57 were done in dogs and 13 in cats. Nineteen animals had colitides; six of these cases were Boxer dogs with chronic ulcerative histiocytic colitis. Marked ulcerative colitis of undetermined etiology was detected in a German Shepherd dog and a Beagle hound. The remaining colitides were also of undetermined etiology, but varied in severity and in types of cellular inflammation. Histoplasmosis was detected on histologic examination of a specimen taken with the mucosal biopsy capsule from a dog with severe enterocolitis.

Neoplasia of the colon was documented in one cat and three dogs. A space-occupying mass detected on a barium colonogram in the cat was diagnosed as lymphoma from biopsies taken during colonoscopy. Two dogs with diffuse mucosal lymphoma were detected with colonoscopy and biopsy. The third dog had a stricture in the ascending colon on upper gastrointestinal series; an adenocarcinoma was revealed on colonoscopy. One dog, suspected of having neoplasia of the ileum on upper gastrointestinal films, was observed at colonoscopy to have an intussusception (Plate I, Fig. 6). Colonoscopy was used to evaluate medical treatment in two dogs with lymphosarcoma of the colon and in one dog for recurrence of carcinoma after resection.

Helminth parasites involving the colon can be individually discerned and grasped with the biopsy forceps for identification. Whipworms have been found in the cecum and colon of dogs, and *Ancylostoma spp.* was identified in the colon of one dog.

Complications. No perforations or complications due to either colonoscopy or biopsy have occurred in my practice in over 100 consecutive procedures. This number of cases is very low, however. Perforations during colonoscopy occur at the rate of about 3 per 1000 in humans.[46]

As more colonoscopies are performed in veterinary medicine, it is likely that serious complications, probably perforation, peritonitis, and hemorrhage, will occur. Training, experience, and understanding of anatomy as well as pathology will not only contribute to the value of colonoscopy but also prevent complications.

Part IX. Proctoscopy

GERALD F. JOHNSON

Examination of the anus, rectum, and distal colon of the dog and cat is easy to perform and often yields valuable information when performed with the proper equipment. All clinicians should be able to perform this procedure, but too often it is neglected when indicated. Indications for proctoscopy are similar to indications for colonoscopy, excluding lesions beyond the reach of the proctoscope.

Proctoscopy is the examination of the rectum with an endoscope. Either flexible fiberoptic or rigid tube endoscopes can be used for this purpose. Because of the relatively simple anatomy of the carnivore, however, much or all of the descending colon in addition to the rectum can be visualized using rigid tube proctoscopes. The vast majority of diseases affecting the colon and rectum of the dog and cat are within reach of the standard 25-cm rigid proctoscope. The more distal rectal and anal lesions can be better examined with a shorter rectal speculum or anoscope. Radiographic examinations are usually deferred if the signs or findings indicate that the lesion is in the distal colon or rectum.

Instrumentation. Rigid proctoscopes are made in various diameters and lengths. For small animal veterinary use, the standard 25-cm model provides adequate length, although at least two diameters of 16 mm and 8 mm (inside diameter) are advantageous because of the varying size of the animals. The material of which the proctoscope is made is not so important as the view provided. A high-intensity light source is beneficial, and basically two types of lighting, proximal and distal, are incorporated in the proctoscopes. The distal lighting provided by circumferentially arranged, incoherent-fiber light bundles within the wall is preferred. The proctoscope should permit the insufflation of air with a hand bulb and have a hinged or detachable window that establishes a closed system (Fig. 8–7). The window,

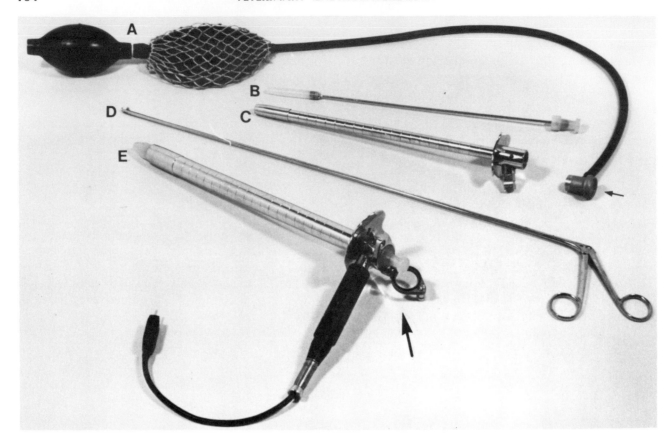

Figure 8–7.   Pictured from top to bottom are: rubber bulb for air insufflation (A), obturator for small proctoscope (B), small proctoscope (C), biopsy forceps (D), and large proctoscope with obturator in place and light source attached (E).
The detachable window (small arrow) of small proctoscope is attached to the hose of the rubber bulb. The large proctoscope has a hinged window (large arrow).

often a magnifying lens, releases the insufflated air when it is opened. This can be a problem in maintaining the view of a selected site, but permits the passage of swabs or biopsy instruments which, unfortunately, also partially block one's vision.

Flexible fiberoptic endoscopes of 60 to 90 cm in length, designed for examination of the rectum and sigmoid colon of humans, are available for use in small animals. Several pediatric prototype endoscopes have been used in dogs and cats to examine the rectum and descending colon. Compared to rigid tube proctoscopes, these instruments provide a better overall wide angle view from a distance and a better close-up view. The lesion and the extent of its involvement in the rectum and colon (even those within reach of the rigid proctoscope) can be better appreciated with flexible, fiberoptic endoscopes. More accurate biopsy of selected sites is obtained because the view is not obscured by forceps, and the volume of insufflated air is maintained. Anoscopes or specula can be of a larger diameter and

are shorter, and are used with proximal or spot lighting (Fig. 8–8). They are equipped neither with windows nor for air insufflation. Anoscopes and specula provide a good direct view and access to distal lesions.

Accessory equipment should include swabs, suction apparatus, and biopsy instruments. Cotton balls used with alligator forceps of adequate length serve well as swabs.

Preparation and Restraint of the Patient. In general, the endoscopy and biopsy procedures will be safer and more helpful in diagnosis if the bowel is cleansed. Preparation may be extensive, including a liquid diet with little or no residue for 24 hours, followed by a 24-hour fast and laxative to simplify administration of the enema several hours prior to examination. Enemas should be avoided immediately prior to the examination. However, with obstructive signs such as tenesmus, stricture, diverticula, or mass lesions, cleansing of the bowel can be done after chemical restraint with the aid of a

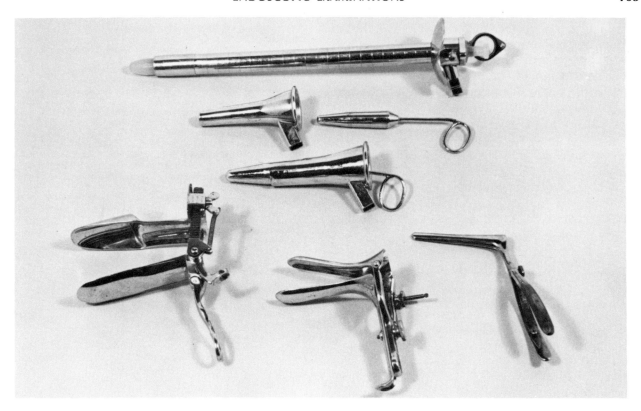

Figure 8–8. A standard-sized proctoscope with obturator in place is shown on the top. Below it are various specula for examination of anorectal lesions.

gentle stream of water at body temperature from a tube attached directly to a tap.

Restraint can vary depending on the animal's ability to tolerate the discomfort caused by the proctoscope and the anticipated duration of the procedure. Drugs such as oxymorphone and phenothiazine tranquilizers or barbiturates with or without inhalation anesthesia can be used. Adequate restraint, however, is a prerequisite for careful examination.

Technique and Normal Findings. With the patient positioned on a table of adequate height, the examiner can be seated on a comfortable stool with instruments readily accessible on an instrument stand or tray. The position of the animal varies, depending on the preference of the examiner and location of the lesion. Either sternal or lateral recumbency can be used. When using rigid proctoscopes, elevation of the hindquarters causes colonic fluid to flow more cranially in the transverse colon, thus facilitating examination.

Valuable information can be obtained by performing a digital examination prior to insertion of the endoscope. The rectal mucosa and deeper structures should be palpated and anal sacs gently evacuated to be certain their contents are not abnormal. The ventral aspect of the sacrum, the urethra, and the vagina or prostate, as well as the lateral and dorsal aspects should be palpated.

Rigid proctoscopes should first be lubricated and grasped between the index and middle fingers with the thumb on the obturator. The obturator is in place only to facilitate passage of the proctoscope through the anal sphincters. When this is done, the obturator is removed and the endoscopist then looks through the proctoscope before advancing it further and while insufflating air.

Rectal mucosa is pinkish-grey and thus is paler than colonic mucosa. Numerous lymphoid nodules (2 to 3 mm diameter) are present in the mucosa. They have umbilicated centers and may be mistaken for small ulcers.

Biopsy should be done nearly every time that proctoscopy is performed. There are two types of cutting forceps, the angulated cup-type and the straight; either of these can be used. The angulated cup-type is advantageous in the biopsy of the relatively flat rectum of dogs and cats, a surface that lacks folds and haustrations. This type is also safer than the straight cutting forceps. Mucosal lesions should be gently grasped and tented up with the intention of obtaining only mucosa and submucosa. Snare forceps are advantageous in the biopsy of raised and polypoid masses. For diffuse mucosal disease, the suction biopsy instrument is safer than forceps biopsy instruments, and better biopsy specimens are obtained (see Colonoscopy).

Pathologic Findings. Lesions observed at proctoscopy include inflammation, erosion, ulcer, mass, stenosis, and, rarely, a foreign body. It is sufficient to say that knowledge of colonic and rectal diseases and their gross pathology is invaluable when interpreting findings as seen through the endoscope. Biopsy results should always be correlated with visual observations. If the lesion appears neoplastic, but the biopsy specimen is interpreted as being benign, it may be wise to repeat the procedure.

Complications. It is important to detect the presence of rectal diverticula due to perineal hernias by digital examination in order to avoid perforation of the rectum when the proctoscope is inserted. The only two perforations occurring with rigid proctoscopy in my practice from 1968 to 1976 were associated with failure to detect rectal diverticula prior to proctoscopy.

Another important point is to remove the obturator as soon as the proctoscope tip passes the anal sphincters. The instrument should not be advanced unless the lumen can be seen. This avoids perforation of the bowel wall when diverticula or areas of compromised bowel are encountered. The proctoscope should not be advanced against resistance nor should it be used to dilate strictures.

When biopsying the colon with forceps, care should be taken to avoid perforation, which would lead to peritonitis. In the dog, especially in the male, the peritoneal cavity extends very far caudally to the third coccygeal vertebra as the rectovesical excavation ventrally and the pararectal fossa laterally.[47]

REFERENCES

1. Kato, H., and Matsushima, S.: Experimental study for rapid sterilization of the flexible fiberoptic bronchoscope. Chest 66:723, 1974.
2. Cook, W. R.: Procedure and technique for endoscopy of the equine respiratory tract and eustachian tube diverticulum. Equine Vet. J. 2:137, 1970.
3. Johnson, J. H.: Endoscopy of the pharynx, larynx, and guttural pouch in the horse. VM/SAC 66:47, 1971.
4. Johnson, J. H., and Merriam, J. G.: Equine endoscopy. Vet. Scope 19:2, 1975.
5. Atkins, J. P.: Chapter 9, Esophagoscopy in the study of esophageal affections. In Gastroenterology. Vol. 1, 2nd ed. Edited by H. L. Bockus. Philadelphia, W. B. Saunders Co., 1966, p. 133.
6. Boyce, H. W., and Palmer, E. D.: Techniques of Clinical Gastroenterology. Springfield, Illinois, Charles C Thomas Publishers, 1975.
7. O'Brien, J. A.: Esophagoscopy. Vet. Clin. North Am. 2:99, 1972.
8. Katz, S., Boyle, C. C., Sherlock, P., and Winawer, S. J.: Gastric exfoliative cytology—a rapid method. Am. J. Gastroenterol. 60:157, 1973.
9. Heinkel, K.: Correlation of gastroscopy, gastric photography, and biopsy in diagnosis. Gastrointest. Endosc. 16:81, 1969.
10. van der Gaag, I., Happi, R. P., and Wolvekamp, W. Th. C.: Investigation of the Dog Stomach. In Proceedings, Netherlands Small Animal Veterinary Association, Amsterdam, 1974, p. 60.
11. Johnson, G. F., and Twedt, D. C.: Endoscopy and laparoscopy in the diagnosis and management of neoplasia in small animals. Vet. Clin. North Am. 7:77, 1977.
12. Murray, M., McKeating, P. J., and Lauder, I. M.: Peptic ulceration in the dog: a clinico-pathological study. Vet. Rec. 91:441, 1972.
13. Barrett, B.: Editorial: new instruments, new horizons, new hazards—the impaction theory. Gastrointest. Endosc. 16:142, 1970.
14. Nielson, S. W., and Bishop, E. J.: The duct system of the canine pancreas. Am. J. Vet. Res. 15:266, 1954.
15. Straus, E., Johnson, G. F., and Yalow, R. S.: Canine Zollinger-Ellison syndrome. Gastroenterology 72:380, 1977.
16. Dalton, J. R. F., and Hill, F. W. G.: A procedure for the examination of the liver and pancreas in the dog. J. Small Anim. Prac. 13:527, 1972.
17. McCune, W. S., Short, P. E., and Moscovitz, H.: Endoscopic cannulation of the ampulla of Vater: a preliminary report. Ann. Surg. 167:752, 1968.
18. Falkenstein, D. B., Abrams, R. M., Kessler, R. E., Jones, B. D., Johnson, G. F., and Zimmon, D. S.: Endoscopic retrograde cholangiopancreatography in the dog: a model for training and research. Gastrointest. Endosc. 21:25, 1974.
19. Kobayashi, M., Nakada, M., Taguchi, T., Nagashima, H., Miynao, K., Shimamoto, M., and Tsuneoka, K.: Retrograde cholangiography using a duodenoscope. Naika 27:629, 1971.
20. Oi, I., Kobayashi, S., and Kondo, T.: Endoscopic pancreato-cholangiography. Endoscopy 2:103, 1970.
21. Tagaki, K., Ikeda, S., Nakagawa, Y., Sakaguchi, N., Takahashi, T., Kumakura, K., Maruyama, M., Sumeya, N., Nakano, H., Takada, T., Takekoshi, T., and Kin, T.: Retrograde pancreatography and cholangiography by fiber duodenoscope. Gastroenterology 59:445, 1970.
22. Cotton, P. B.: Progress report—cannulation of the papilla of Vater by endoscopy and retrograde cholangiopancreatography (ERCP). Gut 13:1014, 1972.
23. Waye, J. D.: Endoscopic visualization of the pancreatic and biliary ducts. Mt. Sinai J. Med. N.Y. 42:35, 1975.
24. Zimmon, D. S.: The clinical value of endoscopic retrograde cholangiopancreatography. Bull. N. Y. Acad. Med. 51:472, 1975.
25. Classen, M., and Safrany, L.: Endoscopic papillotomy and removal of gall stones. Br. Med. J. 4:371, 1975.
26. Nakajima, M., Akasaka, Y., Fukumoto, K., Mitsuyoshi, Y., and Kawai, K.: Peroral cholangiopancreatography (PCPS) under duodenoscopic guidance. Am. J. Gastroenterol. 66:241, 1976.
27. Getty, R.: Sisson & Grossman's The Anatomy of the Domestic Animals. 5th ed. Philadelphia, W. B. Saunders Co., 1975.
28. Nebel, O. T., Siluis, S. E., Rogers, G., Sugawa, C., and Mandelstam, P.: Complications associated with endoscopic retrograde cholangiopancreatography. Results of the 1974 A/S/G/E survey. Gastrointest. Endosc. 22:34, 1975.
29. Nadeau, O. C. and Kampmein, P. F.: Endoscopy of the abdomen: abdomenoscopy. Surg. Gynecol. Obstet. 41:259, 1925.
30. Edwards, D.: Personal communication, 1977.
31. Feldman, E. C., and Ettinger, S. J.: Percutaneous transthoracic liver biopsy in the dog. J.A.V.M.A. 169:805, 1976.
32. Lettow, E.: Die Blinde Leberpunktion nach Menghini beim Hund. Berl. Munch. Tieraerztl. Wochenschr. 76:273, 1963.
33. Lettow, E.: Laparoscopic examinations in liver disease in dogs. Vet. Med. Rev. 2:159, 1972.
34. Jones, B. D.: Personal communication, 1976.
35. Hegstrom, G. J., Zoeckler, S. J., and Keil, P. G.: Peritoneoscopy. Gastroenterology 25:243, 1953.
36. Royer, M., Colombato, L. O., and Mazure, P. A.: Peritoneoscopic cholangiography with manometric control. Gastroenterology 26:626, 1954.
37. Hogan, M. T., Watne, A., Mossburg, W., and Castaneda, W.: Direct inspection into the gallbladder in dogs using ultrasonic guidance. Arch. Surg. 111:564, 1976.
38. Berci, G., Morgenstern, L., Shone, J. M., and Shapiro, S.: A direct approach to the differential diagnosis of jaundice: laparoscopy with transhepatic cholecystocholangiography. Am. J. Surg., 126:372, 1973.

39. Akuda, K., Tanikawa, K., Emura, T., Kuratomi, S., Jinnouchi, S., Uruba, K., Sumikoshi, T., Kanda, Y., Fukuyama, Y., Musha, H., Mori, H., Shimokawa, Y., Yakushiji, F., and Matsuura, Y.: Nonsurgical percutaneous transhepatic cholangiography: diagnostic significance in medical problems of the liver. Am. J. Dig. Dis. *19*:21, 1974.
40. Geyer, S.: Die Laparoskopische Darstellung des Pankreas des Hundes. Tieraerztl. Praxis *1*:433, 1973.
41. Ewing, G. O., Suter, P. F., and Bailey, C. S.: Hepatic insufficiency associated with congenital anomalies of the portal vein in dogs. J.A.A.H.A. *10*:463, 1974.
42. Patnaik, A. K., Hurvitz, A. I., and Johnson, G. F.: Canine gastrointestinal neoplasms. Vet. Pathol. *14*:547, 1977.
43. Patnaik, A. K., Liu, S. K., and Johnson, G. F.: Feline intestinal adenocarcinoma. Vet. Pathol. *13*:1, 1976.
44. Panish, J. F.: Colonoscopy. *In* Endoscopy. Edited by G. Berci. New York, Appleton-Century-Crofts, 1976, p. 300.
45. Overholt, B.: Colonoscopy: a review. Gastroenterology *68*:1308, 1975.
46. Schaer, M., Cavanagh, P., Hause, W., and Wilkins, R. J.: Iatrogenic hyperphosphatemia, hypocalcemia, and hypernatremia in a cat. J.A.A.H.A. *13*:39, 1977.
47. Miller, M.E., Christensen, G. C., and Evans, H. E.: Anatomy of the Dog. Philadelphia, W. B. Saunders Co., 1964.

SUGGESTED READINGS

Gastroscopy

Berci, G. (Ed.): Endoscopy. New York, Appleton-Century-Crofts, 1976.
Bockus, H. L.: Examination of the patient. Disorders of the esophagus and stomach. *In* Gastroenterology, Vol. 1, 3rd ed. Edited by Bockus, H. L. Philadelphia, W. B. Saunders Co., 1974.

Laparoscopy

Berci, G. (Ed.): Endoscopy. New York, Appleton-Century-Crofts, 1976.
Boyce, H. W.: Chapter 10, Laparoscopy. *In* Diseases of the Liver, 4th ed. Edited by L. Schiff. Philadelphia, J. B. Lippincott Co., 1975, p. 272.
Palmer, E. D., and Boyce, H. E., Jr.: Techniques of Clinical Gastroenterology. Springfield, Illinois, Charles C Thomas Publisher, 1975.
Vilardell, F., and Marti-Vicente, A.: Peritoneoscopy (laparoscopy). *In* Gastroenterology, Vol. IV, 3rd ed. Edited by Bockus, H. L. Philadelphia, W. B. Saunders Co., 1976, p. 65.

SOURCES OF INSTRUMENTS

Part II

V-902-A, American Cystoscope Makers, Inc., 300 Stillwater Ave., Stamford, CT 06902.
ACMI Colonscope, F9-S, ibid.
Olympus Gastrointestinal Fiberscope, Model GIF, type D2, Olympus Corp. of America, 2 Nevada Drive, New Hyde Park, NY 11040.

Part III

Flexible Fiberoptic Endoscope. VGS-60, American Optical, Southbridge, MA. Distributed by: Western Serum Company, Inc., 2318 S. Industrial Park Drive, Tempe, AZ 85282.
George P. Pilling & Son Co., Delaware Drive, Fort Washington, PA 19034.

Part IV

Olympus GIF-P with accessories and Gomco suction pump. Olympus Corporation of America, ibid.

Part VI

Olympus JF-B Duodenoscope, Olympus Corporation of America, ibid.

Part VII

Wolf Laparoscope, Richard Wolf Medical Instrument Corp., 7046 Lyndon Ave., Rosemont, IL 60018.
Needlescope, Dyonics, Woburn, MA 01801.
Laparoscope, Karl Storz Endoscopy America, Inc., 658 South San Vicente Blvd., Los Angeles, CA 90048.
Laparoscope, Eder Instrument Co., 5100 N. Ravenwood Ave., Chicago, IL 60640.

Chapter 9

THE EXPLORATORY LAPAROTOMY

J. THOMAS VAUGHAN

The exploratory laparotomy, when conducted as a systematic, intraoperative search for abdominal lesions, can furnish the greatest amount of diagnostic evidence of any phase of the examination, while at the same time providing the opportunity for definitive correction of problems. Experience gained from necropsies is of great help, but recognition of lesions spread out on the postmortem floor is no substitute for a knowledge of pathologic anatomy in situ. The same system employed so faithfully in collecting the medical case history and in performing the physical and laboratory examination should be applied to the surgical investigation of the abdominal organs. This, then, is an appeal to the veterinarian to use a routine in exploring this largest and most complex of the body compartments.

THE APPROACH

Conduct of the laparotomy varies greatly with the species. Surgical approaches through the lateral walls of the abdomen have greater application, understandably, in the equine and the bovine. However, exploration through the flank in these species is limited in exposure by the grid incision through heavy musculature. Primarily for this reason, such exploratory procedures are most useful when there is a high degree of certainty as to the nature and location of the problem prior to entry. When greater exposure is required by the size of the lesion, the expectation of a wide field of dissection or the uncertainty of the preoperative diagnosis, a ventral approach is often preferred, be it midline or paramedian.

A considerable advantage of the ventral laparotomy is the extensile incision. For example, an initial midline incision in the central abdomen can be extended cranially or caudally to facilitate dissection and exposure of the lesion after entering the abdomen. Such approaches afford even greater exposure in the small animal species due to the relatively shallow abdomen. In the large animal, much of the search must be conducted by blind palpation, virtually at arm's length, correlating fingertip findings with anatomic relationships in the mind's eye. This places a premium on an accurate command of both normal and pathologic anatomy, especially in the larger species.

THE SEARCH

In organizing the search, one must first classify the products of disease that can be recognized at exploratory laparotomy:

 I. Distentions
    a. acute or chronic
    b. primary or secondary
    c. solid, fluid, or gas
 II. Effusions
    a. serous
    b. hemorrhagic
    c. purulent
    d. gastroenteric
    e. biliary
    f. urinary
    g. uterine
 III. Discolorations
    a. congestive
    b. hyperemic (inflammation or strangulation)
    c. hemorrhagic
    d. icteric
    e. cyanotic
    f. ischemic
    g. gangrenous
 IV. Deposits
    a. fibrin
    b. ingesta
    c. miliary neoformations
 V. The Lesion per se
    a. inflammatory lesion
    b. obturation obstruction
    c. displacement
    d. perforation or rupture
    e. luminal deformity
    f. neoplasm
    g. angiopathy
    h. congenital anomaly

Upon incising the peritoneum, the great temptation is to plunge into the abdomen forthwith. This urge must be resisted long enough to study the distribution pattern of distended bowel, to assess the color, odor, and character of any effusions, to note the significance of readily discernible discolorations of viscera or peritoneal surfaces, as well as noting deposits characteristic of peritonitis, intestinal rupture, or neoplasia. After having made these observations, one proceeds with the examination according to the species and the indications for the laparotomy.

Distentions. Distentions must be qualified according to duration and course as well as content. Acute distentions of the small intestine due to obstruction are predominantly fluid-filled, as are the acute gastric dilatations caused by enterogastric reflux secondary to intestinal obstructions. Acute distentions of the cecum and large intestine in the horse contain large amounts of gas, causing the tympany characteristic of large intestinal obstructions in all herbivores. In ruminants, distentions of the stomach and forestomachs due to displacements, torsions, and impactions overshadow intestinal problems and, thus, receive special attention. In horses, primary gastric dilatation is usually associated with engorgement, but gastric volvulus is rare, in contrast to large dogs in which acute gastric dilatation is frequently associated with gastric volvulus.[1]

By noting the distribution pattern of intestinal distention, the general location of the blockage should be apparent. In the horse, if part of the small intestine is distended, but not all, likelihoods include volvulus, entrapment through a mesenteric or omental rent, internal hernia, restricting adhesion or fibrous band, or perhaps a pedunculated lipoma. If all of the small intestine is distended, but none of the large intestine, ileocecal intussusception should be suspected. If the cecum and both ventral limbs of the large colon are distended, an impaction of the pelvic flexure or left dorsal colon is suspected. If both limbs of the left colon are distended, but not the right dorsal, a torsion of the left colon or incarceration by the suspensory ligament of the spleen may have occurred. If all of the large colon is distended but none of the small colon, a case is made for an impaction of the transverse colon. If the small colon is distended, an impaction of the small colon may exist.[2]

In the bovine, patterns of gastrointestinal distention are so characteristic, and methods of physical examination (such as percussion, auscultation, and palpation per rectum) so revealing that the location and nature of the obstruction are often known

sufficiently well to dictate the choice and site of abdominal incision. Many of the surgical diseases of the ruminant stomachs are associated with advanced pregnancy and with displacement of abdominal organs by the gravid uterus. Fluid and gaseous distention of the displaced or twisted abomasum produces detectable zones of tympany either to the left or to the right of the rumen. These displacements are accessible from both lateral and ventral approaches. Acute and primary distentions of the small intestine in cattle are typified by jejunal intussusception, oftentimes palpable per rectum on physical examination. Other possibilities include strangulated hernias. Distention of the cecum and of the spiral colon are usually due to torsion, and are commonly diagnosed on the basis of percussion and auscultation at the right flank and by palpation per rectum of the typical gaseous distention in the pelvic inlet and/or the right quadrants of the abdomen. Laparotomy through the right flank or the right paramedian approach is chosen on the basis of the same patterns of distention.[3,4]

In the canine and feline, the sequence of bowel segments is the same except for length and complexity. The abdominal cavity is shallower, and the limbs of bowel more easily exteriorized for inspection. The ventral midline is preferred by many for easy access and generous exposure.[3,5]

In addition to what has been said in reference to the diagnostic value of patterns of gastrointestinal distention, it is important to stress the usefulness of decompression of these distentions to facilitate exploratory laparotomy. Tympanitic segments of cecum and great colon in the horse, and rumen, abomasum, and cecum in the cow are effectively decompressed by machine suction via enterocentesis. Suction applied to bowel filled with fluid or solid ingesta is largely ineffectual in herbivores due to the fiber content. Evacuation in these instances usually requires enterotomy and manual manipulation. Progressive motility in exposed bowel is nonexistent. Hence, intestinal drainage via operative means is at best a compromise in the herbivore, and adynamic ileus in the postoperative period is often a problem.

Effusions. The majority of patients examined at exploratory laparotomy will have benefitted from an abdominocentesis for effusion during the preoperative workup. Cytologic study, microbiologic culture, and chemical tests are used to characterize the fluid specimen. However, much information can be gained at surgery by observing gross appearance (color, transparency, viscosity, particulate content, fibrin, and odor) and by correlation with other findings. Expected correlates would include: serous effusion in congestive heart failure and chronic passive congestion of the liver, blood-tinged serous effusion with acute intestinal volvulus, and hemorrhagic effusion in ruptured spleen, purulent effusion and fibrin with peritonitis, food and fiber in gastroenteric perforation, bile and urine accumulation with rupture of the respective bladder, and uterine fluids in rupture of the uterus.

Discolorations. Discolorations of abdominal organs or adjacent body wall are valuable clues to the diagnosis. Segmental strangulation of small intestine produces a telltale congestion of the affected bowel that advances rapidly through the spectrum of reds from an angry pink to a dark liver color within a matter of hours. Thromboembolism of the ileocecocolic artery in the horse, with resultant infarction of ileum, cecum and ascending colon produces the unmistakable grey-green pallor of gangrene of the bowel. Multiple paintbrush ecchymoses under the visceral peritoneum identify the region of a strangulation obstruction of the jejunum. A patch of grey on a greater curvature (antimesenteric border) of the small colon indicates advancing ischemic necrosis occurring in the intestinal wall overlying a chronic fecalith obstruction. A diffuse cyanotic visceral bed heralds the presence of shock. When icterus is detected, a cause should first be sought in the liver and extrahepatic biliary system.

There are notable occasions, however, when discolorations of viscera are not to be expected in the exploratory examination. Prompt operation very early in the clinical course may precede any conspicuous color changes. This is a favorable prognostic sign. Concealed incarcerations of the intestine occur in internal hernias, such as diaphragmatic and epiploic hernias, and in ileocecal intussusceptions, where the intussusceptum is effectively concealed by a normal-appearing intussuscipiens (the cecum). In such cases as these, other criteria must be used for detection of the lesion, since absence of color change is an unreliable basis for decision-making.[2]

Deposits. Perhaps the most common of the serosal and subserosal deposits are fibrin and nodules due to parasitic larval migrations. These may range in distribution from a few isolated foci to such a great number as to give a nodular or shaggy appearance to the bowels. These may constitute an incidental finding, but may point to a less obvious but more serious problem such as verminous arteritis. Certainly, the evidence of past parasitism of clinical proportions in a horse should dictate the careful palpation of the cranial mesenteric artery for size and patency and for pathologic changes.

Peritonitis from causes other than parasites may produce substantial adhesions that obstruct or otherwise interfere with visceral function. Immature fibrinous adhesions and deposits indicate existing or recent peritonitis and may be attended by a purulent or at least turbid peritoneal effusion. Mature fibrous adhesions are evidence of past bouts with peritonitis, but may cause clinical, obstructive lesions.

Deposits of ingesta found on exploratory examination are of grave significance since they indicate either perforation or rupture of the bowel. In isolated instances where the contamination is fairly well localized and the opening in the gut wall can be found and repaired promptly, the patient may survive. The majority of such cases will develop generalized peritonitis with fatal issue.

Multiple, miliary neoformations suggest either diffuse microbial infections such as miliary tuberculosis, or disseminated neoplasia such as mesothelioma or lymphosarcoma. Here, again, careful presurgical cytologic examination of the abdominocentesis specimen is frequently diagnostic in such cases.

METHODOLOGY

In tracing sections of bowel it is generally held that manipulation of the empty segments from distal to proximal is less traumatic than palpating distended bowel. It is also less time-consuming and less fatiguing to the surgeon. In the equine and bovine species, the large intestinal limbs are easily distinguished by their conspicuous identifying characteristics. Not so the greater extent of the small intestine, and in order to start at a known location to ensure progress in the proper direction, the ileum is used as a reference point.

The ileum of the horse is located by exteriorizing the cecum and turning it backward to reveal the dorsal band which bears the ileocecal fold. Tracing this fold downward into the lesser curvature of the cecum will lead shortly to the ileum, which is also exteriorized for visual confirmation. If the problem is with the terminal jejunum or ileum, as is so often the case in small intestinal obstructions, the diagnosis is in hand within minutes after entering the abdomen. Efforts to duplicate this tactic by blind palpation (groping) are nowhere near so reliable or expeditious. The ileum is instantly recognizable by its unique antimesenteric fold and also by its marginal/segmental blood supply as compared to the arcuate pattern found in the jejunum. Therefore, the search is started at this point and continued proximally until the obstruction is reached. In tracing the bowel, an effort should be made to keep track of the length of bowel examined by stripping off a foot at a time, returning the examined bowel to the abdomen as adjacent bowel is brought forth. In this way, if one examines only 10 meters of equine small intestine without finding pathologic change, it is evident that the duodenum has not been reached since the length of the small intestine (in a 450-kg horse) is as much as 21 meters (ca. 70 feet).

It might be rightly argued at this point that much trauma is done and time wasted by stripping many feet of intestine looking for an obstruction that could be found more directly by other means. This may be true in cases where the problem is in the proximal small bowel. Therefore, to retreat slightly to the initial steps of the examination, if the inspection of the ileum and terminal jejunum are unproductive, it may be advantageous to go then to several checkpoints that are sites of common problems. A gentle sweep of the entire abdominal cavity can be made starting with the pelvic cavity and the inguinal rings in the male or the gravid uterus in the pregnant female. Working to the left, the spleen and splenic ligaments are checked; then, the stomach and diaphragm. Moving from left to right, the pylorus and duodenum can be followed to the dorsal area of the fourteenth rib in the right hypochondriac region to check the epiploic foramen. As the duodenum inclines around the mesenteric root from right to left (in the region of the ileum), the cranial mesenteric artery and its branches are close by. It is convenient, in this region, to pass the hand anterior to the mesenteric root and palpate the transverse colon, where antemortem diagnosis can be made only by careful and systematic palpation during exploratory operation. Access to the transverse colon (and also the cranial mesenteric artery) can be expedited by picking up a section of small colon from the left caudal abdomen and following it proximally to the transverse colon. The correct direction in tracing the small colon is quickly determined by observing the gradient of fecal ball formation, harder masses distally, softer proximally.

The senses should be trained to be perceptive of unnaturally hard masses, tense bands, twisted mesenteries, fluid distentions of small intestine, and tympanitic large intestine. A common mistake is to palpate dry, doughy contents in the large intestine in the absence of tympany, and to equate it with impaction (reminiscent of the consistency of an impacted rumen in the cow). Mindful that obstructed large intestine is usually tympanitic (unless in the very early stages), the finding described is typical of the character of large colon contents when the fluid supply from the small intestine has been impeded by an obstruction upstream.

In the bovine, the abomasum may displace to the left of the rumen as far forward as the diaphragm and reticulum and as far posteriorly as the left paralumbar fossa, deflecting the rumen medially and completely away from the lateral wall. Abomasal displacements to the right may be located in the right hypochondriac quadrant between the liver and the thoracic wall, occasionally extending caudally to the paralumbar fossa. Abomasal torsions may be 180° in either clockwise or counterclockwise directions. In addition to the expected abomasal distention and thrombosis, there is also omasal distention. The liver is displaced medially in this case also. Ruminal torsion is rare but has been documented. Cecal dilatation and torsion produce a fullness in the right paralumbar fossa with resonant and fluid sounds detectable on auscultation and percussion.[3,4]

Other pathologic findings on laparotomy in the bovine include: abscesses, adhesions, foreign bodies, hematomas, eventrations, hernias, segmental atony, ulcers, lymphosarcoma, actinomycosis, fat necrosis, obstructions of the bile duct, perimetritis, pyelonephritis, rupture of the urinary bladder, vesical calculi, and torsions, and rupture of the uterus.[3,4]

In the canine where size permits, a ventral (extensile) incision is made large enough to admit the hand. No definitive repair other than hemostasis is attempted until the exploratory has been completed. The falciform ligament is divided to permit palpation and inspection of the liver, gallbladder, bile ducts, and diaphragm. Starting in the left dorsal quadrant of the cranial region of the abdomen, the stomach is palpated from cardia to pylorus, then the spleen and the left lobe of the pancreas. Returning to the pylorus, the duodenum is palpated on the right side, extending distally to the duodenocolic fold. Traction permits exteriorization of the descending duodenum, enabling examination of the right lobe of the pancreas and of the cecum lying just dorsal to the duodenum. At the same time, the right kidney and ureter, and in the female, the right ovary and uterine horn are examined. The mesoduodenum acts as a net to hold the abdominal organs away from the right abdominal wall. In the caudal abdomen, the bladder and urethra and other abdominal components of the genital tract are palpated, i.e., uterus and prostate. Moving to the left side of the caudal and middle abdominal regions, the descending colon is examined and the mesocolon is used to displace viscera away from the left abdominal wall. The left kidney and ureter are examined as well as the left ovary and uterine horn in the female. Finally, the greater omentum is drawn cranially and the entire intestinal tract is inspected.[5,6,7,8]

In the feline, the bladder and colon are examined first, then the uterus and ovaries (in the female) followed by the cecum, visceral lymph nodes, and the small intestine. The spleen is lifted up for examination. The intestines are exteriorized sufficiently to visualize the kidneys and adrenals. Then, the stomach is palpated, and afterward, the pylorus, duodenum, and pancreas. The posterior rib cage is elevated to inspect the liver, gallbladder, and diaphragm. Gentle pressure is applied to the gallbladder to test the patency of the bile ducts.[9]

The foregoing discussion is sufficient to emphasize the need for a routine in the exploratory laparotomy. With specialization and refinement of skills, it is inevitable that the individual will personalize the method, departing somewhat from these descriptions. However, certain truths and principles will prevail. Even if experience is limited to a single species, one is soon impressed with the seemingly endless variety of lesions. As astute as surgical judgment may become, it is impossible to predict the exact nature of more than a few problems, but it is possible to know the normal anatomy and to recognize something gone awry.

Exploratory dissection of lesions is usually best initiated in normal, undisturbed tissue planes or areas of uninvolved organ parts, palpating, visualizing, and mobilizing from distal or peripheral to proximal or central. Diseased organs should be exteriorized when possible. The blood supply should be respected and preserved whenever feasible, and when division or ablation is necessary, the main arterial supply should be controlled before venous occlusion. Of course, when malignancy is suspected, and when en bloc resection is indicated, channels of venous drainage and regional lymphatics would have to be ligated early in the course of dissection.

Proper relationships of organs should be maintained or reestablished by gentle manipulation, lifting instead of pulling, avoiding inordinate or unnecessary tension on mesenteries, exposure of visceral surfaces, desiccation of tissues, abrasion of wound margins, or soilage from internal bowel contents or external body surfaces. Do not waste time after the patient is anesthetized and the abdomen is opened. Paralytic ileus and shock parallel operative time, trauma, hemorrhage, and contamination. In addition to preparedness in the surgery and competency on the part of the team, conservation of time and motion during the exploratory procedure is greatly served by a careful preoperative investigation, so that the surgeon enters the abdomen with reasonable expectations. In this way, an exploratory laparotomy is not a substitute for but a supplement to a clinical examination.

REFERENCES

1. Wingfield, W. E., and Hoffer, R. E.: Chapter 10, The stomach. *In* Current Techniques in Small Animal Surgery. Edited by M. J. Bojrab. Philadelphia, Lea & Febiger, 1975, p. 112.
2. Vaughan, J. T.: Surgical management of abdominal crisis in the horse. J.A.V.M.A., *161*:119, 1972.
3. Fox, Francis H.: Chapter 10, The digestive system. *In* Bovine Medicine and Surgery. Wheaton, IL, American Veterinary Publications, 1970, p. 430.
4. Hofmeyr, C. F. B.: Chapter 11, The digestive system. *In* Textbook of Large Animal Surgery. Edited by F. W. Oehme anf J. E. Prier. Baltimore, MD, The Williams & Wilkins Co., 1974, p. 399.
5. Archibald, J., and Summer-Smith, G.: Chapter 12, Abdomen. *In* Canine Surgery. Edited by J. Archibald. Santa Barbara, CA, American Veterinary Publications, 1974, p. 553.
6. Greiner, T., and Christie, T.: The cecum, colon, rectum, and anus. *In* Current Techniques in Small Animal Surgery. Edited by M. J. Bojrab. Philadelphia, Lea & Febiger, 1975, p. 126.
7. Grier, R. L.: Chapter 11, The intestines. *In* Current Techniques in Small Animal Surgery. Edited by M. J. Bojrab. Philadelphia, Lea & Febiger, 1975, p. 119.
8. Leonard, E. P.: Fundamentals of Small Animal Surgery. Philadelphia, W. B. Saunders Co., 1968, p. 144.
9. Leighton, R. L.: Chapter 21, Surgical procedures of the head, thorax, abdomen, genitals and skin, 2nd ed. *In* Feline Medicine and Surgery. Edited by. E. J. Catcott. Santa Barbara, CA, American Veterinary Publications, 1975, p. 562.

Chapter 10

PRINCIPLES OF SYMPTOMATIC THERAPY IN GASTROINTESTINAL DISEASE

H. FRED TROUTT

Gastrointestinal problems in animals can and will show a diversity of client complaints and clinical signs, as described in Chapter 2. After the physical examination has been completed, one or more problems are usually identified and decisions are made about diagnostic effort and symptomatic therapy.

In reality, therapy of gastrointestinal disorders is an alterable process conducted at the current level of definition of the problem. The more precisely the problem is defined, the more complete the treatment plan (Rx) and the more specific the therapy. Because the ultimate resolution of problems to one or more etiologic diagnoses may be delayed for hours or even days, symptomatic or life-support therapy is essential during the interim. Even if cause is never established, symptomatic therapy can be and often is the key factor in re-establishing homeostatic mechanisms, thus permitting survival of the patient.

Because of the time-pressures of practice, the veterinarian may hurriedly develop the diagnosis (Dx) and begin treatment immediately. Later, the clinician may suffer the acute embarrassment of realizing that both the Dx and Rx are inappropriate because of hasty and ill-founded decisions.

It is advisable, even with gastrointestinal problems requiring immediate intensive care, to collect both clotted and anticoagulant-treated blood samples before beginning therapy. This does not mean that therapy must be delayed pending the results of analysis. However, this approach does offer the opportunity to adjust the Rx later, based on the expanded data base. If the signs are obscure, not life-threatening, and if the patient is stable, it may be entirely prudent to defer all treatment until laboratory analysis is completed.

The clinician must constantly weigh what is medically feasible against what is economically possible, given the prevailing market value or intrinsic value of the patient. These concerns are of importance in all branches of veterinary practice, but are especially so in food animal practice where gastrointestinal disorders are often of herd magnitude, requiring comprehensive and innovative approaches to defining and alleviating the problem and preventing its recurrence.

SYMPTOMATIC TREATMENT

Certain principles should be adhered to in symptomatic therapy of gastrointestinal disorders. These principles are functional; i.e., they are designed to correct the abnormal physiologic function without regard to primary cause. Symptomatic treatment sustains life while diagnostic effort and specific therapy continue. The healing process is usually enhanced by symptomatic treatment.

Relieve Abdominal Distention. The most immediately life-threatening gastrointestinal problem encountered by the veterinarian is acute abdominal distention. Whether encountered in the individual horse, cow, or dog, or as a herd problem in ruminants, rapid action is called for. Gaseous distention requires immediate relief because of its labile character. Fluid distentions are less life-threatening because they increase in severity less rapidly. Solid masses are usually approached at a more measured diagnostic pace.

Physical examination is usually adequate to differentiate gas from liquid or solid (tissue). Observation at a distance, percussion and auscultation, external and rectal palpation, and passage of a tube into the rumen or stomach are the techniques used most often. If free gas is present in stomach or rumen, detection of and relief of gas will occur simultaneously when a tube is passed. Trocarization of the rumen at the left paralumbar fossa is acceptable treatment if the patient is in extremis. If a small trocar or large hypodermic needle is used on the dog with acute gastric dilatation, one must avoid the spleen and other solid organs. Paracentesis abdominis with a large needle will usually aid in detection of and, if advisable, removal of peritoneal fluid.

Correct Fluid and Electrolyte Loss or Imbalance. Diarrhea, vomiting, and sequestration of fluid frequently cause dehydration and electrolyte imbalances. These pathophysiologic changes can be life-threatening, especially if the changes take place rapidly. This is of special importance in the young, which are most susceptible to depletion of extracellular water.

The composition of fluid and the route of administration are based on site of loss or sequestration, serum electrolyte concentration, and acid-base status, as discussed in Chapter 6.

Minimize Contemporary Fluid and Electrolyte Loss. Schemes for fluid and electrolyte therapy must include provisions for fluid maintenance requirements as well as contemporary fluid losses. In many instances, even when adequate replenishment and maintenance therapy are provided, contemporary fluid loss is ignored and a life-threatening situation is left unresolved or may even be exacerbated. Certain practices and procedures can be used in treatment plans to reduce contemporary losses. These include:

1. *Resting the gastrointestinal tract.* The continued intake of food containing osmotically active nutrients and providing direct irritative stimuli tends to increase the severity of vomiting and diarrhea. Fasting the patient for 24 hours or longer is frequently advisable. The intake of liberal amounts of water by animals that are vomiting is likely to perpetuate the problem. However, this can be circumvented or minimized by providing cool water repeatedly in very small volumes, or in the form of ice cubes. Parenteral fluid therapy is an essential accompaniment to resting the gastrointestinal tract; deprivation of water is justifiable only if adequate fluid therapy is being used.

2. *Using the intravenous route.* The intravenous administration of fluid and electrolyte solutions offers certain advantages for patient management. This route permits the rapid dispersion of fluid and electrolytes throughout the extracellular fluid and allows for more precise administration of calculated dosage.

3. *Using the subcutaneous route.* This method for fluid administration is inadequate for replacement of fluid deficits, although it has some merit in maintenance fluid therapy. Only isotonic fluids should be used subcutaneously.

4. *Using the oral route.* Orally administered solutions are most frequently used in the treatment of diarrheal disease in food animal patients. With this approach, an attempt is made to repair deficits and replace contemporary losses. Orally administered electrolyte solutions should contain appropriate concentrations of glucose and sodium. Glucose facilitates the active transport of sodium ion or amino acid and water across the intestinal epithelium into the blood. For practical purposes, the concentration of glucose and sodium in oral electrolyte solutions should be such as to provide 20 to 50 g of glucose and 120 to 140 mEq of sodium per liter of solution.

To minimize contemporary losses, orally administered solutions must contain those elements that are lost from the body. As an example, in diarrhea, considerable amounts of sodium, bicarbonate, chloride, and potassium are lost and must be replaced. To facilitate the preparation of oral solutions, a number of commercial products are available to the clinician.

5. *Correcting abnormal gastrointestinal motility.* Contemporary losses may result from either hypomotile or hypermotile gastrointestinal activity. The correction of hypomotile conditions may be approached, with caution, through the parenteral administration of parasympathomimetic agents or by the use of oral laxative or purgative preparations. The hypomotile rumen sequesters fluid rather than resulting in direct loss from the body. Frequently, the simple administration of warm water by stomach tube is sufficient to effect enhanced ruminoreticular activity in the bovine. Hypermotile activity can be treated with a variety of compounds (see Chapter 18). When hypermotile activity is considered to be the result of gastrointestinal mucosal inflammation, withholding all food and water seems to be the best approach.

In gastrointestinal disease, the use of motility-altering drugs must be approached with caution and then only after a diagnostic plan has been synthesized and at least partially implemented. Depending on the clinical situation, the use of some agents may be contraindicated. Often the treatment plan for diahhrea in calves "automatically" includes the use of an anticholinergic or parasympatholytic drug. The cause of the diarrhea may be a strain of *E. coli* that produces intestinal flaccidity; the anticholinergic drug would therefore actually augment and worsen the pathophysiologic process by delaying the evacuation of both bacteria and toxin from the gut.

Alleviate Visceral Pain. In gastrointestinal disease, visceral pain may be an important component of the disease process. Alleviation of such pain should receive medical priority but may be difficult to accomplish. Every effort must be made to identify and remove its cause. Prior to the removal of the cause, the parenteral administration of analgesic and sedative agents, such as meperidine hydrochloride, dipyrone, and xylazine is indicated.

Provide Nutritional Support. In the treatment of digestive disease, the Rx must often include provisions for the nutritional support of the patient by supplying energy (calories), protein, vitamins, and minerals. The adequacy with which these substances can be supplied and effectively utilized depends on the nature of the problem, its duration, the species of animal involved, and the innovativeness of the clinician.

A caloric deficit will exist in patients experiencing an acute gastrointestinal disorder, especially when this is associated with fluid loss. On a short-term basis, the animal can usually cope with this deficit by utilizing hepatic glycogen reserves and then mobilizing adipose tissue stores. However, in diseases that are more severe and persistent, especially those characterized by fever, pronounced tissue catabolism, and loss of body weight, the demand for both calories and protein can be immediate and substantial.

When possible, nutritional support is best accomplished via the oral route. Anorectic animals of all species can be given nutrients and water by force-feeding or gavage, although vomiting may be difficult to control in dogs and cats following force-feeding. For the equine and bovine patient, a gruel or slurry preparation of the usual ration can be mixed and administered by nasal or oral intubation. In companion animals, such products as commercial pet foods mixed with water in a blender, human baby foods, and human liquid diets can be used. These preparations may be administered two to three times daily with the aid of a large syringe or squeeze bulb attached to tubing of appropriate size and length. Regardless of the species, ease of digestion and minimal gas production are factors to consider in selection of ingredients.

Adjust Rumen and Gastric pH. The development of optimal intraruminal biochemical reactions and the establishment of suitable populations of bacteria and protozoa necessary to provide these reactions depends to a large extent on the maintenance of a relatively narrow range (6.2 to 7.4) of pH.

Protracted anorexia as a consequence of a digestive disorder, a systemic illness, or starvation will depress numbers of rumen organisms. To facilitate the correction of the primary problem or to promote convalescence, it is necessary for the clinician to use means that will enhance the repopulation of the rumen microflora. This can be aided by the administration, by stomach tube, of rumen fluid obtained from healthy animals at the time of slaughter. This approach is often not feasible. However, on the farm, the clinician can obtain sufficient rumen fluid from animals fed a similar ration by using a stomach tube connected to a small aspirator pump. Alternatively, regurgitated boluses can be retrieved from the mouths of healthy, ruminating cattle, squeezed out into a small volume of warm water (37°C), and pumped into the patient's rumen, although it is difficult to obtain an adequate inoculum by this method. When no rumen fluid can be obtained, growth of rumen organisms can be enhanced by obtaining hay chaff from feed bunks or mangers, suspending this in warm water, and administering the suspension by pump or funnel through a stomach tube. Commercial preparations consisting of rumen organisms, yeasts, and substrates necessary to promote the growth of these organisms are available, but seem to offer limited benefit.

For energy purposes, the ruminant depends on the intraruminal production of acetic, propionic, and butyric acids from digestible roughage, with acetic acid predominating. The ingestion of excessive carbohydrate can increase the intraruminal molar concentration of propionic and butyric acids, enhance the production of lactic acid, increase the total acid concentration, reduce intraruminal pH, and depress the numbers of rumen bacteria and protozoa, especially gram-negative bacteria. The net effect of these events is the production of a digestive disorder that can vary from simple indigestion to that severe form classified as rumenitis.

The veterinarian can facilitate the formulation of treatment plans for digestive disturbances in ruminants by simply including the measurement of rumen pH as part of the Dx. A small volume (5 to 10 ml) of rumen fluid can easily be obtained by passing a stomach tube into the rumen and closing off the exterior end. The tube can then be withdrawn and the volume of retained fluid allowed to run into a test tube or small plastic bag. The pH of this specimen, devoid of saliva, can then be determined using commercially available pH indicator paper having a pH range of 4.0 to 9.0. Indeed, a few drops of the fluid can be placed on a glass slide and examined microscopically for protozoa content. If a microscope is not available, the specimen, without shaking, can be examined through direct light to ascertain "brownian activity," which is roughly correlated with numbers of protozoa present.

The pH within the rumen should be adjusted to between 6.2 and 7.4 if it is outside that range. A number of commercially available antacid antiferment agents may be used. The alkalizing agents—magnesium hydroxide, magnesium oxide, or magnesium sulfate—are some of the usual components of these preparations. Sodium bicarbonate (baking soda) can also be used. The amount of alkalizing agent appropriate to the size of the animal should be mixed with warm water to facilitate delivery into the rumen. Two to four liters of water should be used, in most instances. Elevated rumen pH, as might occur from excessive ammonia production, can be depressed by solutions of vinegar or reagent acetic acid. As much as 1 L of 5% acetic acid or its equivalent of vinegar may be needed for effect. After administration of any pH-adjusting solution, the rumen pH should be re-evaluated.

The indications for the usefulness of gastric pH adjustment in companion animals do not appear to be as clear as in man or ruminants. However, based on the definition of the medical problem, which could include analysis of gastric contents at gastroscopy, the clinician may choose to use certain antacids symptomatically in companion animals. These include aluminum salts, calcium carbonate, magnesium oxide, or magnesium hydroxide.

Alleviate Tenesmus. Tenesmus, or involuntary straining, is a clinical sign that is often a manifestation of intrapelvic lesions of the genitourinary tract, less often by an irritative or obstructive lesion of the distal colon or rectum, and occasionally by a neurologic disease. The clinician must define the underlying problem, and if possible, correct it. Symptomatic therapy to alleviate tenesmus must be instituted if possible. Treatments that may be useful include sedation, epidural anesthesia, and rectally administered topical anesthetics.

SPECIFIC EXAMPLES OF SYMPTOMATIC THERAPY

The initial treatments (Rx) described next provide an example of how one might begin treating the patients described in Chapter 5. In addition a complete first-day medical management system (Dx, Rx, and CE) for a field case of neonatal diarrhea in a calf is described under DIARRHEA.

Weight Loss

Case History
   A 9-year-old, 500-kg castrated male Thoroughbred Hunter (Chapter 5).
   1. Weight Loss
      Rx: None

2. Occasional Abdominal Pain
   Rx: Confine to box stall   ☑
        Observe closely for pain   ☑

Discussion
   The problems are of some duration and the Thoroughbred is not acutely ill at the time of examination. There is no evidence of anorexia and the caloric intake for this animal is adequate. The life of the horse does not appear to be in jeopardy. Pain is not detected at this examination. The problem is of a chronic nature that must be defined more thoroughly prior to the establishment of a specific therapeutic plan. Confinement and close observation are in order while awaiting the results of the initial diagnostic effort.

Abnormal Prehension and/or Mastication

Case History
   A crossbred 400-kg Hereford-Angus cow (Chapter 5).
   1. Rapid Weight Loss
      Rx: See dehydration, #5   ☑
   2. Abnormal Prehension
      Rx: None
   3. Ulcers of Lips and Oral Mucous Membranes
      Rx: Procaine penicillin 20,000 IU/kg
           b.i.d. IM   ☑
   4. Ptyalism
      Rx: None
   5. Dehydration, 8%
      Rx: 25 L tepid H_2O (per stomach tube) with
           1 package (227 g) commercially available electrolyte preparation   ☑

Discussion
   The Rx outlined in the case history provides replacement fluid by a physiologic route, promoting rumen activity. Penicillin combats intercurrent bacterial infection in the mouth. Administration of water by stomach tube presumes that the pharynx is not obstructed or severely ulcerated. If severe pharyngeal lesions absolutely preclude passage of the stomach tube, intravenous administration of a balanced electrolyte solution is the best alternative.

   Since the cow will continue to lose weight until she begins to eat and drink, one might add ground grain and protein concentrate to the tepid water and siphon the slurry into the rumen. However, this carries some risk for iatrogenic digestive upset, since the cow is presently on lush grass only. Three or four protein concentrate boluses in place of the slurry might be a suitable compromise for initial treatment.

Dysphagia

Case History

A 4-year-old 20-kg male Bassett (Chapter 5).

1. Dysphagia
   Rx: None
2. Dehydration, 10%
   Rx: Lactated Ringer's solution, 1 L, IV   ☑

Discussion

Venoclysis can be established at the time that anesthesia is induced. One liter of fluid will replace about one-half of the deficit. Only a small contemporary loss (ptyalism) is occurring, and the maintenance requirement is approximately 1370 ml/24 hr, as calculated by the caloric requirement method (Body weight, $kg^{0.75}$ (metabolic body size) $\times$ 145 kcal/kg MBS = $20^{0.75} \times 145$ = 1370 kcal/day). Maintenance water requirement equals 1 ml/kcal.

The oropharyngeal examination will be completed while the fluid infusion is continuing. Additional medical treatments will probably be given, based on the results of that examination. If it is apparent that the patient will not be able to drink water for some time, fluid therapy can be continued to provide the maintenance volume as well. Reassessment of the patient's fluid balance is done several times daily.

Nutrient therapy will almost certainly be needed while the patient is recovering from the effects of the oropharyngeal lesion. While the nutrient formulation to be used will depend partially on the diagnosis and response to therapy, the quantity of calories has been calculated above (1370 kcal/day). High-energy canned dog food can be slurried with water in an electric food blender and delivered to the stomach via tube 3 to 4 times daily. Again depending on the diagnosis, a pharyngostomy feeding tube may be placed to facilitate nutrient therapy and to reduce irritation to the inflamed oropharynx.

Vomiting

Case History

A 6-year-old, 22-kg (obese), spayed female Cocker Spaniel (Chapter 5).

1. Vomiting
   Rx: Atropine sulfate, 0.044 mg/kg
       t.i.d. SC   ☑

2. Abdominal Pain
   Rx: Meperidine HCl, 11 mg/kg t.i.d. IM   ☑
       Gentamicin, 5 mg/kg b.i.d. IM   ☑
3. Dehydration, 8%
   Rx: 0.9% NaCl solution, 1.0 L IV   ☑
       $NaHCO_3$:____mEq/L (based on
       plasma bicarbonate determination)   ☑

Discussion

Atropine is chosen as an antiemetic to avoid the hypotension associated with phenothiazine-derivative tranquilizers. It also reduces pancreatic exocrine secretion. Meperidine HCl has a rather brief duration of measurable analgesic effect, but has been clinically useful in enhancing rest in patients with a syndrome of vomiting, abdominal pain, and dehydration. Gentamicin has a broad spectrum of antibacterial activity. In this instance there is a concern that resident clostridia in pancreas and liver may proliferate as a consequence of pancreatic necrosis, and that bacteria in static, inflamed loops of bowel may invade damaged tissue and cause abscess formation.

Isotonic saline solution is selected as the initial hydrating solution. When 1 liter of fluid has been infused, perhaps in 60 to 90 minutes, the patient's status can be reassessed. Contemporary loss will be more readily estimated after this brief interval of intensive care, and that loss plus the fluid maintenance requirement ($22^{0.75}$ kg $\times$ 145 kcal/kg = 1450 kcal/day, 1 ml H_2O/kcal) may be included in subsequent calculations of volume replacement fluid.

Bicarbonate ion is added on the basis of plasma bicarbonate determination. If the latter test is not available, one might select a balanced isotonic electrolyte solution if the animal appears to be in shock. Acetate and gluconate are metabolized more readily than lactate and are preferred as components of the electrolyte solution. Whichever solution is chosen, additional bicarbonate ion may be indicated if acidosis is severe. The advantage of having the laboratory data on serum concentration of Na^+, K^+, Cl^- and plasma HCO_3^- is that fluid therapy may be more carefully adapted to the needs of the patient. Additionally, some vomiting dogs are alkalotic, and having electrolyte and HCO_3^- values may help the veterinarian avoid the choice of a fluid infusion with components (e.g., HCO_3^-) that are actually contraindicated because alkalosis exists.

Diarrhea

Case History
A 3-year-old Quarter Horse filly (Chapter 5).
1. Diarrhea
    Rx: 1. 4 L mineral oil via stomach tube   ☑
        2. Reduce grain intake to 4
            pounds/day; free choice access
            to hay   ☑
        3. Fresh clean water ad libitum   ☑
        4. Provide fresh water with electro-
            lytes ad libitum   ☑
        CE Client observe horse closely
            while diagnostic workup is
            done. Parasites, bacterial infec-
            tion, and overfeeding are prob-
            able causes.   ☑
2. Depression
    Rx: None

Discussion

There is some concern for grain overload as a cause of the diarrhea; thus the mineral oil is given. The oil promotes evacuation of the bowel. Reducing the grain intake sharply is of importance because it reduces the amount of carbohydrate that enters the cecum and colon. Thus the osmotic load of the large intestine is reduced.

This patient has a large water requirement because of diarrhea. Water must be provided free choice. At times, clients will deprive such animals of water in the mistaken belief that water deprivation will facilitate control of the problem. Water deprivation will only worsen the dehydration, hypovolemia, and metabolic acidosis. Any lessening of diarrhea is hard-won at the expense of further dehydrating the patient. Adding electrolytes to a second volume of fresh water makes electrolytes available on a free-choice basis.

Drug treatment for the diarrhea is probably not indicated until the diagnostic workup has been advanced further. Additional antibiotic treatment for the respiratory disease should be deferred for a day or two while the diagnostic workup for diarrhea is done.

Case History
A 5-day-old, 50-kg Holstein heifer calf.
Neonatal diarrhea is extremely common in calves. This case illustrates how the veterinarian who is knowledgeable about management factors in such a case can provide complete, comprehensive veterinary service.

A 5-day-old Holstein heifer calf weighing approximately 50 kg (110 lb), confined in an elevated wooden crate in a calf-barn with eight other calves, now has profuse diarrhea and is weak.

Narrative History

"We found this calf with watery scours this morning about 7:30 a.m. (it is now 5:30 p.m.) when we were feeding. Diarrhea was just running out of her. She got up slow to suck the bottle but didn't take much of the milk replacer. I gave her a 'scour tablet' (300 mg neomycin sulfate) and took the water out of the crate, thinking she'd come around. This afternoon (4:00 p.m.) when we fed, she didn't get up; we lifted her to the bottle but she kept lying down and wouldn't suck at all."

Direct Questions

Question: "Was this morning the first time you noticed the diarrhea?"

Answer: "No, last night when I checked the calves, I saw that this one was a little 'loose'."

Q: "Did any of the other calves have diarrhea?"

A: "No, I don't believe they did."

Q: "What was the color of the bowel movement last night?"

A: "Well, I'd say it was whitish-yellow."

Q: "Did you see any solid material in it?"

A: "No, it was just a puddle."

Q: "Did it contain any blood?"

A: "I didn't see anything that looked like that."

Q: "Did you take the calf's temperature either last night or today?"

A: "No."

Q: "Who usually feeds the calves and when?"

A: "Usually my wife or I do right after we've finished milking. Yesterday, we had problems with the vacuum pump, and the kids fed them."

Q: "Did you tell them how to feed?"

A: "We were kind of busy, but they help out all the time and know how to do it."

Q: "Where do your cows usually calve?"

A: "Right out in the dry cow pasture. We had to deliver this calf. It was overdue and I had moved the cow into an empty pen in the heifer shed."

Q: "After you delivered the calf, did you help her nurse or give her colostrum?"

A: "No, I wiped her off and made sure she was breathing good. By the time I got cleaned up, the cow was licking her, and she was struggling to get up. She seemed strong, so I left them alone and went to bed."

Q: "When did you move her into the calf barn?"

A: "The following morning after we fed the calves. The cow's udder looked like the calf had nursed, so I put the calf in the barn and gave her a shot of vitamin A."

Q: "In the past, would you say that diarrhea in your calves has been a problem?"

A: "No, we don't have that much of it; we generally do a pretty good job raising calves."

Physical Examination

The depressed calf is lying in sternal recumbency in the crate with her head directed into her left flank. Her tail and rear quarters are obviously wet, as are the floors of the crate and barn immediately behind her. Neither blood nor mucus is observed. Respiratory rate is within normal limits, but an increase in the depth of respiration is evident. Rectal temperature is 39°C (102.2°F). Heart rate is greater than 100 beats per minute and cardiac sounds are loud. With gentle prodding, the calf does rise only to lie down immediately. To facilitate further examination, the calf is removed from the crate and, with assistance, it walks to a corner of the barn.

The skin over the lateral cervical area just anterior to the scapula lacks elasticity. The eyes are slightly retracted into the orbit, and the conjunctival mucous membranes are congested. The color of the oral mucous membranes is normal. Insertion of a finger into the calf's mouth, which feels "cottony," elicits a weak sucking reflex. Her legs are cool, but body surfaces over the thorax, abdomen, and dorsum are warm. The abdomen is normal to auscultation but gentle ballottement and lifting with simultaneous auscultation elicit distinct fluid sounds.

The following problems are identified:
1. Diarrhea
2. Metabolic acidosis (by inference from diarrhea and deep respirations)
3. Dehydration—10%
4. Weakness
5. Depression
6. Inappetence

The first three problems are each of potentially life-threatening severity and will form the working problem list.

1. Diarrhea
   Dx: Fecal culture and antibacterial
   sensitivity   ☑
   CBC   ☑
   BUN   ☑
2. Dehydration
   Dx: Total plasma protein   ☑
   Serum protein electrophoresis   ☑
3. Metabolic Acidosis
   Dx: Serum electrolytes, and plasma
   bicarbonate   ☑

Assessment

The history suggests that the diarrhea may have occurred because of the ingestion of excess food, i.e., an osmotic diarrhea, but rotavirus or coronavirus infection must be considered. However, no other calves have developed diarrhea as yet. At the time of examination the role of a bacterial agent, whether as a primary or secondary cause, is strongly considered. Additionally, the history of isolation tends to reduce the probability of viral or parasitic causes. Fecal culture and antibacterial sensitivity are justified because other calves may become ill subsequently.

Enteropathogenic *E. coli* are common causes of diarrhea in calves and one can prospectively search out the extent of drug resistance by appropriate culture techniques. The CBC increases the data base for interpreting the possibility of bacterial cause or intercurrent infection. The PCV, BUN, and total serum proteins are useful in assessing water balance. Failure of transfer of passive immunity (colostral immunoglobulins) may be inferred from a low total serum protein value. Serum protein electrophoresis provides more precise information concerning the gamma globulin status of the calf. Serum electrolyte determinations are used to determine electrolyte deficits or excesses (osmolality of extracellular fluids). In particular, the bicarbonate determination is employed as an index of acid-base status. Because of the requirement to determine PCO_2 and blood pH as rapidly as possible after collection of blood, these two tests were not done in this case.

Other tests would yield more data right on the premises:
1. plasma bicarbonate determination using a commercially available kit* and

---

* Harleco CO₂ Apparatus Set (64887), Harleco, A Division of American Hospital Supply Corp. Gibbstown, N. J. 08027, distributed through Scientific Products.

2. plasma protein concentration with a total-solids refractometer as an index of gamma globulin values and adequacy of intake of colostrum.

Treatments are listed in original order to maintain consistency for this discussion. However, dehydration is the most important problem for the short term, and fluid therapy should be started immediately.

1. Diarrhea
   Rx: Antibiotic IM   ☑
       Antibacterial p.o.   ☑
       B-complex vitamins IV   ☑
   CE: Management instructions to client   ☑
       a. Withhold milk replacer for 24 hours
       b. Give oral electrolyte solution p.o.
       c. Provide comfort zone for calf
          (1) Bedding   ☑
          (2) Heat lamp   ☑
       d. Confirm appointment for return call and reevaluation
2. Dehydration, 10%
   Rx: Intravenous Fluid
       a. Deficit repair   5.0 L   ☑
       b. Maintenance   2.5 L/12 hr   ☑
       c. Contemporary losses   1.0 L/12 hr   ☑
3. Metabolic Acidosis
   Rx: 270 mEq/NaHCO₃ in IV fluid during
       first 2 hours (see Table 23–4)   ☑

Discussion

Physical examination indicated reduced skin turgor (elasticity), bilateral ocular retraction, cool extremities, and relative dryness of the oral mucous membranes, associated with a weak sucking reflex. These findings are consistent with a clinical impression that the calf is approximately 10% dehydrated. In clinical practice, it is entirely appropriate to express the degree of dehydration in terms of percent body weight. This allows the clinician to calculate immediately the volumes of fluid necessary to effect rehydration. This calculation is accomplished by applying the formula:

Body weight × estimated % dehydration = volume (L)

Utilizing this formula for this calf:

$$50 \text{ kg} \times 0.10 = 5.00 \text{ L} = 5,000 \text{ ml}$$

Hence, to correct the estimated fluid losses in this calf, approximately 5.0 L of an appropriate rehydrating solution must be administered.

In animals experiencing diarrhea, depending on the duration and nature of that diarrhea, there can be significant fecal losses of sodium, potassium, chloride, calcium, magnesium, and bicarbonate. Therefore, because of the type of losses associated with a diarrhea, the solution selected to replace water and electrolyte deficits should be isotonic or mildly hypertonic, containing those electrolytes lost. Additionally, because bicarbonate is lost from extracellular fluid into the feces, the patient with a diarrhea may be metabolically acidotic. The extent of the metabolic acidosis will depend on the severity of the diarrhea and the degree of dehydration. This calf is considered to be acidotic because of profuse fluid diarrhea, 10% dehydration, and the increased depth of respirations.

For this field situation, lactated Ringer's solution was used as the rehydrating solution. This solution is similar in composition to extracellular fluid with regard to sodium, potassium, calcium, and chloride. However, it contains 28 mEq/L of lactate which, if metabolized, provides the same effect as bicarbonate. An acetate-containing fluid would be preferable, since such solutions are considered to be the fluid of choice to restore extracellular deficits when metabolic acidosis is present, or when doubt exists as to the metabolic state. However, for the therapy of metabolic acidosis it is also advantageous to provide bicarbonate directly, as was done in this case. Also, with advanced dehydration in calves, retarded hepatic perfusion may minimize the metabolism of lactate. For these reasons, and with concern for the possible vitamin deficits present, bicarbonate and B-vitamins were added to the rehydrating solution. On an empirical basis, 270 mEq of a commercially available sodium bicarbonate solution is given in the initial hours of therapy. The B-vitamins are administered because of their loss in the fluid feces. Thiamine is particularly indicated to facilitate tissue metabolism of lactate and one may elect to give more thiamine than is contained within the dose of B-complex vitamins.

It must be recognized that this calf could have been transiently hyperkalemic because of H^+ displacing intracellular K^+ into the extracellular fluid, even though total body K^+ was probably depleted due to fecal loss.[1] Because of the danger of cardiotoxicity due to hyperkalemia, the potassium solution for intravenous use should be administered at a rate not to exceed 0.5 mEq/kg/hr.[2]

It is estimated that this calf would require an additional 2.5 liters (approximately 50 ml/kg body weight) of fluid and electrolyte solution to meet maintenance requirements during the ensuing 12 hours. Also, it is estimated that the volume of fluid that might be lost within the next 12 hours as the result of continuing diarrhea will be 1.0 liter.

Hence, the total volume of fluid and electrolytes to be administered over the initial period of therapy is:

For dehydration		5.0 L
For maintenance		2.5 L/12 hr
For continuing losses		1.0 L/12 hr
	Total	8.5 L

It is recognized that, for optimal benefit, the total volume of fluid to effect deficit repair (rehydration) should be administered over a 48-hour period. Eighty percent of the calculated deficit (5.0 L × 0.8 = 4.0 L) plus all of the volumes for maintenance and continuing losses would be administered during the initial 24-hour period. During the second 24-hour period, 20% of the calculated deficit (1.0 liter) and all of the needs for maintenance and continuing losses would be given. However, this plan was not considered feasible for this field situation, because hypovolemic shock was imminent; so in order to restore plasma volume as quickly as possible, 3 liters of the modified lactated Ringer's solution were administered intravenously, with careful monitoring, over a 35-minute period. It has been proposed[2] that isotonic fluids, with a composition similar to extracellular water, can be infused into animal patients with adequate cardiovascular and renal function at a rate of 90 ml/kg/hour, a rate faster than that used here.

The calf was then confined to a small stall ("comfort zone," approximately 2 by 4 feet) constructed from bales of hay and bedded with straw. This comfort zone was made so that the calf could not turn around in it. An indwelling catheter was inserted into the right jugular vein and taped to the calf's neck. The catheter was connected by latex tubing, associated drip-chamber, and screw-type clamp to a glass container (3.8 L) of lactated Ringer's solution suspended above the calf. The flow was adjusted to provide a rate of 30 ml/kg/hour or 1500 ml/hr (30 ml/kg × 50 kg). The client was advised that initial fluid therapy would be done in approximately 3.5 hours and was instructed how to disconnect and remove the catheter.

For additional fluid and electrolyte therapy, a commercial electrolyte preparation containing dextrose was dispensed with instructions for mixing. To this volume of solution, the client was instructed to add one level tablespoonful of sodium bicarbonate (baking soda) at each feeding to provide additional bicarbonate intake. Approximately 1.3 L of this solution was to be administered orally, with the aid of a bovine esophageal feeding tube, at 11 p.m. and the same amount at 8 a.m. the following morning. The remaining 1.3 L with two level tablespoonsful of sodium bicarbonate was dissolved in a 10-liter pail of water and offered as the only source of drinking water.

In order to rest the intestine by minimizing the opportunity for increased intraintestinal osmotic pressure and direct mucosal irritation, the client was specifically instructed not to feed the calf milk or milk replacer. Apprehension on the part of the farmer as to "starving" the calf was at least partially alleviated by a brief description of the possible pathophysiologic consequences associated with feeding; i.e., a worsening of diarrhea, and by the statement that the clinical condition of the calf would be reevaluated the next morning. At this juncture, it was learned that the milk replacer contained both neomycin and chlortetracycline.

A heat lamp was carefully and safely arranged over the calf's comfort zone to reduce chilling. The calf received an intramuscular injection of a broad-spectrum antibiotic. It was administered to counteract the suspected coliform infection and to forestall potential complications such as polyarthritis and meningitis resulting from a gram-negative bacteremia. A like volume was dispensed to the client with instructions to administer it subcutaneously at 11 p.m. A nitrofuran preparation suspended in a small volume of lactated Ringer's solution was given orally by intubation. This preparation was also dispensed with instructions to incorporate it into the fluid and electrolyte solution given at 11 p.m.

The use of oral antibacterial preparations in cases such as this is debatable. However, it was incorporated into the Rx because:
1. The cause of the diarrhea was considered to be an infectious bacterial agent.
2. The calf had been previously exposed to two antibiotics as feed additives; i.e., neomycin and chlortetracycline. These agents could have influenced alteration of the bacterial flora of the intestine, particularly the induction of resistance factors.
3. There was no history of previous treatment with a nitrofuran.
4. Nitrofurans have antibacterial activity against gram-negative organisms.

In the vast majority of diarrheal diseases in calves, symptomatic therapy routinely includes the use of orally administered antibacterial preparations which may include a number of ingredients, including antispasmodics. Veterinarians and producers frequently ascribe a high degree of effectiveness to antispasmodics in controlling diarrhea. However, transient removal of the ration-substrate, e.g., milk or milk replacer, for approximately 24 hours and oral administration of an electrolyte solution containing dextrose is fully as effective. With respect to diarrhea caused by certain enteropathogenic serotypes of *E. coli,* intestinal flaccidity may be a factor in the pathogenesis of the diarrhea. In these circumstances, antispasmodic agents could be contraindicated. This needs investigational clarification.

Experience indicates that oral antibacterials seem most effective when given early in the course, before the diarrhea is severe. However, experience also indicates that oral antibacterial preparations need not be used routinely to effect control. Whether the clinician decides to use symptomatic oral antibacterial therapy or not, the decision should be made from a data base that includes adequate history, thorough physical examination, knowledge of the pathophysiologic mechanisms involved, and concern for potential consequences.

Abdominal Pain

Case History

A two-year-old 500-kg Quarterhorse stallion (Chapter 5).

Comment

It is assumed that reflux of gastric contents did not occur on passage of the stomach tube.

Rx: 1. Administer via stomach tube:
Mineral oil, 4 L　　　　　☑
2. Dipyrone, 7500 mg IV　　☑
3. Confine to box stall　　☑
4. Wrap legs　　　　　　☑
CE instructions to owner　☑
a. Observe closely　　☑
b. Prevent rolling　　☑
c. Contingency plan as problem is more defined:　☑
Establish plan to combat shock　☑
Consider need to control infection　☑
Consider need for surgical intervention　☑

Discussion

The agents advocated for administration by stomach tube are used primarily to promote movement of fecal material and to facilitate diminution of intestinal gas. The volume administered should be adjusted so that overdistention of stomach does not occur. Because the causes of the problems have not yet been defined, extreme caution must be exercised in the selection of chemical agents that will stimulate intestinal motility. Mineral oil is a mild, safe laxative that does not irritate the intestine nor is it absorbed from the intestine.

The control of pain is essential and the analgesic selected should have little, if any, hypotensive effect.

Efforts must be exerted to prevent the patient from rolling, which could precipitate an intestinal crisis; hence the animal should be confined and continually observed. The legs are wrapped to minimize edema of the limbs. Traditionally horses demonstrating evidence of abdominal pain (colic) are "walked." This approach often leads only to fatigue of both the patient and the handler.

With problems similar to this one, the clinician often vacillates between a course of immediate surgical or medical intervention, and a course that essentially "bides time" while awaiting resolution of the problem. In these situations, repeated evaluation of the patient's physical condition is essential. It is advocated that as the decision process evolves, the veterinarian should be planning for alternative medical-surgical therapies. Hence, the concern for listing contingencies as a portion of the plan for client education.

Abdominal Distention

Case History

A 400-kg feedlot steer (Chapter 5).

The physical examination may make it possible to localize the cause of abdominal distention to either the digestive or urinary tract. If the urinary system is intact, as observation suggests, one will provide symptomatic therapy while the digestive tract is investigated further.

The following treatment plan is used, with variations to fit individual cases, as initial therapy for rumenitis with metabolic (lactic) acidosis.

1. Abdominal Distention
Rx: Rumenotomy　　　　　　　☑
Re-inoculate the rumen　　　☑
10 L lactated Ringer's IV　　☑
480 mEq (40 gms) NaHCO$_3$ in Ringer's solution　　　☑

454 g NaHCO₃ in rumen ☑

Dexamethasone 20 mg IM ☑

Antihistamine IV ☑

Oxytetracycline 4 g IV ☑

Thiamine HCl 2 g IV ☑

2. Depression

   Rx: See dexamethasone, above

3. Anorexia

   Rx: Grass hay and fresh water, free choice ☑

   CE: Advise client as to follow up treatments and make arrangements for reevaluating the patient. ☑

Discussion

The client will have made the decision to treat or slaughter the steer when the physical examination is completed. One should, in such instances, defer antibiotic treatment for those few minutes that it takes most clients to make that decision.

The decision to treat the patient having been made, the Rx outlined previously is carried out to minimize or reverse the metabolic aberrations associated with severe rumenitis.

Rumen acidity is drastically increased initially because of increased molar concentrations of the volatile fatty acids and then by the increased production of lactic acid. The concentration of hydrogen ions produced is, in large measure, responsible for an increase in intraruminal osmotic pressure. Elevated rumen osmotic pressure in turn is responsible for dehydration. Histamine is produced, at times in relatively large concentrations. As populations of gram-positive bacteria proliferate, gram-negative populations diminish and endotoxin is released. Lactates are absorbed but slowly from the rumen.

The net effect from the overall process on the patient is dehydration, acidosis, and a tendency to develop endotoxic shock. Chemical rumenitis with infectious sequelae can develop early in the disorder.

The sequence of biochemical and pathologic events forms the basis of the treatment plan. Thiamine hydrochloride (1 g IV) is employed in an attempt at favorably influencing the tissue metabolism of absorbed lactates. After rumenotomy and the use of alkalizing agents such as sodium bicarbonate, rumen inoculation is essential in order to re-establish the microbial flora and to facilitate convalescence.

REFERENCES

1. Donawick, W. J., and Christie, B. A.: Clinicopathologic Conference. J.A.V.M.A. *158*:501, 1971.
2. Finco, D. R.: General guidelines for fluid therapy. J.A.A.H.A. *8*:166, 1972.

Section Two

GENERAL TOPICS
IN
VETERINARY GASTROENTEROLOGY

Chapter 11

COMPARATIVE ANATOMY

WESLEY D. ANDERSON
BETTINA G. ANDERSON

ORAL CAVITY AND ASSOCIATED STRUCTURES

The oral cavity is the first portion of the alimentary tract. It communicates with the exterior at the *rima oris* or oral orifice where it is encircled by the upper and lower lips which form the margins of the rima oris and meet laterally at the *angle of the mouth*.

The oral cavity is divided by the upper and lower teeth and the alveolar processes of the maxilla and mandible into the *vestibule* and the *oral cavity proper*. In the vestibule there is a small eminence located opposite the crown of one of the upper cheek teeth through which the duct of the parotid gland opens; and located in the ventral midline of the vestibule is a fold of mucous membrane, the *frenulum*, which extends from the upper and lower lips to the adjacent gum.

The oral cavity and pharynx are best examined in the living animal or in the non-embalmed state. When studying this region of the body using embalmed specimens, median and parasagittal sections provide the most meaningful type of exposure.

In the at-rest state the upper and lower teeth are likely to be separated slightly from each other, the tongue at least partially in contact with the palate. The vestibule is then obliterated by the lips and cheeks, which lie against the teeth and gums.

The oral cavity communicates caudally with the *pharynx* through the *isthmus faucium*, which is merely the dividing line between mouth and pharynx.

The *cheek* is that lateral portion of the oral cavity that extends back from and is continuous with the lips. Many small glands are located in the mucous membranes of the lips, termed *labial glands*, and in the cheeks, termed *buccal glands*. These tiny glands empty their secretions directly into the space of the vestibule.

The muscle of the cheek is the *buccinator*. It is strengthened by a firm fascial layer, with the sub-cutaneous tissue and skin external to it and mucous membrane located internal to the buccinator muscle. External to the buccinator muscle at the rostral border of the masseter muscle lies a pad of fat, the *buccal* or *suctorial fat pad*.

The Floor of the Mouth

Although the term "the floor of the mouth" may be used to mean different things, in all cases it applies to the floor of the oral cavity proper and does not include the vestibule. The floor of the mouth consists of the *tongue*, its downward reflections of *mucous membrane*, and the *muscles and associated structures* that fill the mandibular space. All structures combined are usually spoken of as the "lingual region."

The Tongue

The tongue, situated in the front of the mouth between the two mandibular rami and supported by the sling-like arrangement of the mylohyoid muscle, has a shape which in general corresponds to that of the lower jaw. It consists of a mucosa which contains cornified, stratified squamous epithelium and a carpet of papillae which are projections of the submucosa and lamina propria covered by the epithelial cells (Figs. 11–1 and 11–2).

The *dorsum of the tongue* is the upper flat surface which is in contact with the palate when the mouth is closed. In the dog it has a well-developed *median sulcus*, which extends from the caudal *root* over the *body* (forming the bulk of the tongue) and terminates near the *apex* or rostral free portion of the tongue. The sulcus is only present on the apex of the equine tongue, and instead of a depression, there is a raised ridge on the tongues of bovine and porcine species. The cord-like palpable *lyssa*, the "worm under the tongue" of the dog, is of historic rather than clinical interest.

Mucous Membrane, Papillae, and Taste Buds. The mucosa is thickest on the dorsum of the tongue

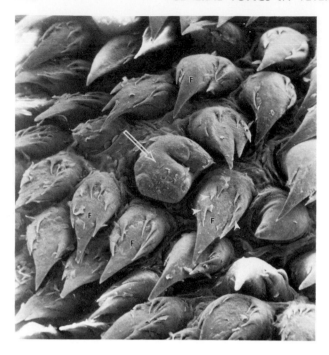

Figure 11–1. Scanning electron micrograph (65×) of the *dog* tongue shows caudally directed filiform (F) papillae each with major and minor apices (arrow heads). A fungiform papilla (arrow) is centrally located.

where the greatest contact with food occurs. There are numerous papillae, named for their shapes, chiefly located on the dorsum of the tongue, but some are also located on its lateral surfaces.

Filiform and fungiform papillae appear in all species. The filiform papillae cover the greater part of the dorsum and body of the tongue (Figs. 11–1 to 11–3). In the bovine species, fungiform papillae are especially prominent on the sides of the tip of the tongue and are found on the dorsum scattered among the numerous filiform papillae. In the horse, the fungiform papillae are scattered over the dorsum of the apex and the lateral surfaces of the body.

The *foliate papillae* are found along the lateral surface of the root of the tongue just rostral to a thick fold of mucosa which connects the root of the tongue with the ventral surface of the soft palate, called the *palatoglossal arch*. They are prominent in the horse, dog, and pig and rudimentary in cattle. In the horse, the foliate papillae form a rounded eminence about an inch long which is indented by a transverse fissure, while in the dog the papillae are in two groups of eight to twelve each, located on the dorsolateral surface at the base of the tongue.

Vallate (circumvallate) papillae are present in all species but are most numerous in those that lack

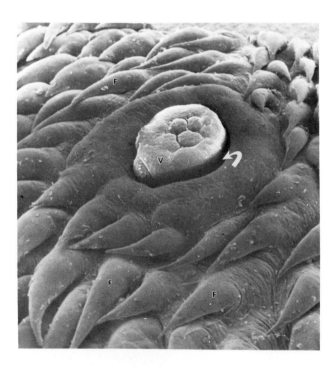

Figure 11–2. A scanning electron micrograph (62×) of the tongue of the *dog*. Filiform papillae (F) encompass a large vallate (V) papilla. The lingual epithelium around the papilla is raised such as to leave it surrounded immediately by a deep furrow (arrow).

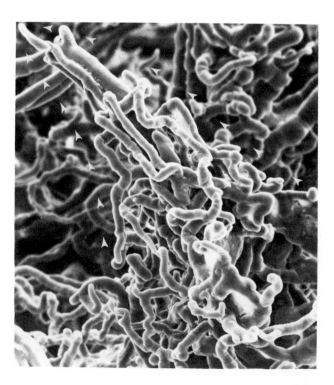

Figure 11–3. A scanning electron micrograph (400×) from a methyl methacrylate cast of the *cat* tongue. The cast demonstrates the core of vessels located within each filiform papilla (outlined in arrows).

foliate papillae. In the dog they number four to six and are present in the form of an inverted letter V on the dorsum of the tongue at the junction of the caudal one-third with the rostral two-thirds of the tongue (Fig. 11–2). The papilla at the apex of the V is absent in the dog. The vallate papillae in the horse are only two or three in number and are also located on the dorsum of the root of the tongue. In the bovine species, there are eight to seventeen vallate papillae on the prominence of the dorsum of the root of the tongue.

Conical and lenticular papillae are scattered among the smaller and more pointed filiform papillae as large, broad, cornified structures. The *conical* papillae have pointed tips directed toward the pharynx, while the *lenticular* papillae have rounded or flattened tips and are present only in ruminants.

Neuroepithelial cells associated with taste are called *taste buds* and are present in the crypts of some papillae. They are present on the dorsal surfaces of fungiform papillae, on the sides and dorsal surfaces of the vallate papillae, and on the free surfaces and the epithelial surface facing the crypts of the foliate papillae. Taste buds are usually not described for the filiform papillae.

Frenulum Linguae. The *frenulum linguae* is a fold of mucous membrane that passes from the ventral portion of the free part of the tongue, the apex, downward to its attachment on the floor of the mouth.

Muscles of the Tongue. The *intrinsic muscles* of the tongue are those that have their entire course within the substance of the tongue, and consist of a system of fibers that are not attached to the bones of the head. The fibers course in longitudinal, perpendicular, and transverse directions. Although they are four in number, they are grouped together and called merely intrinsic muscles of the tongue. The function of the intrinsic muscles of the tongue is to alter the shape of the tongue, such as rotating its tip upward and sideways, to make the dorsum concave or convex, to narrow and elongate the tongue, or to flatten and broaden it.

The *extrinsic muscles* of the tongue are three pairs located on each side of the tongue, originating from the skeleton and entering the tongue from behind and below. The muscles blend with the fibers of the intrinsic muscles inside the tongue. A thin, median *lingual septum* divides the tongue into symmetrical halves.

The *genioglossus* is a flat, fan-shaped muscle that lies next to the median plane and is separated from its fellow on the opposite side by the lingual septum. Its ventral margin is tendinous and extends from the incisive part of the mandible to the hyoid bone. From the tendinous margin the muscle bundles enter the tongue from below in a fan-shaped fashion. The action of the caudal portion of the genioglossus is to protrude the tongue, while the rostral part may retract the tongue or assist in curling it downward as in drinking.

The *styloglossus* muscle is long and slender and originates as a flat tendon from the ventral end of the stylohyoid bone. The muscle enters the tongue from behind, runs forward in the lateral part, and ends at the apex of the tongue. When the two styloglossus muscles act together, they shorten the tongue and elevate its apex; when acting singly, the tongue is rotated laterally.

The *hyoglossus* muscle lies ventrolateral to the root of the tongue and is inserted between the genioglossus medially and the styloglossus laterally. The hyoglossus originates from the basihyoid bone and its lingual process (when present) and also from the thyrohyoid bone. Its fibers enter the root of the tongue from behind and extend into the apex. Contraction of the hyoglossus causes the tongue to be drawn caudally. With the hyoid bone fixed, simultaneous action of the hyoglossus and genioglossus muscles will depress the tongue.

Innervation of the Tongue. The *hypoglossal nerve* is motor to all intrinsic and extrinsic muscles of the tongue.

General sensory innervation to the mucosa of the tongue is chiefly by way of the following nerves: the lingual branch of the *trigeminal nerve* innervates the rostral two-thirds of the tongue; sensory fibers in the *glossopharyngeal nerve* supply most of the caudal one-third of the tongue; and the *vagus nerve* supplies small portions of the caudal surface of the tongue.

Gustatory fibers are special visceral afferent fibers which mediate taste. They have their nuclei of origin in the nucleus of the fasciculus solitarius in the medulla oblongata and pass to taste buds in the caudal one-third of the tongue by traveling in the *glossopharyngeal nerve* and to the taste buds in the rostral two-thirds by fibers of the chorda tympani portion of the *facial nerve*.

Salivary Glands (Fig. 11–4)

These glands drain into or near the floor of the mouth, even though they are not all located therein.

Parotid Gland. The parotid gland in all species more or less fills the *retromandibular fossa,* the depression caudal to the ramus of the mandible and ventral to the wing of the atlas. It is least extensive in the dog and cat and far more extensive in the

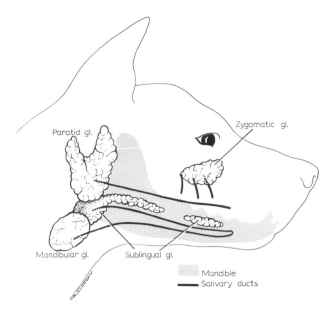

Figure 11–4. Salivary Glands of the Dog.

horse. Dorsally, the gland is in contact with the base of the ear and ventrally it extends into the intermandibular space or into the neck region for varying distances.

The color of the parotid gland depends on its functional state and will change with the amount of blood present in the gland. It does, however, always remain a lighter shade of red than the adjacent skeletal muscles.

Shape. The parotid gland of carnivores is small and triangular. The apex is directed ventrally and covers only a small portion of the mandibular gland. Preauricular and postauricular processes of the basal portion surround the base of the auricular cartilage. In the horse the gland fills the retromandibular fossa completely. Its dorsal end is at the base of the ear; the ventral end is wider and fills the angle between the linguofacial and external jugular veins. In cattle the gland is somewhat club-like in its appearance and the thicker end is directed toward the ear.

Relations. The relations of the parotid gland become important in surgical procedures involving the gland. In all species, the lateral surface of the gland is covered by fascia and by the parotidoauricularis muscle. The medial surface is closely related to a number of important structures, especially the common carotid artery and external jugular vein and their branches. In addition, branches of the facial and trigeminal nerves, lymph nodes, and the hyoid apparatus with its related muscles are all in the vicinity.

In the dog the parotid gland is related medially to the facial nerve, maxillary artery and vein, and parotid lymph node.

In the horse, the ventral border of the gland follows the linguofacial vein and the maxillary vein passes through the gland. Medially, the gland is related to both carotid arteries, cranial nerves VII, IX, X, and XII, and several groups of lymph nodes (parotid, medial and lateral retropharyngeal and the cranial cervical nodes).

Parotid Duct. The *parotid duct* is formed by the union of numerous radicles within the parotid gland.

The parotid duct has a different course in small animals as compared to the large animal species. In the dog it extends across the surface of the masseter muscle between the dorsal and ventral buccal branches of the facial nerve and enters the vestibule of the buccal cavity by passing through the buccinator muscle and buccal mucosa near the fourth upper cheek tooth.

In the large animal species the duct extends along the medial surface of the mandible and around its ventral border in company with the facial artery and vein. Subsequently it ascends along the rostral edge of the masseter muscle and passes under the facial vessels to open into the buccal vestibule opposite the upper third cheek tooth in the horse and the fifth in cattle.

Sublingual Gland. The *sublingual gland* in all species lies between the mylohyoideus muscle and the lateral surface of the tongue. It is divided into caudal and rostral parts. In the dog, the *caudal (monostomatic)* part overlies the rostral belly of the digastricus muscle and is closely associated with the duct of the mandibular salivary gland. This portion is absent in the horse. The *rostral* part of the sublingual gland is called *polystomatic* since it discharges directly by means of a number of ducts which open on the floor of the oral cavity; the openings of ducts are grossly visible and are located on a fold of mucous membrane.

Mandibular Gland. In the dog, the *mandibular gland* is round and closely associated with the caudal part of the sublingual gland. In the equine species, this gland is elongated and semilunar in shape. It extends from the atlantal fossa rostrally and ventrally to the intermandibular space.

In cattle, the gland extends from the atlantal fossa to the basihyoid much as in the horse, almost touching the ventral end of the gland of the opposite side.

The *mandibular duct* passes rostrally from the mandibular gland, crosses the digastricus muscle, and then passes deep to the mylohyoid muscle to open on the *caruncula sublingualis*, located on either side of the ventral attachment of the median frenulum of the tongue.

Zygomatic Gland. In the dog, a large, well-defined *zygomatic salivary gland* is present in the rostral part of the pterygopalatine fossa. Superficially it is covered by the zygomatic arch, masseter and temporalis muscles. The gland may have as many as five ducts which open near the last upper cheek tooth, one of which is nearly as large as the parotid duct.

Buccal Glands. In the horse, the buccal glands are in two rows. The *dorsal* glands lie on the outer surface of the buccinator muscle and are partially hidden by the masseter muscle, while the *ventral* buccal glands extend from the angle of the mouth to under the masseter. The small ducts of the buccal glands open between the papillae on the oral mucosa of the cheek. In carnivores the dorsal buccal glands are represented by the zygomatic glands.

In cattle the buccal glands may be divided into three groups; *dorsal, middle,* and *ventral.* The dorsal group extends from the angles of the mouth a short distance under the masseter muscle. The middle glands are loosely arranged along the dorsal border of the ventral glands, which extend from the angle of the mouth at the level of the lower cheek teeth to the rostral edge of the masseter.

CLINICAL CONSIDERATIONS—SALIVARY GLANDS

In the dog, cysts are said to be the most common lesions affecting the salivary glands. They result from blockage of a portion of the duct system and may occur in the floor of the mouth (called a ranula) or within the parenchyma of the gland, necessitating surgical excision of the involved tissues in the subcutis ventral to the mandible, or in the cranial cervical region.

The Roof of the Mouth

Hard Palate

The hard palate intervenes between the nasal and oral cavities and is necessary for proper swallowing. The hard palate is bounded laterally and rostrally by the upper dental arch. Its thick mucosa is rich in venous plexuses; it is continuous laterally with the gums and caudally with the mucous membrane of the soft palate. The hard palate is divided into two symmetrical halves by a median palatine raphe which usually takes the form of a shallow groove; however, in the dog, the median raphe forms a slight ridge.

On either side of the palatine raphe are the transversely directed palatine ridges. In the horse,

the ridges of the hard palate are concave caudally and have a gradual rostral slope and a steeper caudal slope. In the bovine species, the crests are studded with caudally directed cornified papillae, and rostrally the incisors and upper canine teeth are replaced by a modification of the hard palate, the *dental pad.* The number of palatine ridges differs with the species: the dog has 6 to 10 pairs, cattle 15 to 20, and the horse 16 to 18. In the horse, the palatine ridges extend to the soft palate, while in other species the caudal portion of the hard palate is smooth.

Generally speaking, the *mucosa* of the hard palate is without glands; however, palatine glands are found in the caudal portion of the hard palate in the dog and in ruminants. The palatine mucosa may be more or less pigmented (black) in all domestic animals. The central prominence just behind the upper incisors in non-ruminants, or just behind the dental pad in ruminants, is the *incisive papilla.* Two minute openings of the incisive ducts are found on the papilla in most species except the horse.

The hard palate functions in the separation of nasal and oral cavities and with its ridges, it assists the tongue during prehension and mastication and also in moving the bolus into the oropharynx.

Soft Palate

The soft palate extends into the pharyngeal region, dividing its rostral portion into a nasal part, the *nasopharynx,* and an oral part, the *oropharynx.* The most caudal part of the soft palate usually lies against the ventral surface of the apex of the epiglottis. The *uvula,* well developed in primates, is not prominent in domestic animals, although a rudimentary one may be seen in ruminants and swine.

The two mucosal folds that connect the root of the tongue with the soft palate form the palatoglossal arch, while the palatopharyngeal arch is located more caudally and attaches the free border of the soft palate to the pharynx. Between the two arches is a fossa in which lies the *palatine tonsil.*

Muscles of the Soft Palate. The palatine muscles are composed of muscle bundles extending on each side of the midline from the palatine bones to the caudal border of the soft palate. When they contract, they shorten the soft palate.

The *levator veli palatini muscles* extend from the petrous part of the temporal bone and the auditory (eustachian) tube to the caudal midline of the soft palate where they unite. Their action is to raise the soft palate during swallowing.

The *tensor veli palatini muscles* also extend from the petrous part of the temporal bone and the lateral lamina of the auditory tube as well as the pterygoid bones, around the hamulus of the pterygoid bones. Their tendons end by expanding into an *aponeurosis* of the soft palate and function in tensing the soft palate.

CLINICAL CONSIDERATIONS—PALATE

Due to the length of the soft palate in the horse, its elevation above the level of the opening into the larynx is a difficult process; therefore nasal breathing is virtually obligatory in this species.

The Fauces

The aperture by which the mouth or oral cavity proper communicates with the pharynx is called the *isthmus faucium* or the *pharyngeal aditus* and its lateral walls are spoken of as the *fauces*. Its dorsal wall is the caudal portion of the soft palate, while on the lateral pharyngeal wall is the palatoglossal arch and ventrally the root of the tongue.

The Pharynx

The pharynx is a funnel-shaped, musculomembranous passage that connects the oral cavity with the esophagus and the nasal cavity with the larynx. The concave *roof* of the pharynx is related to the base of the cranium and to the rectus capitis ventralis and longus capitis muscles.

In the dog and cat, the pharynx extends caudally as far as the second cervical vertebra, while the pharynx of the horse is expanded from the base of the cranium by the guttural pouches. The pharynx of ruminants is relatively short and does not extend caudally beyond the base of the skull.

The lateral walls of the pharynx are related to the stylohyoid and pterygoid muscles, and also to the guttural pouches in the horse. The floor of the pharynx extends from the root of the tongue over and around the laryngeal entrance to about the level of the cricoid cartilage of the larynx.

Divisions (Fig. 11–5)

The rostral portion of the pharyngeal cavity is divided by the soft palate into dorsal and ventral channels, the *nasal part, nasopharynx* and the *oral part, oropharynx* respectively. The narrower, caudal portion of the pharyngeal cavity is the *laryngeal part* or *laryngopharynx*.

Mucous Membrane and Fasciae

The *mucous membrane* lining the nasopharynx is similar to that of the respiratory region of the nasal cavity. It is vascular and slightly folded; it contains

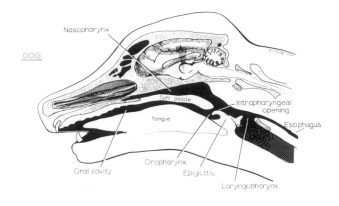

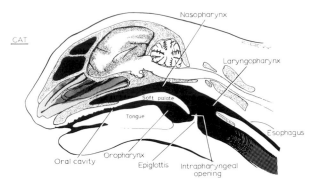

Figure 11–5. Divisions of Pharynx—median sagittal section. (Modified from Nickel et al.[1])

glands and regional accumulations of lymphoid tissue; and it has a ciliated pseudostratified columnar epithelium. In acute and chronic catarrhal disease, it secretes an obnoxious serous or mucoid discharge from its many glands. The mucosa of the oropharynx and laryngopharynx is similar to that of the oral cavity in that it contains glands but it has a stratified squamous epithelium. At the entrance to the esophagus, the mucosa overlies extensive venous plexuses. The *fascia* between the mucosa and the pharyngeal muscles is thin, while the fascia on the outside of the pharyngeal muscles is much thicker.

The Oropharynx. Although this portion of the pharynx is a part of the alimentary canal, it also serves as a passageway for air when the animal coughs or breathes through its mouth. The oral part of the pharynx extends from the pharyngeal entrance at the level of the palatoglossal arch, to the base of the epiglottis. Its roof is formed by the soft palate and its floor is the root of the tongue. When the animal breathes through its nose, which it does most of the time, the ventral surface of the soft palate is in contact with the root of the tongue and the lumen of the oropharynx is obliterated. During swallowing, however, the palate is lifted away from the tongue and the bolus can pass through the oropharynx.

The Nasopharynx. The nasal part of the pharynx is part of the respiratory channel. It lies dorsal to the soft palate and extends from the conchae (turbinates) to the epiglottis. In the bovine species, the nasal septum is continued into the nasopharynx as the *pharyngeal septum*, which divides the dorsal part of the nasopharynx into right and left recesses. The pharyngeal septum is high in the calf and somewhat lower in adult cattle.

Auditory Tube and Guttural Pouch (Horse). The auditory tubes connect the nasal part of the pharynx with the tympanic cavity, the cavity of the middle ear. The pharyngeal openings or ostia of the auditory tubes are small slits located in the caudal part of the nasopharynx, and close to the pharyngeal ostia are patches of lymphoid tissue called *pharyngeal* or *tubal tonsils*. When the pharyngeal (tubal) tonsils are enlarged in children, they are referred to as *adenoids*.

In the horse, and all members of the family Equidae, the ventral part of the auditory tube is extensively dilated and is called the *guttural pouch.** Each pouch is a large mucous sac situated between the base of the cranium and the atlas above, and the nasopharynx below. Medially the two pouches are in apposition in part but are to some extent separated by the intervening ventral straight muscles of the head. Each pouch is related dorsally to the base of the cranium, the atlanto-occipital joint capsule and the ventral straight muscles, and ventrally the two pouches lie on the pharynx and the origin of the esophagus. Each guttural pouch communicates with the pharynx through the pharyngeal ostium of the auditory tube, and its mucous membrane is in direct continuity with the mucous membrane of the auditory tube. The average capacity of each pouch is about 10 fluid ounces, but the two pouches are often unequal in size.

The inner lining of the guttural pouch is a delicate mucous membrane which is in general rather loosely attached to the surrounding structures, and its epithelium is pseudostratified columnar with cilia, similar to that of the respiratory system. The mucous membrane is supplied with glands, chiefly of the seromucous and serous type, and also contains numerous lymph nodes, especially in the foal.

CLINICAL CONSIDERATIONS—GUTTURAL POUCH

Because of the similarity in the morphology of the mucous membrane in the auditory

---
*Officially called the *diverticulum of the auditory tube*.

tube and the nasopharynx, inflammation of the pharynx and auditory tube may extend into the guttural pouch. Swelling of the auditory tube and the location of its pharyngeal ostium in the nasopharynx often interfere with drainage during inflammatory processes. The pouch may be entered surgically for purposes of drainage through Viborg's triangle. The triangle is located by compressing the external jugular vein to distend the linguofacial vein, which is the ventral boundary of the triangle. Then palpate the ramus of the mandible and the tendon of the sternocephalicus muscle, which are the rostral and dorsal boundaries respectively of the triangle.

The Laryngopharynx. The laryngopharynx is common to both the respiratory and digestive channels. It is the caudal continuation of the oral part of the pharynx and extends from the base of the epiglottis to about the level of the cricoid cartilage. In the dog, the laryngopharynx is unusually long and much of it overlies the larynx. It contains the rostral parts of the larynx which project rostrodorsally from the floor; on each side of the base of the epiglottis are the *piriform recesses* which continue the floor of the oropharynx around the entrance into the larynx.

CLINICAL CONSIDERATIONS—LARYNGOPHARYNX

In the normal breathing position, the soft palate lies apposed to the dorsum of the tongue. The rostral portion of the larynx protrudes through the intrapharyngeal opening, thus largely obliterating the laryngopharynx. Liquids such as milk or saliva in the newborn may pass from the mouth to the esophagus through the piriform recesses without the normal swallowing movements.

Pharyngeal Muscles

The pharyngeal muscles are striated and are grouped as either pharyngeal constrictor or pharyngeal dilator muscles. They function in the swallowing reflex, and therefore are not entirely under direct voluntary control. Except for the caudal stylopharyngeus, which is a dilator, the pharyngeal muscles are constrictors and are all inserted dorsally on the pharyngeal raphe.

Although the pharyngeal constrictors can be subdivided into distinct muscles, common usage is to call them merely *rostral, middle,* and *caudal pharyngeal constrictor muscles.*

The *rostral pharyngeal constrictors* are the palatopharyngeus and the pterygopharyngeus muscles. The *palatopharyngeus* lies medial to the tensor veli palatini muscle. Most of its fibers arise from the soft palate and sweep obliquely upward and backward over the pharynx to the mid-dorsal line. The *pterygopharyngeus* arises from the hamulus of the pterygoid bone, passes backward lateral to the levator veli palatini muscle, and continues over the pharynx to be inserted on the mid-dorsal raphe.

The *middle pharyngeal constrictor* is the hyopharyngeus. The *hyopharyngeus* attaches to the caudal end of the thyrohyoid bone and the fibers of both sides pass over the larynx and pharynx to insert on the dorsal raphe of the pharynx.

The *caudal pharyngeal constrictors* are the thyropharyngeus and the cricopharyngeus muscles. The *thyropharyngeus* lies on the larynx and pharynx just caudal to the hyopharyngeus muscle. It arises from the thyroid cartilage. The fibers spread out over the dorsal surface of the pharynx and insert on the median dorsal raphe of the pharynx, just caudal to the hyopharyngeus muscle. The *cricopharyngeus* lies on the larynx and pharynx immediately caudal to the thyropharyngeus muscle. It arises from the lateral surface of the cricoid cartilage and passes upward to be inserted on the median dorsal raphe.

The *dilator of the pharynx* is the *stylopharyngeus*. It arises from the medial surface of the dorsal third of the stylohyoid, passes rostroventrally between the hyopharyngeus and the caudal pharyngeal constrictors, and ends in the lateral wall of the pharynx.

Innervation

The nerves to the pharynx are derived from the pharyngeal plexus formed by the union of the glossopharyngeal and vagus nerves. The vagus and glossopharyngeal nerves are motor to all the muscles of the pharynx except the stylopharyngeus and to most of the soft palate with the exception of the tensor veli palatini muscle. The stylopharyngeus is innervated by the glossopharyngeal nerve, and the tensor veli palatini is innervated by the trigeminal nerve.

The sensory supply to the pharyngeal mucosa is by way of the trigeminal, glossopharyngeal and vagus nerves. The trigeminal and glossopharyngeal nerves innervate the mucosa of the nasal part of the pharynx, while the glossopharyngeal supplies the oral part and the vagus the laryngeal part of the pharynx.

Lymphatic Tissue of the Pharynx (Tonsils)

Lymphatic tissues are found as more or less organized accumulations in several places in the pharyngeal mucosa. These accumulations may take the form of diffuse, unorganized lymphocytic infiltrations, which appear in certain areas only to disappear later; or they may take the form of permanent solitary lymph nodules, or of small or large aggregates of such lymph nodules which may be surrounded by a connective tissue capsule. When large numbers of lymph nodules combine with diffuse lymphatic tissue, they form independent lymphatic organs known as *tonsils*.

There are two types of tonsils: follicular and nonfollicular. In the *follicular tonsils*, the lymphatic follicles may be present singly, separated from each other by connective tissue as is the case in the *lingual tonsil* of the horse; on the other hand, the follicles may be closely packed into a solid mass of lymphatic tissue which usually lies exposed on the wall of the pharynx. Only the *tonsillar sinus* of the *palatine tonsil* in ruminants, however, opens on the pharyngeal wall; the rest of the tonsil lies embedded in the wall of the pharynx.

The *nonfollicular tonsils* have their lymphatic portions deep to the epithelium of the pharynx, either lying within a tonsillar fossa or just under the mucosa of the pharyngeal wall.

The Five Groups of Tonsils in Animals. The *lingual tonsil* is located in the mucosa of the root of the tongue. In the dog and cat, there are no tonsillar follicles, only areas of diffuse lymphoid tissue and solitary nodules; while in the bovine and equine species, there are numerous large tonsillar follicles with distinct fossulae.

The *palatine tonsils* are located either on or in the lateral wall of the oropharynx. These tonsils are follicular in *large animal* species; they are absent in the pig. In the dog, the palatine tonsil is a nonfollicular, cylindrical mass on the lateral wall of the oropharynx lodged in a tonsillar fossa and covered medially by a semilunar fold. In the bovine species, the palatine tonsil is a follicular, spherical tonsil, embedded in the lateral wall of the oropharynx in the underlying musculature and connective tissue. The fossulae open into a branching tonsillar sinus. In the horse, the palatine tonsil is a large follicular tonsil lying on the surface of the pharyngeal wall between the base of the epiglottis and the palatoglossal arch.

The *tonsil of the soft palate* lies on the ventral surface of the soft palate. In the dog, only small amounts of diffuse lymphoid tissue or isolated lymph nodules are noticeable; while in the equine and bovine species, flat follicular tonsils, median in position, are found.

The *pharyngeal tonsil* is located in the roof of the nasopharynx. In the dog it is a flat nonfollicular tonsil between the openings of the auditory tubes. In the bovine species it is an irregularly raised nonfollicular tonsil on the caudal end of the pharyngeal septum, while in the horse it is a follicular tonsil between the openings of the auditory tubes.

The *tubal tonsil* lies in the lateral wall of the pharyngeal opening of the auditory tube. This tonsil is absent in the dog, flat and nonfollicular in ruminants, and present only as small amounts of diffuse lymphoid tissue in the horse.

CLINICAL CONSIDERATIONS—TONSILS

Both follicular and nonfollicular tonsils have a connective tissue capsule and are well supplied with blood vessels. They have efferent lymphatics, which carry lymph away from the tonsil toward more centrally located lymph nodes. The tonsils, more than the solitary lymph nodes, are an important defense against microorganisms; they produce lymphocytes which participate in the production of antibodies.

Functional Anatomy of Swallowing[1] (Fig. 11–6)

Deglutition, or swallowing, is a complex activity which causes a bolus of food to be transferred from the oral cavity through the pharynx into the esophagus and finally into the stomach. This se-

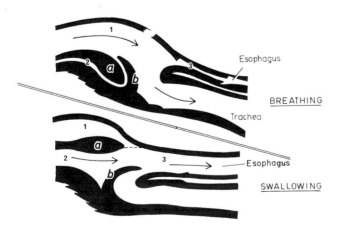

Figure 11–6. Pharyngeal cavity of dog during nasal breathing and swallowing—schematic sagittal section. (Modified from Nickel et al.[1])

quence of events may be divided into two *stages,* the first of which is voluntary and the second reflex.

During the first, *voluntary stage* of deglutition, the bolus or fluid is pressed into the oropharynx by a wavelike pressure of the tongue caudally progressing against the palate. The successful accomplishment of this action requires that the mouth be closed. The passage of the bolus is facilitated by the caudally directed filiform papillae and by the palatine ridges.

The second, *involuntary* or *reflex stage* of deglutition begins as the bolus enters the oropharynx. In order to convey the bolus toward the esophageal entrance, the pharynx must change its shape in such a way as to prevent the escape of the bolus through any of the other pharyngeal openings such as the nasopharynx or the larynx, or to re-enter the oral cavity.

The first action that occurs in this space is the elevation of the soft palate by the levator veli palatini and tensor veli palatini muscles. The oropharynx is then tightly closed by the raised root of the tongue pressing against the ventral surface of the soft palate. For this to occur the hyoid bone is moved forward and upward by the hyoid muscles and the digastric and rostral pharyngeal constrictor muscles.

The forward and upward movement of the hyoid apparatus also draws the larynx cranially. As the larynx moves forward with the hyoid bone, the cranial parts of the larynx are tucked under the elevated root of the tongue and the epiglottis is pressed like a lid over the laryngeal aditus. With the forward movement of the larynx, the esophageal entrance is dilated and pulled toward the oncoming bolus. If the bolus is fairly liquid, it is divided by the epiglottis and much of it passes along the piriform recesses. If the bolus is coarse or insufficiently insalivated, it passes directly over the epiglottis and is pressed into the esophagus by the action of the pharyngeal constrictors. Liquids or semifluid boluses may be propelled by the plunger-like action of the tongue with such force that they are hurled through the pharynx and even through the esophagus, making active constriction of these structures superfluous.

After swallowing, the soft palate, the hyoid bone, and the larynx return to their normal breathing positions, and air can once again pass freely through the intrapharyngeal opening into the larynx.

THE TEETH

Teeth are derived from epithelial and connective tissues and are hard, white or yellowish structures implanted in the alveoli of the bones of the jaws. Functionally the teeth serve mainly as organs of prehension and mastication.

Structure of Simple (Brachydont) Teeth (Fig. 11–7)

The *pulp* is the soft, gelatinous tissue located in the central part of the tooth, the *pulp cavity*. The pulp contains vessels and nerves which enter or leave through the apical foramina located at the *apex of the root*. The *dentin*, which is modified bone, forms the bulk of the tooth, while the *enamel*, the hardest substance of the body, covers the dentin from the neck of the tooth to the exposed tip. The portion of the tooth referred to as the *cementum*, is a bone-like tissue without haversian canals which covers the dentin at the level of the root. The root of the tooth is attached to the alveolus by a connective tissue periodontal membrane.

Each simple tooth has three parts: the *crown*, which is the exposed part of the tooth; the *root*, the embedded part of the tooth; and the *neck*, the demarcation between these two parts which is located at the gum line.

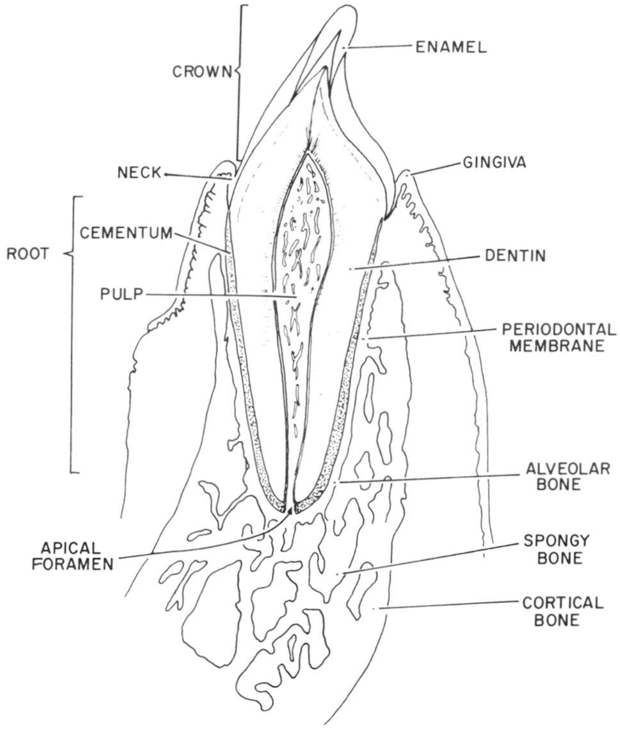

Structure of Complex (Hypsodont)*
Teeth in the Horse

Although reference is found in the literature to the "crown," "reserve crown," and "neck" of equine teeth, there is no clear, distinct demarcation between the crown, neck, and root in this species. Instead there is merely a long *body* and a very short *root* or *roots*. The body of the hypsodont tooth has a free portion, which protrudes from the gum, and an embedded portion, commonly called the "reserve crown." With wear of the occlusal surface, the "reserve crown" erupts from the gum line and is then the free portion of the body of the tooth. The root is usually short and has within it an apical foramen or foramina.

In addition to the differences between simple and complex teeth mentioned previously, in the horse the incisor, premolar, and molar teeth have cementum and enamel extending the entire length of the tooth. Also in hypsodont teeth the enamel and cementum are invaginated into the central part of the equine incisor teeth forming the *infundibulum* or "cup." The infundibulum is also present as rostral and caudal infundibula on the occlusal surfaces of premolar and molar teeth. The presence or absence of infundibula of the lower incisor teeth in the horse is used as a guide in estimating age. With age, the

Figure 11–7.   Sagittal Section of Dog Canine Tooth.

occlusal surface wears away and with it also the infundibulum.

Surfaces of Simple and Complex Teeth

The *buccal* (vestibular) *surface* is the outer or lateral surface, while the *lingual surface* is the inner, *medial surface* related to adjacent teeth, and the *occlusal* (mastication) *surface* is the surface facing the opposite dental arch. The *labial surface* is that surface facing the lips.

Incisor Teeth

The incisor teeth are located in the rostral part of the mouth and have their roots embedded in either the incisive bone or mandible. Each tooth possesses one root in all species.

In ruminants* only lower incisors are present. They have a distinct neck and a loose periodontal membrane which allows a small amount of movement within the alveoli. In the horse, the incisor teeth are complex teeth, with invaginated enamel and cementum forming infundibula.

The incisor teeth of the pig are separated somewhat from each other and the upper incisors are

---

*From the Greek meaning "high crowned." Prism-shaped teeth with high crowns, as in the horse.

---

*Upper incisors are not present in ruminants and are replaced by a *dental pad*.

smaller than the lower ones. The incisor teeth of the dog have tubercles on the occlusal surface; the upper incisors have three tubercles, of which the central is the highest, while the lower incisors have two tubercles.

Canine Teeth

The canine teeth (a term not specific for this species) are located behind the incisors in the interdental space. The upper canine tooth is situated at the junction of the incisive and maxilla bones, while the lower canine tooth is relatively closer to the corner incisor. Each canine tooth has a single, long root.

In the male horse, there are four canine teeth, while in the mare they are usually absent or rudimentary. In the ruminant the canine teeth are absent.* In the male pig, the canines or *tusks* are greatly developed and project out of the mouth, while in the sow they are much smaller.

Premolar and Molar Teeth ("Cheek Teeth")

Located caudal to the canine teeth, the premolar and molar teeth, commonly referred to collectively as "cheek teeth," are embedded in the maxilla of the upper jaw and the mandible of the lower jaw.

The Horse. The upper and lower cheek teeth are divided into four premolar (the first of which generally does not develop) and three molar teeth.

Occasionally a rudimentary first upper premolar is present, commonly referred to as the "wolf tooth." When present, it is usually small and drops out when the animal is young, and is not replaced. The first premolar in the lower jaw does not erupt. The second premolar is the first well-developed cheek tooth. In the upper jaw, the last three or sometimes last four cheek teeth project into the maxillary sinus.† The first and last upper cheek teeth have three roots while the rest have three or four. The first five lower cheek teeth have two roots and the last one commonly has three. The vestibular edges of the upper cheek teeth and the lingual edges of the lower cheek teeth are prominent and sharp and may interfere with mastication.

Ruminants and Swine. The cheek teeth of the ruminant resemble those of the horse, but are smaller and also differ in that they progressively increase in size from the first to the sixth. The cheek teeth of the pig have complex tuberculate crowns and the first premolar of both jaws is small; in the

lower jaw a space exists between the first and second premolar, while in the upper jaw the first premolar is close to the second.

Dog. There are four premolar teeth on each side in the upper and lower jaw. The premolars have all erupted by 4 to 5 months, and by 5 to 6 months all but the first premolar has been replaced. The first cheek tooth is the second premolar because the first premolar is not replaced in the permanent dentition. In the upper jaw, the first cheek tooth has one root; the second and third have two; and the rest have three. In the lower jaw, the first and last cheek teeth have one root and the rest have two. The *carnassial* or sectorial teeth are the upper fourth premolar and the lower first molar. They are the largest cutting teeth of the upper and lower jaw and are adapted for tearing the food. The upper carnassial tooth may become involved with root abscesses.

Dental Formulae (Table 11–1)

The teeth are arranged in upper and lower dental arcades or arches. As the teeth of the two sides of each jaw are usually similar in number and character, it is possible to express their arrangement in a dental formula. The domesticated animals, like man, have two sets of teeth. The teeth of the first set appear during early life and are known as *deciduous* or temporary teeth, and are later replaced by the *permanent teeth*. The molar teeth in domesticated animals do not have deciduous predecessors.

THE ESOPHAGUS

The esophagus is a muscular tube which functions to convey swallowed food and drink from the laryngopharynx to the stomach. Its anatomic features are described in Chapter 21.

---

*Some authors consider the fourth incisors in the lower jaw as canine teeth; however, this is not generally the accepted concept.
†Of importance when surgically removing infected cheek teeth in the horse.

Table 11–1. Dental formulae for permanent teeth in domestic animals

Horse	$2 \left(I\frac{3}{3} \ C\frac{(1)}{(1)} \ PM \ \frac{3 \text{ or } 4^*}{3} \ M\frac{3}{3} \right)$
Cow Sheep Goat	$2 \left(I\frac{0}{4} \ C\frac{0}{0} \ PM \ \frac{3}{3} \ M\frac{3}{3} \right)$
Pig	$2 \left(I\frac{3}{3} \ C\frac{1}{1} \ PM \ \frac{3}{3} \ M\frac{3}{3} \right)$
Dog	$2 \left(I\frac{3}{3} \ C\frac{1}{1} \ PM \ \frac{4}{4} \ M\frac{2}{3} \right)$
Cat	$2 \left(I\frac{3}{3} \ C\frac{1}{1} \ PM \ \frac{3}{2} \ M\frac{1}{1} \right)$

*Four if P_1, the wolf tooth, develops.

ABDOMINAL AND PERITONEAL CAVITIES, MESENTERIES, AND OMENTA IN DOMESTIC ANIMALS

Abdominal Cavity

The abdomen is the region of the body which extends from the caudal portion of the diaphragm to the inlet of the pelvis. It possesses two cavities, the *abdominal cavity*, which is defined as the space enclosed by the fascial lining of the abdominal wall, the transversalis fascia; and within the abdominal cavity is the abdominal portion of the *peritoneal cavity*. The remainder of the peritoneal cavity is located within the caudal extension of the abdominal cavity proper, the *pelvic cavity*.

The *abdominal cavity* contains the gastrointestinal tract and its accessory organs (liver, gallbladder, and pancreas) and the spleen, as well as some of the urogenital organs such as kidney, ureter and variable amounts of the urinary bladder, endocrine glands (suprarenal) and nerve plexuses. Its cranial boundary is the muscular and tendinous sheet which separates the abdomen from the thoracic cavity, the diaphragm; laterally and ventrally it is bounded by muscles and aponeuroses, forming the abdominal wall; and dorsally by the sublumbar muscles, lumbar vertebrae and intervertebral discs.

Peritoneal Cavity

The *peritoneal cavity* is merely the space between the *parietal* and *visceral peritoneum*, and contains no organs but rather just enough peritoneal fluid to lubricate the two serosal surfaces mentioned previously. This cavity, however, is the more important of the two (abdominal and peritoneal) to the veterinarian; in order to gain access surgically to the organs of the abdomen, the abdominal cavity must first be entered; and then by cutting the "glistening" parietal peritoneum, the peritoneal cavity is entered. Since the abdominal cavity does not have a serous lining, it is not subject to infections as is the peritoneal one (peritonitis), nor can it serve to absorb injected fluids as can the peritoneal cavity. The peritoneal cavity is the largest of the four serous cavities into which the primitive celomic cavity of the body is subdivided. It, and the digestive organs with which it is associated, largely fills the abdominal cavity.

The supporting walls of the peritoneal cavity are therefore those of the abdominal and pelvic cavities; the diaphragm cranially, structures associated with the pelvic floor caudally, and the muscular and bony walls of the abdomen and pelvis in between. A thin layer of connective tissue with a mesothelial surface lines the peritoneal cavity and is called *peritoneum*. Similar layers line the other celomic derivatives, the two pleural cavities and the pericardial cavity.

The *peritoneum* may be conveniently thought of as forming a closed sac, with its dorsal wall invaginated by the digestive system. The part that remains in contact with the body wall is the *parietal peritoneum;* the remainder is the *visceral peritoneum*. The peritoneum may be divided in two additional parts; that which lies directly on the gut, the *serosa*, and a double-walled fold, the *mesentery*, which extends from the parietal peritoneum to the serosa and transmits vessels and nerves to the gut.

From what has been said concerning the peritoneal cavity, it should be clear that no organ is actually within it. The distinction between a *retroperitoneal organ* (literally, one behind the peritoneum) and organs *with mesenteries* refers to the extent to which they are surrounded by the cavity. Those organs that have a mesentery are almost completely surrounded by the cavity, and the only possible surgical approach to them is through the peritoneal cavity. Those that are retroperitoneal are adjacent to the cavity only on their ventral surfaces; they can be approached surgically without entering the peritoneal cavity, although often the peritoneum is so tightly attached to their ventral surfaces that a transperitoneal approach is necessary.

CLINICAL CONSIDERATIONS—PERITONEAL CAVITY

The size of the peritoneal cavity is usually exaggerated in diagrams for clarity; actually, the digestive tract is so long and convoluted that it largely fills the abdominal cavity, and the walls of the peritoneal cavity are everywhere in contact with each other. Thus, unless it is enlarged by an accumulation of fluid or by opening during an operation, the cavity is slit-like throughout and contains only enough fluid to moisten its walls. It is not so much the size of the peritoneal cavity but, rather, the enormous surface of its walls that is important. This warm, moist surface provides not only an excellent breeding ground for certain types of bacteria, but also a large area through which toxins can be absorbed, a combination accounting for the seriousness of peritonitis.

The Mesentery

That portion of the *mesentery* that extends from the gastrointestinal tract to the dorsal abdominal wall is the *common dorsal mesentery* (also called "great mesentery") and the site where it attaches is the *root of the mesentery;* the mesentery that extends from the stomach, duodenum, and liver to the ventral abdominal wall in the fetus is the *ventral mesentery.* This mesentery in the adult is reduced in size and its remains are called the *falciform ligament.*

The subdivisions of the common dorsal mesentery are named according to the organs to which portions of the mesentery attach. They are: mesogastrium, mesoduodenum, mesentery proper (jejunum, ileum), mesocolon and mesorectum. The mesocolon is further subdivided according to the part to which it attaches (e.g., the *ascending mesocolon* attaches to the ascending colon).

The mesentery has been defined as a double layer of peritoneum enclosing blood vessels, nerves, and a variable amount of fat and extending from the gastrointestinal tract to the partietal peritoneum; another double layer of peritoneum which also carries vessels and nerves (and fat deposits) but passes from the stomach to another abdominal organ is the *omentum.*

Greater and Lesser Omenta and Omental Bursa

In all species of animals, the *omentum* is divided into the *greater* and *lesser* omenta. The *lesser omentum,* a derivative of ventral mesogastrium, is merely a double layer of peritoneum enclosing vessels, nerves, and a variable amount of fat, which extends from the lesser curvature of the stomach and first part of the duodenum to the porta of the liver (porta hepatis). The term *ligament* (actually it is a *visceral ligament* as compared with collagenous ligaments in the limbs and back which extend between bones and are relatively avascular) is applied to portions of both the lesser and greater omenta.

The *greater omentum* is a derivative of the dorsal mesogastrium of the fetus. It has three subdivisions named for organs to which it is attached.

1. The part of the greater omentum extending between the stomach and spleen is the *gastrosplenic (gastrolienal) ligament.*

2. That part from the stomach to the diaphragm is the *gastrophrenic ligament.*

3. The part of the greater omentum extending from the diaphragm to the spleen is the *phrenicolienal ligament.*

The *lesser omentum* may be divided into two ligaments: the *hepatogastric,* extending, as the name suggests, from liver to stomach; and the *hepatoduodenal,* from liver to duodenum.

The *omental bursa* is merely a space located within the peritoneal cavity itself, but separated from it except for one opening, the *epiploic foramen,* which is situated dorsocranially between the liver and the duodenum with the caudal vena cava located dorsally and the portal vein below.

Abdominal Regions[2] (Fig. 11–8)

The abdomen can be divided into nine regions by extending two imaginary transverse planes and two sagittal planes through the body (Fig. 11–8).

The cranialmost transverse plane extends through the caudal borders of the costal arches just in front of the umbilicus. The caudalmost transverse plane passes from one side of the abdomen to the other at the level just ahead of the wing of each ilium. The two sagittal planes extend from approximately each mid-inguinal region in straight lines cranially through the costal arches.

As a result of subdividing the abdomen in this manner, nine regions become apparent. They are:

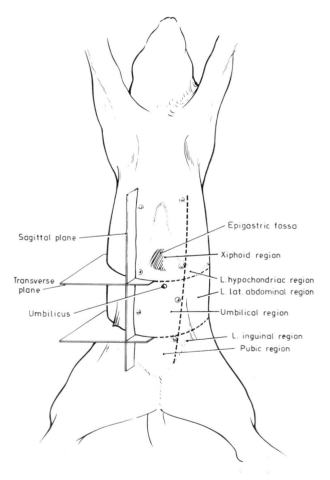

Figure 11–8. Regions of the Abdomen. (Redrawn from Miller et al.[2])

right and left hypochondriac regions and xiphoid region; right and left lateral abdominal regions and umbilical region; right and left inguinal regions and pubic region.

ALIMENTARY CANAL AND ACCESSORY DIGESTIVE ORGANS IN DOMESTIC ANIMALS WITH SIMPLE STOMACHS

The *liver* lies chiefly on the right side of the abdomen and against the diaphragm. The *gallbladder*, a green-colored structure shaped like a small pear, is partially hidden between the right and left lobes of the liver. It is not present in the horse.

The *spleen* (lien) lies on the left side of the body protected in part by the ribs and is in contact with the stomach and diaphragm. The spleen is attached to the greater curvature of the stomach by a portion of the greater omentum, the *gastrosplenic (gastrolienal) ligament*.

The *stomach*, which may be filled with ingesta or empty and contracted, is situated chiefly in the xiphoid region. It is connected to the liver by the *lesser omentum*, and extending from the lower border of its greater curvature is the *greater omentum*.

The *small intestine* can be exposed by reflecting the portion of the greater omentum which covers it. The small intestine is divided into three parts: (1) *duodenum*, most proximally; (2) *jejunum;* and (3) *ileum*.

The *large intestine* is divided into *cecum, colon, rectum,* and *anal canal*. The *cecum* is generally considered to be the first part of the colon; however, in the dog and cat, it is a diverticulum of the colon as the ileum communicates directly with the ascending colon. The cecum of the horse is a large structure approximately 1 meter (3 feet) long and occupies a large area on the right side of the abdominal cavity. The cecum of *cattle* arises at the ileocolic junction and ends blindly to the right of the pelvic inlet.

The *colon* in all species of animals is divided into *ascending, transverse, descending,* and *sigmoid* portions. In the dog and cat, it is the least complicated of all the species, while in the horse, the huge ascending colon is modified into the *great colon,* which in turn is divided into a right and left dorsal and ventral colon and associated flexures. The coils of the descending (small) colon in the horse lie dorsal to the left portions of the great colon and are closely associated with the small intestine. In ruminants the ascending colon is also modified producing a spiral colon of considerable length (nearly 10 meters long in cattle). It is in the form of coils and loops located between the layers of mesentery to the left of the cranial mesenteric vessels. In swine, the colon is also spiral; the coils adhere together and extend from the xiphoid caudally into the right and left lateral regions.

DEVELOPMENT OF THE STOMACH AND INTESTINE OF SIMPLE STOMACH DOMESTIC ANIMALS (Fig. 11–9)[3]

In early development, the gut is a simple tube approximately the same length as the abdominopelvic cavity. It is suspended from the dorsal abdominal wall by a double fold of peritoneum, termed the *dorsal mesentery*. The *ventral mesentery* is shorter than the *dorsal mesentery* and attaches only the stomach to the ventral abdominal wall. Early in development, the digestive tract becomes too long for the abdominal cavity and thus bulges into that part of the coelom which lies in the base of the umbilical cord, forming a simple loop at this point. The first stage in rotation of the stomach and intestinal tract is a 90° rotation to the right. Although the intestine will continue to undergo further rotation, this is the only rotation that the stomach will normally undergo. The distal colon likewise essentially undergoes no further rotation. The second stage in rotation involves principally the midgut loop, small intestine, and the future ascending and transverse colon. As room develops in the abdominal cavity, the loop of gut that has protruded at the umbilicus will gradually return into the abdominal cavity and in the process will undergo an additional rotation of 180° to the right, thus making a total rotation of 270° for that portion of the intestinal tract mentioned previously and 90° rotation for the stomach and distal portion of colon. The intestinal tract now assumes its normal postnatal position of cecum and ascending colon on the right, transverse colon crossing to the left and descending colon on the left side of the body. Anomalous or abnormal development can result in: (1) abnormal narrowing of a tubular structure, or *stenosis;* (2) transposition of one or more parts to opposite sides of the body, situs inversus; (3) lack of development, *congenital intestinal atresia;* (4) sacculation of ileum, a persistent yolk sac, known as *Meckel's diverticulum*.

Postion and Form of the Stomach, Duodenum, and Pancreas

The Stomach (Fig. 11–10)

The stomach is an irregular dilatation of the digestive tube which lies caudal to the diaphragm and the liver and mostly to the left of the midline.

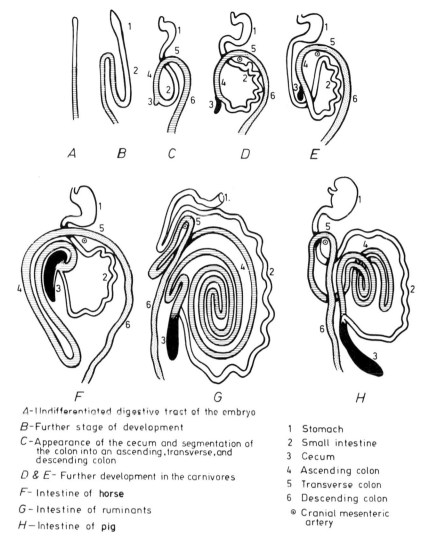

A—Undifferentiated digestive tract of the embryo

B—Further stage of development

C—Appearance of the cecum and segmentation of the colon into an ascending, transverse, and descending colon

D & E— Further development in the carnivores

F— Intestine of **horse**

G—Intestine of **ruminants**

H—Intestine of **pig**

1 Stomach
2 Small intestine
3 Cecum
4 Ascending colon
5 Transverse colon
6 Descending colon
⊚ Cranial mesenteric artery

Figure 11–9.   Schematic Representation of the Development of the Intestine. (From Kitchell et al., 1960—unpublished.[3])

The stomach is divided into several parts: a cardiac part, a fundus, a body, and finally, a pyloric part. In swine there is an exaggerated muscular portion which protrudes into the pyloric canal called the torus pyloricus.

Curvatures and Surfaces. The stomach has greater and lesser curvatures and parietal and visceral surfaces. The *greater curvature* of the stomach is its most ventral portion and is related to the spleen, while its *fundus* is related to the left kidney. Caudally, the stomach is related to the left lobe of the pancreas and the greater omentum, which separates it from the coils of the intestine. The cranial surface of the stomach is designated the *parietal surface,* and the caudal surface is its *visceral surface.*

Position and Attachments. When examining the stomach, one notes that it lies caudal to the liver and cranial to the coils of the small intestine; also that the attachment of the greater omentum is from the dorsal body wall ventrally to the greater curvature of the stomach and onto the pyloric extremity of the duodenum, where the greater omentum is continuous with the mesoduodenum. When the stomach is pulled away from the visceral surface of the liver, the lesser omentum may be seen; and when the liver is pulled away from the diaphragm, the remnants of the falciform ligament below the caudal vena cava, and on the ventral body wall cranial to the umbilicus, are visible. On the right side, the caudal free border of the lesser omentum can be seen extending from the liver to the pyloric extremity of the intestine. Just above this free

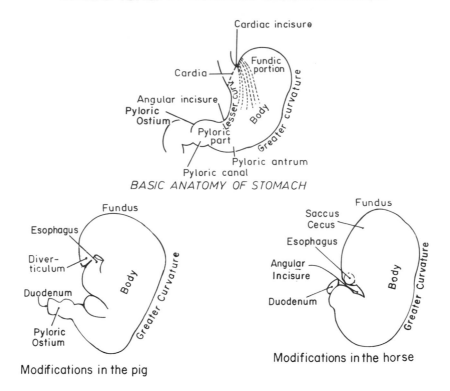

Figure 11–10.   General Form of the Stomach in Nonruminant Animals.

border, between the liver and the place where the greater omentum and mesoduodenum are continuous, is the *epiploic foramen*.

External Surface (Fig. 11–10). *Horse* (Fig. 11–10). The equine stomach is generally similar externally to the stomach of other simple stomach quadrupeds. The chief difference in the equine stomach is in the expanded fundus, the "saccus cecus," and in the *angular incisure*, that notch on the lesser curvature which is more pronounced in the horse than in other simple stomach animals.

Pig (Fig. 11–10). The stomach of the pig differs externally from the dog and horse in that there is a *gastric diverticulum of the fundus*. The diverticulum projects to the right, and is separated from the fundus of the stomach by an annular groove.

Dog and Cat. The non-engorged stomach has a semilunar shape with greater and lesser curvatures. The *greater curvature* extends from the junction of stomach with the esophagus to the junction with the duodenum. The concave *lesser curvature* of the stomach has an indentation called the *angular incisure*. The *fundus* is the portion of the stomach which protrudes upward from the body and joins the cardiac part, and the *body* of the stomach is its central portion; the *cardiac part* of the stomach is that portion closest to the esophagus. The pyloric

part of the stomach is that portion near the duodenum and consists of the *pyloric antrum and pyloric canal*. The *pylorus* is the sphincteric termination of the stomach which joins the duodenum, and the opening at the pylorus is called the *pyloric ostium*.

CLINICAL CONSIDERATIONS—STOMACH, DOG AND CAT

The shape and position of the stomach of the dog and cat is dependent upon the degree of fullness; when the stomach is relatively empty, it lies in the intrathoracic portion of the abdominal cavity and is not palpable. After a meal, the full stomach is stretched so that it makes contact with the ventral abdominal floor and can be palpated. Distention of the stomach usually results in displacement of the spleen and left kidney caudally, the small intestine and liver to the right, and the diaphragm becomes displaced cranially.

Internal Structure. The Horse (Fig. 11–11).[4] In the stomach of the horse, there are four mucosal regions, two of which are distinct: a prominent, whitish *esophageal* cutaneous region; a less distinct

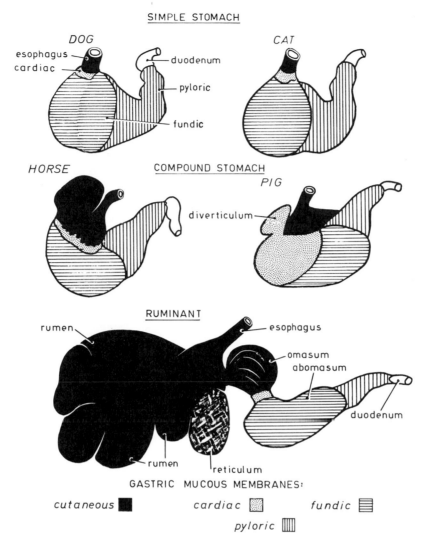

SIMPLE STOMACH

DOG

esophagus
cardiac
duodenum
pyloric
fundic

CAT

HORSE

COMPOUND STOMACH

PIG

diverticulum

RUMINANT

rumen
esophagus
omasum
abomasum
duodenum
rumen
reticulum

GASTRIC MUCOUS MEMBRANES:

cutaneous ■   cardiac ▨   fundic ▤

pyloric ▥

Figure 11–11. Variations in Gastric Mucosa in Stomachs of Domestic Animals. (After Krölling and Grau.[4])

cardiac region; and the *fundic* and *pyloric* gland regions. The latter two regions appear somewhat similar grossly as dark reddish mucosal surfaces. The two prominent regions of the stomach are separated by a ridge of mucosa, called the *margo plicatus.*

The Pig (Fig. 11–11). *Internally,* the mucosal surface of the pig stomach can be divided into four regions based on the color and character of the mucosa.

1. The *esophageal* (cutaneous) region, a glandless, esophageal-like mucosal surface around the cardia extends dorsally to the margin of the stomach diverticulum, laterally to the margins of the cardiac gland region, and downward to the angular incisure.

2. The *cardiac gland* region occupies a narrow strip at the junction of the glandular and nonglandular mucosa in all domestic animals except in the pig, where it covers nearly one-half of the stomach, including the diverticulum.[5]

3. The *fundic gland* region, which occupies what is commonly called the body of the stomach, is a reddish-brown area characterized by the increased thickness of the mucosa.

4. The *pyloric gland* region, in contrast to the reddish fundic gland region, is light in color with more rugae than in the other portions.

Dog and Cat. The outer layer of the stomach wall is the *tunica serosa.* It is covered with visceral peritoneum and has marked elasticity. Deep to the serosa is the *tunica muscularis,* with its several muscle layers, followed by the *tunica submucosa* and the innermost layer, the *tunica mucosa*. The outer *longitudinal muscle layer* is continuous with the longitudinal muscle layer of the esophagus and the duodenum, and is also continuous along the lesser and greater curvatures with narrow *external oblique fibers*. The *circular layer* of muscle fibers lies deep to the longitudinal layer and covers all of the stomach except the fundic portion. The circular smooth muscle fibers are well developed as they encircle the pylorus and here the fibers are called the *pyloric sphincter*. The circular muscle fibers are also thickened in the central portion of the pyloric part of the stomach producing a division into the pyloric antrum and pyloric canal. *Internal oblique fibers* are found in the area of the cardiac incisure and arch across the dorsal portion of the cardia contributing to the formation of a weak *cardiac sphincter* at this location.

***Mucous Membrane and Glands*[5]** (Fig. 11–11). The glandular mucous membrane of the stomach, which is in the form of irregular folds called rugae, is continuous with that of the esophagus at the cardiac ostium and with the duodenum at the pyloric ostium. The *rugae* play a role in the digestive processes by greatly increasing the surface area of the stomach.

The gastric mucous membrane in the dog as in other nonruminant animals is divided into esophageal, cardiac, fundic, and pyloric zones.

Duodenum and Pancreas

The *duodenum* is formed by the terminal part of the foregut and the cranial portion of the midgut. The junction of the two parts is located directly distal to the origin of the hepatic and pancreatic buds. As the stomach rotates, the duodenum takes on a U-shaped loop, rotates to the right, and comes to lie high in the dorsal abdomen. During early development the lumen of the duodenum may temporarily be obliterated, but under normal conditions the lumen is re-established shortly afterwards.

The *pancreas* arises as two outgrowths, one from the dorsal surface of the duodenum, called the *dorsal pancreas*; the other, the *ventral pancreas*, arises from the common bile duct near the entrance of the duct into the duodenum. During the process of growth and clockwise rotation of the gut, the dorsal and ventral pancreata and their ducts are brought together, with the ventral pancreas coming to lie cranial to and closely adherent to the dorsal pancreas (Fig. 11–12[6]).

The relative growth of these two pancreatic primordia varies in some species. For example, in

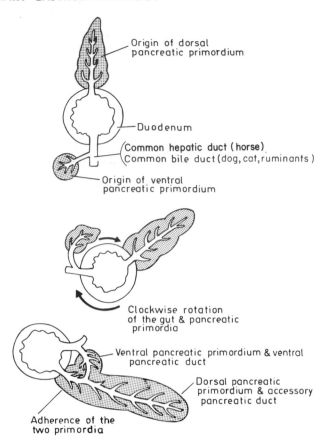

Figure 11–12. Development of the Pancreas. In the dog and horse both primordia develop, while in the cow and pig only the dorsal pancreatic primordium does, and in the sheep, goat, and cat, the ventral primordium develops. (Redrawn from Hollinshead.[6])

the dog and the horse both dorsal and ventral primordia remain. After rotation and fusion of the pancreas the two ducts also remain, but in most cases communicate with each other within the gland. These two ducts are named the pancreatic and accessory pancreatic ducts. The *pancreatic duct*, which originates from the ventral primordium, opens into the lumen of the descending part of the duodenum on the major duodenal papilla with the common bile duct (ductus choledochus). The *accessory pancreatic duct*, from the dorsal primordium, opens into the duodenal lumen on the *minor duodenal papilla*, just a few centimeters distal to the major papilla (dog). In the *horse* both papillae and both pancreatic ducts are located close together.

In cattle and swine, only the dorsal pancreatic primordium develops fully; therefore, there is only one pancreatic duct, and it opens into the duodenal lumen distal to the entrance of the common bile duct of the minor duodenal papilla.

In sheep, goat, and cat, the situation is again different and here only the ventral pancreatic primordium and its duct persist. The duct of the ventral pancreas is called the *pancreatic duct* and opens into the duodenum close to the common bile duct on the major duodenal papilla.

Form and Relations. In all animal species, the *duodenum* is the first and the shortest segment of the small intestine, and because of its relatively short mesentery, the duodenum is the least movable portion of the small intestine. Its name, which means "twelve," refers to the fact that in man the duodenum is approximately 12 fingerbreadths long. In the dog, this is also the approximate length of the duodenum, while in the horse, it is three to four times as long (1 meter). The duodenum is a particularly important organ because it receives the openings of the common bile and the pancreatic ducts.

The duodenum is described as having four parts. These are: (1) the *cranial part;* (2) the *descending part* passing downward below the right kidney; (3) the *transverse part* running to the left across the vertebral column; and (4) the *ascending part,* which turns upward to the duodenojejunal flexure. The four parts are frequently referred to by number instead of name.

The cranial portion of the duodenum is fairly mobile, moving up or down with the pyloric end of the stomach. Depending upon the position of the stomach, the first part of the duodenum may lie cranial to the pancreas or caudal to it. The remainder of the duodenum is relatively fixed in position, and its terminal part is the *duodenojejunal junction.*

The *pancreas*[7] extends almost transversely across the front of the vertebral column. It is divided into a *right lobe,* a *body,* and *left lobe* (tail). The right lobe is held close to the duodenum not only by connective tissue but by vessels that the two share, and it is separated from the left lobe by the *pancreatic incisure* or body in which the cranial mesenteric vessels lie.

Pancreatic Ducts and Common Bile Duct (Fig. 11–13 and Table 11–2). As discussed in the development of the pancreas, there are usually two

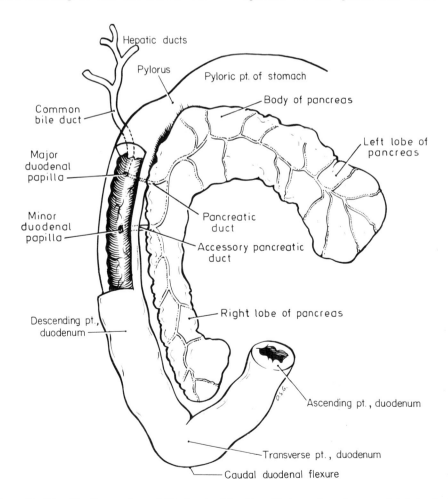

Figure 11–13. The Pancreatic and Bile Ducts of the Dog. (Redrawn from Evans and deLahunta.[7])

Table 11–2. Comparison of pancreatic ducts of dog, horse, and cattle

Pancreas	Official Name	Synonym	Location of Ostium of Duct in Descending Portion of Duodenum

Ventral pancreas	Pancreatic duct	• Duct of Wirsung
		• Chief pancreatic duct
			Dog
			  —on major duodenal papilla with common bile duct
			Horse
			  —in hepatopancreatic ampulla with common hepatic duct
			Cattle
			  —ventral pancreatic duct not usually developed

Dorsal pancreas	Accessory pancreatic duct	• Duct of Santorini
		• Dorsal pancreatic duct
			Dog
			  —on minor duodenal papilla approx. 2.8 cm caudal to major duodenal papilla
			Horse
			  —on small papilla across lumen from opening of pancreatic and common hepatic ducts
			Cattle
			  —at caudal end of right lobe of pancreas approx. 30 cm caudal to opening of common bile duct

pancreatic ducts in the dog* and horse, while only one is some of the other species. When two ducts are present, the one that opens on the major duodenal papilla is called the *pancreatic duct*,† and the duct that opens on the minor duodenal papilla is the *accessory pancreatic duct*.‡ When a single pancreatic duct is present, whether it develops from the ventral pancreatic primordium as in the cat, sheep, and goat or from the dorsal primordium as in cattle or swine, common usage has been merely to call it the *pancreatic duct*, even though in those animals with only a single pancreatic duct, the ducts are not homologous with one another.

As previously mentioned, the common bile duct is formed by the union of the cystic duct and the hepatic ducts. This union occurs at a location cranial and dorsal to the first part of the duodenum. The common bile duct, or the common hepatic duct as it is called in the horse, passes caudally in the lesser omentum above the duodenum and pancreas, and penetrates the wall of the duodenum on its mesenteric border. The intramural course of the common bile duct is variable in length according to species, and the duct terminates by opening into the lumen of the duodenum on the tip of the major duodenal papilla with the pancreatic duct. Examination of the tip of the major duodenal papilla may reveal a single duct in the sheep and goat and

usually a double opening for the two ducts in other species. When the common bile duct opens very close to or in common with the pancreatic duct, there is a dilated area known as the *hepatopancreatic ampulla*, or diverticulum duodeni, as it has been called in the horse (Fig. 11–14). The hepatopancreatic ampulla is encased in tiny bands of smooth muscle called the *sphincter of the hepatopancreatic ampulla* or sphincter of Oddi.

The Spleen

The primordium of the spleen appears early as a mesenchymal condensation between the two layers of the mesogastrium but later, due to its relatively

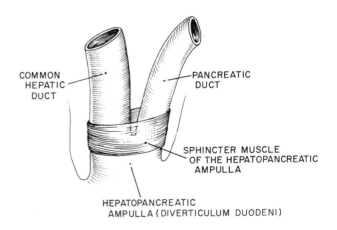

Figure 11–14. Hepatopancreatic Ampulla and Sphincter of Horse.

---

*In the majority of *cats*, only a single pancreatic duct is present.
†Duct of Wirsung, the ventral pancreatic duct or chief pancreatic duct.
‡Duct of Santorini or the dorsal pancreatic duct.

rapid growth, the spleen bulges into the left part of the peritoneal cavity. With the formation of the omental bursa, a portion of the dorsal mesogastrium, which is located between the spleen and dorsal midline, fuses with the dorsal abdominal wall. The remaining part of the dorsal mesogastrium connects the spleen to the kidney and is known as the *lienorenal ligament*. The connection between the spleen and stomach is formed by the *gastrolienal ligament*. In all domesticated species, the spleen continues to remain in an intraperitoneal position.

The spleen of the domestic animals varies in shape and attachment, but nearly always is present on the left side of the body under cover of the last ribs. The degree of fullness of the stomach in the non-ruminant animals will influence the position and palpability of the spleen.

In all species, the spleen has a parietal surface which is opposed to the diaphragm, and a visceral which contacts adjacent viscera, namely intestine, stomach, and kidney. The spleen also has a dorsal end or extremity and ventral end, as well as cranial and caudal margins and a hilus for blood and lymph vessels entering and leaving the spleen.

Arterial Supply and Venous Drainage of the Liver, Stomach, Pancreas, Duodenum, and Spleen

Celiac Artery (Fig. 11–15)

The celiac, cranial, and caudal mesenteric arteries provide the blood supply to the gastrointestinal tract. The origins of the branches of the *celiac artery* are schematically illustrated in Figure 11–15. The three major branches of the celiac artery are the common hepatic, left gastric, and splenic. The *common hepatic artery*, after giving off a *proper hepatic artery* or *arteries*, terminates by supplying a portion of the lesser curvature of the stomach by way of the *right gastric artery* and portions of the greater curvature of the stomach, the duodenum, and pancreas as the *gastroduodenal artery*. On both lesser and greater curvatures of the stomach, branches of the common hepatic artery enter into

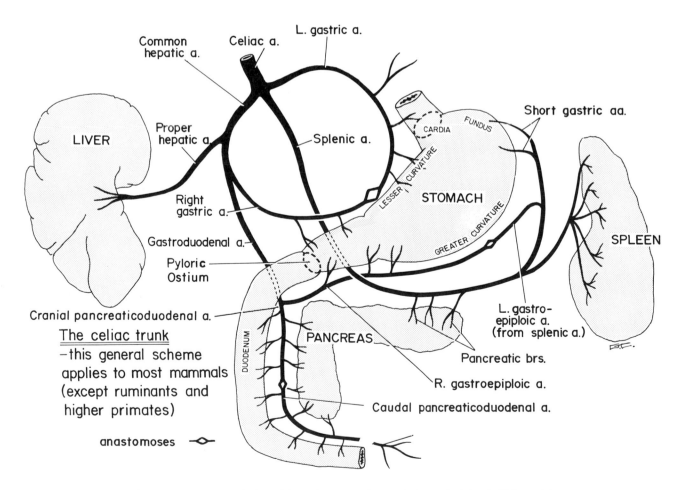

Figure 11–15. General Plan of the Celiac Artery in Simple Stomach Animals (Schematic).

anastomotic connections with the other two branches of the celiac trunk.

The *splenic artery,* the largest of the three branches of the celiac, has three named branches.

1. Because the artery is closely associated with the body and left lobe of the pancreas, the splenic artery gives off *pancreatic branches* to this portion of the gland.

2. As the splenic artery passes across the visceral surface of the fundus of the stomach, it gives off *short gastric arteries.*

3. The artery supplies *left gastroepiploic* branches to the greater curvature of the stomach.

These gastroepiploic branches usually establish anastomotic connections along the stomach's greater curvature with the right gastroepiploic artery, a branch of the gastroduodenal, and thus re-establish a connection between the common hepatic and splenic arteries.

The *left gastric artery,* the smallest of the three branches of the celiac, supplies the cardiac part and portions of the lesser curvature of the stomach. The only named branches of the left gastric are *esophageal* branches, which supply the terminal part of the esophagus and also pass through the esophageal hiatus to supply portions of the thoracic esophagus. The left gastric establishes anastomotic connections along the lesser curvature of the stomach with the right gastric, a branch of the (common) hepatic artery.

CLINICAL CONSIDERATIONS—ARTERIAL SUPPLY

The duodenum, the body and right lobe of the pancreas share for the most part the same vessels, and for this reason the duodenum is usually surgically removed when the right lobe of the pancreas is resected. The common blood supply for duodenum and pancreas is through two arcades that lie on or slightly embedded in the ventral and dorsal surfaces of the pancreas, a variable distance from the duodenum. The cranial ends of the arterial arcades are both derived from the gastroduodenal artery, while the caudal ends usually have a common stem from the caudal mesenteric artery. The right lobe of the pancreas thus derives its blood supply from the cranial and caudal pancreaticoduodenal arteries, while the majority of the left lobe is supplied by pancreatic branches of the splenic artery.

Venous Drainage

Blood from the visceral organs of the abdomen is collected by a number of tributaries of various sizes to form a major trunk, the *portal vein.* The connotation of a "portal system" is that the major vessel begins in a capillary bed, in this case the capillaries of the intestine and other abdominal splanchnic organs, and ends in a capillary system, the liver.

The venous drainage of the pancreas and duodenum in general follows its arterial supply. There are venous arcades within that parallel the arterial ones, which in turn empty into the cranial and caudal pancreaticoduodenal veins. The cranial pancreaticoduodenal vein drains into the gastroduodenal and then directly into the portal vein, while the caudal pancreaticoduodenal vein empties into the caudal mesenteric vein and thence into the portal. There are pancreatic tributaries from the left lobe of the pancreas that drain into the splenic vein in all species.

In the case of the rectum, there are two routes for venous drainage:

1. Blood can enter the portal vein by way of the cranial rectal veins.

2. Blood from the caudal rectum can bypass the portal vein in draining into the caudal rectal veins, tributaries of the internal iliac veins, which in turn drain into the caudal vena cava.

Portal Vein (Fig. 11–16). The major tributaries of the portal vein in the domestic animals are: (1) the *splenic vein,* which receives the left gastroepiploic, short gastric, left gastric, and pancreatic veins; (2)

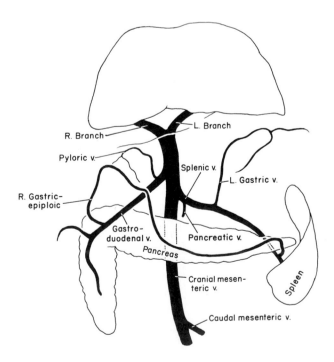

Figure 11–16. Formation of Portal Vein in Simple Stomach Animals (Schematic).

the *cranial mesenteric vein*, which in most species is the largest of the portal tributaries and is closely associated with the artery of the same name; (3) the *caudal mesenteric vein*, which is formed by the cranial rectal and left colic veins, and is the smallest of the tributaries of the portal vein; and (4) the *gastroepiploic vein*.

CLINICAL CONSIDERATIONS—PORTAL VEIN

The portal vein after its formation in the mesojejunum, lies deep in the abdomen and continues cranially closely associated with the common hepatic artery and common bile duct;* its course is toward the porta hepatis enwrapped in the lesser omentum. While in the lesser omentum, the portal vein and common hepatic artery form the ventral boundary of the epiploic foramen. When hemostasis is required following liver trauma, it is at the epiploic foramen that the artery and vein may be compressed by digital pressure. The surgeon inserts one finger into the epiploic foramen and exerts compression with thumb and finger to stop blood flow to the liver temporarily.

Lymphatic Drainage

In general, lymphatic vessels of the digestive tract tend to follow the blood vessels so that drainage is through a converging series of lymphatics and lymph nodes in which the chief nodes lie close to the aorta; thus, by the time lymph from the digestive tract has reached the nodes about the aorta, it has passed through several sets of regional nodes.

The cranial and caudal mesenteric lymph node groups (lymphocentrum) are scattered throughout the common dorsal mesentery and are grouped together and commonly classified as *mesenteric lymph nodes*. The *cranial mesenteric lymph nodes* are located close together along the course of the cranial mesenteric vessels and take the names of major vessels such as: *jejunal lymph nodes, ileocolic lymph nodes, cecal lymph nodes*, and *colic lymph nodes*.

The lymphatic drainage of most of the transverse colon, all of the ascending colon, cecum, ileum, and jejunum is into the nodes of the cranial mesenteric group, then into the *intestinal lymphatic trunk(s)* and from the trunks into the *cisterna chyli*. The *caudal mesenteric lymph nodes* likewise are found along the branches and tributaries of the caudal mesenteric vessels. The lumbar lymph nodes re-

ceive lymph from the kidneys, suprarenal glands, gonads, and pelvic limbs, and all efferent lymphatics from the lumbar nodes drain into the cisterna chyli.

Lymphatic drainage from the rectum and anal canal is considered to be into the *internal iliac lymph nodes*. Efferent lymphatics from these nodes pass to *medial iliac nodes* and from there into the cisterna chyli.

Lymphatics of the Liver, Stomach, Spleen, Duodenum, and Pancreas. The lymphatic vessels draining the above organs accompany branches of the celiac artery, and the lymph vessels and nodes form a diverging pattern which tends to converge upon the *celiac lymph node group* located around the base of the celiac artery. Lymphatic drainage from the liver and hepatic ducts is into *hepatic lymph nodes* which lie along the course of the common hepatic artery and its branches and the portal vein. The hepatic lymph nodes also receive lymph from portions of the stomach, duodenum and pancreas and adjacent omentum.

The *gastric lymph nodes* are most abundant in the area of the lesser curvature of the stomach and cardia along the course of the left gastric vein and artery. The gastric nodes drain portions of the stomach, distal esophagus, and adjacent omentum as well as portions of the liver. Efferent lymphatic vessels from the mediastinum and lungs pass through foramina in the diaphragm and enter gastric lymph nodes.

The *splenic lymph nodes* lie along the splenic artery and vein and receive efferent lymph vessels from the spleen, the greater curvature area of the stomach, and the adjacent greater omentum.

Lymphatic Trunks. Efferent lymphatic vessels from regional visceral lymph nodes form thin-walled lymphatic trunks which eventually come together as the cisterna chyli. The *cisterna chyli*, which can be considered to be the caudal expanded part of the thoracic duct, lies in the cranial portion of the abdomen approximately between the right side of the aorta and the right crus of the diaphragm.

In general, lymph from the stomach, liver and gallbladder, pancreas, duodenum, and spleen passes into efferent vessels which course to the celiac lymph nodes and leave these nodes as the *celiac lymphatic trunk(s)*. Efferent lymph vessels from cranial mesenteric nodes, which represent lymph drainage from the jejunum, ileum, cecum, ascending and transverse colon, join together to form the *intestinal lymphatic trunk(s)*. The *lumbar lymph trunks*, usually two in number and located along the dorsal surface of the aorta, are formed by

---

* In species without a gallbladder, the duct is the common hepatic duct.

efferent lymph vessels coming from medial iliac nodes and also lymph nodes around the caudal part of the aorta. All of the previously described lymphatic trunks and lesser ones, such as the visceral, jejunal, gastric, and hepatic trunks, come together and empty their contents into the cisterna chyli.

The Liver

This largest gland of the body, the liver, is obliquely positioned on the right abdominal surface of the diaphragm, extending from the area of the right kidney downward to near the floor of the abdomen. The liver extends cranially as far as the seventh rib and thus receives protection from the caudal part of the bony thorax.

Lobes of the Liver (Figs. 11–17 through 11–20, Table 11–3)

Most animals have four lobes of the liver. They are: (1) *right lobe*, (2) *left lobe*, (3) *caudate lobe*, and (4) *quadrate lobe*. In addition, each lobe, except the quadrate lobe, may be subdivided into sublobes.

Ligaments of the Liver

The ligaments of the liver are formed by the reflection of the peritoneum from the diaphragm onto the liver. They are: (1) *right* and (2) *left triangular ligaments* which attach the liver to the diaphragm; (3) the *coronary ligament*, which like the triangular ligaments attaches the liver to the diaphragm but is composed of two laminae which meet below the caudal vena cava to form the (4) *falciform ligament*. The falciform ligament is the remnant of the ventral mesentery into which the

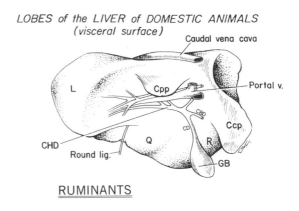

LOBES of the LIVER of DOMESTIC ANIMALS
(visceral surface)

RUMINANTS

Figure 11–18. Lobes of the Liver of Ruminants—visceral surface. (Redrawn from Nickel et al.[1])

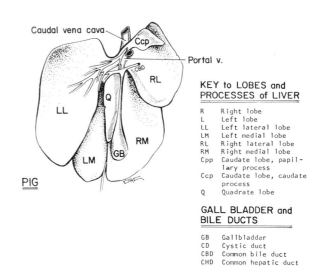

KEY to LOBES and PROCESSES of LIVER

R   Right lobe
L   Left lobe
LL   Left lateral lobe
LM   Left medial lobe
RL   Right lateral lobe
RM   Right medial lobe
Cpp Caudate lobe, papillary process
Ccp Caudate lobe, caudate process
Q   Quadrate lobe

GALL BLADDER and BILE DUCTS

GB   Gallbladder
CD   Cystic duct
CBD Common bile duct
CHD Common hepatic duct

Figure 11–19. Lobes of the Liver of Pig—visceral surface. (Redrawn from Nickel et al.[1])

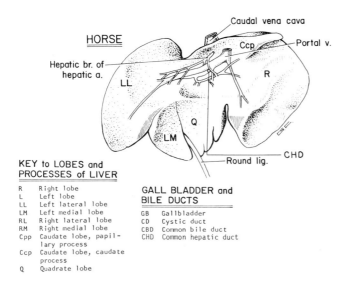

HORSE

KEY to LOBES and PROCESSES of LIVER

R   Right lobe
L   Left lobe
LL   Left lateral lobe
LM   Left medial lobe
RL   Right lateral lobe
RM   Right medial lobe
Cpp Caudate lobe, papillary process
Ccp Caudate lobe, caudate process
Q   Quadrate lobe

GALL BLADDER and BILE DUCTS

GB   Gallbladder
CD   Cystic duct
CBD Common bile duct
CHD Common hepatic duct

Figure 11–17. Lobes of the Liver (Visceral Surface) of Horse. (Redrawn from Nickel et al.[1])

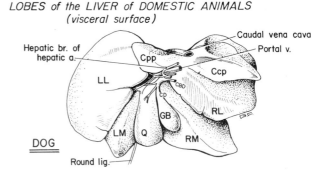

LOBES of the LIVER of DOMESTIC ANIMALS
(visceral surface)

DOG

Figure 11–20. Lobes of the Liver of Dog—visceral surface. (Redrawn from Nickel et al.[1])

Table 11-3. Summary of lobes and sublobes of the liver in domestic animals

Species	Right Lobe		Left Lobe		Caudate Lobe		
	R. Med. Lobe	R. Lat. Lobe	L. Lat. Lobe	L. Med. Lobe	Caudate Process	Papillary Process	Quadrate Lobe
Dog	*	*	*	*	*	*	*
Horse	1	1	*	*	*	—	*
Ruminants	1	1	1	1	*	*	*
Pig	*	*	*	*	*	*2	*

* = Present.
— = Absent.
1 = Not clearly separable into medial and lateral sublobes.
2 = Occasionally absent.

liver grew during embryonic development. In both the young and the adult it extends from the ventral surface of the liver to the diaphragm and to the ventral abdominal wall and umbilicus. The (left) umbilical vein, a very large vessel in the fetus and newborn, carries blood from the placenta to the fetus. The umbilical vein can be found in the edge of the falciform ligament before it joins the portal vein within the substance of the liver. After birth the vein becomes largely or entirely obliterated and cordlike, and is then called the (5) *round ligament* of the liver. The (6) *hepatorenal ligament* is a peritoneal fold of variable thickness in the different species which passes from the right kidney to the liver, usually the caudate process of the caudate lobe.

Surfaces and Impressions of the Liver
(Figs. 11–17 through 11–20)

The liver has two surfaces: diaphragmatic (parietal) and visceral. The *diaphragmatic surface* lies chiefly against the diaphragm and is convex in shape. It has one named impression, the *sulcus for the caudal vena cava.*

The *visceral surface*, as its name implies, is the caudal one which fits against various visceral organs, giving their names to the depressions in the surface of the liver. They are: (1) *esophageal* impression; (2) *gastric* impression, large in the liver of the dog and horse; (3) *omasal* impression on the papillary process of the caudate lobe of the liver of ruminants; (4) *reticular* impression on the distal part of the left lobe of the liver of ruminants; (5) *duodenal* impression; (6) *renal* impression or fossa; (7) *colic* impression; (8) *cecal* impression (equine); and (9) *suprarenal* (adrenal) impression.

The *porta hepatis* is that depression on the visceral surface of the liver through which blood vessels, such as the portal vein and hepatic arteries,

enter the liver, and where the hepatic bile ducts leave the liver.

Gallbladder and Duct Systems

The gallbladder is a sac in which bile is stored and concentrated during those times when it is produced more rapidly than it is needed for the digestive processes occurring in the small intestine. The gallbladder lies on the visceral surface of the liver in the *fossa for the gallbladder*, which in the dog and cat is located between the quadrate and right medial lobes of the liver. The capacity of the gallbladder in the dog is approximately 5 to 15 ml, depending on the size of the breed. The gallbladder has a *fundus*, which is the blind protruding end, a *body, neck*, and a *cystic duct*. In those species possessing a gallbladder, the cystic duct extends from the neck of the gallbladder to a junction with the *common hepatic duct*. The union of ducts results in the formation of the common bile duct (ductus choledochus). In animals that do not possess a gallbladder, the hepatic ducts from the lobes of the liver come together to form a common duct which in general has the same course to the duodenum as the common bile duct. The *common bile duct* courses through the lesser omentum, enters the duodenal wall where it has an intramural course within the wall of the descending duodenum, and ends at the *major duodenal papilla* with the pancreatic duct. The course and termination of the common bile duct are discussed with the pancreatic ducts.

Duct System—Horse (see Fig. 11–14). Bile leaves the liver by way of the right and left *hepatic ducts* as there is no gallbladder in the horse. The hepatic ducts converge at the ventral part of the portal fissure to form the common hepatic duct.

The *common hepatic duct* carries bile to the duodenum at which site it is joined by the pancreatic duct. As in species possessing a gallbladder, the conjoined two ducts in the horse, hepatic and pancreatic, pass obliquely through the duodenal wall and open into the lumen at the *hepatopancreatic ampulla* (diverticulum duodeni). A valve-like arrangement formed by smooth muscle fibers encircling the ampulla in a sphincteric fashion (see Fig. 11–14) prevents reflux of ingesta from the intestine into the hepatic or pancreatic ducts.

Small Intestine

The small intestine is separated into fixed and mesenteric portions. The first part of the small intestine is suspended by a relatively short mesentery and is called the duodenum. In all species the *duodenum* is divided into cranial, descending, transverse, and ascending parts. The *cranial duodenal flexure* is located between the cranial and descending parts, the *caudal flexure* between the descending and transverse parts, and the *duodenojejunal flexure* marks the transition to jejunum. The other parts of the intestine, *jejunum* and *ileum,* make up the majority of the small intestine. The duodenum extends from the right hypochondriac region into the right lateral abdominal region and then descends into the umbilical region (see Fig. 11–8). The large loop of small intestine is the jejunum and ileum, and the greater portion of this loop is the jejunum, while only the terminal part which joins the large intestine is the ileum; the division between small intestine and large intestine is at the *ileocecal ostium* and *valve* (ilial papilla).

The Horse (Table 11–4). The small intestine is approximately 20 to 30 m long and as in other species is separated into a *fixed* part, composed of duodenum (to which the pancreas is closely attached), and a *mesenteric* portion (jejunum and ileum), which makes up the rest of the small intestine.

The *jejunum,* measuring about 20 to 25 meters long, is in the form of coils suspended by the extensive mesojejunum from the dorsal abdominal wall.

The jejunum is located chiefly in the dorsal part of the abdomen to the left of the median plane as far forward as the liver and caudally into the inguinal region, but may be found anywhere in the abdominal cavity or interspersed among coils of the small colon.

The *ileum,* only about 1 m long, has a thicker muscular wall than the jejunum. A double fold of peritoneum extending from ileum to cecum (ileocecal fold) marks the transition from jejunum to ileum. The ileum courses from its origin in the left flank, across the midline and passes dorsally to join the lesser curvature of the cecum. Here the ileum protrudes into the base of the cecum forming the *ileal papilla*. The ileal papilla contains a plexus of veins, which when engorged increase the ileal protrusion and narrow the ileal ostium, thus preventing reflux of contents from cecum into the ileum.[8]

The Pig. The *small intestine* is approximately 15.2 to 18.3 meters in length, from its origin to the ileocecal ostium, and is divided into the less moveable *duodenum* and the bulk of the intestine, the jejunum and ileum. The *jejunum* and *ileum* are in the shape of tightly arranged intestinal coils which on the left side lie dorsal to the large intestine and extend from the stomach back to the pelvic inlet; on the right side of the abdominal cavity, they lie on the caudal abdominal floor apposed to the right flank.

Dog and Cat (Fig. 11–21). The small intestine lies on both sides of the abdomen and has a length of 1.80 to 4.80 meters in the dog and about 1.3 meters in the cat. The duodenum lies to the right of the median plane. The *jejunum,* consisting of up to eight loops of gut, covered below and on the sides by greater omentum, occupies the space between the stomach and liver and the pelvic inlet. The *jejunum* is continuous with the duodenum at the duodenojejunal flexure and with the ileum at a poorly defined jejunoileal junction. The *ileum* opens into the proximal part of the ascending colon at the *ileal ostium* at approximately the level of the first or

Table 11–4. Comparison of Intestinal Length Among Domestic Animals

| Species | Intestinal Lengths | | |
	Small Intestine	Large Intestine	Total Length
Horse	21.3M (70 ft)	7.6M (25 ft)	28.9M (95 ft)
Dog	3.96M (13 ft)	0.76M (2.5 ft)	4.7M (15 ft)
Cow	39.6M (130 ft)	11.3M (37 ft)	50.9M (167 ft)
Pig	15.2–19.8M (50–65 ft)	3.7–4.6M (12–15 ft)	19.8–24.4M (65–80 ft)
Man	6.1M (20 ft)	1.8M (6 ft)	7.9M (26 ft)

Modified from Nickel et al., 1973.[1]

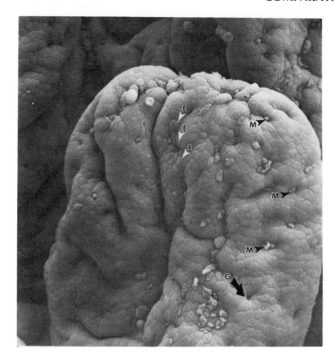

Figure 11–21. Scanning electron micrograph (430×) of the luminal surface of the *dog* jejunum. An individual villus shows numerous goblet cell openings (G), some of which are blocked by small amounts of mucus (M). Individual epithelial cells are evident (E).

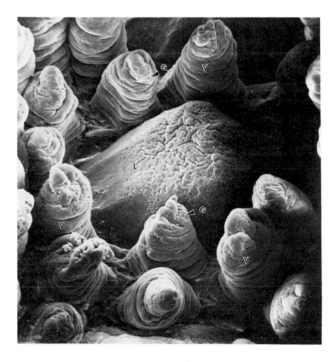

Figure 11–22. Scanning electron micrograph (80×) of the inner surface of the *dog* duodenum. Long, slender mucosal villi (V) project into the lumen. Goblet cell openings (G) appear as indentations in the bulging epithelium. Villi surround a small mass of lymphoid tissue (L).

second lumbar vertebra. Surrounding this orifice is a projection of the ileum into the ascending colon, the *ileal papilla,* formerly called the "ileocecal valve." The name change was justified on the basis that the term "valve" implies a passive flap-like closure, a structure that does not correspond to the ileal papilla in the dog or cat.

Lymphoid Tissue in the Intestine (Fig. 11–22). Many areas of lymphoid nodules, called Peyer's patches, are scattered throughout the small intestine, and in some species also in the large intestine. The lymph nodes found in the common dorsal mesentery are related to tributaries of the cranial mesenteric vein and are thus called the *cranial mesenteric lymph node* group, and those nodes in the mesentery of the jejunum are *jejunal lymph nodes.*

FUNCTIONAL AND CLINICAL CONSIDERATIONS— EQUINE SMALL INTESTINE

The long mesojejunum allows for freedom of mobility of the jejunum and also increases the chances for volvulus, intussusception, or incarceration of the jejunum. Potential sites for incarceration of gut are the epiploic foramen and inguinal canal.

A potential cause of colic in the horse is associated with changes in the normal emptying pattern of the ileum. With contraction and shortening of the ileum, ileal contents are delivered by intermittent squirts into the cecum against a higher gradient of pressure. Normally active, muscular contraction assisted by venous engorgement of the ileal papilla effectively closes the ileal ostium to reflux of ingesta from the cecum into the ileum. Interference with the normal sphincteric function of the papilla can be a cause of colic.

Large Intestine—Horse (Fig. 11–23)

The Cecum. The cecum of the horse[9] is a large organ located to the right side of the median plane. It is approximately 1.25 meters (4 feet) long and extends from the area below the right sublumbar region along the floor of the abdominal cavity to near the xiphoid cartilage of the sternum. The cecum has a base, body, and an apex. The *base* is the caudal curved blind end which has connected to it the terminal portions of the ileum and large colon and is also attached to the ventral surface of the right kidney. The long *body* extends downward and forward resting mostly on the parietal peritoneum of the ventral abdominal wall. The *apex* is the pointed

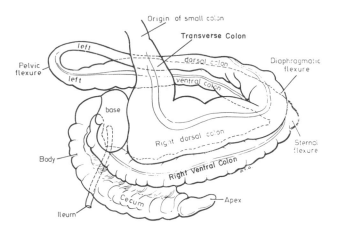

Figure 11–23. Cecum and Large Colon of Horse. (Redrawn from Getty.[9])

cranial portion which lies approximately 10 to 12.5 centimeters (4 to 5 inches) caudal to the xiphoid cartilage.

The *cecum* has four *teniae ceci*, which are longitudinal fibromuscular bands extending along the surfaces of the cecum. As a result of the teniae, four rows of *haustra* or *sacculations* are produced in the cecal wall.

The Colon. The complex colon of the horse is divided into the *great colon*, a derivative of the ascending colon, *transverse colon*, *small colon*, and *sigmoid colon*.

Great Colon. This large, double, U-shaped structure with an average capacity of about 80 liters consists of two parallel limbs with a terminal flexure. Beginning at the cecocolic ostium the *right ventral colon* extends cranially and makes a bend to the left called the *sternal flexure*. It extends caudally as the *left ventral colon* to the pelvic inlet. Here it turns cranially and its curvature at this point is the *pelvic flexure*. The luminal diameter in this area is much reduced and is a common site of intestinal obstruction in the horse. The *left dorsal colon* is the cranial continuation from the pelvic flexure to the *diaphragmatic flexure,* thence to the right as the *right dorsal colon*. The *transverse colon* is the continuation of the right colon, and the *small colon*, which is comparable to the descending colon in the dog, extends from the transverse colon to the sigmoid colon.

Longitudinal bands of smooth muscle, the *teniae coli,* are present on the great and small colon of the *equine* intestine. Four bands are present on the ventral part of the great colon whereas the pelvic flexure and left dorsal colon have but one band, and

the diaphragmatic flexure and right dorsal colon have three bands.

Small Colon. The small colon is a derivative of the *descending colon*. It begins at the termination of the transverse colon, and extends for a distance of 3.5 meters. Its approximate diameter in an average-size horse is 7.5 to 10 centimeters. In the living animal its shape is in the form of coils which lie between the stomach and the pelvic inlet above the left dorsal colon, in and among the small intestinal loops. The small colon is attached by *colic mesentery* to the sublumbar region and also to the terminal part of the duodenum by a fold of peritoneum, the *duodenocolic ligament*. The small colon has two large *teniae coli* and two rows of *haustra (sacculations),* while no teniae are present in the equine rectum.

Large Intestine—Dog and Cat

The large intestine is divided into the *cecum, colon, rectum,* and *anal canal*. Due to the rotation of the gut, the colon is divided into three parts. They are: (1) *ascending colon*, which lies to the right side of the origin of the cranial mesenteric artery from the aorta; (2) *transverse colon*, which extends to the left of the median plane and in front of the cranial mesenteric artery; and (3) *descending colon*, which extends caudally toward the rectum and anal canal and lies to the left of the cranial mesenteric artery. The rectum is the most caudal portion of the large intestine and passes as a relatively straight tube which terminates as the short *anal canal*.

The flexuous *cecum* of the dog is approximately 2.5 to 15.0 centimeters long and is attached by peritoneum to the ascending colon and the ileum and is a direct caudal continuation of the ascending colon. Although the cecum begins as a caudally directed organ, its blind end is usually rotated so that it points cranially; in both cat and dog, the cecum communicates only with the ascending colon as the ileal papilla in both species opens into the colon. The cecum in the cat is not corkscrew-shaped but rather a short, comma-shaped, caudal diverticulum of the ascending colon.

The *colon* of both dog and cat is relatively uniform in diameter throughout its length and does not have the teniae coli or haustrae which the horse and pig colon possess. The *ascending colon*, which joins the transverse colon at the right colic flexure, is its shortest portion. The *transverse colon* lies between the cranial mesenteric artery and the stomach, and at the left colic flexure is continued as the descending colon. The *descending colon* is longer and has a

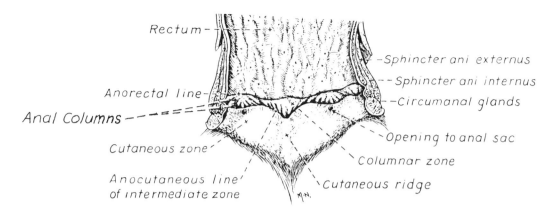

Figure 11–24. Canine Anal Canal (Longitudinal section—view into bottom half of opened tube). (From Miller et al.[2])

greater diameter than the other segments of the colon. It terminates at about the seventh lumbar vertebra and near the pelvic inlet as the rectum. The relatively short *rectum* in the dog has a mesorectum for part of its course and at the *ampulla recti,* its widest part, the rectum is retroperitoneal. The rectum lies dorsal to the urinary bladder. In the male dog and cat, other organs that lie ventral to the rectum are the ductus deferens connected by the genital fold, the prostate gland and the pelvic portion of the urethra, and in the male cat the bulbourethral glands. Lying below the rectum in the female dog and cat is the body and cervix of the uterus and the vagina.

The short *anal canal* (Fig. 11–24) is the terminal part of the colon and has a mucous membrane lining which can be grossly divided into three zones. The *columnar zone,* more distinct in dog than in cat, has dark mucosa arranged in longitudinal folds called anal columns between which lie depressions termed *anal sinuses* which produce a lipid material in the dog and cat and a mucous secretion in the pig. The *intermediate zone,* or anocutaneous zone, is a thin line of tissue and, like the columnar zone, is covered by stratified squamous epithelium. The *cutaneous zone* blends with the anal skin and is covered by fine hairs and is discolored a bluish-red. The *circumanal glands* are located in this zone in both dog and cat. The two *anal sacs (paranal sinuses)* are located on either side of the anal canal between the inner smooth muscle, internal and sphincter muscle, and the outer striated muscle or external anal sphincter. Each anal zone has a duct which opens to the exterior at the level of the anocutaneous junction.

The *glands of anal sacs* (glands of paranal sinuses) lie within the wall of the anal sacs and discharge their secretions into the sacs. The glands are of the sebaceous and apocrine type in the cat and only the apocrine type in dogs.[3]

CLINICAL CONSIDERATIONS—ANAL SACS

The anal sac duct is subject to occlusion in the dog but rarely in the cat, and occlusion of the duct is followed by engorgement of the anal sacs with accompanying pain and sometimes abscessation and rupture to the exterior.

Arterial Supply and Venous Drainage of the Intestine

Cranial Mesenteric Artery. The *cranial mesenteric artery* (Fig. 11–25) is the chief artery to the intestine in all quadrupeds and in man. Like the celiac artery, the cranial mesenteric is at first difficult to locate and identify because it is surrounded by a dense plexus of autonomic and sensory nerves, called the *cranial mesenteric plexus and ganglia.* The cranial mesenteric artery arises just caudal to the origin of the celiac and descends in the common dorsal mesentery. In its central location in the dorsal mesentery, the cranial mesenteric artery is axial during the development and rotation of the intestinal tract. In general, the artery supplies branches to the following structures: a portion of the pancreas, duodenum, jejunum, ileum, cecum, ascending colon, transverse colon, and portions of the descending colon.

CLINICAL CONSIDERATIONS—ARTERIOLES OF THE INTESTINE (Figs. 11–26 through 11–30)

When methyl methacrylate casts of arterioles of the small intestine are examined by electron microscopy, the transition of the arteriole to capillary is characterized by the presence of a single precapillary sphincter.[10]

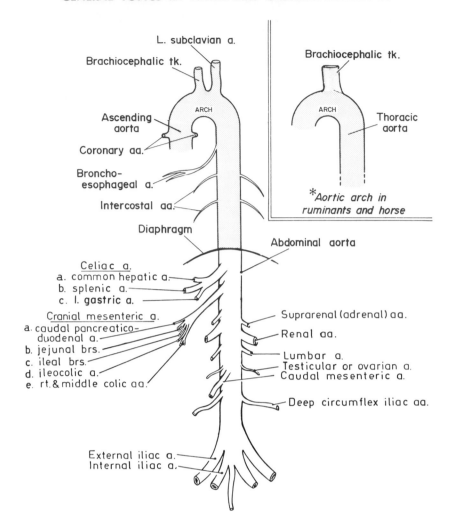

Figure 11–25. Aorta and Branches in Dog and Cat (Schematic).

The Horse (Fig. 11–31).[11] The branches of the cranial mesenteric artery in the horse are the caudal pancreaticoduodenal artery, jejunal arteries, right colic, middle colic, and ileocolic arteries.

The *caudal pancreaticoduodenal artery*, usually one of the first branches from the cranial mesenteric, supplies the distal portion of the right lobe of the pancreas, and also the descending, transverse, and ascending parts of the duodenum. It establishes anastomotic connections with the celiac artery by way of the cranial pancreaticoduodenal artery.

Fifteen to twenty *jejunal arteries* arise and pass between the layers of the mesojejunum. Each artery terminates near the mesenteric border of the gut by bifurcating into right and left branches which will anastomose with adjacent branches to form a series of arterial arches or arcades, and they in turn give

rise to many vasa recta (straight arteries). The vasa recta enter the mesenteric border of the jejunum, penetrate the tunica adventitia, and send tiny branches to the antimesenteric border of the gut to anastomose with similar vessels coming from the opposite side.

The right colic and middle colic arteries usually arise by a common trunk from the cranial mesenteric. The *right colic*, formerly dorsal colic artery, is a large vessel which supplies blood to both the right and left portions of the dorsal colon. At the pelvic flexure, the right colic artery may anastomose with the colic branch of the ileocolic artery. Examination of the pelvic flexure of the large colon indicates that its blood supply is not as extensive as the other portions of the large colon, indicating that potentially there may be greater likelihood of ischemia of

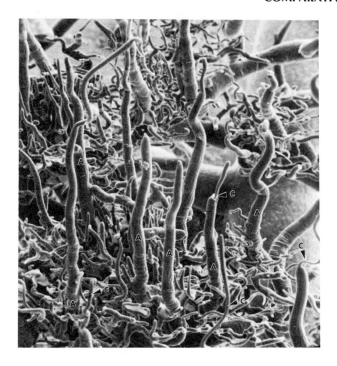

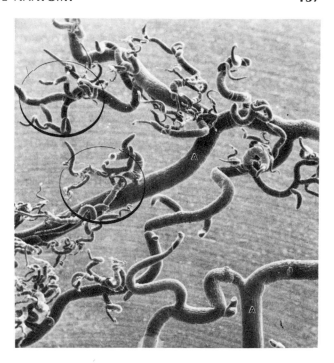

Figure 11–26. Scanning electron micrograph (70×) of arterioles, capillaries, and venules of the *dog* duodenum prepared by injection of methyl methacrylate. Rising arterioles (A) terminate as capillaries (C).

Figure 11–28. Scanning electron micrograph (45×) of small blood vessels in the descending colon of the *dog* prepared from a methyl methacrylate cast. These vessels are typically short, tortuous branches from small arteries (A). Circled areas are enlarged in Figures 11–29 and 11–30.

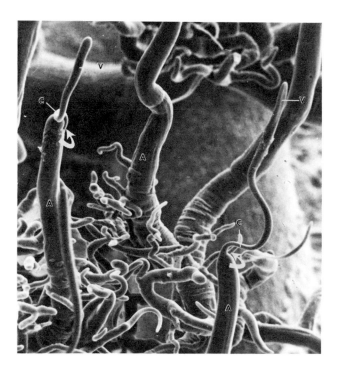

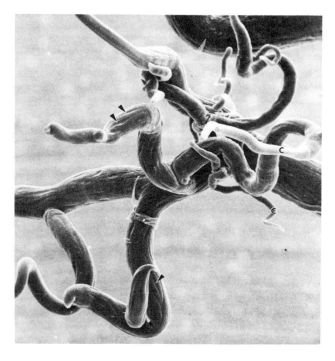

Figure 11–27. Scanning electron micrograph (150×). Arterioles, capillaries, and venules of the duodenum of the *dog*, prepared from a methyl metacrylate cast. Arterioles (A) terminate abruptly (arrows) as capillaries (C), which are continued as venules (V).

Figure 11–29. Scanning electron micrograph (175×) of small blood vessels in the descending colon of the *dog* prepared from a methyl methacrylate cast. Small arteries of the colic region demonstrate deep, furrowed impressions (arrows) made by the endothelial cells. (C) capillaries.

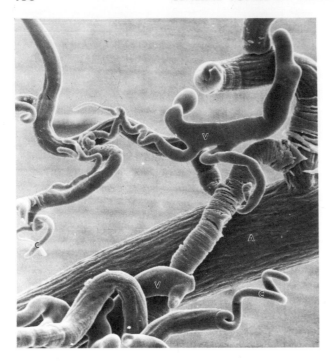

Figure 11–30. Scanning electron micrograph (185×) of small arteries (A), capillaries (C), and veins (V) of the descending colon of the *dog* prepared from a methyl methacrylate cast.

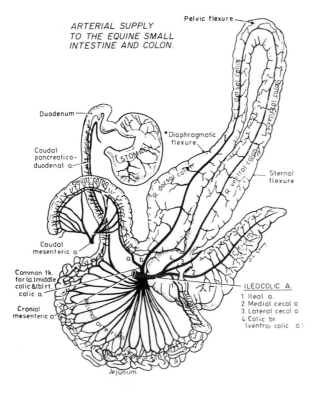

Figure 11–31. Arterial Supply to the Equine Small Intestine and Colon. (Modified from Hopkins—unpublished.[11])

this flexure occurring in infestations of *Strongylus vulgaris.*

The *ileocolic artery,* formerly called the right branch of the cranial mesenteric artery, is the continuation of the cranial mesenteric in the horse. It has four major sets of branches which supply blood to the cecum, ventral colon, and ileum. The branches are the ileal arteries, medial and lateral cecal arteries, and the colic branch.

CLINICAL CONSIDERATIONS—EQUINE COLIC

In the horse, the cranial mesenteric artery is frequently enlarged due to disease of its wall caused by the parasite *Strongylus vulgaris.* This parasite appears to have an affinity for the cranial mesenteric artery and as a result of larval migrations into the wall, vascular damage occurs. Tissue destruction is particularly serious because of disruption of the intima which results in thrombus formation. Emboli are dislodged and carried down the vessel to produce obstruction of smaller arteries and arterioles.

When segments of the gut are made hypoxic in this manner, acute abdominal signs appear, such as severe abdominal pain, rolling on the ground, stretching, fever, and possibly death of the animal. These signs are commonly associated with colic in the horse due to emboli from a diseased cranial mesenteric artery.

Another common abnormality associated with the cranial mesenteric artery is the progression of the condition discussed above, viz., continued destruction of the arterial wall to the point where the arterial blood pressure expands the artery laterally, producing an aneurysm which may rupture causing death of the animal.

Caudal Mesenteric Artery (Fig. 11–31). The *caudal mesenteric artery* supplies that portion of the intestine from the left colic flexure to the cranial rectal region. The caudal mesenteric has three named branches or sets of branches: *left colic, sigmoid arteries,* and *cranial rectal artery.* In the *dog,* the terminal branches of the colic artery are as shown in Figures 11–28 through 11–30.

Venous Drainage of Jejunum, Ileum, and Colon. The venous drainage of the majority of the small intestine and the colon is by way of tributaries which empty into the caudal and cranial mesenteric veins. The mesenteric veins are joined by the splenic to form the portal vein.

ALIMENTARY CANAL AND ACCESSORY DIGESTIVE ORGANS IN DOMESTIC RUMINANT ANIMALS

The Omentum

Greater Omentum

The greater omentum is an important storage area for fat which is usually deposited first along the small vessels between the peritoneal layers, and is often present in such large amounts that the whole omentum becomes thickened and opaque.

The *greater omentum* of the adult ruminant[12] can be traced from its attachment to the sublumbar musculature on the left side of the abdomen as two layers of peritoneum which pass directly onto the rumen. The attachment of the greater omentum is along the right longitudinal groove of the rumen, into the caudal ruminal groove between the caudal blind sacs and then forward along the left longitudinal groove in close proximity to the reticulum. The greater omentum passes under the rumen and reticulum to the greater curvature of the abomasum and distally to the mesoduodenum.

The greater omentum (Fig. 11–32) has superficial and deep walls or layers. The *superficial wall* extends from the greater curvature of the abomasum, the cranial and descending parts of the duodenum along the floor of the abdomen to the left longitudinal groove. The *deep wall* of the greater omentum attaches to the right longitudinal groove of the rumen and joins the superficial wall in the rumen's caudal groove. From the right longitudinal groove, the superficial wall drops down to the floor of the abdomen and then upward to the descending duodenum, forming a double sling-like suspension for the intestines.

The *omental bursa* is merely the space between the two walls of the greater omentum, the peritoneal surface of the ventral sac of the rumen and a portion of the liver. The entrance to the omental bursa is the epiploic foramen.

The *supraomental ("intestinal") recess* is the part of the peritoneal cavity located dorsal to the greater omentum which is open caudally and contains within it most of the intestinal mass; some of the intestinal mass, however, will project caudally out of the recess and lie near the pelvic inlet.

Lesser Omentum

The *lesser omentum*, in ruminants as in simple stomach species, extends between the visceral surface of the liver and the lesser curvature of the stomach or abomasum as it is called in ruminants. The lesser omentum is divided into two ligaments: (1) the *hepatogastric ligament*, which extends from the liver to the abomasum; and (2) the *hepatoduodenal ligament*, which extends from liver to duodenum.

CLINICAL CONSIDERATIONS—OMENTUM

One of the important features of the omentum is that like other serosal surfaces it has a tendency to adhere to inflamed abdominal organs, and in doing so helps to assist body defense mechanisms in controlling the spread of infection. The surgeon uses this fact of nature by suturing portions of the omentum around a repaired piece of intestine or stomach to help prevent leakage of contents from the sutured gut.

In order to expose the intestines on the right side of the peritoneal cavity, the *superficial wall* of the greater omentum must be first incised. This opens the omental bursa and exposes the deep wall of the greater omentum. Incisions through the deep wall expose the intestinal mass.

Abdominal Organs

In the living animal, abdominal and pelvic organs do not assume constant form and position, a false concept that may have been obtained by remembering only what was learned about the disposition of abdominal organs in embalmed animals. In some cases, however, abdominal organs, or portions of them, do not normally change in position because they are anchored by connective tissue or visceral ligaments. This is the case with the liver, which is

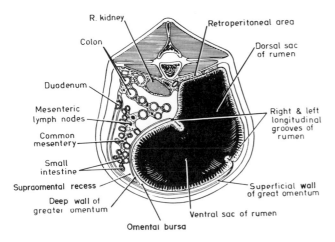

Figure 11–32. Transverse Plane Through Bovine Rumen Showing Walls of Greater Omentum—viewed from the cranial portion of abdomen. (Modified from Dyce and Wensing.[12])

attached to the diaphragm by visceral ligaments, and also the dorsal sac of the rumen, which is attached by connective tissue to the sublumbar region.

Alimentary Canal

Forestomach and Stomach

The stomach of ruminants is divided into a forestomach and a true stomach. The *forestomach* is composed of reticulum, rumen, and omasum; and the *abomasum* is homologous to the stomach of non-ruminants.

The *rumen* is the largest compartment of the forestomach and occupies the major portion of the abdominal cavity. It extends from the diaphragm to the pelvic inlet almost completely filling the left half and at times part of the right half of the abdominal cavity. On the left side its *dorsal* and *ventral sacs* are subdivided on each side by horizontally situated *longitudinal grooves*.

The *reticulum* is the most cranial compartment of the forestomach and in large ruminants is located generally in the area from ribs 6 to 8, mostly to the left of the median plane.

The *omasum* is a hemispherical structure lying to the right of the median plane at approximately the level of ribs 7 to 11 in cattle, where it is also located close to the liver.

The *abomasum* or true stomach is connected to the forestomach at the omasoabomasal ostium. Because the abomasum resembles the stomach of the dog, horse, or pig, it thus has the same subdivisions; namely, *fundus, body, pyloric portion, lesser* and *greater curvatures*. Although the abomasum is commonly considered to lie on the xiphoid cartilage, i.e., forward on the right floor of the abdominal cavity, when distended with ingesta, the abomasum will extend to the left and lie ventral to the cranial ends of the dorsal and ventral sacs of the rumen.

Spleen. This flat, oblong organ is attached to the craniodorsal end of the twelfth intercostal space (the last one) ventrally and cranially approximately to the middle of the 6–7 intercostal space in large ruminants.

CLINICAL CONSIDERATIONS—UTERUS

In the pregnant cow or ewe, the position of the uterus in the abdominal cavity may greatly affect the position of forestomach, the abomasum, and the intestine. For example, usually in the cow, the enlarging uterus will push forward into the intestinal recess and come to lie between the right surface of the rumen and the greater omentum. As the uterus enlarges, it extends forward displacing the rumen further to the left, the intestines more dorsally and the diaphragm towards the thorax, so that toward term, the pregnant uterus will occupy most of the ventral and right half of the abdomen.

Ruminant Forestomach and Abomasum

Development (Figs. 11–33 through 11–35). Development implies the transition from a point of origin of stomach primordia to the point at which the primordia may be considered "adult" in form. Although it has often been taught that the stomach primordia develop from the esophagus, comprehensive studies by Lewis,[13] Pernkopf,[14] Lambert,[15] and Warner[16] have shown that there is no esophageal contribution to any part of the com-

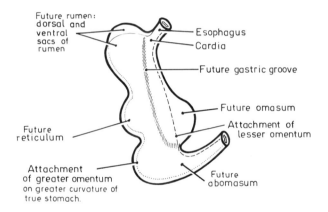

Figure 11–33. Ruminant Stomach: bovine embryo, approximately 15 mm long and 36 days' gestation. (Redrawn from Martin, 1891; Pernkopf;[14] and Warner.[16])

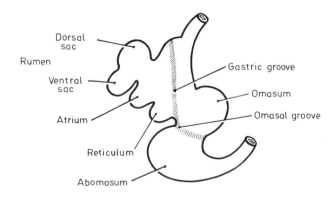

Figure 11–34. Ruminant Stomach: bovine embryo, approximately 25 mm long and 43 days' gestation. (Redrawn from Martin, 1891; Pernkopf;[14] and Warner.[16])

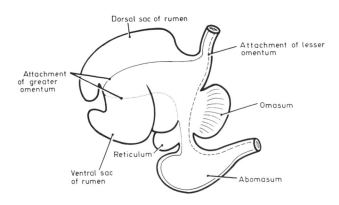

Figure 11-35. Ruminant Stomach: bovine embryo, approximately 43 mm long and 55 days' gestation. (Redrawn from Martin, 1891; Pernkopf;[14] and Warner.[16])

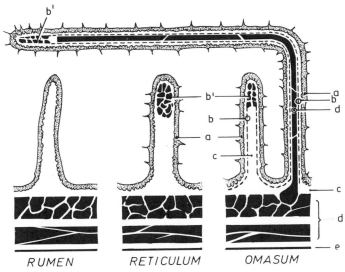

a – epithelium
b – muscularis mucosae
b' – strands of muscularis mucosa
c – submucosae
d – muscularis
e – serosa

Figure 11-36. Composition of the Wall of Forestomach in Ruminants. (After Hrudka, 1975.)

partmentalized stomach including the reticular groove.

In sheep, differentiation of the stomach compartments is described in an embryo measuring only 9 millimeters in length. Also in sheep, by 20 to 24 days, the areas of the future *reticulorumen* and *abomasum* are distinguishable grossly, with the *omasum* being first observed at 43 days; and by 46 days the omasal wall forms laminae, and at 70 days one can distinguish all four components.

Form and Position. The ruminant stomach of cattle or sheep is large and in the adult occupies about three-fourths of the abdominal cavity. The rumen and reticulum are located on the left side of the abdomen, but the ventral ruminal sac, omasum and abomasum are to the right of the median plane.

The forestomach of ruminants is composed of three parts: *reticulum, rumen,* and *omasum.* The axis about which the ruminant forestomach develops is a mucosal depression called the *gastric (esophageal) groove,* which begins at the esophagus and ends at the omasoabomasal ostium. Within the reticulum, the gastric groove is usually referred to as the *reticular groove,* and within the omasum it is called the *omasal groove;* that portion of the gastric groove within the abomasum is the *abomasal groove.*

The Reticulum (Figs. 11-11, 11-36 through 11-39). The reticulum is the smallest and most cranial compartment of the forestomach. It lies between the diaphragm and the rumen and is separated internally from the rumen by the U-shaped *ruminoreticular pillar.* The mucosa of the reticulum is in the form of permanent interconnected folds resembling a honeycomb.[17] This mucosal characteristic is helpful in recognizing the reticulum when

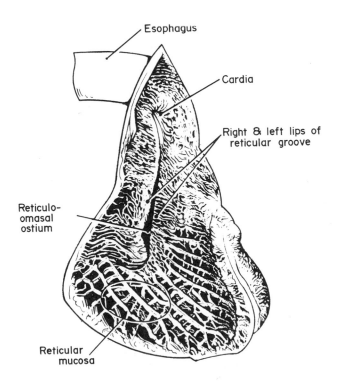

Figure 11-37. Reticular Groove of Cow. (Redrawn from Getty.[9])

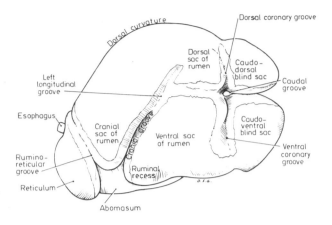

Figure 11–38. Mature Ruminant Stomach: Cow—parietal left surface. (Redrawn from Nickel et al.[1])

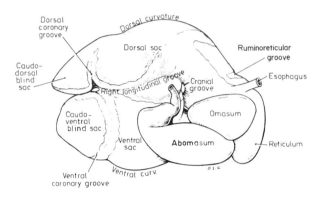

Figure 11–39. Mature Ruminant Stomach: Cow—visceral (right) surface. (Redrawn from Nickel et al.[1])

one blindly enters the interior of the reticulum in rumenotomy procedures.

The *reticular groove* has right and left lips and descends in a spiral fashion to the *reticulo-omasal ostium*, which is located in the depths of the reticular groove. Likewise, when one palpates the reticular groove, one can feel small cornified papillae on its floor. Surrounding the reticulo-omasal ostium the smooth muscle is well developed and is referred to as the reticulo-omasal "sphincter." The sphincter contracts in rumination, thus moving ingesta from the reticulum into the omasum, and is spoken of as the "omasal pump" mechanism.

CLINICAL CONSIDERATIONS—RETICULUM

The convex, diaphragmatic surface of the reticulum lies against the curvature of the diaphragm; also the right surface of the reticulum is in contact with the left lobe of the liver. Foreign bodies such as wire and nails which have been ingested with grain or roughage lodge in the reticulum. Foreign body penetrations of the reticulum can be through the diaphragm and into the pericardial sac, into the caudal lobe of either lung, or also into the liver. Less commonly, foreign bodies within the reticulum penetrate through its left wall into the ventral part of the spleen.

The Rumen (Figs. 11–11, 11–36, 11–38, 11–39). In adult cattle, sheep, and goats, the rumen is the largest compartment of the forestomach. The rumen has a capacity of approximately 150 to 190 liters (40 to 50 U.S. gallons) in the large cow or bull; this amounts to 80% of the total capacity of the entire *ruminant* stomach. Internally the rumen is subdivided by longitudinal and transverse infoldings of the wall called *pillars*. Most of the internal portion of the *dorsal* and *ventral ruminal sacs*, with the exception of the pillars, is characterized by small papillae of variable length. The papillae are long in the cranial ruminal sac, the cranial part of the ventral sac, and in the caudodorsal and caudoventral blind sacs. The papillae of the dorsal sac are short and blunt, which probably corresponds to the fact that this area functions little in absorption of the rumen contents.

As mentioned previously, the ruminal grooves (Figs. 11–38 and 11–39) are represented within the ruminal interior by *pillars*. In front, the *cranial pillar* separates the *cranial sac (ruminal atrium)* above and the cranial part of the *ventral sac* below. The left *ruminal pillar* continues caudally from the cranial pillar and appears as a low fold joining the cranial and caudal pillars. A short *left accessory groove* extends caudodorsal from the cranial pillar, and externally it appears as the *left accessory groove*, which contains the terminal part of the left ruminal artery. The *coronary pillars* extend dorsally and ventrally from each caudal pillar and divide the caudal end of the rumen into *caudodorsal* and *caudoventral blind sacs*.

The Omasum (Figs. 11–11, 11–36, 11–38, 11–39). The *development of the omasum* is in two portions. The base of the omasum with its *omasal groove* develops as a portion of the greater curvature of the true stomach, while the rest of the omasum is a development of the original lesser curvature of the true stomach.[13-16]

In the adult state the omasum has a nearly spherical shape and lies to the right of the median plane. The interior of the omasum has been described as having the appearance of "pages of a book," e.g., being composed of approximately 100 longitudinal folds or *omasal laminae*. One action of the laminae is thought to be rhythmic contraction, effecting the extraction of fluids from the semisolid ingesta incoming from the rumen. The laminae are also concerned with absorption of certain biochemical products of digestion. The muscularis mucosae forms a thick layer just beneath the lamina propria on both sides of the folds of laminae. The inner circular layer of smooth muscle of the lamina muscularis is continued between them into the large omasal folds.

The ostia and grooves of the omasum have been mentioned. They are: the *reticulo-omasal orifice* or *ostium* and the *omasal groove*.

The Abomasum (Figs. 11–11, 11–38, 11–39). The abomasum is the true stomach and homologous to the stomach of the dog, horse, and pig. The position of the abomasum is determined chiefly by the contractions and the fullness of the rumen and reticulum to which it is attached. Generally speaking, the abomasum lies on the abdominal floor to the right of the median plane, and in large ruminants, the abomasum lies opposite the seventh to eleventh ribs.

The abomasum is lined by glandular mucosa in contrast to the rough mucosa in the forestomach. The abomasum is subdivided by a constriction, the *angular incisure*, into a proximal *fundic* portion containing gastric glands, and a distal *pyloric* part having pyloric glands. The *omasoabomasal ostium* is surrounded by a cardiac gland zone, and it is here that the *omasal* groove joins the *abomasal* groove. The entire mucosal channel extending from esophagus to abomasum is called the *gastric (esophageal) groove;* it is especially functional in the newborn ruminant during suckling, at which time partial closure of the gastric groove enables ingested milk to bypass the rumen and pass directly from the esophagus into the abomasum.

CLINICAL CONSIDERATIONS—ABOMASAL DISPLACEMENT

There are limits to the normal variations in position of the abomasum, beyond which transgressions produce digestive disturbances which may be severe enough to endanger the life of the animal. When the abomasum is displaced, it is often found on the left side of the abdominal cavity, some-times extending dorsally to the left paralumbar fossa.

Liver and Gallbladder (Fig. 11–18, Table 11–3)

The liver in ruminants lies to the right of and parallel to the median plane and is directed obliquely downward and forward toward the right portion of the diaphragm. The liver has a diaphragmatic surface located next to the diaphragm and a visceral surface which is in contact chiefly with the omasum and reticulum.

Ruminants possess a *gallbladder*, a pear-shaped structure approximately 10 to 13 cm long, lying partly against and attached to the visceral surface of the liver at approximately the level of the tenth or eleventh intercostal space. The duct of the gallbladder is the *cystic duct*, and it joins the common *hepatic duct* to form the regular type *common bile duct*. The *common bile duct*, also called *ductus choledochus*, penetrates the wall of the duodenum approximately 60 centimeters distal to the pylorus in large *ruminants* and approximately 35 centimeters in small *ruminants*.

The Spleen

In ruminants, due to the expansion of the greater curvature of the gastric primordium into the rumen and reticulum, the spleen loses its connection with the greater omentum and can be found directly applied to the left dorsocranial surface of the rumen. Its *parietal (diaphragmatic) surface* lies against the diaphragm, to which it is attached and the *visceral surface* of the spleen lies firmly against the rumen, thus allowing little opportunity for the spleen to rotate upon itself, producing constriction of its vessels as seen in torsion of other organs.

The spleen in adult cattle measures approximately 60 centimeters in length by 2 centimeters thick by 15 centimeters wide, and weighs about 0.9 kg. The spleen extends downward and forward on the left side of the body from the twelfth and thirteenth ribs (its dorsal extremity) to approximately the junction of the middle and lower third of the seventh rib. Thus under normal conditions the spleen is protected by the thoracic cage and does not extend caudally as far as the paralumbar fossa.

The Intestine

The development of the intestine in ruminant animals begins as it does in the simple stomach quadrupeds, and ends as a tubular structure approximately 20 times the length of the body (Fig. 11–9). With the development of the ruminant forestomach, the postnatal intestine will lie chiefly on the right side of the abdomen, with the small intestine taking the form of many short coils within the free margin of the common dorsal mesentery. The position of the coils will be dependent upon the fullness of the rumen and the size of the uterus. The large intestine comes to lie chiefly in the right dorsal part of the abdominal cavity, and here it is related on the left to the rumen and on the right to the lateral abdominal wall from which it is separated by the greater omentum.

In the development of the ruminant colon, the ascending colon becomes modified to form what is essentially a *spiral loop** with the portions of colon tightly adherent to each other. The portion of the ascending colon that enters the spiral loop is quite appropriately named the *proximal loop of the colon,*† and the portion leaving the spiral loop is the *distal loop of the colon.*‡ The spiral loop itself is the most confusing part of this intestinal modification and will be explained in a later paragraph.

Small Intestine (Fig. 11–40). The intestine lies almost entirely to the right of the midline and in the dorsal part of the abdomen. Its capacity is relatively less than the small intestine of other species, and as previously mentioned, the intestine lies in a "sling-like" suspension of the greater omentum, the *supraomental recess.*

Duodenum (Fig. 11–40). The duodenum of adult cattle is approximately 1 meter long. It arises at the pylorus of the abomasum approximately at the level of the ventral end of the right ninth intercostal space or tenth rib. The duodenum extends to the visceral surface of the liver where it takes the form of an S-shape curve, the *ansa sigmoidea,* which with the *cranial duodenal flexure* forms the cranial part of the duodenum. The duodenum then passes caudally high in the sublumbar region as the *descending duodenum,* and near the pelvic inlet it turns cranially at the *caudal duodenal flexure.* Its *ascending part* passes toward the liver again and is continued at the *duodenojejunal flexure* as the jejunum.

The cranial portion of the duodenum is attached to the liver by the *hepatoduodenal ligament,* a part of the lesser omentum, which is not as ligamentous in appearance in the bovine species as it is in some of the other domestic species. Nevertheless, the hepatoduodenal ligament does help to anchor this proximal portion of the duodenum, giving it a constant location and making it invulnerable to torsion. The hepatoduodenal ligament is continued

---

*Ansa spiralis coli
†Ansa proximalis coli
‡Ansa distalis coli

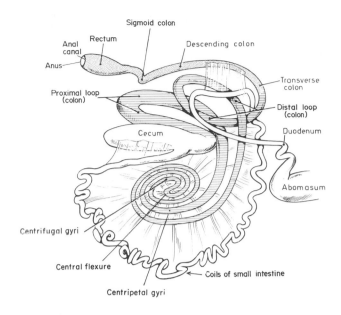

Figure 11–40. Schematic Representation of the Adult Ruminant Intestine. (Redrawn from Dyce and Wensing.[12])

as the *mesoduodenum,* a portion of the common dorsal mesentery, which carries vessels and nerve fibers to and from the duodenum and in addition attaches the duodenum to portions of the liver, pancreas, right kidney, and the cecum.

Pancreatic and Common Bile Ducts. Embryonically it is the dorsal pancreatic primordium that develops in large ruminants, providing for only a single pancreatic duct which opens into the descending duodenum on the minor duodenal papilla. The *pancreatic duct* in cattle is homologous to the *accessory pancreatic duct* of those species (dog, horse) in which both dorsal and ventral primordia develop fully, but because cattle possess only the one duct, it is commonly called the *pancreatic duct* rather than the accessory duct.

The *common bile duct* opens into the lumen of the descending duodenum at the major duodenal papilla, which is located at the ventral portion of the ansa sigmoidea, and the *accessory pancreatic duct* opens approximately 30 to 40 centimeters distally at the minor duodenal papilla. Occasionally there is a second pancreatic duct in large ruminants and when it is present, it enters the duodenum with the common bile duct at the major duodenal papilla. The most common situation in small ruminants, however, is a single pancreatic duct which enters the duodenum with the common bile duct at the major duodenal papilla.

Jejunum and Ileum (Fig. 11–40). As in the other species of domestic animals there is no clear boundary between the jejunum and *ileum*, which together form many short coils within the free margin of the mesentery. The position of these coils depends upon the fullness of the rumen and the size of the uterus, but usually most of the jejunum lies within the recess bounded by the rumen and greater omentum. However, some small intestine may be found behind the rumen and thus against the left flank.

Large Intestine. The *cecum*, a tubular organ with a rounded, blind tip which projects caudally from the intestinal mass, is the first portion of the large intestine, and it is separated from the colon by the entrance of the ileum.

The tip of the cecum when filled with gas is located high in the abdomen, but sinks to the abdominal floor when its contents are heavier. The length of the cecum in cattle is about 75 centimeters, and its diameter is approximately 12 centimeters.

The *colon* is divided into the usual *ascending*, *transverse*, and *descending parts*. The ascending colon is unusually long and, as mentioned in the development of the intestine, it is divided into proximal, spiral, and distal loops. The *proximal loop of the colon* is a direct continuation from the cecum. It is continued ventrally as the *centripetal gyri*, which makes two full turns toward the center of the intestinal mass; the intestine then reverses its direction and at this point it is called the *central flexure*. From the *central flexure* the intestinal coil turns toward the outside and is termed the *centrifugal gyri* and is continued as the *distal loop* of the colon, which passes dorsally and caudally on the surface of the proximal loop to be continued on the transverse body just in front of the cranial mesenteric artery; from here it is continued as the descending colon.

The *descending colon* courses caudally high in the abdomen bound by mesentery to the ascending duodenum. At about the level of the sixth lumbar vertebra, the descending (sigmoid) colon makes a bend and is more movable than the rest of the colon due to its longer mesentery. Unlike the large intestine of the horse and the pig, the ruminant large intestine does not possess teniae coli.

The *rectum* is the intrapelvic portion of the colon. Most of the rectum has a mesorectum, with only its caudal part being retroperitoneal and relatively immovable. The muscular layers are thick with intermittent *transverse folds* produced by circular smooth muscle present. The *anal canal* is the short terminal segment of the bowel which ends at the exterior as the anus. *Rectal columns*, longitudinal mucosal folds, are found for a distance of approxi-

mately 10 cm at the junction of the rectum and anal canal.

A detailed description of the external and internal anal sphincter, and the levator ani and coccygeus muscles of the pelvic diaphragm has been made.[18]

Arterial Supply, Venous and Lymphatic Drainage of the Alimentary Canal and Accessory Digestive Organs in Domestic Ruminants

Arterial Supply[19] (Figs. 11–41 through 11–45)

The arterial blood supply of the forestomach and stomach in the ruminant animals is from the *celiac artery*. The celiac artery, encircled by a dense celiac autonomic plexus, is the first major branch to arise from the abdominal aorta.

A major branch of the celiac artery is the *common hepatic artery*. The common hepatic supplies the liver and gallbladder, duodenum, pancreas, and abomasum. The artery courses through the lesser omentum to a position near the porta hepatis where it divides into right and left hepatic, cystic, gastroduodenal, and right gastric arteries. One of the terminal branches of the common hepatic, the *gastroduodenal artery*, supplies blood to the descending duodenum, and the sigmoid flexure of the duodenum, and to the right portion of the greater curvature of the abomasum. The other terminal branch of the common hepatic artery is the *right gastric*. It supplies blood to the lesser curvature of the abomasum and terminates here by making anastomotic connections with the left gastric artery. It is along both the lesser and greater curvatures of the abomasum that anastomotic connections take place between different branches of the common hepatic artery.

The *right ruminal artery* in both the large and small ruminants usually arises in common with the splenic artery, and when this occurs, the combined vessel has been called the "*splenoruminal*" trunk. The *splenic artery*, the smaller of the two, passes over the dorsal sac of the rumen to the spleen, and the *right ruminal artery* descends to the origin of the right longitudinal groove of the rumen where it is accompanied by a branch of the dorsal vagal trunk. The right ruminal artery and vagal trunk course caudally in the right longitudinal groove of the rumen and supply portions of both dorsal and ventral sacs of this organ. The right ruminal artery terminates by forming anastomotic connections with the left ruminal artery.

The *left ruminal artery* is a large vessel which arises distal to the origin of the "*splenoruminal*" trunk. It frequently serves as an accessory source of

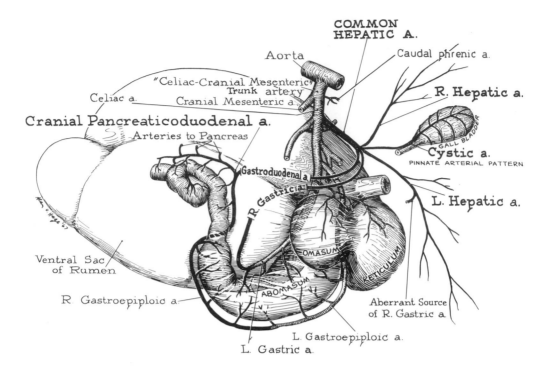

Figure 11-41. Common Hepatic Artery—Sheep. (From Anderson and Weber.[19])

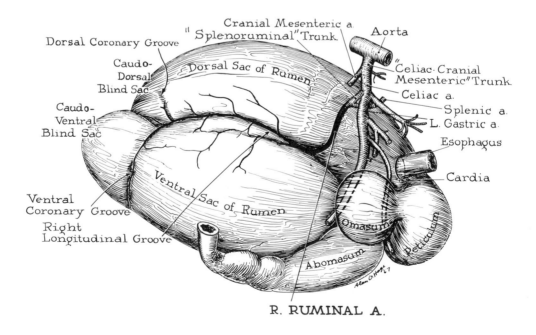

Figure 11-42. Right Ruminal Artery—Sheep. (From Anderson and Weber.[19])

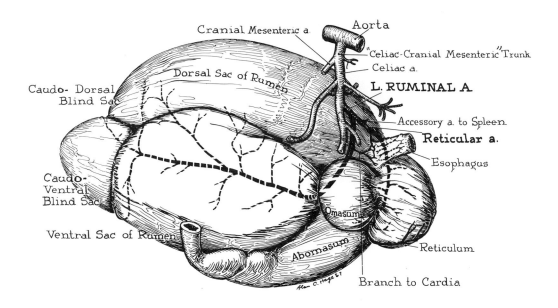

Figure 11–43. Left Ruminal Artery—Sheep. (From Anderson and Weber.[19])

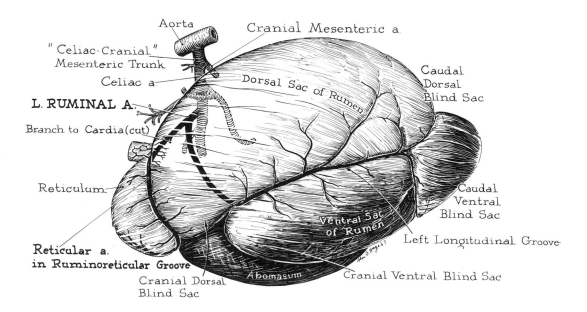

Figure 11–44. Left Ruminal Artery—Sheep. (From Anderson and Weber.[19])

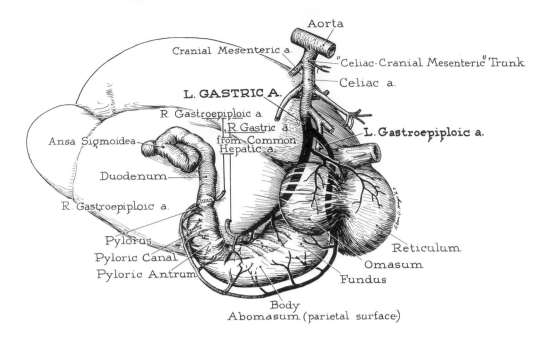

Figure 11–45. Left Gastric Artery—Sheep. (From Anderson and Weber.[19])

blood supply to the spleen and regularly supplies the reticulum and the cranial sac of the rumen (ruminal atrium). In addition the left ruminal artery has esophageal branches which pass through the esophageal hiatus to the distal esophagus. In the well-injected specimen one can trace *vasa nervorum* from these branches into the epineurium of the dorsal and ventral vagal trunks. The *dorsal vagal trunk* also receives vasa nervorum from the phrenic artery, a small branch of the celiac trunk. The left ruminal artery terminates in the ruminoreticular groove deep to the serosa which binds the reticulum and cranial ventral sac* of the rumen together. The artery continues caudally on the right side.

The *left gastric artery* is the continuation of the celiac artery following the origin of the common hepatic, splenic, and ruminal arteries. The left gastric artery provides most of the blood supply to the abomasum. It terminates in both the lesser and greater curvature of the stomach by anastomosing with other branches of the celiac trunk.

CLINICAL CONSIDERATIONS—ABOMASAL DISPLACEMENT

The fact that the abomasum receives blood supply from two major arteries, namely the

common hepatic and the left gastric, may be a factor in preventing ischemia of the organ during periods of severe stretching of organ and vessels when the abomasum is displaced.

Venous Drainage

In simple stomach animals, the portal vein carries blood from the stomach, intestine, and spleen to the liver. In these species, the largest tributaries of the portal vein are the cranial mesenteric and splenic, and the smallest is the caudal mesenteric. In ruminants there are, in addition to the above-mentioned veins, large *ruminal veins* which parallel the arteries. They are *right* and *left ruminal veins, reticular vein*, and *left gastric vein*. The splenic vein joins the right ruminal vein, which in turn unites with the left ruminal vein to form a major venous tributary which returns blood from the forestomach and abomasum to the liver by way of the portal vein.

Lymphatic Drainage

Small lymph nodes are scattered over the surface of the *ruminant* forestomach and stomach. *Right* and *left ruminal lymph nodes* are especially numerous in the two longitudinal grooves of the rumen, and small nodes are found at the curvature of the omasum and abomasum. Efferent lymphatic vessels which leave the lymph nodes of the greater curvature of the abomasum drain into the *hepatic nodes*,

_____
*Ruminal recess

while efferent vessels from the *gastric* nodes of the forestomach, the *reticular, omasal,* and *ruminal* lymph nodes, pass toward the area of the cardia and ruminal atrium into *atrial lymph nodes* and then into the cisterna chyli.

The lymph vessels and nodes of the ruminant intestine are similar to those in the intestine of the simple stomach animals; however, lymphoid tissue appears more abundant throughout the intestinal mucosa in ruminants than in non-ruminants. In ruminants, aggregated nodules of lymph tissue may be as long as 25 cm and extend through the ileocecal ostium into the large intestine.

The efferent lymphatics which drain the *liver* and *gallbladder* run chiefly along the portal vein and hepatic and celiac arteries as the *hepatic lymph trunk(s),* and contribute to the formation of the *cisterna chyli.* Although the principal lymphatic drainage from the liver is into *hepatic lymph nodes* which are found along the course of the hepatic vessels, there is a secondary drainage from the diaphragmatic surface of the liver by way of lymphatics which course in the falciform and triangular ligaments through the diaphragm at the foramen for the caudal vena cava, and then into the *mediastinal lymph nodes.* This alternate route for lymph from the liver into the thorax instead of directly into the cisterna chyli provides a more direct channel for pathogenic organisms and neoplastic cells to reach thoracic organs.

The *splenic lymph vessels and nodes* extend from the hilus of the *spleen* to the gastrosplenic ligament and along the course of the splenic vein and its tributaries.

The *gastric lymph nodes* have efferent vessels which form *gastric lymph trunks* and drain into the cisterna chyli.

The *celiac lymph nodes* lie embedded around the celiac artery, and receive many efferent lymph vessels from the organs supplied by the celiac trunk.

The *cranial* and *caudal mesenteric lymph nodes* are located in the common dorsal mesentery. There are many mesenteric nodes and they are subdivided into that portion of the gut with which they are associated. Thus, there are *jejunal, cecal, right, left and middle colic nodes* whose efferent vessels form *lymphatic trunks* of the same name and course to the cisterna chyli. In addition, there are *intestinal lymph trunks* of indistinct origin in the gut.

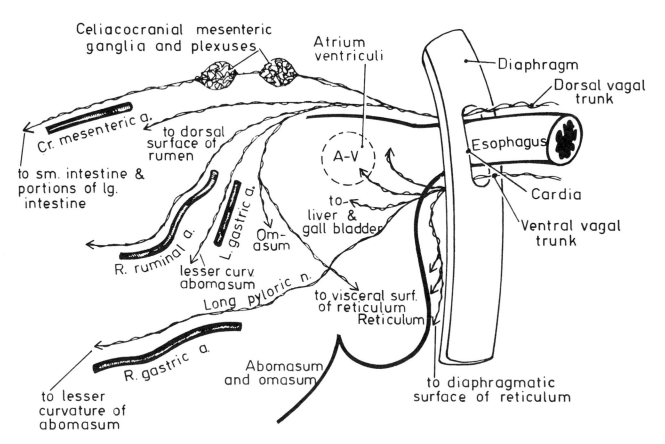

Figure 11–46. Terminations of Vagal Trunks in Ruminants—Schematic. (Modified from Habel.[21])

Innervation of the Ruminant Forestomach and Stomach

Parasympathetic Innervation (Fig. 11–46)

The *vagus nerves* are exceedingly important to the ruminant animal in the control of the muscular contraction cycles of the forestomach and abomasum. In addition, the vagi control acts of regurgitation of the bolus from forestomach to oral cavity for resalivation and remastication. The vagal nerves function in the stimulation of closure of the reticular groove in the younger ruminant during the process of suckling. The vagi also function in stimulating contraction of the abomasum so that its contents may be transferred to the duodenum.

The vagi are arranged similarly in ruminants and non-ruminants so that there are dorsal and ventral vagal trunks which pass through the esophageal hiatus into the abdomen. The *dorsal vagal trunk* innervates a relatively large portion of the stomach in ruminant animals, due to the fact that the areas of the simple stomach normally supplied by the dorsal vagal trunk develop into compartments of the forestomach. As a result the dorsal vagus innervates most of the rumen in the adult. The course of branches of the dorsal vagus is with the right and left ruminal arteries and veins in the two longitudinal grooves of the rumen. Branches of the nerves also pass to the dorsal surfaces and sides of the omasum with the left gastric artery, and terminal branches reach the lesser curvature of the abomasum. In addition to the preceding visceral branches, there are communicating branches with the ventral vagal trunk and important contributions to the celiac plexus.

The *ventral vagal trunk* innervates the liver and gallbladder, cardia, ruminal atrium, and the lesser curvature of the abomasum by way of the *long pyloric nerve*, which parallels the right gastric vessels.

Sympathetic Innervation

The *sympathetic innervation*, which is particularly important in regulating the luminal diameters of arterioles and to a lesser extent the veins of the gastrointestinal tract, is chiefly from the greater splanchnic nerves. The *greater splanchnic* arises as preganglionic fibers from the fifth and sixth segments of the thoracic sympathetic trunk as well as from a variable number of the more caudal segments. The greater splanchnic nerve passes caudally in the abdomen between the crura of the diaphragm and the lateral border of the psoas minor muscle where fibers of the greater splanchnic synapse in the celiac, cranial mesenteric, or aortico-renal ganglia. As previously mentioned, the celiac and cranial mesenteric plexuses form a dense network of fibers around the arteries just ventral to the abdominal aorta, and embedded in the plexuses are the celiac and cranial mesenteric ganglia. These ganglia are sites of synapse for the majority of preganglionic sympathetic fibers which run in the splanchnic nerves. After synapsing, the resultant postganglionic fibers pass with branches of the celiac trunk and cranial mesenteric artery to all parts of the viscera.

CLINICAL AND EXPERIMENTAL CONSIDERATIONS –VAGAL NERVES

The vagal nerves are responsible for tone and contraction of the ruminant forestomach and to a lesser degree the abomasum. Section of both vagi abolishes all motor activity to the forestomach, while section of only the dorsal vagal trunk results in nearly complete, but not always permanent paralysis of the rumen, with a less marked effect on the reticulum.

Division of only the ventral vagal trunk usually results in less of a paralytic effect upon rumen motility than section of the dorsal trunk. Section of the splanchnic (sympathetic) nerves does not affect rumen motility. Bilateral splanchnotomy had no effect on gastric motility in the sheep nor did sectioning of the splanchnic nerves prevent the serious distention of the forestomach which follows sectioning of both vagal trunks.[20] One can assume, based on these experiences, that if both vagi are incapable of transmitting impulses to the ruminant stomach, paralysis of the forestomach will occur even in the presence of normal sympathetic function. Also, the fatal gastric distention which results from complete lack of vagal function is not due to a spasm of the pyloric sphincter resulting from unopposed sympathetic impulses.

REFERENCES

1. Nickel, R., Schummer, A., Seiferle, E., and Sack, W.: The Viscera of the Domestic Mammals. Berlin and Hamburg, Verlag Paul Parey, —New York, Springer-Verlag, 1973.
2. Miller, M. E., Christensen, G. C., and Evans, H. E.: Anatomy of the Dog. Philadelphia, W. B. Saunders Co., 1964.
3. Kitchell, R. E.: Unpublished data.
4. Krölling, O., and Grau, H.: Lehrbuch der Histologie und vergleichenden mikroskopischen Anatomie der Haustiere, 10th ed. Berlin, Paul Parey, 1960.

5. Stinson, A. W., and Calhoun, M. J.: Digestive system. *In* Textbook of Veterinary Histology. Edited by H. D. Dellman and E. M. Brown. Philadelphia, Lea & Febiger, 1976.

6. Hollinshead, W. H.: Textbook of Anatomy, 2nd ed. New York, Harper & Row Publishers, 1974.

7. Evans, H. E., and deLahunta, A.: Miller's Guide to the Dissection of the Dog. Philadelphia, W. B. Saunders Co., 1971.

8. Schummer, A.: Morphologisne Untersuchungen uber die Functionszustande des Ileums. Tieraerztl. Umschau *8*:244, 1953.

9. Getty, R: Sisson and Grossman's The Anatomy of the Domestic Animals, 5th ed. Philadelphia, W. B. Saunders Co., 1975.

10. Anderson, W. D., and Anderson, B. G.: Unpublished data, 1977.

11. Hopkins, G. S.: Unpublished data.

12. Dyce, K. M., and Wensing, C. J. C.: Essentials of Bovine Anatomy. Philadelphia, Lea & Febiger, 1971.

13. Lewis, F. T.: The comparative embryology of the mammalian stomach. Anat. Rec. *9*:102, 1915.

14. Pernkopf, E.: Die Entwicklung des Vorderdarmes, insbesondere des Magens der Wiederkauer. Eine vergleichendembryologische Studie. Z. Gesamte Anat. (Abt. 1) *94*:490, 1931.

15. Lambert, P. S.: The development of the stomach in the ruminant. Vet. J. *194*:302, 1948.

16. Warner, E. D.: The organogenesis and early histogenesis of the bovine stomach. Am. J. Anat. *102*:33, 1958.

17. Hrudka, F.: Unpublished data.

18. Habel, R. E.: The topographic anatomy of the muscles, nerves and arteries in the bovine female perineum. Am. J. Anat. *119*:79, 1966.

19. Anderson, W. D., and Weber, A. T., Normal arterial supply to the ruminants (ovine) stomach. J. Am. Sci. *28*:379, 1969.

20. Duncan, D. L.: The effects of vagotomy and splanchnotomy on gastric motility in sheep. J. Physiol. *119*:157, 1953.

21. Habel, R. E.: Guide to the Dissection of Domestic Ruminants. Ithaca, NY, published by author, 1970.

Chapter 12

COMPARATIVE PHYSIOLOGY OF THE GASTROINTESTINAL SYSTEM

ROBERT A. ARGENZIO

NEUROENDOCRINE CONTROL OF GASTROINTESTINAL FUNCTION

Secretory and motor function of the gut is to a large degree controlled or modulated by the autonomic nervous system and by gastrointestinal hormones. The action and interaction of these two control systems are complex and require an introduction before the specific functions are considered in detail.

Neural Mechanisms

A scheme of the extrinsic and intrinsic fibers of the enteric plexus is shown in Figure 12–1. Nerve fibers arising from enteric neurons and ending ex-

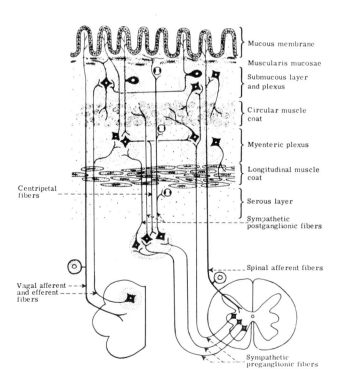

Figure 12–1. Scheme of the extrinsic and intrinsic innervation of the bowel. (Reprinted from Handbook of Physiology, Vol. IV.[1])

clusively in the wall of the gut are termed intrinsic fibers. These fibers are capable of sensory and motor transmission over local reflex arcs. The intrinsic neural plexus also is connected to the central nervous system via the vagi and splanchnic nerves. An exception is the distal colon, which receives parasympathetic innervation via the sacral nerves.[1]

The vagi are primarily composed of afferent fibers (>90%) which convey information to the central nervous system from mechanoreceptors and chemoreceptors. The vagal efferent fibers are (1) preganglionic parasympathetic fibers connecting with secondary parasympathetic cholinergic neurons of the local plexus, (2) fibers that mediate sympathetic responses, and (3) fibers of the non-adrenergic inhibitory system. The postganglionic transmitter of the parasympathetic fibers is acetylcholine (ACH), which is primarily stimulatory to smooth muscle and certain secretory glands. The transmitter of the non-adrenergic inhibitory system is thought to be ATP, which produces inhibition of smooth muscle contraction.[2]

Sympathetic efferent transmission is primarily due to release of catecholamines at postganglionic sympathetic nerve terminals. Epinephrine is primarily inhibitory to smooth muscle, while in the sphincters, the adrenergic system is stimulatory. However, the non-adrenergic inhibitory fibers of the vagus also exert control over the pyloric and reticulo-omasal sphincter. Sympathetic efferent transmission to the blood vessels usually causes constriction. The sympathetic system also contains sensory fibers which convey pain impulses to the central nervous system.[2]

Hormonal Mechanisms

A group of endocrine cells known as the amine precursor uptake and decarboxylation (APUD) cells are present in gastric, intestinal, and pancreatic tissue. These cells are capable of transforming chemical stimuli into a hormonal signal which then activates specific receptor sites. The three well-known gastrointestinal hormones are gastrin, released from the pyloric antrum, and secretin and cholecystokinin-pancreozymin (CCK-PZ), both of which are released from the proximal small intestine. These agents have known specific actions on gastrointestinal function, the most notable of which are acid and pepsin secretion (gastrin), pancreatic HCO_3^- secretion (secretin) and pancreatic enzyme secretion and gallbladder contraction (CCK-PZ). However, these hormones, acting singly or in combination with each other or with neurotransmitters, have a wide variety of effects on gastrointestinal function, the clinical importance of which is only now becoming apparent.[3]

In addition to these three hormones are a group of polypeptides which have been extracted from intestinal mucosa and which have biologic actions. These include enteroglucagon, gastric inhibitory polypeptide (GIP), and vasoactive intestinal peptide (VIP). Several other new hormones have been postulated but will not be considered further here. The major concern with these three new hormones is their stimulation of intestinal secretion. However, acting singly or in combination with the three major hormones, they also have potentiating and inhibitory effects on other systems. For example, there is good evidence that GIP may inhibit gastric acid secretion and gastric motility, from whence its name was derived.[3]

Receptor Sites

These are postulated configurations of organic molecules on cell membranes which bind neural or endocrine transmitters according to their affinity. The efficacy of these agents is determined by their ability to activate the intracellular machinery that brings about the physiologic response. Since a number of chemical transmitters have similar structures and therefore may compete for receptor sites, it can be expected that potentiation or inhibition will occur depending on their relative efficiency and concentration.[3]

For example, VIP has only approximately 17% of the efficacy of secretin on pancreatic HCO_3^- secretion in the dog.[4] Both hormones share the same receptor site and are competitive inhibitors. Thus at high concentrations, VIP is a potent inhibitor of pancreatic HCO_3^- secretion. However, at low secretin concentration, VIP is a weak stimulus to pancreatic HCO_3^- secretion and amplifies the secretin response. This type of control seems to be the rule in the gut. Gastrointestinal hormones do not appear to be capable of exerting feedback control on their

own release.[3] Thus, in the preceding example, secretion by the pancreas is held within reasonable limits should excessive amounts of secretin be released.

MOTILITY

Gastrointestinal motility is discussed from two aspects. The first describes the mechanical events associated with motility patterns of each segment. These events in turn accomplish specific functional purposes which vary considerably among segments. Thus, abnormal motility in specific areas of bowel will predictably affect these processes. Second, control of the motor events is discussed. This control, whether mediated by intrinsic or extrinsic nervous reflexes or by endocrine effects, provides a basis for pharmacologic intervention as well as clues to the underlying cause of abnormal motility.

Mouth and Esophagus

The method of prehension differs considerably among species. In the horse, the lips are the major prehensile organ, while in ruminants, the tongue, and in the pig, the pointed lower lip serves to deliver food into the mouth. The dog and cat obtain food by movements of the head and jaws but fluids are taken in by the tongue. In other animals, liquids are drawn into the mouth by suction.[5]

Mastication of the food accomplishes two purposes. First the grinding action of the molars breaks down the food to expose a greater surface area for digestive enzymes. No other part of the gastrointestinal tract can break down the food as effectively into small particles should the teeth fail in this operation. Second, chewing of the food permits the admixture of saliva, which lubricates the bolus in preparation for swallowing.

Deglutition begins as a voluntary act but becomes automatic as soon as the bolus is presented to the pharynx. Pharyngeal receptors send afferent impulses to the swallowing center in the medulla via the glossopharyngeal, vagus, and trigeminal nerves. Efferent impulses are conducted to the tongue, floor of the mouth, fauces and laryngeal muscles via the fifth to twelfth cranial nerves. During the pharyngeal stage of swallowing, contraction of the laryngeal muscle closes the glottis. Simultaneously, the epiglottis is deflected caudally to cover the laryngeal orifice completely as the larynx is drawn rostrally by the hyoid apparatus. The nasopharynx must also be closed and this is accomplished by elevation of the palate assisted by elevation of the pharynx. The swallowing center specifically inhibits the respiratory center of the medulla during this stage so that respiration is suspended in any stage of its cycle to allow swallowing to proceed. The food is then delivered to the cranial esophagus through the cranial esophageal sphincter, which is relaxed in advance of arrival of the bolus.[5,6]

Functions of the esophagus will be described in Chapter 21.

Control Systems of Gastrointestinal Motility

The basic control system governing smooth muscle motility is the electrical slow wave or basic electrical rhythm (BER).[7] As in many other cell types, smooth muscle exhibits a membrane potential with the intracellular contents negative to the extracellular fluid. The membrane potential undergoes spontaneous depolarizations and repolarizations which are independent of nervous control. These electrical events determine the time and space in which contraction of smooth muscle can occur.[7] Spike discharges or action potentials are associated with muscle contraction, but these can only occur with, and are superimposed on, the electric slow wave (Fig. 12–2). Therefore the slow wave sets the pace for basic motility patterns and its frequency is remarkably constant in specific areas of the gastrointestinal tract.

Whether or not the muscle is to contract is influenced by neural and endocrine factors. The neurotransmitter acetylcholine increases the fre-

quency of action potentials, presumably by increasing the permeability of the membrane to Na^+ and K^+.[8] The entry of Na^+ is responsible for depolarization.[9] Low doses of ACH also increase the velocity of slow wave propagation. Epinephrine leads to hyperpolarization of the membrane. Most likely this is due to either an increase in K^+ or a decrease in Na^+ permeability.[8] Yet, the slow waves and spike discharges can still occur in the stomach and intestine in vitro and after complete neural blockade.[7] Therefore, it appears that while neural and endocrine factors can greatly modulate gastrointestinal motility, the basic motor control originates in the smooth muscle itself.

The forestomachs, however, are totally dependent on extrinsic innervation. Bilateral vagal section at the diaphragm abolishes cyclic forestomach motility as well as the specific reflexes and is followed by death.

Forestomach Motility

Motility of the forestomachs has to accomplish several purposes. First, ingesta must be retained and mixed so that the contents can undergo a relatively slow process of microbial digestion, followed by absorption. Second, some of the contents must be regurgitated, reinsalivated, and reswallowed. Third, large amounts of gas produced in the rumen (2 liters/min/1000-lb animal)[10] must be eructated in an efficient manner, and fourth, the contents must leave the rumen in an orderly and controlled fashion. All of these events are accomplished in complex but coordinated cycles of forestomach motility.

Cyclic Motility and Associated Reflex Events of the Forestomach. Pressure recordings obtained in the forestomach compartments of a cow are shown in Figure 12–3. The cycle is initiated by a biphasic reticular contraction followed by a primary contraction of the dorsal rumen sac. This contraction progresses caudally and ventrally and then cranially. A secondary contraction of the rumen also occurs but this is not associated with every cycle. Primary and secondary contractions of the omasal canal are associated with the corresponding rumen contractions. However, the omasal body contractions are not synchronized with the ruminoreticular cycle but occur at random in any phase of the cycle, or not at all.[11]

The result of the cyclic motor activity of the reticulum and rumen is to mix and circulate the ingested food in the rumen and prepare the contents further for regurgitation, absorption, or passage into the omasum.

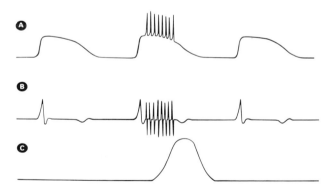

Figure 12–2. Diagram of time relations between slow waves, spike bursts, and contractions. A represents the electromyogram of a single smooth muscle cell, recorded with an intracellular microelectrode. B represents the electromyogram recorded from several such cells by a large extracellular volume-recording electrode. C shows tension in the muscle mass. All three traces are drawn to a common time base. In A, three slow waves appear as a monophasic depolarization from a stable maximal value, the resting membrane potential. In B, the slow waves appear with two components, an initial biphasic spike which represents depolarization, and a secondary slower biphasic signal representing repolarization. The second of the three slow waves bears a burst of spikes, appearing on the plateau of the slow wave. The tension record, in C, shows a contraction beginning during the spike burst, and apparently initiated by it. (From N. Engl. J. Med. 285:85, 1971).

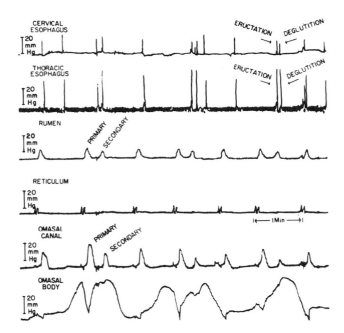

Figure 12–3. Pressure events recorded in esophagus and forestomachs of cow during a normal cycle of motility. (From Sellers.[11])

Also shown in Figure 12–3 are the pressure events recorded in the esophagus during eructation and swallowing.[11] Rise in pressure of the dorsal sac during the primary or secondary contraction is followed by dilation of the cardia and expulsion of gas into the esophagus. The antiperistaltic wave of eructation is immediately followed by a peristaltic wave of deglutition. The number of secondary rumen contractions associated with eructation increases when the intraruminal pressure increases. These contractions appear to originate in the caudo-dorsal blind sac or its associated pillars and occur at a time when the reticulum has relaxed and the cardia is exposed.

Regurgitation (not shown in Fig. 12–3) is also a reflex event coordinated with the ongoing ruminoreticular cycle.[11] An extrareticular contraction, which floods the cardia with ingesta, immediately precedes the biphasic reticular contraction which initiates the cycle. Coinciding with the extrareticular contraction is a negative intrathoracic esophageal pressure of some 40 mm Hg. This is accomplished by an inspiratory effort against a closed glottis, which is the primary driving force for regurgitation. Aspiration of digesta into the caudal esophagus is followed by an antiperistaltic wave of contraction that is approximately twice the rate of waves recorded during deglutition. Regurgitation is followed by mastication for about 1 minute. At the end of the cycle of rumination, the bolus is reswal-

lowed and this is immediately followed by regurgitation of another bolus. These closely integrated reflex events with the normal cyclic forestomach activity indicate a high degree of central control.

During the consecutive cycles of ruminoreticular motility, food contents containing a high specific gravity are collected in the cranial sac and finally presented to the reticulo-omasal orifice. During the second reticular contraction, a negative pressure is recorded in the omasal canal. At the height of this reticular contraction, the reticulo-omasal orifice opens and reticular contents are aspirated into the omasal canal. Contraction of the omasal canal is associated with closure of the reticulo-omasal orifice, and contents are forced into the body of the omasum.

The major volume flow to the abomasum occurs with omasal body contractions. The omasum is a two-stage pump. The first stage consists of aspiration of reticular contents and is coupled to the ruminoreticular cycle. The second stage of contraction is probably stimulated by distention of the omasum; however conditions in the abomasum also affect omasal motility. The omasum selectively retains particles and propels liquid rapidly to the abomasum; thus it may also serve as a filter.

Control of Forestomach Motility. The rumen and reticulum receive postganglionic muscarinic excitatory innervation via the vagus nerves. Since the vagus is composed primarily of afferent fibers, much attention has been paid to reflex pathways controlling forestomach motility. It is now well established that the basic control of ruminoreticular motility involves vagovagal reflexes integrated in the gastric centers of the medulla.[12]

Afferent stimulation from buccal, pharyngeal, esophageal, gastric, and intestinal receptors all affect the frequency of contractions of the reticulorumen.[13] Both inhibitory and excitatory neurons are involved in the overall integration and coordination of the ruminoreticular cycle and its associated reflexes.

Two types of receptors have been identified as sending information to the gastric center over afferent pathways.[12] The first of these are *tension receptors*, located in greatest density around the reticular groove. These receptors send a tonic afferent input to the medulla which is primarily excitatory. However, receptors in the abomasum responding to distention inhibit gastric center neurons, thereby inhibiting primary cycle contractions of the reticulorumen. In this way the abomasum prevents an overload while its contents are being prepared for delivery into the duodenum.

The second type of receptors which have been recently identified are termed *epithelial receptors.* Those localized in the reticulorumen respond to both mechanical and chemical stimulation and are mainly inhibitory. Acids, alkali, and hyper- and hypo-osmotic solutions are capable of eliciting a response. In fact, volatile fatty acid concentrations which are normally present in the rumen are capable of providing a tonically active afferent input to the gastric centers which exert a reflex inhibition on the reticulorumen. Although the afferent input via the tension receptors is the dominant reflex, this tonic inhibition is probably important as a means of prolonging digesta retention for microbial digestion.

Abomasal acidity is, on the other hand, a potent stimulus for reticulorumen contractions. These mucosal receptors are also tonically active and exert an excitatory influence on the gastric centers.[12]

Gastric Motility

Motor activity of the stomach, while not as complex as that of the forestomach, must accomplish a number of important functions. For convenience, the stomach may be functionally divided into three zones. The dorsal portion, the fundus, is involved with storage of the contents and adaptation to volume so that excessive pressure does not develop. The body serves as a mixing vat, and the antrum is concerned with propulsion of the contents to the duodenum.[14] The stomach also selectively retains its contents until they undergo a degree of digestion and reach a critical size for removal. This latter function is also controlled by the antrum and probably the pyloric sphincter. Therefore the antrum is not simply a peristaltic pump since the contractions also serve to mix the ingesta and delay the passage of solid particles. For example, the pig stomach selectively retains particles according to their size. Fifty percent of larger particles (2 mm × 2 cm O.D.) were retained in the stomach for at least 60 hours, while approximately 50% of the small (2 mm × 2 mm) particles had left the stomach by 8 hours. Liquid marker left the stomach with a half time of approximately 2 hours.[15] A similar pattern of emptying applies to the horse, whereas in the dog fluid and particulate markers leave at comparable rates.[15] Therefore the antrum and/or pyloric sphincter may be more selective in herbivores and omnivores which would provide time for the coarser food material of the diet to be broken down, facilitating both small and large bowel digestion.

Control of Gastric Motility. The maximum frequency of antral contractions is regulated by the gastric slow wave initiated somewhere on the greater curvature by a pacemaker. The slow wave spreads distally with increasing velocity and voltage so that in the terminal antrum the velocity is highest and vigorous contractions, if present, occur. The pacemaker generates a new signal at constant intervals whether or not the muscle contracts. The mechanical response to the slow wave depends upon the participation of neural reflexes as well as antral and duodenal hormones.[16]

Most of the reflexes controlling gastric emptying are inhibitory. The only known natural stimulus to increase gastric motility is distention which stimulates gastric mechanoreceptors. The meal leaves the stomach as an exponential function of the square root of the volume suggesting that volume per se determines the rate of leaving. However, recent evidence indicates that this may be a function of the caloric density rather than volume.[17]

Although inhibition of gastric emptying is largely controlled by the proximal small bowel, recent evidence suggests that volatile fatty acid (VFA) in the abomasum may inhibit motility.[18,19] This may be a direct effect of these acids on the smooth muscle rather than neural reflex inhibition.[19] However, while the spike potentials and contractions were abolished, the frequency of the slow wave was unaffected.[18]

The primary inhibitory control of gastric emptying is the enterogastric reflex. Four sets of receptors in the duodenum responding to the chemical composition of the meal send information via neural or hormonal mechanisms to inhibit the rate of gastric emptying. The first of these are osmoreceptors, which have the widest range of stimulus but a low sensitivity. These receptors have been postulated as a vesicle which shrinks or swells depending on the osmolality of the contents. For example, hypertonic solutions of nonpenetrating solutes such as glucose cause the vesicle to shrink and inhibit emptying. Pure water causes the vesicle to swell, but an isotonic solution of NaCl causes the vesicle to swell to a maximum because there is a net movement of NaCl and water into the vesicle. Therefore gastric contents leave at a maximal rate when the duodenum is presented with an isotonic solution of a penetrating solute.[20]

A second set of receptors responds to acid in the duodenum. Strength of the acid is not important since acetic acid is next most effective to HCl. The effectiveness of the acids is determined by their molecular weights, presumably because the smaller anions are capable of diffusing to the receptor more rapidly.[20] The inhibitory response to acid appears to be neurally mediated via an adrenergic mechanism.[21]

The receptors of greatest sensitivity respond to lipids of 12 to 18 carbon atoms. This response in all probability is in part hormonal.[22] Release of cholecystokinin (CCK) from the duodenal mucosa in response to lipid has been demonstrated, and CCK in physiologic doses is inhibitory to gastric emptying.[23] Another "enterogastrone" that may be involved is gastric inhibitory polypeptide (GIP). It is likely that both of these hormones and perhaps neural reflexes mediate the action of lipids.[22]

Digestion products of protein and carbohydrate also inhibit gastric emptying. While this response is primarily due to the osmoreceptor, at least one amino acid, L-tryptophan, inhibits gastric motility via another mechanism which seems to involve release of CCK.[22]

Although a number of gastrointestinal hormones such as gastrin, GIP, and vasoactive intestinal polypeptide (VIP) have been shown to be released during digestion, there is a question as to their physiologic importance in regulation of gastric motility. In most cases pharmacologic doses have been used to study their effects, which nevertheless have the combined effect of inhibiting gastric motility and contracting the pyloric sphincter. Thus it is probable that some of these hormones participate in the overall motor control of the stomach but this area needs further study.

Small Bowel Motility

Motility of the small bowel accomplishes two purposes. First, ingesta is mixed by rhythmic segmental contractions which enable the digestive enzymes to contact the substrates and expose the chyme to a greater surface area for absorption. Second, peristaltic contractions move the ingesta aborally through the small intestine and finally into the large intestine.

Movement through the small intestine is rapid. For example, 60 to 70% of the liquid phase of a meal reaches the cecum within 2 hours in the horse, and this retention primarily occurs in the stomach. The ileocecal junction presents only a minor barrier to flow and is unable to discriminate against particulate matter to nearly the same degree as the pylorus. Yet this junction is competent in preventing ileocecal reflux under normal dietary conditions.[24]

Control of Small Bowel Motility. The most important basic control system for motility in the small bowel is the omnipresent electrical slow wave.[25] The rhythmicity and polarity of contractile movements can be ascribed to properties of the slow wave alone. They are not neurally mediated. Slow waves that are associated with spike discharges are propagated aborally at the same velocity as contractions. Migrating myoelectric complexes (MMC) are associated with propulsion of contents. MMC occur intermittently and their frequency is changed by feedings.[26] The frequency of the slow wave decreases aborally in a stepwise fashion, and each of these steps or plateaus is driven by a pacemaker at the oral end. Furthermore, it is now thought that slow waves are propagated in the same manner as nerve action potentials, i.e., by local circuit currents.[7] This propagation velocity decreases aborally due to an increasing resistance to local circuit current flow. The latter is due to the degree of electrical coupling between cells, which is greater in the proximal intestine. Therefore, peristaltic activity is more prevalent in the upper bowel, and contractile waves travelling short distances or not at all (segmentation) are characteristic of the lower small bowel.[7]

Small bowel motility is mediated by intrinsic and extrinsic innervation which may increase or decrease the excitability of the muscle and thus the probability of spike discharge.[25] The most important intrinsic nervous reflex of the small bowel is the peristaltic reflex. Distention in one segment of the bowel initiates activity above and inhibition below.[25] The receptors for distention activate local reflexes. Extrinsic reflexes also exist, the most important of which is the intestino-intestinal inhibitory reflex. Handling or distention of one part of the bowel may reflexly inhibit motility of the entire small intestine.[27] Both sensory and motor connections involved in this reflex appear to travel through the splanchnic nerves. Reflex inhibition of the small bowel due to stimulation of the peritoneum also may be primarily sympathetic. Vagal afferents conduct stimuli from mechanoreceptors and the efferent innervation is primarily excitatory.[25,28]

Intravenous CCK stimulates contractions in jejunal smooth muscle while secretin inhibits these contractions.[29] The same is true for the colon.[30] This reciprocal action suggests that these hormones may be physiologically involved in the control of both small and large bowel motility.

Large Bowel Motility

The large intestine, particularly of the nonruminant herbivore, is faced with functional problems nearly as complex as those of the forestomach. The diet of these animals is composed in large part of cellulose, which must be degraded by microbial digestion in the large intestine. Furthermore, the large intestine must retrieve critical amounts of electrolytes and water. These two functions are shared to varying degrees by all species but in the horse they have reached maximum development. Thus, like the forestomach, provision must be made for prolonged digesta retention, the elimination of large amounts of gas, and the controlled flow of digesta through the various segments of large bowel.

Types of Contractions and Propulsion of Ingesta. In some animals, such as the horse, ileal contents first enter the cecum and then are propelled into the colon. In others, the proximal colon receives a large portion of ileal ingesta and some of this may be retropelled into the cecum. In the horse, digesta moves from the body of the cecum into the base from which it is transferred into the colon. Two distinct types of mass movement of the cranial portion of the base have been described.[31] The first, occurring more frequently, results in transfer of ingesta. The other occurs after the cranial sac has been largely dilated with gas and when the cecocolic orifice is exposed above the surface of ingesta. Gas transport associated with very little ingesta movement occurs during this latter contraction and is somewhat analogous to eructation in ruminants.

In general, three types of contractile movements have been observed in the colon of most species. The first of these are stationary haustral contrac-tions, which may be similar to segmentation in the small bowel. These contractions are not associated with aboral movement of ingesta but perform a mixing function. The contractions also increase the resistance to flow and therefore zones of high pressure and increased motor activity cannot be equated with aboral flow. There must be a with-drawal of segmental resistance before propulsion can take place. Thus, unlike the small bowel, in-creased motor activity is usually associated with constipation, while diarrhea occurs in a flaccid colon.[32]

The second type of movement which has been observed in a number of species is retrograde flow.[33,34] In the sheep and rabbit and probably some other species this type of motility serves to fill the cecum with proximal colon contents.[33] Particulate matter is selectively rejected by the rabbit cecum and thus the cecum is filled with fluid in which the microbial population can be maintained. This ret-rograde filling of the cecum is not characteristic of the horse, in which the cecum is emptied relatively rapidly and no reflux occurs. Yet retrograde move-ment probably occurs in specific areas of the colon and has the function of mixing the contents and delaying the flow of digesta.

A third type of movement, which has been occa-sionally observed in the distal colon of the dog and also in man, is an aboral mass movement. This

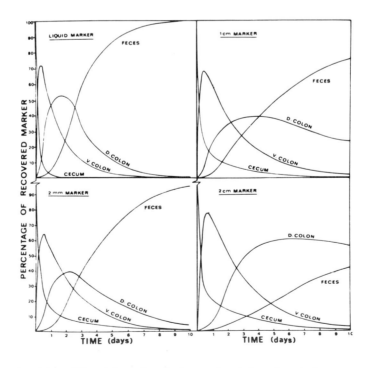

Figure 12–4. Retention of liquid and three different sizes of particulate markers in large intestinal compartments of equine. The area under the curves is equivalent to the mean retention time. Markers were given into the cecum. (From Am. J. Physiol. 226:1035, 1974.)

movement occurs when peripheral resistance is withdrawn and very little force, e.g., gravity, is adequate to effect movement over long distances.[32] However, strong ring-like contractions which are peristaltic in nature, have been observed to sweep over the distal colon.

Figure 12–4 shows the movement of fluid and various sizes of particles through the equine large intestine. First, it is apparent that both fluid and particles are rapidly emptied from the cecum but retained in the two segments of large colon. Second, the dorsal colon selectively retains particles to a greater degree than the ventral colon. From this, it may be inferred that resistance to flow increases in the aboral direction and the major points of resistance were found to be cecocolic junction < pelvic flexure < dorsal-small colic junction. Contents were well mixed in each of these compartments but no retrograde flow between the compartments was demonstrated. Third, although the exponential nature of the retention curves suggests that the volume of the segment determines the rate of outflow, the volume can increase three- to fourfold over that present after an overnight fast without provoking diarrhea. Therefore distensibility as well as resistance account for the prolonged retention of digesta.

A similar pattern of motility but less resistance and distensibility is present in the pig.[15] The major resistance to flow occurs at the flexure of the spiral colon and at the centrifugal-terminal colonic junction. Thus, the two segments of spiral colon are the major sites of digesta retention. In contrast, the major retention of digesta occurs in the cecum and proximal colon of the sheep and very little mixing or delay occurs in the spiral colon.

Control of Large Bowel Motility. Electrical slow waves in the colon differ in a number of respects from those of the stomach and small bowel. First, colonic slow waves seem to be generated in the circular muscle layer and spread to the longitudinal layer, while the reverse is true in gastric and small bowel muscle. Second, cholinergic and adrenergic drugs are capable of affecting slow wave frequency and duration. Third, the frequency gradient of the slow wave is the reverse of that in the small bowel.[35]

Pacemaker zones have been described in various species in which electrical activity and contractile movements are propagated in both directions. This activity seems to be more prevalent in the proximal colon. Migrating spike complexes have been described in the left ventral colon of the horse which were propagated both orally and aborally.[36] These electrical events suggest that retardation of flow in these areas may not be simply a matter of anatomic resistance.

Migrating spike complexes have been demonstrated in the distal colon of the cat and other species.[35] They do not seem to be associated with slow waves but are attended by strong contractions of the circular muscle and are usually propagated aborally. These events may be the electrical correlate of the mass movement.[35] While the mass movement may be under the control of the pelvic and sympathetic nerves, the migrating spike complexes occur in vitro in the species that have been studied (e.g., cat), which indicates that, as in the stomach and small bowel, the extrinsic nerves serve mainly to modulate the basic inherent motor activity.

Defecation. Defecation is both a voluntary and a reflex act. Impulses resulting from distention in the rectum convey information to the cortex, which may then initiate the voluntary mechanism of increased intra-abdominal pressure and relaxation of the pelvic floor and external anal sphincter. However, much of the control is reflex, mediated via a parasympathetic reflex arc in the pelvic nerves. Yet defecation is inefficient and contraction of the rectum is abnormal without central control.[37]

SECRETION

Secretion of electrolytes and water and digestive enzymes is an active energy-requiring process which is brought under control by the neuroendocrine system. Salivary glands, gastric mucosa, exocrine pancreas, liver, and intestine all are capable of secreting large volumes of their respective fluids. Since intestinal absorption and secretion are not easily separable events, these will be considered together in a later section.

Control Systems of Secretion

It is now becoming clear that activation of a secretory process by neural or endocrine transmission requires the participation of an intracellular catalytic unit which engages the cellular machinery to bring about the response. Two such systems which have recently been brought to light are the cyclic nucleotides; cyclic adenosine 3′,5′-monophosphate (cyclic AMP) and cyclic guanosine 3′,5′-monophosphate (cyclic GMP). One or both of these nucleotides have been demonstrated to be involved with salivary, gastric, pancreatic, small intestinal and colonic secretion.[38]

Besides a number of gastrointestinal hormones and neurotransmitters which are capable of modulating these nucleotides, several other agents are now known to be involved. Thus, prostaglandins, *Vibrio cholerae* and *E. coli* enterotoxins, and bile acids are a few agents that raise intracellular concentrations of cAMP. This process is of such clinical importance in the intestine that the mechanism will be discussed in detail in Chapter 14 and will not be considered further here. However, it should be kept in mind that regulation of synthesis and degradation of these nucleotides by endogenous agents may apply to other secretory tissues besides the intestine and therefore may be a means of physiologic control.

Salivary Secretion

The salivary glands of mammalian species perform a number of functions dependent on a wide variety of environmental conditions. Therefore, the salivary composition, secretory flow and control systems can be expected to vary accordingly.

Function of Saliva in Non-Ruminants

In all mammalian species, one of the prime functions of saliva is facilitation of mastication and deglutition. This function is of particular importance in the horse fed roughage, and secretory flows of as high as 50 ml/min have been recorded in the 150-kg pony during mastication.[39] In the dog and cat, salivary secretion has the special function of evaporative cooling. In fact, regulation of body heat by this means is as effective in these animals as evaporation of sweat in man. Thus, the parotid gland of the dog, under intense parasympathetic stimulation, is capable of secreting at 10 times the rate (per gram gland) of the parotid gland in man.[40] Obviously, this is an important route of fluid loss in these species.

Function of Saliva in Ruminants

Normal rumen function critically depends on salivary secretion. Microbial digestion in the forestomach requires two environmental conditions which are brought about by the saliva. First, a fluid medium must be provided for the microflora. Since the forestomach has no secretory glands, this fluid comes solely from salivary secretion. Thus, in ruminants, the parotid gland spontaneously secretes a fluid which is not under control of the secretory nerves.[40] Second, because of the large quantities of acid produced in the rumen, the salivary glands must provide a highly buffered medium to maintain an optimal rumen pH. Therefore, the salivary glands of the cow secrete from 100 to 200 liters/day of a fluid rich in sodium bicarbonate and sodium phosphate buffers. Approximately 2 times the Na^+

content of the extracellular fluid (ECF) volume of these animals passes down the esophagus each day, and at any one time, half the Na^+ content of the ECF is sequestered in the forestomach.[41]

When the animal is eating or ruminating, the volume of secretion increases some fourfold due to the influence of the secretory nerves.[40] Thus, it can be expected that renal and circulatory function and acid-base balance can be changed dramatically by eating.

Composition of Saliva

The basal salivary secretion from the submaxillary and parotid glands of non-ruminants, including the horse, is markedly hypotonic. For example, at low rates of flow, saliva from the dog has the following electrolyte composition (mEq/L): Na^+ 10, K^+ 10, Cl^- 10, HCO_3^- 5, $PO_4^\equiv$ <1, pH 7.4.[40] As the salivary flow increases, saliva approaches isotonicity primarily as the result of an increase in Na^+, Cl^-, and HCO_3^-. The K^+ concentration remains approximately constant and thus the $Na:K$ ratio varies directly with the rate of flow.

In contrast, the saliva of ruminants is isotonic at any rate of flow. The normal composition of parotid saliva of sheep is (mEq/L): Na^+ 160 to 180, K^+ 4 to 10, HCO_3^- 90 to 140, $HPO_4^=$ 10 to 70, Cl^- 10 to 20, pH 8.2.[41] Besides the tonicity, two other distinguishing features of ruminant saliva are present. First, the basal secretion of $PO_4^\equiv$ is remarkably high (70 mEq/L). Second, as the rate of secretion increases, the concentration of $PO_4^\equiv$ decreases and is reciprocated by an increase in HCO_3^- (not Cl^-). Thus, the salivary output of ruminants ensures a powerful neutralizing capacity for forestomach digestion.

Secretory Process

The water of saliva is transferred from the plasma secondary to active solute transport by the acini. The generally accepted view is that this primary secretion has a composition similar to the plasma. Therefore, the marked changes observed in salivary composition appear to be due to modification of the secretion in the salivary ducts. Thus, as salivary flow increases, the hypotonic salivas of non-ruminants approach isotonicity and more closely resemble the primary secretion, presumably owing to saturation of the reabsorptive process along the ducts.[42]

Control of Secretion

The primary control of salivary secretion appears to be exerted solely by the nervous system. The parasympathetic fibers contribute a dense secretory innervation mediated by the release of ACH. Although the sympathetic system supplies vasoconstrictor fibers to the glands, sympathetic stimulation results in marked differences in response depending on the species or gland. The increase in secretory rate is brought about by both central stimulation and reflex stimulation from mechanoreceptors in the mouth and stomach.

While the autonomic nerves appear to govern primarily the secretory flow, it is now established that secretions of adrenal hormones have profound effects on the Na:K ratio of ruminant saliva.[41] For example, if Na is withheld from a sheep for 48 hours, urinary Na^+ excretion ceases, but in addition, salivary Na^+ concentration decreases from 180 to 60 mEq/L and is reciprocated by an increase in K^+. Thus, the normally large urinary excretion if K^+ is transferred to the saliva in order to conserve Na^+. Salivary flow is also reduced by about 50% probably as a result of decreased blood flow through the gland. This remarkable change in the Na:K ratio is due to an increased level of circulating aldosterone, which is now known to induce synthesis of enzymes responsible for active Na^+ transport. Therefore, aldosterone may act by inducing ductular reabsorption of Na^+ in exchange for K^+; however, the precise mechanisms responsible for alteration of the secretory fluid are not firmly established.

Gastric Secretion

The stomach secretes HCl and pepsinogen into the lumen and gastrin into the blood. The complex control of these secretions is regulated centrally as well as reflexly from mechanical and chemical receptors in the stomach and duodenum.

Mucosal Zones and Secretions

Gastric mucosa of most species consists of one nonsecretory zone and three secretory zones. The distribution of these zones differs considerably among species and warrants special consideration.[43] The nonglandular mucosa is a stratified squamous epithelium which constitutes the entire forestomach of ruminants. This mucosa invades a small zone of the pig stomach from the esophagus, but in the horse, it occupies the entire cranial half of the stomach.

The cardiac glandular mucosa occupies a thin zone in the cranial portion of the dog stomach and in the ruminant abomasum, while in the pig, this region occupies the cranial half of the stomach. A thin belt of cardiac mucosa is interposed between the cranial nonglandular and caudal glandular re-gions of the horse stomach. In the pig, this mucosa secretes a fluid similar to the plasma except for a HCO_3^- concentration approximately four times that of plasma.[44] Therefore, this secretion has the property of a powerful buffer.

The proper gastric or oxyntic zone occupies the cranial two-thirds of the dog stomach and ruminant abomasum, while a smaller zone (slightly less than 1/3) is present in the pig and horse stomach. This mucosa secretes HCl from the parietal cells and pepsinogen from the chief cells.

The remaining secretory mucosa, i.e., pyloric, secretes mucus and contains the gastrin cell which upon appropriate stimulation releases gastrin into the blood.

Gastric Mucosal Barrier

Hydrogen and chloride ions are actively secreted by the oxyntic zone in concentrations that are approximately 150 mN. Carbonic anhydrase activity is high in these cells. It catalyzes the hydration or hydroxylation of CO_2 to HCO_3^- and H^+. Thus for each H^+ secreted into the lumen, one molecule of HCO_3^- diffuses into the blood.

Since the gastric juice contains a H^+ ion concentration approximately 3×10^6 times greater than the plasma, there must exist means of preventing the back-diffusion of H^+ into the mucosal cells. This barrier is due primarily to the apical cell walls and tight junctions which normally allow little passive ionic diffusion. The mucous secretion of the stomach is a very weak barrier and cannot be equated with the gastric mucosal barrier.[45]

Once the gastric barrier is broken, Na^+, K^+, and protein leak into the lumen and H^+ into the cell.[45] The barrier can be broken by a number of agents, one of which is weak organic acids, e.g., VFA. In the carnivore, VFA are relatively unimportant as a weak acid source in the stomach, but in the omnivore, e.g., pig, high concentrations have been recorded, and in the horse stomach concentrations as high as 100 mEq/L are normally present.[46] These acids are a result of varying degrees of microbial digestion which occurs in the stomach of these species. Similarly, the abomasum is presented with variable concentrations of VFA which escape absorption from the forestomach. Since these acids are lipid soluble at a low pH, they can rapidly gain entrance into the mucosal cell. Fortunately, additional barriers to back-diffusion of acid are present in the pig and horse stomach, while in the dog, 100 mM acetate results in extensive ulceration. As previously indicated, cardiac mucosa of the pig stomach provides a degree of buffering capacity.

Thus, within the first 4 hours after feeding, the pH of the proximal portion of the pig stomach is between pH 5 and 6. The horse stomach, which has only a small zone of cardiac mucosa, is protected by other means. This seems to be due to the extremely efficient barrier of the stratified squamous mucosa. Although the analogous mucosa of the forestomach is capable of rapidly absorbing VFA, the stratified squamous mucosa in the horse is relatively impermeable to these organic acids under comparable conditions.[46]

In addition to these mucosal barriers, the secretion of saliva, particularly in the horse, provides a means of neutralizing acid. Thus, the acidity of the horse stomach is maintained between pH 4 and 6 when the animal is fed a conventional pelleted hay-grain diet.

Phases of Gastric Secretion

Gastric secretion of acid is dependent on the release of ACH at the oxyntic cell or the release of gastrin from the pyloric gland area which then stimulates the oxyntic cell to secrete acid. The release of gastrin is under direct cholinergic control and it can be brought about by vagal or local intramural cholinergic reflex pathways. Release of gastrin is also stimulated by an "enterogastrone" released from the duodenum. Thus the cephalic, gastric, and intestinal phases of H^+ secretion have both neural and hormonal components which are related and which potentiate each other.[45]

The cephalic phase of acid secretion occurs due to central stimulation, e.g., sight, taste, smell, chewing, and swallowing. Therefore the response is mediated entirely by the vagus via (1) direct cholinergic stimulation of the oxyntic glands and (2) cholinergic release of gastrin from the pyloric glands.[47] Intracellular hypoglycemia is another cephalic stimulant acting on the vagal centers in the medulla. The cephalic phase appears to be unimportant for abomasal secretion in ruminants.

The gastric phase involves both direct cholinergic stimulation of the oxyntic glands and cholinergic release of gastrin from the pyloric glands.[47] The stimuli for the release of ACH are mechanical or chemical agents acting locally. Mechanoreceptors in the fundus and antrum responding to distention activate long (vagovagal) reflexes which bring about the release of acid and pepsin. Local cholinergic reflexes in the antrum and fundus responding to mechanical or chemical stimulation also cause release of gastrin. The protein component of the food is probably responsible for the chemical activation.

However, the most potent stimuli for acid production by the abomasum are the VFA themselves. Acidification to pH 1 to 2 counteracts both vagal and local reflexes, but deacidification alone cannot stimulate the release of gastrin without vagal or local stimuli.[47]

The intestinal phase is activated by duodenal acidification, fat and hypertonic solutions, which liberate an enterogastrone which inhibits gastric acid secretion.[45] Both CCK and secretin are liberated from the duodenum; however, species differences are involved in the response. For example, in the cat, CCK is a full agonist of gastrin on H^+ secretion, so CCK stimulates H^+ secretion in this species. In the dog, CCK is a partial agonist and competitive inhibitor of gastrin on H^+ secretion.[45] Secretin also inhibits H^+ secretion in the dog. In addition to these two hormones, there is now good evidence to suggest that GIP is probably physiologically involved in the inhibition of gastric acid and pepsinogen secretion and may be the primary enterogastrone.[48]

Secretion of Pepsinogen and Intrinsic Factor. Secretion of pepsinogen from the chief cells is stimulated by the same general stimuli as for H^+, except that secretin enhances pepsinogen secretion.[45] Thus, the strongest stimulants for pepsin secretion are the cholinergics. Pepsinogen is converted autocatalytically to pepsin in the presence of an acid pH, and this is necessary for the initiation of gastric protein digestion.

The secretion of intrinsic factor is correlated with the secretion of H^+ and is secreted from the same cell. Intrinsic factor interacts with vitamin B_{12} forming a complex which binds to specific receptors in the ileum and facilitates vitamin B_{12} absorption.

Pancreatic Secretion

The prime function of the exocrine pancreas is to anticipate and neutralize the diverse spectrum of material presented to the proximal duodenum from the stomach. Large quantities of buffer must be secreted in an attempt to rectify the acid pH of inflowing gastric contents. Enzymes that are capable of breaking down undigested carbohydrate, protein, and fat are delivered by the pancreas into the duodenum. In omnivores and nonruminant herbivores; e.g., pig and horse, the pancreas further provides a large portion of the fluid and buffering capacity required by the large intestine for microbial digestion. Thus, in these animals, pancreatic secretion may be analogous to salivary secretion in ruminants.

Electrolyte Composition and Volume of Juice

Sodium and potassium concentrations in pancreatic fluid approximate the plasma and are independent of the rate of flow. The remarkable electrolyte feature is the concentration of HCO_3^-, which can reach 150 mM at high rates of flow. A reciprocal decrease in Cl^- concentration accompanies the increase in HCO_3^-.[49] An exception to this general situation is found in the horse, in which the HCO_3^- concentrations never exceed 60 to 70 mEq/L at maximum flow rates.[39] This seems to imply that pancreatic juice in this species would not be capable of the high degree of neutralization required by the large bowel. However, the situation appears to be rectified in the distal small intestine.

The pancreas is capable of producing large volumes of fluid. In the dog this may reach 2 to 3 ml/min[49] and in the 150-kg pony as high as 10 ml/min.[39] However, the sheep pancreas is not capable of secreting large volumes and under the same degree of stimulation secretes at only one fifth to one tenth the rate of the dog. Only 300 to 400 ml/day are secreted by the sheep pancreas into the duodenum.[50]

Mechanisms of Electrolyte and Water Secretion

While the mechanism of secretion is not firmly established, one widely held view is that the centroacinar cells and ductular cells actively secrete an isotonic HCO_3^- solution.[49,51] This solution is altered as it moves along the collecting system by passive exchange of HCO_3^- for Cl^-. Thus at low rates of flow, the opportunity for this exchange would be greatest. Bicarbonate of the primary secretion is derived in part from the blood and in part from the CO_2 resulting from metabolism of the cell. High activity of carbonic anhydrase is present in the ductular epithelium. Thus, the secretory cell of the pancreas is the reverse of the gastric parietal cell. While the parietal cell secretes H^+ into the lumen and HCO_3^- into the blood, the centroacinar and ductular cells secrete HCO_3^- into the lumen of the acini and ducts. The net result is that at high secretory rates, sufficient buffer to neutralize the acid gastric contents is delivered into the proximal small bowel.

Pancreatic Enzyme Secretion

Two groups of proteolytic enzymes of pancreatic juice are secreted as the inactive proenzyme. The first of these are endopeptidases which cleave bonds that occupy internal positions of the protein molecule. These are trypsinogen, which is activated to trypsin in the lumen of the small bowel, and chymotrypsinogen, which is activated to chymotrypsin. The exopeptidases are carboxypeptidase A and B, which are activated in the small bowel lumen by trypsin.[52] Lipase appears to require bile acids, at least in part, for activation. Amylase is secreted as the active enzyme.

Neural Control of Pancreatic Secretion

All secretory nerves to the pancreas are cholinergic. Cholinergic stimulation also enhances the effect of secretin on the pancreas.[53]

In most species, the effect of cholinergic stimulation is a profound increase in the enzyme output. For example, in the dog, cat, and sheep vagal stimulation increases primarily enzyme secretion with only a small increase in electrolytes and H_2O.[50,53] In contrast, vagal stimulation in the horse and pig results in a profuse flow of electrolytes and water.[39,53] In these species, the pancreas receives a secretory innervation comparable to the salivary glands. The resting pancreatic secretion in the horse is already profuse and continuous, but upon vagal stimulation a fivefold increase in flow occurs. While cholinergic stimulation in the pig also increases the output of enzymes, the content of digestive enzymes in horse pancreatic juice is extremely small and raised only slightly with vagal stimulation. Thus, the horse pancreas is capable of only one twentieth the rate of enzyme output by the pancreas of the pig (per unit weight of pancreatic tissue).

The *cephalic* and *gastric phases* of pancreatic secretion are controlled primarily by the nerves.[53] The vagus has a direct action on the glands of the pancreas. There are also cholinergic reflex arcs between the stomach and pancreas which lead to pancreatic secretion following fundic distention.[52] However, vagal stimulation also releases gastrin, which is capable of stimulating the pancreas to secrete enzymes. Therefore, cholinergic stimulation and cholinergic release of gastrin potentiate each other's effect on the pancreas.

Hormonal Control of Pancreatic Secretion

Aside from the release of gastrin, at least two hormones which act on the pancreas are released from the small intestine. The first of these is secretin, which is released primarily in response to acid perfusing the duodenum.[52] Secretin stimulates the pancreas to secrete HCO_3^- and H_2O; thus its effect is to neutralize the acid gastric contents. Very little stimulation of enzyme secretion can be attributed to secretin alone.

Cholecystokinin-pancreozymin (CCK-PZ), on the other hand, is released in response to protein and fat in the duodenum and elicits enzyme secretion from the pancreas. The products of protein and fat digestion are much less effective in releasing secretin than is HCl.[52]

Most of the evidence suggests that the release of these two hormones, as in the case for gastrin, is brought about by excitation of afferent nerve endings in the mucosa responding to mechanical or chemical stimulation. Transmission occurs over a short reflex arc containing a cholinergic synapse or nerve ending and stimulates the release of the intestinal hormones.[54] Unlike gastrin, however, direct vagal stimulation does not appear to be involved.

Endocrine Interactions on the Pancreas

As previously mentioned, the effect of gastrin on the pancreas is to stimulate enzyme secretion. Gastrin and CCK are full agonists of pancreatic enzyme secretion and partial agonists of pancreatic HCO_3^- secretion. The opposite is true for secretin.[3] Thus, the effect of secretin plus CCK results in a powerful potentiation of H_2O and electrolyte secretion, and it appears that only small amounts of secretin are released under normal conditions.

A third enteric hormone, VIP, has been shown to be a potent inhibitor of secretin-induced pancreatic secretion in the dog. Typical competitive inhibition was demonstrated, indicating that secretin and VIP share a common receptor site.[4]

Biliary Secretion

Secretion of bile by the liver provides (1) a source of bile salts required for lipid absorption in the small intestine, (2) an excretory route for certain endogenous metabolites and drugs, and (3) additional buffer to neutralize acid in the proximal small bowel.[55]

Bile Formation and Secretion

There are two components of bile secretion. The first is active transport of bile acids from the hepatocyte into the bile canaliculus. Bile salts are synthesized in the liver from cholesterol and the bile is a major route of cholesterol excretion.[56] These bile salts are conjugated with either taurine or glycine, which reduces their pK and prevents the formation of protonated bile acids that would have limited H_2O solubility. Lipid soluble substances, e.g., cholesterol and lecithin, are incorporated into micelles formed by the bile salts thereby making them water soluble.

The mechanism for uptake and excretion of bile acids by the hepatocyte is separate from that involved with other organic acids such as bilirubin.[57] Thus, competitive inhibition of bile acid uptake and excretion by endogenous compounds or drugs does not usually occur. Active bile acid transport into the canalicular lumen induces a choleresis owing to the osmotic effect of the bile acids. Therefore, the bile salts that are recirculated from the intestine and taken up by the hepatocyte are a prime stimulus of hepatic bile flow.

The second component of bile secretion involves the ductular epithelium and constitutes 40 to 70% of the basal bile secretion.[57] This component is the non-bile acid-dependent secretory mechanism. Active Na^+ transport is involved and the bile ducts also contribute buffer to the duodenum by secreting a HCO_3^- rich fluid.

Control of Bile Secretion

The bile salts themselves primarily govern the bile flow from the hepatocyte into the canaliculus. However, the non-bile acid secretory flow is directly under hormonal control. Both gastrin and secretin cause a choleresis by acting on the ductular epithelium, and the final anion content of hepatic bile will therefore depend on the relative contribution of the two components of biliary secretion.

In the sheep, for example, the output of electrolytes and HCO_3^- delivered into the duodenum is three to five times greater than from the pancreas. Bile flow in these animals amounts to 500 to 1550 ml/day. Thus, the liver of the sheep is much more important than the pancreas in neutralization of H^+ in the proximal duodenum.[50]

Role of the Extrahepatic Biliary Tract

Hepatic bile can be further modified in species that possess a gallbladder epithelium and, upon contraction, a concentrated solution of bile salts may be delivered into the duodenum. The bile salts themselves are only poorly absorbed by the gallbladder because of the alkaline pH (approximately 8) and because they are ionized. The amount of electrolyte and water absorbed depends on the length of time bile stays in the gallbladder.

In the continuously fed sheep, the gallbladder empties relatively frequently and delivers a dilute, buffered solution to the small bowel. On the other hand, the duodenum of the dog fed only once or twice a day is presented with a highly concentrated solution of gallbladder bile.

Contraction of the gallbladder is primarily under hormonal control.[58] Release of CCK from the small intestinal mucosa in response to lipid and amino acids causes powerful contractions of the gallbladder and relaxes the sphincter of Oddi. However, if bile salts plus amino acids and fat are present in the duodenum, CCK release is inhibited. Therefore, the bile acid dependent portion of bile flow is indirectly under hormonal control. In the horse, bile can be expected to be secreted continuously into the duodenum.

DIGESTION AND ABSORPTION OF CARBOHYDRATE, FAT, AND PROTEIN

The process of digestion can conveniently be divided into a dietary phase and four functional phases, each of which has its own specialized processes. Some substrates do not require a specialized mechanism for each stage, while others do. Therefore, once these functional and anatomic relationships are known, maldigestion and malabsorption can be traced to one of these systems by appropriate diagnostic techniques. The first stage consists of the diet and its relationship to the four functional phases and is discussed in Chapter 14. The second is the intraluminal stage, which consists of microbial or pancreatic enzyme hydrolysis of the dietary substrates. The biliary phase must also be included in this stage of digestion for fat. The third is the mucosal stage, which requires two steps in the case of carbohydrates and proteins. Hydrolysis by intestinal brush border enzymes is step 1, and the absorption across the mucosal membrane of the epithelial cell by specialized transport processes is step 2. The intracellular stage consists of further enzymatic hydrolysis, metabolism, or transformation of the entering substrates. The final pathway involving the gut is transport of the digestive end-products across the serosal membrane of the enterocyte into the capillaries or lymphatic system for delivery to the general circulation.

Forestomach Digestion

No mammalian enzymes are secreted by the forestomachs. Therefore, all forestomach digestion of carbohydrate, protein, and fat results from the action of microbial enzymes and from microbial transformation of the ingested substrates. Microbial digestion is quite different from mammalian enzymatic digestion for three reasons. First, cellulose and other polysaccharides having beta-linked glucose polymers cannot be broken down by mammalian systems, but are readily attacked by microbial enzymes. Second, essential amino acids can be

synthesized by the microflora. Third, water-soluble B vitamins are synthesized by the microbes. Thus microbial digestion can supply energy, protein, and vitamins to the body from sources that mammalian systems cannot utilize.

The forestomach is also capable of absorption, but development of the papillae and thus a functional surface area is dependent on diet. It is now well established that the end-products of microbial carbohydrate digestion, especially butyrate and propionate, are responsible for this development.[59] Therefore, an active microbial digestion must be established prior to maximal absorptive function.

Ruminal Phase of Carbohydrate Digestion

Dietary carbohydrate may be in the form of complex polysaccharides, such as starch or cellulose, or in the form of simple sugars, e.g., lactose or sucrose. The relative amounts of soluble versus insoluble carbohydrate are dependent on the proportion of grain or hay in the ration. Despite the type of carbohydrate that is fed, the end-products arising from microbial fermentation are the same, although the rates at which they are produced and the relative proportion of each are dependent on diet. The adult ruminant depends on these end products for 70 to 80% of its energy supply.

Dietary carbohydrate entering the rumen is fermented first to hexose and then chiefly to three volatile fatty acids: acetate, propionate, and butyrate (Fig. 12–5). A typical fermentation balance for the rumen is given as 57.5 $(C_6H_{12}O_6) \longrightarrow 65$ acetic acid + 20 propionic acid + 15 butyric acid + 60 CO_2 + 35 CH_4 + 25 H_2O.[60] Under normal conditions only small amounts of lactate and other organic acids are formed. Coincident with VFA production is the evolution of large amounts of gas, mainly CO_2 and CH_4.

The relative proportion of the three VFAs produced is in the order of acetate > propionate > butyrate. For example, in sheep weighing 45 to 69 kg and being fed 800 g/day of alfalfa pellets, 3.3 moles of acetic acid, 0.9 moles of propionic acid, and 0.6 moles of butyric acid were formed in the rumen each day.[61] These proportions differ somewhat from the typical fermentation just cited, but the rank order is the same.

The VFAs are produced in the acid form and hence must be rapidly neutralized, or absorbed and neutralized by the tissue or plasma buffers. Fortunately, the large quantity of salivary HCO_3^- and $PO_4^{\equiv}$ delivered into the rumen is capable of neutralizing some of this acid. However, the quantity is not sufficient to deal with the total amount of acid

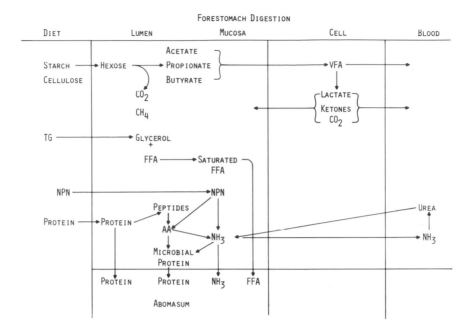

Figure 12–5. Phases of forestomach digestion. TG, triglyceride; NPN, non-protein nitrogen; FFA, free fatty acid; AA, amino acids; VFA, volatile fatty acids.

produced. For example, it has been calculated that 10 liters of sheep saliva would bring 3.3 moles of fatty acid to a pH of only 4.5.[62] Therefore, there must exist other means of neutralization, which is accomplished primarily by the rapid absorption of undissociated acid.

It can also be calculated that the 10 L of saliva containing a HCO_3^- concentration of 110 mM would evolve approximately 25 L of CO_2 if all of the HCO_3^- were neutralized. However, at the usual pH of the normal rumen, somewhat less CO_2 is evolved. Thus, rumen gas is produced in two ways, i.e., by the neutralization of the acid products of microbial metabolism and by the fermentation process itself.

Approximately 90% of the VFA produced in the rumen is directly absorbed into the rumen epithelium.[61] The absorption of VFA across the mucosal membrane into the cell appears to be a diffusion process and thus depends primarily on the concentration gradient between rumen and intracellular contents. As would be expected, the rate of absorption increases as the pH of rumen contents decreases and a greater proportion of the VFA is present in the un-ionized form.

Once the VFA enter the epithelial cell, a large proportion is metabolized to ketone bodies, lactate and CO_2. For instance, of the VFA produced in the rumen of sheep fed alfalfa pellets (in the preceding example), only 2.3 moles of acetic acid, 0.44 moles of propionic acid, and 0.05 moles of butyric acid are transported unchanged into the portal blood. Thus

approximately 30, 50, and 90% of these three VFAs produced in the rumen never reach the general circulation for use by the body tissues.[61]

Fat Digestion

Dietary fats are primarily in the esterified form as mono- and diglycerides if the animal is grazing, while triglycerides predominate if concentrates are the major portion of the ration.[63]

Extensive hydrolysis of the esterified lipids and phospholipids occurs in the rumen under the action of microbial lipases. A portion of the glycerol thus formed is fermented to propionic acid and absorbed. The remaining free fatty acids are then progressively hydrogenated to the saturated form.

Absorption of long-chain fatty acids from the rumen is of no quantitative significance. Thus, most of the non-esterified fatty acids are delivered to the abomasum and thence to the small bowel for further digestion and absorption.

Protein Digestion

Use has been made of the fact that rumen microbes can synthesize essential amino acids from nonprotein nitrogen (NPN) sources such as urea, while deriving the carbon skeleton from fibrous carbohydrate sources such as cellulose. Unfortunately, synthesis of microbial protein from these sources is a complex process requiring optimal balances of available carbohydrate and nitrogen.

Thus, one of the problems encountered in modern-day feeding practice is NH_3 toxicity.

Extensive breakdown of ingested protein occurs in the rumen. Approximately two thirds of the intact dietary protein is degraded by the action of proteolytic microbial enzymes, yielding peptides and amino acids which in turn are attacked by deaminases to yield free ammonia. However, under normal dietary conditions only 30% of the dietary N is converted to NH_3 and the remaining 70% either passes intact to the intestine or is converted to peptides and amino acids which are then directly synthesized into microbial protein.[64] The free NH_3 formed may also be used by the microbes to synthesize microbial protein, which is then delivered to abomasum and intestine and digested. While excess NH_3 is absorbed into the portal blood or transferred to the intestine, absorbed NH_3 can be recycled to the rumen for further use by the microbes in the following way.

Absorption of NH_3 is a passive process and therefore depends only on the pH of the rumen contents and the concentration gradient of NH_3 between rumen content and blood. At a low rumen pH, proportionately more of the ammonia is trapped in the rumen as NH_4^+, while at a high pH, the lipid soluble form diffuses into the circulation down its concentration gradient. Normally, the liver is capable of immediately removing NH_3 from the portal blood and converting it to urea. The urea thus formed may then re-enter the rumen via the saliva or by diffusion from the blood across the rumen wall (a large portion of urea also enters the intestine from the blood). The excess urea is excreted in the urine. Once in the rumen, ureases of microbial origin rapidly convert the urea to NH_3, which can then be utilized by the bacteria.[64] Thus, the urea concentration in the rumen is kept at low levels and establishes a steep concentration gradient for urea between blood and lumen. In the protein deficient animal, this mechanism is of importance in that the proportion of urea recycled to the forestomach increases while the amount excreted by the kidney decreases. Therefore, nitrogen is conserved for protein synthesis by an enterosytemic circulation.

Small Bowel Digestion

Apart from forestomach digestion, the principal digestive and absorptive mechanisms of carbohydrate, fat, and protein are conferred upon the proximal small bowel. Salivary amylase initiates starch digestion in the pig stomach, emulsification of fats takes place in the stomach, and some of the protein is hydrolyzed by the action of pepsin and HCl. However, pepsin is not essential for protein digestion.

Carbohydrate Digestion

Only soluble carbohydrates having the α-glucose linkage are digested in the small bowel. The *luminal*

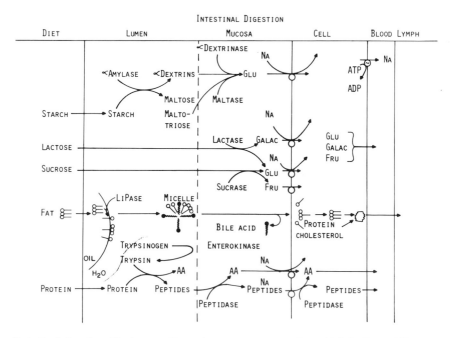

Figure 12–6.   Phases of intestinal digestion. Circles on cell membranes represent carriers which facilitate diffusion (fructose) or are capable of transporting sugars or amino acids and peptides against their respective chemical gradients.

phase of digestion consists of enzymatic hydrolysis of these α linkages by the pancreatic enzyme α-amylase (Fig. 12–6). In non-ruminants, with the possible exception of the horse, tremendous amounts of pancreatic amylase are delivered into the duodenum, and the lumen phase of starch digestion is usually complete by the time ingesta has reached the distal duodenum.[65] Thus, in these animals, the rate-limiting step is distal to the lumen. However, the calf is unable to utilize starch owing in part to low levels of pancreatic amylase.[66,67,68] This low activity persists in the adult bovine and is important, due to the fact that in feeding practices where intake of grain is high, as much as 35 to 40% of the starch may reach the abomasum and small bowel.

The final products of starch digestion in the lumen consist of maltose (glucose–glucose), maltotriose (glucose–glucose–glucose), and α-dextrins consisting on the average of eight glucose molecules. No free glucose is formed by pancreatic amylase hydrolysis.[69]

The *mucosal phase* of carbohydrate digestion consists of two steps. The first is hydrolysis of the α-dextrins and disaccharides by oligosaccharidases in the brush border of the intestinal epithelial cell. The second is absorption of the monosaccharides thus produced across the mucosal membrane into the cytoplasm of the cell.

The brush border enzymes together with their products are shown in Figure 12–6. Important exceptions to this scheme exist in neonatal animals and in ruminants,[66,67,68] in which low levels of maltase are present. Sucrase is absent in intestinal mucosa of ruminants. Thus, while the young calf can readily utilize lactose and its hydrolytic products, glucose and galactose, it has limited ability to utilize maltose and is unable to utilize sucrose or starch.[67] In contrast, the neonatal pig has the ability to break down starch far in excess of what is normally fed, but the amount of maltose that is hydrolyzed is very small compared to the amounts of starch broken down to maltose.[70] The activity of both sucrase and maltase increases up to 4 to 5 weeks of age in the pig. In most species, lactase activity progressively decreases with age. Therefore, in general, the activity of these enzymes slowly adapts to the type of substrate presented to the brush border for digestion.

Only after the disaccharides are cleaved into monosaccharides are they available for absorption. Absorption of glucose and galactose across the mucosal membrane is an active transport process requiring the presence of Na^+. Fructose absorption is facilitated by a carrier mechanism but, unlike glucose and galactose, it cannot be absorbed against its chemical gradient into the epithelial cell. There appears to be little absorption of fructose per se in the calf, and the active transport system for glucose becomes rudimentary in the adult ruminant, again implying a substrate-sensitive change.[71]

A small portion of glucose and the other monosaccharides may be metabolized during the intracellular and transport phase; e.g., 14% of glucose is metabolized to lactic acid in the dog. Due to the active accumulation of glucose by the cell, the concentration of intracellular glucose is greater than in the blood. Thus, glucose can simply diffuse down the concentration gradient into the portal blood from which it is delivered to the liver or peripheral tissues for storage or utilization.[72]

Fat Digestion

The *lumen phase* of fat digestion is a highly specialized process requiring the participation of both pancreatic and biliary secretions.[73] In adult ruminants, lipolysis has already occurred to a large extent in the forestomach so pancreatic lipase is not a limiting factor.[63] Low pancreatic lipase activity is present in the neonatal calf but milk fat undergoes appreciable hydrolysis in the abomasum, catalyzed by a lipase (pregastric esterase) that is secreted in the pharyngeal region.[74] In non-ruminants, fat, primarily triglyceride, is delivered into the duodenum in an emulsion. Pancreatic lipase acts at the water-oil interface of these emulsion droplets, releasing a 2-monoglyceride and two free fatty acids from the 1 and 3 positions of the triglyceride. These products, as in the case of triglyceride, are water insoluble but are amphipaths, i.e., part polar and H_2O soluble and part non-polar and lipid soluble.[75]

The monoglycerides and free fatty acids are brought into solution by the action of bile acids. These acids act as a detergent and bring the H_2O-insoluble material into solution by forming a negatively charged polymolecular aggregate called a micelle. The H_2O insoluble material is dissolved in the non-polar interior of the micelle. In the conversion of fats from an emulsion to a micelle, the diameter of the particles is reduced 100 times and the surface area increased over 10,000-fold.[73] The micelles act as a transport vehicle from the emulsion particle to the brush border of the jejunal epithelium. Here the fat is released and diffuses across the lipid membrane into the cell.

During the intracellular and transport phase of fat digestion, the free fatty acids are resynthesized to triglyceride by intracellular enzymes.[73] Synthesis of phospholipid and protein in combination with cholesterol forms lipoproteins, including chylomicrons. Formation of the chylomicron, which is analogous to the micelle, facilitates transport of H_2O-insoluble triglyceride. These chylomicrons and lipoproteins are then transported across the serosal membrane of the cell, by an as-yet unknown process (without the protein coat, fat is unable to leave the cell). From here they diffuse into the central lacteal and are carried by the lymphatic system to the thoracic duct and enter the general circulation.

Enterophepatic Circulation of Bile Salts. The bile salts themselves are not absorbed in the jejunum with the fat but are carried on to the ileum where they are then absorbed by a specific active transport process requiring Na^+. In the absence of bile salts, absorption of fat and fat soluble vitamins is seriously impaired and cholesterol absorption is absent. In fact, the quantities of bile salts needed far exceed the normal production rate by the liver and thus must be recycled to the intestine for further use. The active transport system of the ileum is so efficient that approximately 95% of the bile salts are reabsorbed into the portal circulation and returned to the liver where they are re-secreted.[76]

Before secretion, bile acids are conjugated with either glycine or taurine in hepatic microsomes. However, nonabsorbed bile acids which reach the colon are deconjugated by microbial action and some of these are reabsorbed. Therefore, a small portion of unconjugated bile acids also participate in the enterohepatic circulation under normal conditions.

Protein Digestion

Although pepsin hydrolysis of protein begins in the stomach and lasts 1 to 2 hours because of the acid pH, most of the dietary protein is hydrolyzed in the duodenum and upper jejunum.[65] Activation of pancreatic pro-enzymes by the mucosal enzyme enterokinase takes place at the brush border. Enterokinase activates the proenzyme trypsinogen to trypsin,[77] which then activates the remaining trypsinogen as well as the other pancreatic proenzymes. The main products of protein hydrolysis are neutral and basic amino acids and oligopeptides (Fig. 12–6). With protein as with carbohydrates, the *mucosal phase* of digestion consists of hydrolysis and absorption. However, only about 20% of the peptides are hydrolyzed to amino acids by the brush border enzymes. Active transport systems for neutral and basic amino acids and also for some di- and tripeptides are present in the mucosal membrane and, as in the case for glucose, require the presence of the

sodium ion.[77] Mucosal uptake of peptides and amino acids involves separate mechanisms and because of rapid uptake of peptides, the absorptive capacity of the small intestine is considerably greater for oligopeptide/amino acid mixtures than for mixtures of free amino acids alone.

During the intracellular and transport phase of protein digestion, approximately 90% of the peptides that were not hydrolyzed by either pancreatic or brush border enzymes are hydrolyzed inside the cell by intracellular peptidases. The remaining 10% diffuse across the serosal membrane into the portal circulation. These peptides are not capable of being metabolized by the general body tissues and are excreted in the urine. The bulk of the amino acids also diffuse into the blood, yet a significant portion is used for synthesis of intestinal proteins. A much smaller amount are deaminated and enter the tricarboxylic acid cycle where they are used for energy metabolism by the enterocyte.[77]

Large Bowel Digestion

In ruminants and non-ruminant herbivores, the large intestine is thought to act primarily as a functional reserve to extract the remaining energy from the thus-far undigested carbohydrates. Despite the efficiency of forestomach digestion, as much as 15% of the soluble carbohydrate still reaches the colon under conditions of high grain feeding and as much as 30% of the cellulose in diets of high fiber.[78] In omnivores, but less so in carnivores, significant amounts of undigested carbohydrate reach the colon. In the horse the primary energy supply to the body is derived from large intestinal microbial digestion of both soluble and insoluble carbohydrate. As much as 50% of the soluble carbohydrate of the ration reaches the large intestine of the horse and virtually all of the insoluble carbohydrate is presented to the large bowel for digestion.[79]

The process of microbial fermentation in the large intestine is for the most part identical to forestomach digestion. Similar motility, digestive, absorptive, and secretory functions exist. Unlike the forestomach, however, no means are available to deal with the overflow of fermented products, and the ability of the colon to deal with these products is continuously challenged under a wide variety of nutritional conditions.

While the colon of omnivores and herbivores normally can effectively digest and absorb carbohydrate, the situation for protein is by no means as clear. Microbial protein produced in the forestomach can subsequently be digested in the small bowel, but in the case of the large bowel, means would have to exist in the colon for proteolytic activity and absorption of amino acids. Despite the obvious importance of this process, especially to the horse, the question of whether microbial protein can be hydrolyzed and absorbed from the large intestine remains to be answered.

INTESTINAL TRANSPORT OF IONS AND WATER

One of the prime functions of the lower small intestine and colon, quite apart from their capacity to digest and absorb nutrients, is the reabsorption of isotonic secretions delivered to the proximal small bowel. Although these secretions are required primarily for digestion, large quantities of fluid are also presented to the intestine during fasting. Therefore, recovery of these fluids by the distal intestine is critical in maintenance of the extracellular fluid volume. In addition to its absorptive ability it is now well established that the intestine is capable of secreting large volumes of isotonic fluid. While this could bring about massive fluid and electrolyte losses, controlled small bowel secretion in some species, e.g., herbivores, may be the rule. The demonstration that the mucosal cAMP system is central to a number of secretory states implies that a certain degree of secretion may be normal and under physiologic control.

For these reasons, it is important to understand the underlying mechanisms of ion transport as well as the volume and composition of fluid residing in various regions of the gut lumen. These factors provide a rational approach to supportive treatment and a prediction of clinical manifestations of intestinal malfunction.

Much of the work in recent years has concentrated on the transport properties of the epithelial cell membranes rather than considering the mucosa as a single rate limiting barrier.[80] This is important for two reasons. First, physiologic and pathologic factors influencing absorption may be of quite different nature if the process is near the lumen rather than near the blood side of the epithelium. Second, the pharmacologic control of the mechanism is dictated by the nature and location of these processes in relation to the transporting cell itself.

Passive Forces Governing Absorption

Several passive forces are known to influence intestinal absorption of ions and water. The permeability characteristics of the epithelial cell membrane, osmotic pressure and electrochemical potential gradients, solvent drag and the hydrogen ion gradient—each is of importance in the absorptive process.

Permeability Characteristics

The epithelial cells lining the gut present the only barrier between lumen contents and blood. The opposing membranes of these cells (mucosal and serosal plus lateral membranes) are the major barriers to transcellular ion and H_2O movement. However, it is now becoming apparent that a large percentage of passive flow of many small ions and water occurs via extracellular routes, i.e., the tight junctions.[81] Thus, the passive forces moving ions and water across the mucosa may be of quite different magnitude and orientation depending on the route of penetration.

The mucosal membranes are lipoidal in nature but are penetrated with water-filled pores. As a first approximation, it can be assumed that lipid-soluble substances can cross the membrane rapidly, while diffusion of water or water-soluble ions are restricted by the size of the pores. The effective pore radius differs considerably in different segments of the bowel.[81] The stomach possesses a relatively tight epithelium, while mucosa of the proximal small bowel is quite pervious. This high permeability of proximal intestine decreases appreciably along the jejunum and ileum reaching a low value at the ileocecal junction. The epithelium of the colon is also tight, restricting the passive movement of water-soluble substances as small as urea. Therefore, it can be anticipated that flows of H_2O and ions in response to a given force will be of greater magnitude in the proximal intestine.

The Osmotic Pressure Gradient

It is now well established that flow of H_2O across the mucosa is secondary to development of osmotic pressure gradients.[80-83] The osmotic pressure difference ($\Delta\pi$) across a perfectly semipermeable membrane (permeable to H_2O but not to solute) can be predicted by the relation $\Delta\pi = RT\Delta C$, where C is the molar concentration, R the gas constant, and T the absolute temperature. However, the effective $\Delta\pi$ decreases inversely with the permeability of the membrane to solute. Thus, from simply a permeability standpoint a solute of given radius would be expected to exert a greater effective $\Delta\pi$ in the stomach and colon than in the proximal small bowel.

Although H_2O has been observed to flow across the mucosa against adverse osmotic gradients, it is now established that local intercellular osmotic gradients set up by net solute transport are responsible for these flows.[84] The process of bulk fluid transfer must be examined in terms of forces moving solute across the mucosal barriers as well as hyper- or hypotonic solutions within the gut lumen.

Solvent Drag

If an osmotic or hydrostatic pressure is applied across a membrane, water may flow from the higher to lower potential. If the permeability of the membrane is such as to allow solute penetration, e.g., proximal small bowel, then solute may beome entrapped in the solvent stream. In these conditions, solute may even be transported against the electrochemical potential gradient. This mechanism of solute transport has been termed "solvent drag."[80]

The Electrochemical Potential Gradient

The two physical factors governing diffusion of charged ions across the membrane, aside from those previously mentioned, are the concentration gradient of the ion and the electrical potential difference across the membrane.[80] The electrochemical potential ($\mu_1 - \mu_2$) of an ion at equilibrium can be predicted from the equation: $\mu_1 - \mu_2 = RT \ln (C_2/C_1) + ZF (\psi_1 - \psi_2)$, where C_2/C_1 is the concentration gradient between side 2 and side 1, Z the charge of the ion, F the Faraday constant and $\psi_1 - \psi_2$ the electrical potential difference. The effect of the electrical potential difference (PD) is to accelerate the flux of an ion toward the side of the membrane having the opposite electrical sign. It must be emphasized that the transepithelial PD (blood/lumen) is the algebraic sum of the potential differences, opposite in sign and arranged in series across both the mucosal and serosal membranes of the cell (Fig. 12–7).[82] Most cells have a low Na$^+$ and high K$^+$ concentration and are electrically negative with respect to the exterior solutions. For example, the concentration and electrical gradient may favor diffusion of Na$^+$ across the mucosal border, as in Figure 12–7, yet the energy to move Na$^+$ from cell to blood would be much greater than predicted from consideration of the transepithelial concentration and electrical gradients alone. Many passive ion flows seem to occur via the extracellular pathway. These flows will be directly influenced by the transepithelial electrochemical potential.

The Hydrogen Ion Gradient

The movement of weak electrolytes, e.g., most drugs and fatty acids, across the mucosa is primarily a result of factors governing their lipid solubility.[80] Due to the large molecular radius of most of these compounds, the un-ionized form of the electro-

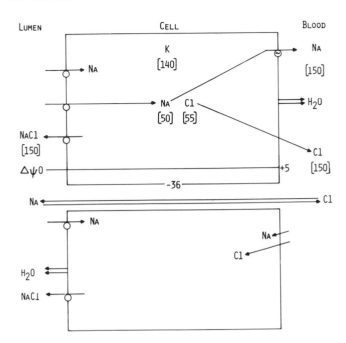

Figure 12–7. Small intestinal absorptive cell which is also capable of secretion. Transmembrane and transepithelial electrochemical potentials for Na$^+$ and Cl$^-$ are shown for upper absorptive cell. Na$^+$ can diffuse down its transmembrane electrochemical potential into the cell from the lumen while Cl$^-$ must be actively transported into the cell. A Cl$^-$ independent Na$^+$ influx process (Na$^+$–H$^+$ exchange?) is also present. A coupled NaCl efflux process is present at the mucosal border but this is normally overwhelmed by the more powerful NaCl influx process. The process coupling the influx of Na$^+$ and glucose is not operating due to the absence of glucose in the lumen. At the opposing cell membrane, Na$^+$ must be actively transported from cell to blood while Cl$^-$ transport into the blood can be explained by passive diffusion. Intra- and extracellular concentrations are shown in brackets. Passive net movements of Na$^+$ and Cl$^-$ (between cells) are driven by the transepithelial electrochemical potential difference of 5 mV. In the lower cell, in which intracellular levels of cAMP are raised, the NaCl influx process is abolished while the Cl$^-$-independent Na$^+$ influx is preserved. However, Na$^+$ is simply recycled back into the lumen. Chloride can now diffuse into the cell from the blood and is actively transported into the lumen via the coupled NaCl efflux process. The serosal border of the cell is much more permeable to Cl$^-$ than Na$^+$, while the reverse is true for the extracellular pathway. (Modified from Schultz,[82] and from Field.[85])

lyte would be expected to penetrate the membrane barrier at a much greater rate. The ratio of the ionized to un-ionized form of the weak acid or base may be predicted from the Henderson-Hasselbach equation: $pH = pK + \log \frac{\text{(unprotonated)}}{\text{(protonated)}}$. Thus the rate of penetration depends upon the pK of the electrolyte and the pH of the opposing solutions. As in the preceding cases, the intracellular environment can greatly modify the distribution of the electrolyte between lumen and plasma.

Carrier-Mediated Transport

Three types of mucosal transport are identified: facilitated diffusion, secondary active transport, and primary active transport.

Facilitated Diffusion

In many instances the rate of diffusion of a solute may be too rapid to be explained by the preceding forces even though the solute may be moving in the direction of its electrochemical potential. In such cases, it has been postulated that the membrane possesses "carriers" which can bring about the movement of the solute more rapidly than would be predicted from the membrane permeability alone.[80] This type, facilitated diffusion, does not require metabolic energy and cannot effect transport of the solute against the electrochemical potential gradient. The transport of fructose into the cell is an example of this process.

Secondary Active Transport Systems

The concept of carrier-mediated transport introduces two other processes which are of importance in the intestine. These processes also may not depend directly on metabolic energy of the cell but are coupled to the free energy available from the electrochemical gradient of a passively diffusing solute. The first of these is *exchange diffusion*, in which a molecule on one side of the membrane, e.g., Na^+, is exchanged for a molecule of the same species on the other side.[80] If the carrier can accommodate a species of similar structure, e.g., H^+, then net transport against the electrochemical gradient may occur. Similarly, an exchange process of Cl^- for HCO_3^- seems to be present in a number of epithelia.

The second type of carrier-mediated transport, *co-transport* or *coupled transport*, is of importance in the absorption of certain sugars and amino acids as well as electrolytes.[72] The carrier requires the presence of Na^+ together with the partner ion or nonelectrolyte, e.g., glucose, at the mucosal border. The driving force is the electrochemical gradient for Na^+, and the carrier can bring about the transfer of glucose from a lower to higher chemical potential. Thus the cell is capable of accumulating glucose, which in turn is free to diffuse down its concentration gradient into the blood.

There is little doubt that the presence of glucose greatly augments Na^+ absorption in the small bowel via this mechanism.[85] Similarly, a coupled transport of Na^+ and Cl^- is brought about by the small intestine, but via a separate carrier system (Fig. 12–7). In this case, Cl^- is transported against an electrochemical gradient into the cell and this probably is but another manifestation of an active process deriving its energy from the electrochemical Na^+ gradient.[85]

Primary Active Transport

In the previous examples of ion transport, it is obvious that establishment of the transcellular Na^+ gradient requires that the intracellular Na^+ concentration be maintained at low levels. This is generally believed to be due to a carrier located at the serosal or lateral membranes which is capable of transporting Na^+ from cell contents to blood. This process appears independent of coupling to other passive flows but may be coupled to transport of K^+ from the plasma into the cell. In either case, the net transfer of one or both of the ions is against the electrochemical potential (Fig. 12–7). This process requires a direct source of metabolic energy and has been associated with the presence of Na–K activated ATPases located at the serosal or lateral membranes of most transporting epithelia.

Absorption from the Intestine

The net flux of intestinal absorption is the sum of *secretion* and *absorption*. Several important components are present in this dynamic process.

The Enterosystemic Cycle

Quantitatively, the absorption of electrolytes and H_2O is of particular importance in the herbivore because of the much larger volumes of salivary and pancreatic secretions presented to the intestine for absorption. Also apparent is the fact that the organs concerned with microbial digestion, e.g., rumen and colon, require a highly buffered fluid environment. Therefore, in the case of the large intestine, a precarious balance between digestion and absorption must be handled at maximum efficiency.

The cycle of fluid into and out of the gut during a 24-hour period in the 100-kg pony is shown in Figure 12–8. The sum of the parotid, biliary, and pancreatic secretions amounts to approximately 30 liters per day, which is roughly 1.5 times the extracellular fluid volume. To this must be added unknown amounts of gastric and small intestinal secretions. Of this, 14 liters are presented to the large intestine from the ileum. However, a further net addition of about 7 liters is delivered to the large colon from the blood. The daily fecal output of 1 liter per day indicates an efficiency of 95% in the reabsorptive capacity of the large intestine under normal feeding conditions. Therefore, while the

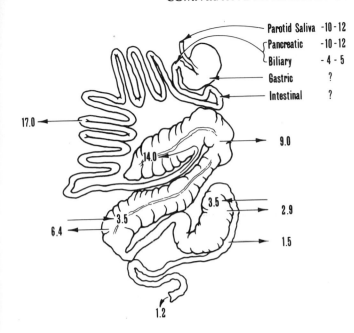

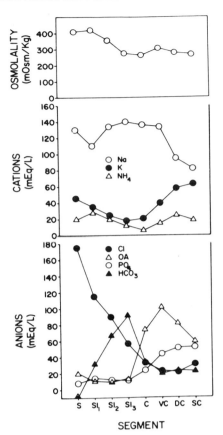

Figure 12–8. Enterosystemic cycle of fluid (liters/24 hours) in the 100-kg pony. Endogenous secretions into the small bowel amount to at least 30 liters/day and in the colon 7 liters/day. Thus, the animal must reabsorb approximately 40% of its own weight during a 24-hour period. The reserve capacity of the colon is probably at least twice that shown, so that normally 95% of the fluid presented to the large bowel is effectively reabsorbed. (Figures for net secretion and absorption adapted from Argenzio et al.[79] and from Alexander and Hickson.[39])

Figure 12–9. Osmolality and concentrations of cations and anions along gastrointestinal tract of 160-kg ponies. OA, organic acids (lactate and VFA). Symbols for segment represent: S, stomach; SI₁, SI₂, SI₃, proximal, middle, and distal thirds of small bowel; C, cecum; VC, DC, SC, ventral, dorsal, and small colon. (From Argenzio.[79])

small intestine of the pony may process larger volumes of fluid, its efficiency in reabsorption is less than that of the colon. Furthermore, the pony's colon has considerably more reserve capacity than its small bowel due not only to its large volume capacity, but also to a more efficient absorptive process.

Water Movement and the Transmucosal Osmotic Gradient

The mean osmotic pressure of gastric contents in the pony is considerably higher than the plasma over a 12-hour period (Fig. 12–9). Values as high as 700 mOsm/kg are present in the stomach 4 hours after feeding a conventional pelleted hay-grain ration.[79] Since the epithelium of the stomach is tight and little absorption takes place, these solutes should be capable of exerting a high effective osmotic pressure. Fortunately, the normal stomach mucosa is also relatively impermeable to H_2O and large gradients of osmotic pressure are not capable of eliciting bulk flow of H_2O from the plasma.[81]

The proximal intestine, however, is quite permeable to water but large flows of water from the plasma are prevented for three main reasons.[81]

First, as previously discussed, gastric emptying is largely controlled by osmoreceptors in the duodenum. Thus, the hypertonic gastric contents are delivered slowly to the proximal small bowel. Second, the carriers in the small intestinal mucosa are capable of rapidly transporting solute from the lumen of the intestine, so the effective osmotic pressure of the contents is lower than that expected from the measured osmolality. Third, the contents are diluted with isotonic secretions. Thus, the jejunum equilibrates the osmolality of its contents with the blood and presents the ileum and colon with an isotonic fluid. Although the mean colonic osmolality approximates that of the plasma, large fluctuations due to microbial activity were present throughout the day.[79] Unlike the stomach, water moves into and out of the lumen in response to these osmotic gradients. Yet it is apparent from an examination of Figures 12–8 and 12–9 that the large flows of H_2O from lumen to blood cannot be explained by transmucosal osmotic pressure differences alone. In the normal situation the major driving force for net water movement is the local osmotic gradient (presumably at the intercellular space) set up by active solute transport.

Ion Absorption from Small Bowel

The Na^+ concentration in small bowel contents approximates the plasma (Fig. 12–9). In most species there is an electrical potential across the small intestine of some 5 to 10 mv (blood positive), indicating that the transmucosal movement of Na^+ is directed against an electrical potential.[84] Referring again to Figure 12–7, it is evident that the cell to plasma movement is directed against a much steeper gradient than the transmural PD would indicate.

The principal mechanism responsible for Na^+ absorption in the jejunum seems to be carrier-mediated co-transport across the mucosal border coupled with glucose, amino acids, or Cl^-. The ATPase-dependent pump on the lateral or serosal membrane establishes the gradient for this reaction (Fig. 12–7). However, recent evidence in the human jejunum suggests the contrary; i.e., actively transported sugars and amino acids are capable of inducing an osmotic bulk H_2O flow which in turn carries Na^+ and other small ions across the highly permeable jejunal mucosa.[81] Thus, solvent drag may also be a major determinant of ion absorption in the jejunum.

There is also evidence for special carrier mechanisms in the jejunum and ileum for transport of Na^+, H^+, Cl^-, and HCO_3^-.[81] A Na^+–H^+ exchange process has been postulated to be present in the jejunum which transports Na^+ from lumen to blood in exchange for H^+. Functionally, this process would also result in reabsorption of pancreatic HCO_3^-, since the secreted H^+ would react chemically with HCO_3^- producing CO_2, which in turn could freely diffuse into the blood. In the ileum, both a Na^+–H^+ and a Cl^-–HCO_3^- exchange have been postulated. If both ion exchanges functioned at the same rate, Na^+ and Cl^- would be absorbed at equal rates and net transport of HCO_3^- would be unobserved. Referring to Figure 12–9, the striking reciprocal relationship of Cl^- and HCO_3^- concentrations along the small bowel of the pony suggest that a Cl^-–HCO_3^- exchange process may be of major importance in this animal. Obviously, the concentration of these two ions in the ileum cannot be explained by the electrochemical PD alone. Such a neutral anion exchange would be advantageous to this animal since Cl^- could be absorbed without the accompanying absorption of H_2O and the cecum would be presented with large volumes of highly buffered fluid.

No evidence for active transport of K^+ has been demonstrated in the small bowel and as can be seen from Figure 12–9, the concentration of K^+ along the small intestine is decreasing in accordance with the electrochemical PD.

The end result of the small intestine absorptive process is not only to reabsorb certain solutes by specific transport mechanisms but to alter the fluid composition in such a way as to deliver a fluid rich in HCO_3^- to the cecum. Most of the Cl^- secreted into gastric contents has been effectively reabsorbed by the time the ingesta reaches the terminal small bowel.

Small Bowel Secretion

Referring once again to Figure 12–7, a small intestinal cell secreting NaCl into the lumen is shown in the lower part of the figure. A comparison of the two cells indicates that (1) the coupled influx of NaCl is abolished and therefore a preexistent secretory process is unmasked or stimulated and (2) the major net secretion from blood to lumen can be attributed to Cl^-. Although it is not as yet clearly established whether the secretory process is simply unmasked (as shown) or enhanced, two facts are apparent. First, a normal absorptive process is abolished and second, the intestine is capable of net active secretion, quite apart from the existing passive forces, e.g., electrochemical gradients.[85] The choice of whether Cl^- or HCO_3^- is secreted seems to depend on the region of bowel, the relative affinity to the carriers, and the concentration gradients involved.

These transport alterations are induced by an increase in intracellular cAMP.[85] The cAMP system is specific for this coupled NaCl process and does not interfere with the Na^+ transport system at the serosal border. There simply is no available Na^+ to transport. The Na^+-glucose coupled absorptive process at the mucosal border is also left intact. Thus, the presence of glucose can reverse the direction of net Na^+ transport across the brush border, and active Na^+ absorption at the serosal membrane is restored.

Ion Absorption from Forestomachs and Colon

While the forestomach and colon are at opposing ends of the alimentary tract, they are faced with similar acid-base and electrolyte problems. Both must retrieve critical amounts of Na^+ and H_2O, both are presented with large volumes of highly buffered fluid, and both digest carbohydrates into their constituent volatile fatty acids, which must be rapidly neutralized and/or absorbed. Although the stratified squamous epithelium of the rumen is structurally quite different from the simple columnar epithelium of the colon, recent evidence suggests a similarity in function of these two types of epithelia.

The electrical potential difference (PD) across both the rumen epithelium of the sheep[86] and the ventral colon of the pony[87] is about 40 mv (blood positive). Thus, it is apparent from the concentration of Na^+ in the rumen (100 mM) and from Figure 12–9, that Na^+ is absorbed against a combined steep electrical and chemical PD. There is also an appreciable decrease in the concentration of Na^+ along the colon suggesting that the process is efficient and that very little back flux (leak) of Na occurs.

The mechanisms responsible for active Na^+ absorption in the rumen or colon have not been localized but they seem to involve both electrogenic Na^+ absorption and either a neutral, coupled NaCl absorption or a Na^+–H^+ exchange such as has been postulated for the ileum.[88] Chloride also is actively absorbed from rumen and possibly colonic contents, but the concentration of Cl in the colon (Fig. 12–9) can be almost entirely explained by the electrochemical PD. However, an active accumulation of HCO_3 occurs in both the rumen and colon which appears to be dependent in part on the presence of Cl in the lumen.[87–89] In all likelihood, this involves a Cl^-–HCO_3^- exchange mechanism similar to that in the ileum. In direct contrast to the rumen, the omasum appears to secrete Cl^- while absorbing CO_2 (HCO_3^-). The suggestion was put forth that this mechanism would prevent the large production of gas which would presumably occur if HCO_3^- were delivered into the acid contents of the abomasum.[90]

The direct secretion of HCO_3^- into the rumen or colon would be of importance in the neutralization of the VFA produced there. The amount of HCO_3^- in ruminant saliva or ileal contents of the pony is not sufficient to neutralize the total acid produced in these organs. For example, it has been estimated that the total VFA production in the cecum of a pony amounts to some 7 moles/day, while the amount of HCO_3^- entering the cecum/day would only be about 1 mole (Figs. 12–8 and 12–9). As can be seen from Figure 12–9, the HCO_3^- concentration is markedly reduced in cecal contents due to the chemical reaction of HCO_3^- with the VFA ($NaHCO_3$ + HA $\longrightarrow$ NaA + CO_2 + H_2O). Thus CO_2 is produced from the reaction, which accounts in part for the high pCO_2 in rumen and large intestinal contents.

The concentrations of both K^+ and $PO_4^\equiv$ increase along the colon, but there is no evidence for active secretion of these ions. The electrical gradient would favor the accumulation of K^+ in the lumen but it would take a PD of about 60 mv to explain the terminal small colon concentration. It appears that both K^+ and $PO_4^\equiv$ are poorly absorbed by the colon, and the increased concentration can be explained in part by the more rapid absorption of Na^+ and H_2O which would concentrate these two ions in the lumen.[79]

The absorption of volatile fatty acids from the forestomach has received considerable attention owing to the importance of the VFA as an energy source in ruminants. However, the large intestinal production of VFA is by no means insignificant and even in non-herbivorous animals, the VFA constitute the major anions in colonic digesta.

With regard to the pH of large intestinal contents (approximately 6.5), it is apparent that more than 90% of the VFA are present in the dissociated form and a slow rate of absorption would be expected. A similar situation is present in the forestomach. Indeed, in vitro studies of both rumen and colonic epithelium have demonstrated that at least one membrane is impermeable to the dissociated form of the acid. Yet, the VFA are rapidly absorbed by the forestomach as well as from the colon of the species that have been examined.

Studies with the isolated rumen and the colon of the pony have shown that hydration of CO_2, within either the lumen solution or mucosal cell, provides the hydrogen ions to form the more permeable undissociated acid.[86,87] Further studies of the goat colon have provided evidence of an interaction of VFA and Na^+. At a physiologic pH (6.2) and pCO_2 (300 mmHg), the VFA induce a twofold increase in Na^+ absorption.[91]

Augmentation of Na^+ absorption by VFA does not appear to be shared by the forestomach of ruminants or proximal colon of the horse. Yet from a teleologic point of view, the forestomach and proximal colon of these animals must maintain a fluid environment to supply microbial digestion. For example, in vitro studies indicate that the small (distal) colon of the pony actively transports Na^+ at a rate six times that of the ventral colon.[87]

While an overall description of ion absorption in the colon is not presently available, it is apparent that this organ makes a substantial contribution to the reabsorption of electrolytes and H_2O in the normal animal. Equally important is the fact that the products of microbial metabolism, e.g., H^+, CO_2, are directly involved with these absorptive processes. Therefore, normal absorptive function of the large bowel depends not only on the underlying transport mechanisms but also upon an optimal environment for microbial fermentation.

Large Bowel Secretion

Cyclic AMP-mediated secretion is also present in the colon. The $Cl^-–HCO_3^-$ exchange process is abolished and active Cl^- secretion is elicited.[89] As in the small bowel, the active Na^+ absorptive process at the serosal membrane is preserved.

Control of Intestinal Ion Transport

Among the gastrointestinal hormones known to stimulate small bowel secretion are gastrin, CCK, GIP, VIP, and enteroglucagon. Evidence is now accumulating to suggest that prostaglandins and cholinergic stimulation also cause the bowel to secrete, while adrenergic stimulation enhances absorption. Aldosterone also enhances colonic Na^+ absorption. It is likely that these agents are physiologically involved in regulation of intestinal ion transport but this point has yet to be demonstrated conclusively. Of these agents, only prostaglandins, VIP, and catecholamines exert an influence on cAMP metabolism. The mechanisms by which these and other exogenous agents act and their influence in diarrhea will be considered in detail in Chapter 14.

REFERENCES

1. Schofield, G. C.: Chapter 80, Anatomy of muscular and neural tissues in the alimentary canal. *In* Handbook of Physiology, Alimentary Canal, Sect. 6, Vol. IV, Washington, D.C., Am. Physiol. Soc., 1968, p. 1579.
2. Christensen, J.: Movements of the small intestine. *In* Gastrointestinal Disease. Edited by M. H. Sleisenger and J. S. Fordtran. Philadelphia, W. B. Saunders Co. 1973, p. 216.
3. Makhlouf, G. M.: The neuroendocrine design of the gut. Gastroenterology 67:159, 1974.
4. Konturek, S. J., Thor, P., Dembinski, A., and Krol. R.: Comparison of secretin and vasoactive intestinal peptide on pancreatic secretion in dogs. Gastroenterology 68:1527, 1975.
5. Hill, K. J.: Chapter 17, Prehension, mastication, deglutition, and the esophagus. *In* Dukes' Physiology of Domestic Animals, 8th ed. Edited by M. J. Swenson. Ithaca, NY, Comstock, 1970, p. 351.
6. Doty, R. W.: Chapter 92, Neural organization of deglutition. *In* Handbook of Physiology, Alimentary Canal, Sect. 6, Vol. IV. Washington, D. C., Am. Physiol. Soc., 1968, p. 1861.
7. Bortoff, A.: Myogenic control of intestinal motility. Physiol. Rev. 56:418, 1976.
8. Schatzmann, H. J.: Chapter 105, Action of acetylcholine and epinephrine on intestinal smooth muscle. *In* Handbook of Physiology, Alimentary Canal. Sect. 6, Vol. IV. Washington, D.C., Am. Physiol. Soc., 1968, p. 2173.
9. Gillespie, J. S.: Chapter 102, Electrical activity in the colon. *In* Handbook of Physiology, Alimentary Canal, Sect. 6, Vol. IV. Washington, D.C., Am. Physiol. Soc., 1968, p. 2093.
10. Dougherty, R. W.: Eructation in ruminants. Ann. N.Y. Acad. Sci. 150; Art. 1:22, 1968.
11. Sellers, A. F., and Stevens, C. E.: Motor functions of the ruminant forestomach. Physiol. Rev. 46:634, 1966.
12. Leek, B. F., and Harding, R. H.: Sensory nervous receptors in the ruminant stomach and the reflex control of reticulo-ruminal motility. *In* Digestion and Metabolism in the Ruminant. Edited by I. W. McDonald and A.C.I. Warner. Armidale, Univ. of New England Publ. Unit, 1975, p. 60.
13. Titchen, D. A.: Chapter 129, Nervous control of motility of the forestomach of ruminants. *In* Handbook of Physiology, Alimentary Canal, Sect. 6, Vol. V. Washington, D.C., Am. Physiol. Soc., 1968, p. 2705.
14. Code, C. F., and Carlson, H. C.: Chapter 93, Motor activity of the stomach. *In* Handbook of Physiology, Alimentary Canal, Sect. 6, Vol. IV. Washington, D.C., Am. Physiol. Soc., 1968, p. 1903.
15. Clemens, E. T., Stevens, C. E., and Southworth, M.: Sites of organic acid production and pattern of digesta movement in the gastrointestinal tract of swine. J. Nutr. 105:759, 1975.
16. Cooke, A. R., and Christensen, J.: Motor functions of the stomach. *In* Gastrointestinal Disease. Edited by M. H. Sleisenger and J. S. Fordtran. Philadelphia, W. B. Saunders Co., 1973, p. 115.
17. Hunt, J. N., and Stubbs, D. F.: The volume and energy content of meals as determinants of gastric emptying. J. Physiol. 245:299, 1975.
18. Bolton, J. R., Merritt, A. M., Carlson, G. M., and Donawick, W. J.: Normal abomasal electromyography and emptying in sheep and the effects of intraabomasal volatile fatty acid infusion. Am. J. Vet. Res. 37:1387, 1976.
19. Svendson, P.: Experimental studies of gastrointestinal atony in ruminants. *In* Digestion and Metabolism in the Ruminant. Edited by I. W. McDonald and A.C.I. Warner. Armidale, Univ. of New England Publ. Unit, 1975, p. 563.
20. Hunt, J. N., and Knox, M. T.: Chapter 94, Regulation of gastric emptying. *In* Handbook of Physiology, Alimentary Canal, Sect. 6, Vol. IV. Washington, D.C., Am. Physiol. Soc., 1968, p. 1917.
21. Cooke, A. R., and Clark, E. D.: Effect of first part of duodenum on gastric emptying in dogs: response to acid, fat, glucose, and neural blockade. Gastroenterology 70:550, 1976.
22. Cooke, A. R.: Control of gastric emptying and motility. Gastroenterology 68:804, 1975.
23. Debas, H. T., Farooq, O., and Grossman, M. I.: Inhibition of gastric emptying as a physiological action of cholecystokinin. Gastroenterology 68:1211, 1975.
24. Argenzio, R. A., Lowe, J. E., Pickard, D. W., and Stevens, C. E.: Digesta passage and water exchange in the equine large intestine. Am. J. Physiol. 226:1035, 1974.
25. Reference deleted.
26. Ruckebusch, Y., and Bueno, L.: The effect of feeding on the motility of the stomach and small intestine in the pig. Brit. J. Nutr., 35:397, 1976.
27. Kosterlitz, H. W.: Chapter 104, Intrinsic and extrinsic nervous control of motility of the stomach and the intestines. *In* Handbook of Physiology, Alimentary Canal, Sect. 6, Vol. IV. Washington, D. C., Am. Physiol. Soc., 1968, p. 2147.
28. Smith, J., Kelly, K. A., and Weinshilboum, R. M.: Pathophysiology of post operative ileus. Arch. Surg. 112:203, 1977.
29. Farrar, T., and Ramirez, M.: The effect of gastrointestinal hormones on small intestinal motility. *In* Gastrointestinal Motility. Edited by L. Demling and R. Ottenjann. Stuttgart, Georg Thieme Verlag, 1971, p. 192.
30. Dinoso, V. P., Jr., Meshkin Pour, H., Lorber, S. H., Gutierrez, J. G., and Chey, W. Y.: Motor responses of the sigmoid colon and rectum to exogenous cholectystokinin and secretin. Gastroenterology 65:438,1973.
31. Dyce, K. M., and Hartman, W.: A cinefluoroscopic study of the caecal base of the horse. Res. Vet. Sci. 20:40, 1976.
32. Connell, A. M.: Chapter 101, Motor action of the large bowel. *In* Handbook of Physiology, Alimentary Canal, Sect. 6, Vol. IV. Washington, D.C., Am. Physiol. Soc. 1968, p. 2075.
33. Pickard, D. W., and Stevens, C. E.: Digesta flow through the rabbit large intestine. Am. J. Physiol. 225:1161, 1972.
34. Hukuhara, T., and Neya, T.: The movements of the colon of rats and guinea pigs. Jpn. J. Physiol. 18:551, 1968.
35. Christensen, J.: Myoelectric control of the colon. Gastroenterology 68:601, 1975.
36. Young, K., Bolton, J. R., Beech, J., and Merritt, A. M.: Relation between migrating spike complexes and motility of the equine colon. Chicago, Proc. Conf. Res. Workers Anim. Dis., 1976.
37. Sleisenger, M. H.: Physiology of the colon. *In* Gastrointestinal

Disease. Edited by M. H. Sleisenger and J. S. Fordtran. Philadelphia, W. B. Saunders Co., 1973, p. 229.

38. Kimberg, D. V.: Cyclic nucleotides and their role in gastrointestinal secretion. Gastroenterology 67:1023, 1974.

39. Alexander, F., and Hickson, J. C. D.: The salivary and pancreatic secretions of the horse. In Physiology of Digestion and Metabolism in the Ruminant. Edited by A. T. Phillipson, Newcastle upon Tyne, England, Oriel, 1970, p. 375.

40. Schneyer, L. H., and Schneyer, C. A.: Chapter 33, Inorganic composition of saliva. In Handbook of Physiology. Alimentary Canal, Sect. 6, Vol II. Washington, D.C., Am. Physiol. Soc., 1968, p. 497.

41. Blair-West, J. R., Coghlan, J. P., Denton, D. A., and Wright, R. D.: Chapter 38, Effect of endocrines on salivary glands. In Handbook of Physiology, Alimentary Canal, Sect. 6, Vol. II. Washington, D.C., Am. Physiol. Soc., 1968, p. 633.

42. Burgen, A. S. V.: Chapter 35, Secretory processes in salivary glands. In Handbook of Physiology, Alimentary Canal, Sect. 6, Vol. II, Washington, D.C., Am. Physiol. Soc., 1968, p. 561.

43. Stevens, C. E.: Transport across rumen epithelium. In 5th Alfred Benzon Symp., Transport Mechanisms in Epithelia. Edited by H. H. Ussing and N. A. Thorn. Copenhagen, Munksgaard, 1973, p. 10.

44. Holler, H.: Studies of the secretory activity of the glands in the cardiac zone of the pig stomach. I. Volume and rhythm of secretion properties of glands. Zentralb. Veterinaermed. 17A:685, 1970.

45. Walsh, J. H.: Control of gastric secretion. In Gastrointestinal Disease. Edited by M. H. Sleisenger and J. S. Fordtran. Philadelphia, W. B. Saunders Co., 1973, p. 144.

46. Argenzio, R. A., Southworth, M., and Stevens, C. E.: Sites of organic acid production and absorption in the equine gastrointestinal tract. Am. J. Physiol. 226:1043, 1974b.

47. Grossman, M. I.: Chapter 47, Neural and hormonal stimulation of gastric secretion of acid. In Handbook of Physiology, Alimentary Canal. Sect. 6, Vol. II. Washington, D.C., Am. Physiol. Soc., 1968, p. 835.

48. Grossman, M. I.: Candidate hormones of the gut. Gastroenterology 67:730, 1974.

49. Janowitz, H. D.: Chapter 52, Pancreatic secretion of fluid and electrolytes. In Handbook of Physiology, Alimentary Canal, Sect. 6, Vol. II. Washington, D.C., Am. Physiol. Soc., 1968, p. 925.

50. Caple, I. W., and Heath, T. J.: Biliary and pancreatic secretions in sheep: their regulation and roles. In Digestion and Metabolism in the Ruminant. Edited by I. W. McDonald and A. C. I. Warner. Armidale, Univ. of New England Publ. Unit. 1975, p. 91.

51. Brandborg, L. L.: Pancreatic physiology. In Gastrointestinal Disease. Edited by M. H. Sleisenger and J. S. Fordtran. Philadelphia, W. B. Saunders Co., 1973, p. 359.

52. Janowitz, H. D., and Banks, P. A.: Normal functional physiology of the pancreas. In Disorders of the Gastrointestinal Tract; Disorders of the Liver; Nutritional Disorders. Edited by J. M. Dietschy. New York, Grune and Stratton, 1976, p. 193.

53. Thomas, J. E.: Chapter 54, Neural regulation of pancreatic secretion. In Handbook of Physiology, Alimentary Canal, Sect. 6, Vol. II. Washington, D.C., Am. Physiol. Soc., 1968, p. 955.

54. Harper, A. A.: Chapter 55, Hormonal control of pancreatic secretion. In Handbook of Physiology, Alimentary Canal, Sect. 6, Vol. II. Washington, D.C., Am. Physiol. Soc., 1968, p. 969.

55. Boyer, J. L.: Bile formation and secretion. In Disorders of the Gastrointestinal Tract, Disorders of the Liver, Nutritional Disorders. Fdited by J. M. Dietschy. New York, Grune and Stratton, 1976, p. 22.

56. Admirand, W., and Way, L. W.: Bile formation and biliary tract function. In Gastrointestinal Disease. Edited by M. H. Sleisenger and J. S. Fordtran. Philadelphia, W. B. Saunders Co., 1973, p. 352.

57. Erlinger, S., and Dhumeaux, D.: Mechanisms and control of secretion of bile water and electrolytes. Gastroenterology 66:281, 1974.

58. Banfield, W. J.: Physiology of the gallbladder. Gastroenterology 69:770, 1975.

59. Moir, R. J.: Chapter 126, Ruminant digestion and evolution. In Handbook of Physiology, Alimentary Canal, Sect. 6, Vol. V. Washington, D.C., Am. Physiol. Soc., 1968, p. 2673.

60. Bryant, M. P.: Normal flora-rumen bacteria. Am. J. Clin. Nutr. 23:1440, 1970.

61. Bergman, E. N., and Wolff, J. E.: Metabolism of volatile fatty acids by liver and portal-drained viscera in sheep. Am. J. Physiol. 221:586, 1971.

62. Ash, R. W., and Dobson, A.: The effect of absorption on the acidity of rumen contents. J. Physiol. 229:997, 1963.

63. Leat, W. M. F., and Harrison, F. A.: Digestion, absorption and transport of lipids in the sheep. In Digestion and Metabolism in the Ruminant. Edited by I. W. McDonald and A. C. I. Warner. Armidale, Univ. of New England Publ. Unit, 1975, p. 481.

64. Nolan, J. V.: Quantitative models of nitrogen metabolism in sheep. In Digestion and Metabolism in the Ruminant. Edited by I. W. McDonald and A. C. I. Warner. Armidale, Univ. of New England Publ. Unit, 1975, p. 416.

65. Gray, G. M.: Mechanisms of digestion and absorption of food. In Gastrointestinal Disease. Edited by M. H. Sleisenger and J. S. Fordtran. Philadelphia, W. B. Saunders Co., 1973, p. 250–257.

66. Huber, J. T.: Development of the digestive and metabolic apparatus of the calf. J. Dairy Sci. 52:1, 1968.

67. Siddons, R. C., Smith, R. H., Henschel, M. J., Hill, W. B., and Porter, J. W. G.: Carbohydrate utilization in the pre-ruminant calf. Br. J. Nutr. 23:333, 1969.

68. Toofanian, F.: Small intestinal infusion studies in the calf. Br. Vet. J. 132:215, 1976.

69. Nerri, F. O.: Normal mechanisms of carbohydrate absorption. In Disorders of the Gastrointestinal Tract; Disorders of the Liver; Nutritional Disorders. Edited by J. M. Dietschy. New York, Grune and Stratton, 1976, p. 35.

70. Walker, D. M.: The development of the digestive system of the young animal. II. Carbohydrase enzyme development in the young pig. J. Agric. Sci. 52:357, 1959.

71. Scharrer, E.: Developmental changes of sugar and amino acid transport in different tissues of ruminants. In Digestion and Metabolism in the Ruminant. Edited by I. W. McDonald and A. C. I. Warner. Armidale, Univ. of New England Publ. Unit, 1975, p. 49.

72. Crane, R. K.: Chapter 69, Absorption of sugars. In Handbook of Physiology, Alimentary Canal, Sect. 6, Vol. III. Washington, D.C., Am. Physiol. Soc., 1968, p. 1323.

73. Johnston, J. M.: Chapter 70, Mechanism of fat absorption. In Handbook of Physiology, Alimentary Canal, Sect. 6, Vol. III. Washington, D.C., Am. Physiol. Soc., 1968, p. 1353.

74. Moore, J. H., and Noble, R. C.: Foetal and neonatal lipid metabolism. In Digestion and Metabolism in the Ruminant. Edited by I. W. McDonald and A. C. I. Warner. Armidale, Univ. of New England Publ. Unit, 1975, p. 465.

75. Westergaard, H.: Normal mechanisms of lipid absorption. In Disorders of the Gastrointestinal Tract; Disorders of the Liver; Nutritional Disorders. Edited by J. M. Dietschy. New York, Grune and Stratton, 1976, p. 38.

76. Weiner, I. M., and Lack, L.: Chapter 73, Bile salt absorption, enterohepatic circulation. In Handbook of Physiology, Alimentary Canal, Sect. 6, Vol. III, Washington, D.C., Am. Physiol. Soc., 1968, p. 1439.

77. Nervi, F. O.: Normal mechanisms of protein absorption. In Disorders of the Gastrointestinal Tract; Disorders of the Liver; Nutritional Disorders. Edited by J. M. Dietschy. New York, Grune and Stratton, 1976, p. 38.

78. Ulyatt, M. J., Dellow, D. W., Reid, C. S. W., and Bauchop, T.: Structure and functions of the large intestine of ruminants. In Digestion and Metabolism in the Ruminant. Edited by I. W. McDonald and A. C. I. Warner. Armidale, Univ. of New England Publ. Unit, 1975, p. 119.

79. Argenzio, R. A.: Functions of the equine large intestine and their interrelationship in disease. Cornell Vet. 65:303, 1975.

80. Curran, P. F., and Schultz, S. G.: Chapter 65, Transport across membranes: general principles. In Handbook of Physiology, Alimentary Canal, Sect. 6, Vol. III. Washington, D.C., Am. Physiol. Soc., 1968, p. 1217.

81. Fordtran, J. S.: Diarrhea. In Gastrointestinal Disease. Edited by M. H. Sleisenger and J. S. Fordtran. Philadelphia, W. B. Saunders Co., 1973, p. 291.

82. Schultz, S. G.: Chapter 3, Principles of electrophysiology and their application to epithelial tissues. In Gastrointestinal Physiology, MTP International Review of Science, Vol. 4. Edited by E. D. Jacobson and L. L. Shanbour. London, Butterworths, 1974, p. 69.

83. Diamond, J. M.: Chapter 115, Transport mechanisms in the gallbladder. In Handbook of Physiology, Alimentary Canal, Sect. 6, Vol. V. Washington, D.C., Am. Physiol. Soc., 1968, p. 2451.

84. Schultz, S. G., and Curran, P. F.: Intestinal absorption of sodium chloride and water. In Handbook of Physiology, Alimentary Canal, Sec. 6, Vol. III. Washington, D.C., Am. Physiol. Soc., 1968, p. 1245.

85. Field, M.: Intestinal secretion. Gastroenterology 66:1063, 1974.

86. Ash, R. W., and Dobson, A.: The effect of absorption on the acidity of rumen contents. J. Physiol. 169:39, 1963.

87. Argenzio, R. A., Southworth, M., Lowe, J. E., and Stevens, C. E.: Interrelationship of Na, HCO₃ and volatile fatty acid transport by equine large intestine. Am. J. Physiol. *223*:E469, 1977.

88. Chien, W-J., and Stevens, C. E.: Coupled active transport of Na and Cl across forestomach epithelium. Am. J. Physiol. *223*:997, 1972.

89. Frizzell, R. A., Koch, M. J., and Schultz, S. G.: Ion transport by rabbit colon. I. Active and passive components. J. Membr. Biol. *27*:297, 1976.

90. von Engelhardt, W., and Hauffe, R.: Role of the omasum in absorption and secretion of water and electrolytes in sheep and goats. *In* Digestion and Metabolism in the Ruminant. Edited by I. W. McDonald and A. C. I. Warner. Armidale, Univ. of New England Publ. Unit, 1975, p. 216.

91. Argenzio, R. A., Miller, N., and von Engelhardt, W.: Effect of volatile fatty acids on water and ion absorption from the goat colon. Am. J. Physiol. *229*:997, 1975.

Chapter 13

MICROFLORA, MUCOSA, AND IMMUNITY

DWIGHT C. HIRSH

The gastrointestinal tract contains a vast number and variety of microorganisms. In the colon, there are 10^{11} organisms per gram of feces.[1] It has been estimated that 400 to 500 different species may be represented, many of which have not yet been cultured.[2]

The microbial flora that inhabits the gastrointestinal tract serves at least a threefold purpose: first, it provides a source of energy from ingested materials; second, it serves as a host-defense barrier in the prevention of disease by agents seeking entry via the intestinal tract; and third, the microbial inhabitants condition the immunologic components of the gastrointestinal tract to respond to antigenic materials in a highly efficient manner.

NORMAL MICROFLORA OF THE GASTROINTESTINAL TRACT

The gastrointestinal tract of the animal is sterile at birth. Within minutes of birth, the canal is flooded with microorganisms acquired from the immediate environment. The most important contributor to this microbial environment is the dam.

The flora of the gastrointestinal tract changes as the newborn's diet changes from milk to solid food. This change in flora is dramatically different depending upon the character and nature of the food ingested and takes place in a sequential manner.[3-6] Herbivores, such as cattle and sheep, develop a rumen with flora and fauna that are quite distinct from the rest of the domestic species, though in many ways similar to the colon and cecum of non-ruminant herbivores. Omnivores and carnivores are much the same with respect to the flora of their gastrointestinal tract.

The Rumen. This area is sterile at birth in the so-called "pre-ruminant" herbivore, as is the rest of the gastrointestinal tract. The rumen itself is very small in size. The development of the rumen and its flora and fauna depend a great deal upon the diet of the animal.[7] In general terms, however, during the first weeks the flora consists of streptococci (*S. bovis* is the main organism), *Lactobacillus* spp.,

coliform types (*Escherichia coli-Enterobacter*), *Clostridium perfringens,* and *Bacteroides* spp.[8,9] Ciliate protozoans make their appearance by 8 to 14 days of age.[7] With time, more and more of the flora and fauna of the rumen are acquired. The sources of the microorganisms that inhabit the rumen have been shown to be the "environment." The main contributors to this environment are other ruminant animals.[7] Direct contact or ingestion of fomites contaminated with rumen organisms is the mechanism whereby the rumen flora is acquired.[7]

Once the microflora and fauna have become established in the rumen, it can be looked upon as a large continuous culture system.[7,10-13] It is here that the ingested cellulose, starch, and other carbohydrates, lipids, and protein are converted into energy for use by the animal. The system is buffered in a narrow range (pH 6 to 7) by $NaHCO_3$ and urea in the saliva. The microbial action in the absence of oxygen creates an extremely anaerobic environment, with an oxidation-reduction potential of less than -400 mv.

The number and kinds of microorganisms living in this environment are varied depending on the type of food ingested. In general, there are about 10^9 to 10^{10} bacteria/g of contents and 10^5 to 10^6 protozoa/g.

The most numerous facultative anaerobes are *Streptococcus bovis* (10^5 to 10^7/g) and the coliforms (*Escherichia coli-Enterobacter*) at concentrations of 10^3 to 10^5/g of contents. Thus, the facultative microorganisms comprise only about 1 to 2% of the rumen flora. The most numerous type of microorganism in the rumen is the obligate anaerobes. These organisms make it possible for the rumen to do its work. Of the 10^9 or so obligate anaerobes, there are only 6 to 10 dominant genera with no one species dominating under normal conditions. Most are gram-negative non-spore-forming microorganisms. The predominate anaerobic bacteria will be discussed in groups, depending upon the role played in the fermentation process:

1. Cellulose digesters: Members of the genus *Bacteroides (B. succinogenes* and *B. ruminicola)*

199

and *Butyrivibrio* (also one of the major producers of butyric acid in the rumen). These break down cellulose (and hemicellulose) to the fatty acids: acetic, formic, butyric, succinic, propionic, and lactic.

2. Starch digesters: *S. bovis* and *B. amylophilus* are examples of the predominate starch digesters. These organisms liberate amylases that break down starch. A major end-product of fermentation by *S. bovis* is lactic acid.

3. Mono- and disaccharide fermenters: All polysaccharide-digesting bacteria (see above) plus members of the genus *Lactobacillus* will ferment mono- and disaccharides. Lactobacilli do not exist in the normal rumen in large numbers.

4. Acid utilizers: The nonvolatile fatty acids, lactic and succinic, and the volatile fatty acid, formic, are degraded by members of genus *Bacteroides* (*B. succinogenes*) and *Megasphaera* (*M. elsdenii*). This activity helps maintain the pH of the rumen near neutrality (pH 6 to 7).

5. Proteolytic strains: Members of the genera *Succinovibrio*, *Butyrivibrio*, and *Megasphaera* are proteolytic. These organisms break down protein into peptides and amino acids. The amino acids are used for microbial protein, NH_3, volatile fatty acids, and/or CO_2. Because of the polysaccharide nature of the diet, proteolytic strains are not numerous (10^7 or so per gram of contents).

6. Miscellaneous: Methanogenic bacteria (*Methanobacterium*, 10^8/g) convert CO_2 and H_2 to CH_4, which is eructated (with a concurrent loss of energy); lipolytic bacteria split fats into glycerol and fatty acids.

What has been outlined in the preceding six items is a general overview of the bacterial components of the rumen. Protozoa also exist in the rumen along with the bacteria. These organisms are anaerobic and most occur only in the rumen. Both ciliates and flagellates are present. The ciliates are the most numerous with the predominant species belonging to the following genera: *Entodinium*, *Diplodinium*, *Epidinium*, *Ophryoscolex*, *Dasytricha*, and *Isotricha*. The protozoa are sensitive to acid (pH ≤ 5.5) and exist in the rumen in concentrations of 10^3 to 10^6/ml of rumen contents. Although the protozoa ingest insoluble carbohydrates, such as starch and cellulose, and digest them internally, their presence does not seem to be essential to the fermentation process taking place in the rumen. They do apparently make some contribution to the nutrition of the host since they are digested in the abomasum. Rumen bacteria have been shown to be ingested by protozoa. This may account for the higher number of bacteria observed in the rumen of defaunated animals.

Carbohydrates, in the form of cellulose, hemicellulose, starch, and mono/disaccharides are fermented to H_2, formate, succinate, lactate, butyrate, acetate, propionate, and CO_2. Formate is rapidly degraded to CO_2 and H_2 by the carbohydrate fermenters, methanogenic species, and the polysaccharide digesters. The methanogenic species use H_2 to reduce CO_2 and synthesize CH_4. Succinate is decarboxylated to form propionate and CO_2 by the carbohydrate fermenters and the acid-hydrolyzers. Lactate is metabolized to acetate, propionate, butyrate, CO_2, and H_2 by the acid hydrolyzers. The volatile fatty acids, acetate, propionate, and butyrate are absorbed across the rumen epithelium and provide the animal with a major energy source. Carbon dioxide (50 to 70% of the gaseous environment of the rumen) and CH_4 (representing the difference) is eructated.

The proteolytic species of microorganisms in the rumen hydrolyze dietary protein to peptides and amino acids, which are either catabolized to NH_3 or incorporated by the microflora into microbial protein (structural protein). The ammonia liberated in this process is utilized by the microbial flora as their main nitrogen source. If there is an excess of NH_3, it is absorbed into the blood stream and then changed to urea in the liver. The urea is either excreted by the kidneys or returned to the rumen via the saliva. Once back in the rumen, urea is split into NH_3 and CO_2 by bacterial ureases.

The proteins that have been incorporated into bacterial cell components are made available to the host when the bacteria themselves are digested by the various acidic and enzymatic processes that occur in the abomasum and small intestine.

Thus, the only by-products of the diet that escape are CO_2, CH_4, and NH_3 (as urea) and approximately 15 to 30% of the total digestible dry matter. All the rest in the form of volatile fatty acids and microbial protein are utilized by the host.

At weaning, the flora of the gastrointestinal tract (abomasum to rectum) is predominately anaerobic (95 to 99%). The composition of the flora is shown in Table 13–1.[14–16] It is worthy of note that members of the family Enterobacteriaceae (notably *E. coli*) can be found throughout the small intestine.[8,9]

Flora of Cecum and Colon. Before the flora of the non-ruminant is discussed, some comment concerning the cecum and colon and their function in pigs and horses is appropriate. The cecum and colon contain a flora and fauna much like that seen in the rumen, though on a much lesser scale. The most

Table 13–1. Microbial Flora of the Gastrointestinal Tract of the Normal Bovine

	No. of Viable Microorganisms/Gram of Contents*				
		Small Intestine			
	Abomasum	Anterior	Posterior	Cecum	Feces
Total	6–8	>7	6–7	8–9	9
Anaerobes (excluding *Lactobacillus*)	7–8†	NA‡	5–6	8–9	6–9
Enterobacteriaceae (mainly *E. coli*)	3–4	0–7	5–6	4–5	5–6
Enterococci	6–7	2–3	3–4	4–5	4–5
Yeasts	2–3	0	0–3	2	0
Lactobacillus spp.	7–8	3–5	5–6	5	5–6

*Expressed as $\log_{10} (x+1)$ of the number of organisms cultured (x).
†*Bacteroides spp.* most frequent.
‡Not available.

important members are the cellulose digesters; these occur as $>10^6$/g of content.[17] In the horse, the volatile fatty acids produced in the cecum account for 30% of the digestible energy intake.[18]

Flora of the Non-Ruminant. As in the calf, the predominant genera in the young piglet are *E. coli, C. perfringens,* streptococci, lactobacilli, and *Bac-*teroides.[8,9] *E. coli* can be cultured from all segments of the small intestine.[8,9] As the pig grows older and more solid food is ingested, the flora changes to one that is predominantly anaerobic in nature. The composition of the flora at weaning is as seen in Table 13–2.[11,19–21]

The predominant species of bacteria found in the

Table 13–2. Microbial Flora of the Gastrointestinal Tract of the Normal Porcine

	No. of Viable Microorganisms/Gram of Contents*				
		Small Intestine			
	Stomach	Anterior	Posterior	Cecum	Feces
Total	3–8	3–7	4–8	4–11	10–11
Anaerobes (excluding *Lactobacillus*)	7–8†	6–7	7–8	7–11	10–11
Enterobacteriaceae (mainly *E. coli*)	3–5	3–4	4–5	6–9	6–9
Enterococci	4–6	4–5	6–7	7–10	7–10
Yeasts	4–5‡	4	4	4	4
Lactobacillus	7–9	6–7	7–8	8–9	8–9
Spirochetes	NA§	NA	NA	NA	8

*Expressed as $\log_{10} (x+1)$ of the number of organisms cultured (x).
†*Eubacterium spp., Peptostreptococcus spp., Veillonella spp., Clostridium perfringens, Propionibacterium spp.,* and *Bacteroides spp.*
‡Mostly *Candida albicans* and *C. slooffii.*
§Not available.

Table 13–3. Microbial Flora of the Gastrointestinal Tract of the Normal Canine

	No. of Viable Microorganisms/Gram of Contents*				
		Small Intestine			
	Stomach	Anterior	Posterior	Cecum	Feces
Total	>6	>6	>7	>8.5	10–11
Anaerobes (excluding *Lactobacillus*)	1–2	>5	4–5	>8.5	10–11
Enterobacteriaceae (mainly *E. coli*)	0.8–5	2–4	4–6	7–8	7–8
Enterococci	0.8–6	5–6	5–7	8–9	9.3
Staphylococcus aureus	0.4	NA†	1.4	NA	4–5
Lactobacillus spp.	4–5	3–5	4–6	8–9	9
Spirochetes (relative amounts)	1+	1+	1+	2+(4+colon)	0

*Expressed as $\log_{10} (x+1)$ of the number of organisms cultured (x).
†Not available.

Table 13–4.   Microbial Flora and Fauna of the Gastrointestinal Tract of the Normal Equine

| | Stomach | Small Intestine | | Cecum | Feces |
		Anterior	Posterior		
Total	7–9	NA†	7–8	8–9	8–9
Anaerobes (excluding *Lactobacillus*)	6–8	NA	6–7	8–9	8–9
Enterobacteriaceae (mainly *E. coli*)	3–5	3–4	4–6	3–4	3–5
Enterococci	6–7	5–6	5–6	6–7	5–6
Yeasts	0	0	0	0	0–3
Lactobacillus spp.	4–6	4–5	4–5	5–6	5–4
Protozoa	0	NA	0	2–3	0

No. of Viable Microorganisms/Gram of Contents*

*Expressed as $\log_{10}(x+1)$ of the number of organisms cultured (x).
†Not available.

gastrointestinal tract of newborn puppies are *E. coli*, *C. perfringens*, streptococci, lactobacilli, *Bacteroides*, and *Staphylococcus aureus*.[8] Yeasts are not usually found. The flora at weaning is as shown in Table 13–3.[11,22–24]

The kitten, like the calf and piglet, harbors *E. coli*, *C. perfringens*, streptococci, lactobacilli, and *Bacteroides* in its digestive tract.[8] Yeasts are occasionally found in the kitten (*Candida* sp.). They can be found throughout the tract in numbers ranging from 10^3 to 10^5/g of contents.[8]

The foal has not been examined in detail with respect to normal flora. The adult horse has been studied to some degree. What is known about the flora is shown in Table 13–4.[10,11]

RELATION OF NORMAL MICROFLORA TO STRUCTURE AND FUNCTION OF THE GASTROINTESTINAL TRACT

The microbial flora influences the anatomic structures that line the gastrointestinal tract. Epithelial cell renewal has been shown to be faster in animals that have acquired a microbial flora.[25–27] Likewise the crypts are longer and there is more surface area in normal intestine as compared to the germ-free state.[25] The microbial flora also aids or stimulates the formation of lymphatic tissue that lies beneath and in the tract. Specifically, the formation of lymphoid nodules takes place very rapidly once the flora begins to be established.[25,28,29] As will be seen, these nodules contain cells that can respond specifically to antigenic determinants that are presented to the animal via the gastrointestinal tract. Most of these cells will respond with the production of antibody that is aptly suited to perform its function in the milieu of the lumen of the intestinal tract.

In addition to the changes in the lymphoid system

that take place following the acquisition of the microbial flora, changes occur in the activity of the cells belonging to the reticuloendothelial system. Macrophages from conventional animals have been shown to digest phagocytosed materials more efficiently than macrophages taken from germ-free animals.[28] Macrophage mobilization and subsequent participation in immune-related phenomenon have been shown to be increased in animals possessing a microbial flora.[28]

In addition to anatomic changes in the tract, functional activity has also been shown to be related to the microbial flora. If germ-free and conventional animals are compared with respect to the transit time of non-absorbable substances, it will be seen that these substances move through the tract at a significantly faster rate when a microbial flora is present.[30] This increase in peristaltic activity may appear to be a detriment, for by decreasing the peristaltic activity (e.g., by removing the normal flora), the absorption of otherwise poorly absorbed substances, e.g., xylose, increases.[31] But more important, the peristaltic activity of the small bowel is a host defense mechanism that sweeps microorganisms that do not belong there (i.e., pathogens) distally into a more noxious environment.

NORMAL FLORA AS AN ECOSYSTEM

The flora of the gastrointestinal tract is remarkably stable. Fluctuations in numbers of bacteria that occur as the result of various stimuli are transient. Following the removal of such disruptive influences, the flora returns to the state that existed prior to the change.[32,33] Because of this stability, it has been postulated that the relationship between the normal host and its flora is optimal. In other words, each location or site along the gastrointestinal tract is especially suited for a particular species

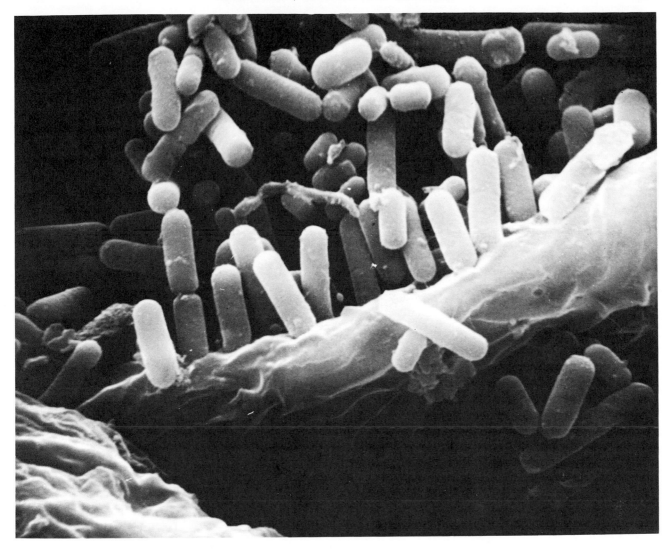

Figure 13–1. Scanning electron microscopic view (900×) of indigenous lactobacilli attached to the keratinized stratified squamous epithelium in the murine stomach. (Photograph generously provided by Dwayne C. Savage, Department of Microbiology, University of Illinois, Urbana.)

of microorganism. Each particular strain of microbe occupies a particular site or niche, to the exclusion of all others (Fig. 13–1). This can be exemplified from the following observation. If calves are fed a strain of *E. coli* isolated from another unrelated calf, the strain is eliminated within 24 to 28 hours. This occurs even if the number of "foreign" *E. coli* fed is in the range of 10^{10} to 10^{11} microorganisms (Table 13–5).[34] If microorganisms with pathogenic potential are likewise excluded from the tract, then it can be said that the relationship between the host and its flora results in a primary defense barrier against bacterial species with pathogenic potential. It is this barrier and how it is formed that will now be discussed.

In order to understand better how the stabilized, normal microbial flora acts as a barrier to pathogenic bacterial species, it is necessary to describe in general terms the events leading up to a disease process caused by a pathogenic bacterium. In general, bacterial pathogens go through a two-step process in the initiation of a disease state. The first step is attachment of the pathogen to the epithelial cells of the gastrointestinal tract; the second, an activity that results in the production of the disease state.

Bacterial pathogens attach to a so-called "target cell" as a first step in producing disease, in most instances. The concept of a target cell was formulated because disease produced by various

Table 13–5. Potential for a Bovine *Escherichia coli* to Colonize 1-Week-Old Calves

No. *E. coli* Fed*	Days After Feeding		
	2	4	6
10^3	<0.01	<0.01	<0.01
10^6	<0.01	<0.01	<0.01
10^9	0.3	0.5	<0.001
10^{11}	1	0.02	<0.0004

Median Percentage of Total Coliforms Represented by the Fed *E. coli* (feces)

*Calves fed a nalidixic acid resistant strain of *E. coli* in 100 ml of milk.

pathogenic species of bacteria almost always occurs at a particular site along the gastrointestinal tract. Following attachment to the target cell, the bacterial pathogen multiplies on the epithelial cell.

After attachment and multiplication, the pathogen may act in one of the following ways in order to produce disease, depending upon the genetic information possessed by that species of microorganism:

1. Produce a toxin (e.g., neonatal diarrhea of calves and pigs).
2. Invade and kill the target cell (e.g., salmonella gastroenteritis).
3. Invade and enter the lymphatics, ultimately gaining entry into the blood stream (e.g., colisepticemia in calves).

By definition, a strain of bacteria is called enteropathogenic if, after attachment to the target cell, disease results. Enteropathogenic strains of bacteria can be invasive or noninvasive. Of the three basic mechanisms listed above, 2 and 3 are characteristic of invasive strains. The noninvasive pathogens usually produce disease by the liberation of a toxin, and are termed enterotoxigenic strains.

The *normal microbial flora* acts as a defense barrier either by making the target cell unavailable to the pathogen, or by creating an environment that is detrimental to the pathogen. In other words, if the normal inhabitants of the gastrointestinal tract are secure in their niche, then species of bacteria with pathogenic potential may not be able to compete successfully with them for a site of attachment. Without a site of attachment, the pathogen is swept distally by peristalsis, away from the susceptible target cell. If, for instance, newborn animals are first fed a non-toxin-producing bacterial strain that has the same target cell as a toxin-producing strain, no disease will result following ingestion of the

toxigenic strain.[35,36] Thus, anything that results in an upset in the balance between host and normal flora may give a pathogen easier access to its target cell, or allow it to multiply to high enough numbers so that competition for the target cell is easier.

The mechanisms whereby members of the normal flora establish their particular niche, and thereby exclude other species of bacteria as well as potential pathogens, can be divided into bacterial properties and host properties.

Bacterial Properties

Structures on the surface of microorganisms living in the gastrointestinal tract are probably one of the most important of all the bacterium properties that are involved in the establishment of the ecosystem. These structures are important because it is through these that the microorganism comes in intimate contact with the host.

Adhesin is a term used by some to describe surface structures that account for the "stickiness" certain bacteria have for certain epithelial cells (Fig. 13–2). Hypothetically, it is these adhesins that stick a particular microbe in its niche so that it will not be swept away by peristalsis. Adhesins may be classified under three general categories: fimbria, agglutinins, and capsules.

Fimbria are whisker-like protrusions on the surface of a microorganism. Chemically, they are protein. The most well-studied fimbrial structure relative to the gastrointestinal tract is the K-88 antigen. Though this antigen is used by enterotoxigenic *E. coli* to stick to toxin-sensitive cells of the small intestine, it can be hypothesized that similar structures may be present on the surface of microorganisms comprising the normal flora. K-88 antigens have an affinity for certain substrates found on or as part of the epithelial cells of the distal small intestine (jejunum and ileum).[37–40] Similar structures with different site specificity may well account for the locational stability of the normal flora.[41,42]

Agglutinins, so-named because they will agglutinate red blood cells, are a group of substances found on the surface of various microorganisms occupying the gastrointestinal tract. These substances have not been defined chemically. Experimentally, bacteria possessing these substances have been shown to also adhere to the brush border of rabbit intestinal cells.[43] It can, therefore, be theorized that certain agglutinins have affinity for various substrates throughout the tract.

Capsules, chemically polysaccharide in nature, are sticky, especially for the surface of epithelial

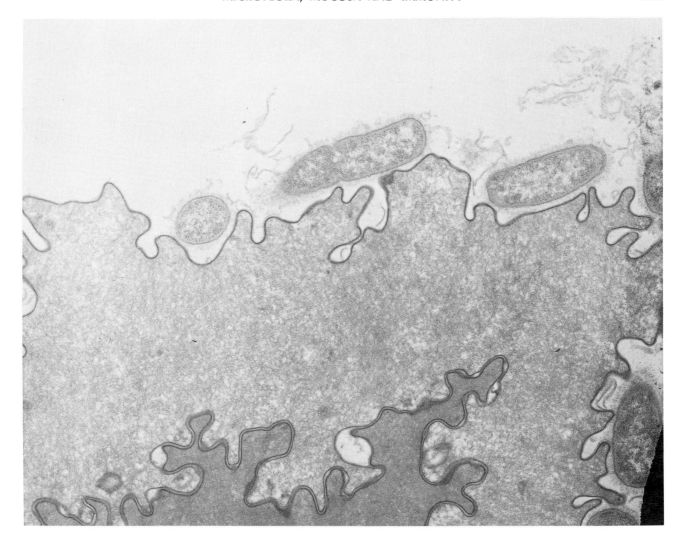

Figure 13–2. Transmission electron microscopic view (28,000×) of indigenous lactobacilli attached to the keratinized stratified squamous epithelium in the murine stomach. Note the electron dense "fuzzy" material that represents some type of "adhesin." (Photograph generously provided by Dwayne C. Savage, Department of Microbiology, University of Illinois, Urbana.)

cells. Though proof of specificity is lacking, it is hypothesized that some capsular types will stick to certain cell surfaces. An example of the possible specificity of capsular antigens is seen in the specific adherence of certain capsular types of *E. coli* and urinary bladder epithelial cells.[44] Again, it is tempting to speculate upon the same sort of specificity occurring in the gastrointestinal tract.[45]

Aside from these three general categories, there are many other ways that bacteria may adhere to an epithelial surface.[46,47]

Metabolic By-products. The secretion of certain substances into the immediate environment may be important in keeping population size in check, in addition to making conditions undesirable for other competing species of microorganisms. Three

classes of bacterial metabolic by-products have greater or lesser influence on gut bacteria: (1) bacteriocins, (2) fatty acids, and (3) deconjugated bile salts.

Bacteriocins are proteins secreted by bacteria that possess the requisite genes, usually located on a plasmid. The bacteria that do not possess these genes are killed by these proteins, whereas those that do possess the genes are immune.[48] For the purposes of this discussion interest will focus on those bacteriocins secreted by the enteric bacteria—called colicins. Since their discovery, colicins were hypothesized to be a substance that would be primarily responsible for the stability of the gastrointestinal flora. Unfortunately, this has been very difficult to prove experimentally. In fact, the bulk of the evidence seems to indicate that colicins do not appear to be very active in vivo.[49,50]

The fatty acids, especially acetic and butyric, are powerful stabilizing influences in the gastrointestinal tract. These substances are secreted as a metabolic by-product of the species of obligate anaerobes that live in the tract. These substances do not act alone, however. To be most effective, the fatty acids work in concert with the pH and oxidation-reduction potential (Eh) of the bowel. When the pH is between 5 and 6 (the normal pH of the large intestine) and the Eh approximately -200 mv or less (the normal Eh of the large intestine is approximately -500 mv), the fatty acids present are extremely toxic to members of the family Enterobacteriaceae.[51-57] It is probably the fatty acids in cooperation with the pH and Eh that are responsible for the precipitous drop that occurs in the numbers of enterics following the colonization of the large bowel with anaerobes. Even more spectacular than the preceding are the effects of these particular by-products upon members of the family Enterobacteriaceae that possess pathogenic potential. An animal with a normal gut (0.0025 N in fatty acids, particularly butyric and acetic, pH 5 to 6, Eh <-200 mv) would have to ingest approximately 10^6 *Salmonella typhimurium* to become infected. If an animal is first treated in such a way as to eliminate the producers of the fatty acids (this results also in an increase in pH and Eh) and then given *S. typhimurium*, the number of microorganisms needed to infect is <10![58-62]

Free bile acids, e.g., deoxycholic and cholic, under certain conditions of concentration and pH are inhibitory to members of the flora of the large bowel. This flora will deconjugate the conjugated bile acids, e.g., taurocholic acid, as it moves distally in the small intestine.[63-65] The resulting deconjugated acid is toxic at concentrations of 1 to 2 mmoles/liter and pH 5.8, the conditions of the terminal ileum.[66] Though the phenomenon as described probably does not play a role at the level of the niche, it has been postulated to be the mechanism whereby retrograde bacterial colonization in the upper small gut by large bowel organisms is prevented.

Nutritional Factors. The last bacterial property to be discussed is that of nutrition. Nutritional substrate availability is probably a mixture of host and bacterial properties. In its simplest terms, nutritional substrate availability means that some strains of bacteria eat what others need. It has been shown that keen competition occurs for fermentable carbon sources under highly anaerobic conditions.[67] If an invader can successfully compete for a carbon source with an inhabitant of a particular niche, then the invader will take over the niche.

Host Properties

Epithelial surfaces and the substances bathing them are the structures in most intimate contact with the microorganisms living in the gastrointestinal tract. The nature of the substances within the cell membrane or within the substances secreted by the epithelial cells is presently under study. The most probable sites for bacterial adhesion appear to be the brush border and the overlying mucous gel.

Peristalsis has been used throughout the discussion as a mechanism whereby microorganisms that are not anchored would be swept distally. In the small bowel, peristaltic activity plays a major role in host defense of the intestinal tract.[68] The size of a population of pathogenic species of bacteria in the small intestine has been shown to be related directly to whether disease will result.[69] The most important regulator of the size of this population is peristaltic activity since there are few other metabolic regulators such as those that exist in the large bowel (Eh, fatty acids, and pH). The normal flora contributes to the defense of the small bowel by stimulating peristalsis.[30]

It is known that the local *immune response* at an epithelial cell surface will prevent the binding of pathogenic microorganisms.[70-73] Presumably this is a result of antibody made against antigenic determinants on the surface of the pathogen. Since the pathogen can no longer stick to the epithelial cell, it will be swept distally away from the target cell. This immunologic phenomenon is easily understood in terms of host response to a pathogen. But what about the response to the normal flora? In other words, can the immunologically competent animal recognize pathogen from non-pathogen?

There is experimental evidence that suggests that animals do not form much of an immune response to antigenic determinants possessed by members of their own flora.[74,75] There is a great deal of similarity between the antigenic determinants on the surface of epithelial cells that line the intestinal tract and the microorganisms that live there.[76] If this is so, it is unlikely that an immune response will be made against the normal flora. But even if an immune response were made against the members of the normal flora, only those organisms that must adhere to an epithelial surface will be affected. And these can be influenced only if their numbers are small.[77]

On the other hand, the microorganisms can change under the influence of an immune response.

It has been shown, for instance, that certain species of epithelial cell "dwellers" constantly change surface antigenic determinants, presumably under antibody pressure.[78,79] Conceivably these sorts of changes would occur until antibodies were no longer made, i.e., when the determinants on the surface of the microbe were similar to the determinants on the surface of the epithelial cells.

One might ask why this change of surface antigenic determinants could not occur with the pathogenic species of microorganism. Perhaps it could, except that it has been shown that antibody and bacterial antagonism work in a synergistic manner.[77] A pathogenic microorganism (in small numbers) would have to contend with both an immune response and bacterial antagonism to be able to adhere to a target cell.

All of the factors discussed have been hypothesized to account for the stability of the normal flora which acts as a primary protective barrier to block selective adsorption of pathogenic species of bacteria to their target tissue. The next question one might ask, then, is how can the ecosystem be changed to favor microorganisms with pathogenic potential?

DISRUPTION OF THE NORMAL MICROFLORA

The newborn animal would be the most susceptible to disease since it has no established niches and all target cell sites are unoccupied. This is exactly what happens when the newborn animal does not receive colostrum. Colostrum contains the antibodies that are specific for surface structures on potential pathogens, assuming that the dam has been optimally exposed to the pathogens. Combination of these antibodies to these surface structures blocks attachment of the pathogen to its target cell.[72]

Antimicrobial drugs can interfere with the normal defense barrier of the gastrointestinal tract to such a degree that serious illness can result secondary to antimicrobial treatment. This reaction occurs because the bulk of the normal microbial flora (prokaryotic) is inhibited or killed by the commonly used antibacterial agents. However, two segments of the normal flora may not be affected as seriously as the rest—yeasts and fungi, and members of the family Enterobacteriaceae.

Members of the family Enterobacteriaceae may acquire the genes necessary either to inactivate an antimicrobial drug or to become resistant directly, e.g., a decrease in permeability to a certain antimicrobial.[80] Those genes that are acquired are on pieces of DNA measuring in size from approximately 1 or 2 to 80 × 10⁶ daltons. Microorganisms possessing them have a distinct advantage in an antimicrobial environment. The pieces of DNA upon which the resistance genes reside belong to a family of genetic elements called plasmids. Plasmids exist inside the bacterial cell membrane in the cytoplasm and are unassociated with the chromosomal DNA. In fact, plasmid DNA replicates autonomously and for the most part is not controlled by chromosomal DNA. Most plasmid DNA that carries genes for antimicrobial resistance (R plasmids) is transmissible. This means that R plasmids and their antimicrobial resistances can be passed, by conjugation, from one bacterium to another. This can be done at any time but is very efficient during log phase growth. Thus, a resistant bacterium can pass antimicrobial resistance to any member of the family Enterobacteriaceae and, providing the particular plasmid that is transmitted is compatible with the new host cell, the recipient will also be resistant. R plasmids may carry variable numbers and/or combinations of resistance genes. Bacteria possessing R plasmids are resistant to two or more antimicrobial agents. In my experience, the median number of resistance genes is 3 or 4. Thus, selections of a resistant bacterium through the use of antimicrobial drugs (either prophylactically or therapeutically) results in the selection of a bacterium resistant to other antimicrobials as well. Over the years, the environmental pool of the R plasmids has grown tremendously. The reasons for this growth are beyond the scope of this chapter, but the fact remains that most of the members of the family Enterobacteriaceae (pathogen and nonpathogen alike) possess R plasmids. Thus, since most of the enteric pathogens belong to the family Enterobacteriaceae, antimicrobials will select for these bacteria at the expense of other nonenterobacteriaceae, especially the obligate anaerobes. If this latter group of microorganisms is removed, so also is a powerful regulatory substance, i.e., the fatty acids.

Yeasts and fungi can also be affected by antimicrobial agents, albeit indirectly. These microorganisms are kept in check, as are the Enterobacteriaceae, by the low pH, low Eh, and volatile fatty acids.[51,81] Antimicrobial agents, by removing the producers of the volatile fatty acids, also remove an important restraint on the growth of yeasts and fungi. In addition, some evidence suggests that yeasts (especially of the genus *Candida*) are affected directly by antimicrobials in such a manner as to make them more invasive.[82-85] The mechanism by which this occurs is not understood.

Stress, be it nutritional or emotional, appears to increase the likelihood of disease of any kind, but especially intestinal disease. Experimentally, stress will result in a change in the normal intestinal flora.[86] These changes, at least in experimental animals, are related to a decrease in the anaerobic component of the normal flora. Subsequently, the numbers of coliform bacteria increase greatly. What appears to be occurring is a change in the major regulatory mechanism of the intestinal tract, the fatty acid production. Most if not all enteric pathogens belong to the family Enterobacteriaceae. Without fatty acid control these pathogens are able to grow to numbers that would allow for successful competition for attachment to a target cell site. The key question appears to be: Why did the population of anaerobic bacteria drop? The answer to this question is not known. One possibility may be substrate availability for the anaerobic species. It is known that the amount of mucin secreted into the gastrointestinal tract can be decreased by the administration of corticosteroids.[87] If the stress were of sufficient magnitude and chronicity to result in an increased concentration of corticosteroids that would be sufficient to decrease mucin production, conceivably the numbers of anaerobic bacteria that utilize the mucin as an energy source would also be reduced.[88,89]

IMMUNITY OF THE GASTROINTESTINAL TRACT

Most species of animals have a lowered ability to respond immunologically to externally introduced antigens at birth. This is not because they lack the ability to do so, but because of immunologic immaturity and, perhaps, partial immunosuppression. In those species studied, a specific immune response in utero can be generated toward antigenic determinants carried by certain antigens. The maturation of the propensity of an animal to respond to certain antigenic determinants progresses in a sequential fashion, starting in utero.[90-93] The sequence depends upon the species of animal. It has been found that the response of the fetus is not of the same magnitude, by any means, as that seen after birth but it is sufficient to abort disease following infection by certain agents, e.g., bovine viral diarrhea.[94]

The lowered ability to respond to antigen determinants presented neonatally may in part be because of increased levels of corticosteroids found in the fetal and neonatal circulation and in part to the relative immaturity of certain elements of the immune system.[95-99] Whatever the reason, the neonate is at risk. The antigenic determinants that place the animal at risk are for the most part carried by species of bacteria with pathogenic potential whose target cell resides in the intestinal tract.

Passive Immunity

Protection of the neonate from such insults is acquired from the dam in the form of antibodies. It must be stressed that it is not just antibody per se, but antibody with specificity for antigenic determinants possessed by the pathogen. Thus, the dam must have been exposed to those antigenic determinants. This protection is passed to the offspring prenatally, postnatally, or both, depending on the species of animal. Horse, ruminant, and pig acquire no immunoglobulins from the dam prenatally, whereas 5% of the passively acquired immunoglobulins are passed prenatally in the dog and 95% postnatally.[100] In man and rabbits, it is acquired entirely prenatal.[100] There are, therefore, two modes of transfer of maternal antibody, placental and intestinal.

Passage of antibody across the placenta depends upon the placentation and/or the possession of appropriate receptors for the Fc portion of IgG.[100] The placentation and receptors of human, dog, cat, and rabbit are sufficient for passage of all (human and rabbit) or part (dog and cat) of passively acquired immunity. Only IgG is acquired by transplacental passage. Acquisition of antibody after birth is a process that starts with the ingestion of colostrum and continues with the ingestion of milk until weaning. The most abundant immunoglobulin in colostrum is IgG, followed by IgA and IgM.[101,102] In ruminants, this immunoglobulin (IgG_1) is selectively absorbed from the plasma of the dam and concentrated in the mammary gland.[103,104] In horses, pigs, and dogs there is probably no selective absorption of IgG from plasma to milk, but IgG is still predominant.[100,105-107]

Immunoglobulins acquired neonatally protect the newborn in two ways: (1) they provide circulating antibody to help prevent systemic disease, and (2) they provide antibody at the level of the intestinal epithelial cell to block subsequent attachment of potential pathogenic microorganisms to target cells. In order to provide protection in the systemic circulation of the newborn, colostral antibodies must be able to cross the epithelial boundary of the intestinal tract and gain entrance, intact, into the lymphatics and blood vascular system. During the first 24 to 48 hours, depending on the species, the epithelial cells of the small intestine will absorb Ig from the lumen of the bowel. This absorption is relatively nonselective as far as isotype of immunoglobulin is concerned.[100,108-110] Diet or feeding practices may influence absorption time.[108] The mechanism behind the phenomenon is not known, but one reasonable hypothesis is as follows: Ig adsorbs to receptors for Fc at the base of the microvilli of the small intestine.[111] A pinocytic vesicle then forms with the Ig attached to the pinocytic vacuole wall. The Ig as such passes through the epithelial cell to the lamina propria. The receptors are present only during the time of absorption of Ig. Pinocytic events that take place after the receptor is gone, or in those species of animals where intestinal absorption of Ig does not occur (human, rabbit), result in the fusion of the pinocytic vesicle (containing the Ig) with a lysosome and the ultimate enzymatic degradation of the immunoglobulin protein.[100] The basis for cessation of absorption (closure) is unknown. It may be related to epithelial cell turnover and/or plasma corticosteroid concentration.[112,113]

Immunoglobulins acquired in colostrum are exposed to enzymatic processes in the oral cavity and gastrointestinal tract of the newborn. The most labile in terms of enzymatic degradation is IgG, whereas IgA and IgM are less labile because of their association with secretory component (SC).[114-117] However, colostral secretions have been shown to contain a trypsin-inhibitory factor.[118,119] This factor, and others like it, have been postulated to account for the survival of IgG (and IgM not associated with SC) during the first day or two after birth. In addition, the enzymatic activity of the pancreatic and intestinal secretions of the neonate are only a fraction of what they ultimately will be. In conjunction with enzyme inhibitors in colostrum, trypsin inhibitor serves to protect enzymatically labile immunoglobulins. After the first days of lactation, the concentration of colostral IgG and IgM falls drastically, whereas the concentration of IgA falls relatively little.[101-107] As a result, the major immunoglobulin in the milk of all species except the ruminant is IgA. In the ruminant, IgG (IgG_1 in bovine) remains the most concentrated, four to eight times that of IgA, as compared to 20 to 30 times more concentrated than IgA in colostrum. Whether IgG_1 in mammary secretions is as resistant to enzymatic cleavage as IgG_1 found in intestinal secretions, as recently reported, remains to be proven.[120] This change in emphasis suits the situation beautifully. IgG is no longer able to cross the epithelial surface of the intestinal tract and the enzyme-inhibitors are no longer being secreted.

However, the intestinal tract is still vulnerable to attack by pathogenic species of microorganisms, for two reasons. One, the normal microflora of the gastrointestinal tract has not yet been established (48 hours of age) and competition among microorganisms for ecologic niches is still going on at a great pace. Second, the immune system of the neonate may not be competent enough to respond to the antigenic determinants of a potential pathogen, depending on the determinant and the species of animal. If the neonate is able to respond, it will take time for enough specific antibody to be made in order to block adsorption of the pathogen to a target epithelial cell in the intestine. Thus, the change in the immunoglobulin isotype is fortuitous, IgA being aptly suited for survival in the milieu of the gastrointestinal tract. If the IgA antibody molecules are of the correct specificity, they would be able to prevent disease by blocking attachment of pathogenic bacteria to target epithelial cells.

Active Immunity—General

The immune response to antigens presented to the animal by way of the gastrointestinal tract is in many ways similar to, but in some ways different from the response to antigens presented parenterally. The similarities of the response encompass the cells involved and the end-products (antibody and cell-mediated immunity). The dissimilarities are seen in the traffic patterns that stimulated cells take after contact with antigen and in the major type of antibody that is made (IgA).

Three key cell types are involved with the initiation and elicitation of the immune response: macrophages, B cells, and T cells.

Macrophages. These are large phagocytic cells that arise in the bone marrow, traverse the peripheral circulation as monocytes, and reside in the tissues as wandering phagocytic cells.[121] Aside from their phagocytic activities, these cells appear to play an important role in the initiation of the immune response.[122-124] In particular, macrophages somehow enable the immune response to proceed in the most efficient fashion; i.e., a maximal immune response per unit of antigen.[125,126] How this procedure occurs is not understood. Some contend that macrophages "process" antigen in such a way as to make the antigen more presentable to the other cells of the immune system, the T and B cells.[127] Whether processing occurs or not is beside the point, for without the participation of the macrophage, most responses to antigens are weak and meager, and with some antigenic systems, immunologic tolerance may result.[128,129]

The macrophage pool includes the dendritic macrophages that adhere to the reticular fibers of lymph nodes. These cells not only trap antigen but also serve the same role as the tissue macrophages.[130,131] The phagocytic cells of the spleen have a similar function. The Kupffer cells of the liver, on the other hand, do not appear to act beyond the function of phagocytic cells. There is some evidence that a cell type in the liver may serve to store antigen.[132-134] Whether this storage function is a property of the Kupffer cell or the hepatocyte is not known.

The T Cell. The second cell participating in the immune response, arises in the bone marrow. In order to function to its fullest capacity, it must first travel to the thymus where it acquires properties that enable the observer to determine that it is a T cell; i.e., it displays certain membrane antigens. After leaving the thymus, T cells travel to peripheral lymphoid tissues and accumulate in T-dependent areas of the spleen (periarteriolar cuff of the white pulp) and lymph nodes (diffuse cortex and corticomedullary junction).[135] There are at least three subpopulations of T cells: (1) T-helper cells, (2) T-suppressor cells, and (3) the T cell subpopulation that is involved in cell-mediated immunity. It is not yet entirely clear whether the T-helper cell and the T cell involved with cell-mediated immunity are the same or are two separate subpopulations.

T-helper cells are those T cells that cooperate with the macrophage (containing the "processed" antigenic determinants) and the B cell, the end result being the formation of antibody specific for the antigenic determinants (in or on the macrophage) by cells of the B cell line.[136-138] How the T cell does this is not known. A T cell specific for the antigen will recognize a portion of the antigen (an antigenic determinant) via a receptor on the surface of the T cell in a manner somewhat analogous to a lock and key. The receptor recognizing antigenic determinants has not as yet been defined, but its existence is well documented. Once the correct contact is made, the helper T cell stimulates the B cell (also associated with other antigenic determinants via a receptor) to undergo blastogenesis, divide, and finally make antibody specific for the antigenic determinant recognized by the B cell.[139] At the same time the B cell is dividing (cloning), the T helper cells are doing the same. This enlarging population, in addition to aiding the B cell to clone, also regulates the size of the B cell clone. The expanded clone of T cells, after antigens have left the system, remain as a "memory" compartment waiting for contact with the same antigenic determinant again. When this contact occurs, a response characteristic of a secondary response will arise; i.e., more antibody in a shorter length of time.

The T cells involved with cell-mediated responses (tumor and graft rejection, macrophage activation) may be different from the T helper cell population. After specific stimulation by macrophage-associated antigenic determinants, T cells will contribute to the immune response in other ways in addition to acting as a helper cell. One of the major ways is through the cell-mediated response (CMI), so-called because certain states of immunity can only be transferred with cells (T cells). Thus, tumor immunity is the result of specific T cells recognizing specific non-self antigenic determinants on the surface of tumor cells.[140] T cells then respond by the liberation of substances called lymphokines which have detrimental effects on the tumor cell or on the non-self cell in the case of an allograft.[141,142] An analogous T cell response may occur in viral infections, in which viral-determined antigenic determinants (non-self) are exhibited by the infected cell.

T cell-mediated immunity is also important in diseases caused by certain infectious agents. The classics are *Brucella, Listeria, Mycobacterium, Salmonella,* and *Toxoplasma.*[143-148] These organisms reside quite happily inside macrophage cells. Antibody, though specifically made against antigenic determinants on the microbial cell surface, cannot bind with them because of the intracellular location of the microbe. The T cell, however, following contact with antigenic determinants on the macrophage surface, will liberate lymphokines that will "soup-up" the macrophages to kill the bacteria living in their cytoplasm in an efficient manner.

The third subpopulation of T cells is the T suppressor cell.[149,150] This subpopulation, recognized relatively recently, has been called by some the regulatory cell type. Instead of aiding the immune response, this subpopulation turns it off. T suppressor cells, like T cells in general, take part in the immune response in a specific fashion; i.e., they recognize specific antigenic determinants. Thus, it can be said that the magnitude of an immune response is dependent upon the relative proportions of T suppressor cells and T helper cells (CMI T cell). How the T suppressor cell works is not understood.

B Cells. Like macrophages and T cells, B cells are a population of lymphocytes that arise in the bone marrow.[138] But unlike macrophages and T cells, they travel to a site in the body that has yet to be identified. This site is analogous to the bursa of Fabricius in birds and in mammals is called the bursal equivalent, thus the epithet *B* cell. Before they can realize their full potential, B cells must go to this bursal equivalent. Candidate bursal equivalents include the gut-associated lymphoid tissue, fetal liver, lymphoid follicles, or the bone marrow itself.[150-153]

Following induction to further differentiation in the bursal equivalent, they become full-fledged B cells with certain characteristics that enable the observer to distinguish them from T cells; i.e., receptors for complement, immunoglobulins on their surface, and most important, the ability to make antibody following exposure to antigen.[154,155] After leaving the bursal equivalent, B cells travel to B dependent areas of the spleen (germinal centers in white pulp) and lymph nodes (germinal centers).[134] The B cell possesses antigenic-determinant-recognizing receptors on their surface that have been defined in considerable detail.[156] These receptors are immunoglobulins in nature and in fact contain the combining site of the same specificity of the antibody the cell will ultimately make.[157-159]

The Primary Immune Response. The B cell cooperates with the helper T cell and with the antigenic determinants on the surface of the macrophage. The B cell, after receiving a signal from the T helper cell along with a signal from its own surface via the combination of receptor and antigenic determinant, undergoes blastogenesis, division, and production of antibody.[138] The helper T cell continuously controls the B cell clone size. In addition, the helper T cell will signal the B cell to stop making IgM, the immunoglobulin that the B cell will make initially, and make another isotype (depending on where the cell is located, this might be IgG, IgA, or IgE).[160] Some of the B cell clones will stop their cloning process and, like the T helper cells, remain as memory cells. It is doubtful that memory cells per se are evolved, but rather the cloning process is interrupted because of the lack of antigen and T helper cell signals. Other B cells, probably those that were first stimulated by the newly arrived antigen, will differentiate all the way to plasma cells. The prime function of these cells is to produce antibody, and by this time, almost all the antibody that they will make will be IgG, IgA, or IgE.

The immune response against antigens introduced parenterally takes place in organized lymphoid tissues (lymph nodes and spleen). Antigens finding their way into the systemic circulation will be phagocytosed by macrophages (RE cells) of the spleen and presented to appropriate T and B cells in the white pulp. Antibodies to specific antigenic determinants are made here, along with memory B cells, memory T cells, and T cells that are part of the CMI response.

The same sort of activity will be found when antigen is introduced into the tissue spaces. Depending upon their physical state (particulate versus soluble antigens), either the antigen will come in contact with and be phagocytosed by macrophages at the site of antigen deposition, then to be taken to the draining lymph node, or, as is the case of most soluble antigens, the antigen will diffuse to the afferent lymphatic and be filtered out by the dendritic macrophages of the lymph node. It is in the cortex of the lymph node that specific T and B cells come in contact with the antigenic determinants and triggering of the immune response takes place.

Shortly after the primary immune response, some memory B and memory T cells leave the lymph node (via the efferent lymphatics) or spleen (via the splenic vein or efferent splenic lymphatic) and become distributed throughout the body.[161-163] Those cells in lymphatic channels get back into the blood via the thoracic duct by way of the posterior vena cava near the thoracic inlet.[161,164-166] Once in the blood stream, these cells can go to any lymphoid tissue in the body via the various post-capillary venules of lymph nodes, which possess a special type of endothelial lining (tall endothelial cells).[167,168] Lymphoid cells wishing to gain entrance into the lymph node do so by passing between the high endothelial cells and thereby find themselves in the cortex of the lymph node.

The end result is that after a primary immune response, every lymphatic structure in the body becomes seeded with T cells and B cells specific for the antigenic determinant on the antigen that first elicited the primary response. Thus, the same antigen introduced a second time will come in contact with an expanded population (relative to the first exposure) of lymphocytes specific for the determinant on the antigen. The response is therefore quicker because recruitment of virgin B and T cells is not necessary, and the response is more vigorous because more cells are responding.

Active Immunity—Intestinal

Antigens that contact the animal by way of the gastrointestinal tract elicit the production of IgA antibody and other isotypes, as well as stimulating cell-mediated immunity. The manner in which the immune system accomplishes this is somewhat different from that seen with parenterally introduced antigens because the gastrointestinal tract is unique in regard to exposure to antigenic materials. Being a long tube, it possesses an enormous surface area that is in contact with a variety of antigens, yet the initial antigenic stimulus is localized at a particular site. To be effective, the immune response must be triggered locally, but at the same time it must be able to "protect" a relatively large surface area.

In addition to the previous considerations, the products of the immune response must be able to function along the entire length of the tract. Thus, antibodies that find their way into the lumen must be able to withstand the enzymatic assaults of proteolytic enzymes that exist there. The antibodies must also be able to function at a site that possesses no phagocytic cells and in a milieu that is anticomplementary.

Before discussing how the animal does this, it would be best to review the microanatomy of the gastrointestinal tract with emphasis on cells and cell types involved in the immune response. Macrophages, lymphocytes, and plasma cells are found in great numbers throughout the length of the gastrointestinal tract.[169] These cells are found in the lamina propria as diffuse collections of cells, or as nodules with germinal centers, or as a collection of nodules with a unique association with the epithelial surface (Peyer's patches).

The diffuse collections of these immunocytes can be found in the lamina propria from stomach to rectum. Some lymphocytes can be seen between the columnar epithelial cells (interepithelial lymphocytes).[170] The lymphoid cell types are both B and T cells. Nonlymphoid cells include macrophages, some eosinophils, and rare mast cells.[169] At one time it was thought that the interepithelial cells represented old and retired lymphocytes being excreted into the intestinal lumen. This is not the case.[170,171,177] They are primarily T cells, and their presence seems to be dependent upon antigen in the gut.[172] Their function is not known at present.

The Lymphoid Nodule. This nodule, the surrounding cells, and the relation of the nodule to the epithelial surface deserve special note. The nodules are found scattered throughout the length of the tract. Groups of nodules occur as Peyer's patches near the terminal end of the small intestine. These nodules arise in the lamina propria and extend down through the muscularis mucosa into the submucosa.[173] The epithelial cells lining the mucosal surface over the lymphoid nodule change from columnar to cuboidal.[169] The cell type overlying the lymphoid nodules requires special mention. These cells, recently termed M cells (membranous epithelium) lack microvilli and glycocalyx, and possess no terminal webs.[174,175] M cells, unlike adjacent columnar cells with interlocking tight junctions and terminal webs, permit the passage of substances from the luminal surface through the cytoplasm into

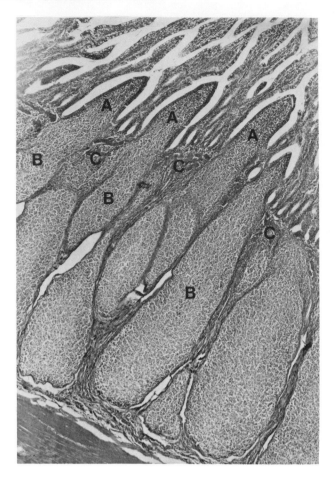

Figure 13–3. Cross section through a Peyer's patch showing the dome (A), follicle (B), and T-dependent area (C). The lumen of the bowel is at the top. (H and E section of canine ileum, 11×.)

the lamina propria.[174,176] It has been hypothesized that M cells are immature columnar cells.[177]

The nodule itself is divided into three areas (Fig. 13–3): dome, T-dependent area, and follicle.[178,179] The dome-follicle complex contains almost exclusively B cells, whereas the interfollicle area contains T cells.[179] Macrophage-type cells are present in the nodule, though there does seem to be debate on this subject.[180,181] Also, there is always the possibility that the M cell may function immunologically like a macrophage-type cell.[174]

As suggested earlier, Peyer's patches may be the mammalian bursal-equivalent.[152] At present, evidence is accumulating that this may not be the case. Indeed, Peyer's patches appear to behave more like a secondary lymphoid structure (e.g., a lymph node) rather than a primary one (e.g., the thymus or bursa of Fabricius).[180,182–186] Thus, Peyer's patches will be discussed as a secondary lymphoid structure.

Absorption of Antigenic Materials. Antigenic materials can be absorbed intact from the gastrointestinal tract. Some antigens are not only absorbed but also stimulate lymphoid cells located in tissues peripheral to the intestinal tract,[187,188] This has been shown to be a size-related phenomenon.[187] Questions about the site where these materials are absorbed has led to a great deal of research. Apparently antigenic material can be absorbed from the gastrointestinal tract in two ways. The major route is through pinocytic vacuoles of the M cell.[174] Another, though minor, is through the columnar epithelium.[189,190] In the latter instance, there is a balance between what is digested within the pinocytic vacuole and what is not digested.[100] After the intestine attains closure, most of the macromolecules that enter the columnar cells are digested before they reach the lamina propria.[100]

The Primary Immune Response. Whichever way the antigenic material gains entrance to the lamina propria, macrophage cells phagocytose (pinocytose) the antigen and initiate the immune response.[191,192] The M cell itself may act directly in this capacity. Very close associations between M cells and lymphocytes in nodules have been observed.[174]

If the antigen is invasive (e.g., *Salmonella*), macrophages may phagocytose, process, and present antigenic determinants to appropriate B and T cells in the nodule or mesenteric lymph node.

The next step in the immune response is poorly understood. Macrophages probably initiate the response. The T and B cells that form the "triplex" are specific in that they have receptors that "fit" an antigenic determinant. The triplex probably forms in the nodule, but there is little evidence of triplex formation in the mesenteric lymph node. It is at this stage that similarities between immune responses to parenterally introduced antigens and antigens absorbed via the gastrointestinal tract ends. The majority of the B cells that are stimulated in Peyer's patches will ultimately differentiate into plasma cells that will secrete IgA.[193-196] There is little support for the hypothesis that these B cells will first secrete IgM, then switch to IgA (or IgM, then switch to IgG and then to IgA).[197] There is no evidence that indicates a significant number of IgG producing cells are precursors to the IgA secreting cell. Immediate precursors of IgA producing cells do not contain IgM on their surface. Unlike B cells elsewhere in the body, those in mouse Peyer's patches are enriched with a large population of B cells with antigen-recognizing receptors composed of IgD only (instead of a mixture of IgD with IgM or IgG).[198] It is postulated that it is these IgD-bearing cells that will produce IgA following contact with the appropriate antigenic determinant and T helper cell. Animals born without a thymus (no T cells) will have no IgA secreting cells in the lamina propria.[169] The minor population of B cells in the nodule with IgD and IgM on their surface will be those that will first produce IgM, then switch to IgG production.[160]

T and B cells undergo blastogenesis and division following stimulation by antigen. Most of the division is observed with the T cell population.[182] After stimulation, the T and B cells leave the nodule and travel via afferent lymphatics to the mesenteric lymph nodes, then through these nodes to the thoracic duct.[199] After a brief stay in the spleen, these cells will "home" to the lamina propria of the intestinal tract. Although it is not an exclusive pathway, four to five go to the intestinal tract for every cell that goes elsewhere.[193-196,200-202] They finish differentiating to plasma cells in the lamina propria and secrete IgA.[203] Smaller numbers of IgM- and IgG-secreting lymphocytes find their way to the intestinal tract. Stimulated precursors of IgA cells taken from peripheral lymphoid tissue or spleen do not "home" to the lamina propria of the gastrointestinal tract.[193-195]

The homing phenomenon is poorly understood. It does not seem to be dependent upon antigen, since antigen-free grafts of intestinal tissue placed under the kidney capsule will serve as "homing devices" for the IgA-containing lymphocytes.[204] Likewise it does not appear to be related to IgA on the surface, secretory component on the basal side of the epithelial cell surface, or on B or T cells.[205] Whatever the nature of this attraction, it is efficient indeed, for what started at a single locus (a lymphoid nodule) ended as a generalized deposition of antibody-forming cells along the entire length of the gastrointestinal tract.

Immunoglobulins of Intestinal Secretions. In all of the domestic species except the ruminants, IgA is the major immunoglobulin in intestinal secretions, followed by IgM, and then IgG.[101,102,106,206,207] Very little, if any, IgE is found in intestinal secretions.[208] This is reflected in the relative numbers of IgA-, IgM-, and IgG-secreting plasma cells in the lamina propria.[105,107,209,210] All of the IgA found in intestinal secretions comes from local production, whereas IgM and IgG come from both local production and passive diffusion from serum.[102,107,207]

In sheep, the most concentrated immunoglobulin in intestinal secretions is IgA followed closely by IgG_1, IgG_2, and IgM (in decreasing order of amounts).[101,211] Sixty percent of the plasma cells in the lamina propria are IgA-secreting cells.[212] There are considerably fewer IgG$_1$- and IgM-secreting cells with only an occasional cell secreting IgG$_2$.[212] Ninety percent of intestinal IgA is made locally in sheep.[211,213] It has been shown that all of the IgG$_2$ found in the intestinal secretions comes from plasma, whereas 94 and 97% of IgG$_1$ and IgM, respectively, come from plasma.[211] IgG$_1$, unlike in the mammary gland, does not appear to be selectively absorbed from plasma, although there is disagreement upon this point.[211,214]

In the bovine, IgA is a minor immunoglobulin in intestinal secretions.[101,215] The predominant immunoglobulin is IgG, as reflected in the greater numbers of IgG-secreting plasma cells in the lamina propria.[215] Most of the IgG is synthesized locally with the remainder coming from the plasma.[216] Unlike the sheep, bovine IgG$_1$ appears to be selectively absorbed from the plasma and secreted into the intestinal lumen.[215]

The plasma cells that home to the lamina propria of the gastrointestinal tract secrete antibody (IgA, IgM, IgG) into the tissue space beneath the epithelial cells lining the tract. IgA is the most unique of these isotypes, for it is not only the most concentrated (ruminant excluded), but also aptly suited to function in the biochemically hostile environment of the intestinal tract. IgA is made as a 7S monomer inside a plasma cell. Two 7S monomers are hooked together to form an 11S dimer. The sedimentation coefficient of the dimer is slightly different depending upon the species of animal. The plasma cell hooks the two monomers together with a protein called J-piece.[217] The immunoglobulin is then secreted from the cell and enters the lamina propria. From here it can enter the lymphatics, and in all domestic species studied (ruminant, pig, dog) this dimer comprises almost all of the IgA found in the serum.[101,105,207] But the major function of the IgA that is secreted is to impart immunity to the mucosal surface of the gastrointestinal tract. It must, however, get to the luminal side of the epithelium and in addition must be able to withstand the rather harsh proteolytic environment of the intestinal lumen.

The following hypothesis has been proposed.[113] The IgA dimer gets to the lumen by attaching to a glycoprotein (molecular weight of 48,000 to 80,000 daltons, depending on species) that lies on the basal surface of the epithelial cells.[102] This glycoprotein is called secretory component (SC). SC is found on the basal surface of epithelial cells in the villi of the large intestine and in the gland openings and crypt cells of the small intestine.[113,218] Following attach-

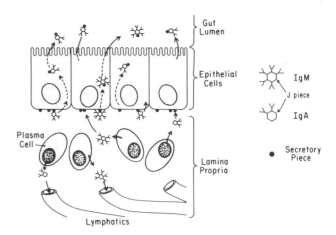

Figure 13–4. Schematic representation of the secretion and transport of IgA and IgM from the lamina propria of the gastrointestinal tract to the lumen.

ment, the IgA-SC complex is interiorized in keeping with the fluid-mosaic model of cell membranes.[219] The complex is transported to the luminal side of the epithelial cell and is exteriorized by the same process.[218] In this case SC stays attached to the dimer. This complex is now called secretory IgA (sIgA). The SC of sIgA imparts relative resistance to proteolytic cleavage by the enzymes in the intestinal tract.[116] The mechanism of inhibition is not understood.

IgM molecules are formed in the lamina propria as they are anywhere else in the body; i.e., five 7S monomers are joined together with J-piece. IgM that is secreted into the lamina propria of the gastrointestinal tract will also come in contact with SC on the basal side of the epithelial cell (Fig. 13–4). Approximately 60 to 75% of the IgM in the lamina propria will form a complex with SC that is stable enough to be transported to the luminal surface of the tract.[113–115] The rest is secreted with SC in a rather loose association. The attachment of SC to IgM apparently is not the same as IgA, but the end result is a relative resistance to proteolytic cleavage.[116]

The IgG of the bovine that gains entrance to the intestinal lumen has been shown to be relatively resistant to proteolytic degradation.[118] This finding is rather new and awaits confirmation. How IgG gets to the lumen is not known, since IgG does not possess SC. As far as is known, the rest of Ig isotypes and subclasses do not appear to have any special resistance to breakdown by gastrointestinal proteolytic enzymes.

The mucosal surface of the gastrointestinal tract is anticomplementary and does not possess phagocytic cells. However, IgA when bound to an antigenic determinant does not fix complement and has been shown to be a very poor opsonizing antibody (probably due to the lack of receptors on phagocytic cells for the Fc portion of IgA).[102] Then how does IgA or any other immunoglobulin impart immunity at this site? Protection elicited by immunoglobulin in the intestinal tract seems to involve the interaction between the antigen (microorganism) and the epithelial cell. In order to produce disease most if not all pathogens must first attach to a target cell; interruption of this attachment aborts disease. It is not clear how this blockage occurs. It may be as simple as a steric interference. On the other hand, it may also involve the epithelial cell (the target cell) itself since metabolic inhibitors abrogate the blocking mechanism.[70–73]

The role of the stimulated T cell, aside from acting as a T-helper or T-suppressor, is hard to quantitate. Though most of the lymphocytes in the lamina propria are B cells, there are significant numbers of T cells. Cell-mediated immune responses in the gastrointestinal tract would be involved with tumor rejection and immunity against certain pathogens, such as *Salmonella*, that gain entry into the lamina propria.[145–148]

Another function of immunoglobulin is to prevent the absorption of food antigens. Food antigens, when bound to specific immunoglobulins, are not absorbed into the body.[220,221] It is thought by some that this plays an important role in preventing food antigens from stimulating peripheral lymphoid tissue which would result in a rise in circulating antibody with the concomitant risk of immune-complex mediated disease.

How immunologic memory operates at the level of the gastrointestinal tract has not been studied to any great degree. Antigens absorbed for the second (or more) time would come in contact with memory B and T cells still in the originally stimulated nodule. However, to be effective the antigen would also have to come in contact with memory B and T cells that arose from the originally stimulated nodule and are now spread throughout the gastrointestinal tract in the lamina propria. Presumably the small amount of intact antigen that makes its way through the columnar epithelium would be enough to trigger the cells to finish differentiation to plasma cells, with the resultant production of antibody.

REFERENCES

1. Moore, W. E. C.: Current research on the anaerobic flora of the gastrointestinal tract. *In* The Use of Drugs in Animal Feeds (Proceedings Symposium). Natl. Acad. Sci., Washington, D.C. 1969, p. 107.

2. Moore, W. E. C., and Holdeman, L. V.: Human fecal flora: the normal flora of 20 Japanese-Hawaiians. Appl. Microbiol. 27:961, 1974.

3. Dubos, R. J., Schaedler, R. W., Costello, R., and Hoet, P.: Indigenous, normal, and autochthonous flora of the gastrointestinal tract. J. Exp. Med. 122:67, 1965.

4. Lee, A., and Gemmell, E.: Changes in the mouse intestinal microflora during weaning: role of volatile fatty acids. Infect. Immun. 5:1, 1972.

5. Lee, A., Gordon, J., Lee, C. J., and Dubos, R. J.: The mouse intestinal microflora with emphasis on the strict anaerobes. J. Exp. Med. 133:339, 1971.

6. Savage, D. C., Dubos, R. J., and Schaedler, R. W.: The gastrointestinal epithelium and its autochthonous bacterial flora. J. Exp. Med. 127:67, 1968.

7. Hungate, R. E.: The Rumen and its Microbes. New York, Academic Press, 1966.

8. Smith, H. W.: The development of the flora of the alimentary tract in young animals. J. Pathol. Bacteriol. 90:495, 1965.

9. Smith, H. W.: The bacteriology of the alimentary tract of domestic animals suffering from *Escherichia coli* infection. Ann. N. Y. Acad. Sci. 176:110, 1971.

10. Bryant, M. P.: Bacterial species of the rumen. Bacteriol. Rev. 23:125, 1959.

11. Bryant, M. P.: Normal flora—rumen bacteria. Am. J. Clin. Nutr. 23:1440, 1970.

12. Glesecke, D.: Comparative microbiology of the alimentary tract. *In* Physiology of Digestion and Metabolism in the Ruminant. Edited by A. T. Phillipson. Newcastle upon Tyne, Oriel, 1970, p. 306.

13. Hungate, R. E., Bryant, M. P., and Mah, R. A.: The rumen bacteria and protozoa. Ann. Rev. Microbiol. 18:131, 1964.

14. Kern, D. L., Slyter, L. L., Leffel, E. D., Weaver, J. M., and Oltjen, R. R.: Ponies vs steers: microbial and chemical characteristics of intestinal ingesta. J. Anim. Sci. 38:559, 1974.

15. Smith, H. W.: Observations on the flora of the alimentary tract of animals and factors affecting its composition. J. Pathol. Bacteriol. 89:95, 1965.

16. Ward, A. C. S., Waldhalm, D. G., Frank, F. W., Meinershagen, W. A., and DeBose, D. A.: *Escherichia coli* populations at various intestinal levels of steers. Am. J. Vet. Res. 35:953, 1974.

17. Davis, M. E.: Cellulolytic bacteria in some ruminants and herbivores as shown by fluorescent antibody. J. Gen. Microbiol. 39:139, 1965.

18. Glinsky, M. J., Smith, R. M., Spires, H. R., and Davis, C. L.: Measurement of volatile fatty acid production rates in the cecum of the pony. J. Anim. Sci. 42:1465, 1976.

19. Salanitro, J. P., Blake, I. G., and Muirhead, P. A.: Isolation and identification of fecal bacteria from adult swine. Appl. Environ. Microbiol. 33:79, 1977.

20. Tannock, G. W., and Smith, J. M. B.: The microflora of the pig stomach and its possible relationship to ulceration of the pars oesophagea. J. Comp. Pathol. 80:359, 1970.

21. Mitsuoka, T., and Kaneuchi, C.: Ecology of the Bifidobacteria. Am. J. Clin. Nutr. 30:1799, 1977.

22. Gelbart, S. M., Larson, C. H., Paez, J. E., and Greenlee, H. B.: Effect of deworming medication on the microbial flora of the upper gastrointestinal tract of dogs. Lab. Anim. Sci. 26:640, 1976.

23. Leach, W. D., Lee, A., and Stubbs, R. P.: Localization of bacteria in the gastrointestinal tract: a possible explanation of the intestinal spirochaetosis. Infect. Immun. 7:961, 1973.

24. Pindak, F. F., Clapper, W. E., and Sherrod, J. H.: Incidence and distribution of spirochaetes in the digestive tract of dogs. Am. J. Vet. Res. 26:1391, 1965.

25. Abrams, G. D.: Effects of the indigenous microbial flora on the mechanisms of host resistance. *In* Resistance to Infectious Disease. Edited by R. H. Dunlop and H. W. Moon. Saskatoon, Modern Press, 1970, p. 129.

26. Reddy, B. S., and Wostmann, B. S.: Intestinal disaccharidase activities in the growing germfree and conventional rats. Arch. Biochem. Biophys. 113:609, 1966.

27. Lesher, S., Walburg, E. E., and Sacher, G. A.: Generation cycle in the duodenal crypt cells of germfree and conventional mice. Nature 202:884, 1964.

28. Bauer, H., Paronetto, F., Burns, W. A., and Einheber, A.: The enhancing effect of the microbial flora on macrophage function and the immune response. J. Exp. Med. 123:1013, 1966.

29. Crabbe, P. A., Bazin, H., Eyssen, H., and Heremans, J. F.: The normal microbial flora as a major stimulus for a proliferation of plasma cells synthesizing IgA in the gut. Int. Arch. Allergy 34:362, 1968.

30. Abrams, G. D., and Bishop, J. E.: Effect of the normal microbial

flora on gastrointestinal motility. Proc. Soc. Exp. Biol. Med. *126*:301, 1967.

31. Heneghan, J. B.: Influence of microbial flora on xylose absorption in rats and mice. Am. J. Physiol. *205*:417, 1963.

32. Sears, H. J., Brownlee, J., and Uchiyama, J. M.: Persistence of individual strains of *Escherichia coli* in the intestinal tract of man. J. Bacteriol. *59*:293, 1950.

33. Sears, H. J., Janes, H., Saloum, R., Brownlee, I., and Lamoreaux, L. F.: Persistence of individual strains of *Escherichia coli* in man and dogs under various conditions. J. Bacteriol. *71*:370, 1956.

34. Hirsh, D. C., and Wiger, N.: Unpublished observation.

35. Davidson, J. N., and Hirsh, D. C.: Use of the K-88 antigen for *in vivo* bacterial competition with porcine strains of enteropathogenic *Escherichia coli*. Infect. Immun. *12*:134, 1975.

36. Davidson, J. N., and Hirsh, D. C.: Bacterial competition as a means of preventing neonatal diarrhea in the pig. Infect. Immun. *13*:1773, 1976.

37. Arbuckle, J. B. R.: The localization of *Escherichia coli* in pig intestine. Med. Microbiol. *3*:333, 1970.

38. Bertschinger, H. U., Moon, H. W., and Whipp, S. C.: Association of *Escherichia coli* with the small intestinal epithelium. I. Comparison of enteropathogenic and non-enteropathogenic porcine strains in pigs. Infect. Immun. *5*:595, 1972.

39. Hohmann, A., and Wilson, M. R.: Adherence of enteropathogenic *Escherichia coli* to intestinal epithelium *in vivo*. Infect. Immun. *12*:866, 1975.

40. Gibbons, R. A., Jones, G. W., and Sellwood, R.: An attempt to identify the intestinal receptor for the K-88 adhesin by means of a haemagglutination inhibition test using glycoproteins and fractions from cow colostrum. J. Gen. Microbiol. *86*:228, 1975.

41. Suegara, N., Morotomi, M., Watanabe, T., Kawai, Y., and Mutai, M.: Behavior of microflora in the rat stomach: adhesion of lactobacilli to the keratinized epithelial cells of the rat stomach *in vitro*. Infect. Immun. *12*:173, 1975.

42. Wagner, R. C., and Barrnett, R. J.: The fine structure of prokaryotic-eukaryotic cell junctions. J. Ultrastruct. Res. *48*:404, 1974.

43. Freter, R.: Studies of the mechanism of action of intestinal antibody in experimental cholera. Tex. Rep. Biol. Med. *27*:299, 1969.

44. Eden, C. S., Hanson, L. A., Jodal, U., Linberg, U., and Akerlund, A. S.: Variable adherence to normal human urinary tract epithelial cells of *Escherichia coli* strains associated with various forms of urinary tract infection. Lancet *2*:490, 1976.

45. Fuller, R., and Booker, B. E.: Lactobacilli which attach to the crop epithelium of the fowl. Am. J. Clin. Nutr. *27*:1305, 1974.

46. Nagy, B., Moon, H. W., and Isaacson, R. E.: Colonization of porcine small intestine by *Escherichia coli*: ileal colonization and adhesion by pig enteropathogens that lack K88 antigen and by some acapsular mutants. Infect. Immun. *13*:1214, 1976.

47. Falkow, S., Williams, L. P., Seaman, S. L., and Rollins, L. D.: Increased survival in calves of *Escherichia coli* K-12 carrying an Ent plasmid. Infect. Immun. *13*:1005, 1976.

48. Davis, B. D., Dulbecco, R., Eisen, H. N., Ginsberg, H. S., and Wood, W. B.: Microbiology. 2nd ed. Hagerstown, MD, Harper & Row Publishers, 1973.

49. Craven, J. A., Miniats, O. P., and Barnum, D. A.: Role of colicins in antagonism between strains of *Escherichia coli* in dual-infected gnotobiotic pigs. Am. J. Vet. Res. *32*:1775, 1971.

50. Ikari, N. S., Kenton, D. M., and Young, V. M.: Interaction on the germfree mouse intestine of colicinogenic and colicin-sensitive microorganisms. Proc. Soc. Exp. Biol. Med. *130*:1280, 1969.

51. Bergeim, O.: Toxicity of intestinal volatile fatty acids for yeasts and *Escherichia coli*. J. Infect. Dis. *66*:222, 1940.

52. Bergeim, O., Hanszen, A. H., Pincussen, L., and Weiss, E.: Relation of volatile fatty acids and H₂S to the intestinal flora. J. Infect. Dis. *69*:155, 1941.

53. Hentges, D. J.: Inhibition of *Shigella flexneri* by the normal intestinal flora. II. Mechanism of inhibition of coliform organisms. J. Bacteriol. *97*:513, 1969.

54. Hentges, D. J., and Maier, B. R.: Inhibition of *Shigella flexneri* by the normal intestinal flora. III. Interactions with *Bacteroides fragilis* strains *in vitro*. Infect. Immun. *2*:364, 1970.

55. Koopman, J. P., Janssen, F. G. J., and VanDruten, J. A. M.: Oxidation-reduction potentials in the cecal contents of rats and mice. Proc. Soc. Exp. Biol. Med. *149*:995, 1975.

56. Meynell, G. G.: Antibacterial mechanisms of the mouse gut. II. The role of Eh and volatile fatty acids in the normal gut. Br. J. Exp. Pathol. *44*:209, 1963.

57. Wostmann, B. A., and Bruckner-Kardoss, E.: Oxidation-reduction potentials in cecal contents of germ-free and conventional rats. Proc. Soc. Exp. Biol. Med. *121*:1111, 1966.

58. Bohnhoff, M., and Miller, C. P.: Enhanced susceptibility of *Salmonella* infections in streptomycin-treated mice. J. Infect. Dis. *111*:117, 1962.

59. Bohnhoff, M., Miller, C. P., and Martin, W. R.: Resistance of the mouse's intestinal tract to experimental *Salmonella* infections by oral inoculation. J. Exp. Med. *120*:805, 1964.

60. Bohnhoff, M., Miller, C. P., and Martin, W. R.: Resistance of the mouse's intestinal tract to experimental *Salmonella* infection. II. Factors responsible for its loss following streptomycin treatment. J. Exp. Med. *120*:817, 1964.

61. Miller, C. P., and Bohnhoff, M.: Change in the mouse's microflora associated with enhanced susceptibility to *Salmonella* infection following streptomycin treatment. J. Infect. Dis. *113*:59, 1963.

62. Miller, C. P., and Bohnhoff, M.: A study of experimental *Salmonella* infection in the mouse. J. Infect. Dis. *111*:107, 1962.

63. Floch, M. H., Binder, J. J., Filburn, B., and Gershengoren, W.: The effect of bile acids on intestinal microflora. Am. J. Clin. Nutr. *25*:1418, 1972.

64. Gilliland, S. E., and Speck, M. L.: Deconjugation of bile acids by intestinal lactobacilli. Appl. Environ. Microbiol. *33*:15, 1977.

65. Shimada, K., Brickness, K. S., and Finegold, S. M.: Deconjugation of bile acids by intestinal bacteria: review of the literature and additional studies. J. Infect. Dis. *119*:273, 1969.

66. Percy-Robb, I. W., and Collee, J. G.: Bile acids: a pH dependent antibacterial system in the gut? Br. Med. J. *3*:813, 1972.

67. Ozawa, A., and Freter, R.: Ecological mechanisms controlling growth of *Escherichia coli* in continuous flow cultures in the mouse intestine. J. Infect. Dis. *114*:235, 1964.

68. Dixon, J. M. S.: The fate of bacteria in the small intestine. J. Pathol. Bacteriol. *79*:131, 1960.

69. Abrams, G. D., and Bishop, J. E.: Effect of the normal microbial flora on the resistance of the small intestine to infection. J. Bacteriol. *92*:1604, 1966.

70. Fubara, E. S., and Freter, R.: Protection against enteric bacterial infections by secretory IgA antibodies. J. Immunol. *111*:395, 1973.

71. Reed, W. P., and Cushing, A. H.: Role of immunoglobulins in protection against shigella-induced keratoconjunctivitis. Infect. Immun. *11*:1265, 1975.

72. Rutter, J. M., Jones, G. W., Brown, G. T. H., Burrows, M. R., and Luther, P. D.: Antibacterial activity in colostrum and milk associated with protection of piglets against enteric disease caused by K88 positive *Escherichia coli*. Infect. Immun. *13*:667, 1976.

73. Williams, R. C., and Gibbons, R. J.: Inhibition of bacterial adherence by secretory immunoglobulin A: a mechanism of antigen disposal. Science *177*:697, 1972.

74. Berg, R. D., and Savage, D. C.: Immune responses of specific pathogen-free and gnotobiotic mice to antigens of indigenous and non-indigenous microorganisms. Infect. Immun. *11*:320, 1975.

75. Foo, M. C., and Lee, A.: Immunological response of mice to members of the autochthonous intestinal flora. Infect. Immun. *6*:525, 1972.

76. Foo, M. C., and Lee, A.: Antigenic cross-reaction between mouse intestine and a member of the autochthonous microflora. Infect. Immun. *9*:1066, 1974.

77. Shedlofsby, S., and Freter, R.: Synergism between ecologic and immunologic control mechanisms of intestinal flora. J. Infect. Dis. *129*:296, 1974.

78. Corbeil, L. B., Schurig, G. G. D., Bier, P. J., and Winter, A. J.: Bovine venereal vibriosis: antigenic variation of the bacterium during infection. Infect. Immun. *11*:240, 1975.

79. Sack, R. B., and Miller, C. E.: Progressive changes of vibrio serotypes in germ-free mice infected with *Vibrio cholerae*. J. Bacteriol. *99*:688, 1969.

80. Falkow, S.: Infectious Multiple Drug Resistance. London, Pion Limited, 1975.

81. Nishikawa, T., Hatano, H., Ohnishi, N., Sasaki, S., and Nomura, T.: Establishment of *Candida albicans* in the alimentary tract of germ-free mice and antagonism with *Escherichia coli* after oral inoculation. Jpn. J. Microbiol. *13*:263, 1969.

82. Huppert, M., Cazin, J., and Smith, H.: Pathogenesis of *Candida albicans* following antibiotic therapy. III. The effect of antibiotics on the incidence of *C. albicans* in the intestinal tract of mice. J. Bacteriol. *70*:440, 1955.

83. Huppert, M., and Cazin, J.: Pathogenesis of *Candida albicans* following antibiotic therapy. II. Further studies on the effect of antibiotics on the *in vitro* growth of *Candida albicans*. J. Bacteriol. *70*:435, 1955.

84. Sellig, M. S.: Mechanisms by which antibiotics increase the incidence and severity of candidiasis and alter the immunological defenses. Bacteriol. Rev. 30:442, 1966.

85. Simonetti, N., and Strippoli, V.: On the action mechanism of the increase in virulence of Candida albicans caused by antibiotics and its regulation. Antibiotica 7:23, 1969.

86. Tannock, G. W., and Savage, D. C.: Influence of dietary and environmental stress on microbial populations in the murine gastrointestinal tract. Infect. Immun. 9:591, 1974.

87. Arnthorsson, G., Johnson, L., Lylander, G., and Wikstrom, S.: Gastric secretion of mucous related to adrenocortical activity. A histochemical study in the rat. Scand. J. Gastroenterol. 6:65, 1971.

88. Hoskins, L. C., and Zamcheck, N.: Bacterial degradation of gastrointestinal mucins. I. Comparisons of mucous constituents in the stools of germ-free and conventional rats. Gastroenterology 54:210, 1968.

89. Savage, D. C., McAllister, J. S., and Davis, C. P.: Anaerobic bacteria on the mucosal epithelium of the murine large bowel. Infect. Immun. 4:492, 1971.

90. Gibson, C. D., and Zemjanis, R.: Immune response of the bovine fetus to several antigens. Am. J. Vet. Res. 34:1277, 1973.

91. Jacoby, R. O., Dennis, R. A., and Griesemer, R. A.: Development of immunity in fetal dogs: humoral responses. Am. J. Vet. Res. 30:1503, 1969.

92. Osburn, B. T.: Immune responsiveness of the fetus and neonate. J.A.V.M.A. 163:801, 1973.

93. Schultz, R. D., Wang, J. T., and Dunne, H. W.: Development of the humoral immune response of the pig. Am. J. Vet. Res. 32:1331, 1971.

94. Braun, R. K., Osburn, B. I., and Kendrick, J. W.: The immunological response of the bovine fetus to bovine viral diarrhea virus. Am. J. Vet. Res. 34:1127, 1973.

95. Osburn, B. I., Stabenfeldt, G. H., Ardans, A. A., Trees, C., and Sayer, M: Perinatal immunity in calves, J.A.V.M.A. 164:295, 1974.

96. Reade, P. C.: The development of bactericidal activity in rat peritoneal macrophages. Aust. J. Exp. Biol. Med. Sci. 46:231, 1968.

97. Richardson, M., Conner, G. H., Beck, C. C., and Clark, D. T.: Prenatal immunization of the lamb to brucella: secondary antibody response in utero and at birth. Immunology 21:795, 1971.

98. Bryant, B. J., Shifrine, M., and McNeil, C.: Cell-mediated immune response in the developing dog. Int. Arch. Allergy 45:937, 1973.

99. Gerber, J. D., and Brown, A. L.: Effect of development and aging on the response of canine lymphocytes to phytohemagglutinin. Infect. Immun. 10:695, 1974.

100. Brambel, F. W. R.: The transmission of passive immunity from mother to young. In Frontier of Biology. Edited by A. Neuberger and E. L. Tatum. Amsterdam, North Holland Publishing Co., 1970.

101. Lascelles, A. K., and McDowell, G. H.: Localized humoral immunity with particular references to ruminants. Transplant. Rev. 19:170, 1974.

102. Vaerman, J. P.: Comparative immunochemistry of IgA. Res. Immunochem. Immunobiol. 3:91, 1973.

103. Mach, J. P., and Pahud, J. J.: Secretory IgA, a major immunoglobulin in most bovine external secretions. J. Immunol. 106:552, 1971.

104. Pierce, A. E., and Feinstein, A.: Biophysical immunological studies on bovine immune globulins with evidence for selective transport within the mammary gland from maternal plasma to colostrum. Immunology 8:106, 1965.

105. Porter, P., and Allen, W. D.: Classes of immunoglobulins related to immunity in the pig. J.A.V.M.A. (Spec. Suppl.) 160:511, 1972.

106. Reynolds, H. Y., and Johnson, J. S.: Quantitation of canine immunoglobulins. J. Immunol. 105:698, 1970.

107. Vaerman, J. P., Querinjean, P., and Heremans, J. F.: Studies on the IgA system of the horse. Immunology 21:443, 1971.

108. Kraehenbuhl, J. P., and Campiche, M. A.: Early stages of intestinal absorption of specific antibodies in the newborn. An ultrastructural, cytochemical, and immunological study in the pig, rat, and rabbit. J. Cell. Biol. 42:345, 1969.

109. Lecce, J. G.: Absorption of macromolecules by neonatal intestine. Biol. Neonatorum 9:50, 1966.

110. Porter, P.: Transfer of immunoglobulin IgG, IgA, and IgM to lacteal secretions in the parturient sow and their absorption by the neonatal piglet. Biochim. Biophys. Acta 181:381, 1969.

111. Guyer, R. L., Koshland, M. E., and Knopf, P. M.: Immunoglobulin binding by mouse intestinal epithelial cell receptors. J. Immunol. 117:587, 1976.

112. Daniels, V. G., Hardy, R. N., Malinowska, K. W., and Nathanielsz, P. W.: Adrenocortical hormone and absorption of macromolecules by the small intestine of the young rat. J. Endocrinol. 52:405, 1972.

113. Halliday, R.: The effect of steroid hormones in the absorption of antibodies by the young rat. J. Endocrinol. 18:56, 1959.

114. Brandtzaeg, P.: Mucosal and glandular distribution of immunoglobulin components: immunohistochemistry with a cold ethanol-fixation technique. Immunology 26:1101, 1974.

115. Brandtzaeg, P.: Human secretory IgM: an immunochemical and immunohistochemical study. Immunology 29:559, 1974.

116. Eskeland, T., and Brandtzaeg, P.: Does J chain mediate the combination of 19S IgM and dimeric IgA with the secretory component rather than being necessary for their polymerization? Immunochemistry 2:161, 1974.

117. Lindh, E.: Increased resistance of immunoglobulin A dimers to proteolytic degradation after binding of secretory component. J. Immunol. 114:284, 1975.

118. Laskowski, M., Kassell, B., and Hagerty, G.: A crystalline trypsin inhibitor from swine colostrum. Biochim. Biophys. Acta 24:300, 1957.

119. Laskowski, M., and Laskowski, M.: Crystalline trypsin inhibitor from colostrum. J. Biol. Chem. 190:563, 1951.

120. Newby, T. J.: Aspects of the Local Immune System of the Ox. Ph.D. Thesis, University of Bristol, 1975. Quoted in Newby, T. J., and Bourne, F. J.: Immunology 31:475, 1976.

121. Pearsall, N. N., and Weiser, R. S.: The Macrophage. Philadelphia, Lea & Febiger, 1970.

122. Argyris, B. F., and Plotkin, D. H.: Effect of antimacrophage serum on antibody production and phagocytosis in mice. J. Immunol. 103:372, 1969.

123. Mosler, D. E.: A requirement for two cell types for antibody formation in vitro. Science 158:1573, 1967.

124. Mosler, D. E., and Coppleson, L. W.: A 3-cell interaction required for the induction of the primary immune response in vitro. Proc. Natl. Acad. Sci. 61:542, 1968.

125. Gallily, R., and Garvey, J. S.: Primary stimulation of rats and mice with hemocyanin in solution and absorbed on bentonite. J. Immunol. 101:924, 1968.

126. Hirsh, D. C., Amkraut, A. A., and Steward, J. P.: Effect of carrier modification on the cellular and serologic responses of the rat to the TNP hapten. I. Dependence of the immunogenicity of the antigen upon processing by macrophages, as well as distribution and retention of the antigen. J. Immunol. 108:765, 1972.

127. Rosenthal, A. S., Lipsky, P. E., and Shevach, E. M.: Macrophage-lymphocyte interaction and antigen recognition. Fed. Proc. 34:1743, 1975.

128. Dresser, D. W., and Mitchison, N. A.: The mechanism of immunological paralysis. Adv. Immunol. 8:129, 1968.

129. Frei, P. C., Benacerraf, B., and Thorbecke, G. J.: Phagocytosis of the antigen, a crucial step in the induction of the immune response. Proc. Natl. Acad. Sci. 53:20, 1965.

130. Nossal, G. J. V., Ada, G. L., and Austin, C. M.: Antigens in immunity. II. Immunogenic properties of flagella, polymerized flagellin, and flagellin in the primary response. Aust. J. Exp. Biol. Med. Sci. 42:283, 1964.

131. Nossal, G. J. V., Ada, G. L., and Austin, C. M.: Antigens in immunity. IV. Cellular localizations of ^{125}I- and ^{131}I-labelled flagella in lymph nodes. Aust. J. Exp. Biol. Med. Sci. 42:311, 1964.

132. Campbell, D. H., and Garvey, J. S.: The fate of foreign antigen and speculations as to its role in immune mechanisms. Lab. Invest. 10:1126, 1961.

133. Garvey, J. S., and Campbell, D. H.: The retention of ^{35}S-labeled BSA in normal and immunized rabbit liver tissue. J. Exp. Med. 105:361, 1957.

134. Garvey, J. S., and Campbell, D. H.: Autoradiographic investigation of tissue after primary and multiple antigenic stimulation of rabbits. Nature 209:1201, 1966.

135. Miller, J. F. A. P., and Mitchell, G. F.: Thymus and antigen reactive cells. Transplant. Rev. 1:3, 1969.

136. Claman, H. N., and Chaperon, E. A.: Immunologic complementation between thymus and marrow cells—a model for the two-cell theory of immunocompetence. Transplant. Rev. 1:92, 1969.

137. Taussig, M. J., and Munro, A. J.: Antigen-specific T-cell factor in cell cooperation and genetic control of the immune response. Fed. Proc. 35:2061, 1976.

138. Playfair, J. H. L.: The role of antibody in T-cell responses. Clin. Exp. Immunol. 17:1, 1974.

139. Williamson, A. R., Zitron, I. M., and McMichael, A. J.: Clones of B lymphocytes: their natural selection and expansion. Fed. Proc. 35:2195, 1976.

140. Cerottini, J-C., and Brunner, K. T.: Cell-mediated cytotoxicity, allograft rejection, and tumor immunity. Adv. Immunol. 18:67, 1974.

141. Rosenau, W., and Tsoukas, C. D.: Lymphotoxin. Am. J. Pathol. *84*:580, 1976.
142. Lawrence, S. H., and Landy, M.: Mediators and Cellular Immunity. London, Academic Press, 1969.
143. Anderson, S. E., Bautista, S., and Remington, J. S.: Induction of resistance to *Toxoplasma gondii* in human macrophages by soluble lymphocyte products. J. Immunol. *117*:381, 1976.
144. Blanden, R. V., Lefford, M. J., and Mackaness, G. B.: The host response to Calmette-Guerin bacillus infection in mice. J. Exp. Med. *129*:1079, 1969.
145. Collins, F. M., Blanden, R. V., and Mackaness, G. B.: Infection immunity in experimental salmonellosis. J. Exp. Med. *124*:601, 1966.
146. Mackaness, G. B.: The immunological basis of acquired cellular resistance. J. Exp. Med. *120*:105, 1964.
147. Mackaness, G. B.: The influence of immunologically committed lymphoid cells on macrophage activity *in vivo*. J. Exp. Med. *129*:973, 1969.
148. Zinkernagel, R. M.: Cell-mediated immune response to *Salmonella typhimurium* infection in mice: development of nonspecific bactericidal activity against *Listeria monocytogenes*. Infect. Immun. *13*:1069, 1976.
149. Baker, P. J.: Homeostatic control of antibody responses: a model based on the recognition of cell associated antibody by regulatory T cells. Transplant. Rev. *26*:3, 1975.
150. Waldmann, T. A., Broder, S., Krakauer, R., MacDermott, R. P., Durm, M., Goldman, C., and Meade, B.: The role of suppressor cells in the pathogenesis of common variable hypogamma-globulinemia and the immunodeficiency associated with myeloma. Fed. Proc. *35*:2067, 1976.
151. Abdou, N. I., and Richter, M.: Cells involved in the immune response. VI. The immune response to RBC in irradiated rabbits after administration of normal, primed, or immune allogeneic rabbit bone marrow cells. J. Exp. Med. *129*:757, 1969.
152. Cooper, M. D., Pevey, D. Y., Gabrielson, A. E., Sutherland, D. E. R., McKneally, M. F., and Good, R. A.: Production of an antibody deficiency syndrome in rabbits by neonatal removal of organized intestinal lymphoid tissue. Int. Arch. Allergy Appl. Immunol. *33*:65, 1968.
153. Owen, J. J. T., Cooper, M. D., and Raff, M. C.: *In vitro* generation of B lymphocytes in mouse foetal liver, a mammalian "bursa equivalent." Nature *249*:361, 1974.
154. Basten, A., Miller, J. F. A. P., Sprent, J., and Pye, J.: A receptor for antibody on B lymphocytes. I. Method of detection and functional significance. J. Exp. Med. *135*:610, 1971.
155. Dukor, P., Bianco, C., and Nussenzweig, V.: Bone marrow origin of complement-receptor lymphocytes. Eur. J. Immunol. *1*:491, 1971.
156. Warner, N. L.: Membrane immunoglobulins and antisera receptors on B and T lymphocytes. Adv. Immunol. *19*:67, 1974.
157. Dutton, R. W., and Eady, J. D.: An *in vitro* system for the study of the mechanism of antigenic stimulation in the secondary response. Immunology *7*:40, 1964.
158. Julius, M. H., Masuda, T., and Herzenberg, L. A.: Demonstration that antigen-binding cells are precursors of antibody-producing cells after purification with a fluorescein-activated cell sorter. Proc. Natl. Acad. Sci. *69*:1934, 1972.
159. Wigzell, H., and Andersson, B.: Cell separation on antigen coated columns. Elimination of high rate antibody-forming cells and immunological memory cells. J. Exp. Med. *129*:23, 1969.
160. Vitetta, E. S., and Uhr, J. W.: Immunoglobulin-receptors revisited: a model for the differentiation of bone marrow-derived lymphocytes is described. Science *189*:964, 1975.
161. Boak, J. L., Mitchison, N. A., and Pattison, P. H.: The carrier effect in the secondary response to hapten-protein conjugates. III. The anatomical distribution of helper cells and antibody-forming cell-precursors. Eur. J. Immunol. *1*:63, 1971.
162. Strober, S.: Initiation of antibody responses by different classes of lymphocytes. V. Fundamental changes in the physiological characteristics of virgin thymus independent ("B") lymphocytes and "B" memory cells. J. Exp. Med. *136*:851, 1972.
163. Strober, S., and Dilley, J.: Biological characteristics of T and B memory lymphocytes in the rat. J. Exp. Med. *137*:1275, 1973.
164. Gowans, J. L., and Uhr, J. W.: The carriage of immunological memory by small lymphocytes in the rat. J. Exp. Med. *124*:1017, 1966.
165. Ellis, S. T., and Gowans, J. L.: The role of lymphocytes in antibody formation. V. Transfer of immunological memory to tetanus toxoid: the origin of plasma cells from small lymphocytes, stimulation of memory cells *in vitro* and the persistence of memory after cell transfer. Proc. R. Soc. Lond. *83*:125, 1973.
166. Smith, J. B., Cunningham, A. J., Lafferty, K. J., and Morris, B.: The role of the lymphatic system and lymphoid cells in the establishment

of immunological memory. Aust. J. Exp. Biol. Med. Sci. *48*:57, 1970.
167. Gutman, G. A., and Weissman, I. L.: Homing properties of thymus-independent follicular lymphocytes. Transplantation *16*:621, 1973.
168. VanEwijk, W., Brons, N. H. C., and Rozing, J.: Scanning electron microscopy of homing and recirculating lymphocyte populations. Cell. Immunol. *19*:245, 1975.
169. Parrott, D. M. V.: The gut-associated lymphoid tissues and gastrointestinal immunity. *In* Immunological Aspects of the Liver and Gastrointestinal Tract. Edited by A. Ferguson and R. N. M. MacSween. Baltimore, University Park Press, 1976.
170. Meader, R. D., and Landers, D. F.: Electron and light microscopic observations on the relationship between lymphocytes and intestinal epithelium. Am. J. Anat. *121*:763, 1967.
171. Parrott, D. M. V., and Ferguson, A.: Selective migration of lymphocytes within the mouse small intestine. Immunology *26*:571, 1974.
172. Ferguson, A., and Parrott, D. M. V.: The effect of antigen deprivation on thymus-dependent and thymus-independent lymphocytes in the small intestine of the mouse. Clin. Exp. Immunol. *12*:477, 1972.
173. Copenhaver, W. M., Bunge, R. P., and Bunge, M. B.: Bailey's Textbook of Histology, 16th ed. Baltimore, The Williams & Wilkins Co., 1971.
174. Owen, R. L.: Sequential uptake of horseradish peroxidase by lymphoid follicle epithelium of Peyer's patches in the normal unobstructed mouse intestine: an ultrastructural study. Gastroenterology *72*:440, 1977.
175. Owen, R. L., and Jones, A. L.: Epithelial cell specialization within human Peyer's patches: an ultrastructural study of intestinal lymphoid follicles. Gastroenterology *66*:189, 1974.
176. Cornell, R., Walker, W. A., and Isselbacher, K. J.: Small intestinal absorption of horseradish peroxidase. A cytochemical study. Lab. Invest. *25*:42, 1971.
177. Guy-Grand, D., Griscelli, C., and Vassalli, P.: The gut associated lymphoid system: nature and properties of the large dividing cell. Eur. J. Immunol. *4*:435, 1974.
178. Faulk, W. P., McCormick, J. N., Goodman, J. R., Yoffey, J. M., and Fudenberg, H. H.: Peyer's patches: Morphologic studies. Cell. Immunol. *1*:500, 1971.
179. Waksman, B. H.: The homing pattern of thymus-derived lymphocytes in calf and neonatal mouse Peyer's patches. J. Immunol. *111*:878, 1973.
180. Kagnoff, M. E., and Campbell, S.: Functional characteristics of Peyer's patch lymphoid cells. I. Induction of humoral antibody and cell mediated allograft reactions. J. Exp. Med. *139*:398, 1974.
181. Levin, D. M., Rosenstreich, D. L., and Reynolds, H. Y.: Immunologic responses in the gastrointestinal tract of the guinea pig. I. Characterization of Peyer's patch cells. J. Immunol. *111*:980, 1973.
182. Friedberg, S. H., and Weissman, I. L.: Lymphoid tissue architecture. Ii. Ontogeny of peripheral T and B cells in mice: evidence against Peyer's patches as the site of generation of B cells. J. Immunol. *113*:1477, 1974.
183. Joel, D. D., Hess, M. W., and Cottier, H.: Magnitude and patterns of thymic lymphocyte migration in neonatal mice. J. Exp. Med. *135*:907, 1972.
184. Joel, D. D., Hess, M. W., and Cottier, H.: Thymic origin of lymphocytes in developing Peyer's patches of newborn mice. Nature [New Biol.] *231*:24, 1971.
185. Muller-Schoop, J. W., and Good, R. A.: Functional studies of Peyer's patches: evidence for their participation in intestinal immune responses. J. Immunol. *114*:1757, 1975.
186. Henry, C., Faulk, W. P., Kuhn, L., Yoffey, J. M., and Fudenberg, H. H.: Peyer's patches: immunologic studies. J. Exp. Med. *131*:1200, 1970.
187. Bernstein, I. D., and Ovary, Z.: Absorption of antigens from the gastrointestinal tract. Int. Arch. Appl. Immunol. *33*:521, 1968.
188. Perrotto, J. L., Hang, L. M., Isselbacher, K. J., and Warren, K. S.: Systemic cellular hypersensitivity induced by an intestinally absorbed antigen. J. Exp. Med. *140*:296, 1974.
189. Walker, W. A., Cornell, R., Davenport, L., and Isselbacher, K. J.: Mechanism of horseradish peroxidase uptake and transport in adult and neonatal rat intestine. J. Cell. Biol. *54*:195, 1972.
190. Warshaw, A. L., Walker, W. A., and Isselbacher, K. J.: Small intestinal permeability of macromolecules. Transmission of horseradish peroxidase into mesenteric lymph and portal blood. Lab. Invest. *25*:675, 1971.
191. Bienenstock, J., and Dolezel, J.: Peyer's patches: lack of specific antibody-containing cells after oral and parenteral immunization. J. Immunol. *106*:938, 1971.
192. Hunter, R. L.: Antigen trapping in the lamina propria and production of IgA antibody. J. Reticuloendothel. Soc. *11*:245, 1972.
193. Craig, S. W., and Cebra, J. J.: Rabbit Peyer's patches, appendix and

popliteal lymph node B lymphocytes. A comparative analysis of their membrane immunoglobulin components and plasma cell precursor potential. J. Immunol. *114*:492, 1975.

194. Craig, S. W., and Cebra, J. J.: Peyer's patches: an enriched source of precursors for IgA-producing immunocytes in the rabbit. J. Exp. Med. *134*:188, 1971.

195. Guy-Grand, D., Griscelli, C., and Vassalli, P.: Gut-associated lymphoblasts and intestinal IgA plasma cells. *In* The Immunoglobulin A System. Edited by J. Mestecky and A. R. Lawton. New York, Plenum Press, 1974.

196. Williams, A. F., and Gowans, J. L.: The presence of IgA on the surface of rat thoracic duct lymphocytes which contain internal IgA. J. Exp. Med. *141*:335, 1975.

197. Jones, P. P., Craig, S. W., Cebra, J. J., and Herzenberg, L. A.: Restriction of gene expression in B lymphocytes and their progeny. II. Commitment to immunoglobulin heavy chain isotype. J. Exp. Med. *140*:452, 1974.

198. Vitetta, E. S., McWilliams, M., Phillips-Quagliata, J. M., Lamm, M. E., and Uhr, J.: Cell surface immunoglobulin. XIV. Synthesis, surface expression, and secretion of immunoglobulin by Peyer's patch cells in the mouse. J. Immunol. *115*:603, 1975.

199. Mann, J. D., and Higgens, G. M.: Lymphocytes in the thoracic duct, intestinal and hepatic lymph. Blood 5:177, 1950.

200. Hall, J. G., and Smith, M. E.: Homing of lymph-borne immunoblasts to the gut. Nature 226:262, 1970.

201. Halstead, T. E., and Hall, J. G.: The homing of lymph-borne immunoblasts to the small gut of neonatal rats. Transplantation *14*:339, 1972.

202. Parrott, D. M. V., Tilney, N. L., and Sless, F.: The different migratory characteristics of lymphocyte populations from a whole spleen transplant. Clin. Exp. Immunol. *19*:459, 1975.

203. Hall, J. G., Parry, D. M., and Smith, M. E.: The distribution of lymph-borne immunoblasts after intravenous injection into syngeneic recipients. Cell. Tissue Kinet. 5:269, 1972.

204. Ferguson, A.: Secretion of IgA into "antigen-free" isografts of mouse small intestine. Clin. Exp. Immunol. *17*:691, 1974.

205. McWilliams, M., Phillips-Quagliata, J. M., and Lamm, M. E.: Characteristics of mesenteric lymph node cells homing to gut associated lymphoid tissue in syngeneic mice. J. Immunol. *115*:54, 1975.

206. Reynolds, H. Y., and Johnson, J. S.: Canine immunoglobulins. IV. Coproimmunoglobulins. J. Immunol. *104*:888, 1970.

207. Vaerman, J. P., and Heremans, J. F.: Origin and molecular size of immunoglobulin-A in the mesenteric lymph of the dog. Immunology *18*:27, 1970.

208. Waldman, R. H., Virchow, C., and Rowe, D. S.: IgE levels in external secretions. Int. Arch. Allergy Appl. Immunol. *44*:242, 1973.

209. Brown, P. J., and Bourne, F. J.: Distributions of immunoglobulin containing cells in alimentary tract, spleen, and mesenteric lymph nodes of the pig demonstrated by peroxidase-conjugated antiserums to porcine immunoglobulins G, A, and M. Am. J. Vet. Res. *37*:9, 1976.

210. Vaerman, J. P., and Heremans, J. F.: Distribution of various immunoglobulin containing cells in canine lymphoid tissue. Immunology *17*:627, 1969.

211. Cripps, A. W., Husband, A. J., and Lascelles, A. K.: The origin of immunoglobulin in intestinal secretion of sheep. Aust. J. Exp. Biol. Med. Sci. *52*:711, 1974.

212. Lee, C. S., and Lascelles, A. K.: Antibody producing cells in antigenically stimulated mammary glands and in the gastrointestinal tract of sheep. Aust. J. Exp. Biol. Med. Sci. *48*:525, 1970.

213. Quin, J. W., Husband, A. J., and Lascelles, A. K.: The origin of the immunoglobulins in the intestinal lymph of sheep. Aust. J. Exp. Biol. Med. Sci. *53*:205, 1975.

214. Curtain, C. C., and Anderson, N. A.: Immunocytochemical localization of the ovine immunoglobulins IgA, IgG_1, IgG_{1A}, and IgG_2: effect of gastrointestinal parasitism in the sheep. Clin. Exp. Immunol. *8*:151, 1971.

215. Newby, T. J., and Bourne, F. J.: The nature of the local immune system of the bovine small intestine. Immunology *31*:475, 1976.

216. Curtain, C. C., Clark, B. L., and Duffy, J. H.: The origins of the immunoglobulins in the mucous secretions of cattle. Clin. Exp. Immunol. *8*:335, 1971.

217. Morrison, S. L., and Koshland, M. E.: Characterization of the J chain from polymeric immunoglobulins. Proc. Natl. Acad. Sci. *69*:124, 1972.

218. Poger, M. E., and Lamm, M. E.: Localization of free and bound secretory component in human intestinal epithelial cells. A model for the assembly of secretory IgA. J. Exp. Med. *139*:629, 1974.

219. Singer, S. J., and Nicolson, G. L.: The fluid mosaic model of the structure of cell membranes. Science *175*:720, 1972.

220. Walker, W. A., Isselbacher, K. J., and Block, K. J.: Intestinal uptake of macromolecules: effect of oral immunization. Science *177*:608, 1972.

221. Walker, W. A., Wu, M., Isselbacher, K. J., and Block, K. J.: Intestinal uptake of macromolecules. III. Studies on the mechanism by which immunization interferes with antigen uptake. J. Immunol. *115*:854, 1975.

Chapter 14

PATHOPHYSIOLOGY OF DIARRHEA

ROBERT A. ARGENZIO
SHANNON C. WHIPP

Diarrhea is defined as passage of feces containing an excess of water. While this description accurately defines the clinical condition, it is misleading from the outset as to the cause of diarrhea. It is now well established that all net water movement is secondary to net solute movement and the establishment of local or transmural osmotic gradients. No convincing evidence has been presented to date to implicate the contrary. Therefore, the ultimate cause of any diarrhea must be examined from the standpoint of (1) secretion of a solute in amounts which can reverse the normal absorptive process into one of net secretion, or (2) failure to absorb a solute which is normally transported by a specific mechanism.

Overwhelming evidence is now available which demonstrates conclusively that both the small and large intestine are capable of net secretion. The absorptive (or secretory) surface of the small bowel mucosa is so great (200 m² in man) that only a small net secretion, e.g., 1 μl/cm²/hr, would result in a net volume of 48 liters delivered to the colon in 24 hours. Such massive secretory diarrheas are not uncommon in man or animals. Intestinal absorptive failure can also result in large fecal volumes.

Although primary concern has recently been directed to secretory mechanisms of the small bowel mucosa, the fact is that large volumes of endogenous secretions are presented to the intestine for absorption. This is particularly true of herbivores, as was discussed in Chapter 12. Thus, the 100-kg pony must reabsorb the fluid equivalent of 40% of its own weight during a 24-hour period.

While endogenous secretion depends in part on whether the animal is eating, large volumes are still secreted during fasting. In fact, secretion by the salivary glands, pancreas, and liver continues whether or not the animal has diarrhea and whether or not the fluids are sequestered in the lumen due to obstruction. Therefore, it can readily be calculated, from the figures presented in Chapter 12, that complete failure of the distal intestine of the pony to absorb these endogenous secretions would result in death within 12 hours, due to severe contraction of the plasma volume and drastic reduction in arterial pressure.

Large fluxes of solute and water traverse the intestinal mucosa in opposite directions, while the net flux is usually a relatively small component of these two opposing undirectional fluxes. The net flux, however, must be driven by a force, whether active or passive. Passive driving forces in the intestine include electrical and chemical potentials, and osmotic or hydrostatic pressure gradients across the mucosa. Therefore, changes in passive driving forces effecting small changes in the large bidirectional fluxes may result in large changes or reversal of the net flux. The active forces are due to active solute transport processes within the epithelial cell itself, and these are primarily responsible for the net absorptive flux under normal conditions. Thus, the pathogenesis of fluid loss can be examined from the standpoint of passive driving forces and active driving forces.

FLUID LOSS BY PASSIVE MECHANISMS

There are three mechanisms by which fluid can be lost from the intestine as a result of altered passive driving forces. These are (1) permeability changes, (2) osmotic diarrhea, and (3) deranged intestinal motility.

Permeability Changes

The normal passive permeability of the intestinal mucosa to ions and water depends to a large degree on the region of bowel. The jejunum is a high conductance epithelium with very little resistance to passive movements of certain small ions and water. Although the Na⁺ pump at the baso-lateral border of the epithelial cell works against a steep electrochemical gradient, the process is inefficient because Na⁺ leaks back into the lumen.[1] However, this recirculation of Na⁺ normally accomplishes two purposes. First, active transport processes which

220

are coupled to Na^+ for transcellular transport, e.g., Cl^-, glucose, amino acids, are ensured of a continuous driving force for the carriers. Second, these actively transported solutes induce a net water flow which may transport additional small solutes across the permeable mucosa by solvent drag.[2]

It is now well established that the major, if not the sole, pathway for passive Na^+ movement from blood to lumen is via the extracellular shunt pathway (e.g., lateral intercellular spaces and tight junctions).[1] This passage is cation selective and while Cl^- passage is thereby restricted, Na^+ moves freely through the channel. Thus, the small electrical potential across the small bowel mucosa augments the leak of Na^+ from blood to lumen while Cl^- is conserved.

In contrast to the small bowel, the epithelium of the colon is normally so tight that even Na^+ backflux is restricted. Osmotic equilibration is also much slower in the colon than in the small bowel. Thus, Na^+ is conserved by the colon, and impressive electrochemical and osmotic gradients across colonic mucosa can be established.[2]

From these considerations, it is readily apparent that permeability changes will have markedly different effects depending on the region of bowel that is damaged.

Reduced permeability of the mucosa results from a loss in surface area, e.g., loss of villi or selective damage to the brush border. The brush border carriers are primarily responsible for transcellular permeability. A reduction in permeability of the extracellular pathway, e.g., by cell swelling (anisotonic solutions) or fusion of the lateral membranes, results in decreased passive permeability. Therefore, the manifestations of reduced permeability will largely depend on which pathway is involved as well as the segment of bowel.

In the proximal small bowel, a reduction in surface area, e.g., transmissible gastroenteritis of pigs, results in malabsorption.[3] A reduction in hydrolysis of disaccharides and decreased active transport of solutes by the brush border enzymes may be primarily responsible. On the other hand, the influence of solvent drag may be lost in the presence of increased resistance through the extracellular shunt pathway. This effect is also associated with other diseases characterized by villus atrophy, illustrating that the remaining mucosa is not normal.[2]

A gross reduction in colonic surface area, e.g., lymphosarcoma and granulomatous colitis, results in a decrease in transcellular ion and water absorption. Thus, decreased permeability of either the small or large intestine can result in malabsorption of ions and water. In the proximal small bowel, malabsorption of carbohydrates, proteins, and fats can also be expected to contribute to the diarrheal fluid.

Increased transcellular permeability may be associated with damage to the mucosal cell membranes, and it has recently been suggested that the diarrhea associated with hydroxylated long-chain fatty acids may in part be due to this mechanism.[4] These fatty acids are capable of inducing diarrhea in both the small and large bowel. The tight junctions of the small bowel do not appear to be damaged, and the pathway of fluid loss seems more likely to be transcellular. While it is apparent that membrane damage could effectively reduce absorption, frank net secretion is present in the isolated, perfused small bowel lumen and, therefore, a driving force other than osmotic pressure must be present. Since the electrochemical gradients across the small bowel are not sufficient to induce massive net secretion, an alternative driving force may be the capillary or tissue hydrostatic pressure, although recent evidence suggests that an active secretion is present.[5]

Increased permeability of the tight junctions or cell membranes with accompanying fluid secretion could intuitively be expected to result from invasive bacterial and enteric viral diseases. This is not always the case and other mechanisms for many of these infectious diarrheas must be sought. The presence of blood or protein in the diarrheal fluid suggests an exudative process with gross damage to the epithelium. However, more subtle changes are probably common and these will be examined from the standpoint of driving forces.

Increased extracellular permeability is thought to be associated with intraluminal bile acids and the observed fluid loss may be due in part to increased permeability of the tight junctions.[6] These permeability changes would theoretically be more pronounced in the colon owing to the normally tight epithelium and the large transepithelial driving forces which are present. Thus, the presence of 3 mM deoxycholate in the colonic lumen abolishes the steep concentration gradient for Na^+ and Cl^-. Massive net Na^+ secretion occurs and this appears to be due to diffusion of Na^+ through damaged tight junctions. Therefore, not only is the normally effective net Na^+ absorption abolished, but also net Na^+ secretion is elicited due to the concentration and electrical gradients which exist. Secretion could be expected to continue until these gradients themselves are attenuated. However, even in the absence of electrochemical gradients, net secretion continues and while this may be a result of the tissue hydrostatic pressure, it is more likely the result of an active secretory process.

Tissue Pressure as a Mechanism for Intestinal Secretion. Under normal conditions, the filtration coefficient of the membrane is far too low to account for large secretory flows driven by hydrostatic pressure gradients. However, when the existing inter- and extracellular channels are open, as in the preceding cases, hydrostatic pressure may be high enough to cause secretion. Furthermore, it is now known that elevated tissue pressure can, of itself, bring about dramatic increases in mucosal permeability.[7]

Capillary dynamics are contrasted with two pairs of intestinal cells in Figure 14–1. The cells on the left are normal and absorbing NaCl and water. In this case, the hydrostatic pressure of the intercellular channel is high because of the Na^+ pumping and tight junctions, and this pressure effectively opposes the hydrostatic tissue pressure and forces fluid across the basement membrane into the capillary. While the absorptive mechanisms of the opposite set of cells are also normal, the effective hydrostatic pressure of the intercellular channel is abolished because of the wide open tight junctions. Therefore, net absorption is difficult or impossible.[8]

In order for net secretion to occur via this mechanism, the tissue colloid osmotic pressure must become negligible in opposing secretion. This may occur if the epithelial channels are large enough to allow protein to move freely. Dilution of the tissue colloid osmotic pressure by the transcapillary filtrate and the intestinal absorbate occurs, but this augments removal by the capillary rather than increasing the tissue hydrostatic pressure. Thus, in the absence of gross increases in permeability it is difficult to see how significant net secretion can occur under conditions of normal tissue pressure, although net absorption can effectively be abolished.

It is also evident from Figure 14–1 that a number of conditions such as arteriolar dilation, increased capillary permeability (inflammation), raised venous pressure, lymphatic obstruction, extracellular volume expansion, or decreased plasma colloid osmotic pressure may increase the net capillary filtration and thereby may increase the tissue hydrostatic pressure.[7,9,10] In fact, elevation of the venous pressure sufficient to raise the tissue pressure to only 4 or 5 cm H_2O not only elicits secretion but also produces an increase in the permeability of the membrane to molecules as large as the plasma proteins.[7] Therefore, it should be kept in mind that any disorder affecting fluid dynamics in the capillary and subepithelial fluid compartment may well alter fluid transport by the intestinal mucosa.

Osmotic Diarrhea

Osmotic diarrhea can be caused by (1) the presence of nonabsorbable solutes in the gut lumen or (2) intraluminal production of osmotically active particles. Either of these conditions can theoretically result in tremendous driving forces for water movement, but these forces are considerably modified by the hydraulic conductivity of the epithelium.

Nonabsorbable Solutes. If a membrane is strictly impermeable to a solute but freely permeable to water, even small differences in concentration across the membrane are capable of producing large pressure gradients. For example, if the concentration of an impermeable solute on side one of the membrane was 0.25 M and that on side two 0.3 M, the driving force for water movement from side one to side two would be 912 mm Hg. However, if the membrane was equally permeable to the solute as to water, the osmotic driving pressure would be zero.[11]

From these considerations, it is apparent that while the measured luminal osmotic pressure may be equal to or even less than the plasma, its effective osmotic pressure may, in fact, be far greater than the plasma if the solutes of the fluid are less permeable than those of plasma. The reverse is likewise true. Thus, if the measured osmolality of a $MgSO_4$ solution were 300 mOsm, it would act as a bulk cathartic due not only to retention of its

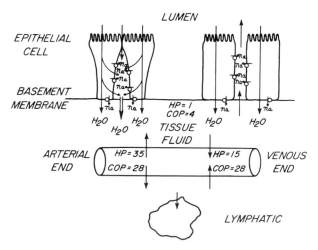

Figure 14–1. Effect of increased extracellular permeability on net absorption by intestinal epithelial cells. (Modified from Rummel and Wanitschke.[8] Values of hydrostatic (HP) and colloid osmotic pressures (COP) are from Guyton, 1966.)

osmotic equivalent of water, but also to net solute and water movement from blood to lumen.

The osmotic pressure of luminal contents can be raised by two mechanisms. The first is by microbial breakdown of large particles, e.g., starch, in the forestomach or large intestine to smaller particles, e.g., VFA.[12] Second, enzymatic hydrolysis of carbohydrates and proteins in the proximal intestine results in an increase in the number of osmotically active particles.

Referring back to the typical fermentation balance cited in Chapter 12 (57.5 glucose $\rightarrow$ 65 acetic acid + 20 propionic acid + 15 butyric acid + 60 CO_2 + 35 CH_4 + H_2O), it can be seen that the microbial fermentation of glucose immediately raises the theoretical osmotic pressure approximately threefold. However, a number of additional considerations must be taken into account. First, the production of CO_2 does not appreciably raise the effective osmotic pressure in the lumen since CO_2 is rapidly absorbed. Second, the HCO_3^- buffer system reacts immediately with the organic acids via the following reaction: $NaHCO_3 + HA \rightarrow NaA + CO_2 + H_2O$. Thus, the effective osmotic pressure of the solution is, in fact, reduced by the buffer system since an anion (HCO_3^-) with restricted permeation characteristics is converted to CO_2. Third, the normal mucosa of the rumen and large intestine is highly permeable to VFA and as the VFA are absorbed, HCO_3^- accumulates once again in the lumen.

These factors indicate that as long as sufficient HCO_3^- buffer is present and the membrane remains permeable to CO_2 and VFA, establishment of the full theoretical osmotic pressure is impossible at any rate of acid production. This is not true of the phosphate buffer system. Thus, it is fortunate that the HCO_3^- to $PO_4^{\equiv}$ ratio of ruminant saliva is directly proportional to salivary flow; i.e., high rates of salivary flow are associated with increased HCO_3^- concentration.

Luminal Acidification. Obviously, an overproduction of fermentation products may far exceed the capacity of the HCO_3^- buffer system and result in luminal acidification and hyperosmolality. As the pH decreases and approaches the pK of the organic acids, a number of sequential events are brought about.[13] The VFA-producing organisms are destroyed and replaced by lactic acid bacteria, which thrive at a low pH. Lactic acid itself is absorbed at a low pH, as are the other organic acids, but far less rapidly than CO_2 and at only one tenth the rate of VFA. The acidification also damages the epithelium leading to increased permeability and rapid solute

and water movement from blood to the lumen. Partial buffering results in the formation of sodium salts of D- and L-lactate, which are even less well absorbed than lactic acid. Thus, once the VFA are replaced by lactate, the effective osmotic pressure increases dramatically.

These conditions are commonly brought about by an overload of rapidly fermentable carbohydrate to the rumen or large intestine. The situation in the rumen is almost entirely due to grain engorgement. Lactic acid production, hyperosmolality, and acidification result and these effects may overwhelm the intestine provoking an osmotic diarrhea.

The cause of osmotic diarrhea in the large intestine can also result from an overload of dietary carbohydrate. However, a far more important situation is due to malabsorption of digested carbohydrate by the small intestine, and delivery of large amounts of carbohydrate to the large intestine.

Osmosis Due to Malabsorption. Enzymatic hydrolysis in the lumen of the small bowel results in the production of disaccharides, long-chain fatty acids, and peptides. Of these, only carbohydrate malabsorption is clinically important in the pathogenesis of osmotic diarrhea. Long-chain fatty acids, even when ionized, are insoluble in water and an alternative mechanism must be postulated for the diarrhea associated with steatorrhea.[14]

In the case of carbohydrate, three stages occur prior to absorption into the mucosal cell, each of which may be responsible for osmotic pressure production. The first is pancreatic enzyme hydrolysis of starch into smaller saccharides in the bulk lumen contents, which raises the theoretical osmotic pressure. Second, disaccharidases in the brush border further increase the osmolality by splitting the disaccharides into monosaccharides, and finally the monosaccharides are transported into the cell.

Of the primary disorders of carbohydrate or protein digestion, only disaccharidase deficiency seems to be of major importance in malabsorption-induced osmotic diarrhea. Glucose-galactose malabsorption appears to be a rare disease, at least in man, and enterokinase deficiency is also of infrequent occurrence.[14] Obviously, any mucosal disease of the small bowel may secondarily result in malabsorption owing to damage or loss of the brush border and its enzymes.

In the normal situation, the effective osmotic pressure of intestinal contents is not appreciably raised by pancreatic or brush border hydrolysis owing to the rapid absorption of the monosaccharides by the transport carriers.[2] However, if disaccharidase deficiency is present, absorption by the carriers is impossible and these disaccharides, therefore, are capable of exerting their full theoretical osmotic pressure. Thus, carbohydrate malabsorption can induce diarrhea in four ways. First, by exerting an osmotic pressure in the lumen, disaccharides retain an osmotic equivalent of water. Second, they prevent the absorption of other solutes which are normally absorbed by solvent drag or coupled to active transport systems, e.g., Na^+, and these solutes also retain an osmotic equivalent of water. Third, the increase in effective osmotic pressure of the disaccharides and nonabsorbed solutes may initiate bulk solute and water flow from blood to lumen, and fourth, the disaccharides are fermented in the colon and may overwhelm the colonic buffering capacity.

Aside from congenital disaccharidase deficiency, the development of these enzymes also depends to a large degree on the age of the animal and adaptation to the presence of substrate. Therefore, it would not seem surprising that many of the diarrheas in young animals, or in adult animals subjected to abrupt dietary changes, can be directly attributed to disaccharidase deficiency.

Although the mechanisms of fluid losses during viral diarrheas have not been clearly defined, the best evidence available at the present time suggests that passive mechanisms are involved. It is known, for example, that activity of adenyl cyclase in intestinal mucosal cells is unchanged by infection with the Norwalk agent,[15] transmissible gastroenteritis (TGE) virus,[16] or human rotavirus (HRV).[17] The enteritis viruses tend to cause selective damage to the intestinal epithelium[18] (Fig. 14–2). The character and the severity of the digestive and malabsorptive defects induced will vary with the agent because of the characteristic predilection for certain areas of the intestinal epithelium. Thus, although there is no evidence for active secretory mechanisms, absorptive defects accompany infection with some viral agents. A defect in glucose-mediated sodium absorption has been identified in the jejunum of pigs infected with TGE virus.[19] Decreased activity of Na-K-ATPase and several brush border enzymes has been reported.[20,21] Selective destruction of the villous epithelium without damage to crypt epithelium results in an increased rate of migration of crypt cells up the villus. The enzymic changes that occur are compatible with repopulation of the villus with relatively immature crypt cells.[21] Thus, these changes result in a malabsorptive state which may lead to an osmotic and fermentative diarrhea.

Deranged Intestinal Motility

Although primary disorders of motility have long been thought to be of major concern in the pathogenesis of diarrhea, it is now abundantly clear that this assumption is no longer tenable.[22] Increased intestinal transit cannot, except for one specific instance discussed next, result in an increase in the luminal volume. On the other hand, motility plays an important role secondary to increased luminal volumes brought about by other specific causes. Thus, treating the symptoms of increased motility may well aggravate the primary cause of diarrhea.

Furthermore, increased motor activity cannot, in many instances, be equated with an increase in intestinal transit, thereby complicating the situation further. This is particularly true of colonic motor activity, which displays a combination of propulsive, segmental, and antiperistaltic activity. Therefore, it is far more useful to examine the consequences of deranged intestinal transit first and then, when possible, relate these to primary motor dysfunction.

Increased Gastric Emptying. An abnormal increase in the rate of delivery of hypertonic gastric contents to the proximal small bowel can be expected to result in osmotic movement of water from blood to the lumen. This condition, known as the dumping syndrome, is usually a complication following gastric or duodenal surgery including vagotomy and pyloroplasty.[23] The increased luminal volumes provoke small bowel motility via the peristaltic reflex

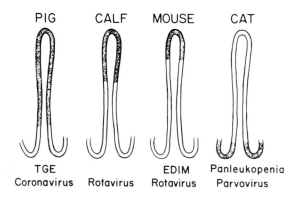

PIG   CALF   MOUSE   CAT

TGE   EDIM   Panleukopenia
Coronavirus   Rotavirus   Rotavirus   Parvovirus

Figure 14–2. Predilection for different parts of intestinal epithelium among different viruses. The coronavirus of TGE infects villous epithelium and spares crypt epithelium. The rotaviruses of calves and mice infect only the most mature villous epithelium. In contrast, the parvovirus of feline panleukopenia infects only the immature, proliferating crypt epithelium. EDIM = Epizootic diarrhea of infant mice. (From Moon.[18])

and often result in diarrhea. In some instances, the amount of fluid lost seriously compromises the blood volume and promotes vasomotor reflexes. However, it is now known that vasomotor symptoms are also precipitated by the release of vasoactive substances from the intestinal mucosa. The release of these agents appears to be due to the presence of hypertonic glucose solutions in the proximal small bowel.

Increased Small Bowel Transit. An increase in the rate of small bowel transit cannot, by itself, produce an increase in luminal volume. Although net absorption may be reduced owing to insufficient mucosal contact time, the relation between transit and absorption has not been well documented. It is known from perfusion studies that as the rate of flow along the intestine increases, the percentage of water absorbed decreases and the absolute volume required to produce diarrhea decreases.[14] In addition, a decrease in absorption alone has a similar effect because of the large volumes of endogenous secretions.

Specific causes of increased small bowel motility have been even less well studied. While it has been suggested that bacterial enterotoxins as well as invasive bacteria stimulate small bowel motility,[24] the effects of these agents on ion transport mechanisms and possibly on intestinal permeability are of far greater importance. If increased motility does, in fact, occur as a primary event, it would appear to offer a protective mechanism to the small bowel mucosa.

Decreased Small Bowel Transit. This abnormality may result in local stasis which is conducive to bacterial growth. Conditions that promote bacterial overgrowth in the small bowel, e.g., diverticula, partial obstructions, ileocecal reflux, or primary hypomotility are collectively known as the blind- or stagnant-loop syndrome.[25] In addition, the stasis may allow pathogens to proliferate.

Abnormal bacterial overgrowth in the small bowel can provoke diarrhea in two ways. First, certain bacteria are capable of hydrolyzing conjugated bile acids, which results in fat malabsorption. Second, these bacterial or colonic bacteria can hydroxylate fatty acids, which are known to evoke diarrhea either by mucosal damage or by alteration of ion transport mechanisms, or both.

While the causes of primary small bowel hypomotility are obscure, it is known that scleroderma of man produces pseudo-obstruction of the bowel by decreasing motor activity.[26] Furthermore, surgical procedures, e.g., vagotomy, or resections that disrupt the normal slow wave propagation can be expected to alter small bowel motility and decrease small bowel transit.

Increased Colonic Transit. The prime functions of the colon are (1) reabsorption of electrolytes and water, and (2) microbial digestion, both of which depend to a large degree on delayed colonic transit. Absorption studies in the goat[27] and horse[28,29] have provided preliminary evidence of the relation between transit and absorption. First, osmotic equilibration between actively transported solutes and passive water flow is extremely slow due to the tight colonic epithelium. Second, as the rate of flow along the colon increases, the percentage of solutes and water absorbed decreases, as would be expected, and proportionately more H_2O is delivered in the feces. Third, normal microbial digestion is necessary for efficient colonic absorption of solute and water, and this is impossible in the face of markedly increased transit.

The normal colonic digestive cycle in the horse fed twice daily is characterized by high luminal volumes during 8 of the 12 hours between meals. Only during the last 4 hours does significant net absorption take place. Thus, a mean fluid transit time of approximately 2 days is featured in the large intestine of this species. Therefore, increased colonic transit will likely be characterized by maldigestion, malabsorption, and diarrhea.

Unfortunately, specific causes of deranged colonic motility in animal species are largely unidentified. In man, the irritable colon syndrome,[30] an apparent motor abnormality, is characterized by a loss of segmental resistance, which is entirely consistent with the view that hypomotility, rather than hypermotility, of the colon is associated with diarrhea.

FLUID LOSS BY ACTIVE MECHANISMS

Studies on the pathogenesis of cholera in man focused attention on the mammalian small intestine as a secretory organ. Through those studies it has become apparent that the ability to secrete, i.e., induce net transfer of electrolytes and water from blood to gut lumen, is a normal characteristic of the small intestine and colon. In fact, it has been suggested that net fluid and electrolyte secretion may be the natural functional state of the nonruminant herbivore. If true, this should focus attention on the colon of the horse as a prime candidate for diarrheagenic mechanisms since the horse is a highly developed non-ruminant herbivore. Whether more than one secretory mechanism is operational in the small intestine and colon is not known. It is known that a variety of bacterial exotoxins, gastrointestinal hormones, and other agents are capable of stimulating intestinal secretion.[31,32] Since diarrhea results when the rate of intestinal secretion exceeds the capacity to reabsorb, agents capable of stimulating intestinal secretion are potentially diarrheagenic. The only well-defined intestinal transport system known to elicit active secretion of electrolytes and water does so via activation of the enzyme adenyl cyclase.[33,34] Accordingly, this system will be discussed in detail before considering secretory diarrheal syndromes.

Cyclic adenosine monophosphate (cAMP) functions as an intracellular "second messenger" mediating the effects of a large number of hormones in a variety of cell types. More recently, activity of this messenger has been shown to be affected by a variety of bacterial exotoxins, particularly in intestinal mucosa. Physiologically, intracellular concentrations of cAMP are modulated by enzyme activity, being increased by adenyl cyclase and decreased by specific nucleotide phosphodiesterase.[33] Adenyl cyclase is located in the cell membrane. Receptors through which agents activate adenyl cyclase are located on the exterior surface of the cell membrane. Part of the specificity of cellular response to different hormones resides in the binding specificity of these receptors. Activated adenyl cyclase increases intracellular conversion of adenosine triphosphate (ATP) to cAMP, which activates a class of enzymes known as protein kinases. Activation occurs through binding of cAMP to a regulatory subunit freeing the catalytic portion of the protein kinase. The activated kinase phosphorylates endogenous substrates, which in turn elicit the physiologic responses. In this chain of events, there are several steps at which toxic or pharmacologic intervention can theoretically induce intestinal secretion and diarrhea. To date, the only step that has been well defined as a bacterial diarrheagenic mechanism is the activation of adenyl cyclase.

In the case of intestinal epithelia, one of the physiologic responses elicited by a rise in cAMP is net secretion of electrolytes from blood to gut lumen. This is achieved primarily by active secretion of Cl^- with an associated passive net secretion of Na^+. Since small intestinal absorption and secretion tend to be isosmotic with the fluid of origin, net electrolyte secretion is accompanied by appropriate water movement from blood to gut. This mechanism does not appear to involve impaired Na^+ absorption by either the active Na^+ pump in the lateral or serosal membrane or facilitated transport involving non-electrolytes.

Although the interrelationships are not clear at this time, there is evidence suggesting an active electrolyte secretory mechanism which does not involve adenyl cyclase. Secretion can be induced with a compound known to stimulate the entry of Ca^{++} into mucosal cells; Ca^{++} ionophore A23187.[35] Similarly the "non-cAMP" intestinal secretogogues, serotonin and acetylcholine, induce an increase in intracellular Ca^{++}. These three agents have also been associated with increased intracellular cyclic guanosine monophosphate (cGMP) in other tissues. More recently, secretion induced by the heat-stable enterotoxin of enteropathogenic *Escherichia coli* has also been associated with increased intracellular cGMP.[36] Thus, evidence for a mechanism is emerging which may explain the action of "non-cAMP" secretogogues.

Secretory Diarrhea of Bacterial Origin

Several enteric bacteria release exotoxins, termed enterotoxins, which are capable of stimulating active secretion by the small intestine. *Vibrio cholerae* causes an acute, fulminating diarrhea in man and does so in the absence of any apparent pathologic change in the intestine.[34] Since the enterotoxin of *V. cholerae*, choleragen, is the most thoroughly studied and is the classic example of a pure "secretory" diarrhea, it is useful as a model with which to compare other bacterial enterotoxins. Cholera toxin (CT) is a protein enterotoxin (MW 84,000) which binds to mucosal receptors in the brush border with high affinity and results in activation of adenyl cyclase. Its activity is characterized by a delayed onset of action and a prolonged duration of action. After exposure of small intestinal mucosa to CT, decreased net absorption can be detected within 30 to 60 minutes but maximum secretion is not observed until 3 or 4 hours. The delayed onset of action is thought to be related to dissociation of a toxin subunit from the catalytic site of the adenyl cyclase complex at the intracellular surface of the cell membrane. The delayed onset of secretion correlates well with activation of adenyl cyclase and increased cAMP concentrations. Furthermore, *in vitro* studies of electrolyte transport changes induced by CT mimic the effects of cAMP on ileal mucosa. Although the primary effect is activation of an active Cl^- secretory system, the net effect *in vivo* is net secretion of Na^+, HCO_3^-, and water into the intestinal lumen. Quantitatively, this mechanism is capable of stimulating fluid losses totaling up to 20% of the body weight in 24 hours. The obvious result is rapid dehydration, acidosis, and death.

One other characteristic of CT deserves mention. Most of the hormone-adenyl cyclase interactions are characterized by a high degree of specificity. In contrast, CT is quite promiscuous in its ability to mate with cell-surface receptors activating adenyl cyclase. It stimulates adenyl cyclase in adrenal tissue, fat cells, ovary, platelets, thymocytes, thyroid, and several other tissues. In each case it evokes the response characteristic of the tissue, e.g., steroidogenesis in adrenal tissue. It appears that CT is not absorbed from the gastrointestinal tract, however, so the intestinal affect appears to be the only one of significance in the pathogenesis of cholera in humans.

Enterotoxigenic *Escherichia coli* (ETEC) strains are of more immediate veterinary interest since they induce neonatal diarrhea in a number of animal species as well as neonatal and adult humans.[37] ETEC's are known to produce two types of enterotoxins capable of inducing an acute fulminating diarrhea in the neonate. Both appear to do so by stimulating an active intestinal secretory system and like CT, they do so in the absence of any detectable lesions in the intestinal mucosa.

One type of ETEC enterotoxin, heat-labile toxin or LT, is characterized as a large molecular weight, immunogenic compound which loses its biologic activity when heated to 100° C for 15 minutes. The second type, heat-stable toxin or ST, is characterized as a small molecular weight, non-immunogenic compound which does not lose its biologic activity after heating to 100° C for 15 minutes.

Since LT and ST have only recently been purified, most studies on the physiopathology induced by these two enterotoxins have been done with crude preparations. However, several valid points can be made about their activities. In general, LT follows the pattern of CT, whereas ST does not, although both induce an active intestinal secretion.

The host response evoked by ST differs from that evoked by LT and CT in several respects.

1. ST is characterized by a rapid onset and a short duration of action whereas LT, like CT, has a delayed onset and a prolonged duration of action.

2. LT, like CT, tends to be ubiquitous in its ability to activate adenyl cyclase in that it does so in several extraintestinal tissues, whereas ST is not known to have any extraintestinal biologic activity.

3. The secretory response to LT, like CT, can be correlated with a rise in adenyl cyclase activity in intestinal mucosa. In contrast, attempts to demonstrate a rise in intestinal adenyl cyclase activity in tissues stimulated with ST have failed. However,

recent evidence suggests that the secretory effects of ST may involve cGMP.[36]

4. The binding characteristics of the two ETEC toxins differ. Although LT is rapidly bound by pig and rabbit ileal mucosa, binding of ST to intestinal mucosal components has not been demonstrated. However, it should be further noted that the binding characteristics of LT differ also from those of CT. Finally, there is marked species variation in responsiveness of intestinal mucosa to these two toxins. Pig jejunum tends to be relatively more sensitive to the effects of ST than to those of LT, whereas rabbit jejunum tends to be more responsive to LT than to ST. Conversely, the infant mouse responds to ST but not to LT. These differences may reflect specificities of receptor-enterotoxin interactions as well as activation of different secretory mechanisms.

Although the literature of veterinary medicine has described no other diarrheal syndromes which have a well-defined intestinal secretory component, such descriptions are to be anticipated. Enterotoxins capable of stimulating intestinal secretion have been described from a variety of enteric bacteria. These include *Clostridium perfringens* type A, *Enterobacter cloacae*,[38] *Klebsiella pneumoniae*,[39] *Bacillus cereus*,[40] *Shigella flexneri, Shigella dysenteriae*,[31,41] and *Salmonella enteriditis*.[42] There has also been one report of a diarrhea-producing toxin obtained from a blue-green algae, *Microcystis aeruginosa*.[43] The latter observation is pertinent since *Microcystis* is widely distributed in water sources.

Of the enterotoxins other than CT and the ETEC toxins, only those from *Bacillus cereus, Clostridium perfringens*, and *Shigella dysenteriae* have been reported to activate adenyl cyclase. However, infection of rabbit ileal loops with *Salmonella typhimurium*[44] has been reported to result in secretion with an associated rise in adenyl cyclase activity and cAMP concentrations. Although the studies on the pathogenesis of shigellosis and salmonellosis have been done with pathogenic isolates obtained from diarrheal disease in man,[31,44,45] these studies have important significance for veterinary medicine. First, in contrast to the cholera and *E. coli* models, the pathogenesis of these two diseases involves colonic secretion as well as secretion by the small intestine. For reasons discussed previously, the concept of colonic secretion may have particular significance in non-ruminant herbivores. Second, both of these diseases are associated with invasion and destruction of the mucosal epithelium. Nevertheless, attempts to demonstrate altered permeability and passive fluid losses as the mechanisms involved in the pathogenesis of the associated diarrhea have failed. Despite the obvious tissue damage, it appears that the primary mechanism involved in the fluid losses observed with these diseases is an active secretion from the colon. Similar mechanisms should be considered in the pathogenesis of infectious diseases associated with colitis in domestic animals.

Secretory Diarrhea of Endocrine Origin

Recently, several gastrointestinal hormones have been reported to be capable of stimulating intestinal secretion or inhibiting intestinal absorption. These include secretin, calcitonin, glucagon, gastrin, vasoactive intestinal polypeptide, and gastric inhibitory polypeptide, among others.[46-48] Although the mechanisms and physiologic significance of these actions are poorly defined at this time, this concept has obvious implications relative to control of absorption and secretion. It also furnishes another potentially diarrheagenic mechanism. This mechanism has been implicated in the watery diarrhea associated with a variety of pancreatic and non-pancreatic tumors. In this case, it appears that vasoactive intestinal polypeptide is the agent and that it is mediating its effects through the cyclic AMP system.

Another class of agents involved is the prostaglandins. Some of these derivatives of arachidonic acid are also capable of stimulating intestinal secretion. These provide a diarrheagenic mechanism which has been implicated as causing the watery diarrhea associated with medullary carcinoma of the thyroid, which induces high circulating levels of prostaglandins. These compounds also stimulate secretion via the cAMP system. In addition to intestinal secretion secondary to ectopic tumor secretion, these systems provide another potential mechanism for microbial stimulation of secretory diarrhea. For example, the intestinal secretion associated with salmonellosis appears to be mediated by prostaglandin stimulation of adenyl cyclase.

SYSTEMIC EFFECTS OF DIARRHEA

The relative amount of solute to water lost to the bowel as well as the specific electrolyte losses depends on the pathogenesis of the diarrhea and the transport processes which are involved. The problem of fluid balance can be categorized from the pathogenetic factors known at present into (1) isotonic fluid loss, or (2) hypotonic fluid loss. The problem of acid-base equilibrium depends on intestinal, renal, and skeletal muscle transport processes associated with Na^+, H^+, Cl^-, HCO_3^-, and K^+.

Solute and Water Depletion. Active secretory processes as well as secretory filtration (due to hydrostatic pressure gradients), inhibition of absorption, and increased intestinal transit can, for all practical purposes, be classified under isotonic fluid loss. Active solute secretion, at least in the small intestine, is accompanied by an approximately isotonic equivalent of water. Similarly, inhibited absorption, whether due to permeability changes, specific transport processes, or an increased rate of intestinal transit, prevents the absorption of isotonic secretions delivered into the proximal small bowel.

On the other hand, an osmotic diarrhea may elicit water movement from the plasma in greater proportion than solute, resulting in a hypotonic fluid loss. The type of fluid loss and fluid shifts in the body also depend on whether the animal is eating or drinking. For example, ingested water may be retained owing to an increased secretion of antidiuretic hormones.[2]

An isotonic fluid loss into the bowel lumen depletes the extracellular compartment alone. Serum Na^+ and osmolality may be normal, but serum protein and hematocrit are increased unless an exudative process is present. The decreased blood pressure may cause the glomerular filtration rate to drop and volume receptors elicit the secretion of aldosterone, which augments Na^+ reabsorption in an attempt to bring the extracellular volume back to normal.

In contrast, loss of proportionally more water than solute from the extracellular fluid into the gut causes a shift of water from the intracellular to extracellular compartment until osmotic equilibration is achieved. In this case, serum Na^+ and osmolality may be elevated. Osmoreceptors, as well as volume receptors, stimulate the release of antidiuretic hormone and aldosterone in an attempt to bring about normal osmolality and volume.

Thus, a patient may present with low, normal, or elevated serum osmolality depending on the pathogenesis of the diarrhea, the animal's opportunity to drink, and the degree of compensation which is present.

Changes in Acid-Base Equilibria. The plasma composition of normal calves and calves with diagnosed enteric colibacillosis[49,50] is shown in Table 14–1. A third group of calves with spontaneous diarrhea is also shown and, as will be discussed in the next section (Fecal Electrolyte Analysis), the pathogenesis of these two diarrheas is most likely of quite different origin. Despite the different mechanisms of the diarrhea, the acid-base status is remarkably similar. Thus, an extracellular acidosis is present,

Table 14–1. Plasma composition of normal and diarrheic calves

	Normal	E. coli* Diarrhea	Spontaneous† Diarrhea
Na⁺	143	138	134
K⁺	4.8	7.4	7.1
HCO₃⁻	26.4	13.7	10.1
pH	7.38	7.08	6.99
PCV	36.9	45	51.7
BUN	11.4	50.1	68

*From Tennant et al., 1972.[50]
†From Fisher and De la Fuente, 1972.[49]

and the increased hematocrit and BUN suggest hypovolemia and renal failure. The third feature common to both of these diarrheas is the elevation in plasma K⁺ concentration.

Extracellular acidosis is present in all the calves in the preceding example. The underlying causes of acidosis are complex and depend only in part on the pathogenetic mechanism involved.[50] Thus, secretion of HCO₃⁻ into the gut (*E. coli* diarrhea) or absorption of acid into the blood (fermentative diarrhea) both acidify the extracellular fluids and lower the plasma HCO₃⁻ concentration. Acidosis also can occur secondary to hypovolemia and decreased tissue perfusion of the skeletal muscle. In the face of O₂ lack, anaerobic metabolism of muscle becomes significant and lactic acid accumulates in the extracellular fluids. Furthermore, when renal failure is present, because of the low arterial pressure, H⁺ excretion by the renal tubules decreases. Therefore, a number of factors acting alone or in combination may participate in the development of acidosis.

Intracellular acidosis develops as a compensatory mechanism after an onset of extracellular acidosis. The elevated plasma K⁺ concentrations which are characteristic of hypovolemia and acidosis are believed to result, at least in part, from an exchange of extracellular H⁺ for intracellular K⁺ in skeletal muscle.[51] Thus, the intracellular muscle compartment acts as a buffer for the extracellular fluid, at the expense of hyperkalemia. Cardiotoxic effects occur when hyperkalemia is severe and may, in fact, be the ultimate cause of death in diarrhea-induced acidosis.

FECAL ELECTROLYTE ANALYSIS

Routine clinical diagnostic procedures will not be considered in this chapter. Rather, the use of fecal electrolyte analysis will be discussed. Although this procedure has yet to find practical use in veterinary

medicine, the rapidly expanding knowledge of intestinal pathophysiology suggests that fecal electrolyte analysis may become useful in diagnosis and treatment of particularly difficult cases.

Normal Composition of Feces. Figure 14–3 shows a fecal ionogram of a 160-kg pony and compares these values to the electrolyte composition of the plasma. Large variations, due to time after feeding, diet, and species, are present, and the values shown in the figure are useful from a descriptive standpoint only. For example, fecal PO₄⁼ concentrations are usually much lower in most species.

Composition of the feces is the end result of the overall processes of intestinal absorption and secretion. The values in Figure 14–3 indicate that the normal feces primarily reflect colonic function, except for the low Cl⁻ concentration which is brought about by the small bowel. Thus, steep concentration gradients are maintained between feces and plasma; a high K⁺ and low Cl⁻ and HCO₃⁻ are present. The major anions of feces are organic, derived primarily from bacterial metabolism of carbohydrate. Furthermore, the feces of the pony are approximately isotonic with plasma, but a pH of 6.5 is normal.[52]

Three aspects of normal feces require further consideration. First, the low HCO₃⁻ concentration suggests a minor loss of HCO₃⁻ in the feces. However, this low HCO₃⁻ is due to the reaction of

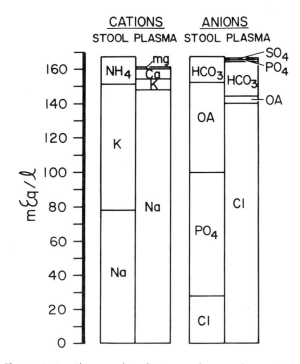

Figure 14–3. Plasma and stool ionogram for normal pony. (Values are from Dittmer[57] and Argenzio et al.[52])

organic acids with the HCO_3^- buffer system as discussed previously. Therefore, measurements of bicarbonate in feces are of no help in assessing HCO_3^- loss and acid-base balance. The value of $Na^+ + K^+ - Cl^-$ is of much greater value in determining the loss of base.[2] Second, the high concentrations of K^+ and $PO_4^{\equiv}$ which are present are not due to colonic secretion but are a result of the more rapid absorption of other solutes and water.[52] Therefore, these two ions are primarily of dietary origin. Third, the isotonicity of the feces is due in part to the prolonged large intestinal transit which allows osmotic equilibration between actively transported solutes and passive water absorption.

Electrolyte Changes in Feces During Diarrhea. Active secretory diarrheas of the small bowel, e.g., *E. coli* enterotoxin, are characterized by fluids which resemble the electrolyte composition of the particular segment involved.[53] Thus, it can be expected that as fecal volumes increase, the composition of the feces will approach that of the affected bowel. If the ileum is primarily involved, a higher HCO_3^- concentration is usually present. It is necessary to keep in mind that the pathophysiology of these secretory diarrheas has been primarily examined in man and dog and several laboratory animals. In adult animals, particularly the horse, sheep, goat, and pig, where colonic absorption has been shown to be of major significance, the fecal composition will also reflect the compensatory ability of the colon. For example, while the normal ileal outflow of a 70-kg goat is approximately 3 liters per day, perfusion studies indicate that the colon of this animal can absorb at least four times this amount.[20] Therefore, unless massive small bowel secretion is present, some compensation by a normal colon can be expected. If colonic transit is rapid, hypotonic stools may result.

Massive fluid losses are also present in diseases such as transmissible gastroenteritis of pigs or viral enteritis of calves.[54] These diseases are characterized by villus atrophy and fluid loss is presumably due to malabsorption and osmotic diarrhea rather than active secretion. Diarrheal feces resulting from carbohydrate malabsorption in man are characterized by hypertonicity and an acid pH due to metabolism of the unabsorbed carbohydrate by colonic bacteria. Similarly, grain overload in cattle is characterized by hyperosmolality and lactic acid in the feces. The use of indicator strips to estimate pH of fresh feces is a useful adjunct to the diagnostic workup.

Diarrhea associated with steatorrhea suggests colonic secretion secondary to unabsorbed bile acids and fatty acids. As previously indicated, the steep Na^+ and Cl^- concentrations across colonic mucosa are abolished and the fecal ionic composition may approach that of the plasma. If small bowel disease is responsible, osmotic diarrhea may be superimposed on colonic secretion.

Table 14–2 shows the electrolyte composition of feces from two groups of calves with spontaneous diarrhea. In a third group of calves, diarrhea was induced by sucrose feeding and in the fourth group, a diagnosis of primary enteric colibacillosis was made. The fifth and sixth columns of the table present data obtained from isolated jejunal loops of the calf and pig in which *E. coli* enterotoxin was introduced. In studies in which Cl^- was measured, HCO_3^- was estimated as $Na^+ + K^+ - Cl^-$. In the isolated loop studies, HCO_3^- was also measured directly and as can be seen, the two values are in good agreement.

The low Na^+ and Cl^- concentrations in the sucrose-fed calves and the low Na^+ concentration in the first group of calves with spontaneous diarrhea are entirely consistent with the presence of nonabsorbable, osmotically active solute in the gut lumen.

Table 14–2. Comparison of fecal electrolytes from diarrheic calves and intestinal fluid of calves and pigs in presence of *E. coli* enterotoxin

	Spontaneous* Diarrhea	Spontaneous† Diarrhea (Transmissible)	Sucrose† Feeding	*E. coli*‡ Diarrhea	Jejunal‡ Loop— Calf	Jejunal§ Loop— Pig
Na^+	42	146	97	122	148	147
K^+	13	14	31	16	11	5
Cl^-		96	8		95	103
$Na^+ + K^+ - Cl^-$		64	120		64	49
HCO_3^-					66	40

*From Fisher and De la Fuente, 1972.[49]
†From Lewis and Phillips, 1972.[55]
‡From Tennant et al., 1972.[50]
§From Moon et al., 1971.[56]

In striking contrast, the feces and secreted jejunal fluid of calves with colibacillosis and that of the second group of calves resemble the plasma, except for a HCO_3^- concentration approximately twice that of plasma. In further marked contrast between these two diarrheas, of obviously different pathogenetic origin, is the concentration of "HCO_3^-" in the feces.

The plasma electrolyte composition for the *E. coli* calves and the first group of calves with spontaneous diarrhea was also presented in Table 14–1. The plasma values give no indication of different pathogenetic mechanisms, although the fecal Na^+ concentrations strongly suggest quite different mechanisms. On the other hand, the feces of the second group of calves are almost identical to the jejunal loop fluid and feces of calves infected with enteropathogenic *E. coli*. This remarkable agreement, between two separate studies, points to a common pathogenesis, i.e., active small bowel secretion.

Since the pathophysiology of most diarrheas in animals has yet to be examined, further speculation at the present time is clearly unwarranted. At present, electrolyte analysis of feces cannot be considered for specific diagnostic use. Rather, it provides a tool for speculation as to the pathogenesis of diarrhea. As more diarrheal diseases are classified in terms of their pathophysiology, fecal analysis may become an important means of obtaining rapid and relatively inexpensive information for both diagnosis and treatment.

REFERENCES

1. Schultz, S. G.: Principles of electrophysiology and their application to epithelial tissues. International Review of Physiology. Gastrointestinal Physiology, Vol. 4. Edited by E. D. Jacobson and L. L. Shanbour. Baltimore, University Park Press, 1974, p. 69.
2. Fordtran, J. S.: Diarrhea. *In* Gastrointestinal Disease. Edited by M. H. Sleisenger and J. S. Fordtran. Philadelphia, W. B. Saunders Co., 1973, p. 291.
3. Kent, T. H., and Moon, H. W.: The comparative pathogenesis of some enteric diseases. Vet. Pathol. *10*:414, 1973.
4. Nell, G., Forth, W., Rummel, W., and Wanitschke, R.: Pathway of sodium moving from blood to intestinal lumen under the influence of oxyphenisatin and deoxycholate. Arch. Pharmacol. *293*:31, 1976.
5. Cline, W. S., Lorenzsonn, V., Benz, L., Buss, P., and Olsen, W. A.: The effects of sodium ricinoleate on small intestinal function and structure. J. Clin. Invest. *58*:380, 1976.
6. Bright-Asare, P., and Binder, H. J.: Stimulation of colonic secretion of water and electrolytes by hydroxy fatty acids. Gastroenterology *64*:81, 1973.
7. Yablonski, M. E., and Lifson, N.: Mechanism of production of intestinal secretion by elevated venous pressure. J. Clin. Invest. *57*:904, 1976.
8. Rummel, W., Nell, G., and Wanitschke, R.: Action mechanisms of antiabsorptive and hydragogue drugs. *In* Intestinal Absorption and Malabsorption. Edited by T. Z. Csaky. New York, Raven Press, 1975, p. 209.
9. Guyton, A. C.: Medical Physiology, 2nd ed. Philadelphia, W. B. Saunders Co., 1966.
10. Granger, D. N., Mortillaro, N. A., and Taylor, A. E.: Interactions of intestinal lymph flow and secretion. Am. J. Physiol. *232*:E13, 1977.
11. Fordtran, J. S., and Locklear, T. W.: Ionic constituents and osmolality of gastric and small intestinal fluids after eating. Am. J. Dig. Dis. *11*:503, 1966.
12. Bond, J. H., Jr., and Levitt, M. D.: Fate of soluble carbohydrate in the colon of rats and man. J. Clin. Invest. *57*:1158, 1976.
13. Dunlop, R. H.: Discussion of paper by G. Dirksen. *In* Physiology of Digestion and Metabolism in the Ruminant. Edited by A. T. Phillipson. Newcastle upon Tyne, England, Oriel Press, 1970, p. 626.
14. Phillips, S. F.: Diarrhea: a current view of the pathophysiology. Gastroenterology *63*:495, 1972.
15. Levy, A. G., Widerlite, L., Schwartz, C. J., Dolin, R., Blacklow, N. R., Gardner, J. D., Kimberg, D. V., and Trier, J. S.: Jejunal adenylate cyclase activity in human subjects during viral gastroenteritis. Gastroenterology *70*:321, 1976.
16. Butler, D. G., Gall, D. G., Kelly, M. H., and Hamilton, J. R.: Transmissible gastroenteritis. Mechanisms responsible for diarrhea in acute viral enteritis in piglets. J. Clin. Invest. *53*:1335, 1974.
17. Davidson, G. P., Gall, D. G., Petric, M., Butler, D. G., and Hamilton, J. R.: Human rotavirus enteritis induced in conventional piglets. Intestinal structure and transport. J. Clin. Invest. *60*:1402, 1977.
18. Moon, H. W.: Mechanisms in the pathogenesis of diarrhea: a review. J.A.V.M.A. *172*:443, 1978.
19. McClung, H. J., Butler, D. G., Kerzner, B., Gall, D. G., and Hamilton, J. R.: Transmissible gastroenteritis. Mucosa ion transport in acute viral enteritis. Gastroenterology *70*:1091, 1976.
20. Kelly, M., Butler, D. G., and Hamilton, J. R.: Transmissible gastroenteritis in piglets: a model of infantile viral diarrhea. J. Pediatr. *80*:925, 1972.
21. Kerzner, B., Kelley, M. H., Gall, D. G., Butler, D. G., and Hamilton, J. R.: Transmissible gastroenteritis: sodium transport and the intestinal epithelium during the course of viral enteritis. Gastroenterology *72*:457, 1977.
22. Binder, H. J., and Donowitz, M.: A new look at laxative action. Gastroenterology *69*:1001, 1975.
23. Smith, F. W., and Jeffries, G. H.: Late and persistent postgastrectomy problems. *In* Gastrointestinal Disease. Edited by M. H. Sleisenger and J. S. Fordtran. Philadelphia, W. B. Saunders Co., 1973, p. 822.
24. Grady, G. F., and Keusch, G. T.: Pathogenesis of bacterial diarrheas. N. Engl. J. Med. *285*:831, 891, 1971.
25. Donaldson, R. M., Jr.: The blind loop syndrome. *In* Gastrointestinal Disease. Edited by M. H. Sleisenger and J. S. Fordtran. Philadelphia, W. B. Saunders Co., 1973, p. 927.
26. Christensen, J.: Movements of the small intestine. *In* Gastrointestinal Disease. Edited by M. H. Sleisenger and J. S. Fordtran. Philadelphia, W. B. Saunders Co., 1973, p. 216.
27. Argenzio, R. A., Miller, N., and von Engelhardt, W.: Effect of volatile fatty acids on water and ion absorption from the goat colon. Am. J. Physiol. *229*:997, 1975.
28. Argenzio, R. A., Lowe, J. E., Pickard, D. W., and Stevens, C. E.: Digesta passage and water exchange in the equine large intestine. Am. J. Physiol. *226*:1035, 1974.
29. Argenzio, R. A., Lowe, J. E., Southworth, M., and Stevens, C. E.: Interrelationship of Na, HCO_3 and volatile fatty acid transport by equine large intestine. Am. J. Physiol. *223*:E469, 1977.
30. Ritchie, J. A.: Colonic transport in the irritable colon syndrome. *In* Gastrointestinal Motility. Edited by L. Demling and R. Ottenjann. New York, Academic Press, 1971, p. 104.
31. Donowitz, M., and Binder, H. J.: Effect of enterotoxins of *Vibrio cholerae*, *Escherichia coli*, and *Shigella dysenteriae* type 1 on fluid and electrolyte transport in the colon. J. Infect. Dis. *134*:135, 1976.
32. Turnberg, L. A.: Absorption and secretion of salt and water by the small intestine. Digestion *9*:357, 1973.
33. Kimberg, D. V.: Cyclic nucleotides and their role in gastrointestinal secretion. Gastroenterology *67*:1023, 1974.
34. Sharp, G. W. G.: Action of cholera toxin on fluid and electrolyte movement in the small intestine. Ann. Rev. Med. *24*:19, 1973.
35. Bolton, J. E., and Field, M.: Ca ionophore-stimulated ion secretion in rabbit ileal mucosa: relation to actions of cyclic 3',5'-AMP and carbamylcholine. J. Membr. Biol. *35*:159, 1977.
36. Hughes, J. M., Murad, F., Chang, B., and Guerrant, R. L.: Role of cGMP in the action of heat-stable enterotoxin of *Escherichia coli*. Nature *271*:755, 1978.
37. Moon, H. W.: Pathogenesis of enteric diseases caused by *Escherichia coli*. Adv. Vet. Sci. *18*:179, 1974.
38. Klipstein, F. A., and Engert, R. F.: Partial purification and properties of *Enterobacter cloacae* heat-stable enterotoxin. Infect. Immun. *13*:1307, 1976.
39. Klipstein, F. A., and Engert, R. F.: Purification and properties of *Klebsiella pneumoniae* heat-stable enterotoxin. Infect. Immun. *13*:373, 1976.

40. Melling, J., Capel, B. J., Turnbull, C. P. B., and Gilbert, R. J.: Identification of a novel enterotoxigenic activity associated with *Bacillus cereus*. J. Clin. Pathol. *29*:938, 1976.
41. Charney, A. N., Gots, R. E., Formal, S. B., and Giannella, R. A.: Activation of intestinal mucosal adenylate cyclase by *Shigella dysenteriae* 1 enterotoxin. Gastroenterology *70*:1085, 1976.
42. Koupal, L. R., and Deibel, R. H.: Assay, characterization, and localization of an enterotoxin produced by *Salmonella*. Infect. Immun. *11*:14, 1975.
43. Aziz, K. M. S.: Diarrhea toxin obtained from a waterbloom-producing species, *Microcystic aeurginosa* kutzing. Science *183*:1205, 1974.
44. Giannella, R. A., Gots, R. E., Charney, A. N., Greenough, W. B., and Formal, S. B.: Pathogenesis of Salmonella-mediated intestinal fluid secretion. Gastroenterology *69*:1238, 1975.
45. Kinsey, M. D., Dammin, G. J., Formal, S. B., and Giannella, R. A.: The role of altered intestinal permeability in the pathogenesis of Salmonella diarrhea in the Rhesus monkey. Gastroenterology *71*:429, 1976.
46. Rayford, P. L., Miller, T. A., and Thompson, J. C.: Secretin cholecystokinin and newer gastrointestinal hormones. N. Engl. J. Med. *294*:1093, 1157, 1976.
47. Said, S. I., and Faloona, G. R.: Elevated plasma and tissue levels of vasoactive intestinal polypeptide in the watery-diarrhea syndrome due to pancreatic, bronchiogenic and other tumors. N. Engl. J. Med. *293*:155, 1975.
48. Barrington, E. J. W., and Dockray, G. J.: Gastrointestinal hormones. J. Endocrinol. *69*:299, 1976.
49. Fisher, E. W., and De la Fuente, G. H.: Water and electrolyte studies in newborn calves with particular reference to the effects of diarrhea. Res. Vet. Sci. *13*:315, 1972.
50. Tennant, B., Harrold, D., and Reina-Guerra, M.: Physiologic and metabolic factors in the pathogenesis of neonatal enteric infections in calves. J.A.V.M.A. *161*:993, 1972.
51. Lewis, L. D., and Phillips, R. W.: Diarrheic induced changes in intracellular and extracellular ion concentrations in neonatal calves. Ann. Res. Vet. *4*:99, 1973.
52. Argenzio, R. A., and Stevens, C. E.: Cyclic changes in ionic composition of digesta in the equine intestinal tract. Am. J. Physiol. *228*:1224, 1975.
53. Hendrix, T. R., and Paulk, H. T.: Intestinal secretion. International Review of Physiology, Gastrointestinal Physiology II, Vol. 12. Edited by R. K. Crane. Baltimore, University Park Press, 1977, p. 257.
54. Halpin, C. G., and Cuple, I. W.: Changes in intestinal structure and function of neonatal calves infected with reovirus-like agent and *Escherichia coli*. Aust. Vet. J. *52*:438, 1976.
55. Lewis, L. D., and Phillips, R. W.: Water and electrolyte losses in neonatal calves with acute diarrhea. A complete balance study. Cornell Vet. *62*:596, 1972.
56. Moon, H. W., Whipp, S. C., and Baetz, A. L.: Comparative effects of enterotoxins from *Escherichia coli* and *Vibrio cholerae* on rabbit and swine small intestine. Lab. Invest. *25*:133, 1971.
57. Dittmer, D. S.: Blood and other body fluids. Washington, D.C., Federation of American Societies for Experimental Biology, 1961, p. 35.

Chapter 15

FEEDING, NUTRITION, AND GASTROINTESTINAL DISORDERS

DAVID S. KRONFELD

There are all possible combinations of faulty feeding, gastrointestinal disturbances, and malnutrition; i.e., any one may occur primarily and lead to either one or both of the other two. A poor diet when fed in a way that allows the animal to accommodate will eventually be manifested by poor performance and nutritional disease. If fed improperly, however, even a sound diet may induce digestive disturbances, such as flatus and diarrhea. In my experience, feeding management is more often awry than the diet, so in the long run much time is saved if feeding management is checked before the diet is evaluated.

NUTRITION AND DIETETICS

Nutrition is a broad, integrative subject, more like medicine than biochemistry. It aims to provide food energy and essential nutrients in amounts and proportions that will enable an animal to sustain a desired level of performance. The total amounts of energy and nutrients provided each day constitute the ration (calories or grams per day per animal). This ration includes components of feeding man-

agement in addition to the diet, which is a description of the food (amounts of ingredients or nutrients per unit weight of food as fed, on a dry matter basis, or on an energy basis). The difference between diet and ration is not trivial; I regret the hours that I have wasted evaluating diets before looking at feeding management, especially actual consumption, changes in intake from day to day, and the way in which the food is offered. One should look at the big picture before focusing any attention on the diet (Fig. 15–1).

"Nutritional problems" as described by clients are likely to represent digestive disturbances more often than any genuine nutritional disease (Fig. 15–2). Veterinarians tend to be pulled into this point of view. Two common examples are the calf improperly fed a perfectly sound milk replacer, or the dog abruptly introduced to a canned product rich in protein and fat. The milk replacer and canned dog food may have ideal compositions and be thoroughly tested by their manufacturers and still be liable to faulty feeding management. The consequences are presented to us as poor nutrition, and

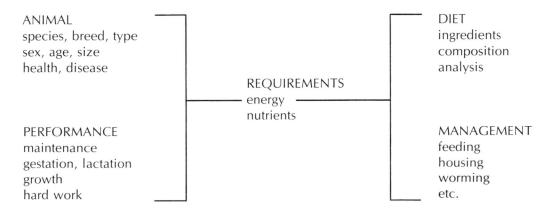

ANIMAL
species, breed, type
sex, age, size
health, disease

PERFORMANCE
maintenance
gestation, lactation
growth
hard work

REQUIREMENTS
energy
nutrients

DIET
ingredients
composition
analysis

MANAGEMENT
feeding
housing
worming
etc.

Figure 15–1. This scheme represents a general approach to nutrition and dietetics. The type of animal and desired level of performance combine to determine the required intake of food energy and essential nutrients. This requirement must be met by the diet and the feeding program.

233

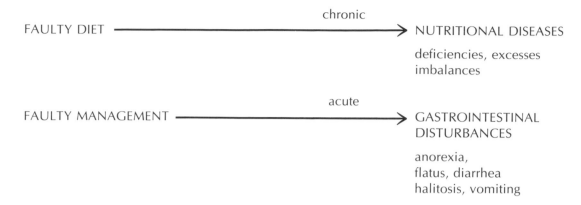

Figure 15–2. This image should be a starting point for any diagnostic algorithm in the field of feeding, gastrointestinal disturbances, and nutrition.

we are asked to examine the diet, but they are more accurately regarded as manifestations of faulty feeding, and it is more useful to look first at the way the food is fed than at its composition.

FEEDING MISMANAGEMENT

Faulty feeding practices usually lead fairly soon to digestive disturbances. Malnutrition does not develop if the connection is identified promptly by the feeder or the animal. If the gastrointestinal disturbance persists, however, it may lead to multiple deficiencies. Among the first to develop are deficiencies of several B vitamins. These in turn may cause diarrhea. In calves, for example, diarrhea attends deficiencies of thiamine, riboflavin, pantothenic acid, nicotinic acid, and folic acid.[1] The vicious cycle of diarrhea causing B vitamin deficiencies which perpetuate the diarrhea was first well described in human pellagra, beri beri, and riboflavin deficiency.[2]

In a classic example of feeding mismanagement in research, pups were introduced abruptly and ad libitum to a highly palatable diet of meat and meat by-products.[3] They presumably ate too much and developed diarrhea, which persisted until multiple deficiencies were manifested. The most dramatic lesion was inadequate mineralization of bone, osteoporosis.

This was interpreted to mean that the diet was deficient in calcium. While it is conceded that muscle meat alone is deficient in calcium, there may have been enough bone scraps in the meat by-product portion of the mixture to provide adequate calcium. In any event, no analysis of the food was presented. In my opinion, the calcium deficiency was more reasonably attributable to diarrhea initi-

ated by deliberately improper feeding, resulting in poor assimilation of calcium.

OVERFEEDING

The consequences of overfeeding are partially dependent upon age. The very young usually develop diarrhea. Older growing animals may accommodate digestively but seem prone to develop more skeletal problems when overfed. They may also become obese, and this is the sure fate of mature animals that are overfed.

Feeding too much colostrum or milk may cause diarrhea. One often sees recommendations that very young animals should be fed about 10% of their body weight in the form of milk. That should be the aim after a few days of life, but a young animal taken away from its mother on the first or second day should be given only 5% of its body weight per 24 hours in the form of colostrum or about 7% as milk. It is better to underfeed than overfeed during any dietary transition, including this first great step into extrauterine life.

The daily intake of the very young should be divided into four or five meals. The number of feedings per day is diminished progressively to two a day for herbivores and omnivores, perhaps once a day for carnivores. In the latter case, the number of daily feedings should be increased again when the nutrient requirements increase greatly, for example, for lactation or very hard work in the cold.

Colostrum contains about 17% solids, milk about 13%. So any colostrum fed after 2 or 3 days should be diluted about two parts to one of safe water. In dairy herds, excess colostrum may be preserved for 2 to 4 weeks by fermentation. The soured colostrum is diluted prior to feeding. It is very useful food for calves from 2 days to 2 months of age.

Milk replacers for calves are made in two energy densities, about 5% fat for replacement heifers, but more fat, up to 20%, for vealers. Also, some products are more suitable for very young calves because they contain less plant materials, while others are best kept for calves at least 3 weeks old because they contain more plant fiber. Replacers are sensitive to cooking, especially those containing more grain and grain by-products. The efficiency of digestion of raw starch is poor. It improves with cooking, reaches maximum, then declines as insoluble polymers are formed with amino acids (the browning or Maillard reaction). We are dependent upon quality assurance of manufacturers for optimal cooking and digestibility of all cereal products, especially those fortified with protein, e.g., milk replacers and pet foods.

Despite the great opportunities for choosing an inappropriate type of milk replacer or a poor manufacturer, one should first rule out faulty management in any nutritional problem involving milk replacers. Though labels carry explicit instructions, the portions seem small, so the temptation is to overfeed out of sympathy for the calf. If only this kindness were to be expressed in attention to proper mixing and cleanliness! All too often, the utensils are dirty. The mixing process often leaves lumps which are wet on the outside but dry on the inside. These internally dry lumps carry undesirable amounts of nutrients to the lower bowel where they are likely to foment unrest in the indigenous population of microorganisms. When confronted with unthrifty or sick calves fed milk replacer, I ask to see the whole procedure of feeding, and encourage the help through the whole lot before evincing any displeasure with dirty utensils, incomplete mixing, overfeeding, and poor choice of type of replacer. Only then do I become concerned about the manufacturer. The dairyman and his employees usually find this very frustrating because they would like to begin by accusing the manufacturer of producing a flawed product.

Commercial products are available for feeding the young of most species. Most companies provide feeding instructions for their products which should be followed assiduously. The most common aberration is overfeeding, with resultant diarrhea.

An appropriate correction to overfeeding in the young is to recommend dilution of the milk or further dilution of the soured colostrum or milk replacer for calves, or the evaporated milk or Esbilac (Borden Co.) for pups. The intention is to diminish the intake of solids but not water. Young animals conserve water poorly and become dehy-

drated rapidly if they receive too small a volume of water or too great an amount of solids. Remember, however, to put a time limit on any recommendations for dilution of milk or milk substitute. Usually a week is enough; the ration should be built back to full strength during the second week. Otherwise, the young animals will soon be underfed. We have seen many pups, calves, and foals suffering from such secondary persistent underfeeding which results from inadequate communication between practitioner and client.

Bone abnormalities may develop in growing animals which are overfed. The overfeeding may be complicated by malnutrition, and sometimes it is difficult to decide whether the diet should be changed or only its intake restricted. In one study, pups were accommodated to a highly palatable mixture of cereal, meat, and meat by-products.[4] They eventually developed excessive mineralization of bone, osteopetrosis, and hypertrophic osteodystrophy. The lesions were attributed to the diet being rich in protein, energy, calcium, and phosphorus. Actually the diet approached the ideal in these respects in my judgment even though it is possible to fault it for containing 14 times the NRC recommendation for vitamin D.[4] This would overwhelm the first defense against a high calcium intake by forcing a high efficiency of absorption from the intestine. I would rank the combination of a very high vitamin D content and a moderately high calcium content behind the unrestricted feeding as a contributory factor to the overmineralization of bone, because the lesion did not develop in control pups whose intake was restricted to the usually recommended amount, about twice maintenance. This suggested that the primary fault lay in feeding management rather than the diet.

The authors blamed the diet, however, not only in the original publication but also in many subsequent presentations to practitioners and the public. For example, they recommended that the "best selling" puppy chow be avoided because it contained too much protein and calcium, basing their reasoning on the preceding study. In fact, the "best selling" puppy chow is thoroughly tested and its label carries sound feeding instructions. For veterinarians to warn the public against its use is ridiculous, especially on the basis of the preceding study.

Case Histories

Secondary Nutritional Hyperparathyroidism in Bull Calves
    We were called to examine a group of very rapidly growing Angus bull calves.[5] They were on

lush pasture near the southern tip of the Maryland peninsula. They were production tested, with an average daily gain of about 4 lb in body weight. They were very well grown, in full condition, perhaps tending to be obese. Swellings about the hocks and knees were palpated and regarded as bony overgrowths or exostoses. A grain concentrate was fed free choice, but we could estimate the average intake per calf. The client regarded the diet as perfect and the lesions were attributed initially to overfeeding. Assuming a pasture intake commensurate with daily gain, the daily intakes of calcium and phosphorus were 46 g and 39 g respectively. These estimates easily met the NRC minimum requirements for beef calves of this age and size, namely, 20 g calcium and 15 to 21 g phosphorus.[6] The British ARC[7] recommends intakes related to average daily gain but only up to 1 kg (2.2 lb) per day. We extrapolated this regression to 4 lb/day and found it to be 60 g calcium. The ARC estimate assumes 45% efficiency of absorption of calcium. We have found an efficiency of only 27% in beef calves in our laboratory; using this value, the estimated calcium requirement would be 100 g/day. So we diagnosed the disorder as secondary nutritional hyperparathyroidism due to a calcium deficiency, despite the fact that the calcium intake was far above the NRC recommendation. The bull calves responded favorably to the increased calcium intake.

Epiphysitis in Overfed Young Horses

Yearling horses in our region often develop epiphysitis. This disorder has been attributed to rapid growth and overfeeding.[8] When we evaluated the ration of young horses with epiphysitis, we repeatedly found that they were fed 50% to 150% more than the NRC recommendations for horses of their age and weight.[9] So we used to promulgate the notion that overfeeding causes epiphysitis. Recently, we evaluated rations fed to young horses on 10 nearby establishments among which only two were troubled with epiphysitis or splints. All 10 were grossly overfeeding weanlings and yearlings according to the NRC standards. It is difficult for us to recommend against this "overfeeding" when the horse breeders are pleased with the results, and the products realize gratifying prices in the sale ring. What would happen if we were to cut the ration back to the NRC recommendations, and the yearlings were to fail in the sales?

In this situation, we heed the performance objective. If the young ones are destined for the sale ring,

we bring the diet in line with NRC recommendations for contents of essential nutrients, usually allowing margins up to 50% above the minimum requirements. This diet is then fed according to the eye of the feeder; in practice, it is overfed, but we disclaim responsibility for this aspect. If the horses are to be retained by the owners for racing or other use, then we do recommend restricting the daily intake to no more than 25% above the NRC recommendation for age and projected mature weight.[9] This example illustrates the difference between the diet and the ration. In both cases, we recommend a smooth growth curve, because there is at least a reasonable suspicion that slumps followed by compensatory rapid growth may induce disproportionate growth of bones and tendons, hence dysflexia.

Overfeeding in Ruminants

Ruminants allowed free abrupt access to highly palatable feeds may overconsume and develop enterotoxemia or intraruminal acidosis. Enterotoxemia may occur in overfed sheep of any age but is most common in lambs fed lush young pasture or with grain supplements. Overeating, especially if associated with a sudden change of diet, allows the escape of undigested or partially digested, readily fermentable material into the small intestine. This favors a rapid growth of *Clostridium perfringens D*.[10] Its epsilon toxin increases the permeability of the intestinal wall, enhancing absorption of the toxin, which causes sudden death. In the field, enterotoxemia may overlap with ruminal acidosis. Experimentally these disorders may be differentiated by vaccination against enterotoxemia or by feeding sodium bicarbonate to prevent acidosis. Hyperglycemia and glycosuria characterize enterotoxemia but not acidosis.

Excessive acidity in the rumen has several adverse effects.[11] The protozoa become pale in a few hours and usually disappear within a day. Their rupture may release sufficient foam-stabilizing materials to favor the development of frothy bloat. Antiprotozoal agents, copper sulfate and dioctyl sulfosuccinate have been found as effective as poloxalene, a plurionic detergent, in the prevention of frothy bloat in cattle, in one study.[12]

Protozoa usually constitute 20 to 50% of the microbial mass in the rumen. This amount is about 10% of rumen contents. Protozoa engulf bacteria and smaller food particles. Compared to bacteria, protozoa produce more gas and their protein has a higher digestibility and biologic value. Only 20 to 30% of the protozoal growth rate in the rumen is accounted for by the numbers of protozoa which pass into the omasum; the fate of the remainder is uncertain.

Protozoa are the most sensitive ruminal microorganisms to any abrupt change in conditions, e.g., a decrease in available nutrients following underfeeding or a drop in pH following refeeding or overfeeding. Their rapid obliteration lowers the overall fermentative power of the rumen for 24 or 48 hours before compensatory bacterial growth repairs the deficit. Re-establishment of the protozoal population takes longer. The host suffers a decline in available nutrients even if it continues to eat. More often, its food intake decreases. This is usually ascribed to mild acidosis but recent studies have also implicated a protein/energy imbalance.[13]

Most studies of defaunated ruminants have indicated a slight depression of performance compared to controls. On the other hand, protozoal instability appears to be the first limit on the robustness, flexibility, and versatility of the rumen system. So there is renewed interest in formulating rations which eliminate protozoa.[13]

Protozoa are usually pale and few or absent in sick ruminants. We commonly try to re-establish them by infusions of rumen contents from healthy animals. This procedure deserves more serious study.

The next most vulnerable microorganisms in the rumen are gram-negative bacteria which utilize lactic acid. Like the protozoa, these disappear during underfeeding due to lack of nutrients and during overfeeding due to excess acidity. Lysis releases endotoxins from some of these bacteria. The possible contribution of these endotoxins to grain engorgement syndromes or laminitis remains poorly defined but very interesting.[11,14] Among the most hardy of rumen microorganisms are the cocci and gram-positive bacilli which generate lactic acid. They persist during underfeeding and generate lactate upon refeeding. And they operate after the lactate utilizers decline during the development of increasingly acidic conditions in the rumen following the ingestion of soluble carbohydrates.

Excessive intraruminal acidity, probably beginning at about pH 5.5, induces deterioration of the rumen wall. This may be transient or progressive, and patchy or diffuse. The least damage may allow entry of microorganisms into the portal blood. Spicules of hair may penetrate the weakened wall and facilitate invasion. Some pathogenic organisms, e.g., *Fusobacterium necrophorum*, establish foci of infection in the liver with the eventual development of telangiectasis ("sawdust liver"), and multiple liver abscesses.[11] Condemnations of livers

for these lesions are about 10% in the United States and sometimes reaches 95% for particular feedlots. Control is achieved with antibiotics, such as chlortetracycline, which probably acts at the liver, or buffers, such as sodium bicarbonate or dolomitic limestone.

If patches of rumenitis occur around the cardia, or in the lower esophagus due to regurgitation of acidic material, there may be inhibition of the eructation reflex and an accumulation of gas in the rumen and reticulum. This form of free-gas bloat[15] occurs in feedlots when the fiber content of the diet is low (6 or 7%) and intake is unrestricted. It is not amenable to treatment with anti-frothing agents, such as poloxalene. It is managed by gathering susceptible calves into a separate pen, feeding them a diet containing 9 to 10% fiber, and avoiding overfeeding.

In this situation, the less concentrated diet has several beneficial effects. Roughage stimulates salivary flow, partly through the scabrous reflex on the anterior wall of the reticulum and partly through increasing chewing time. Salivary bicarbonate neutralizes acids produced by fermentation. This tends to preserve protozoa from rupture. Also, mucin in saliva acts as an anti-foaming agent. So roughage tends to minimize some causes of both free-gas and frothy bloat.

Laminitis. Laminitis occurs in 1 to 10% of ruminants fed diets rich in soluble carbohydrates, e.g., starch in grains or sugar in bagasse. The acute vascular lesions of the laminae appear to be due to local release of inflammatory factors, e.g., histamine from degranulating mast cells. Many possible causes of this local injury have been suggested but none conclusively established.[11] Ruminal histamine has been discounted because the base dissociates at pH 5 and is poorly absorbed. Other vasoactive amines, e.g., tyramine, produced by decarboxylation of amino acids in the rumen, would also be poorly absorbed. Endotoxins released from lysed bacteria may be more likely to reach the laminae in sufficient amounts to provoke injury. Allergic reactions have been suggested for this and every other poorly understood disease. Deficiencies of thiamine and methionine have been suspected and prompted therapeutic tests which have yielded inconsistent results.

Laminitis in ponies and horses is also usually associated with a change in diet or digestion. Young grass is rich in soluble carbohydrates and protein, which may respectively influence the thiamine requirement or amine supply. It may be precipitated by low fiber diets intended for the preparation or aftercare of surgical patients. It may follow the administration of certain drugs, e.g., trichlorfon, thiabendazole, or dexamethasone. Despite these associations, mechanistic links between diet or drugs and laminitis in horses or ruminants remain obscure. Incidence of the condition can be minimized by conservative feeding management if diets rich in soluble carbohydrates and proteins but low in fiber are used.

Polioencephalomalacia. A conditioned thiamine deficiency has been implicated in polioencephalomalacia or cerebrocortical necrosis. This disease occurs most commonly but not exclusively in calves and lambs fed diets rich in soluble carbohydrates. Its clinical course may run for 2 days to 2 weeks. Even recumbent, convulsing, comatose animals with severe dyspnea and nystagmus may respond dramatically to massive intravenous doses (1 or 2 g) of thiamine, though some remain blind or partially decorticate.

High carbohydrate diets apparently favor the growth of bacteria which have a thiaminase.[11] This exchanges the thiazole moiety for another base, e.g., nicotinamide or histamine. These analogs are thought to have anti-thiamine activity, especially in phosphorylative reactions, hence to lead to the accumulation of pyruvic and eventually lactic acid. Type I thiaminase has an optimal pH of 5.8–6.5. Note the vicious cycle: soluble carbohydrate yields acid which enhances thiaminase activity which hinders utilization of carbohydrate.

Ruminal D-lactic Acidosis. The disorders mentioned so far in connection with a hyperacidic rumen (protozoal instability and anorexia, telangiectasis and liver abscesses, bloat, laminitis, and polioencephalomalacia) are usually regarded as ancillary to a central overfeeding problem, ruminal D-lactic acidosis,[16] which is caused by an overload of soluble carbohydrates, e.g., sugars from fruit or starch from grain. The rapid and altered fermentation leads to relatively less acetic and propionic acids, the usual satiety signals, and to the accumulation of lactic acid. Some of this is in the D-form as well as the usual L-isomer, which is present only in small concentrations as a metabolic intermediate under most circumstances. There are many consequences. The proliferation of small molecules in the rumen liquor draws water from the blood, leading to hemoconcentration and hypovolemic hypotension. D-lactic acid is removed from blood much more slowly than the L-form, so it accumulates and induces metabolic acidosis. In addition, there may be overtones of enterotoxemia in some cases,[10] endotoxins in others, or accumulation of amines

and other toxins.[14] But the milder syndromes that follow overfeeding of soluble carbohydrates are usually attributable to moderate acidosis, while more severe syndromes reflect both severe acidosis and hypotension.

Preventing adventitious engorgement with grain or fruits is usually a matter of care with fences and gates. On the other hand, overfeeding of rations rich in soluble carbohydrates is often deliberate, intended to attain maximal growth rate or milk production. This is a common debasement of the principle of challenge feeding or the provision of a ration that should enable the animal to fulfill its genetic potential. The "Catch 22" of challenge feeders is to declare those individuals who fail when fed a superabundance of the "ideal" diet to be genetically undesirable.

Overfeeding After Transport. Calves and lambs often lose about 5% body weight in transit. Two or three weeks are required to make up this shrink. In haste to revert this loss, most feedlot operators use starters containing only about 10% fiber. A veterinarian more concerned with health and disease than with immediate gains may prefer more fiber. The compromise may turn in several directions. One is the use of roughage substitutes, such as oyster shells or plastic ticklers designed to remain in the rumen. Another is to add buffers, like dolomitic limestone, cement dust, or sodium bicarbonate, about 1%.

A new approach is to use antibiotics which influence predominance among bacterial species in the rumen.[17] Both capreomycin and oxamycin maintain higher pH levels. Oxamycin appears to facilitate conversion of lactate to acetate. Capreomycin enhances conversion of lactate to propionate. Both acetic and propionic acids are absorbed more rapidly than lactic acid. More propionate relative to acetate (or lactate) appears to confer greater efficiency of metabolism in host tissues.

Overfeeding the Postpartum Dairy Cow. The dairy cow usually fasts for 4 to 16 hours on the day of calving. Then she starts to eat abruptly. Most dairy nutritionists, with an eye on production, recommend feeding the grain concentrate (about 17% fiber) free choice. I think that this leads too often to slight engorgement, depression of appetite for half a day or more, then overeating again. This cyclic feeding is averted if the cow is fed grain by hand, say about 10 pounds per day prepartum, then increasing by 1 to 2 pounds per day, depending on the size and production potential of the cow, for a week. She can then be allowed ad libitum intakes with little fear of acidosis.

Overfeeding and Obesity. Obesity is the inevitable result of persistent overeating. Paradoxically, its main gastrointestinal consequence is a diminished ability to increase food intake at times of need, such as late gestation and early lactation. The fat ewe (or bitch, cow, or goat) is the most likely to develop pregnancy toxemia. The fat cow is most susceptible to ketosis as well as all the maladies that attend parturition and the rising and peak phases of lactation. Pregnancy toxemia and lactation ketosis involve fatty changes in the liver.

For many years, obesity was regarded as a sign of weak will in humans, but recent studies have shown that fat adolescent girls eat less than thin girls. Similarly fat cows and ewes eat less than thin ones. Many observations in various species suggest the existence of a negative influence of plethoric fat cells on food intake. This may be humoral but any such juice has eluded chemical characterization. It may be neural but the morphology remains obscure. It may be mechanical when fat accumulating in the mesentery and omasum usurps abdominal space and compresses the digestive tract. This factor becomes more important during pregnancy when the conceptus also occupies space at the expense of the gut. It has been shown in sheep that 1 kg of conceptus exerts an effect equivalent to a decreased food intake of 100 g dry matter per day.[18] This occurs just at the time when fetal requirements are burgeoning. Rate of passage of materials through the gut is more rapid during late pregnancy, probably because the gut is compressed by conceptus. This compression would be exacerbated by accumulation of abdominal fat. Any acceleration in transit time tends to diminish the efficiency of digestion. So fat animals have a double disadvantage in late pregnancy, a lower food intake and faster transit. There is a compensatory process, hypertrophy of the intestinal mucosa, villi, and absorptive surface.[19] This is obviously beneficial in general but not quantitatively adequate to counteract the nutritional imbalances which develop during late gestation in animals, especially those which are too fat.

Many fat sheep develop fatty livers and intermittent ketosis late in gestation without showing any clinical signs.[20] These fatty livers are indistinguishable grossly from those of ewes which develop pregnancy toxemia.[21] All hepatic cells are distended with fat.

Two fatty changes have been described in livers of fat cows exhibiting ketosis.[22] One is a fine stippling of fat near the periphery of the cells, actually near the surfaces where fat would enter the cells from the hepatic arterioles and portal venules. This is thought to represent incoming fat derived from stores in adipose tissues. The second abnormality consists of large fat globules in cells near the central venule, i.e., the surface where fat leaves the cell. This change is typical of a lipotroph deficiency, an inability to attach triglycerides to lipoproteins for release into blood. In severe cases, these fat globules extend throughout the cell and displace any faint stippling that may have preceded extensive accumulation of fat. Cows with fatty livers of this nature may have Bromsulphalein half-times of 10 to 20 minutes. We treat these cows with methionine, 20 g intravenously, or its hydroxy analog, 40 g per os, and have observed consistent reductions in Bromsulphalein removal within a few days but have conducted no comparative trials. Other lipotrophic agents may be expected to exert similar effects and several have been found effective in the treatment of ketotic cows in some trials though not most; included in this group are acetyl-methionine, cysteamine, and choline.[23]

Obesity in pregnant mares and ponies may predispose them to develop anorexia and hyperlipemia toward the end of gestation or just after parturition. This condition resembles pregnancy toxemia in several respects but fat tends to accumulate in the blood rather than the liver.

To avoid these problems of relative hypophagia and fat mobilization in pregnant or lactating animals which were overfed before mating or early in pregnancy, we recommend a general plan of feeding for breeding in all species. The female is prepared for mating by first assuming a thin condition, then is brought gradually up in condition before and during estrus. During pregnancy, weight gain is restricted for the first two thirds by keeping food energy intake down to maintenance. Then food energy intake is raised progressively by increasing the energy density and palatability of the diet, the amount offered, and the frequency of feeding, so that it reaches 150% of maintenance.

The Fat Cow Syndrome. The fat cow syndrome alludes to the collection of health and production problems that afflict overweight cows during parturition and the rising and peak phases of lactation.[24] Overfeeding leads eventually to hypophagia relative to the demands of lactation and to a fatty liver. Dairy cows lose from 10 to 25% of their body weight during the first 6 to 12 weeks of lactation, then gain weight progressively until calving. During the declining phase of lactation, which lasts 6 months or more, the adipose tissue of the cow appears to compete more effectively than the mammary gland for blood-borne lipogenic substances. With typical North American dairy rations, it is difficult to avoid marginal or deficient provision of protein if energy intakes are curtailed sufficiently to control the tendency of the cow to gain weight. The grain concentrate may be fed *ad libitum* or perhaps one part to three of milk during the rising and peak phases of lactation. Once production is declining, it should be restricted to one part concentrate for four or five of milk. Now a different concentrate should be used, one which contains a higher protein content, especially if corn silage is the staple. These cows run the gauntlet between protein deficiency and energy excess.

The fat cow syndrome is usually presented at one of three stages. Cows gaining weight during the sixth or seventh month of lactation may abruptly dry up. We have seen this problem often in the field and simulated it by feeding a high fat diet, using fat protected from ruminal fermentation by coating it with formaldehyde-treated protein.[25] More commonly, we are called to freshening herds of fat cows which have a high incidence of dystocia, retained placenta, and downers. The third presentation is a high incidence of ketosis during the rising and peak phases of lactation. All of these stages involve fatty livers.

Unfortunately, by the time one is called to a fat cow or ewe, it is too late to act directly on the obesity. That must wait until the next pregnancy of the ewe or the next lactation-pregnancy of the cow. Meanwhile, every ewe should be examined repeatedly for the prodromal signs of pregnancy toxemia, e.g., detachment from the group and an awkward gait. This disease in ewes responds well to therapy only during its earlier stages.[26]

Similarly, the diet of the fat cow postpartum must aim to offset her lower food intake. This is no time to curtail her energy intake, because that would surely lower her production. So the intervention is paradoxical; she is too fat, but we must strive to provide her with a diet of the highest energy density and palatability. The obesity must wait until the declining phase of lactation before attempt is made to correct it. Meanwhile both practitioner and client must mount a campaign to treat promptly every disorder of parturition and early lactation, for seriousness of most of these disorders increases with their duration.

Overfeeding and Gastric Dilatation. Acute gastric dilatation has been associated with overfeeding or engorgement in many species.[27] It occurs most commonly in greedy, rapid feeders, especially those which engorge on grain. Lead feeding of grain concentrates has been associated with a high incidence of abomasal displacement in dairy cattle.[28] Rapid fermentation of starch generates volatile fatty acids which appear to inhibit abomasal motility and mobility. Thus gas accumulates and the organ may become trapped out of its usual position.

A similar disorder may occur in dogs, though its etiology has not yet been demonstrated convincingly. In one group of 33 afflicted dogs, 20 had been fed dry predominantly cereal dog foods, four table scraps, and nine unknown diets.[27] Distending gas may be derived from fermentation or swallowed air. This may be swallowed while gulping food or water, or it may be trapped in the expanded cereal dog food. (Manufacturers of the best-selling dry dog foods advertise that caloric contents of a cupful of the best-selling expanded chow is nearly half that of the best-selling dog meal; dog foods vary much more in the amount of air present and added by the manufacturers than in the amount of water.) Irrespective of the source of gas, commonly recommended ways to avoid gastric dilatation are to feed less dry cereal-based dog foods to individuals which bloat, or to feed one of the less palatable dry products continuously when expense is an overriding factor. Success of these recommendations has not been demonstrated by critically conducted trials, and it is by no means assured.

In the horse, engorgement on grain may cause acute gastric dilatation within 4 to 6 hours. This is manifested as colic, i.e., abdominal pain. Vomiting would indicate location of the distention in the stomach rather than the small intestine, and it is often a forerunner of gastric rupture. Other causes of colic may be distentions of lower sections of the abdominal tract. These are more likely to attend changes in the diet, inadequate hydrolytic digestion, hence increased fermentation in the large intestine. However, colic in horses, like gastric dilatation in dogs, has been the subject of much comment about feeding management and diets, but all too little systematic investigation.

UNDERFEEDING AND REFEEDING

One should discriminate between too little food offered and too little food consumed. If the latter occurs, there may still be some extrinsic cause, such as an unpalatable ingredient in the diet or a threatening presence in the environment, but the likelihood of intrinsic factors contributing to poor consumption must never be neglected. In other words, if enough food is offered but too little consumed, the animal should be subjected to a thorough physical examination for organic disease. By the same token hypophagia and anorexia should be ruled out before seriously embarking on the workup of a supposed malabsorptive disorder.

Cats are far more sensitive than dogs to any threat in their environment. Perhaps this stems from their evolution as solitary predators, eating alone with no fellows to protect them. In contrast, dogs hunted and ate as a pack and they are much less concerned about being attacked while they are eating. Even so, both dogs and cats appreciate regular meals of the same type at the same place at the same time, day after day. If more than one pet is kept in the home, feeding bowls should be at least 3 feet apart. If dogs and cats are fed at the same time, it may be necessary to put the cat in a separate room or at a higher level, perhaps on a bench, in the same room. When working as a student in a boarding cattery, I observed dozens of cats that refused to eat for a few days or a week. They were hard to woo into a feeling of security in a strange environment. When they began refeeding, they would always develop diarrhea.

Underfeeding occurs most commonly in dogs during lactation. A major cereal dog food company advises owners to feed their dog only dry food, 2% of its body weight for maintenance and three times that much in lactation. This type of dog food is the least palatable, so the poor bitch may not consume 6% of her body weight. It is also the least digestible, so she is bound to produce more abundant watery feces if she does consume 6%; indeed, one should expect diarrhea. In either case, she is not likely to produce enough milk for a medium or large litter, so some pups may have to be removed in order to avoid underfeeding all of them. This situation can be avoided or ameliorated by mixing some canned meat and meat by-products fortified with vitamins and minerals into the ration; this will increase palatability, energy density, digestibility, and the efficiency of utilization of absorbed nutrients. The positive influence of protein intake on milk production was first demonstrated in the bitch.[29]

Dogs may also be underfed when subjected to repeated prolonged strenuous work, especially under cold environmental conditions. Again, more meat and meat by-products, especially fat, are needed to reach energy requirements of five to seven times maintenance. Such diets have very low contents of carbohydrate. Fat becomes important not only in raising the energy density but also in preventing diarrhea. The last point is not well documented, but I have found in several instances that diarrhea in dogs fed zero carbohydrates and less than 20% fat (dry basis) has abated when dietary fat is increased above 25%.

Grazing animals are often underfed when the nutritional value of pastures declines in the fall and winter. This happens to virtually all dairy cows in New Zealand, when the number of cows per acre is chosen to control the peak growth rate of the pasture during spring and early summer. In contrast, the number of horses on breeding farms is restricted to the carrying capacity during the season of slowest pasture growth, and the excess during the other seasons is removed by nonselective grazers, e.g., sheep or motor mowers.

As the summer wears on, pasture plants pass their peak in contents of digestible energy, protein, vitamin A, and phosphorus. Grazing wears down the sward, and carrying capacity declines. Numbers of animals must be reduced, or supplements must be provided. In much of North America, horse farms cannot carry their stock on pasture alone. We receive innumerable requests to suggest a number of horses per farm or per acre. Any such recommendations would have to be based on a comprehensive evaluation of the farm, its management, and its objectives. Every year, in late fall or winter, we see gaunt ponies and horses on chewed-out pastures. The owners have often provided vitamin and mineral supplements instead of food energy. They want worming medicine or antibiotics and refuse to believe that their well-loved pets are underfed. Like the fasting cats mentioned previously, these starved equids tend to develop diarrhea when refed, then voluntarily go off feed again. We try to start them on good quality grass hay, perhaps with a sprinkle of moistened oats. A horse weakened to the point of recumbency may start to eat better if supported in a sling.

The diarrhea which attends the refeeding of a starved animal has not been studied in any depth. I presume that it is not unlike the diarrhea which follows an abrupt change in diet; neither hydrolytic enzymes nor, presumably, fermentative bacteria are present in suitable amounts and proportions for efficient digestion.

ABRUPT CHANGES IN DIET

The advantages of changing diets slowly have been well-recognized in the feeding of ruminants. Abrupt changes of any sort threaten the protozoa, and then the lactate-utilizing bacteria. The consequences of abruptly increasing soluble carbohydrate intake were discussed in conjunction with general overfeeding because both conditions lead to excessive intraruminal acidity. Bloat, laminitis, and acute D-lactic acidemia are the most likely to attend a sudden starch or sugar overload. Chronic acidosis, cyclic feeding, liver abscesses, and polioencephalomalacia tend to be associated with accommodation to starch and sugar, followed by prolonged feeding. Full accommodation of the rumen to a new diet takes from 3 days to 3 weeks.

Abrupt increases in soluble protein or nonprotein nitrogen, such as urea, lead to an accumulation of ammonia in the rumen, then in the blood.[46] This is exacerbated if protozoa form a high fraction of the ruminal biomass. The liver's reserve capacity for handling ammonia is limited, and if blood ammonia concentration rises above about 0.5 mg/dl, central nervous system signs of depression and seizures may occur. Ammonia absorption may be impeded by the administration of vinegar or other mild acids; the base dissociates at a lower pH. This problem may be minimized eventually by formulating diets which balance soluble ammonia precursors against insoluble protein and soluble carbohydrates which favor microbial utilization of ammonia and hinder its absorption.

Pancreatic protease, amylase, and lipase are adaptive enzymes.[30] Their activities and rates of synthesis and release are influenced by the diet. Most studies of these changes have been conducted on rats and humans and are poorly documented in regard to rates of changes. Though times required for enzymic adaptations to dietary changes are of great practical importance in animals, they must usually be estimated by inference from accommodation periods allowed by research workers and from clinical histories of animals which exhibit changes in feces and flatus following a change in diet.

The rate of intraluminal hydrolysis by pancreatic enzymes is usually rate limiting in the digestion and absorption of fats and proteins (except perhaps the most soluble). Brush border peptidases and disaccharidases are usually present in abundance, except lactase after weaning. The rate limiting step in the digestion of starch and most disaccharides is hexose transport. For lactose, it is hydrolysis. Thus the digestion of fats, proteins, and lactose is more vulnerable than that of starch to changes in diet. Deficiencies in hydrolysis lead to excesses in fermentation. In my experience with dogs following 4-day changeovers from cereal to meat or vice versa, another 4 to 11 days pass before the feces assume their final character. I think that this reflects microbial changes in the large intestine as well as adaptations of pancreatic enzymes but have found no critical pertinent data in the literature.

Abrupt introduction of milk to an animal unaccus-

tomed to it will occasionally, by no means always, cause diarrhea. This is usually ascribed primarily to a low activity of intestinal lactase.[31] Unhydrolyzed lactose is thought to hold water in the lumen of the large intestine, so causing an osmotic diarrhea. The young of all mammalian species, with the exception of a few Pacific pinnipeds whose milk contains no lactose, have abundant intestinal lactase though genetic deficiencies have been observed in infants and baby pigs. Otherwise lactase activity is high at birth and declines after weaning. Whether continued milk drinking will diminish this progressive decline in intestinal lactase activity is an issue clouded by such disparate factors as racial bias and neglect of changes in microbial degradation of lactose. I expect that this situation will be resolved by further studies of fermentative digestion of lactose. Production of short-chain fatty acids which are readily absorbed across the wall of the cecum and, perhaps, other parts of the large intestine should constitute an adequate accommodation to lactose. On the other hand, a fermentation yielding lactic acid which has a much lower pK and is poorly absorbed from a neutral medium should lead to osmotic diarrhea.

If milk is fed continuously after weaning or is re-introduced gradually, most animals utilize it effectively. Warnings that dogs and cats should not be fed milk is unfortunate, for milk is one of the best supplements for inexpensive cereals. Its safety in the majority of animals depends on feeding management, which allows time for digestive adaptation.

An abrupt increase in fat intake leads immediately to steatorrhea. The response of pancreatic lipase is more rapid to unsaturated fats than to saturated fats.[30] This had led to a common belief that unsaturated fats are more readily digested, but dogs, for example, can accommodate to huge intakes of predominantly saturated fat in a few days.[32] Pancreatitis may be precipitated by engorgement with fat[33] and is more readily induced experimentally in dogs fed a diet containing 40% fat than in dogs fed diets high in protein or carbohydrate.[34]

Pancreases in general but especially proteases are reduced by underfeeding or specific deficiencies of protein or selenium. Dipeptidases and procarboxypeptidase located at the brush border or inside intestinal mucosal cells are reduced by deficiencies of protein and zinc, respectively.[30] Intraluminal hydrolysis remains rate limiting for protein assimilation, however, so these effects probably contribute little if anything to growth-depressing actions of these nutrient deficiencies. Any sudden load of dietary protein is hydrolyzed slowly and much of it passes on to the large intestine where it is subjected to fermentation or putrefaction with the production of abundant foul-smelling flatus and, quite often but not invariably, diarrhea. Thus, the digestive disturbances which follow the abrupt change from a predominantly cereal diet to one rich in protein and fat are due primarily to slow hydrolysis in the small intestine and secondarily to increased fermentation in the large intestine.

Pancreatic amylase declines to only about 10% of its usual activity in rats when carbohydrates provide 25% or less of food energy. (It is also very low in ruminants, although it has not been studied in ruminants fed regimens which favor starch bypass.) Sucrase and maltase activities in the mucosal brush border also decline during carbohydrate deprivation. Though it has not been shown that hydrolytic activity falls below the rate of hexose transport during carbohydrate deprivation, this would explain the watery feces or diarrhea which develops in dogs or cats following an abrupt shift from a predominantly meat diet to cereal. Starch escaping hydrolysis would be fermented in the large bowel. The outcome would depend on the predominant end-product, acetic or lactic acid. The latter is poorly absorbed and would induce osmotic diarrhea. Otherwise, the feces may simply be more abundant, paler, softer, and foamy. The extent to which they become smaller, denser, and darker within a week or two depends on the amount of food fiber and heat-damaged protein in the pet food.

The dog is probably the most adaptable of all domesticated species in regard to the diversity of feedstuffs which it will ingest. It can be enticed to tackle almost anything its master provides, especially if the master displays a willingness to compete for its consumption. This ingestional adaptability developed during the brief period of dog's association with men. The first signs of this are hunting scenes in the Magdalene Caves drawn about 20,000 years ago. Women learned to cook cereal grains about 10,000 years later, food energy became suddenly abundant, and the population explosion began. Another 10,000 years brought the present century when we suddenly began to feed predominantly cereal diets to dogs. From a taxonomic point of view, the dog remains a carnivore. Its gastrointestinal structure and function emphasize simple hydrolytic digestion suitable for raw feedstuffs of mainly animal origin.

For half a century, people experienced difficulties in introducing dogs to cereal diets and were admonished to do this gradually, "especially when changing from a moist or canned product to a meal-type ration," according to the first subcommittee on Canine Nutrition of the National Research Council.[35] Market preferences changed in the 1960s back toward canned moist products, especially those containing mainly meat and meat by-products. A widely acknowledged epidemic of digestive upsets was associated with this resurgence of "all-meat" dog foods. Going beyond these digestive upsets, all the ills that may attend the prolonged feeding of 100% skeletal muscle were attributed to canned products containing 95% meat and meat by-products.[36] This suggestion was propagated uncritically,[37,38] but the only published epidemiologic data do not support that claim.[39] Following many interviews with practitioners, I have concluded that veterinarians were seeing only digestive upsets that were not accompanied by nutritional diseases.

NUTRITION AND GASTROINTESTINAL DISEASE

Celiac-Like Disease in Dogs

Celiac disease or gluten-sensitive enteropathy is well described in humans and has been hypothesized to occur in dogs and other animals, though this is not thoroughly established. A disorder resembling celiac disease has been observed in dogs.[40,41] Clinical signs are persistent diarrhea, steatorrhea, pale bulky feces, cramps, flatulence, poor growth, or weight loss. These are attributable to malabsorption and partial fermentation of nutrients. Malabsorption initially affects fat assimilation but soon includes all nutrients. The clinical consequences are highly variable; almost any form of nutritional deficiency may become manifested. For this reason, gluten enteropathy is included on the initial differential diagnosis of every malnourished dog that has been fed grains which contain gliadins. These are polyamine proteins from which gluten, a peptide, arises during digestion. Proteins of wheat, rye, barley, oats, and maize contain 30 to 55% gliadins, but rice contains only 1 to 5%. Antigliadin serum from wheat-sensitized patients usually cross-reacts with rye, barley, and oats but not maize or rice; these observations on humans are not consistent,[42] however, so any cross-reactions would have to be studied carefully in animals suspected of having celiac disease.

Celiac disease is characterized by a reduction in the activities of eight intestinal peptidases and disaccharidases and, perhaps secondarily, pancreatic insufficiency.[30] The villi subside, and the flat mucosal surface of the duodenum and jejunum takes on a mosaic appearance. Plasma cells infiltrate the lamina propria and suggest an abnormal immune response.[40] It has responded to restricting the animals to diets containing no cereals except rice or, perhaps, maize (corn). Improvement should occur within a day or two in regard to the character of the feces though manifestations of nutritional deficiencies may take weeks or months to subside.

High Fat Intake and Pancreatitis

The association between a high fat intake and pancreatitis in dogs has some enigmatic features. Chronic pancreatitis has been induced experimentally by feeding a diet containing 77% fat and only 8% protein.[43] The fibrotic changes in the pancreas were just as likely due to protein deficiency as fat excess and may also have partially reflected associated cirrhotic changes in the liver. Experimental induction of acute hemorrhagic pancreatitis by injection of bile and trypsin into the pancreatic duct occurs more readily in dogs fed 40% fat than in others fed 87% carbohydrate or 88% protein.[34] The high fat diet did not increase the volume or enzyme content of pancreatic juice. On the other hand, dogs fed a "1000 calorie, mainly carbohydrate, diet" were far less susceptible to induced acute pancreatitis than those fed a "standard 1400-calorie diet," and this difference was associated with diminished activities of proelastase and trypsinogen in the pancreases of underfed dogs.[44] Epidemiologic data from the author's practice* show no increase in the incidence of pancreatitis associated with an increase in the use of canned meat and meat by-products, i.e., diets that contain 20 to 30% fat on a dry matter basis.[39] In our studies on racing sled dogs, no differences in serum amylase were found after feeding diets containing 17, 25, or 37% fat for 6 months.[45]

Calcium and Vitamin D

Chronic excesses of dietary fats or oils may impair absorption of fat soluble vitamins. Long-term daily use of mineral oil is a classic example of laxative misuse in man. It produces a deficiency of vitamin D, which ultimately leads to a diminution of calcium binding protein in the intestinal mucosa. Impaired calcium absorption results in hypomineralization of bone, a major component of rickets.

An excess of vitamin D may overwhelm the body's first defense against a high calcium intake, namely, a decrease in the efficiency of absorption of calcium. Thus the toxicity of vitamin D is partly dependent upon dietary calcium. Dogs have developed bone abnormalities when fed about twice the dietary calcium recommended as the minimum for maintenance in association with about 14 times the minimum for vitamin D.[4] Rats tolerate about 1000 times the vitamin D minimum, humans only about three times. The primary pathogenic effect of vitamin D deficiency or excess is on calcium absorption from the intestine.

Moderate or high calcium intakes by dairy cows for a month or two prepartum may contribute to the development of parturient hypocalcemia.[46] Total calcium transport through the lactating cow's blood averages about 16 g/day. A rate of calcium absorption from the gut less than this is needed to allow any prepartum calcium mobilization from bone.

The calcium drain associated with the onset of lactation usually lowers the plasma calcium concentration to about 8 mg/dl. This slows down ruminal motility, hence stops the delivery of calcium from the rumen to absorptive sites in the intestines. Also, cows usually stop eating for 4 hours or more after calving, and this limits the delivery of calcium to absorptive sites. If calcium absorption has been the main source of blood calcium, its abrupt cessation exacerbates the hypocalcemia. On the other hand, if calcium absorption has been minor and calcium mobilization has been active, then repair of the hypocalcemia is more likely to occur without the development of paresis.

Fluorosis

Fluorosis diminishes calcium absorption from the digestive tract and promotes a reciprocal increase in calcium removal from bones.[47] The well-known lameness and abnormalities of bones and teeth are secondary to the effect on intestinal function.

Calcium and Trace Minerals

Calcium absorption is also decreased by high intakes of fats or oils which form soaps, or of phytin, which is a mixed salt of inositol hexaphosphate. Phytin is degraded in the rumen, but its effects are important in other mammals, e.g., dogs and pigs. It is abundant in soybeans, so it is customary to fortify corn-soy diets with abundant calcium not only because corn is deficient in calcium but also because soybean oil meal is rich in phytin. Excessive dietary calcium tends to impair absorption of copper or zinc, hence induces os-

*University of Pennsylvania, School of Veterinary Medicine, New Bolton Center, Kennett Square, PA 19348

teoporosis and other signs of copper deficiency,[48] or parakeratosis.[49] The latter zinc-responsive condition has been observed in pigs, calves, and dogs. Excess calcium may also induce goiter, but the action seems to be on the thyroid rather than the absorption of iodine from the gut.

Severe diarrhea may or may not attend copper deficiency in cattle.[50] Copper deficiency must be very severe in order to induce diarrhea if there is no concurrent excess of molybdenum. Morphologic changes occur in the small intestine. Partial atrophy of villi occurs in the duodenum and jejunum. Cytochrome oxidase activity is depleted in the epithelial cells of the duodenum, jejunum, and ileum. How these changes relate to the diarrhea remains obscure. More often the diarrhea manifests a copper-responsive imbalance between copper and molybdenum. Excessive molybdenum unaccompanied by copper deficiency (hypocuprosis) may also cause diarrhea. In this disorder, there is no inflammation or other local damage in the intestine. Molybdenosis may disturb bacterial activity in the large intestine. The interaction between dietary sulfur and molybdenum may involve the formation of thiomolybdate in the rumen. Administration of copper sulfate results in the formation of copper thiomolybdate, which is insoluble and apparently innocuous.

The complex interactions between copper, molybdenum, and sulfate have challenged nutritional scientists. Now the gastroenterologist is confronted by the possibility that there may be two different types of diarrhea in cattle; one associated with epithelial damage in the small intestine, the other with bacterial changes in the rumen and large intestine. Fortunately, whatever the pathogenesis, both forms of diarrhea respond favorably to copper administration and subsequent nutritional prophylaxis with copper. Doses are 1 to 2 g of copper sulfate orally per day or 100 to 200 mg of copper glycinate intravenously, depending on the age and size of the cattle. The usual minimum requirement of copper in the diet of cattle is 10 ppm on a dry matter basis, but the copper:molybdenum ratio should be kept above 2:1 as a general rule, occasionally up to 4:1.

ADAPTING TO IMPROVED PASTURES AND GRAIN

The disorders discussed previously arise in general because we are now feeding animals on diets different from those they adapted to during evolution. Cattle would not have grazed for long on copper-deficient pastures. We may presume that postingestational aversion acted during the past millennia much as it does today. Once we oblige them to reside on land deficient in copper, they become subject to persistent diarrhea.

Man's improvement of pastures started in earnest in the 17th century and since than has threatened the health of animals. Agronomists fertilized the soil with nitrogen, phosphorus, and potassium in order to promote maximal production of plant material per acre. The results were swards which had imbalances of carbohydrate and protein, magnesium and potassium, and copper and molybdenum. At the present time, veterinarians and some animal scientists want agronomists to pay attention to animal health as well as plant growth, but I urge that we learn how to manage animals better on pastures, and how to supplement properly whatever plants are grown.

Undoubtedly the greatest change in food history was the domestication of cereals about 10,000 years ago. Suddenly a new food energy source became available which was much less expensive in terms of time and effort than any staple in the past. Man and other omnivores, especially rats, adapted readily; their populations exploded. Only in the past century, and mainly in North America, have we tried to accommodate herbivores and carnivores to predominantly grain diets. Our efforts have been extremely successful in some species. For example, the "research" (actually much practical trial and error) done on the use of cereal grains as the main constituents of pet foods has yielded products so widely accepted by animals and owners alike that they are now the most common foods for dogs and cats, at least in the United States.

The formulation of whole rations for ruminants based on grain has been less successful. Most of the feeding problems encountered in these animals in North America are attributable to the overfeeding of grain, i.e., bloat, rumenitis, cyclic feeding, liver abscesses, laminitis, D-lactic acidosis, and, in dairy cows, abomasal displacement, milk fat depression, and the "fat cow syndrome."

Current efforts to improve rations for ruminants focus on the need to bypass the rumen with materials which are digested readily by hydrolysis. This includes the starch from grains as well as high-quality protein and fat. Fermentation should be restricted to materials that require it for their utilization, such as cellulosic materials and nonprotein nitrogen. Successful bypass of grain through the rumen will eliminate gastrointestinal problems due to feeding high-grain diets to cattle.

REFERENCES

1. Anonymous: Nutrient Requirements of Dairy Cattle. Washington, D.C., National Academy of Sciences, 1971.
2. Bean, W. B., and Spies, T. D.: Vitamin deficiencies in diarrheal states. J.A.M.A. *115*:1078, 1940.
3. Goddard, K. M., Williams, G. D., Newberne, P. M., and Wilson, R. B.: A comparison of all-meat, semi-moist, and dry-type dog foods as diets for growing beagles. J.A.V.M.A. *157*:1233, 1970.
4. Hedhammar, A., Wu, F. M., Krook, L., Schryver, H. F., deLahunta, A., Whalen, J. P., Kallfelz, F. A., Nunez, E. A., Hintz, H. F., Sheffy, B. E., and Ryan, G. D.: Overnutrition and skeletal disease. An experimental study in growing Great Dane dogs. Cornell Vet. *64*(Suppl. 5):1, 1974.
5. Kronfeld, D. S.: The calcium requirement of calves growing from 400 to 1000 lb in 150 days. *In* Preconditioning Seminar. Edited by D. R. Gill and G. Crenshaw. Laramie, WY, University of Wyoming, 1968.
6. Anonymous: Nutrient Requirements of Beef Cattle. Washington, D.C., National Academy of Sciences, 1970.
7. Anonymous: The Nutrient Requirements of Farm Livestock. Number 2, Ruminants, Technical Reviews and Summaries. London, U.K. Agricultural Research Council, 1965.
8. Rooney, J. R.: The Lame Horse. New York, A. S. Barnes, 1974.
9. Anonymous: Nutrient Requirements of Horses. Washington, D.C., National Academy of Sciences, 1973.
10. Bullen, J. J., and Scarisbrick, R.: Enterotoxemia of sheep: experimental reproduction of the disease. J. Pathol. *73*:495, 1957.
11. Brent, B. E.: Relationship of acidosis to other feedlot ailments. J. Anim. Sci. *43*:930, 1976.
12. Davis, J. D., and Essig, H. W.: Comparison of three bloat-preventing compounds for cattle grazing clover. Can. J. Anim. Sci. *52*:329, 1972.
13. Leng, R. A.: Factors influencing net protein production by the rumen microbiota. *In* Reviews in Rural Science III. Edited by T. M. Sutherland and R. A. Leng. Armidale, Australia, University of New England Publishing Unit, 1976, p. 85.
14. Dougherty, R. W., Coburn, K. S., Cook, H. M., and Allison, M. J.: Preliminary study of appearance of endotoxin in circulatory system of sheep and cattle after induced grain engorgement. Am. J. Vet. Res. *36*:831, 1975.
15. Pounden, W. D., Frank, N. A., Sanger, V. L., and King, N. B.: Feedlot bloat associated with rumenitis and esophagitis. J.A.V.M.A. *137*:503, 1960.
16. Dunlop, R. H., and Hammond, P. L.: D-lactic acidosis of ruminants. Ann. N. Y. Acad. Sci. *119*:1109, 1965.
17. Beede, D. K., and Farlin, S. D.: Effects of capreomycin disulfate and oxamycin on ruminal pH, lactate and volatile fatty acid concentrations in sheep experiencing induced acidosis. J. Anim. Sci. *45*:393, 1977.
18. Graham, N. M., and Williams, A. J.: The effects of pregnancy on the passage of food through the digestive tract of sheep. Aust. J. Agric. Res. *13*:894, 1962.
19. Fell, B. F., Campbell, R. M., and Boyne, R.: Observations on the morphology and nitrogen content of the alimentary canal in breeding hill sheep. Res. Vet. Sci. *5*:175, 1964.
20. Kronfeld, D. S.: A comparison of normal concentrations of reducing sugar, volatile fatty acids and ketone bodies in the blood of lambs, pregnant ewes and nonpregnant adult ewes. Aust. J. Agric. Res. *8*:202, 1957.
21. Snook, L. C.: Fatty infiltration of the liver in pregnant ewes. J. Physiol. *97*:238, 1939.
22. Kronfeld, D. S., Simensen, M. G., and Dungworth, D. L.: Liver glycogen in normal and ketotic cows. Res. Vet. Sci. *1*:242, 1960.
23. Kronfeld, D. S., and Emery, R. S.: Acetonemia. *In* Bovine Medicine and Surgery. Edited by W. J. Gibbons, E. J. Catcott, and J. F. Smithcors. Wheaton, IL, American Veterinary Publications, 1970, p. 350.
24. Kronfeld, D. S.: Energy problems in dairy cows, with additional thoughts on dairy fat in human diets. DVM Newsmagazine *6*:2, 1974.
25. Donaghue, S., and Kronfeld, D. S.: Metabolic responses in dairy cows fed protected tallow. Fed. Proc. *36*:1140, 1977.
26. Kronfeld, D. S.: Pregnancy toxemia. *In* Bovine Medicine and Surgery. Edited by W. J. Gibbons, E. J. Catcott, and J. F. Smithcors. Wheaton, IL, American Veterinary Publications, 1970, p. 377.
27. Van Kruiningan, H. J., Gregoire, K., and Meuten, D. J.: Acute gastric dilatation: a review of comparative aspects by species, and a study in dogs and monkeys. J.A.A.H.A. *10*:294, 1974.
28. Robertson, J. M.: Left displacement of the bovine abomasum: epizootiologic factors. J.A.V.M.A. *29*:421, 1968.
29. Daggs, R. G.: Studies on lactation. I. Production of milk in the dog as influenced by different kinds of food proteins. J. Nutr. *4*:443, 1931.
30. Snook, J. T.: Adaptive and nonadaptive changes in digestive enzyme capacity influencing digestive function. Fed. Proc. *33*:88, 1974.
31. Weijers, H. A., van de Kamer, J. H., Dicke, W. K., and Ijsseling, J.: Diarrhea caused by deficiency of sugar splitting enzymes. Acta Paediatr. *50*:55, 1961.
32. Hill, F. W. G., and Kidder, D. E.: Fat assimilation in dogs estimated by a fat-balance procedure. J. Small Anim. Pract. *13*:23, 1972.
33. Anderson, N. V.: Pancreatitis in dogs. Vet. Clin. North Am. *2*:79, 1972.
34. Haig, T. H.: Experimental pancreatitis intensified by a high fat diet. Surg. Gynecol. Obstet. *131*:914, 1970.
35. Anonymous: Nutrient Requirements of Dogs. Washington, D.C. National Academy of Sciences, 1952.
36. Anonymous: "All meat" petfoods are gone forever. Newsletter to Veterinarians. Topeka, KS, Mark Morris Associates, 1969.
37. Price, D. A.: Dogs need more than meat. J.A.V.M.A. *156*:681, 1970.
38. Newberne, P. M.: Reply to a letter on all-meat dog food. J.A.V.M.A. *159*:138, 1971.
39. Kronfeld, D. S.: Some nutritional problems in dogs. *In* Canine Nutrition. Edited by D. S. Kronfeld. Philadelphia, University of Pennsylvania School of Veterinary Medicine, 1972, p. 26.
40. Kasarda, D. D.: Celiac disease: malabsorption of nutrients induced by a toxic factor in gluten. *In* Protein Nutritional Quality of Foods and Feeds, Part 2. Edited by M. Friedman. New York, Marcel Dekker, 1975, p. 566.
41. Strombeck, D. R.: Dietary management of gastrointestinal disorders. *In* Diet and Disease in Dogs. Edited by D. S. Kronfeld and D. G. Low. Irvine, CA, University of California, 1975.
42. Kronfeld, D. S.: Diet and drugs for diarrhea. DVM Newsmagazine *8*(2):12, 1977.
43. Lindsay, S., Entenman, C., and Chaikoff, I. L.: Pancreatitis accompanying hepatic disease in dogs fed a high fat, low protein diet. Arch. Pathol. *45*:635, 1948.
44. Goodhead, B.: Importance of nutrition in the pathogenesis of experimental pancreatitis in the dog. Arch. Surg. *103*:724, 1971.
45. Kronfeld, D. S., Hammel, E. P., Ramberg, C. F., and Dunlap, H. L.: Hematologic and metabolic responses to training in racing sled dogs fed diets containing medium, low or zero carbohydrate. Am. J. Clin. Nutr. *30*:419, 1977.
46. Kronfeld, D. S.: Parturient hypocalcemia in dairy cows. Adv. Vet. Sci. *15*:133, 1971.
47. Ramberg, C. F., Phang, J. M., Mayer, G. P., Norberg, A. I., and Kronfeld, D. S.: Inhibition of calcium absorption and elevation of calcium removal rate from bone in fluoride treated calves. J. Nutr. *100*:981, 1970.
48. Hartley, W. J., Kater, J. C., and Mackay, A.: Goitre and low copper status in a litter of meat fed puppies. N. Z. Vet. J. *11*:1, 1963.
49. Tucker, H. F., and Salmon, W. D.: Parakeratosis or zinc deficiency disease in the pig. Proc. Soc. Exp. Biol. Med. *88*:613, 1955.
50. Underwood, E. J.: Trace Elements in Human and Animal Nutrition, 4th ed. New York, Academic Press, 1977.

Chapter 16

GASTROINTESTINAL FUNCTION TESTING

A. M. MERRITT and J. HAROLD REED

Function tests may be thought of as probes into the biochemical "milieu internale" of the animal. They are the medical equivalent of exploratory surgery, in a sense. Gastrointestinal function tests are employed primarily as an aid in the diagnosis and prognosis of chronic disorders of stomach and small bowel. Tests of the status of the pancreas and liver are described in their respective chapters.

The usual order of species will be altered in this paragraph, since the bulk of function tests apply to the dog. Gastrointestinal function tests for companion animals are discussed first, followed by those for the pig.

Part I. Function Tests for Dogs, Cats, and Horses

A. M. MERRITT

The decision to apply a specific gut function study to the case at hand should be made only after history, clinical findings, and routine laboratory studies have been evaluated. If possible, the patient should be allowed to adjust to the hospital environment before any special diagnostic studies are done. During this period, the animal's general attitude, appetite, water consumption, defecation pattern, and fecal consistency should be closely observed. As a general rule, the studies described herein would be done primarily in cases of a chronic nature. Before beginning a test, the clinician and client must squarely face the issue of whether the expense of the test is warranted when balanced against the severity of the disease. Also, it is possible that the results of the study will not improve the chances of making a definitive diagnosis.

Tests that are dynamic in nature, as are most gut function tests, are subject to considerable variability around a mean, even within a normal population. Therefore the specific point delineating between normal and abnormal is sometimes difficult to estab-

lish precisely, again emphasizing that the results of a test are only as useful as the completeness of the clinical evaluation to that point, or the adherence to the specific protocol for the test. One should be grateful for those results that are clearly normal or abnormal!

The tests described herein are most easily applied to animals with simple stomachs. The ruminants present problems, particularly for tests involving feeding of a test substance, in that most of the substances commonly used lose their identity by rumen microfloral transformation or degradation.

The state of development of gastrointestinal function testing in veterinary medicine is still fairly rudimentary for a number of reasons, but it is the intention of this chapter to discuss procedures currently in use and to stimulate thinking about new approaches. One of the many challenges in the application of a gut function test to an animal problem, whether the test is unique to veterinary medicine or currently in use in human medicine, is the development of a protocol that is least traumatic to both animal and clinician. For example, where sequential blood samples are necessary for an absorption (tolerance) study, anxiety induced by repeated venipuncture might distress the patient to the point that gastric emptying is slowed and the test invalidated. Placement of a venous catheter before commencement of the study would avoid such a problem.

TESTS OF GASTRIC FUNCTION

Acid Secretion

The rate of gastric acid secretion, under either "basal" (fasting, non-stimulated) or stimulated conditions, is measured in humans when gastric disease is suspected. Histamine dihydrochloride or the histamine analog, betazole, are the stimulants most commonly used since standard dose-response relationships have been established. Gastric acid hypersecretion and duodenal ulceration occur in patients with a gastrin-producing tumor in the pancreas (Zollinger-Ellison syndrome).[1,2] Those with low basal secretion and showing no response to histamine usually have a chronic gastritis and are regarded as "achlorhydric"; they are often anemic since intrinsic factor (IF) production is depressed.

Ulceration of the glandular portion of the stomach occurs commonly enough in domestic animals, often related to some stressful event. To date, however, gastric secretory studies have not been done in such cases, probably for one of a number of reasons: (1) an antemortem diagnosis of ulceration was never made, (2) long-term gastric intubation of domestic animals through either nose or mouth is difficult or impossible, (3) routine procedures for testing have never been established in some species and for others (pig, dog, cat) have not been applied clinically.

At present gastric acid analysis probably has its most potential benefit in canine medicine. Säteri has described a technique for chronic gastrointestinal intubation which is time-consuming but effective.[3] Alternatively, gastric intubation via pharyngostomy is relatively simple in the dog. Finally, if histamine is used as a stimulant, the procedure could be accomplished while the dog is under anesthesia, but this method would not be valid for evaluating basal secretory activity.

Ideally, for a gastric secretory study, a tube should be placed in the most dependent portion of the stomach and all the gastric contents should be collected for the entire duration of the study. Practically, this cannot be done unless an animal will tolerate a nasogastric tube or has a pharyngostomy.

If orogastric intubation is the only alternative, a single sample will provide a lot of information and constant drainage for any length of time will be just that much better.

A method for performing a histamine study in a dog might be:

1. Fast for 18 hours, with no water for 6 hours prior to commencement of study.
2. Pretreat with an antihistamine such as chlorpheniramine maleate, 1 mg/kg body weight intramuscularly, 30 minutes prior to commencement of the study. This will not block the effect of histamine on the stomach but will reduce its other side effects.
3. Intubate to collect a pre-stimulation sample. Leave the tube in place as long as it is tolerated. Try to remove as much of the stomach contents as possible. If the tube is tolerated, discard this initial collection, wait up to 15 minutes, and aspirate as much of the contents as possible. If the animal "fights" the tube, the initial sample will have to suffice.
4. Remove the tube (or leave in place if convenient) and give the dog a single *subcutaneous* injection of histamine at a dose of 0.32 mg of *base* per kilogram body weight. This dose should stimulate the stomach to secrete acid at a maximal rate;[4] i.e., induce a "maximal histamine response" (MHR). Histamine is commercially available as the HCl salt and 2.75 mg of histamine dihydrochloride = 1.0 mg histamine base.
5. One hour after histamine injection collect another gastric sample, again for up to 15 minutes if possible. The gastric juice, particularly after stimulation, should be clear and nearly colorless.
6. To analyze the samples for acid content, mix 1 ml of juice with 10 ml of distilled water and titrate with 0.1 N NaOH to pH 7.
   a. *HCl concentration* in mEq/L = ml 0.1N NaOH used × 100
   b. *HCl output* in mEq/time = [HCl concentration (mEq/L ÷ 1000] × (ml juice collected/time).
      Example: Collect 25 ml of juice in 5 minutes with an HCl concentration of 100 mEq/L

$$\frac{100 \text{ mEq/L}}{1000} \times 25 = 2.5 \text{ mEq output/5 minutes}$$

   c. The pH of the samples is best determined by a pH meter and the values may quite

Table 16–1. Comparative Histamine-Induced Gastric Acid Secretion

| Animal | Interdigestive (Basal) Acid Output | Histamine Dose* | | Maximal Acid Output (mEq/kg/15 min) |
		IV Infusion (mg/kg/min)	SC Injection (mg/kg)	
Dog	Virtually nonexistent	1.6[5]	0.32[4]	0.5[5]
Cat	Virtually nonexistent	1.6[5]	0.32	0.35[5]
Miniature Pig	Spontaneously variable	1.0–2.0[6]	0.32	0.32[6]
Human	Spontaneously variable	0.1–0.2[7]	0.014[8]	0.12[7]

*Expressed as histamine base.

accurately indicate acid concentration if the juice is not contaminated. In samples that contain food, bile, or blood, pH will not be very reliable.

Since the dog has been one of the most commonly used animals in gastrointestinal research, there is a plethora of data available for this species, collected primarily from gastric fistula preparations. It must be emphasized that a well-fasted dog or cat in an environment that has no association with feeding, should secrete very little acid in the basal state[5] (Table 16–1). It would probably be impossible to achieve this state under clinical conditions but, suffice it to say, carnivora should not secrete much acid unless they are stimulated. If the acid concentration of prestimulation samples is > 100 mEq/L and output > 0.5 mEq/15 minutes, something such as a mast cell tumor,[9] a toxic agent with cholinergic effects, or a gastrin-producing tumor[10,11] of the pancreas should be considered.

Normally, dogs given the dose of histamine recommended should have a peak acid output of 0.5 to 0.6 mEq per kilogram body weight per 15 minutes, with a concentration of 135 to 140 mEq/L, occurring between 45 and 75 minutes after administering the drug.[4] There have been a few cases of so-called "achlorhydria" described in dogs, the diagnosis being based primarily upon a history of chronic vomiting, body wasting, and high pH of the vomitus. Unless some sort of secretory challenge study is done on such patients, with failure to respond to a stimulus, a clinical diagnosis of achlorhydria cannot be substantiated.

A method for assessing gastric acid secretory capacity in dogs without passing a tube has been described.[12] Essentially, it involves oral administration of a carboxylic cation-exchange combined with a dye, azure A carbacrylic resin (Diagnex Blue). In the presence of gastric acid the dye is released, absorbed from the intestine, and cleared into the urine. Needless to say, this test indicates only whether the stomach can secrete acid after histamine is given and does not give quantitative information. Pyloric obstruction, malabsorption syndromes, diarrhea, or renal disease may yield false results concerning gastric acid secretion, since each of these disorders interferes with absorption or excretion of the dye.

Tests of Gastric Emptying

The routine way of grossly evaluating gastric-emptying rate in small animals is through sequential radiographs following a radiopaque meal. The evaluation is crude because manipulation of the animal and medication used for restraint can potentially alter the animal's gastric motility. Likewise, if the meal is not of a standard osmolarity, comparisons will be invalid since the osmolarity of contents entering the duodenum has a strong effect on gastric emptying rate.[13] This technique is still helpful, however, especially in situations where retention is prolonged.

Reduced gastric emptying rate will also interfere with carbohydrate absorption studies because the meal will not be delivered to the small intestine at the usual rate and the plasma concentration curve will be "flatter" than normal. This has been documented in the dog[14] and should be applicable to other species where such tests are used. Without some other indication of emptying rate, however, such as radiology, it would be difficult to decide whether a flat curve was indicative of gastric or small intestine disease.

Diseases where there is a partial obstruction of the upper duodenum, either mechanical or functional in nature, may interfere with gastric emptying and may cause reflux of hepatic and pancreatic secretions into the stomach as well. In carnivora, such lesions also commonly cause vomiting. In horses, vomiting is rare, but the installation of a nasogastric tube into patients so affected usually results in the reflux of large quantities of fluid through the tube. The fluid may be bile-stained and have a basic pH. If analysis of this fluid reveals a very high bicarbonate concentration, duodenal obstruction or ileus should be high on the list of probable diagnoses. The point is that gastric contents, collected either as vomitus or via a stomach tube, should be analyzed as thoroughly as possible with special regard to pH, gross microscopic examination of centrifuged precipitate, electrolyte concentration, and cytology.

TESTS OF SMALL INTESTINAL ABSORPTIVE CAPACITY

These tests are based on measurements of single food constituents or other substances administered orally and detected in plasma or urine after absorption.

Fat

Since dietary long-chain triglycerides require more steps in processing than other nutrients before they can appear in the circulation, they are most likely to be malabsorbed in cases of small intestinal, pancreatic, or biliary dysfunction. The easiest way to assess fat absorptive capacity is to do a fat balance study. At present this technique is most applicable to the carnivora, and most of the data available to date concerns dogs. Fat balance implies an exact knowledge of fat intake and an exact measurement of fecal fat output. Valid comparisons with established norms can be made only after the patient has been stabilized on the test diet. The influence of amount of dietary fat on amount of fecal fat has been well demonstrated in dogs[15] and in humans.[16] Both studies suggest that the most accurate way to express the results of a fat balance study is in terms of percent assimilation. For instance, normal dogs weighing between 10 and 15 kg, assimilated 95 to 96% of ingested animal fat, whether they ate 100 or 600 g of fat per day.[15] This indicates that normal dogs have a great capacity to process and absorb large quantities of dietary fat. Another study suggests, however, that results should be expressed as g output per kilogram body weight per day, since diet composition may affect assimilation.[17]

The usual clinical procedure for doing a fat balance study is to feed the patient a given quantity of food of known fat composition and expect a fecal output of less than x grams of fat per day on this diet. The standard method for humans is to give a diet containing 100 g of fat and to collect all the feces produced for a 48- to 72-hour period after the patient has been equilibrated on the test diet for at least 3 days. No medication is given during this time, if at all possible. If the patient excretes less

than 6 g of fat per day in the feces, fat absorption is considered normal. This method is applied without respect to differences in body size. Because there is such a wide range of sizes in the canine species, it has been suggested that the standard diet for dogs on a clinical fat balance study be a canned, preferably all-meat, dog food that contains 8 to 9% crude fat, fed in the amount of 50 g dog food per kilogram body weight per day.[17]

1. Feed canned food (Alpo, Ken-L-Ration, or Puss 'N Boots) at rate of 50 g/kg body weight per day for at least 48 hours prior to fecal collection.
2. Collect total fecal output for 24 hours by use of either metabolism cage or run. A small amount of urinary contamination of the feces will probably not invalidate the results.
3. Store all collected feces in a 4°C refrigerator, or freeze if analysis is not to be done for a few days.
4. Analyze feces for fat concentration according to the technique of Van de Kamer et al.[18] Multiply the concentration × weight of total fecal collection in grams.

Fecal fat output should also be expressed in terms of body weight for comparison and should be less than 0.3 g/kg/day on this diet[17,27] (Table 16–2). Even this value, however, probably overestimates normal output for very large dogs.

For humans, it is a fairly easy matter to collect all material defecated in a 72-hour period. For dogs, any long-term collection of feces is burdensome and it has been suggested that a 24-hour collection is accurate enough for clinical purposes, providing the dog is well established on the test diet.[17] A

Table 16–2. Fecal Analysis of Dogs with Chronic Diarrhea Grouped According to a Diagnosis of Pancreatic Insufficiency (PI), Small Intestinal Malabsorption (IM), Colitis (C), or Other Non-Malabsorptive Intestinal Disease (OT)[27]

Group	N	Fecal Wt (gm/kg/day)	Fecal Fat (gm/kg/day)	Fecal Trypsin (mg/kg/day)
PI	20	34.4 ± 4.5	2.08 ± 0.36	0.49 ± 0.22
IM	6	43.0 ± 8.0	1.14 ± 0.11	15.12 ± 1.94
C	10	11.9 ± 1.1	0.19 ± 0.02	4.07 ± 1.77
OT	17	13.2 ± 2.0	0.18 ± 0.03	4.58 ± 1.30
Normal	14	8.5 ± 1.1	0.24 ± 0.06	4.96 ± 2.34

Fed approximately 50 g/kg body weight of canned meat-type dog food while study was conducted.

metabolism cage or run may be used, depending somewhat upon the consistency of the feces. A small amount of urinary contamination is of no concern. A bigger problem when dealing with dogs, especially those with pancreatic disorders, is that they may be coprophagic.

The routine method for analyzing feces for fat content is the technique of Van de Kamer et al.[18] The simplest procedure described by these authors measures all fatty substances, whether triglycerides or fatty acids, of the medium- and long-chain (C_{10} to C_{18}) types. Van de Kamer's further refinement has been modified by Thompson et al.[19] to differentiate triglycerides from fatty acids, thus giving some indication of whether a steatorrhea is due to true malabsorptive disease (fatty acids predominate in feces) or to maldigestion (more triglycerides than fatty acids present in the feces). This is not usually done, however, since there are more definite ways of distinguishing malabsorption from maldigestion. The Van de Kamer procedure as originally described may provide an underestimation of the amount of fecal fat; the issue revolves around the saponification procedure.[20] The fact remains, however, that most of the data available for comparative purposes, concerning either humans or animals, has been generated using the original Van de Kamer procedure.

Other tests have been described for dogs which involve the feeding of a long-chain triglyceride and visually examining the plasma for the presence of turbidity a few hours later. Feeding 3 ml/kg body weight of corn oil to normal dogs and visually comparing the turbidity of plasma taken before and 2 and 3 hours after administration results in an obvious increase in plasma turbidity (alimentary hyperlipemia). This suggests that the animal can absorb at least some fat.[21] The failure of turbidity to develop suggests that perhaps the dog did not absorb the fat, but it does not discount the possibility that (1) gastric emptying had been delayed, or that (2) the intensity or incident angle of light was poor and the turbidity not seen. This test does not distinguish maldigestion from malabsorption unless lipase is added and incubated with the test meal. Another technique quantitates the degree of lipemia with spectrophotometry using peanut oil as the test fat.[22] This is at least an improvement over the visual determination, especially in terms of sensitivity at the lower end of the scale, but is still subject to errors not related to fat absorption per se. Still, this technique has some merit as a screening procedure in that it is much easier to do, especially in a clinical practice situation, than a fat balance study.

A third and even more quantitative fat tolerance procedure has been described for use in dogs. Linseed oil is used as the test substance because it is present in only small amounts in the diet of most species and is rich in polyunsaturated fatty acids (PFA), which are relatively easy to measure in plasma.[23] After a 12-hour fast, a baseline heparinized blood sample is collected and the patient is fed 1.5 g linseed oil/kg body weight, mixed in 25 g of canned food. Further plasma samples are taken at 1, 2, 4, and 6 hours after feeding and analyzed for PFA. Dogs with pancreatic insufficiency have a significantly lower pretest plasma PFA concentration (75 ± 25 mg/dl) than do normals (143 ± 37 mg/dl), as well as having very little rise in plasma concentration after feeding linseed oil. This procedure is reported to be more advantageous than the fat balance study for the veterinary practitioner because: (1) it avoids the problems of dealing with coprophagic dogs; (2) the plasma PFA analysis is relatively uncomplicated;[23] and (3) the diagnostic benefit is "double-barrelled;" pancreatic insufficient dogs have a lower "basal" plasma PFA concentration as well as a reduced response to linseed oil. Hydrolyzed ("digested") linseed oil has been used to see whether a distinction between malabsorption and maldigestion can be made but results have been inconclusive.

In another attempt to avoid the messy business of collecting fecal material, a system of assessing fat absorption by the oral administration of I^{131}-labelled triolein and oleic acid has been described.[24,25] Since both the fatty acid and the triglyceride are labelled with the same isotope, they have to be given a few days apart to get meaningful results. The technique requires sequential blood sampling and the ready availability of a gamma counter. Ostensibly one can differentiate between maldigestive and malabsorptive components of the steatorrhea with this test in that the triolein will be preferentially malabsorbed if the case is an uncomplicated pancreatic insufficiency. These principles have been demonstrated in the dog.[25] The isotopic techniques have been evaluated in comparison with the usual quantitative analysis. It has been concluded that: (1) measurement of quantitative fecal radioactivity is much more accurate than blood peak radioactivity; (2) the error increases when feces are counted in the presence of steatorrhea; and (3) the radioactive tests do not give an accurate indication of degree of steatorrhea.[24] This would suggest that feces must be collected even with the labelled fat procedure. Therefore, it seems better to do just the quantitative analysis and avoid the problems and equipment needed for handling, measuring, and disposing of isotopes.

A simple way of qualitatively assessing the amount of split (digested) versus neutral (undigested) fat in the feces has been found to be quite accurate in distinguishing pancreatic insufficiency, in which neutral fats predominate, from other causes of steatorrhea in humans.[26] Split fats are detected by vigorously mixing a 3-mm diameter pellet of feces with a drop of 36% acetic acid on a glass slide. A drop of Sudan III is added, a coverslip is applied, and the mixture is brought to a boil 3 times. When examined microscopically, the split fats appear as orange globules that form sheaths and spicules upon cooling. For humans on a fat tolerance study, split fats are considered positive when 10 or more globules of 20 to 40 μ or larger are seen per hpf. Neutral fats are detected by Sudan III without boiling and using the preceding criteria. There was an excellent correlation in humans between the amount of split fat and the degree of steatorrhea,[26] but the cause of the fat malabsorption (e.g., villous atrophy, stagnant loop) obviously could not be determined. If positive only for neutral fats, it strongly suggested that the patient had pancreatic insufficiency.

In my opinion, the best way to assess a carnivore's or omnivore's ability to assimilate fat is to do a balance study. Adjunct tests will need to be done to indicate whether steatorrhea is due to maldigestion or malabsorption, but experience with dogs suggests that very high fecal fat outputs are usually related to pancreatic insufficiency[27] (Table 16–3). In ruminants, and perhaps in horses, where dietary fat is totally transformed by gastrointestinal microorganisms, tests other than fat balance may be necessary to indicate pancreatic or intestinal dysfunction.

Carbohydrate

The two sugars that have been used most frequently to assess small bowel absorptive function are D-glucose and D-xylose. At present D-glucose is more popular with veterinary practitioners because it is easier to measure. D-xylose is more sensitive, however, since it does not normally appear in plasma in measurable amounts and is not as subject to changes in the metabolic state of the animal.

Essentially, the test involves the oral administration of a standard amount of the sugar, either drunk ad libitum by the patient or instilled via stomach tube, and subsequent documentation of the sugar's appearance in the plasma over the next 3 or 4 hours.

The plasma concentration usually peaks 60 to 90 minutes after administration. This technique relies on organs other than the small intestine to function normally in order for the plasma concentration curve to attain the expected configurations (Figs. 16–1 and 16–2). A full stomach will retard movement of the test meal into the intestine, for example. Second, gastric emptying rate can be slowed considerably by excessive excitement (perhaps associated with administration of the test substance), hypertonicity of the test meal,[13] excessive abdominal pain, or small intestinal obstruction. Third, small intestinal transit time can be affected by such things as obstructions, drugs that alter intestinal motility, toxemias, and abdominal pain. Fourth, reduced intestinal blood flow will affect the rate of appearance of the sugar in the general circulation. Fifth, overgrowth of certain bacteria within the small bowel lumen may metabolize the sugar directly and this would be reflected in a lower than normal peak concentration.[28] Finally, the sugar may be rapidly sequestered in ascitic fluid, also resulting in a lower than normal peak.[29]

Figure 16–1 illustrates several of the points discussed previously. Horse A had a chronic cirrhotic partial obstruction of the mid-duodenum, characterized clinically by periodic bouts of colic with reflux of duodenal contents into the stomach. The

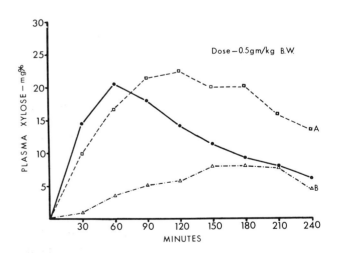

Figure 16–1. Equine xylose absorption. Disorders other than a primary intestinal malabsorption that can influence the results of a xylose absorption study are illustrated. The unbroken line indicates the mean values for 10 normal horses. Horse A had a chronic partial obstruction of the mid-duodenum; her values are consistent with an increased intestinal transit time where the xylose was in contact with the absorptive mucosa for a longer than normal time period. Horse B had a gastrojejunostomy to bypass a pyloric stenosis; his values are consistent with a "blind loop" syndrome where overgrowth of bacteria within the small intestine could have metabolized the xylose before it was absorbed.

The procedure for conducting a carbohydrate absorption test is quite simple.

1. Fast (allow water free choice)
   a. Dogs and Cats—overnight
   b. Horses—24 hours (muzzle)
2. Catheterize jugular or cephalic vein and draw blood sample into heparinized tube.
3. Feed or instill by stomach tube 0.5 g/kg body weight of d-xylose as a 10% solution. Do not give any other food along with the xylose if at all possible. Withhold water for 2 hours after xylose administration.
4. Collect heparinized blood samples every 30 minutes for 4 hours (cats 3 hours) after feeding the d-xylose.
   NOTE: If d-xylose is to be measured directly, there is no need to process the blood samples immediately. If a test measuring all reducing substances is to be used (e.g., a ferrocyanide technique), blood samples must be centrifuged immediately and the plasma must be harvested and frozen.
5. D-xylose can be measured directly using a modified method of Frankel[11,12] or by a technique described by Roe and Rice.[13]

The patients should have a relatively empty stomach; for dogs and cats a 12- to 18-hour fast suffices. In horses, a 24-hour fast is necessary. The animals may drink water free choice during the fast but it should be withheld during the test. If possible, an indwelling catheter should then be inserted into the jugular or cephalic vein. A pretest blood sample is drawn, and catheter patency is maintained with heparinized saline solution for further sampling. Ideally the sugar should be in a 5% solution which is isosmolar (300 mOsm/L) and should be emptied from the stomach at an optimum rate.[13] This concentration is not practical, however, since it requires a volume that is undesirably large. A 10% solution provides a more convenient volume with clinically useful results. One should avoid giving the sugar with any other food. Blood samples are then collected every 30 minutes for 3 or 4 hours after administration of the sugar. As mentioned before, the plasma concentration usually peaks in 60 to 90 minutes so that if time and/or money are constraints, a pretest blood sample and two others at the times stated above will give an accurate curve in most cases. The possible exception to this concerns the observation that ponies given glucose had a peak plasma concentration 3½ hours after dosing if fasted 36 hours, while a peak was attained at 1 hour

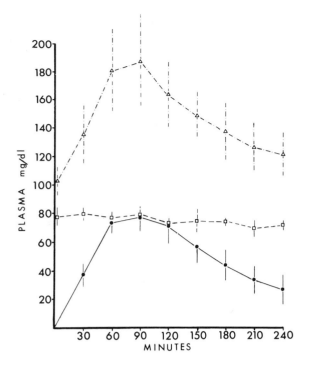

Figure 16–2. Plasma xylose concentration measured by the orcinol method[42] [●———●], plasma glucose concentration measured by the glucose oxidase method [□- - -□], and total plasma reducing substances measured by the potassium ferricyanide method [△—·—·△] in five normal fasted dogs given 0.5 g of xylose per kilogram body weight per os. The vertical lines are standard deviations (S.D.). The potassium ferricyanide method is used commonly in autoanalyzers to measure plasma glucose concentration. This figure suggests that a diagnostic xylose absorption study may be done in dogs using potassium ferricyanide as the reagent, since xylose administration does not influence the fasting plasma glucose concentration. The heparinized samples must be centrifuged and the plasma harvested immediately for the results to be accurate.

xylose absorption study presented in Figure 16–1 was conducted during a nonsymptomatic interval. The results suggest that the xylose could get out of the stomach at the usual rate, as demonstrated by a fairly normal rate of increase in the plasma concentration but was held up in the duodenum during its absorption, as shown by the sustained high concentration. Horse B had a partial obstruction of the duodenum near the pylorus that was manifested clinically by persistent mild colic and partial anorexia. A gastrojejunostomy was surgically created which gave the animal substantial relief. The abnormally low plasma concentration curve in this case might reflect the effects of the surgical procedure, where bypassing the duodenum resulted in the loss of a significant amount of absorptive surface and created a "blind loop" in which intestinal flora overgrew.

if fasted for 12 hours.[30] This occurred independent of transit time.

Glucose is more attractive to the practitioner than xylose because it is easier to obtain and measure. It is also sufficient for identifying cases with severe small intestinal mucosal damage, or more rarely, a specific D-glucose malabsorption. Its use has been well-demonstrated in dogs,[31] horses,[32] and pigs.[33] When given at a dose of 1.5 to 2.0 g/kg body weight, the peak plasma glucose concentration should be at least double that of the fasting value, and should decline rapidly. As suggested, it is not a very specific indicator of malabsorption, however, and its metabolic kinetics are at the whim of numerous metabolic aberrations.

Xylose is desirable because it is not normally present in measurable quantities in the plasma. It was thought at one time that xylose absorption from the intestine was strictly through passive diffusion. More recent studies have shown that some of this pentose is absorbed actively,[34,35,36] perhaps using the same carrier systems as glucose does since competitive inhibition between the sugars can be demonstrated.[37] Once in the plasma, about 50% of the xylose is metabolized, the pathway for which is not known, and the other 50% is excreted into the urine.[38,39]

The usual method for assessing xylose absorption in humans involves a quantitative 5-hour urine collection, instead of measurement of plasma concentration. However, false positive results (i.e., indicating malabsorption) have been seen due to renal dysfunction. Even though quantitating urinary output may be more integrative than the measurement of plasma concentration, the latter is much easier for the veterinary practitioner.

The normal dog appears to have a great capacity to absorb xylose. A positive dose/response relationship has been shown between peak plasma concentrations and doses up to 2.0 g/kg without any indication that the system was saturated with even the highest dose.[40] A working normal value for dogs after a dose of 0.5 g/kg body weight is a peak plasma concentration of greater than 45 mg/dl above baseline; in my experience, the mean peak concentration is considerably higher than this value (Fig. 16–2). Cats appear to be similar to dogs with respect to peak plasma concentration.

Dose/response studies of xylose absorption in horses suggest that 0.5 g/kg is fairly close to, if not exceeding, its transport maximum (TM) in the small intestine.[41] This dose produces a mean peak plasma concentration of only about 20 mg/dl in this species;

the difference between normal and abnormal is large enough, however, to make the test diagnostically useful.

Various techniques have been developed for measuring xylose directly,[42,43] and these must be used on horse plasma since the difference between basal and peak plasma concentrations is relatively small. For the carnivores it may be more practical to measure total plasma reducing substances (many autoanalyzers do this).

This is quite accurate, since administration of the xylose does not significantly affect plasma glucose levels, as illustrated in Figure 16–2.

Protein

It stands to reason that conditions which result from malabsorption of fats and carbohydrates will also affect absorption of nitrogenous substances. In fact, changes in fecal fat and fecal nitrogen outputs closely parallel each other in health and disease.[44,45,46] About half of the nitrogen in feces of normal animals is derived from dietary sources while the other half is endogenous from mucosal cell turnover and plasma leakage.[47] Thus, increased fecal nitrogen output may be due to pancreatic insufficiency, primary malabsorption, or increased plasma protein loss. In contrast to fecal fat, differential analysis cannot be done on fecal nitrogen to distinguish whether its increase is due to maldigestion or malabsorption; the usual battery of challenge tests and fecal enzyme measurements is necessary to make the distinction. Special tests involving the use of radioisotopes are necessary to determine whether excessive leakage of plasma protein into the bowel lumen is involved.

If protein malabsorption or loss is severe and prolonged, the plasma albumin concentration will be depressed. Other causes of hypoalbuminemia such as protein-losing nephropathy, chronic liver disease, or malnutrition can be assessed with relative ease in contrast to the studies necessary to distinguish between protein (nitrogen) maldigestion, malabsorption, and/or hypersecretion.

TESTS OF DIGESTIVE COMPETENCE

Most tests of digestive activity within the intestinal tract are helpful when it has been demonstrated that absorptive capacity is probably normal. For instance, in a test that relies on the appearance of products of digestion in the plasma or urine, a false positive result (i.e., indicating maldigestion) could be obtained if the products were malabsorbed, even though digested adequately.

Fat

The combined use of orally administered ^{131}I oleic acid and triolein, mentioned under absorptive studies, was designed to test for fat digestive versus absorptive competence. Failure of ^{131}I to appear in the plasma after giving the triolein would suggest a deficiency of bile salts and/or pancreatic lipase, whereas if ^{131}I failed to appear after giving the oleic acid, small intestinal disease resulting in malabsorption is present and no definitive impressions could be gained regarding digestive function. The efficacy of using these isotopes has already been discussed.

With regard to measurement of fat in the feces, methods have been described for measuring triglycerides and fatty acids separately.[19] Presumably, if triglycerides predominate, the steatorrhea is more likely due to maldigestion than malabsorption. Not only are the analytic techniques difficult, expensive, and time-consuming, but a large overgrowth of bacteria within the bowel might decrease the triglyceride:fatty acid ratio in the feces.

Carbohydrates

Starch. The oral administration of starch is an extremely simple and useful test for demonstrating the presence of pancreatic amylase, again assuming that the small intestinal mucosa is fully capable of absorbing hexoses. The use of starch tolerance in dogs has been well documented.[48] A dose of 3 g/kg body weight is given via stomach tube and sequential blood samples for measurement of glucose concentration are taken every 30 minutes for 2½ hours after dosing. If pancreatic amylase has been secreted in sufficient quantity, the fasting plasma glucose concentration should rise to about 125 to 130 mg/dl within the hour. The following summarizes the suggested protocol for a starch tolerance test in dogs.

1. Fast overnight but allow water free choice.
2. Weigh starch at 3 g/kg body weight and add 1.5 ml of hot water/3 g and mix to give a clear, readily flowing gel.
3. Catheterize jugular or cephalic vein (to keep catheter open, fill with a small amount of heparinized sailine solution and plug between samples). Collect a control blood sample into a fluoride/oxalate tube.
4. Feed the starch warm to prevent gel formation; instillation by stomach tube will probably

be necessary. Do not mix starch with other food.
5. Collect blood samples in fluoride/oxalate tubes at every 30 minutes for 2½ hours after feeding. Submit to the laboratory for glucose determination. A rise in the plasma glucose concentration to 125 to 130 mg/dl within the first hour is normal.[48]

Lactose. Chronic milk intolerance has been identified in both cats and dogs (see Chapter 23). As with humans, it is necessary to establish whether the gastrointestinal disturbance is due to deficiency of the enzyme lactase or hypersensitivity to the casein in the milk. A lactose tolerance test will distinguish between these and, to date, such a test has been applied to dogs[49] and horses.[50] The principle is the same as the starch tolerance test; give lactose orally and measure changes in plasma glucose. Again, monosaccharide absorptive capacity must also be evaluated if the results of the lactose test are abnormal.

Horses over 3 years of age do not digest lactose and this corresponds to the observation that neutral β-galactosidase normally disappears from the equine small intestinal mucosa around this age.[51] In horses less than 3 years old a lactose dose of 1 g/kg body weight, given as a 20% solution, caused the fasting plasma glucose concentration to rise from 80 to 150 mg/dl within 1 hour.[50] Similar results occurred in 14 ponies given 0.5 g/kg body weight even though their ages ranged from 1 to 14 years.[30]

Lactose intolerance has been described in several adult dogs with chronic diarrhea.[49] They were tested with 2 g lactose per kilogram body weight as a 12.5% solution. In normal dogs, the plasma glucose peaked at 127 mg/dl 90 minutes after dosing while there was no change in the lactose-deficient animals.[49] The effects of age-maturation on β-galactosidase activity in the small intestine in dogs has not been reported, but since many older dogs eat food mixtures which contain milk products and do not have digestive disturbances, one assumes that in most cases the intestine remains capable of producing these enzymes throughout life. There is substantial evidence to suggest that the degree of β-galactosidase activity in the intestine has no relationship to the amount of milk products in the diet, however.[52]

Proteins

Specific challenge tests for gastrointestinal protein digestive capacity are few, even in human medicine. Orally administered gelatin has probably been used most frequently. One of the breakdown products of gelatin hydrolysis is the amino acid hydroxyproline, which is quite stable and apparently not metabolized in the body. The protocol for the test in humans[53] is to place the patients on a hydroxyproline-deficient diet for 3 days prior to the test, collecting all the urine produced on the final day as a baseline. Subjects are then fasted overnight, a control blood sample is drawn in the morning, and 25 g of gelatin are fed in a warm sweet carbohydrate-based vehicle. Blood samples are taken hourly and urine specimens collected every 2 hours, for 8 hours after feeding. Total hydroxyproline in urine and serum is measured. For clinical purposes, measurement of urine output alone will suffice, assuming that renal function is normal, although for animals it may be more convenient to collect blood than urine. The indications from the results in humans are that the test may be more helpful in identifying pancreatic insufficiency than small intestinal mucosal disease,[54] suggesting that the hydroxyproline is a by-product of the pancreatic phase of gelatin digestion.

Measurement of proteolytic enzyme activity in feces has been used extensively as an indicator of pancreatic function in both human and veterinary medicine. The commonly used techniques for indicating presence or absence of activity are well known to veterinary practitioners, involving the digestion of gelatin in x-ray film or in a test tube. Nine parts of 5% $NaHCO_3$ are well mixed with one part feces and centrifuged. The supernatant is placed in a small test tube into which a strip of x-ray film is placed, or 1 ml is added to 2 ml of a warm (37°C) 7.5% gelatin solution.[55] Either preparation is incubated for 1 hour at 37°C or for 2 hours at room temperature. If proteolytic enzyme activity is sufficient, the gelatin emulsion of x-ray film will be liquefied, and the gelatin solution will not gel again after refrigeration for 20 minutes. Both tests are basically qualitative although the gelatin tube test is reported to be more sensitive[56] and may be semiquantitated if time is taken to make serial fecal solutions and match the results with a standard curve which has been derived using known concentrations of trypsin.

These relatively crude qualitative methods have been superseded by highly refined and specific assays for fecal trypsin and chymotrypsin.[57] These assays allow fecal enzyme output to be calculated and some interesting findings have already been reported:

1. In humans, measuring chymotryptic activity may provide a more sensitive indication of pancreatic secreting status than does tryptic activity.[58,59]

2. Normal dogs have extremely variable fecal trypsin output from one day to the next.[60,61]

3. Dogs with intestinal mucosal disease and malabsorption have significantly higher fecal trypsin output than normal[24,49] (Table 16–3).

4. Normal horses and cattle have no measurable tryptic or chymotryptic activity even when the sensitive assays are used, in my experience.

Thus, the highly sophisticated and sensitive assays have advantages over the qualitative methods primarily in that their indication of absence of activity is more reliable than the usual qualitative procedures,[27,62] and that very high outputs can be recognized which may help substantiate the diagnosing of small intestinal mucosal disease with malabsorption. Their major disadvantage is their intricacy and need for considerable equipment. Thus, it is unlikely that they will be adopted as routine veterinary hospital procedures except in an institutional setting.

A technique has now been described for use in humans; it combines maximal peptide stimulation of the pancreas, followed by purgation to expel the enzymes before too much degradation occurs.[63] The fecal enzyme output apparently correlates well with direct measurement of pancreatic secretion as collected by duodenal suction.[64] It is possible that peptide stimulation and purgation could be applied successfully to the carnivora, thus avoiding the need for duodenal intubation.

DIRECT TEST FOR ASSESSING PANCREATIC SECRETORY FUNCTION

While very severe steatorrhea, absence of proteolytic enzymes in the feces, and abnormal starch tolerance are all indicative of pancreatic exocrine insufficiency, such evidence is indirect. Measuring pancreatic secretory capacity directly is definitive, but also rather difficult. The principle involves the placement of the tip of a tube passed via nose or mouth into the duodenum near the opening of the pancreatic duct. Secretin and/or cholecystokinin (CCK) are then given parenterally and the duodenal contents are aspirated continuously for 45 to 60 minutes. The contents are analyzed for bicarbonate concentration and enzyme activity which, when multiplied by the volume of the aspirate, provides an output value. Secretin is most commonly used since it stimulates volume and bicarbonate output,

Table 16–3. Pancreatic Secretin/CCK Responses of Normal and Pancreatic Insufficient Conscious Dogs with Intraduodenal Intubation; After Säteri[23]

	Volume		Bicarbonate				Amylase			
	Control ml/kg/20'	Secretin* ml/kg/20'	Control mEq/L	mEq/kg/20'	Secretin* mEq/L	mEq/kg/20'	Control μ/ml	μ/kg/20'	CCK† μ/ml	μ/kg/20'
Normal	0.58 ± 0.40	0.71 ± 0.33	23.9 ± 17.8	11.3 ± 10.8	60.1 ± 20.5	40.0 ± 15.5	1672 ± 1504	652 ± 474	2583 ± 1495	2112 ± 1331
Pancreatic insufficient	0.22 ± 0.22	0.28 ± 0.28	5.3	1.2	18.5 ± 20.6	6.4 ± 9.8	12 ± 29	2 ± 5	7 ± 12	4 ± 8

mean ± S.D.

* Secretin dose—1 clinical unit/kg body weight, pulse dose intravenously.
† CCK dose—1.5 CHR units/kg body weight, pulse dose intravenously.

thus making aspiration easier. It has been assumed that if the pancreas can secrete electrolytes and water normally, it ought to be able to produce adequate enzymes. This is probably true 99% of the time but sometimes quantitation of enzyme secretory capacity might be desirable and CCK must then be given. If CCK is to be used, it must be administered in conjunction with secretin since, when given alone, it does not stimulate much water and electrolyte secretion and the enzymes would be retained in the duct system or secreted erratically.

The "secretin test" has been used for many years in human medicine where the patient can cooperate in the placement of the tube into the duodenum.[65,66] A technique has been developed for placing a tube into the duodenum of a dog.[3] It involves anesthetizing the animal, passing the tube with a mercury bag on the end into the stomach, and then, through a rather intricate procedure, passing the other end of the tube through a nasal passage in retrograde fashion. The dog is then allowed to wake up and is periodically checked radiographically until the mercury bag is determined to be in the duodenum. The development of this technique resulted in a study of direct challenge testing of the pancreas in the conscious dog without prior placement of intestinal cannulas, i.e., a potentially clinically useful technique.[23] Both normal and sick animals have been tested and an abridgement of the results is shown in Table 16–3.

TESTS FOR EXCESSIVE PLASMA PROTEIN LOSS INTO THE BOWEL ("PROTEIN-LOSING ENTEROPATHY")

In the middle 1960s there was considerable interest in human gastroenterology regarding protein-losing enteropathies (PLE) and the identification thereof. First, the hypoproteinemia seen in conjunction with some gastrointestinal diseases could be rationally explained when liver and kidney function were normal. Then there was the thought that if patients so afflicted could be identified, greater understanding of endogenous protein kinetics and the pathogenesis of the patient's enteric disease would be at hand. Some of these dreams came true and now there is a list of more than 60 enteric diseases in people in which excessive loss of plasma protein into the bowel occurs.[67] Yet the etiology and/or pathophysiology of most of these diseases still is not known.

Hypoproteinemia and edema associated with a gastrointestinal disturbance suggest that PLE is present. The excessive loss of protein may not be reflected in the plasma concentration, however, unless increased intake and synthesis cannot keep up with the loss. Documentation of PLE may not be necessary if it has already been shown to occur in the specific disease condition presented. On the other hand, if a new pathologically and clinically manifested enteric disease were described in an animal, knowing whether excessive plasma protein loss was an essential part of the disease might be helpful in future diagnosis and therapy of the problem. Therefore, while PLE is usually not definitive enough in itself for making a specific diagnosis, knowing that excessive protein loss is occurring in association with some other sign or clinicopathologic manifestation may be definitive.

Documentation of the movement of protein, e.g., albumin, from plasma into gut requires a reliable marker. Ideally, the marker should remain firmly attached to the protein under study while in the plasma, must not be secreted into the intestinal tract unless bound to protein, and must be totally nonabsorbable by the intestine. Radioactive isotopes are the most useful markers, but none is ideal. Some tagged colloids of similar molecular size to plasma macromolecules have been used, such as iodine[131]-polyvinyl pyrollidine, copper[67]-ceruloplasmin, and iron[59]-dextran, with limited success.[68] Chromium[51]-albumin is more popular and physiologic since it involves a protein that is in abundance in the blood; but it is useful only for measuring protein secretion into the intestine and not endogenous albumin kinetics since it elutes in significant quantities to plasma transferrin over the course of a study.[69] Conversely, I[131]- or I[125]-albumin is stable in plasma but poor for gastrointestinal studies since iodine is both secreted and absorbed in the gastrointestinal tract. Thus if one desires to know both the amount of albumin moving from plasma into gut lumen and the effects of this movement on endogenous albumin kinetics, a double isotope study using [51]Cr- and ^{125}I-labelled albumin is indicated.[70]

Successful accomplishment of these kinds of studies requires cooperative animals and methods of restraint, caging, and training whereby there is no chance that urine and feces will be mixed. In the early part of the study in particular, the urine is always very radioactive since even the best prepared injections contain free isotope which is cleared through the kidney. If the injection is to be ^{51}Cr-labelled albumin, it is best that the albumin be species-specific, although the commercially prepared radiolabelled human albumin[71,72] or just [51]CrCl$_3$[69,71] will suffice if only cumulative percent dose in the feces is being measured. Unfortunately not much control data are available for animals, using either the albumin-labelled material or the radioactive salt (Table 16–4).

For clinical purposes, documentation of the cumulative fecal output of the isotope over 4 to 5 days after injection will suffice in most cases. If obtaining some figure for plasma clearance of albumin into the gut is desired, sequential blood samples must be taken. The "clearance" is an expression of the fraction of the plasma pool lost into the gut per time and this provides more meaningful information about plasma albumin kinetics than cumulative fecal excretion of [51]Cr. For comparison within a species where body sizes vary greatly, normalization by body weight is recommended. Therefore a clearance value would indicate x ml of plasma per kilogram body weight from which all of the albumin was removed per day. This value is usually small.

Clearance is best calculated from data that have been collected from 48 hours after isotope injection to the end of the study. By this time any significant amounts of free ^{51}Cr administered in the injectate will have been removed from the plasma and the calculation is thus:[67]

ml of plasma cleared of protein/day =

$$\frac{\text{radioactivity in the feces in a 24-hour period}}{\text{mean radioactivity/ml serum in the period}}$$

Using *all* data in the study, a more kinetically applicable calculation for clearance is:[67]

$$Cl_{gi} = \frac{Q_t}{\int_{t=o}^{t=n} Q_p \, dt}$$

Cl_{gi} = fraction of plasma pool cleared of protein per day into gastrointestinal tract.

Q_t = cumulative fecal excretion of ^{51}Cr as a fraction of the injected dose.

Q_p = plasma radioactivity as fraction of the injection dose.

Table 16–4. Fecal Loss of Intravenously Injected ^{51}Cr-Albumin in Dog, Horse, and Man

Species	Injection	IV Dose	% Dose ^{51}Cr in Feces	Reference
Canine	^{51}Cr-labelled human albumin	1.47 μCi/kg-bw	1.72 ± 1.41 in 3 days	Finco et al.[70]
Canine	^{51}Cr-labelled canine albumin	2 μCi/kg-bw	5.86 ± 1.06% in 12 days	Kallfelz and Wallace[71]
	[51]CrCl$_3$	2 μCi/kg-bw	7.6 ± 1.1% in 11 days	Kallfelz and Wallace[71]
Equine	^{51}Cr-labelled equine albumin	2 μCi/kg-bw	1.25 ± 0.64% in 5 days	Merritt et al.[72]
Human	^{51}Cr-labelled human albumin	2–4 μCi/kg-bw	<0.7% in 4 days	Waldmann[67]

LOOKING TOWARD THE FUTURE

Vitamin B$_{12}$ Absorption Test

The vitamin B$_{12}$ absorption (Schilling) test is used in human medicine when either achlorhydria and intrinsic factor (IF) deficiency or small intestinal disease is suspected. As mentioned before, IF deficiency is not a recognized clinical entity in veterinary medicine, but more methods for evaluating intestinal function in animals are always welcome. In humans, vitamin B$_{12}$ is preferentially absorbed in the ileum so that its malabsorption indicates ileal disease; whether this would be the case for domestic animals remains to be investigated. Vitamin B$_{12}$ is also malabsorbed in people who have an overgrowth of bacteria in their small intestine[73,74] (stagnant or blind loop syndrome) which presents clinically as a malabsorption syndrome. The intestinal bacteria under these conditions metabolize vitamin B$_{12}$ before it can be absorbed.[74] Thus the Schilling test is helpful in distinguishing this disorder from other kinds of small intestinal diseases that result in malabsorption.

The Schilling test has been applied to dogs under experimental conditions[75] and should be thought of seriously in the future for clinical use in veterinary medicine. In the experimental study, fasted healthy mongrel dogs were given 1 μC of radioactive B$_{12}$ in 100 ml of saline solution via stomach tube, followed in 2 hours by the administration of 1000 μg of non-radioactive B$_{12}$ injected intramuscularly to effect a renal flush. The animals were then placed in a metabolism cage and the urine was collected for 1 day. The cumulative 24-hour urinary output ranged between 15% and 56% of the radioactive dose and averaged 35%.

The "Breath Tests"

The principle behind the breath tests is that a ^{14}C-labelled substance which is known to be metabolized by intestinal bacteria is fed, and that portion of the substance which is broken down is indicated by the amount of $^{14}CO_2$ that appears at a certain time in the expired air of the patient. These tests are relatively easy to perform in any radioisotope laboratory and use only small amounts of stable, safe isotopes. The common breath test used in humans to date involves bile acid metabolism. A bile acid such as cholic acid is fed as a glycine conjugate, the form it would be in if secreted by the liver into the gut. The conjugate is tagged with ^{14}C.[76] Normally most of the conjugated bile acids are absorbed intact from the ileum; the minute amount escaping into the colon is metabolized by colonic bacteria to release $^{14}CO_2$ which is absorbed and exhaled. If there is a sufficient overgrowth of bacteria in the small intestine, the ^{14}C-conjugated bile salts will be deconjugated and metabolized in the small intestine and large amounts of ^{14}C will appear in the exhaled breath within an hour or two of ingestion. ^{14}C-xylose is another substrate being studied in this regard.[77,78]

These and related tests have great promise in veterinary gastroenterology, especially for small animals. Techniques could be developed whereby exhaled gases could be collected, stored, and shipped to a central radioisotope laboratory for counting.

Substrate-PABA Digestion Tests[34]

Two other function studies, involving para-amino benzoic acid (PABA) have been reported. N-benzoyl-L-tyrosyl-aminobenzoic acid, a synthetic peptide, is cleaved by pancreatic chymotrypsin, releasing PABA, which is absorbed and excreted in the urine. In human patients with pancreatic insufficiency, urinary PABA excretion was significantly reduced.[79] Recently, this test has been applied to dogs,[80] and the results look promising in helping to distinguish pancreatic insufficiency from other maldigestive/malabsorptive diseases. At this writing, however, the N-benzoyl-L-tyrosyl-PABA conjugate is not commercially available.

Part II. Function Tests for Pigs

J. HAROLD REED

Information concerning the absorption of carbohydrates by the gastrointestinal tract has been produced as a result of investigations into the nutrition and metabolism of pigs and from work to develop suitable diets for early weaned pigs.[81]

THE ORAL GLUCOSE TOLERANCE TEST

Reproducible results for the oral glucose tolerance test have been reported for the pig.[33,82,83] The procedure involves withholding food and water for 12 hours prior to the test and allowing the pig to drink a solution of glucose voluntarily or administering the test dose by stomach tube. A dose of 1.5 g/kg given as a 20% aqueous solution is satisfactory for pigs weighing 10 to 25 kg, while less glucose (0.75 to 1.0 g/kg) is adequate for older pigs. It is wise to train the pigs to drink glucose prior to the test. Blood is collected easily from the anterior vena cava.[84] Samples taken every 15 minutes for 60 to 90 minutes will be adequate to plot the curve. The

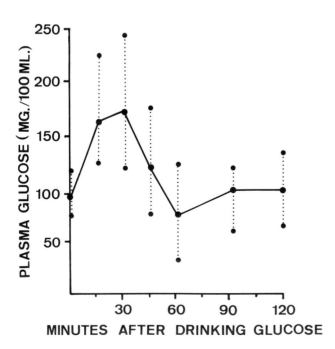

Figure 16–3. The mean oral glucose tolerance curve and the range of values obtained for 18 tests done on 24 pigs weighing 10 to 25 kg. Glucose (20% w/v in water) was given at the dosage rate of 1.5 g/kg.

results of control studies indicate that the fasting plasma glucose concentration of pigs remains stable in spite of the stimulation due to handling and blood collection.[33]

Using this technique, the plasma glucose concentration will be found to peak at 30 minutes and to have returned to the fasting concentration by 60 minutes in most pigs (Fig. 16–3). The degree of hyperglycemia is variable.

D-XYLOSE ABSORPTION TEST

Xylose absorption has had only limited study in the pig. In piglets fed diets containing glucose, fructose, and xylose, xylose was found to disappear from the first half of the small intestine much more slowly than glucose. This was thought to be caused by competition for the common transport system for which xylose has less affinity. Ill effects have been reported to result from feeding xylose to young pigs.[85] This information indicates that the young pig can absorb xylose but that it is not metabolized and that a xylose absorption test could be developed for the pig.

ORAL STARCH TOLERANCE TEST

The digestion of starch and some of its degradation products by newborn pigs has been investigated. After feeding raw starch to 42-day-old pigs, the blood glucose concentration peaked at 1 hour and returned to normal values within 4 hours. After feeding soluble starch to pigs 10 days of age and older, the blood glucose concentration fell to normal in 3 hours. The elevation of blood glucose in the latter group was approximately one-half the value recorded when glucose or maltose was administered.[86]

LACTOSE ABSORPTION TEST

Lactase activity is present at high levels in newborn pigs, but between birth and 8 weeks of age there is a decrease in the amount of lactase activity of the small intestine. In older pigs, the lactase activity is not greatly different from that found in 8-week-old pigs.[87] For piglets 0 to 22 days of age, the oral administration of lactose produced a greater rise in the blood glucose concentration than in older pigs.[88]

ALL DISACCHARIDASES

Simple semiquantitative tests for small intestinal disaccharidase activity have been developed to aid in the diagnosis of transmissible gastroenteritis (TGE) of swine, where villus atrophy is a histologic feature. Presumably, this could be used in the evaluation of enteric coronavirus infection in any species. The reduction in the number of mature absorptive cells results in lowered maltase, sucrase, and β-galactosidase activity.

The test involves incubating 1-g segments of opened small intestine in 4 to 5 ml of buffered 2% maltose, sucrose, or lactose solution at 37°C for 1 hour. The solution is then tested for the presence of glucose using a reagent strip (Clinistix) and the response recorded as "negative, light, medium, or heavy," or "negative, plus 1, plus 2, plus 3, plus 4."[89,90]

REFERENCES

1. Isenberg, J. I., Walsh, J. H., and Grossman, M. I.: Zollinger-Ellison syndrome. Gastroenterology 65:140, 1973.
2. Jeffries, G. H.: Gastritis. In Gastrointestinal Disease. Edited by M. H. Sleisenger and J. S. Fordtran. Philadelphia, W. B. Saunders Co., 1973, p. 560.
3. Säteri, H.: A non-surgical method for collecting pancreatic juice in dogs. Acta Vet. Scand. 4:1, 1963.
4. Marks, I. N., Komarov, S. A., and Shay, H.: Maximal acid secretory response to histamine and its relation to parietal cell mass in the dog. Am. J. Physiol. 199:579, 1960.
5. Emas, S., and Grossman, M. I.: Comparison of gastric secretion in conscious dogs and cats. Gastroenterology 52:29, 1967.
6. Merritt, A. M., and Brooks, F. P.: Basal and histamine-induced gastric acid and pepsin secretion in the conscious miniature pig. Gastroenterology 58:801, 1970.
7. Laurie, J. H., Smith, G. M., and Forrest, A. P.: The histamine infusion test. Lancet 2:270, 1964.
8. Kay, A. W.: Effect of large doses of histamine on gastric secretion of HCl; an augmented histamine test. Br. J. Med. 2:77, 1953.
9. Carrig, C. B., and Seawright, A. A.: Mastocytosis with gastrointestinal ulceration in a dog. Aust. Vet. J. 44: 503, 1968.
10. Jones, B. R., Nicholls, M. R., and Badman, R.: Peptic ulceration in a dog associated with an islet cell carcinoma of the pancreas and an elevated plasma gastrin level. J. Small Anim. Pract. 17:593, 1976.
11. Straus, E., Johnson, G. F., and Yalow, R. S.: Canine Zollinger-Ellison syndrome. Gastroenterology 72:380, 1977.
12. Freudiger, U.: Testing gastric acidity without the use of a stomach tube: dye tests in dogs. Schweiz. Arch. Tierheilkd. 104:85, 1962.
13. Hunt, J. N. and Knox, M. T.: Regulation of gastric emptying. In Handbook of Physiology, Section G.: Alimentary Canal, Vol. 4. Edited by C. F. Code. Washington, D.C., American Physiological Society, 1968, p. 1917.
14. van der Gaag, I., Happé, R. P., and Wolvekamp, W. Th. C.: A boxer dog with chronic hypertrophic gastritis resembling Ménétrier's disease in man. Vet. Pathol. 13:172, 1976.
15. Hill, F. W. G., and Kidder, D. E.: Fat assimilation in dogs, estimated by a fat-balance procedure. J. Small Anim. Pract. 13:23, 1972.
16. Walker, B. E., Kelleher, J., Davies, T., Smith, C. L. and Losowski, M. S.: Influence of dietary fat on fecal fat. Gastroenterology 64:233, 1973.
17. Merritt, A. M., Burrows, C. F., Cowgill, L., and Street, W.: Fecal fat and trypsin in dogs fed a meat-base or cereal-base diet. J.A.V.M.A. 174:59, 1979.
18. Van de Kamer, J. H., ten Bokkel Huinink, H., and Weyers, H. A.: Rapid method for the determination of fat in feces. J. Biol. Chem. 177:347, 1949.
19. Thompson, J. B., Su, C. K., Ringrose, R. E., and Welsh, J. D.: Fecal triglycerides. II. Digestive versus absorptive steatorrhea. J. Lab. Clin. Med. 73:521, 1969.
20. Braddock, L. I., Fleisher, D. R., and Barbero, G. J.: A physical chemical study of the Van de Kamer method for fecal fat analysis. Gastroenterology 55:165, 1968.
21. Anderson, N. V., and Low, D. G.: Juvenile atrophy of the canine pancreas. Anim. Hosp. 1:101, 1965.
22. Brobst, D. F., and Funk, A.: Simplified test of fat absorption in dogs. J.A.V.M.A. 161:1412, 1972.
23. Säteri, H.: Investigations on the exocrine pancreatic function in dogs suffering from chronic exocrine pancreatic insufficiency. Acta Vet. Scand. Suppl. 53:1, 1975.
24. Pimparkar, B. D., Tulsky, E. G., Kalser, M. H., and Bockus, H. L.: Correlation of radioactive and chemical fecal fat determinations in the malabsorption syndrome. Am. J. Med. 30:910, 1961.
25. Kallfelz, F. A., Norrdin, R. W., and Neal, T. M.: Intestinal absorption of oleic acid ^{131}I and triolein ^{131}I in the differential diagnosis of malabsorption syndrome and pancreatic dysfunction in the dog. J.A.V.M.A. 153:43, 1968.
26. Luk, G. D., and Hendrix, T. R.: Microscopic examination of stool as a screening test for steatorrhea (abstract). Gastroenterology 74:1134, 1978.
27. Burrows, C. F., Merritt, A. M., and Chiapella, A.: Determination of fecal fat and trypsin output in the evaluation of chronic canine diarrhea. J.A.V.M.A. 174:62, 1979.
28. Hindmarsh, J. T.: Xylose absorption and its clinical significance. Clin. Biochem. 9:141, 1976.
29. Marin, G. A., Clark, M. L., and Senior, J. R.: Distribution of d-xylose in sequestered fluid resulting in false-positive tests for malabsorption. Ann. Intern. Med. 69: 1155, 1968.
30. Breukink, H. J.: Oral mono- and disaccharide tolerance tests in ponies. Am. J. Vet. Res. 35:1523, 1974.
31. Hill, F. W. G., and Kidder, D. E.: The oral glucose tolerance test in canine pancreatic malabsorption. Br. Vet. J. 128:207, 1972.
32. Roberts, M. C., and Hill, F. W. G.: The oral glucose tolerance test in the horse. Equine Vet. J. 5:171, 1973.
33. Reed, J. H. and Kidder, D. E.: The oral glucose tolerance test in the young pig. Br. Vet. J. 127:318, 1971.
34. Csaky, T. Z., and Ho, P. M.: Intestinal transport of D-xylose. Proc. Soc. Exp. Biol. Med. 120:403, 1965.
35. Levitt, D. G., Hakim, A. A., and Lifson, N.: Evaluation of components of transport of sugars by dog jejunum in vivo. Am. J. Physiol. 217:777, 1969.
36. Bihler, I.: Intestinal sugar transport: ionic activation and chemical specificity. Biochim. Biophys. Acta 183:169, 1969.
37. Annegers, J. H.: Absorption of glucose, galactose, and xylose in the dog. Proc. Soc. Exp. Biol. Med. 127:1071, 1968.
38. Dominguez, R., Goldblatt, H., and Pomerene, E.: Kinetics of the excretion and utilization of xylose. Am. J. Physiol. 119:429, 1936.
39. Wyngaarden, J. B., Segal, S., and Foley, J. B.: Physiological disposition and metabolic fate of infused pentoses in man. J. Clin. Invest. 36:1395, 1957.
40. Hill, F. W. G., Kidder, D. E., and Frew, J.: A xylose absorption test for the dog. Vet. Rec. 87:250, 1970.
41. Bolton, J. R., Merritt, A. M., Cimprich, R. E., Ramberg, C. F., and Street, W.: Normal and abnormal xylose absorption in the horse. Cornell Vet. 66:183, 1976.
42. Frankel, S.: Miscellaneous tests. In Gradwohl's Clinical Laboratory Methods and Diagnosis. Edited by S. Frankel, S. Reitman, and A. C. Sonnenworth. St. Louis, The C. V. Mosby Co., 1970, p. 211.
43. Roe, J. H., and Rice, E. N.: A photometric method for the determination of free pentoses in animal tissues. J. Biol. Chem. 173:507, 1948.
44. Da Costa, L. R.: Tests for intestinal function. Clin. Biochem. 9:136, 1976.
45. Jeffries, G. H., Weser, E., and Sleisenger, M. D.: Malabsorption. Gastroenterology 56:777, 1969.
46. Hayden, D. W., and VanKruiningen, H. J.: Control values for evaluating gastrointestinal function in the dog. J.A.A.H.A. 12:31, 1976.
47. Gray, G. M.: Maldigestion and malabsorption: clinical manifestations and specific diseases. In Gastrointestinal Disease. Edited by M. H. Sleisenger and J. S. Fordtran. Philadelphia, W. B. Saunders Co., 1973. p. 259.
48. Hill, F. W. G.: A starch tolerance test in canine pancreatic malabsorption. Vet. Rec. 91:169, 1972.
49. Hill, F. W. G.: Malabsorption syndrome in the dog: a study of thirty-eight cases. J. Small Anim. Pract. 13:575, 1972.
50. Roberts, M. C.: Carbohydrate digestion and absorption studies in the horse. Res. Vet. Sci. 18:64, 1975.

51. Roberts, M. C., Kidder, D. E., and Hill, F. W. G.: Small intestinal beta-galactosidase activity in the horse. Gut *14*:535, 1973.
52. Welsh, J. D.: Isolated lactose deficiency in humans: report on 100 patients. Medicine *49*:257, 1970.
53. Bronstein, H. D., Haeffner, L. J., and Kowlessar, O. D.: The significance of gelatin tolerance in malabsorptive states. Gastroenterology *50*:621, 1966.
54. Prokop, D. J., Keiser, H. R., and Sjoerdsma, A.: Gastrointestinal absorption and renal excretion of hydroxyproline peptides. Lancet *2*:527, 1962.
55. Jasper, D. E.: A simple diagnostic test for pancreatic enzyme deficiency in dogs. North Am. Vet. *35*:523, 1954.
56. Lorenz, M. D.: Laboratory diagnosis of gastrointestinal disease and pancreatic insufficiency. Vet. Clin. North Am. *6*:663, 1976.
57. Haverback, B. J., Dyce, B. J., Gutent, P. J., and Montgomery, D. W.: Measurement of trypsin and chymotrypsin in stool. Gastroenterology *44*:588, 1963.
58. Dyck, W., and Ammann, R.: Quantitative determination of fecal chymotrypsin as a screening test for pancreatic exocrine insufficiency. Am. J. Dig. Dis. *10*:530, 1965.
59. Moeller, D. D., Dunn, G. D., and Klotz, A. P.: Diagnosis of pancreatic exocrine insufficiency by fecal chymotrypsin activity. Am. J. Dig. Dis. *18*:792, 1973.
60. Frankland, A. L.: An investigation of the trypsin digest test on apparently normal canine feces. J. Small Anim. Pract. *10*:531, 1969.
61. Hill, F. W. G., and Kidder, D. E.: The estimation of daily faecal trypsin levels in dogs as an indicator of gross pancreatic exocrine insufficiency. J. Small Anim. Pract. *11*:191, 1970.
62. Grossman, M. I.: Fecal enzymes of dogs with pancreatic exclusion. Proc. Soc. Exp. Biol. Med. *110*:41, 1967.
63. Goldberg, D. M.: Functional, chemical, and clinical aspects of proteolytic enzymes in the alimentary canal. Clin. Biochem. *9*:131, 1976.
64. Goldberg, D. M., Sale, J. K., Fawcett, N., and Wormsley, K. G.: Trypsin and chymotrypsin as aids in the diagnosis of pancreatic disease. Am. J. Dig. Dis. *17*:780, 1972.
65. Gutierrez, L. V., and Baron, J. H.: A comparison of Boots and GIH secretion on stimuli of pancreatic secretion in human subjects with or without chronic pancreatitis. Gut *13*:721, 1972.
66. Beck, I. T.: Diagnosis of chronic pancreatic disease. Clin. Biochem. *9*:121, 1976.
67. Waldmann, T. A.: Protein-losing enteropathy. *In* Modern Trends in Gastroenterology. Edited by W. I. Card and B. Creamer. London, Butterworth's, 1970, p. 125.
68. Waldmann, T. A.: Protein-losing enteropathy. Gastroenterology *50*:422, 1966.
69. Kerr, R. M., DuBois, J. J., and Holt, P. R.: Use of [125]I- and ^{51}Cr-albumin for the measurement of gastrointestinal and total albumin catabolism. J. Clin. Invest. *46*:2064, 1967.
70. Finco, D. R., Duncan, J. R., Schall, W. D., Hooper, B. E., Chandler, F. W., and Keating, K. A.: Chronic enteric disease and hypoproteinemia in 9 dogs. J.A.V.M.A. *163*:262, 1973.
71. Kallfelz, F. A., and Wallace, R. J.: Studies of albumin metabolism in dogs using ^{51}Cr and ^{125}I-labeled albumin. Personal communication, 1977.
72. Merritt, A. M., Kohn, C. W., Ramberg, C. F., Cimprich, R. E., Reid, C. F., and Bolton, J. R.: Plasma clearance of [51]chromium-albumin into the intestinal tract of normal and chronically diarrheal horses. Am. J. Vet. Res. *38*:1769, 1977.
73. Gianella, R. A., Broitman, S. A., and Zamcheck, N.: Competition between bacteria and intrinsic factor for vitamin B_{12}: implications for vitamin B_{12} malabsorption in intestinal bacterial overgrowth. Gastroenterology *62*:255, 1973.
74. Welkos, S., Toskes, P. P., and Baer, H.: The role of anaerobic bacteria with B_{12} malabsorption of the stasis syndrome. Clin. Res. *25*(3):320A, 1977.
75. Muyshondt, E., and Schwartz, S. I.: Vitamin B-12 absorption following gastric surgery in dogs. Surg. Forum *14*:368, 1963.
76. Fromm, H., and Hofmann, A. F.: Breath test for altered bile-acid metabolism. Lancet *2*:621, 1971.
77. Spivey, J., Lorenz, E., Mauderli, W., and Toskes, P.: Evaluation of carbohydrate metabolism in patients with the blind loop syndrome by a ^{14}C-xylose breath test. Gastroenterology *68*:1001, 1975.
78. Roberts, R. K., Campbell, C. B., Bryant, S. J., and Adams, L.: Xylose-I-^{14}C absorption test: the use of urine serum and breath analysis, and comparison with a colorimetric assay. Aust. N.Z. J. Med. *6*:532, 1976.
79. Arvanitakis, C., and Greenberger, N. J.: Diagnosis of pancreatic disease by a synthetic peptide: a new test of exocrine pancreatic function. Lancet *1*:663, 1976.
80. Strombeck, D. R.: New method for evaluation of chymotrypsin deficiency in dogs. J.A.V.M.A. *173*:1319, 1978.
81. Kidder, D. E., and Manners, M. J.: The development of digestive function in the piglet. *In* The Veterinary Annual. Edited by C. S. F. Grunsell and F. W. G. Hill. Bristol, John Wright, 1972, p. 57.
82. Vinovrski, Z., and Findrik, M.: On the function of insulin in swine during glucose tolerance tests. Vet. Arch. *35*:191, 1965.
83. Telepnev, V. A.: Duodenal glucose tolerance test in pigs. Uchenyi Zapiski Vitebskogo Veterinarnogo Institut. *28*:131, 1976.
84. Carle, B. N., and Dewhirst, W. H.: The collection of blood from the anterior vena cava of the pig. J.A.V.M.A. *101*:495, 1942.
85. Kidder, D. E., Manners, M. J., McCrea, M. R., and Osborne, A. D.: Absorption of sugars by the piglet. Br. J. Nutr. *22*:501, 1968.
86. Cunningham, H. M.: Digestion of starch and some of its degradation products by newborn pigs. J. Anim. Sci. *18*:964, 1959.
87. Manners, M. J., and Stevens, J. A.: Changes from birth to maturity in the patterns of distribution of lactase and sucrase activity in the mucosa of the small intestine of pigs. Br. J. Nutr. *28*:113, 1972.
88. Dollar, A. M., Mitchell, K. G., and Porter, J. W. G.: The utilization of carbohydrate in the young pig. Proc. Nutr. Soc. *16*:12, 1957.
89. Tropping, D., Cross, R. F., and Moorhead, P. D.: Simplified presumptive tests for carbohydrate-hydrolyzing enzymes. Can. J. Comp. Med. *32*:518, 1968.
90. Giles, N., Borland, E. D., Counter, D. E., and Gibson, E. A.: Transmissible gastroenteritis in pigs: some observations on laboratory aids to diagnosis. Vet. Rec. *100*:336, 1977.

Chapter 17

CONCEPTS OF GASTROINTESTINAL PARASITISM AND STRATEGIES FOR DESIGNING CORRECTIVE/CONTROL PROGRAMS

HELEN E. JORDAN and S. A. EWING

This chapter is designed to guide the veterinarian in recognizing, evaluating, and correcting parasitic problems of individual animals and herds. In addition, the generalizations presented should aid in evaluating circumstances conducive to parasitism and in predicting the impact of altering conditions as a part of an effort to circumvent problems.

The material in this chapter, therefore, is presented in two parts. Part I is a generalized discussion of gastrointestinal parasitism and the conditions under which parasitism results in disease or is a potential disease problem. Part II presents a strategy for evaluating parasitism and making decisions concerning control programs for specific situations.

Part I. Concepts

Understanding the biology and ecology of parasites provides the veterinarian with a basis for evaluating both parasitic disease and the potential risk of such disease. This understanding is the foundation for designing appropriate corrective and control programs. The essential requirements for the establishment and perpetuation of parasites and for the development of disease are similar for all species of parasites. In the present discussion, however, only gastrointestinal parasites will be used to illustrate the concepts of parasitism and parasitic disease.

Components of Parasitism

Parasitism like other infectious disease cycles, whether with or without clinical disease, depends upon six essential components: (1) the parasite (an infectious organism); (2) a source of the parasite for a susceptible host. The source is a reservoir (intermediate or definitive host). (3) A method of escape of infective larvae, eggs, cysts, or oocysts from the source; (4) a mode of transmission to a susceptible host; (5) a mode of entry into the new host; and (6) a susceptible host.

The six essential components of parasitism form a chain of successive events that perpetuate the parasite in its host and in succeeding generations of hosts. Life cycles of all parasites, i.e., helminths, protozoans, and arthropods of animals, share these components.

The presence of a parasite in a host does not necessarily result in disease; therefore, the essential components of parasitism are considered separately from parasitic disease to aid in distinguishing between subclinical (asymptomatic) and clinical parasitism.

The Parasite: The parasite must be capable of overcoming the host's defensive barriers. These characteristics include (a) invasiveness, the ability to enter the host and to establish itself, and (b) resistance to the host's local and systemic responses.

The Source or Reservoir: The density of the reservoir host (definitive or intermediate host) population from generation to generation must be sufficient to maintain a parasite species from one generation to the next.

Method of Escape from Source: When the parasite is in an intermediate or definitive host reservoir (the host reservoir may be the same animal in case of re-exposure), either the parasite must pass out of the host or the host must be ingested and the parasite subsequently released within the definitive host.

Transmission to Susceptible Host: When the infective stage from the source remains in the external environment, then environmental factors, inherent biologic factors (e.g., larval motility) and mechanical disturbances by animals or humans contribute to the parasite's escape from the excrement and its consequent availability for a new host.

One can generalize about potential exposure rate and relative prevalence of a parasite on the basis of the mode of transmission. For example, if the parasite such as a strongyle has a direct life cycle, one can expect to find parasites in a population of susceptible animals if the environment becomes contaminated and is suitable for larval development. On the other hand, if an intermediate host is required or a vector is the common mode of transmission, then the prevalence of the intermediate host (or vector) as well as the prevalence of the definitive host would be important in regulating parasitism.

Mode of Entry: The most common mode of entry for gastrointestinal parasites is by ingestion of contaminated food or such aberrant host behavior as coprophagy and/or licking of contaminated surfaces. Ingestion of colostrum containing infective larvae is a common mode of entry into the host for some parasites, e.g., *Ancylostoma caninum* and most species of *Strongyloides.*[1] All species of trichurids, spirurids, tapeworms, flukes, acanthocephalans, and gastrointestinal protozoans (coccidia, *Trichomonas* sp., *Giardia* sp., *Balantidium coli*, and *Entamoeba* sp.) and nearly all species of strongyles, ascarids, and capillarids are acquired by ingestion. Some species enter the host via the intrauterine route, e.g., *Toxocara canis*, and to a lesser extent, *Ancylostoma caninum.*[1]

Another mode of entry for parasites is via skin penetration; however, relatively few species have this capability. These few include filariform larvae of *Strongyloides* species, which gain entrance to their hosts mainly by skin penetration, and most species of hookworms (e.g., *Ancylostoma* sp. and *Bunostomum* sp.) which sometimes can penetrate the skin, particularly of young hosts. Although injection is a common mode of entry for blood protozoans and nematodes inhabiting systems other than the digestive system, parasites that inhabit the alimentary tract do not routinely enter this way. Inhalation is a possible route of entry but would be an accidental mode of entry for gastrointestinal parasites. The infective larval stage of some parasites such as *Habronema* sp. may be deposited on the mucous membranes of the nares, but since the organism actively migrates into the alimentary tract, this is not considered inhalation.

A Susceptible Host: The host must provide the essential nutritional requirements for the parasite and be able to tolerate the parasite. This implies that the host does not interfere with the parasite's metabolism sufficiently to cause either its expulsion or death before it reaches sexual maturity. When a parasite can be supported by only one or a very few host species, the organism is said to be highly host specific, i.e., to have a narrow host range. Host specificity is rarely absolute; it is relative. Nevertheless, a few generalizations regarding host specificity can be made for the gastrointestinal parasites.

Some parasites tend to be much more host specific than others. For example, during the gametogenic phase most coccidian species infect a specific host species and most *Strongyloides* sp. also are highly host specific.[2] At the other extreme, *Trichinella spiralis*, *Trichostrongylus axei*, and *Dipylidium caninum* all have very wide host ranges. Host specificity for most species of parasites ranges between these extremes; most utilize one or two host species which may be referred to as the normal host(s), but cross-infection can and does occur in related hosts.

Clinical Parasitism

Clinical parasitism is a host-parasite relationship in a state of imbalance. A change in the susceptibility of the host and/or a change in the numbers of the parasite creates the imbalance resulting in manifestation of disease.[3]

The essential components of a parasite's life cycle must be met before clinical parasitism can occur. Parasites are not equal in their pathogenic potential. Furthermore, even for a pathogenic species, the numbers of parasites required to produce disease vary with the susceptibility of the host and with the virulence of the specific parasite population. Numerous factors regulate the susceptibility of the host to adverse effects of the parasite.

Pathogenic Potential of a Parasite

The parasite's microhabitat and the mechanism by which the parasite produces harm to the host operate in concert to determine the parasite's pathogenic potential.

Virulence: Parasites injure hosts by a wide variety of mechanisms both direct and indirect: (1) cell and tissue destruction, (2) physiologic alteration of the host's system(s), (3) reducing the host's resistance to other disease agents, (4) mechanically creating openings for secondary invaders, and/or (5) transmitting pathogenic organisms.

Examples of cell and tissue destruction are well documented: (a) exsanguination, a predominant characteristic of a few parasites (*Ancylostoma* sp., *Ostertagia* sp., *Haemonchus* sp., *Bunostomum* sp., and *Strongylus* sp.); (b) pressure atrophy and blockage from mechanical obstruction (intestinal or bile duct blockage that sometimes occurs with many ascarid species); (c) invasion of the cell, typical of the coccidia; and (d) local inflammation such as that caused by both larval and adult *Ostertagia* sp., larval *Oesophagostomum* sp., and immature *Paramphistomum* sp.[4,5,6]

The mechanism of the physiologic alterations associated with the parasites is less well described than are specific cellular destruction and local inflammation. There is evidence that the physiologic changes in the host caused by parasites are an important aspect of clinical parasitism.[7] Physiologic alteration of the host can result from anorexia, maldigestion, malabsorption, fluid and ion loss, local and systemic immunologic responses (hypersensitization) and possibly from absorption of local inflammatory products and of excretions and secretions of parasites.[7,8]

Indirect evidence exists showing that the host's physiologic constituents and processes are altered. For example, hypoproteinemia has been demonstrated in animals infected by a variety of parasites (such as *Ostertagia* sp., *Trichostrongylus* sp., *Fasciola hepatica*, coccidia, and most of the voracious bloodsuckers).[8,9,10,11] Hypoproteinemia occurs when either the necessary nutrients are not available to the host or there is a loss of blood protein. However, parasites may cause hypoproteinemia by different mechanisms, specifically by any of the following: alteration of digestive enzyme activities, gut edema interfering with absorption, competition for nutrients, and exsanguination.[8,9,10,11]

Recent studies on the gastrointestinal topographic changes,[12] altered digestive enzyme activity (as has been shown to occur in *Cooperia* infec-

tions),[13] and other physiologic factors, such as altered pH in *Ostertagia*[14] infections undoubtedly will provide the veterinarian and parasitologist a better understanding of the mechanisms by which parasites alter physiologic function of the host.

Microhabitat: The microhabitat is of primary importance because the function of the cells of one microhabitat may vary markedly from the function of those of another microhabitat in close proximity. For example, the cells in the villus crypt of the small intestine have a different function from those at the tip of the villus, and those at the middle have a different function from those at the other two locations.[5] Furthermore, since the epithelial cells of the villus originate at the base of the crypts, a parasite (such as some species of coccidia) that lives in this microhabitat and destroys or alters these cells has a greater pathogenic potential than one located on or in the cells at the villus tip. On the other hand, a parasite causing local cellular irritation at the tip of the villus would cause less harm than one in the crypts. Therefore, different species may appear superficially to occupy the same location, such as the small intestine, but actually inhabit very different microhabitats. The exact microhabitat of parasites is not often reported in the literature.

Numbers of Parasites and Clinical Parasitism

Mere presence of a potential pathogenic species is not necessarily enough to cause clinical parasitism; sufficient numbers of the parasite must invade a susceptible host to create an imbalance. The numbers required to create an imbalance vary markedly among species of parasites, individual host, and even from one time to another in the same individual.[13] The significance of these factors is clarified by considering the population dynamics of the parasites.

Where man does not alter the environment, parasite burdens tend to reach an equilibrium at which the host population can tolerate the parasite species and allow its perpetuation. However, a rapid shift in conditions (e.g., higher humidity) may enhance survival of stages outside the host and thus improve a parasite's chances to increase its numbers faster than the host can adjust to the change, thereby creating an imbalance detrimental to the host. Through management, man alters the environments of domestic animals and many non-domestic animals, thus often facilitating an increased exposure to pathogenic parasites.

The problem for the veterinarian is to determine

the significance of a potential pathogen existing in a host or population of hosts. Thus one has to determine whether the essential factors favoring the parasite have been altered sufficiently to allow development of clinical parasitism. The interaction of the parasite both with its host and with the external environment must be analyzed in each specific situation.

The factors that influence the numbers of parasites that become established and develop to sexual maturity are (a) opportunity of the host for exposure to the parasite, (b) the biology of the parasite, and (c) the degree of susceptibility of the host.

Exposure Opportunity: Aspects of parasite biology that affect exposure rates of the host include fecundity and type of life cycle. Fecundity of parasite species varies markedly because daily egg output, length of productivity, time of peak production, and total egg production all vary. For example, *Ascaris lumbricoides* has been estimated to have an output of 200,000 eggs/day, *Haemonchus contortus* 5,000 to 6,000/day, and *Fasciola hepatica* 20,000/day.[15] One *Eimeria tenella* oocyst has the theoretical potential of giving rise to 2.5 million second generation merozoites.[15] The maximum number of oocysts potentially shed as a result of exposure to a single sporulated oocyst is specific for the various coccidian species; i.e., the number of merozoites produced in each schizont and the number of times asexual multiple fission is repeated is species-specific, but varies among species.

Parasites that have a direct life cycle tend to be more prevalent and have a wider geographic distribution than those that have an indirect cycle. The type of life cycle is not in itself sufficient to account for parasite burdens of clinical significance. Situations must be analyzed to determine the stages of the life cycle that are either enhanced or hindered by host and environment factors.

External environmental factors influencing egg and/or larval development have a primary role in regulating incidence and prevalence of parasites. Those that hatch may be more accessible to the host due to motility, but they also are more vulnerable to external environmental factors than are those that develop to the infective stage within the egg or cyst or within an intermediate host. For example, all strongyles have direct life cycles, and their eggs hatch in the hosts' external environment. Animals that are naturally gregarious or are forced together by management practices that result in accumulation of feces have great opportunity for exposure. Close grazing also enhances exposure rate. Thus, the strongyles that have direct life cycles and motile

larvae tend to be more accessible to their hosts than are trichurids and ascarids, which also have direct life cycles but whose larvae develop and remain within the egg until it is ingested. On the other hand, larvae exposed to prolonged drying and sunlight would more likely be damaged than eggs similarly exposed.

Likewise, host and environmental factors can either enhance or decrease exposure rate to parasites having indirect life cycles. For example, if the cockroaches that feed on *Physaloptera* sp.-contaminated feces are introduced into a kennel or cattery, or if cattle infected with *Fasciola hepatica* are introduced into a pasture having the suitable molluscan intermediate host (e.g., *Lymnaea* sp.), then exposure opportunity would be enhanced for the definitive host.

Influence of Host Behavior: Both exposure rate (frequency) and dose of the parasite are influenced significantly by the behavior of the animal. For example, *Ollulanus tricuspis*, a trichostrongyle inhabiting the cat's stomach, appears to be transmitted only by feeding on freshly regurgitated material or on stomach contents from an infected cat. Cats normally are considered to be finicky eaters, but they will ingest fresh vomitus when emesis occurs within minutes after ingestion; therefore, the vomitus from an infected cat has much the same characteristics as the original food except that it contains infective *Ollulanus*. Following the introduction of a single infected cat, all or most of the cats in a cattery can become infected if contact is permitted. In general, however, exposure and perpetuation of a parasite do not depend exclusively on the host's behavior; rather, behavior may enhance exposure.

When evaluating the significance of the host's behavior for exposure to parasites, one needs to consider abnormal or unusual behavior as well as normal behavior. For example, dogs are often coprophagous, and are particularly attracted to feces containing blood; some dogs are habitually coprophagic, and thereby at greater risk than other dogs in the same kennel.[16] Consequently, when considering the possible source of infection and the potential for reinfection by parasites with direct life cycles, coprophagic habits should not be overlooked. This behavior is more important with respect to some parasite species than to others. For example, *Entamoeba histolytica* produces severe dysentery in dogs in the United States, but the dog does not pass cysts.[16] Since the cyst is normally the infective stage for this protozoan, the source usually is another host species, viz., man. Transmission from dog to dog can occur, however, if feces containing blood and motile trophozoites are ingested within 3 hours after they are passed. For this reason, dogs, especially in a kennel, must be considered when determining the source of infection and developing a prognosis for canine amebiasis. Other forms of animal behavior such as indiscriminate licking and chewing of objects, cleaning the young, preening, grooming others in the group, and gregarious grazing, all potentially enhance exposure to parasites. Thus, these and other behavior patterns must be considered in identifying the source and determining exposure dose for a parasite. The significance of behavior depends on the degree of contamination of objects and the frequency with which the animal exhibits the behavior. One should also determine which management practices enhance exposure opportunity.

Environmental Factors: Desiccation and direct sunlight (which has detrimental effects in addition to drying) are most deleterious to all stages of parasites; only physical destruction by fire or other agents of high temperature is as damaging to parasitic stages free in the environment. Extremely low temperatures are also detrimental. Some parasite eggs that are protected by relatively thick shells, particularly those of ascarids, trichurids, acanthocephalans, and some tapeworms, can withstand natural environmental extremes for prolonged periods. Therefore, when considering pasture rotation and other management changes, the longevity of specific parasites must be known. Information regarding environmental factors affecting specific parasites is available elsewhere.[17]

Climatic variation has an impact over an entire region. For example, low annual rainfall and long periods of high temperature in arid regions such as Arizona have an adverse effect on thin-shelled eggs and on free-living parasitic larvae. As one might expect, therefore, *Ancylostoma caninum* is extremely rare in the dog population of such regions. On the other hand, canine ancylostomiasis is a persistent problem in regions such as the Gulf Coast and South Atlantic states which have high rainfall, high relative humidity, and mild to hot temperatures most of the year with only a few successive days of ground temperature below 0°C. Other factors such as type and amount of vegetation have an important role in protecting parasites from the effects of desiccation and sunlight. For this reason, rainfall necessary for abundant vegetation enhances a parasite's survival and overshadows the detrimental effects of high temperatures in these southeastern states.

Seasonally, the length of forage may be important

for parasite survival, particularly for free-living parasitic larvae. For example, one study indicated that more larvae survived and calves acquired more strongyles from the tall forage than from short during a dry period, but little difference was shown in either survival or infection rate between the tall and short forage during a wet season.[18] The type of forage also may affect the survival time of free-living parasitic larvae. Calves have been shown to acquire higher worm burdens from contaminated fescue pastures than from crimson clover or winter rye grass pastures.[18,19] This was suggested to be due to difference in nutritive value;[18,19] however, growth characteristics of forage and/or some other factor may contribute to the variation.[20]

The survival of parasites may be altered drastically by changes in management which affect the degree of contamination. Awareness of moisture requirements and protection against detrimental climatic factors afforded parasites by vegetation, snow cover, and other materials is especially relevant in the husbandry of animals. For example, improved pastures are being used in many areas of the United States to increase animal production. This often involves changing from native prairie to Bermuda grass (i.e., straight blade to matted grass), but may instead involve increasing density of native grasses by use of fertilizer. Such vegetative changes tend to enhance a parasite's survival. Furthermore, with improved pastures the numbers of animals are increased per unit of space, and this concentration potentially intensifies pasture contamination and increases exposure opportunity.

Host concentration affects the contamination level and leads to environmental "build up" that provides for early exposure of young animals and overwhelming or continual re-exposure of adults. This condition is referred to as overcrowding. Indicators of overcrowding are overgrazing, in the case of ruminants and horses, and for other species, excessive accumulation of feces that remain in the environment from one season to another. In temperate climates, rain, dungbeetles and other animals tend to disperse feces and there is usually no accumulation of feces unless overcrowding exists.

Most larvae do not survive for more than a few days or weeks on unshaded bare soil, particularly if it is nonporous, like clay; however, very little vegetation or shade is required to protect larvae and thus extend the survival time considerably, particularly on porous soil like sandy loam.[21] In general, thin-shelled eggs and first- and second-stage nematode larvae are more susceptible to the adverse effects of environmental factors than are either third-stage infective larvae or thick-shelled eggs.[21]

Moisture is essential to the development and survival of eggs, larvae, and oocysts; however, resistance to desiccation is not identical for all parasites.[21,22,23,24] *Bunostomum* sp. and some stages of *Fasciola hepatica* are exceedingly susceptible to drying and have short survival periods in the environment (less than 2 months for *Bunostomum* sp. and a few hours for miracidia and cercariae and 4 to 6 months for metacercariae of *F. hepatica*) even under conditions considered optimal. When *Bunostomum* or *Fasciola* is recovered at necropsy, one can be relatively certain that the animal was exposed to a field situation such as a grassy pasture with springs, or a pond with sloping, grassy edges as a source of drinking water, or to poorly draining bottom land that frequently floods.

Another important management factor to consider is movement of animals. A pasture rotation system in which calves immediately follow adults may put highly susceptible animals at high risk. Drainage is also important; topography must be considered in determining rotation; animals should not be placed on land contaminated by drainage of waste from other hosts.

Animal movement from outside is as important as traffic within a population because of introduction of new species or pathogenic strains of parasites into an established host population. For example, one cannot assume that a parasite such as *Fasciola hepatica* will not become established simply because it has not been reported for a region; one must be certain that a suitable snail is not available.

Strain variation of pathogenicity has been reported in particular for *Haemonchus contortus*[25] and *Ostertagia ostertagi*.[26,27] It is good practice to isolate animals, check for parasites, and implement appropriate corrective measures prior to introducing new animals, particularly from a different geographic region.

Feeding practices and water source may strongly influence exposure opportunity. For example, if supplemental hay and concentrates are spread on the ground (not in bunkers) and at the same location each day, the area may soon become highly contaminated. The accumulation of infective material may be enhanced further by climatic conditions (mild daytime temperatures and cool nights) resulting in the accumulation of eggs and larvae that may develop to infective stages at approximately the same time. The source of water, its location, and whether it is maintained relatively free of fecal contamination can either create or restrict exposure opportunity.

Cleaning practices are important. One should consider not only how often and by what method facilities and equipment are cleaned but also how excrement is handled. For example, if dirty litter from a horse stall is piled in the pasture used by horses, the parasite exposure will be increased greatly because the animals will seek out undigested grain in the manure, especially if the pastures are overgrazed.

Attention should be given to the species of hosts maintained together or those which have access to the same environment. For example, horses and cattle are less likely to have cross-infections than are cattle and sheep. Environmental factors are more extensively discussed in references 22 to 24 and 28 to 30.

Biology of Parasite: The presence of adult worms and external seasonal factors as well as immunity influence larval inhibition, particularly for *Ostertagia ostertagi* and *Haemonchus contortus*.[1] Thus infection of a host with parasites tends to inhibit development of subsequently acquired infective larvae, provided that the host is in a good nutritional status and does not receive an overwhelming single dose or large number of larvae in a short time.

There appears to be a seasonal variation in the development time within the host for some of the parasites. For example, *Ostertagia ostertagi* from some parts of the world has been shown to differ in its maturation time depending on the season that the third-stage infective larvae developed.[1] Delayed larval development (hypobiosis) occurs when the eggs hatch and develop during a season of chilly but not freezing nights and warm daytime temperatures. The time required for these infective larvae to develop is prolonged. When ingested, as many as 60% or more are inhibited and remain in the abomasal mucosa for up to 6 months before maturing.[1] Maturation usually occurs the following spring, thus coinciding with the time when the young hosts (then most highly susceptible) are beginning to graze. Furthermore, an adult host harboring large numbers of inhibited larvae may develop clinical parasitism during late winter and early spring even though the host is unlikely to be acquiring large numbers of larvae from the environment. Stress factors (e.g., pregnancy, severe climatic changes, lower quality and/or quantity of feedstuff) may contribute to development of disease. This phenomenon, identified and described by British and Australian workers for *Ostertagia*, is referred to as ostertagiasis Type II.[1] It is not known how widespread this phenomenon is in North America, but there is some evidence that it does occur.[31,32] The inhibition phenomenon is particularly important in the case of two genera, *Haemonchus* and *Ostertagia*, since they are among the most common and most pathogenic parasites of ruminants. Large numbers of inhibited larvae may become adults following use of a highly efficacious drug. Following removal of adults, inhibited larvae may develop in a few weeks and cause recurring problems as severe as or even more pronounced than before the treatment. Also, if re-introduced into a highly contaminated environment, the recently treated host may again develop clinical parasitism much sooner than anticipated.[1] The extent to which this phenomenon occurs among parasites is not known since neither the inhibiting influence of adult worms nor the extent of hypobiosis among the parasites has been investigated extensively.

Veterinarians have observed that introducing parasitized animals from one geographic region into herds harboring the same species in another region may precipitate clinical parasitism in one of the groups. This observation is explained in part by evidence that variation of virulence does occur for some species, e.g., *Haemonchus contortus*.[25]

Intrauterine and colostral transmission influence worm burden and exposure opportunity. Both these modes of transmission assure exposure of the host at a time when it is most susceptible; thus a greater proportion of larvae probably develop to maturity than when exposure occurs later in life. Health care programs, therefore, should include preventive measures which give particular attention to those pathogenic parasites known to be acquired in this manner; viz., *Toxocara canis* (mostly acquired prenatally[33] but colostral transmission[34] does occur), *Ancylostoma caninum* (colostral transmission[35] as well as prenatal[36]), and *Strongyloides* sp. (colostral).[37]

The size of the parasite affects numbers required to cause clinical signs. Two species may be equally efficient blood suckers but owing to size, much fewer numbers are required for one than the other to produce anemia. For example, about one-half as many *Haemonchus contortus* as *Ostertagia circumcincta* are required to produce disease.[38,39]

Host Susceptibility: Many factors influence and regulate the host's susceptibility to any infectious agent. Frequently a combination of factors, rather than any single factor, determines the host's susceptibility to parasites.

Nutritional status of the host is a major, if not the most important, factor regulating the number of parasites that can become established in a host and the physiologic balance or imbalance that results.[40] In general, a host in a good nutritional state will tolerate more parasites without developing disease than a malnourished one. Conversely, a host in a poor nutritional status is usually more susceptible to parasites than when well nourished. Owing to the similarity between clinical signs of malnutrition and those of parasitism, it is often difficult to determine whether one or both exist and if both, which came first. In such situations, both parasite control and feeding of the host must be considered in correcting the problem.

However, a nutritionally deficient host is not always more susceptible to parasites than is a well-fed one. Sheep with cobalt deficiency exposed to the same dose of *Haemonchus contortus* as nondeficient animals had fewer parasites develop to maturity than did the nondeficient sheep.[41]

The host's current diet should be considered separately from its nutritional status because the outcome of parasitism may be different in an animal with an established deficiency than in one having a change in diet. For example, hypoproteinemia is one indicator of malnutrition.[8] Frequently, a host having a heavy worm burden and clinical parasitism exhibits hypoproteinemia.[6,7,9,39] On the other hand, studies of barrows exposed to *Strongyloides ransomi* have shown that fewer worms develop to maturity in animals fed low protein diets than in those on a high protein diet.[42]

In contrast, dogs on a high protein diet have few *Trichomonas* and *Giardia* or lose their infection altogether, but when a high carbohydrate diet is used, parasite numbers increase.[43] Cattle whose diet has been changed from maintenance (hay and minimum concentrates) to full feed (high energy diet), as typical for feeder cattle, show a decrease in egg counts and may lose some of their strongyles.[44,45] The cause of the latter phenomenon has not been studied extensively. The diet itself may affect the parasite, or the parasite may respond to physiologic changes of the digestive system caused by the high energy diet.

Specific dietary components may contribute to protecting the young host against parasitic infections. Available evidence indicates that milk has a protective effect against parasites, perhaps because of a mild purgative or "flushing" effect. One study showed, for example, that piglets fed a milk diet had fewer *Ascaris suum* than those fed rolled oats.[46] In another study, calves fed milk had fewer *Haemonchus placei* than those fed grain and hay in addition to milk.[47]

Although the generalization is valid that a nutritionally deficient host is more vulnerable to gastrointestinal parasites than is a well-fed host, an extremely ill or moribund, nutritionally deficient animal may in fact lose much of its worm burden. Therefore, few worms or even no worms may be recovered at the necropsy of such an animal.[48]

The effect of a host's sex on susceptibility has not been completely elucidated. There is some evidence, however, indicating that sex does influence susceptibility and that males tend to be more susceptible than females to some parasites, e.g., *Toxocara canis*[49] and *Strongyloides ratti.*[50]

As stated previously, the young host generally is more susceptible than the adult. The lack of resistance of the young is considered to be due in part to immunologic incompetence and in part to naivety with respect to the parasite.[51,52,53] This assumption suggests, then, that animals can develop resistance to parasites and become immunized against them. Immunologic response is a dominant influence in the outcome of parasitism. Mechanisms in such immunologic response to helminths, protozoans, and arthropods have not been studied as extensively as for viral and bacterial agents. Nevertheless, some generalizations appear to be valid; one, specifically, is that exposure to small numbers of parasites may stimulate protective immunity.

Immunologic responses may be manifested by the following:[54]

1. Effect on normal development of larvae (e.g., causing larvae to wander, as occurs with *Toxocara canis;* or inhibiting development, as is typical for *Ostertagia* sp.; or developing in sites in the immune animal different from those in the nonimmune, as with *Oesophagostomum*).

2. Reduction of adult size *(Ancylostoma caninum)* and/or modification of anatomic structure (*Cooperia* sp.) of adult worms.

3. Reduction of egg production (typical for *Ancylostoma caninum* and *Ascaris suum*).

4. Expulsion of all adults within a short period, i.e., the so-called "self cure" (e.g., *Haemonchus contortus* and *Oesophagostomum* sp.).

5. After maturation, movement of adult worm from normal location (e.g., *Trichinella*).

There is evidence that hypersensitivity also occurs in many parasitic infections. The effect of this phenomenon on susceptibility has not been studied extensively, but there is some evidence to indicate that an allergic response may restrict the numbers of adults that become established and/or shorten their life span.[55]

Immunity to helminths is short-term. For example, immunity against *Ancylostoma caninum* is approximately 2 to 3 months.[56] Furthermore, protective immunity against parasites is not absolute; this is amply demonstrated for *A. caninum.* When recently infected dogs are re-exposed, some worms will mature, but the numbers which become established are much lower than in a hookworm-naive dog with the same exposure.[54,57]

Stress factors tend to override the protective benefits of good nutritional status and immunity. Significant factors known to be stressful for the hosts and to increase their susceptibility to parasites are as follows:

1. Increased population density of the host (overcrowding).

2. Less than optimal unit space per animal. There is some evidence indicating that each host species requires a minimum unit of space even when individually housed and if this is not provided, the host is more susceptible to a wide variety of disease agents including parasites, even when the animal appears to be in a good state of "health."

3. Increased production demands, i.e., pregnancy, lactation, periods of rapid growth, rapid weight gains, strenuous work or a sudden demand in work following prolonged idleness.

4. Concomitant disease which frequently offsets previous immunity to gastrointestinal parasites. If such a host is in a contaminated environment, sufficient parasites could be acquired to produce disease that otherwise would not have occurred, or parasites previously tolerated by the host might not continue to be tolerated.

5. Sudden temperature change.

6. Competition among the host species. This last factor might contribute to disease by creating imbalance in a host-parasite relationship that was previously asymptomatic.

Drugs, particularly chemotherapeutics and hormones, influence an animal's susceptibility to parasites. Removal of parasites by chemotherapy may result in the host's becoming more susceptible to reinfection. Therapy with hormones, particularly those of the cortisone group, often will increase the host's susceptibility to parasitic infections.[58]

Subclinical Parasitism

Today's subclinical parasitism may be tomorrow's disease problem and/or economic loss.

First, subclinical parasitism may cause discernible harm and economic loss if the host loses its immunity or "resistance." Second, the subclinically parasitized animal is a source of contamination of the environment and a reservoir of potential re-exposure of the same host(s), their progeny, and new additions. This is especially important in confined animals when the subclinical parasitism is caused by parasites having direct life cycles. If rapid exposure occurs or a single large dose is acquired, the "resistance" of the subclinically parasitized host may be offset by the increased parasite burden; disease and/or economic loss may result. For young progeny, exposure may occur prior to development of immunologic competence, and for the susceptible animal recently added to the herd, the dose may be intolerable. Therefore, if subclinical parasitism is not identified and evaluated, its existence may go unnoticed until harm and economic loss have been manifested. Recognition of a problem could come too late for correction, or correction might cost more than control would have earlier. In addition, such an oversight might result in introduction and establishment of a harmful parasite in a new environment. This has occurred with *Fasciola hepatica* in some geographic regions. Therefore, all cases of subclinical or asymptomatic parasitism, as well as of clinical parasitism, should be assessed in a veterinary medical practice.

Parasite Control

Disruption of the parasite's life cycle is the most effective corrective action and control strategy for the management of parasitic infections.

Success is more likely if the weakest link of the parasite's life cycle is attacked; however, the probability of effecting control is increased by attacking more than one point in the life cycle. Treating only for the adult parasite, therefore, is frequently insufficient to correct or control parasitism. The specific parasite, its bionomics, the status of parasitism, and the possible disruption of the parasite's life cycle must be considered in order to implement an effective and economic corrective and control plan.

Preventive health programs are more desirable for the welfare of the animal, the client, and other humans than action delayed until clinical parasitism is manifested. Irreversible harm to the host and costly corrective measures can thus often be avoided by timely implementation of preventive measures. Equally important benefits derive from preventing exposure of succeeding host populations and of humans when zoonotic diseases are involved.

Total eradication of parasites generally is not possible for animals maintained out-of-doors and is not economically feasible in many indoor husbandry operations. Notable exceptions in the United States are eradication of *Trypanosoma equiperdum* and of *Boophilus annulatus*. However, no gastrointestinal parasite of large domestic animals has been eradicated. Preventive parasite programs are possible for most pathogenic parasite species in individual companion animals and in animal colonies reared for research purposes. In reality these programs are directed toward control at a subclinical level or toward monitoring to detect reinfection. Corrective measures thus can be taken before discernible harm has occurred.

Control of subclinical parasitism provides the rationale for routine examination for evidence of gastrointestinal parasites when regular physical examinations are conducted and when herds are monitored at regular intervals.

Sanitation: This preventive measure reduces the host's potential exposure to parasites. Sanitation procedures used to maintain an environment free of helminth and protozoan organisms often differ from procedures for controlling pathogenic bacteria and viruses. Because most persons understand sanitation only as it applies to bacteria and viruses, the veterinarian must give detailed instructions to the client regarding helminths and protozoans.

To determine appropriate corrective sanitary procedures, one must know the relative resistance of external stages of parasites to chemical agents and environmental changes. Thick-shelled helminth eggs, particularly ascarids, are resistant to most of the common antiseptics. For example, ascarid eggs will larvate in 2% formalin solution.[29] Decontaminating a pen, cage, and equipment should therefore include physically removing the parasite from the surfaces and properly disposing of the material that has been removed. Hosing a surface and using common disinfectants do not decontaminate a surface adequately, particularly if it is rough-surfaced, as is concrete. Scrubbing with a stiff-bristled brush with hot water and a strong detergent to loosen debris is one of the best ways to clean pens and equipment. A surface free of all dirt and excrement can be decontaminated with live steam or a flame, but these generally are not practical or available. A small dirt pen can be decontaminated by removing the top 5 to 8 cm of soil.

Obviously there are many situations in which scrubbing or removing the soil is not possible. In these cases, improved sanitation is achieved by preventing contamination of drinking water and feed.

Management Practices: If environmental moisture is decreased, desiccation of parasite life stages is increased; this contributes markedly to reduced chance of exposure. Desiccation is generally more detrimental to the parasite than are chemicals used to disinfect surfaces. Strong dehydrating chemicals (e.g., 10 pounds rock salt or borax/100 square feet) will greatly expedite decontamination of an area.

The external phase of a parasite is limited, and time of survival outside a host varies among the species. Management that reduces accumulation of feces and exposes fecal material and litter to drying creates unsuitable developmental conditions for the parasites.

Generally, if fields are free of parasitized animals for extended periods, infective larvae will decrease drastically. The interval for pasture rotation is not specific, and effectiveness varies with the region and time of year. For example, monthly rotation in a region of mild temperatures and high humidity may result in animals acquiring more parasites than if rotation was not practiced. On the other hand, if the daily temperatures exceed 40°C and rainfall is less than 20 mm monthly, rotation may be sufficient to reduce greatly the larval contamination of a pasture; however, the type of vegetation will have a marked influence on larval survival time.[17] A field kept free of animals for 3 months will be cleared of a large proportion of infective larvae of most ruminant strongyles and canine hookworms.

Diet: The well-nourished host is less likely to develop heavy adult parasite burdens and can tolerate relatively larger parasite numbers without clinical signs than can the animal on an inadequate diet. This cannot be overemphasized.

Strategic Therapy. Anthelmintics are given to control any parasite that is a potential threat to the animal's health. Animals parasitized by organisms that have direct life cycles often require intermittent treatment. However, parasite burden, a very important factor in determining harm and disease, is determined by the exposure rate and dose. Furthermore, chance of exposure can be greatly influenced by management. Selective strategic treatment at a time of year when the environment is least contaminated and/or when management changes have reduced the host's exposure or increased the host's resistance to parasites is more likely to control parasites satisfactorily than is regular routine therapy without consideration of other factors.

Corrective Therapy. The most effective, safest drug should be used, and where indicated, supportive therapy should be employed if that is economically possible. It is not always wise to treat for all parasites at one time or even to treat parasitism first in disease conditions of multiple etiology. Severe anemia, obstruction, or gut perforations caused by parasites should be treated immediately upon diagnosis. Most of the other parasitisms do not require emergency attention, and treatment can be delayed until other acute disease problems are under control. Reduction of parasite burden frequently alleviates clinical signs even though significant numbers of parasites remain in the host. Basing efficacy of a drug solely on clinical improvement can be, therefore, misleading. A follow-up laboratory examination should be made prior to the time that reinfection would be evident if the veterinarian is to evaluate accurately the drugs used.

Supportive therapy is dictated by the type of injury caused by the parasites. For example, marked anemia resulting from canine hookworm infection[59] requires that blood transfusions be administered just prior to and immediately following treatment with anthelmintics, if recovery is to be expected. In addition, hookworms have a very traumatic effect on the gut, and dietary supplementation with high-quality protein, B complex vitamins, and iron that is readily absorbed is indicated.

Part II. Strategies

The veterinarian is faced with a challenging task in identifying specific factors contributing to parasitism and in evaluating their relative significance because of (1) the great number of individual factors contributing to parasitism and disease; (2) the complexity of host/parasite/environment interactions; and (3) the variation of importance for each factor in different field situations as well as at different times in the same situation. This task can be made simpler by an orderly application of steps in the decision-making process, i.e., by applying systematic problem-solving techniques. Following such a strategy helps prevent oversight of pertinent factors, provides a method for separating major from minor factors, helps to put the situation into perspective, assures selection of the best solutions, and provides alternative solutions. Furthermore, one is alerted that conclusions or recommendations may need revision.

Many persons routinely use this systematic process or a modification of it without being aware of what they are doing. It is suggested that by analyzing situations and putting these principles into practice, one's skills in this capacity can be improved. The following strategies using the decision-making process were developed for evaluating clinical observations and laboratory findings that reflect current and potential parasite problems, and for the design of corrective/control programs.

Collect Pertinent Host, Management, and Environmental Data. Take a complete history, make observations, and conduct routine parasitologic and other appropriate laboratory examinations. Evaluate laboratory results (Fig. 17–1). *Avoid interpreting facts prematurely, making conclusions, or suggesting corrective measures until all data have been recorded.* This deliberate approach will help to prevent undue emphasis on less important facts and to avoid oversight of relevant details. A checklist may help to develop skills in making accurate observations and to assure that important points are not overlooked. The checklist should include reminders of types of information to be collected pertaining to (a) host(s), (b) management, (c) environment not influenced by management, (d) miscellaneous data, e.g., neighbor's disease problems and other species of animals on premise. There is danger, however, in relying solely on a checklist because important factors unique to a situation may be overlooked.

Evaluate Relative Impact: Evaluate the impact of each item identified as a contributor to the clinical problem and record the judgment as a quantitative estimate (e.g., 1 to 5 or − to ++++). Avoid drawing conclusions until the evaluation has been completed.

Weighting the importance of each item helps to recall and determine more readily those factors that have the greatest impact on the current situation. It serves to guide re-evaluation, expose errors made in the first analysis, or reveal changing trends that would require revision in the program. When evaluating the relative importance of factors contributing to clinical parasitism, one should attempt to answer the following questions for each factor:

a. Is the parasite burden or the evidence of parasitic disease influenced by this factor, and if so, is it of major or minor importance?

b. Does this factor affect exposure rate and, if so, is it of primary or secondary importance?

c. Does this factor affect the host's susceptibility?

Generate Corrective Solutions. Generate as many corrective solutions as possible for each factor identified as significant. After identifying the factors contributing to existing parasitism and evaluating the relative inportance of each factor to clinical and potential parasitism, generate solutions for each factor. Determine more than one solution for each factor if possible. Since most parasitic diseases are directly related to exposure dose and rate, this aspect should receive particular attention. Explore the possibility for decreasing exposure by (a) altering animal numbers, pasture rotation, feeding regime, drainage, and water source; (b) separation of animals into similar age groups; and (c) strategic use of anthelmintics.

Analyze the Impact of Solutions. When a solution is generated, its impact bears on both the parasite problem and on the client's willingness to implement the solution. One key to obtaining client cooperation and compliance is found in the quantification process. The client will often accede to a more elaborate and costly solution if the probable outcome, when quantified, more nearly helps meet the production goals.

List the Constraints. These should include the cost range the client is willing to pay for drugs, labor, and feeds; availability of labor and facilities; client education; market price of animals or by-products; topography of environment; available space for animals; recent climatic conditions; management practices such as population groupings, feeding practices, and sources of water. This is not an exhaustive list; therefore, one should look for other constraints not mentioned.

Match Solutions with Constraints. The most feasible solutions having the greatest impact on the problem are matched with the identified constraints that can be altered.

Implement the Most Feasible Solutions.

Evaluate and Monitor the Program to Determine when Revision is Needed.

Effective programs will reduce parasitism, lead to improved animal health and increased profit, and prevent recurrence of clinical parasitism. An effective program, therefore, must either prevent or markedly reduce re-exposure to parasites and/or protectively immunize animals. If pathogenic parasite burdens are increased to a point where impairment of health and/or economic loss results, revisions of the program should be made. Continuous

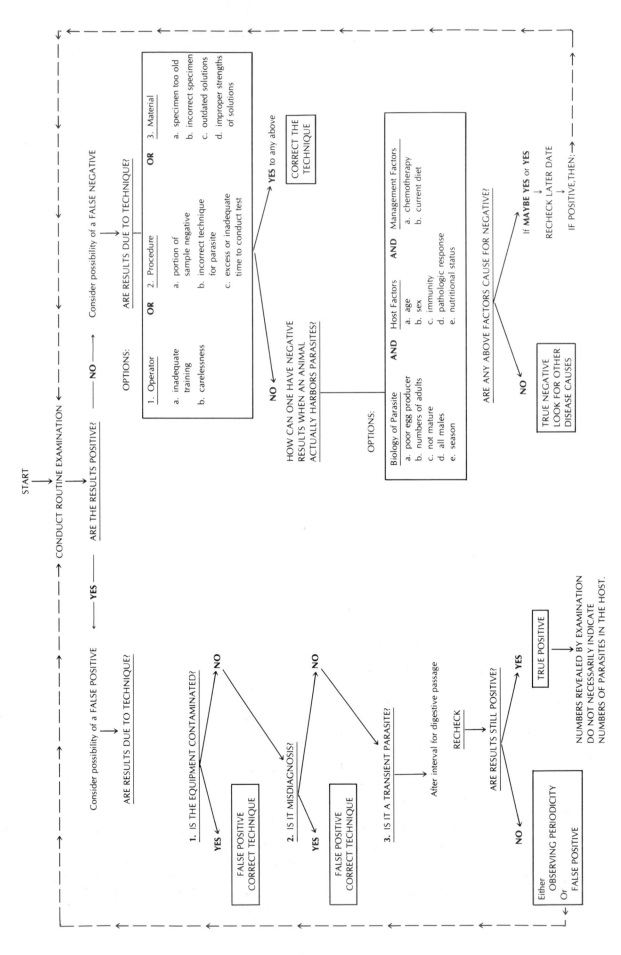

Figure 17–1. Strategy for evaluating parasitology laboratory findings.

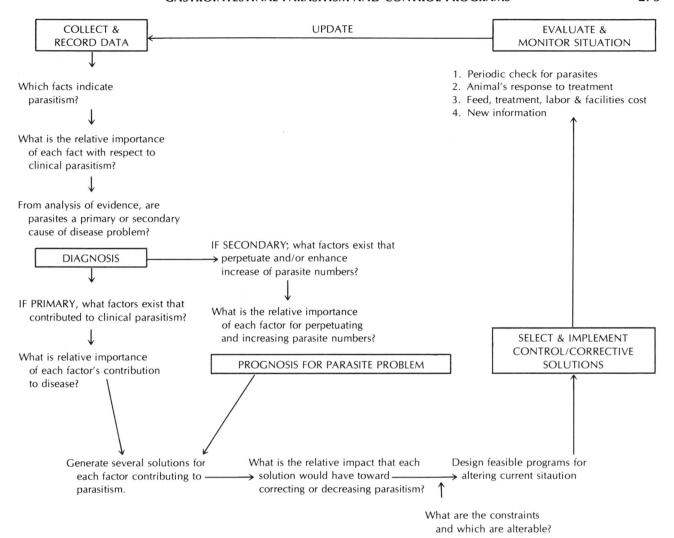

COLLECT & RECORD DATA

UPDATE

EVALUATE & MONITOR SITUATION

1. Periodic check for parasites
2. Animal's response to treatment
3. Feed, treatment, labor & facilities cost
4. New information

Which facts indicate parasitism?

What is the relative importance of each fact with respect to clinical parasitism?

From analysis of evidence, are parasites a primary or secondary cause of disease problem?

DIAGNOSIS

IF SECONDARY; what factors exist that perpetuate and/or enhance increase of parasite numbers?

IF PRIMARY, what factors exist that contributed to clinical parasitism?

What is the relative importance of each factor for perpetuating and increasing parasite numbers?

What is relative importance of each factor's contribution to disease?

PROGNOSIS FOR PARASITE PROBLEM

SELECT & IMPLEMENT CONTROL/CORRECTIVE SOLUTIONS

Generate several solutions for each factor contributing to parasitism.

What is the relative impact that each solution would have toward correcting or decreasing parasitism?

Design feasible programs for altering current sitaution

What are the constraints and which are alterable?

Figure 17–2. Strategy for controlling parasites and correcting parasitism.

monitoring provides a mechanism to evaluate a program's success. Furthermore, timely decisions can be made to change a program that is no longer successful or economically feasible. Monitoring should include:

1. *Parasitologic Examinations.* This includes both an individual animal, or an appropriate sample of a herd if one is dealing with a large population. This examination should be conducted 1 to 2 weeks following treatment and subsequently at regular intervals. The specific interval depends upon the host, production, and frequency of routine treatment. Where a parasite problem persists, more frequent examinations are desirable and should be scheduled with other routine herd health activities.

2. *Study of Feed and Labor Costs.*

3. *Cost and Effectiveness of Anthelmintics.*

4. *Production Records.* Compare changes in production records after entering into a program of parasite control with pre-program records.

This proposed strategy is shown in Figure 17–2.

REFERENCES

1. Michel, J. F.: Arrested development of nematodes and some related phenomena. *In* Advances in Parasitology, Vol. 12. Edited by B. Dawes. London, Academic Press, 1974, p. 279.
2. Baer, J.: Ecology of Animal Parasites. Urbana, University of Illinois Press, 1951.
3. Whitlock, J. H.: Trichostrongylidosis in sheep and cattle. Proc. Am. Vet. Med. Assoc. *127*:123, 1955.
4. Read, C. P.: Parasitism and Symbiology. New York, The Ronald Press Co., 1970.
5. Poynter, D.: Some tissue reactions to the nematode parasites of animals. *In* Advances in Parasitology, Vol. 4. Edited by B. Dawes. London, Academic Press, 1966, p. 321.
6. Horak, I. G., and Clark, R.: Studies on paramphistomiasis. V. The pathological physiology of the acute disease in sheep. Onderstepoort J. Vet. Res. *30*:145, 1963.
7. Mettrick, D. F., and Podesta, R. B.: Ecological and physiological aspects of helminth-host interactions in the mammalian gastrointesti-

nal canal. *In* Advances in Parasitology, Vol. 12. Edited by B. Dawes. London, Academic Press, 1974, p. 183.

8. Mulligan, W.: The effect of helminthic infection on the protein metabolism of the host. Proc. Nutr. Soc. *31*:47, 1972.

9. Barker, I. K.: A study of the pathogenesis of *Trichostrongylus colubriformis* infection in lambs with observation on the contribution of gastrointestinal plasma loss. Int. J. Parasitol. *3*:743, 1973.

10. Ryley, J. F.: Why and how are coccidia harmful to their host? *In* Pathogenic Processes in Parasitic Infections, Vol. 13. Edited by A. E. R. Taylor and R. Muller. Symposia of the British Society for Parasitology. Oxford, Blackwell Scientific Publications, 1975.

11. Baker, N. F., and Douglas, J. R.: Blood alterations in helminth infection. *In* Biology of Parasites. Edited by E. J. L. Soulsby. New York, Academic Press, 1966.

12. Barker, I. K.: The relationship of abnormal mucosal microtopography with distribution of *Trichostrongylus colubriformis* in the small intestines of lambs. Int. J. Parasitol. *4*:153, 1974.

13. Benz, G. W., and Ernst, J. V.: Alkaline phosphatase activities in intestinal mucosa from calves infected with *Cooperia punctata* and *Eimeria bovis*. Am. J. Vet. Res. *37*:895, 1976.

14. Horak, I. G., Clark, R., and Botha, J. C.: The pathological physiology of helminth infestations. I. *Ostertagia circumcincta*. Onderstepoort J. Vet. Res. *32*:147, 1965.

15. Kennedy, C. R.: Ecological Animal Parasitology. New York, John Wiley & Sons, 1975.

16. Jordan, H. E.: Amebiasis *(Entamoeba histolytica)* in the dog. Vet. Med. *62*:61, 1967.

17. Levine, N. D.: Weather, climate, and the bionomics of ruminant nematode larvae. *In* Advances in Veterinary Science, Vol. 8. Edited by C. A. Brandly and E. J. Jungherr. New York, Academic Press, 1963.

18. Vegors, H. H., Baird, D. M., Sell, O. E., and Stewart, T. B.: Parasitisms in beef yearlings as related to forage availability and levels of protein feeding. J. Anim. Sci. *15*:1198, 1956.

19. Vegors, H. H., Sell, O. E., Baird, D. M., and Stewart, T. B.: Internal parasitism of beef yearlings as affected by type of pasture, supplemental corn feeding and age of calf. J. Anim. Sci. *14*:256, 1955.

20. Crofton, H. D.: The ecology of immature phases of trichostrongyle nematodes. Parasitology *39*:17, 1948.

21. Rogers, W. P., and Sommerville, R. I.: The infective stage of nematode parasites and its significance in parasitism. *In* Advances in Parasitology, Vol. 1. Edited by B. Dawes. London, Academic Press, 1968., p. 327.

22. Michel, J. F.: The epidemiology and control of some nematode infections of grazing animals. *In* Advances of Parasitology, Vol. 7. Edited by B. Dawes. London, Academic Press, 1969, p. 211.

23. Michel, J. F.: The epidemiology and control of some nematode infections of grazing animals. *In* Advances in Parasitology, Vol. 14. Edited by B. Dawes. London, Academic Press, 1976, p. 355.

24. Ollerenshaw, C. B., and Smith, L. P.: Meteorological factors and forecasts of helminthic disease. *In* Advances in Parasitology, Vol. 7. Edited by B. Dawes. London, Academic Press, 1969, p. 283.

25. Poeschel, G. P., and Todd, A. C.: Selection for variations in pathogenicity of *Haemonchus contortus* isolates. Am. J. Vet. Res. *33*:1575, 1972.

26. Armour, J. F., Jennings, W., and Urquhart, G. M.: The possible existence of two strains of *Ostertagia ostertagi*. Letter to the Editor. Vet. Rec. *80*:208, 1967.

27. Michel, J. F.: The possible existence of two strains of *Ostertagia ostertagi*. Letter to the Editor. Vet. Rec. *80*:316, 1967.

28. Levine, N. D.: Nematode Parasites of Domestic Animals and of Man. Minneapolis, Burgess Publishing Co., 1968.

29. Soulsby, E. J. L.: Textbook of Veterinary Clinical Parasitology, Vol. I. Helminths. Philadelphia, F. A. Davis Co., 1965.

30. Gordon, H. McL.: Helminthic diseases. *In* Advances in Veterinary Science, Vol. 3. New York, Academic Press, 1957, p. 287.

31. Ciordia, H., Baird, D. M., Neville, W. E., and McCampbell, H. C.: Internal parasitism of beef cattle on winter pastures: effects of initial level of parasitism on beef production. Am. J. Vet. Res. *33*:1407, 1972.

32. Smith, H. J.: Inhibited development of *Ostertagia ostertagi, Cooperia oncophora,* and *Nematodirus helvetianus* in parasite-free calves grazing fall pastures. Am. J. Vet. Res. *35*:935, 1974.

33. Scothorn, M. W., Koutz, F. R., and Groves, H. F.: Prenatal *Toxocara canis* infection in pups. J.A.V.M.A. *146*:45, 1965.

34. Stone, W. M., and Girardeau, M. H.: *Ancylostoma caninum* larvae present in the colostrum of a bitch. Vet. Rec. *79*:773, 1966.

35. Stone, W. M., and Peckham, J. C.: Infectivity of *Ancylostoma caninum* larvae from canine milk. Am. J. Vet. Res. *31*:1693, 1970.

36. Clapham, P. A.: Prepartum infestation of puppies with *Ancylostoma caninum*. Vet. Rec. *74*:754, 1962.

37. Moncol, D. J., and Batte, E. G.: Transcolostral infection of newborn pigs with *Strongyloides ransomi*. Vet. Med. *61*:583, 1966.

38. Lucker, J. T.: Variability in effect of stomach worm, *Haemonchus contortus,* infections in lambs. Proc. Am. Vet. Med. Assoc., 89th Annual Meeting, Atlantic City, 1953, p. 171.

39. Horak, I. G., and Clark, R.: The pathological physiology of *Ostertagia circumcincta* infestation. Onderstepoort J. Vet. Res. *31*:163, 1964.

40. Whitlock, J. H.: The relationship of nutrition to the development of the trichostrongylidoses. Cornell Vet. *39*:146, 1949.

41. Threlkeld, W. L., Price, N. O., and Linkous, W. N.: An observation on the relationship of cobalt deficiency to internal parasites of sheep. Am. J. Vet. Res. *17*:246, 1956.

42. Stewart, T. B., Hale, O. M., and Johnson, J. C., Jr.: Failure of parasitized gilt and barrow pigs on different planes of nutrition to respond alike to a superimposed infection with *Strongyloides ransomi*. J. Parasitol. *55*:1055, 1969.

43. Tsuchiya, H.: The localization of *Giardia canis* (Hegner, 1922) as affected by diet. Am. J. Hyg. *15*:232, 1932.

44. Vetter, R. L., Pope, A. L., Todd, A. C., and Hoekstra, W. C.: Demonstration of a factor in alfalfa hay required for egg production by the stomach worm of sheep. J. Anim. Sci. *19*:1298, 1960.

45. Vetter, R. L., Hoekstra, W. G., Todd, A. C., and Pope, A. L.: Effects on the stomach worm, *Haemonchus contortus,* of feeding lambs natural versus semipurified diets. Am. J. Vet. Res. *24*:439, 1963.

46. Kelley, G. W., Jr., Olsen, L. S., and Hoerlein, A. B.: The influence of diet on the development of *Ascaris suum* in the small intestine of pigs. Am. J. Vet. Res. *19*:401, 1958.

47. Rohrbacher, G. H., Porter, D. A., and Herlick, H.: The effect of milk in the diet of calves and rabbits upon the development of trichostrongylid nematodes. Am. J. Vet. Res. *19*:625, 1958.

48. Georgi, J. R.: Parasitology for Veterinarians, 2nd ed. Philadelphia, W. B. Saunders Co., 1974.

49. Ehrenford, F. A.: Canine ascariasis as a potential source of visceral larva migrans. Am. J. Trop. Med. Hyg. *6*:166, 1957.

50. Katz, F. F.: On a host sex difference in *Strongyloides ratti* intestinal worm burdens in rats. Proc. Pa. Acad. Sci. *41*:30, 1967.

51. Herlick, H.: Age resistance of cattle to nematodes of the gastrointestinal tract. J. Parasitol. *46*:392, 1960.

52. Miller, T. A.: Influence of age and sex on susceptibility of dogs to primary infection with *Ancylostoma caninum*. J. Parasitol. *51*:701, 1965.

53. Smith, H. J., and Archibald, R. McG.: The effects of age and previous infection on the development of gastrointestinal parasitism in cattle. Can. J. Comp. Med. *32*:511, 1968.

54. Jackson, G. J., Herman, R., and Singer, I.: Immunity to Parasitic Animals, Vol. 2. New York, Appleton-Century-Crofts, 1970.

55. Larsh, J. E., Jr., and Weatherly, N. F.: Cell-mediated immunity against certain parasitic worms. *In* Advances in Parasitology, Vol. 13. Edited by B. Dawes. London, Academic Press, 1975.

56. Otto, G. F.: Immunity against canine hookworm disease. Vet. Med. *43*:180, 1948.

57. Soulsby, E. J. L.: Immunity to Animal Parasites. New York, Academic Press, 1972.

58. Michel, J. F.: The effect of cortisone on populations of *Ostertagia ostertagi* of uniform age. Br. Vet. J. *125*:617, 1969.

59. Beaver, P. C., Yoshida, Y., and Ash, L. R.: Mating of *Ancylostoma caninum* in relation to blood loss in the host. J. Parasitol. *50*:286, 1964.

Chapter 18

GASTROINTESTINAL PHARMACOLOGY

LLOYD E. DAVIS
J. DESMOND BAGGOT

Disturbances of gastrointestinal function are probably the most common medical problem seen by the veterinarian. Many of these disorders are self-limiting in nature and are probably best managed by conservative approaches. Because of the high incidence of dysfunction, the practitioner has been presented with numerous medicaments claimed to ameliorate the various disturbances. As a result, one is faced with the problem of evaluating the claims made by various manufacturers. This may be difficult because many of the claims have been based on testimonial or anecdotal evidence rather than on the basis of "blind" trials designed to control observer bias. The difficulty is increased by the fact that many claims are made relative to disorders which are self-limiting in nature, e.g., diarrhea, vomiting or flatulence. In such cases drugs may complicate the clinical picture rather than improve it. In view of these considerations it would seem appropriate to maintain a healthy degree of skepticism relative to claims made for new members of accepted groups of drugs. However, the practitioner should be alert to recognize genuine advances in pharmacology, such as the discovery of the histamine H2 receptor antagonists for decreasing gastric acid secretion.

Part I. Clinical Pharmacology of the Gastrointestinal Tract

LLOYD E. DAVIS

In this part drug dosages for the common domesticated species are tabulated for the convenience of the reader and are intended merely as approximations for initiating therapy. The posology of many drugs has not been studied adequately in most animals of importance to the veterinarian. In any case, the dose and dosage interval should be adjusted by the therapist to the needs of the patient.

The purpose of this section is to describe various drugs which are employed to achieve therapeutic modification of certain gastrointestinal functions. The subject of antibacterial therapy is discussed in Chapter 19.

EMETICS AND ANTIEMETICS

Vomiting is a reflex act, protective in nature, which is limited to carnivorous and omnivorous animals. Isolated occurrences of vomiting are of little medical significance and may subserve this protective function. Protracted vomiting is abnormal and may be deleterious to the patient because of ensuing fluid and electrolyte derangements, altered acid-base balance, and fatigue. Vomiting might cause aspiration pneumonia or gastric rupture and is commonly a great inconvenience to the owner.

Vomiting (emesis) is a reflex act, initiated by a

stimulus transmitted along afferent pathways to an emetic center located in the lateral reticular formation of the medulla oblongata. The emetic center integrates efferent activity resulting in the coordinated act of vomition. The animal salivates profusely; saliva and swallowed air distend the distal esophagus. The diaphragm is depressed which straightens the esophagus. The body, fundus, and cardia of the stomach relax and the pyloric area contracts, the glottis is closed and the soft palate presses against the nasopharynx, the abdominal muscles contract to compress the stomach against the diaphragm while the thorax expands, the cardiac sphincter relaxes, and the gastric contents are ejected. Rectus abdominis contraction and negative pressure in the expanded thorax are major factors in ejecting gastric content.

There are several pathways by which effective stimuli may be conveyed to the emetic center. An understanding of these is a prerequisite for rational therapy of vomiting. Stimulation of the pharynx and fauces is transmitted by afferent nerves in cranial nerve IX. Impulses arising from the heart, stomach, liver and gallbladder, intestines and peritoneum are conveyed to the emetic center via visceral afferent fibers in sympathetic and vagal nerves. Impulses from the kidneys, ureters and urinary bladder are transmitted by visceral afferent fibers in sympathetic nerves. Chemical stimuli and distention are effective in initiating the emetic reflex by this pathway. Treatment with antiemetic drugs may mask clinical signs essential for proper diagnosis in these cases.

Stimuli arising in the semicircular canals are transmitted by way of cranial nerve VIII, the vestibular nucleus, the uvula and nodulus of the cerebellum to the emetic center. The effective stimuli are rhythmic changes in the acceleration of the head (motion sickness) and labyrinthitis.

Vomiting may be initiated by stimuli arising in the cerebral cortex and limbic system of the brain. Psychogenic vomiting as a result of emotional conflicts, visual or olfactory stimuli has its origins in the cerebral cortex. Head injuries, increased intracranial pressure, and nitrogen mustard provoke vomiting by way of the limbic system.

Blood-borne chemical substances will stimulate the chemoreceptor trigger zone (CTZ), which is connected by neural pathways to the emetic center. The CTZ is located in the lateral walls of the third ventricle (area postrema). This area is devoid of the blood-brain barrier, so substances diffuse freely from the capillaries of this region. Vomiting associated with uremia, radiation sickness, digitalis, morphine, apomorphine, bacterial toxins, and certain antibiotics is mediated by this pathway.

Emetic Drugs

Emesis may be useful in the initial treatment of patients which have ingested toxicants. While gastric lavage may be preferred in most cases because it is more thorough, the emetic drugs are convenient for emptying the stomach. As with any drug, good judgment must be exercised in using an emetic. General contraindications include: excessive central nervous depression, prostration, ingestion of corrosives, presence of abdominal pain, hernias or prolapses.

Apomorphine (44 μg/kg, S.C.) is the most reliable emetic for use in the dog. It is a morphine derivative which stimulates the CTZ and is a powerful central nervous depressant. Dosage should not be repeated as the emetic center may be depressed and unresponsive to subsequent doses. Apomorphine may be expected to be ineffective in a patient with medullary depression. Apomorphine should not be given to felines as it produces extreme excitement in these species. It is ineffective in swine.[1] Xylazine (Rompun) is an effective emetic in cats[2] at a dosage of 0.44 mg/kg. This dose is lower than that required for immobilization.

Several drugs may be recommended for the emergency evacuation of the stomach by the client. A teaspoonful of table salt placed in the back of the mouth will stimulate receptors in the fauces and pharynx and initiate vomiting. A tablespoonful of freshly ground mustard seed mixed in tepid water and given orally will stimulate receptors in the gastric mucosa to induce vomiting. Prepared table mustard and mustard powder are ineffective because the oil of mustard is volatile and will be lost from these household preparations. Syrup of ipecac (5 to 20 ml, depending on size) followed by tepid water is usually effective for inducing vomiting in the dog and cat.[3] There is generally a latent period of 15 to 30 minutes before the animal vomits. The dose may be repeated after this time, but if the patient does not vomit, the ipecac should be recovered by gastric lavage. The active alkaloid (emetine) is acutely toxic to the heart, liver, and kidney if sufficient amounts are absorbed.

Copper sulfate and zinc sulfate have been employed as emetics at doses of 50 ml of 1% solutions. They stimulate gastric receptors, have latent periods of 30 to 45 minutes, and are not completely reliable. Care must be taken that the

Table 18–1. Drugs causing vomiting as an undesirable side effect

> Alcohol
> Aminophylline
> Anesthetics
> Antihistaminics
> Bromides
> Chloramphenicol
> Chloroquine
> Digitalis glycosides
> Ergonovine
> Erythromycin
> Estrogens (oral)
> Ferrous sulfate
> Morphine
> Mustargen
> Nicotine
> Nicotinic acid
> Nitrofurantoin
> Penicillin (oral)
> Phenytoin
> Potassium chloride
> Progestogens (oral)
> Salicylates
> Tetracyclines
> Urea
> Veratrine

drugs are in complete solution as the crystals are caustic. These compounds may be useful for inducing vomition in swine as they are inexpensive.

A number of drugs may induce vomiting as an undesirable side effect of therapy. Several drugs which commonly cause vomiting are listed in Table 18–1. Generally, vomiting is not a serious enough problem to force cessation of therapy. Vomiting may be a sign to reduce dosage as in the case of digitalis or salicylate therapy. Some individuals will vomit simply as a result of the mechanics of drug administration.

Antiemetic Drugs

In many cases vomiting is secondary to diseases of visceral organs, infections, or uremia so that use of antiemetic drugs in these disorders is symptomatic and may make diagnosis more difficult. Primary attention should be directed toward accurate diagnosis and treatment of the underlying disorder. Antiemetics are employed in the specific management of vomiting induced by drugs and other foreign chemicals, radiation sickness, motion sickness, and psychosomatic disturbances.

Antiemetic drugs may be considered as having a limited or broad spectrum of activity. Some examples of drugs with a limited spectrum include sedatives which are effective in the control of psychogenic and post-anesthetic vomiting, demulcents which inhibit emesis associated with pharyngitis or gastritis, and drugs effective in the prevention of motion sickness.

Vomiting caused by labyrinthine stimulation is specifically prevented by various antihistaminic drugs. The antiemetic activity of these drugs is independent of their antihistaminic or sedative potencies and appears to have a direct effect on neural pathways arising in the vestibular apparatus. Drugs in this group are listed in Table 18–2. The main differences among the members of this group are their duration of action and the degree of sedation produced. Scopolamine has a rather brief duration of action which makes it less useful in veterinary medical practice. It produces excitement in cats; hence, it should not be used in these species. Dimenhydrinate, diphenhydramine, and promethazine have considerable central nervous system depressant properties, which may be an advantage in an animal traveling for an extended period of time. The principal side effects of this group include drowsiness, xerostomia, blurred vision, and incoordination. Cyclizine or meclizine should not be used in animals following breeding because they have been shown to be teratogenic.[4]

The broad spectrum antiemetics are effective in prophylaxis and treatment of vomiting from all

Table 18–2. Drugs that prevent vomiting caused by stimulation of the vestibular apparatus

Generic Name	Proprietary Name	Duration	Dosage Dog and Cat
L-Hyoscine	Scopolamine	Short	Unsatisfactory response—not to be used in cats
Dimenhydrinate	Dramamine	Intermediate	8 mg/kg, q8h
Diphenhydramine	Benadryl	Intermediate	4 mg/kg, q8h
Cyclizine	Marezine	Intermediate	4 mg/kg, q8h
Meclizine	Bonine	Long	4 mg/kg, s.i.d.
Promethazine	Phenergan	Long	2 mg/kg, s.i.d.

Table 18–3. Broad-spectrum antiemetic drugs

Generic Name	Proprietary Name	Possible Side Effects	Suggested Dosage Dog and Cat
Chlorpromazine	Thorazine	Icterus, agranulocytosis	0.5 mg/kg
Prochlorperazine	Compazine, Darbazine	Extrapyramidal	0.13 mg/kg
Triflupromazine	Vesprin	Icterus, agranulocytosis	0.2 mg/kg
Perphenazine	Trilafon	Extrapyramidal	0.04 mg/kg
Trifluoperazine	Stelazine	Extrapyramidal	0.03 mg/kg
Mepazine	Pacatal	Blurred vision	1.5 mg/kg
Trimethobenzamide	Tigan	Allergic responses	3.0 mg/kg
Diphenidol	Vontrol	Hallucinations	0.4 mg/kg
Metoclopramide	Imperan	Dystonia	0.1 mg/kg

causes except labyrinthine stimulation. For the most part these are phenothiazine derivatives. They block the CTZ at low doses and depress the emetic center at higher doses.[5] These drugs are listed in Table 18–3.

The phenothiazine derivatives have a variety of pharmacologic effects in addition to their antiemetic activity. These include ataraxia, alpha-adrenolytic and anticholinergic actions, and stimulation of the extrapyramidal system. The type of toxic side effects of the phenothiazines varies with the nature of the side-chain. Chlorpromazine and triflupromazine have aliphatic side-chains and are more prone to cause intrahepatic biliary stasis in humans, with jaundice and marrow depression with agranulocytosis. Drugs with a piperazine side-chain (prochlorperazine, perphenazine, and trifluoperazine) are more prone to produce extrapyramidal signs and convulsions with high doses but are less likely to cause hepatitis or agranulocytosis. Phenothiazine derivatives with a piperidine side-chain, such as mepazine, are much less toxic than the other two groups, although it is to be expected that antiemetic therapy with any of the phenothiazines would have a relatively low risk of toxicity because of the low dosage and short-term administration encountered in animal patients. Acute hypotensive reactions may occur on occasion following parenteral administration of these drugs. This is due to blockade of alpha-adrenergic receptors and should be treated with an alpha agonist such as levarterenol (Levophed) or phenylephrine (Neosynephrine). *Epinephrine should not be given in this situation* because of possible reversal (further depression of blood pressure).

Trimethobenzamide is a broad spectrum, non-phenothiazine, antiemetic drug. It suppresses the CTZ without affecting the emetic center and has virtually no other pharmacologic effect in the body. It is effective in the management of vomiting caused by radiation sickness, drugs, infections, anesthesia, and uremia but is without effect in blocking stimuli from viscera or the vestibular apparatus.

Diphenidol is a diphenylmethane derivative which possesses a complete spectrum of antiemetic activity. It appears to be effective in most cases of vomiting and may be the drug of choice for controlling emesis induced by labyrinthitis. It has little anticholinergic, adrenolytic, ataractic, or antihistaminic activity, but it has produced hallucinations and disorientation in human patients. This drug would seem to have promise in veterinary practice, but its use has not been established.

Metoclopramide depresses the CTZ but its main application is to inhibit vomiting associated with gastroduodenal disease. It stimulates gastric emptying and coordinates the pyloroduodenal motility pattern.[6] Large doses may produce dystonia, which may be confused with tetanus or encephalitis.[7]

The veterinarian should consider the various pathways by which the emetic reflex is activated and select the most suitable antiemetic drug based on its mode of action. These drugs are used symptomatically in many cases and should not replace efforts to treat the underlying disease process or to repair the ensuing metabolic deficits.

DRUGS AND GASTROINTESTINAL MOTILITY

Drugs which alter motility do so either by action on autonomic receptors or by direct effects on smooth muscle. The innervation of the gut and chemical mediators associated with gastrointestinal motility were discussed in Chapters 12 and 14. An understanding of normal function is a prerequisite for the intelligent selection of drugs for modifying motility.

Table 18–4. Drugs which modify gastrointestinal motility

Class	Generic Name	Proprietary Name	Increase (+) or Decrease (–) Motility	Suggested Dose					
				Horse	Cow	Sheep and Goat	Pig	Dog	Cat
Cholinergic	Pilocarpine	—	(+)	65–300 mg, SC	65–300 mg, SC	10–30 mg, SC	10–30 mg, SC	0.2 mg/kg, IV	0.5–2 mg, SC
	Arecoline	—	(+)	15 mg, SC	4–8 mg, SC	2–4 mg, SC	—	1.3 mg/kg, oral	1.3 mg/kg, oral
	Carbachol	Lentin	(+)	2–4 mg, SC	4 mg, SC	0.1–0.2 mg	1–4 mg, SC	.05–0.2 mg	0.05–0.1 mg
	Bethanechol	Urecholine	(+)	50 μg/kg, SC	50 μg/kg, SC	50 μg/kg, SC	50 μg/kg, SC	50 μg/kg, SC / 0.25 mg/kg, oral	1 mg, oral
Anticholinesterase	Physostigmine	Stiglyn	(+)	30–120 mg, SC	30–50 mg, SC	5–20 mg, SC	5–20 mg, SC	0.3–2 mg	0.3–0.5 mg
	Neostigmine	—	(+)	1 mg/cwt	1 mg/cwt	0.01–0.02 mg/kg	0.03 mg/kg	10–50 μg/kg	10–50 μg/kg
Anticholinergic	Atropine	—	(–)	0.04 mg/kg	0.08 mg/kg	0.08 mg/kg	0.04 mg/kg	0.04 mg/kg	0.04 mg/kg
	Methscopolamine	Pamine	(–)	20 mg	5 mg/cwt	5 mg/cwt	5 mg/cwt	0.3/1.5 mg/kg	—
	Isopropamide	Darbid	(–)	—	—	—	—	0.2/1.3 mg/kg	0.2–1.0 mg/kg
	Propantheline	Pro-Banthine	(–)	—	—	—	—	0.25 mg/kg	0.25 mg/kg
Musculotropic	Adiphenine	Trasentine	(–)	—	—	—	—	1 mg/kg	—
	Amprotropine	Syntropan	(–)	—	—	—	—	0.7 mg/kg	—
	Carbufluorene	Pavatrine	(–)	—	—	—	—	1.7 mg/kg	—
	Dicyclomine	Bentyl	(–)	—	—	—	—	0.15 mg/kg	—
Opioids	Morphine	—	(–)*	0.1 mg/kg	—	—	—	0.5 mg/kg	0.1 mg/kg
	Camphorated tincture of opium	Paregoric	(–)*	15–30 ml (foals)	15–30 ml (calves)	—	15–120 mg	2–15 ml	—
	Diphenoxylate	Lomotil	(–)*	0.5 mg/kg	0.5 mg/kg	0.5 mg/kg	0.5 mg/kg	0.5–1.0 mg/kg	0.5–1.0 mg/kg
Anti-inflammatory	Methampyrone	Dipyrone	(–), if spasm due to inflammation	2.5–10 g	2.5–10 g	2.5 g	2.5 g	10 mg/kg	10 mg/kg

* Propulsive movement is decreased, but segmental resistance is increased.

Autonomic Drugs

Adrenergic and cholinergic receptors are located throughout the body. Accordingly, it is virtually impossible to specifically treat the gastrointestinal tract with drugs affecting these receptors. Systemic administration of autonomic drugs in gastrointestinal therapy will result in undesired effects on other organs. Conversely, treatment of other organ systems will modify activity of the normal digestive system.

Effects of Adrenergic Drugs. Postganglionic sympathetic nerves innervate the muscularis mucosae, splanchnic blood vessels, mucosal glands, and the intramural nervous plexuses of the gut. They do not directly innervate the longitudinal or circular muscles.[8] Beta adrenergic receptors are located in intramural smooth muscle and alpha receptors are present in the smooth muscle of the blood vessels and myenteric plexuses.[9] Adrenergic drugs and their antagonists have no role in the management of gastrointestinal disorders but their effects often involve the system.

Adrenergic drugs such as epinephrine, levarterenol, isoproterenol, phenylephrine, and methoxamine inhibit gastrointestinal motility by directly inhibiting activity of smooth muscle (β-effect) or by decreasing the release of acetylcholine and decreasing blood flow to the organs (α-effect). The adrenergic drugs will moderate the effects of parasympathetic nerve stimulation on the gut by suppressing the release of acetylcholine by these nerves. However, adrenergics will not antagonize the increased motility produced by cholinergic drugs because these act directly on the smooth muscle.[8]

Sympathetic activity or administration of adrenergic drugs will inhibit motility of the reticulorumen, stomach, small intestine, and colon. This is a factor to be considered in patients that are excited or subjected to pain. Certain drugs may stimulate the release of epinephrine from the adrenal medulla and thus confound the effects of these drugs on the gut.

Effects of Cholinergic Drugs. This group of drugs directly stimulate the cholinergic receptors in the smooth muscle of the gut. They increase gastric emptying and propulsive activity of the intestines and colon. Smooth muscle of sphincters is inhibited. The most commonly used drugs of this group are listed in Table 18–4. For the most part, these drugs act at the muscarinic site with little effect on nicotinic sites (skeletal muscle or ganglia).

The cholinergic drugs all mimic the actions of acetylcholine but the relative effects on organ systems vary considerably. Pilocarpine and arecoline act primarily at muscarinic sites and exert marked effects on the heart, bronchioles, eye, and glands as well as stimulating motility of the gut. The pharmacologic effects of these drugs are readily antagonized by atropine. Carbachol has much less effect on the heart and bronchioles but does stimulate nicotinic sites.[10] This may enhance its effects on the bowel but fasciculation of skeletal muscle and stimulation of epinephrine release from the adrenal medulla may occur. This release of epinephrine may secondarily inhibit activity of the reticulorumen.[11] The effects of carbachol are poorly antagonized by atropine.

Bethanechol is another synthetic choline ester. It has the advantage over other members of the group by virtue of the greater specificity of its actions. It will stimulate the smooth muscle of the gastrointestinal tract and the urinary bladder with minimal effects on the cardiovascular system or bronchioles. It has no nicotinic effects and is readily antagonized by atropine. Neither carbachol nor bethanechol are susceptible to destruction by cholinesterases.

Anticholinesterases. Drugs such as physostigmine and neostigmine reversibly inactivate the enzyme which destroys the cholinergic mediator. As a result, acetylcholine accumulates at the cholinergic receptors and produces its characteristic effects on the tissue or organ. Because of this mechanism of action, the anticholinesterases act at both muscarinic and nicotinic sites. All cholinergic receptors in visceral organs, ganglia, and skeletal muscle are stimulated. There are major differences between the two drugs. Physostigmine contains a tertiary amine which makes the molecule lipid soluble. This allows it to cross cellular membranes readily and it is absorbed following oral administration. Neostigmine is poorly lipid soluble by virtue of its quaternary nitrogen and must be administered parenterally. In addition to its ability to inhibit acetylcholinesterase, neostigmine also directly stimulates the cholinergic receptor.[12]

Panthenol is an alcohol analog of pantothenate. Because pantothenic acid is a precursor of Coenzyme A, panthenol is claimed to increase the formation of acetylcholine and thereby to stimulate smooth muscle in the treatment of atony. Evidence for the mechanism of action and efficacy is poor.[13] Neostigmine and bethanechol remain the best choices of autonomic drugs for increasing motility of the gastrointestinal tract.

Cholinergic or anticholinesterase drugs should not be administered in the presence of mechanical obstruction of the gut, peritonitis, or doubtful viability of the intestinal wall. Whenever these drugs are employed, the therapist must have injectable atropine available to counteract excessive stimulation of the gut.

Anticholinergic Drugs. The anticholinergic drugs occupy the cholinergic receptor at muscarinic sites and prevent the action of acetylcholine on smooth muscle and glands. The cholinergic receptors at ganglia and at skeletal myoneural junctions differ in their configuration so the anticholinergic drugs, by definition, have little effect at these sites. Hexamethonium blocks the receptors at ganglia and tubocurarine competitively blocks acetylcholine at skeletal muscle.

Atropine and scopolamine are prototype antimuscarinic drugs. They will block the effects of parasympathetic stimulation on smooth muscle, glands, and the heart. They cross readily into the central nervous system where they produce excitement (atropine) or sedative (scopolamine) effects. Because of the widespread actions of these drugs on other organ systems, a host of compounds has been synthesized in an attempt to make their effects more specific to the gastrointestinal tract. Derivatives containing a trivalent nitrogen (adiphenine, amprotropine, carbofluorene, dicyclomine) directly inhibit smooth muscle with virtually no antimuscarinic effects elsewhere.[14] The addition of a quaternary nitrogen (methscopolamine, propantheline, isopropamide) prevents central nervous effects because the molecule will not cross the blood-brain barrier. Furthermore, these compounds will block the ganglia of the gut as well as exert antimuscarinic effects.

Inhibition of excessive motility or spasm of the gut by anticholinergic drugs is frequently incomplete as other mediators or autacoids such as serotonin,[15] and histamine[16] may be involved in the abnormal activity of the gut.

Cathartics

The cathartics increase motility of the bowel by directly stimulating the smooth muscle, by activating receptors in the mucosa which reflexly release acetylcholine, or by modifying secretion and absorption of electrolytes and water. The drugs in common use in veterinary medicine are classified in Table 18–5.

The irritant cathartics increase motility of the intestinal tract by directly stimulating smooth muscle in the wall of the bowel and/or by increasing secretion. The most commonly used drugs of this group are the anthraquinone derivatives. These glycosides contain the active principle, emodin. The pharmacologically inactive glycosides in aloin, senna, or cascara are transported to the colon where they are hydrolyzed in the alkaline environment. The emodin is released and stimulates motility of the colon. This accounts for the delay of 6 to 12 hours between ingestion and stimulation of defecation. Danthron (Istizin) is synthetic, nonglycosidic, anthraquinone. Its pharmacologic effects are similar to the glycosides but its use has been associated with "choke" in Shetland ponies. The action of this group most nearly mimics the physiologic act of defecation and is probably preferred for the treatment of simple constipation. These compounds are absorbed to some extent and excreted into the urine and milk. They will color alkaline urine red and acidic urine a dark yellow.

Castor oil is a bland, non-irritating oil which is a triglyceride of ricinoleic acid. Following ingestion, castor oil is hydrolyzed in the small intestine to release ricinoleic acid, which increases secretion of electrolytes and water. Thus, the increased intraluminal volume stimulates motility of the small intestine producing the elimination of liquid feces. Castor oil is relatively nontoxic and self-limiting in its action because the initial fraction which is hydrolyzed increases peristalsis and moves the unhydrolyzed portion through the alimentary canal.

Phenolphthalein is a cathartic commonly used by people. It is odorless, tasteless, and a common constituent of over-the-counter (OTC) laxative preparations. Unfortunately, it is effective only in primates and swine. The basis for these species differences is unknown, but it is possible that the active principle is a metabolite of phenolphthalein. This supposition is supported by the observation that phenolphthalein had no cathartic effect in newborn piglets which were unable to metabolize the drug. By 30 days of age, when drug-metabolizing enzymes had developed,[17] phenolphthalein exerted a purgative effect on the pigs (L. E. Davis—unpublished observations). Phenolphthalein may produce a pruritic skin rash and will confer a red color to alkaline urine.

The irritant cathartics should not be administered to patients with possible obstruction, enteritis or colitis. They should not be given to animals late in pregnancy as they may initiate parturition. Care should attend their use in lactating animals as active fractions are secreted into the milk and may cause purgation in the nursing offspring.

The saline cathartics stimulate motility reflexly by distending the bowel. The magnesium and sulfate ions are poorly absorbed from the gut. Thus, they exert an osmotic effect which causes move-

Table 18–5. Drugs employed as cathartics

Type	Name	Usual Dose						Principal Site of Action
		Horse	Cow	Sheep and Goat	Pig	Dog	Cat	
Irritant	Anthraquinones: Cascara sagrada (aromatic extract)	—	—	—	—	1–4 ml	0.5–1.5 ml	Colon
	Senna	120–150 g	120–150 g	30–60 g	30–60 g	1–8 g	0.1–0.3 g	
	Aloin	2.5–10 g	10–20 g	2–4 g	1–2.5 g	0.5–1 g	50–200 mg	
	Danthron	15–40 g	20–45 g	2.5–5 g	5–20 g	25–45 mg/kg	15–20 mg/kg	
	Castor oil	250–1000 ml	250–1000 ml	50–150 ml	20–150 ml	5–25 ml	3–10 ml	Small intestine
Saline	Magnesium sulfate	250–1000 g	250–1000 g	25–125 g	25–125 g	5–25 g	2–5 g	Small intestine
	Sodium sulfate	250–375 g	500–750 g	60 g	30–60 g	5–25 g	2–5 g	
	Magnesium oxide	—	500 gm	5–10 g	5–10 g	0.5–4 g	0.2–1 g	
	Magnesium hydroxide susp.	1–4 liters	1–4 liters	20–150 ml	10–50 ml	5–10 ml	2–6 ml	
Hydrophilic colloid	Psyllium	—	—	—	—	3–10 g	3 g	Small intestine and colon
	Methylcellulose	—	—	—	—	0.5–5 g	0.5–1 g	
	Bran, dry	0.5–1.5 kg	—	—	—	1–4 g	0.5–2 g	
Emollient	Liquid petrolatum	250–1000 ml	250–500 ml	15–150 ml	25–300 ml	5–30 ml	2–6 ml	Entire tract
	Raw linseed oil	500 ml		100–200 ml	100–200 ml	—	—	
Surfactant	Dioctyl sodium sulfosuccinate	5–15 g	5–15 g	2–5 g	—	2 mg/kg	2 mg/kg	Colon, rumen as defoaming agent
	Dioctyl calcium sulfosuccinate	7–22 g	7–22 g	3–7 g	—	3 mg/kg	3 mg/kg	" "

ment of water from the plasma into the lumen of the intestine until the contained fluid becomes isotonic. The increased volume stretches the mucosa and stimulates mechanoreceptors which reflexly causes an increase in peristaltic activity.

Sodium sulfate (Glauber's salt) is the most effective of the saline cathartics on a molar basis.[18] It is inexpensive and safe but has a very bitter taste. It is best administered by stomach tube in a 6% solution.

Magnesium salts are effective and relatively inexpensive. However, they are absorbed to some extent and may have systemic effects. The magnesium ion depresses the central nervous system, has a curariform effect on skeletal muscle, and prevents the release of acetylcholine from nerve endings. Toxicity is not commonly observed because the catharsis induced by the drugs impairs their absorption and eliminates the ion from the gut. In patients with impaired renal function or with delayed emptying of the gut, as in cases of megacolon or obstruction, magnesium toxicity may occur. The pharmacologic effects of magnesium are antagonized by the calcium ion. Accordingly, toxicity is appropriately treated by the intravenous administration of calcium salts.

Magnesium oxide or magnesium hydroxide magma have a pleasant taste and would be preferred where oral administration is indicated. They are more expensive than magnesium sulfate but are suitable for use in dogs, cats, foals, calves, and piglets. They exert a reliable cathartic effect but their principal use in medicine is as antacids.

The hydrophilic colloids simply imbibe water and provide an increase in the indigestible mass within the lumen of the intestine. The increased bulk stimulates peristaltic activity by way of mechanoreceptors. The use of this group of drugs is undoubtedly the most physiologic method for treating simple constipation. Regimens employing bran or linseed mashes constitute an excellent method for regularizing intestinal function in equine patients.[19] Psyllium (Metamucil) is tasteless and may be added to the feed for dogs and cats for purposes of increasing the fecal volume.

Drugs employed to lubricate the fecal mass in simple constipation or impactions include liquid petrolatum ("mineral oil"), raw linseed oil, and the surfactants. These substances are pharmacologically inert in usual doses. The surfactants may stimulate motor activity of the intestine when administered in high dosage.[20] They are administered orally or may be incorporated in enemata to soften fecal masses in the colon.

The principal untoward reactions of liquid petrolatum are interference with absorption of essential, fat-soluble vitamins,[21] interference with healing of wounds in the anorectal area, staining of household furnishings, interference with normal defecatory reflexes, and foreign body reactions at the gut wall, liver, and mesenteric lymph nodes following absorption.[22] Some of these effects probably will not be important in veterinary therapeutics because liquid petrolatum is not employed on a chronic basis, as it might be in human beings. Liquid petrolatum and surfactants should not be used simultaneously as emulsification of the oil might facilitate its absorption from the gut.[18,23]

There is usually no rational basis for the use of cathartic drugs.[24] Chronic constipation is best corrected by modifying the diet to increase the amount of indigestible fiber. Enemata or the insertion of glycerine suppositories in the rectum will empty the colon of small animals without effect on other segments of the gastrointestinal tract.

Appropriate uses of cathartics include: (1) cleansing the bowel prior to radiographic examinations, colonoscopy, or elective surgery; (2) as an aid to eliminate parasites following administration of a vermifuge; (3) in poisoning to hasten elimination of unabsorbed toxin; (4) to facilitate reduction of impactions of inspissated feces; and (5) to facilitate defecation in patients with prolapses or hernias where straining would be undesirable (use lubricants or surfactants).

Cathartics must not be given to patients showing signs of abdominal pain.

Opioids

The opioids have been used since antiquity to decrease peristaltic activity. Paregoric (camphorated tincture of opium), morphine, oxymorphone, diphenoxylate, meperidine, methadone, and, to a lesser extent, pentazocine decrease propulsive activity, delay gastric emptying, and increase tone of the intestine and sphincters. The decrease in peristalsis occurs because of the spasmogenic effect of the opioids, which prevents the sequential contraction and relaxation characteristic of peristaltic movements. Tone of the colon is increased to the point of spasm, allowing time for desiccation of the feces. Atropine will partially abolish the effects of opioids on intestinal tone but has little effect on the diminished propulsive activity. The spasmogenic action of opioids may involve the local release of serotonin.[25] The narcotic antagonists, nalorphine and naloxone, will reverse the gastrointestinal effects of the opioids.[26]

The drugs of this group which are most commonly used as antidiarrheals are paregoric and diphenoxylate. Effective suppression of motility of the gut can be attained at doses which exert few systemic effects. Diphenoxylate is generally combined with atropine (in Lomotil).

It is questionable whether opioids should be administered for diarrhea except for short-term usage. The fundamental problem in many cases of diarrhea is hypomotility and excessive secretion of fluids and electrolytes into the lumen of the bowel.[27] Thus, indiscriminate use of opioids may aggravate existing problems of hypomotility.

Few drugs specifically stimulate motility of the stomach or the reticulorumen. The extrinsic innervation is similar to that found elsewhere in the gut. Cholinergic stimuli increase motility of the stomach and relax the pylorus whereas adrenergic stimuli inhibit gastric motility. Spontaneous activity of the rumen and reticulum ceases upon transection of the vagi.[28]

Other Drugs

Several drugs have been advocated for use as rumenatorics. Increases in frequency and amplitude were observed following administration of physostigmine,[29] carbachol,[30] and small doses of arecoline.[31] Marked inhibition of ruminal motility follows administration of epinephrine,[29,30] carbachol,[29] high doses of arecoline,[29] histamine,[29,30] and atropine.[32] The conflicting results seen with carbachol can be explained on the basis that the drug exerts both muscarinic and nicotinic effects. In small doses the principal effect is to stimulate the ruminal musculature, whereas, with higher doses, epinephrine is released from the adrenal medulla and inhibits ruminal motility.[33] Veratrine is an alkaloid derived from *Veratrum album* which stimulates reticuloruminal activity at low doses and vomiting at higher doses. The status of this drug for the treatment of ruminal atony has not been established but subcutaneous doses of 40 mg in cattle and 20 mg in sheep have been suggested.[34]

Frequently ruminal stasis is secondary to other disturbances such as ketosis, acid-base disturbances, or infectious diseases. It is generally more rewarding to correct the underlying disturbance rather than to try to stimulate ruminal motility with drugs.

The motility of the stomach of monogastric animals is stimulated by cholinergic and anticholinesterase drugs and inhibited by adrenergic and anticholinergic drugs. Metoclopramide is a p-amino benzoic acid derivative which increases the rate of gastric emptying (see Table 18–3).[35] Its use for this purpose has not been evaluated in the various species of domesticated animals.

DRUGS AND SECRETION

The glands associated with the gastrointestinal tract are under autonomic control and some are influenced by hormones elaborated by cells within the gut; e.g., gastrin, secretin, enterogastrone, and cholecystokinin. The rates of secretion by salivary, gastric and intestinal glands, the pancreas and the liver may be modified by drugs (Table 18–6).

Salivary Secretion

The salivary glands receive both sympathetic and parasympathetic innervation. They contain cholin-

Table 18–6. Drugs that modify secretion of glands

	Drug	Stimulates (+) or Depresses (−)
Salivary	Atropine	(−)
	Propantheline	(−)
	Scopolamine	(−)
	Methscopolamine	(−)
	Pilocarpine	(+)
	Arecoline	(+)
	Physostigmine	(+)
	Neostigmine	(+)
Gastric	Atropine	Partial depression
	Propantheline	(−)
	Cimetidine	(−)
	Metiamide	(−)
	Histamine	(+)
	Betazole	(+)
	Pentagastrin	(+)
Biliary	Bile salts	(+)
	Dehydrocholic acid	(+)
	Sodium dehydrocholate inj.	(+)
	Tocamphyl	(+)
	Ouabain	(+)
	Ethacrynic acid	(+)
	Theophylline	(+)
	Hydrocortisone	(+)
	Phenobarbital	(+)
	Magnesium sulfate	(+)
Pancreatic exocrine	Atropine	(−)
	Propantheline	(−)
	Glucagon	(−)
	Bethanechol	(+)
Intestinal glands	Bethanechol	(+)
	Pilocarpine	(+)
	Prostaglandins (PGA$_2$, PGE$_1$)	(+)
	Levarterenol	(−)
Colon	Bethanechol	(+)
	Atropine	(−)
	Propantheline	(−)
	Levarterenol	(−)
	Neostigmine	(+)

ergic receptors and adrenergic receptors of the alpha type.[36] Pharmacologic alteration of salivary secretion is fairly straightforward. Cholinergic and anticholinesterase drugs are sialagogues, in that they promote the secretion of copious amounts of saliva which is dilute and nonviscid in consistency. Alpha-adrenergic agonists stimulate the secretion of scanty amounts of viscous saliva with a high content of mucin. Histamine will induce increased secretion of saliva but much of this effect is mediated by way of the nerves.[37] The anticholinergic drugs block cholinergic receptors in the glands and produce xerostomia. This may predispose the equine patient to esophageal obstruction ("choke").

Ruminant animals secrete copious amounts of alkaline saliva. Salivary flow in the cow has been computed to be approximately 100 to 200 liters per day.[38]

Cholinergic drugs increase and anticholinergic drugs decrease salivary secretion in ruminants; however, secretion is not abolished as in other species. It has been observed that section of the nerves to the salivary glands of ruminants decreases salivary flow but does not stop it.[39]

Sialagogues have little significance in therapeutics. Their action should be understood as a side effect of systemic therapy with cholinergic drugs and as a sign of anticholinesterase poisoning. The anticholinergic drugs are commonly employed to decrease salivation associated with the administration of general anesthetics.

Gastric Secretion

Four types of secretory cells are found in the gastric glands. They are the zymogenic cells which secrete pepsinogen, the parietal cells which secrete hydrochloric acid and intrinsic factor, mucous cells which secrete mucus responsible for the protective mucous barrier and the argentaffin cells which are believed to secrete serotonin and gastrin.[40] Control of gastric secretion is mediated by the vagus nerves and hormonal influences. Unlike man, gastric secretion is intermittent in the dog and cat.

Secretion of acid, intrinsic factor and pepsinogen is increased by vagal stimulation, gastrin, histamine, betazole, and insulin-induced hypoglycemia. Gastric secretion is decreased by atropine, norepinephrine, vasopressin, cyclic adenosine monophosphate, prostaglandin E_1, and histamine H2 receptor antagonists. Formation of hydrochloric acid is greatly reduced by high doses of carbonic anhydrase inhibitors such as acetazolamide.

The anticholinergic drugs will block gastric secre-

tion which is stimulated by vagal mechanisms (cephalic and gastric phases). They do not abolish gastrin or histamine-induced secretion. This group of drugs is probably less important in veterinary gastroenterology than in the human because gastric secretion in animals is not continuous as it is in human subjects.

Conditions of excessive production of histamine (such as mastocytoma) or gastrin may produce ulceration secondary to increased gastric secretion. This hypersecretion is not blocked by anticholinergic drugs or conventional antihistaminic drugs. Because of a differential blocking effect, histamine receptors are regarded as being of two types: H1 and H2 receptors.[41] Conventional antihistaminic drugs block H1-receptors. The receptors responsible for histamine or gastrin-induced gastric secretion are of the H2 type. The histamine H2-receptor antagonist drugs (burimamide, metiamide, cimetidine) decrease gastric acid secretion induced by histamine or pentagastrin in dogs[42] and cats.[43] These drugs are new additions to our armamentarium and their clinical usage remains to be established in veterinary medical practice. Their structures are illustrated in Figure 18–1. Tentative dosages for the dog and cat are: metiamide (1.5 mg/kg, I.V., used only for investigational purposes because it may cause blood dyscrasia) and cimetidine (0.5 mg/kg, I.V. and 2.0 mg/kg, P.O., q6h).

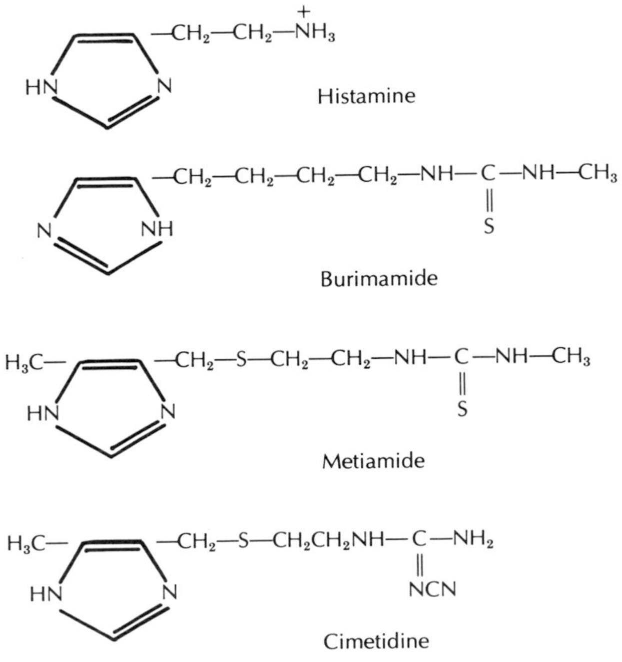

Figure 18–1. Structures of histamine H2-receptor antagonists.

The secretion of mucus by the neck cells of the gastric glands is stimulated by hydrochloric acid, vagal stimulation, serotonin, insulin, and cholinergic drugs. Mucus secretion is decreased by adrenocortical hormones and adrenocorticotrophin. Aspirin, phenylbutazone, and indomethacin reduce the rate of mucus secretion and reduce the concentration of protein-bound carbohydrates. This mucus is more readily digested by pepsin and trypsin.[44] This situation may play a role in the production of acute gastric ulcers which are associated with these anti-inflammatory drugs.[45]

Pancreatic Secretion

Exocrine secretion by the pancreas is regulated by hormonal and nervous stimuli. Secretin released from the duodenal mucosa by HCl stimulates the ducts to secrete water and bicarbonate.[46] Another enzyme, cholecystokinin-pancreozymin (CCK-PZ) released from the duodenum by the presence of peptones, soaps, and certain amino acids stimulates the secretion of enzymes by the pancreatic acini.[47] Vagal stimulation increases secretion of both water and enzymes.[48] Although participation of the sympathetic nerves increases the responsiveness of the pancreas to secretin,[49] it is the cholinergic mechanisms that are most subject to pharmacologic manipulation.

Anticholinergic drugs, such as atropine and propantheline, block vagally induced secretion of the pancreas as well as blocking the release of CCK-PZ from the duodenum.[50] The anticholinergic drugs only partially decrease secretin-induced secretion. Intravenous infusion of glucagon (10 μg/kg/hr) decreases flow and enzyme secretion by the stimulated gland.[51] Bethanechol increases secretion of enzymes by the acini.

Biliary Secretion

The subject of hepatic bile formation has been reviewed.[52] Fundamentally, water flow into biliary canaliculi occurs in response to osmotic gradients.[53] Bile secretion is under the influence of neural, humoral, and vascular factors. Secretion of bile following feeding is increased by vagal stimulation, influences of secretin and pancreozymin, and increased perfusion of the liver with oxygen-rich blood. Bile flow can be regarded as occurring by two processes: bile-acid-dependent and bile-acid-independent flows. Bile-acid-dependent flow is produced by the active secretion of bile acids into the canaliculi where they exert an osmotic effect which increases movement of water.[54] Bile flow in dogs is linearly related to bile acid output.[55] Thus,

the administration of bile salts, dehydrocholic acid, or sodium dehydrocholate injection causes a marked choleresis.

Ox bile extract may be administered to dogs, as tablets, at a dosage of 100 to 300 mg following eating. Sodium dehydrocholate (Decholin) is a partially synthetic compound which can be given intravenously (100 mg/kg in dogs and 3 g in cattle). Tocamphyl (Syncuma) is a non-steroidal choleretic drug which is given orally. Side effects of bile salts include diarrhea and pruritus. Sodium dehydrocholate may produce hypotension, bradycardia, and hyperactivity of skeletal muscle. Chenodeoxycholic acid has been effectively used for dissolving gallstones in human patients.[56]

Bile-acid-independent bile flow is thought to be generated by a sodium pump[52] which is coupled with organic anion transport.[57] This flow is regarded as a hydrocholeresis. It is increased by ouabain[58] and ethacrynic acid.[58,59] Other drugs that increase bile-acid-independent flow are theophylline,[60] hydrocortisone,[61] phenobarbital,[62] etazolate hydrochloride,[60] and glucagon.[60] Other drugs that produce choleresis include aspirin, pilocarpine, choline, acetylcholine, insulin, and histamine.[63]

The gallbladder helps regulate pressure in the biliary system and collects, concentrates, and stores bile until it is released into the duodenum. Emptying of bile into the duodenum is caused by contraction of the gallbladder and relaxation of the sphincter of Oddi at the choledochoduodenal junction. The gallbladder is stimulated to contract by CCK-PZ and by cholinergic drugs. The sphincter of Oddi contains α- and β-adrenergic and cholinergic receptors.[64] It is contracted by acetylcholine and relaxed by epinephrine.[65] Atropine and propantheline relax the sphincter and gallbladder as do nitrates and nitrites. Histamine, morphine, meperidine, and codeine cause spasm of the sphincter and a considerable rise in pressure within the common duct. The spasmogenic effect of the opiates is antagonized by amyl nitrite, theophylline, or nalorphine.[66] Magnesium sulfate in the duodenum causes contraction of the gallbladder and relaxation of the sphincter.

Intestinal Secretion

Glands in the mucosa of the small intestine produce the succus entericus, which is a dilute fluid containing water, electrolytes, mucus, and cellular debris. Their function is under control of neural and humoral influences. Secretin, gastrin, and CCK-PZ stimulate secretion of Brunner's glands in the duodenum.[67] Sympathetic stimulation inhibits secretion and vagal stimulation and cholinergic drugs enhance secretion of intestinal glands. Secretion in the dog and cat is increased by pilocarpine, physostigmine, and bethanechol and decreased by atropine.[68] Cholera toxin causes profuse secretion of water and electrolytes by the intestinal epithelium. The toxin stimulates adenylate cyclase in the cellular membrane which in turn increases the concentration of cyclic-adenosine monophosphate (cAMP). The increased cAMP causes active secretion of chloride and bicarbonate ions into the intestinal lumen accompanied by large volumes of water.[69] Prostaglandins A_2 and E_1 increase bicarbonate, water, and mucus secretion into the intestinal lumen.[70]

Colonic Secretion

The colon serves both absorptive and secretory roles. Water, bicarbonate, potassium, and mucus are secreted by epithelial cells. Secretion is increased by parasympathetic nerves and inhibited by sympathetics. Topically applied irritants (enemata or suppositories) and psychic anxiety increase mucus secretion by colonic mucous cells. Water is absorbed isosmotically from the colon and is dependent on the active absorption of sodium. Aldosterone and adrenocorticosteroids having mineralocorticoid activity enhance the absorption of sodium from the colon. Antidiuretic hormone enhances water absorption from the colon of animals.[71]

MISCELLANEOUS DRUGS FOR GASTROINTESTINAL THERAPY

Drugs and Appetite

Appetite is regulated by glucose concentrations within cells of the median nuclei of the hypothalamus,[72] amino acid concentration in blood, the act of swallowing,[73] gastric distention,[74] and intestinal distention.[75] Disorders of appetite are commonly encountered in veterinary medical practice. Anorexia accompanies many systemic diseases and psychologic disturbances. Overeating with associated obesity is a common problem in companion animals and may be a cause of the fatty liver syndrome in cattle. There are drugs available which modify appetite in animals but disorders are best managed by correcting underlying disease processes, regulating the diet, and educating the owner.

Drugs which have been advocated to enhance appetite include: B vitamins, adrenocorticosteroids, anabolic steroids, and bitters such as nux vomica, quassia, ginseng, and absinthe. The bitters (stomachics) have not been shown to be effective for stimulation of appetite.[76] Vitamin B complex may have some merit in improving appetite and feed consumption in horses[77,78] and may be beneficial in other species with chronic diseases. The steroids may improve appetite secondary to their euphoric effects.

Cyproheptadine (Periactin) is a unique substance which blocks histamine H1 receptors and antagonizes 5-hydroxytryptamine centrally and peripherally. It enhances weight gain, growth, and appetite in human subjects.[79] Side effects include drowsiness, nausea, ataxia, and xerostomia. It has not been subjected to critical evaluation in animal patients with anorexia.

The fundamental problem in the development of obesity is the ingestion of food in excess of the caloric requirement of the animal. Anorectic drugs will appease appetite temporarily as tolerance develops rapidly. Drugs employed for appetite suppression are all sympathomimetic amines such as dextroamphetamine and methamphetamine, which are subject to abuse by human drug users. Newer drugs produce fewer side effects and include fenfluramine (Pondimin), chlorphentermine (Pre-Sate), phenmetrazine (Preludin), and diethylpropion (Tenuate). These agents are no more effective as anorectics than dextroamphetamine,[80] but produce less cardiovascular effects and central nervous excitement and are subject to less abuse by drug users.

Antacids

This group of drugs is employed to neutralize acid in the gastrointestinal tract and to correct metabolic acidosis. Peptic ulcers are reported only occasionally in monogastric animals;[81] antacids may be useful as adjunctive therapy.

Antacids may be systemic or buffered in their actions. Systemic antacids, such as sodium bicarbonate, are absorbed and produce a metabolic alkalosis. They are more useful for correcting metabolic acidosis or for alkalizing the urine than for neutralizing gastric acidity. The buffered antacids such as aluminum hydroxide, magnesium hydroxide, magnesium trisilicate, or calcium carbonate neutralize gastric HCl without modification of the systemic acid-base balance. Calcium carbonate reacts with gastric hydrochloric acid as follows:

$$CaCO_3 + 2HCl \rightleftharpoons CaCl_2 + H_2CO_3 \text{ in stomach}$$
$$CaCl_2 + Na_2CO_3 \rightleftharpoons CaCO_3 + 2 NaCl \text{ in duodenum}$$

Thus, the HCl is neutralized in the stomach and calcium carbonate is regenerated in the duodenum with the hydrogen ion being incorporated into water as CO_2 is lost from H_2CO_3. At the pH of the small intestine there is more than enough carbonate ion in pancreatic secretions to precipitate the calcium and prevent its absorption.

Calcium carbonate and aluminum hydroxide are constipating and are frequently combined with magnesium hydroxide to correct this effect. Untoward side effects are seldom observed with occasional antacid therapy. Intensive therapy over a period of time may result in hypercalcinosis with nephrolithiasis,[82] renal damage from silica deposits,[83] and interaction with other orally administered drugs with resultant interference with their absorption (e.g., tetracyclines).

In simple stomached animals, doses of 0.5 to 1.0 ml/kg of antacid suspension are required every 2 to 4 hours to effectively neutralize gastric acidity.[84] Antacids have been employed in the treatment of ruminal acidosis following excessive consumption of carbohydrates. This practice may cause complications however, because alkalization will increase the absorption of histamine and other basic substances from the gastrointestinal tract.[85]

Carbenoxolone and deglycyrrhizinized licorice increase the rate of healing of gastric and duodenal ulcers in double blind studies of human patients.[86,87] These drugs apparently increase the secretion of gastric mucus and prolong the life span of mucosal cells. They have not been evaluated in animal patients.

DRUGS FOR DIAGNOSIS

Several drugs are employed for diagnosis of abnormalities associated with the gastrointestinal tract. Only their actions on the patient will be discussed; the diagnostic procedures are discussed under appropriate headings elsewhere in the text.

Sulfobromophthalein (Bromsulphalein) is available as a 5% aqueous solution for intravenous administration. This substance is conjugated with glutathione in the liver and the conjugate is excreted in the bile.[88]

The principal side effects associated with the BSP test are rare anaphylactoid reactions and cellular necrosis following extravasation of the drug. Drugs which interfere with the test include: anabolic steroids, morphine, meperidine, radiopaque substances, B vitamins, and amine oxidase inhibitors.

Azuresin (Diagnex Blue) consists of a cation exchange resin to which is adsorbed a blue dye. The use of the resin is described in Chapter 16. Unto-

ward reactions are rare and consist of allergic responses.

Barium sulfate is routinely used as a radiopaque contrast medium for visualizing the esophagus, stomach, intestine, and colon. It is nontoxic, stable, inexpensive, and insoluble in water. Barium sulfate tends to be constipating owing to its adsorbent properties. Administration of a mild cathartic may be advisable following the examination.

A number of organic iodide compounds is available for the roentgenographic visualization of the bile ducts and gallbladder. The insoluble compounds are administered orally, are well absorbed and rapidly excreted in the bile. Water soluble compounds may be given intravenously. Oral compounds for cholecystography include: ipodate calcium (Oragrafin), sodium tyropanate (Bilopaque Sodium), iopanoic acid (Telepaque) and iodoalphionic acid (Priodax). Soluble compounds for intravenous use are ioglycamic acid (Biligram), iodophthalein sodium (Iodeikon), and meglumine iodipamide (Cholografin). The principal adverse reactions observed with the organic iodides include vomiting, urticarial and anaphylactoid reactions, and renal damage. They will interfere with the results of clinical laboratory determinations of protein-bound iodine, albumin, amylase, bilirubin, BUN, cholesterol, and clotting time.[89]

MANAGEMENT OF SEVERE VISCERAL PAIN

Pain is frequently associated with disturbances of the digestive system. Stimuli produced by distention or inflammation of the abdominal organs are conveyed by visceral afferent fibers in sympathetic nerves. Mechanical or chemical irritation of parietal peritoneum initiates impulses which are conveyed by segmental somatic nerves. Pain arising from ischemia, distention, or chemical irritants may be diffuse, agonizing, and of high intensity. Frequently the abrupt onset of pain is the first sign that an animal has a disturbance of the digestive system.

Drugs employed to ease pain are classified into two groups: central-acting and peripheral-acting analgesics. This classification is based on whether the drug modifies the reception and interpretation of pain in the brain or whether it blocks the action of various mediators on pain endings.[90] Peripheral-acting analgesics that are useful in veterinary medicine include the salicylates (aspirin, thiosalicylate) and pyrazole derivatives (phenylbutazone and methampyrone), fenamic acid derivatives (meclofenamic acid, flufenamic acid) and indomethacin.[91] Indomethacin is *absolutely contraindicated* for use in dogs because it is associated with gastrointestinal hemorrhages.[45] These drugs exert anti-inflammatory, antipyretic, and analgesic effects in low-intensity somatic pain. They are ineffective in relieving visceral pain.[92] However, they may be effective in relieving intestinal spasm caused by certain inflammatory mediators;[93] e.g., salicylates suppress prostaglandin activity.

The opioids provide the most effective means of alleviating visceral pain. Morphine is the classic representative of the group and is the most versatile and inexpensive narcotic analgesic. It acts on the central nervous system to raise the pain threshold, decrease the reaction to pain, and promote drowsiness. This relief of pain is selective in that consciousness and other sensory modalities (vision, hearing, touch) are not obtunded. The principal adverse effects are excitement, respiratory depression, bronchiolar constriction, and release of histamine. The effects on the gastrointestinal tract were discussed previously. Species differences in central nervous system response to morphine are noted. Increasing doses produce progressive depression in dogs and rabbits and excitement in cats, horses, and swine. Morphine produces no behavioral effects in ruminant animals, even at rather high dosages, owing to rapid diffusion and sequestration in the rumen.[94] To avoid excitement the dose of morphine should not exceed 0.1 mg/kg in cats[95] or 60 mg (total dose) in the horse.[96] The usual canine dose (1 mg/kg) is probably higher than necessary in most cases. Relief is provided for visceral pain associated with many diseases of dogs at doses of from 0.25 to 0.5 mg/kg. The duration of action is about 6 hours in dogs and cats.[97]

Methadone is a synthetic narcotic which has potency equal to or slightly greater than that of morphine. It produces excellent analgesia without excitement in horses. It is widely used in Europe for the treatment of equine colics and it is now also available to practitioners in the United States. The FDA had restricted its distribution and use to methadone maintenance programs for the treatment of heroin addicts.[98]

Meperidine is a synthetic, narcotic analgesic which is similar to morphine. It is about one tenth as potent as morphine and has too short a duration of action to be of value in the management of visceral pain in horses, dogs, and cats. The duration of action is about 20 minutes in the horse,[99] 2 hours in cats,[95] and about 45 minutes in dogs.[100] Overdoses may produce convulsions so the drug should be administered intramuscularly rather than intravenously.

Oxymorphone is a morphine analog which is about 10 times as potent as morphine. It is less prone to produce excitement in horses and has been used routinely in the management of equine colic. It produces respiratory depression similar to that observed with morphine.

Pentazocine is a narcotic antagonist with agonist activity and a potency about one fourth that of morphine. The main advantage of this compound to the practitioner is that it has a low addiction liability in human beings and hence is not subject to the rigid controls governing the use of the opioids. Pentazocine should be given intramuscularly to decrease the incidence of side effects (hypotension) and because the duration of action is longer than when given intravenously. At a dosage of 3 mg/kg, the duraction of action in ponies was 160 minutes,[99] and the half-lives in the plasma were 97, 22, 84, and 49 minutes in ponies, dogs, cats, and swine, respectively.[101] Pentazocine will antagonize the effects of opioids if given concurrently.

The drug of choice with which to antagonize the effects of the central-acting analgesics is naloxone. This compound occupies opioid receptor sites without initiating any response and will reverse completely the effects of the analgesics within minutes of intravenous administration. The dose recommended is 0.04 mg/kg,[102] which can be repeated at 2- or 3-minute intervals to achieve the desired effect. Naloxone should be kept available by every veterinarian who employs narcotic drugs.

Xylazine is a sedative-analgesic drug which is unique in its actions in that it does not produce excitement in horses and cats. Its analgesic effects have been evaluated in the cecal-distention model for equine colic,[103] in which it was shown to obtund visceral pain. The drug is approved in the United States for use in the horse, dog, and cat.

Xylazine provokes vomiting in dogs and cats,[104] and cardiovascular effects in horses. The cardiovascular disturbances consisted of atrioventricular and sinoatrial block, bradycardia, hypertension followed by prolonged hypotension, and decreased cardiac output.[105] The occurrence of heart block is prevented by atropinization. Rather widespread differences occur among the domesticated species in the susceptibility to the effects of xylazine. Cattle are 10 times as sensitive to a given dose of xylazine as horses, dogs, and cats.[106] Swine are the least sensitive of the common domesticated animals. The dose required to produce effects in swine comparable to those in the horse, dog, and cat is two to three times as great.

Xylazine is limited in value for the management of peristent visceral pain in horses, dogs, and cats

Table 18–7. Drugs employed in the management of severe visceral pain

Generic Name	Proprietary Name	Usual Dose (mg/kg)					Comments
		Horse	Cow	Pig	Dog	Cat	
Morphine	—	0.1	Ineffective	15–120 mg (total)	0.5–1	0.1	Drug of choice for dogs and cats; overdose excites horses and cats
Methadone	Dolophine	0.22	—	—	1.0	—	Useful in horses
Oxymorphone	Numorphan	.02–.03	—	—	0.1–0.2	0.075	
Meperidine	Demerol	1–6.5	Ineffective	1–2	4.4–11	4.4–11	Administer IM, short half-life
Pentazocine	Talwin	1–2	Ineffective	—	1–2.2	—	Administer IM, excitement in cats and swine
Xylazine	Rompun	2–3	0.1–0.2	—	1.0	1.0	Produces cardiac arrhythmias

because of its brief duration of action as compared to the opioids. The duration of effect, following intravenous injection of 1.1 mg/kg in the horse, was 30 to 40 minutes.[107] Analgesia lasts for 15 to 30 minutes in the dog and cat.[108] Intravenously, a dose of 0.1 mg/kg of xylazine produced narcosis in cattle for a period of 1 to 2 hours.[109] Xylazine is not approved by the FDA for use in cattle. It is to be hoped that such approval will be forthcoming as it is the only effective drug available for obtunding severe pain in this species.

It would seem, based on the previous discussion, that morphine would be the most appropriate choice of drug for relieving severe visceral pain in dogs and cats, methadone or oxymorphone in horses, and xylazine in cattle. One must temper this decision regarding use of these drugs by considering the actions of the drug on the gastrointestinal tract together with the pathophysiology of the condition being treated. Suggested dosages of these drugs are listed in Table 18–7.

Part II. Gastrointestinal Absorption and Bioavailability of Drugs

J. DESMOND BAGGOT

Absorption from the gastrointestinal tract is one of the factors which influence activity of a drug following administration by the oral route. Other factors which govern onset, intensity, and duration of pharmacologic response, which are manifestations of drug concentration(s) in the immediate vicinity of the receptor site (biophase), include distribution, biotransformation (or metabolism), and excretion. The dosage form influences mainly the rate and extent of drug absorption.

Pharmacokinetics describes the kinetics of absorption, distribution, and elimination (biotransformation and/or excretion) of a drug and its metabolites in biologic fluids. Appropriate mathe-

matical equations are established to fit the observed data. The derived kinetic constants and quantifiable concepts, such as apparent volume of distribution, are combined in equations which predict dosage regimens. The influence of disease states (uremia, fever, hypoproteinemia) and drug interactions on pharmacologic response can be interpreted in terms of alterations in pharmacokinetic and plasma protein binding parameters. In this way the dosage regimen can be adjusted to obtain the desired pharmacologic (therapeutic) response. Drugs do not create physiologic or biochemical functions; their actions modify ongoing processes. Since pharmacokinetic studies involve measurement of drug concentrations in plasma (or serum), it is essential that some quantitative relationship exists between drug in this fluid and that surrounding the receptor site. Despite the assumptions associated with a compartmental analysis of data, which is the usual technique employed in pharmacokinetics, *in vivo* disposition studies constitute the most efficient means of predicting potential value of a drug product and its dosage regimen. Quantitative measurement of pharmacologic response should be sought whenever possible and related to the drug level-time profile.

Gastrointestinal absorption of a drug involves its passage from the lumen of the alimentary tract across the gastrointestinal mucosa and into the hepatic portal venous blood. Following absorption the drug molecules are conveyed to the liver, an organ highly endowed with drug-metabolizing enzymes, before gaining access to the systemic (or general) circulation. Most drugs are administered as drug products, not drug entities. Drug product means a finished dosage form (e.g., tablet, capsule, solution) that contains the active drug ingredient generally but not necessarily in association with inactive ingredients.[110] The evaluation of a drug product intended for oral administration involves determining its bioavailability, which is defined as the rate and extent to which a drug administered as the particular dosage form (drug product) enters the systemic circulation in an unchanged form.

Two cellular boundaries separate the lumen of the gastrointestinal tract from the blood stream: the epithelial lining of the tract and the capillary endothelium. Since the capillary endothelium at this location is highly porous, the gastrointestinal epithelium must constitute the main barrier to absorption. Animal-cell membranes are composed of phospholipids and protein, but the way in which these molecules are complexed together is really not known.[111] There is now substantial evidence that the major portion of the phospholipids is in bilayer form. According to the fluid mosaic model,[112] the proteins that are integral to the membrane are a heterogeneous set of globular molecules, each arranged in an amphipathic structure.

PASSAGE OF DRUGS ACROSS MUCOSAL MEMBRANES

Since most drugs are organic acids or bases, they exist as both the nonionized and ionized forms in solution. A high degree of lipid solubility is the property of nonionized drug molecules which enables them to traverse mucosal membranes readily.[113] The passive diffusion process is characterized by movement of nonionized drug molecules down a concentration gradient without cellular expenditure of energy. Drug molecules in the ionized form have a low degree of lipid solubility, so that their diffusion across biologic membranes is restricted. Evidence that the gastric epithelium is more permeable to the nonionized form of a drug than to the ionized form was first provided by a study of gastric absorption of some alkaloids (weak organic bases) in the cat.[114] A change in extent of absorption of a weak organic electrolyte following alteration of the pH reaction of stomach contents is evidence that absorption takes place by nonionic diffusion.

The rate and direction of transmembrane movement of a drug are determined by the degree of lipid solubility of the nonionized (diffusible) form of the drug and its concentration on either side of the membrane. Assuming that the gastric mucosal membrane behaves as a simple lipoid barrier which is permeable only to the nonionized lipid-soluble form of a drug, an equilibrium state with equal concentrations of nonionized molecules on both sides of the barrier would eventually be established. The dissociation constant (expressed as pK_a) of a drug and the pH of the environment (solution in which the drug is dissolved) determine its degree of ionization, since according to the Henderson-Hasselbalch equation:

for an acid,

$$pH - pK_a = \log \frac{\text{(conc. of ionized acid)}}{\text{(conc. of nonionized acid)}}$$
Eq. 1

and for a base,

$$pH - pK_a = \log \frac{\text{(conc. of nonionized base)}}{\text{(conc. of ionized base)}}$$
Eq. 2

where pK_a is the negative logarithm of the acidic dissociation constant of the weak acid or base. Since a pH differential exists across the gastric mucosal membrane, unequal concentrations (nonionized plus ionized) of drug will be attained on either side; at equilibrium, there will be a higher total drug concentration on the side of the membrane where the greater degree of ionization takes place. This mechanism is known as ion trapping (Fig. 18–2). The pH gradient across the gastric mucosal barrier is maintained by active (energy-

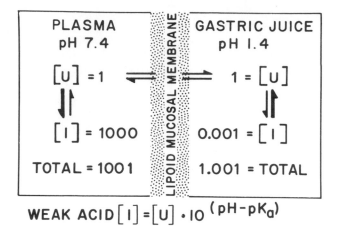

$$\mathrm{WEAK\ ACID}\ [\mathrm{I}] = [\mathrm{U}] \cdot 10^{\,(\mathrm{pH-pK_a})}$$

Figure 18–2. Influence of pH on the distribution of a weak acid between plasma and gastric juice, which are separated by a lipoid barrier. In this figure, [I] and [U] represent the concentrations of the ionized and nonionized forms of the drugs, respectively. It is assumed that the gastric mucosal membrane (barrier) is permeable only to the nonionized form of the compound. (From Baggot: *Principles of Drug Disposition in Domestic Animals*. Philadelphia, W. B. Saunders Co., 1977.)

dependent) secretion of hydrogen ions by the parietal (oxyntic) cells of the mucosa. The primary stimulus for gastric acid secretion is the gastrointestinal hormone gastrin.[115,116]

The equilibrium (theoretical) concentration ratio ($R_{GJ/P}$) of a weak organic electrolyte across the gastric mucosal barrier may be calculated according to the following equation:[117]

for an acid,

$$R_{GJP} = \frac{1 + 10^{(pH_{GJ} - pK_a)}}{1 + 10^{(pH_p - pK_a)}} \qquad \text{Eq. 3}$$

and for a base,

$$R_{GJP} = \frac{1 + 10\,(pK_a - pH_{GJ})}{1 + 10\,(pK_a - pH_p)} \qquad \text{Eq. 4}$$

The term $R_{GJ/P}$ is the ratio of drug concentration in gastric juice to that in plasma water at steady state. It must be realized that while the principles outlined are correct, the system is dynamic; simple reversible equilibrium across the mucosal membrane does not occur until the drug is distributed throughout the body. The preceding equations predict that weak organic acids would be well absorbed from the acidic gastric contents (pH 1 to 2) of dogs and cats, and organic bases would be concentrated in gastric juice. Assuming the pH of gastric juice to be 1.4 and that of plasma 7.4, values of $R_{GJ/P}$ for an acid and a base of pK_a 4.4 are 0.001 and 1000, respectively.

Even though the ruminal mucosa has absorptive capacity,[118,119] any drug administered orally to cattle or sheep would achieve a low concentration in ruminal fluid. The approximate capacities of the adult reticulorumen are 100 to 225 liters in cattle and 6 to 20 liters in sheep and goats. Moreover, a considerably lower pH differential exists across the ruminal mucosa (1 to 2 units) than across the abomasal mucosa (4 to 5 units). Based on these considerations, one would expect less rapid absorption of orally administered organic acids (e.g., salicylates, sulfonamides) in ruminant animals. Repeated oral administration of aspirin to cows (100 mg/kg every 12 hours) maintained serum salicylate levels of 40 to 60 µg/ml after the third dose (Fig. 18–3). This dosage regimen was considered (clinical observation) to provide adequate analgesia for relief of mild arthritic conditions in the cows.[120] The dosage interval for aspirin in cows is based on the rate of absorption (half-time is 2.91 hours) rather than on the half-life (0.54 hour) of salicylate in blood plasma.

The principles that govern passage of weak acids and bases across the gastric mucosa can be applied to absorption of drugs from the small intestine. A low degree of ionization and high lipid solubility of the nonionized form are properties which favor absorption of organic electrolytes.[121]

An effective pH of 5.3 in the microenvironment of the absorbing surface of the intestinal epithelial barrier, rather than the reaction of intestinal contents (pH 6.6), is consistent with observations on

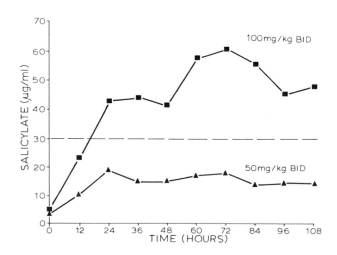

Figure 18–3. Salicylate concentrations in serum of cows after oral administration of aspirin at dosage levels of 50 mg/kg every 12 hours (▲) and 100 mg/kg every 12 hours (■). Each point is the mean serum salicylate level in three animals. Broken line indicates estimated minimum effective serum salicylate concentration (30 µg/ml). (From Gingerich, Baggot, and Yeary.[120])

absorption of organic acids and bases. Detailed studies with a large number of drugs in unbuffered solutions revealed that in the normal intestine, weak acids with pK_a values above 3 and bases with pK_a less than 7.8 were very well absorbed.[122] Moderately strong bases (e.g., ephedrine, pK_a 9.3; amphetamine, pK_a 9.9) are negligibly absorbed from acidic gastric contents, but rapidly from intestinal fluids. Aminoglycoside antibiotics (e.g., streptomycin, kanamycin), highly polar organic bases, are poorly absorbed from the gastrointestinal tract. Absorption of quaternary ammonium compounds, which are always ionized (organic cations), is slow and incomplete, but partial absorption does take place and must be attributed to a mechanism other than nonionic diffusion.

Specialized transport processes are generally thought to be mediated by carriers; that is, membrane components that form a reversible complex with the substance to be transported. Two types of carrier-mediated transport can be distinguished, namely, facilitated diffusion and active transport.[123,124] Features that distinguish specialized transport from passive transfer include saturability and relative selectivity. Two or more substances may compete for combination with the carrier, so that competitive inhibition is characteristic of carrier-mediated transport. Facilitated diffusion requires no cellular energy and transport occurs down a concentration gradient. Translocation of a drug across the membrane takes place at a much faster rate than that associated with passive diffusion. Glucose, for example, is transported into most cells by this process. Facilitated diffusion may be the mechanism of absorption of quaternary ammonium compounds from the gastrointestinal tract.

Active transport, unlike diffusion processes, requires the direct expenditure of energy and the transported substance is transferred against a concentration or electrochemical gradient. Transcellular fluids are formed by the active transport of Na^+ across epithelial cells. Active transport is responsible for the rapid excretion in urine and/or bile of unchanged molecules of certain organic electrolytes as well as polar metabolites of the majority of drugs. Active transport is involved in the intestinal absorption of compounds structurally related to some dietary constituents. The transport of glucose across the gastrointestinal mucosa and renal tubular epithelium is active and can proceed against a concentration gradient.

Pinocytosis is a transport mechanism which, like active transport, requires the expenditure of cellular energy. It differs from active transport in that transfer of the solute is not mediated by combination with a carrier, but by local invagination of the cell membrane and subsequent budding off within the cell interior of a vesicle which contains the solute.[125,126] The capacity of the newborn calf to absorb soluble protein molecules may be attributed to this mechanism. The allergic response to ingested proteins of food and the toxicity of bacterial exotoxins provide evidence that macromolecules are absorbed from the gastrointestinal tract of the human being.

Absorption Parameters

Since passive diffusion is the mechanism of absorption of weak organic electrolytes, certain physicochemical properties (i.e., pK_a, lipid solubility) of a drug, the ambient pH, and concentration of the drug will determine its rate and extent of absorption. A drug will be more rapidly absorbed when given in aqueous solution than in solid dosage form. Absorption from a suspension will usually be more rapid than from a tablet. Either slow or incomplete absorption can make systemic therapy ineffective. Release of drug from a tablet involves disintegration of the dosage form into small particles, deaggregation of the particles, and finally dissolution of the drug in gastrointestinal fluids. The rate of dissolution will be affected by certain characteristics of the drug formulation (i.e., composition of the dosage form). Physiologic variables that greatly influence dissolution include gastric emptying and intestinal transit rate. Dissolution is frequently the rate-limiting factor, in that it is the slowest stage in the overall absorption process.[127] The slower rate of absorption of ampicillin trihydrate in Beagle dogs as compared with the sodium and potassium salts can be attributed to a slower dissolution rate of the hydrated form of the antibiotic.[128] There was no significant difference between the two dosage forms in systemic availability of ampicillin. The gastrointestinal absorption rate of chloramphenicol differs with the crystalline form of the drug. Slow dissolution of sparingly soluble drugs may control not only their rate of absorption but also the duration of pharmacologic response.

Dissolution can be enhanced by using the salt form of a drug (e.g., potassium phenoxymethyl penicillin, phenytoin sodium, propranolol hydrochloride), or by decreasing the particle size—micronization (e.g., spironolactone, griseofulvin), thereby increasing bioavailability of the therapeutic agent. An incompletely absorbed drug, such as griseofulvin,[129] is usually variably absorbed because changes in physiologic factors (gastrointestinal motility and transit rates) can cause pronounced differences in extent of absorption.

One can expect a drug in solution to be well absorbed if it is lipid-soluble, not completely ionized, and is stable (i.e., neither chemically nor enzymatically inactivated) in the gastrointestinal fluids. Penicillin G and erythromycin, for example, are unstable in acidic gastric contents; chloramphenicol is inactivated by rumen microflora. The extent of degradation of orally administered erythromycin will depend on the pH of the gastric fluids, the gastric emptying rate, and the rate of dissolution of the dosage form in the stomach. The dissolution rate may be varied by using different esters of erythromycin, and the bioavailability of the drug will be affected accordingly. The gastrointestinal fluids, including bile, can interact with drug molecules, in some cases solubilizing the drug and in others causing precipitation on the surface of a slowly dissolving complex.[130]

The rate of absorption of a drug is usually reduced and extent of absorption variably affected when the dose is ingested simultaneously with or following a meal. This effect may be attributed to the delaying effect of food on gastric emptying and the diminished accessibility of drug molecules to sites of absorption (mucosal surface). The influence of food intake on the oral absorption of sodium ampicillin (in solution) was evaluated by comparing the concentrations of ampicillin in the serum of the same Beagle dogs when fasted or allowed food ad libitum overnight.[128] The intake of food resulted in a significant reduction in ampicillin concentrations in serum (Fig. 18–4). After food intake, the rate and extent of oral absorption of sodium ampicillin were reduced approximately 40 and 66%, respectively. The rate of absorption of microcrystalline and macrocrystalline nitrofurantoin has been shown to be reduced in the presence of food.[131] However, the overall absorption efficiency of both forms of the drug was markedly increased. Similar situations have been reported for griseofulvin[132] and propoxyphene.[133]

An explanation of the phenomenon is that the increase in drug retention time in the stomach, due to delaying effect of food on gastric emptying, may permit a greater proportion of drug to dissolve in gastric fluids before passing into the small intestine where most absorption occurs.

Tetracycline hydrochloride dissolves rapidly in the acidic gastric environment but the high degree of ionization and poor lipid solubility of the drug make its absorption (by passive diffusion) slow and incomplete. Absorption of the antibiotic is further

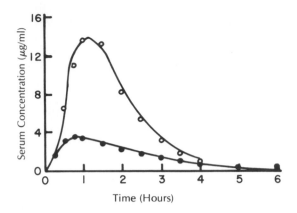

Figure 18–4. Effect of food intake on the oral absorption of sodium ampicillin in beagle dogs. Symbols: ○, sodium ampicillin concentrations in the absence of food; ●, sodium ampicillin concentrations after food intake. (From Cabana, Willhite, and Bierwagen.[128])

reduced if the drug is taken with milk or other source of calcium ions, and by the concomitant administration of aluminum hydroxide gel or sodium bicarbonate. The mechanisms responsible for the decreased absorption appear to be chelation with bivalent cations and an increase in gastric pH.[134,135]

Administration of chlordiazepoxide hydrochloride with a mixture of magnesium and aluminum hydroxides (antacid) reduces the rate of absorption of chlordiazepoxide but does not alter the completeness of absorption or the apparent rate of elimination.[136] Aluminum-containing antacids (e.g., aluminum hydroxide gel) reduce the gastrointestinal drug absorption rate in animals by retarding gastric emptying.[137,138] The trivalent aluminum cation, made soluble when aluminum hydroxide reacts with the hydrochloric acid in gastric contents, apparently interferes with calcium fluxes which occur during excitation-contraction coupling of gastric smooth muscle.[139]

Kaolin, a hydrated aluminum silicate, is an adsorbent used for treatment of diarrhea; it adsorbs drugs and limits gastrointestinal absorption of lincomycin.[140]

Two major factors affecting absorption of a drug are the circulation to the site of absorption and the area of the absorbing surface to which the drug is exposed, in this case the gastrointestinal mucosa. The combination of these histologic factors makes the small intestine the principal site of absorption of all drugs, even weak acids. The rate of gastric emptying is therefore an important determinant of the drug absorption rate. Gastric emptying depends on various physiologic factors, such as autonomic and hormonal activity, and on the volume and composition of the gastric contents. It is also influenced by anticholinergic drugs and morphine,[141] which slow gastric emptying time. In the gastrointestinal tract, drugs modify mainly the various mechanisms that control secretion and motility.[142] Since peristalsis provides close contact between the absorbing surface and the luminal contents, one would expect substances that depress intestinal motility to decrease absorption. This may explain the effect of desipramine on decreasing the absorption of drugs.[143] Following passage across the gastrointestinal mucosal barrier, drug molecules penetrate the capillary endothelium and enter the blood stream (hepatic portal system). There is little uptake of drug molecules by lymphatics, owing to the relatively slow rate of lymph flow.[144] Changes in the intestinal blood flow will alter the rate of absorption of lipid-soluble drugs.[145,146] Ischemia impairs the transport (active) of amino acids across the mucosal epithelium.[147]

Comparative Aspects of Drug Absorption

The domestic animals may be divided, on the basis of dietary habits, into herbivorous (horse, cow, sheep, and goat), omnivorous (pig and primates) and carnivorous (dog and cat) species. The pH gradients between plasma and the gastrointestinal fluids of the various species play an important role in determining the extent of absorption of orally given drug products, and the degree of distribution or excretion into the gastrointestinal tract of parenterally administered weak organic electrolytes.

The physiology of digestion and drug absorption processes are, in general, similar in the dog, cat, and pig, and are not unlike those in the human. The rate of gastric emptying is the most important physiologic factor controlling drug absorption rate, since the small intestine is the site of maximal absorption.

Precise information on physiologic factors that control absorption of drugs in the horse is lacking. The observation that intestinal motility seems to be particularly affected by impairment of the oxygen supply to the tissue[148] suggests that a decrease in the rate of blood flow to the small intestine could significantly reduce the absorption rate of a lipid-soluble drug.

The principal feature of digestive physiology in the ruminant animal is that fermentation continuously takes place in the reticulorumen. Ruminants have alkaline saliva of pH 8.0 to 8.4. The contents of the reticulorumen have an acidic reaction, pH 5.5

to 6.5.[149] After comminution by both microbial digestion and rechewing, the liquid portion of reticuloruminal contents in which small particles of feed are suspended is pumped by the omasum into the abomasum. In dairy cows, the mean retention time of feed particles in the reticulorumen and omasum is of the order of 60 to 80 hours depending upon the nature of the diet.[150] The limited data available suggest a much shorter forestomach retention time for solids in sheep (25 to 40 hours) than in cattle. The reaction of abomasal contents does not vary much and is usually about pH 3.[151]

The nonionized form of organic electrolytes in the water phase of blood plasma passively diffuses into saliva and gastrointestinal fluids. In ruminants, passage of organic acids into alkaline saliva, with a pH differential of one unit, could be of quantitative significance. The flow of mixed saliva in cows, fed in different ways, was estimated to lie between 98 and 190 liters during a 24-hour period.[152] The daily secretion of saliva in sheep was estimated at 6 to 16 liters.[153] The combined bicarbonate (100 to 140 mEq/L) and phosphate (10 to 50 mEq/L) concentrations are always about 150 mEq/L, varying reciprocally. Based on average values of salivary flow and volume of rumen liquid pool (60 liters in cattle and 4.5 liters in sheep), the turnover rate for rumen

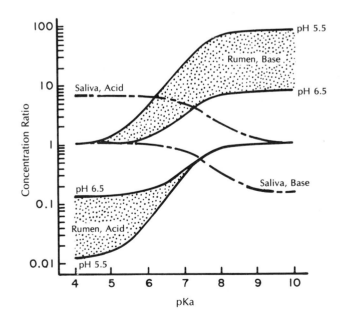

Figure 18–5. Expected equilibrium distribution between saliva or rumen contents and plasma of acids and bases of differing pK_a. Concentration ratio is the ratio of the salivary or ruminal concentration to concentration free in the plasma, calculated separately for acids and bases, for saliva of pH 8.2 and rumen contents over a range of pH 5.5 to 6.5, assuming plasma is pH 7.4. (From Dobson: Fed. Proc. 26:994, 1967.)

liquid was estimated to be 2.0 per day for cattle and 1.1 to 2.2 per day for sheep.[154] Diffusion of organic electrolytes into ruminal fluid, in which organic bases become trapped by ionization, is an important site of their distribution in ruminant species.[155] The concentration of a weak organic electrolyte in ruminal fluid, which is not metabolized by ruminal microflora, will normally reflect the activities of both salivary and ruminal epithelial processes (Fig. 18–5). In the horse, the large intestine is a potential site for accumulation (reservoir) of a fraction of the amount of drug in the body. This aspect of drug distribution should be taken into account in dosage calculations.

PRINCIPLES OF PHARMACOKINETICS

Pharmacokinetics is defined as the mathematical description of concentration changes of drugs within the body. The discipline is concerned with the study and characterization of the time course of drug absorption, distribution, biotransformation, and excretion, and with the relationship of these processes to the intensity and time course of therapeutic and adverse effects of drugs. Interpretation of data derived from pharmacokinetic studies involves the assumptions that some quantitative relationship exists between drug concentration in plasma (or serum) and that at receptor site, and that the action of the drug is rapidly reversible. These assumptions are based on the premise that the intensity of action of the drug is a function of its concentration in the fluid bathing the receptor site. Several studies have shown a good correlation between plasma concentration, tissue concentration, and pharmacologic response to various drugs, in particular cardiac[156] and anti-epileptic[157,158] agents. In contrast, the relation between the amount administered (dose), in particular by the oral route, and the response obtained is highly variable for many drug products. Consequently, plasma concentration rather than dose predicts more accurately the intensity of pharmacologic response of these drugs. Plasma concentration of drugs whose action is not rapidly reversible reveals little about their therapeutic activity. These include drugs that produce a pharmacologic response that greatly outlasts their presence in the plasma (e.g., reserpine, organic phosphate insecticides, many cytotoxic agents).

Drug Disposition

Drug disposition is a term used to describe the simultaneous effects of distribution and elimination (i.e., biotransformation and excretion) processes. A disposition study entails administration of a single dose (intravenous route is most suitable as it bypasses absorption) of drug to a "normal" animal, collection of blood (and urine) samples at predetermined times, and chemical determination or biologic assay of drug concentration or activity in plasma or serum (and urine). A semilogarithmic plot of the plasma drug concentration data versus time shows the pattern of drug disappearance from the blood. Components of the disposition curve are described by least-squares linear regression analysis, the phases of the curve having been separated by the method of residuals or feathering technique. Compartmental analysis, in which the body is conceived as consisting of distinct compartments interconnected by first-order mass transfer constants, is the most common technique employed in pharmacokinetics. Usually these compartments, which are mathematical entities, have no physiologic counterpart. The two-compartment open model (Fig. 18–6) adequately describes the disposition kinetics of many drugs in man and animals.

A drug introduced into the systemic circulation (preferably by intravenous administration) equilibrates very rapidly within the fluids and tissues which comprise the central compartment. This compartment consists of the blood and highly perfused organs (such as the brain for lipophilic drugs) including liver and kidneys. Distribution into the remainder of the available body space, peripheral compartment, takes place more slowly. The peripheral (or tissue) compartment may be considered to

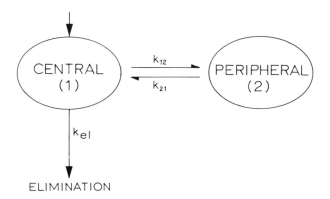

Figure 18–6. Schematic diagram of the two-compartment open model. The dose of drug is introduced into the central compartment where it distributes instantaneously. Distribution between central and peripheral compartments takes place more slowly; k_{12} and k_{21} are first-order rate constants for drug transfer between the two compartments. Elimination, which comprises biotransformation and excretion, is assumed to occur exclusively from the central compartment; k_{el} is the first-order rate constant for drug elimination from the central compartment.

consist of less well perfused tissues, such as muscle, skin, and body fat. The apparent volumes of the central and peripheral compartments for a drug depend upon perfusion of component tissues, partitioning of the drug between plasma and tissues, and the extent of binding to plasma proteins and tissue constituents. While an apparent distribution equilibrium is eventually established, there is only one instant when the system is in equilibrium. The equilibrium condition of no net transfer of drug between the two compartments holds only at that single point in time when the drug concentration in the peripheral compartment has reached a maximum value (Fig. 18–7). An assumption associated with the two-compartment open model is that drug elimination takes place exclusively from the central compartment. The distribution and elimination processes associated with the model are assumed to follow first-order kinetics. Accordingly, the rate of removal of drug from a compartment is proportional to the drug concentration in the compartment.

For most drugs, intravenous injection of a single dose yields a biexponential decline on a semilogarithmic plot of plasma drug concentration as a function of time. The initial steep decline in the plasma level-time profile (disposition curve) represents mainly distribution (by diffusion) of the drug, although elimination is occurring simultaneously.

Once apparent distribution equilibrium is established, the decline in plasma drug concentration is determined mainly by irreversible elimination from the central compartment, appropriately termed the "elimination" phase (Fig. 18–8). The linear (terminal) portion of the disposition curve has a slope which may be defined as $(-)\beta/2.303$ and an extrapolated zero-time intercept, B, in units of concentration. Resolving the biexponential curve into its components by the method of residuals yields a second linear segment, called the distribution phase, with a slope equal to $(-)\alpha/2.303$ and a zero-time intercept of A.[159]

The drug disposition curve is described mathematically by the biexponential expression:

$$C_p = Ae^{-\alpha t} + Be^{-\beta t} \qquad \text{Eq. 5}$$

where C_p is the concentration of drug in the plasma, A and B are "intercept" terms with dimensions of concentration (μg/ml), α and β are hybrid first-order disposition rate constants, expressed in units of reciprocal time (min.$^{-1}$), and e represents the base of the natural logarithm. The derived constants (A, B, α, β) are used to calculate the actual pharmacokinetic rate constants associated with the two-compartment open model (k_{12}, k_{21}, k_{el}) by means of appropriate equations.[160] Determination of the microconstants permits an assessment of the relative contribution of distribution and elimination

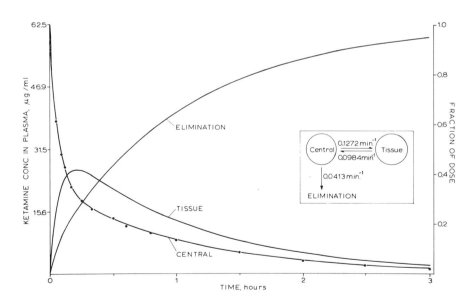

Figure 18–7. Computer-simulated curves of ketamine levels (as fraction of dose) in the central and tissue (peripheral) compartments as a function of time. Curves are based on rate constants derived from measured concentrations of ketamine in plasma (●) of a cat given a single intravenous dose (25 mg/kg) of ketamine hydrochloride. The maximum level (42% of the dose) of the drug was present in the peripheral compartment at 12.5 minutes after administering the dose. At that time the system was in equilibrium. The elimination-time curve is also shown. A scheme of the two-compartment open model with values of the first-order rate constants associated with the model is inset. (From Baggot and Blake. Arch. Int. Pharmacodyn. Ther. 220:115, 1976.)

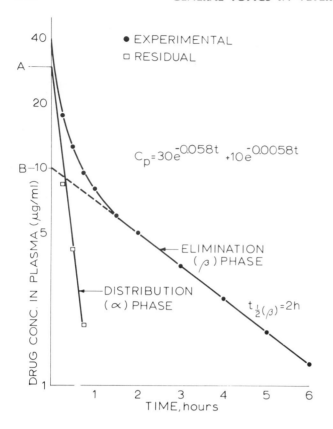

Figure 18–8. Semilogarithmic graph depicting the time course of drug in the plasma after intravenous administration of a single dose (10 mg/kg). The disposition curve is described by the biexponential expression:

$$C_p = 30e^{-0.058t} + 10e^{-0.0058t}$$

where C_p is the concentration of drug in the plasma at time t. The initial plasma drug concentration ($C_p^\circ = 40$ μg/ml) is the sum of A and B.

The half-life of the drug (2 hours) is defined as:

$$t_{1/2(\beta)} = \frac{0.693}{\beta}$$

where β (0.0058 min^{-1}), the overall elimination rate constant, is obtained from the slope of the linear terminal portion (elimination phase) of the disposition curve. (From Baggot: *Principles of Drug Disposition in Domestic Animals.* Philadelphia, W. B. Saunders Co., 1977.)

processes (which may be altered in disease states) to the disposition kinetics of a drug.

The overall elimination rate constant (β) is probably the most important functional pharmacokinetic parameter in a drug disposition study. It is equal to the negative value of the slope of the linear terminal phase of the plot ln C_p *versus* time. The half-life of a drug, which is defined as the time required for the body to eliminate one-half of the drug which is contained therein, is given by the expression:

$$t_{1/2} = \frac{0.693}{\beta} \qquad\qquad \text{Eq. 6}$$

The half-life is a measure of the rate of drug elimination, being the time taken for the plasma (or serum) concentration of the drug to decline by 50% during the elimination phase of the disposition curve. Half-life values of the majority of therapeutic agents are independent of the dose administered, as their overall elimination obeys first-order kinetics. Furthermore, the half-life of a drug, which is eliminated exponentially, is independent of the route of administration. The intravenous injection of a single dose is, however, the only satisfactory procedure on which to base half-life. This parameter is usually an important determinant of the duration of pharmacologic effect and of the optimum dosage regimen. To ascertain whether a drug has linear pharmacokinetic characteristics, the disposition kinetics should be studied at three or more dosage levels. The most important cause of nonlinearity is the limited capacity of certain drug-metabolizing enzyme systems, for example, salicylate elimination in the cat.[161,162]

Volume of Distribution

The volume of distribution is an important concept in the pharmacokinetic characterization of drugs. The parameter is called apparent volume of distribution, V_d, as it does not represent an actual volume and the tissues in which a drug distributes do not all have the same concentration at one time.[163] The value of V_d serves as a proportionality constant relating the drug concentration in the plasma to the total amount of drug in the body after pseudodistribution equilibrium has been attained:

$$C_p \cdot V_d = A_{B(t)} \qquad\qquad \text{Eq. 7}$$

where C_p and $A_{B(t)}$ are the plasma concentration and amount of drug in the body, respectively, at time t. While the apparent volume of distribution provides an estimate of the extent of a drug's distribution, this pharmacokinetic parameter does not distinguish between widespread distribution and high affinity binding with restricted distribution. The nature of distribution must be related to both the value of V_d and physicochemical properties (such as lipid solubility, ionic character of functional groups) which govern diffusion across biologic membranes and binding to tissues. Lipid-soluble organic bases (e.g., amphetamine, quinidine) are widely distributed in the body fluids and tissues, and have large values of V_d which exceed the actual volume of the body (> 1 liter/kg). The low lipid solubility of aminoglycoside antibiotics (polar organic bases) restricts their distribution ($V_d' < 0.3$ liter/kg). While aminoglycosides have a small magnitude of distribution, they are avidly bound to renal tissue, a fact which could never be deduced from the volume of distribution parameter. Organic acids which are predominantly ionized in plasma (e.g., penicillins, salicylates) have small volumes of distribution (< 0.25 liter/kg). The sulfonamides and pentobarbital, weak organic acids which exist as both nonionized and ionized forms in plasma, have values of V_d which may be considered intermediate (0.3 to 0.8 liter/kg).

There are different methods for calculating the apparent volume of distribution. Frequently, V_d is approximated by extrapolation of the terminal linear phase of the drug disposition curve to the y-intercept (B) and substituting this value in the expression:

$$V_{d(B)} = \frac{Dose}{B} \qquad Eq.\ 8$$

The "extrapolation method" for calculating V_d is only valid when disposition kinetics of the drug can be adequately described by a one-compartment open model, i.e., when distribution is instantaneous. When data are best described by two- (or multi-) compartment model, then $V_{d(B)}$ exceeds the magnitude of the parameter calculated by other methods. For drugs which confer upon the body the characteristics of a two-compartment model, the "area" method provides a satisfactory means of calculating volume of distribution:

$$V_{d(area)} = \frac{Dose}{AUC.\beta} \qquad Eq.\ 9$$

$$= \frac{Dose}{(A/\alpha + B/\beta) \cdot \beta} \qquad Eq.\ 10$$

where AUC is the total area under the plasma drug concentration *versus* time curve from $t=0$ to $t=\alpha$. This equation may be employed to calculate V_d after drug administration by any route, provided the dose is completely available systemically.

Volume of distribution, a pharmacokinetic term with no physiologic counterpart, is required for computing the dose that must be administered to provide a desired concentration of drug in the plasma:

Dose   = V_d' × Desired plasma drug conc.
(mg/kg)   (liter/kg)   (mg/liter)

$$Eq.\ 11$$

Table 18–8. Comparison of kinetic parameters for some drugs in the dog and the goat

Drug	Dog		Goat	
	$t_{1/2}$ (hr)	V_d (liter/kg)	$t_{1/2}$ (hr)	V_d (liter/kg)
Salicylate	8.6	0.19	0.8	0.13
Phenol	2.6	1.59	0.5	1.09
Chloramphenicol	4.2	1.77	2.0	1.33
Quinidine	5.6	2.91	0.8	4.86
Amphetamine	4.5	2.67	0.6	3.08
Pentobarbital	3.7	0.58	0.9	0.80
Phenylbutazone	2.6	—	19.0	0.26
Oxyphenbutazone	1.7	—	0.7	—
Tetraethylammonium	0.8	1.04	0.8	4.12

Data from Davis and Jenkins, 1974.[94]

Species differences in V_d are found among domestic animals and can often be attributed to anatomic features of the gastrointestinal tract. Organic bases may have particularly large apparent volumes of distribution in ruminant animals, as these drugs diffuse from plasma into the rumen and become trapped by ionization in ruminal liquor. Values of kinetic parameters, determined in healthy dogs and goats, which are utilized in calculating magnitude and predicting frequency of dosage, are compared (Table 18–8). It may be seen that considerable differences exist between monogastric and ruminant animals in values of $t_{1/2}$ and V_d' for each drug. This table illustrates why it is unwise to extrapolate drug information derived from studies in dogs to the ruminant animal. Furthermore, it explains why the ruminant animal is less susceptible to phenol intoxication,[164] the absence of behavioral effects of amphetamine in goats,[155] and the short duration of pentobarbital anesthesia in ruminants.[161] Efficient biotransformation by microsomal enzymes is the principal factor responsible for short half-life of most foreign chemicals in ruminant animals.[165]

Concept of Clearance

Clearance, defined as the volume of blood completely cleared of drug per unit time, is a measure of the functional ability of an organ to remove the drug. Application of this concept in renal pharmacology includes clearances of inulin and p-aminohippurate, which measure glomerular filtration rate and effective renal plasma flow, respectively. A situation analogous to renal clearance exists for the liver, even though the mechanisms of drug elimination are different. Thus, hepatic clearance is a function of liver blood flow and the ability of the organ to extract the drug from hepatic capillaries. The latter must be a reflection of the overall activity of drug-metabolizing enzymes or other rate-limiting process (such as biliary excretion) involved in elimination. If one considers the body as a whole acting as a drug-eliminating system, then a (total) body clearance, which represents the sum of all clearance processes, can be defined:

$$Cl_B = \beta \cdot V_{d(area)} \qquad \text{Eq. 12}$$

$$= (0.693/t_{\frac{1}{2}}) \cdot V_{d(area)} \qquad \text{Eq. 13}$$

Body clearance is the product of the apparent volume of distribution and the overall elimination rate constant. By rearrangement, the half-life of a drug is seen to depend on clearance and volume of distribution:

$$t_{\frac{1}{2}} = \frac{0.693 \times V_{d(area)}}{Cl_B} \qquad \text{Eq. 14}$$

While one cannot conveniently determine in vivo organ clearances of a drug, the body clearance can be obtained. Body clearance may be estimated by dividing the intravenously administered dose by the total area under the plasma drug concentration versus time curve:

$$Cl_B = \frac{Dose_{(i.v.)}}{AUC} \qquad \text{Eq. 15}$$

and

$$AUC = \int_0^{t^*} C_{pdt} + \frac{C_{p(t^*)}}{\beta} \qquad \text{Eq. 16}$$

where t^* is the time at which the last blood sample was collected, $C_{p(t)}$ the last measured concentration of drug in the plasma, and β the overall elimination rate constant obtained from the linear terminal phase of the semilogarithmic disposition curve. The area under the curve from time zero to t^* can be estimated by using the trapezoidal rule. The contribution of the renal component to body clearance can be separated if the fraction of the intravenous dose which is excreted unchanged in the urine (f_{ex}) is known:

$$Cl_R = f_{ex} \cdot Cl_B \qquad \text{Eq. 17}$$

The difference ($Cl_B - Cl_R$) equals the nonrenal clearance. The body clearance of drugs that are eliminated by metabolism in the liver may be attributed to and will reflect mainly hepatic clearance. For drugs whose disposition kinetics can be described by a two-compartment model, clearance is a more meaningful measurement of drug elimination than half-life, which is a hybrid parameter.[146] Al-

though the AUC, based upon concentrations of drug in the plasma, may be of value for certain pharmacokinetic applications, it may be necessary to derive this estimation from blood concentration data when relating body clearance to organ function.[165]

The dose of a secretory stimulant which elicits one half of the maximal response (D_{50}) is a complex function which is determined by clearance rate as well by the affinity of the stimulant for cellular receptor sites. Differences observed in the D_{50} for gastric acid secretion in man, dog, and cat were proportional to clearance rates; the three species showed an equal sensitivity to human gastrin-17-I at the cellular level.[166]

The clearance rates (ml per kg-min) were 17.5 ± 0.7 (n=8) in man, 48.2 ± 11.6 (n=8) in dogs, and 135 ± 34 (n=4) in cats.

Bioavailability

The biologic performance of a drug from an oral dosage form is usually evaluated by its bioavailability profile, a term which may be defined as the rate and extent to which the drug reaches the systemic circulation intact. A drug administered in solid dosage form encounters three events before entering the systemic circulation: release from dosage form, transport across gastrointestinal mucosal bar-

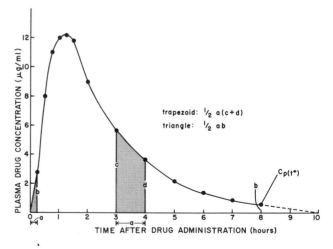

Figure 18–9. Trapezoidal method for estimating area under the curve (AUC). The total area under a curve (plotted on arithmetic coordinates) may be estimated by adding together areas of the trapezoids and triangle at each end of the curve. A better estimate of the area segment under the tail of the curve than that based on the extrapolated triangle is given by $C_{p(t^*)}/\beta'$, where $C_{p(t^*)}$ is the apparent overall elimination of drug in the plasma and β' is the apparent overall elimination rate constant obtained from terminal slope of semilogarithmic plot of plasma drug concentration-time profile (see equation 16). A maximum drug level of 12.2 μg/ml was present in plasma at 1.25 hours. Value of $C_{p(t^*)}$ is 0.6 μg/ml ($t^* = 8$ hours); $\beta' = 0.462$ hour^{-1} (from semilogarithmic plot).

rier, and passage through the liver. Each of these events has the potential to decrease the amount of drug reaching the systemic circulation and the net effect will be reflected in the bioavailability profile. Biophasic availability, in which magnitude and duration of pharmacologic responses are measured, is a more direct measure of biologic performance, but responses are difficult to quantify.

When a single dose of drug is given by the oral route and its concentration in plasma measured for an appropriate period of time, a variation of the plasma concentration curve as shown in Figure 18–9 is obtained. Important features of this curve are the maximum concentration of drug in the plasma (height of peak), the time at which the peak concentration is present, and the area under the curve. The peak height is dependent upon both the rate and extent of drug absorption.

The time at which the plasma level reaches its maximum is a reflection of the rate of absorption. Area under the curve is closely related to the amount of drug that enters the systemic circulation. For best correlation between area under the curve and completeness of absorption, plasma drug concentrations must be determined for a period that is many times longer than the absorption half-time of the drug. This requirement is often limited by sensitivity of the technique for drug assay. The systemic availability (F) of a single oral dose is obtained from the model independent area equation:

$$F \cdot D_{(oral)} = AUC \cdot Cl_B \qquad Eq. 18$$

where AUC represents total area under the curve ($\int_0^\infty C_{pdt}$) and Cl_B, which is equal to $\beta \cdot V_{d(area)}$, is body clearance. Area under the curve is measured by an appropriate numeric integration procedure (trapezoidal method, Fig. 18–8) and is expressed as the product of concentration and time.

One would expect wide differences between monogastric and ruminant species in systemic availability of drug products given by the oral route. Interspecies variation is clearly evident in a comparative study of salicylate absorption, in which sodium salicylate contained in gelatin capsules was administered orally at three dosage rates (18.5, 50 and 133 mg/kg) to dogs, swine, ponies, and goats.[161] Inspection of the plasma salicylate concentration-time curves (Fig. 18–10) shows that a considerably larger amount of salicylate was available systemically in dogs and swine than in the herbivorous

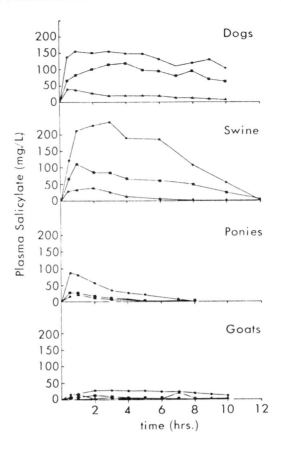

Figure 18–10. Species differences in absorption of sodium salicylate after the oral administration of the drug contained in gelatin capsules. Three dose levels (18.5, 50 and 133 mg/kg) were studied. The data points represent the means from at least four animals. (From Davis and Westfall.[161])

species (ponies and goats). Even though salicylate was promptly absorbed from the digestive tract of dogs and swine, the peak plasma concentrations were only 50% of that resulting from intravenous administration.

The method of corresponding areas is most useful for estimating systemic availability of a drug from an oral dosage form. This method entails comparison of the total areas under the plasma concentration-time curves, plotted on arithmetic coordinates, obtained after oral and intravenous administration of equal doses (in appropriate dosage forms) to the same animals:

$$F = \frac{(AUC)_{oral}}{(AUC)_{iv}} \qquad Eq. 19$$

Should an intravenous preparation not be available, an oral reference standard (usually an aqueous solution or elixir of the drug) may be used for comparison, in which case relative rather than absolute bioavailability is obtained. The method of corresponding areas assumes that clearance is constant over the dosage range of interest.

Absorption of most drugs in monogastric animals is much faster than elimination and the value of β is independent of the route of administration. It is usual that both absorption and elimination processes obey first-order kinetics, except slow-release dosage forms which control supply of drug so that absorption proceeds at a constant rate (zero-order). When the rate of drug elimination in an animal is affected by oral dosage (route-dependent), the overall elimination rate constant, derived from terminal slope of semilogarithmic plot of plasma concentration-time data, is apparent (β'). Under these circumstances a better estimate of F may be obtained by using the corrected areas:

$$F = \frac{(AUC)_{oral} \times \beta'}{(AUC)_{iv} \times \beta} \qquad \text{Eq. 20}$$

This equation takes care of intrasubject variability in the overall elimination rate constant for the drug. Occasionally there may be intrasubject variations in both β and V_d without a change in clearance, as an increase in V_d would be compensated by a commensurate decrease in β. This situation could exist in certain disease states (e.g., fever). So long as clearance in an animal is constant and independent of dose, it is more appropriate to directly compare areas rather than "corrected" areas.

The systemic availability (absolute) of sulfadimethoxine from a suspension of the drug given orally to dogs was calculated by the method of corresponding areas (direct and corrected). The plasma concentration time curves which were obtained after administration of single doses (55 mg/kg) of sodium sulfadimethoxine solution (10%) by the intravenous route and sulfadimethoxine suspension (12.5%) orally to six normal Beagles are shown (Fig. 18–11). Area under the curves was estimated by the trapezoidal rule and systemic availability was calculated for each animal. Values of F obtained, median (range), were 32.8% (22.5 to 80.0) and 48.8% (24.4 to 86.2) when direct and corrected areas, respectively, were used.[167,168]

Bioavailability of drug products intended for oral administration influences the relationship between their dosage and intensity of pharmacologic response or chemotherapeutic activity. The significance of bioavailability profiles rests on there being a direct relationship between the time course

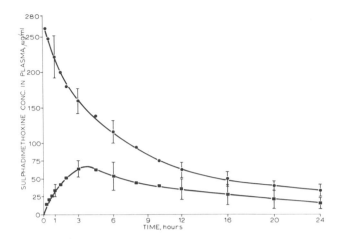

Figure 18–11.   Concentrations (mean ± S.D.) of sulfadimethoxine in the plasma after administration of a fixed dose (55 mg/kg) by the intravenous (●) and oral (■) routes to a group of six dogs. The drug products administered were the injection (10%) and oral suspension (12.5%). (From Baggot, Ludden, and Powers.[167])

of drug in the plasma and the rate of appearance and duration of the requisite concentration of the drug at its site of action (biophase). Since it is usually desirable to maintain an effective level of drug in the body for the duration of therapy, the rate at which a drug becomes available systemically is an important criterion in design of the dosage regimen. While an idea of the absorption rate of a drug from an oral dosage form can be derived from the time at which peak plasma concentration is reached, there is little precise information on drug absorption in domestic animals. Inspection of the mean plasma concentration-time curve (Fig. 18–11) obtained after dosage with sulfadimethoxine suspension shows that a maximum sulfonamide concentration was present at 3.6 hours. The mean half-time of absorption, calculated from the expression $t_{1/2(ab)} = 0.693/k_{ab}$, was 1.94 hours, where k_{ab} is the first-order rate constant of absorption and was obtained by the Loo-Riegelman method.[169] Absorption of sulfadimethoxine was fast when compared with elimination. The half-life of the drug, derived from the slope of linear terminal phase of semilogarithmic disposition curve following intravenous dosage, was 13.2 hours (mean). Bacteriostatic plasma concentrations of the sulfonamide can be maintained by administering the appropriate dose at 24-hour intervals.[167]

Quite a different situation exists with the relative rates of absorption and elimination of salicylate in cows (Table 18–9). The absorption half-time is almost six times the half-life of the drug. Absorption, rather than biotransformation and excretion, con-

Table 18–9. Kinetic constants describing absorption and elimination of salicylate in the cow

Factor	Mean (n = 6)	±	S.D.
Biologic half-life (hr)	0.54	±	0.04
Apparent specific volume of distribution (liter/kg)	0.24	±	0.02
Absorption half-time (hr)	2.91	±	0.37
Elimination half-time after oral dosage (hr)	3.70	±	0.44

Data from Gingerich et al.[120]

trols the rate of elimination of salicylate given orally and is the process upon which the 12-hour dosage interval is based. A doubling of the dosage rate (50 to 100 mg/kg) resulted in twice the amount of salicylate being available systemically, while the rate of absorption remained unchanged. Systemic availability of salicylate following oral administration of aspirin tablets to cows was 70%.[120]

Factors that affect bioavailability of a drug are listed (Table 18–10) and locations at which their effects may be exerted are represented schematically (Fig. 18–12). Differences in bioavailability among different formulations of the same drug may be so great as to result in serious changes in clinical efficacy and adverse effects. After release of drug from an oral dosage form the molecules must be

Table 18–10. Factors influencing bioavailability of oral dosage forms of drugs

Formulation of Drug Product (Drug Release)
  Disintegration time
  Dissolution rate

Physicochemical Properties of Drug (Absorption)
  Lipid solubility
  Degree of ionization (pK$_a$)
  Chemical stability at environmental pH reaction

Physiologic Variables (Absorption)
  Gastric emptying rate
  Intestinal blood flow
  Motility of intestinal tract

Properties of Gastrointestinal Contents (Absorption)
  Hydrogen ion concentration (pH reaction)
  Metabolic activities of intestinal and ruminal microorganisms
  Complexing agents in food
  Drug interactions (kaolin, cholestyramine)
  Bile interaction

Potential Sites of Metabolic Inactivation
  Ruminal microorganisms
  Intestinal bacteria in lumen
  Intestinal mucosa (epithelium)
  Hepatocytes (with wide variety of drug-metabolizing enzymes including microsomal oxidizing system)

Physiologic factors are subject to modification by concurrent administration of other drugs.

stable in the environment within the stomach and small intestine (or reticulorumen of cattle, sheep, and goats), must have sufficient lipid solubility to diffuse through the mucosal barrier and, before entering the systemic circulation, are exposed to drug-metabolizing enzymes in the liver. Microorganisms in the intestinal and ruminal fluids and located within mucosal epithelium are potential sites for metabolic inactivation of drugs. Hydrolytic and reductive reactions are the usual types of metabolic transformations which are mediated by the gut microflora.[170,171]

The columnar epithelial cells of the intestinal mucosa contain a wide variety of enzyme systems capable of metabolizing drugs.[172,173]

Perhaps the most important is glucuronyl transferase, which catalyzes formation of glucuronide conjugates. Oxidation, which is the principal metabolic pathway in the fate of lipid-soluble drugs, is catalyzed by microsomal enzymes, which are associated mainly with smooth-surfaced endoplasmic reticulum of hepatic cells.[174] Biotransformation by enzymes in the intestinal mucosa and by hepatic enzymes preceding drug entry into the systemic circulation ("first-pass effect") may significantly reduce the bioavailability of orally administered drugs, particularly if metabolism is extensive as was found with lidocaine[175] and propranolol.[176] Incomplete systemic availability caused by first-pass effect could be misinterpreted as defective absorption.

ENTEROHEPATIC CIRCULATION

A compound may be excreted by the liver cells into the bile and thus pass into the small intestine. Lipid-soluble compounds may passively diffuse into bile, and polar compounds[177] are actively transported into bile by energy-dependent carrier-mediated processes. The biliary route constitutes a minor pathway compared with glomerular filtration for excretion of lipid-soluble (diffusible) molecules which are in the aqueous phase of blood plasma. On the other hand, it appears that polar compounds, which may be drugs, endogenous substances, or metabolites (in particular glucuronide conjugates), which have molecular weights between 300 and 1000, are likely to be excreted in bile in significant amounts. The fraction of circulating drug that is bound to plasma proteins (usually albumin) is fully available for carrier-mediated excretion processes, both renal and biliary. Imipramine,[178] digitoxin, iodopanoic acid (cholecystographic agent), and steroid hormones are among the compounds which are excreted unchanged in bile.

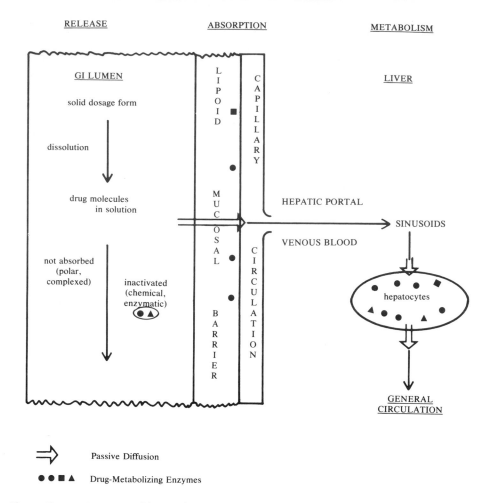

Figure 18-12. Locations of factors that may influence bioavailability of drugs from oral dosage forms.

Both clindamycin and lincomycin are extensively eliminated by hepatic mechanisms.[179,180] The rate of extraction of each antibiotic by the liver and kidneys, expressed as a percentage of the rate of administration (20 mg/kg per hour by continuous intravenous infusion), was studied in dogs.[181] Uptake by the liver accounted for 17 to 28% of infused clindamycin and for 12 to 20% of lincomycin. In contrast, extraction by the kidneys was responsible for 17 to 24% of the administered dose of lincomycin but for less than 5% of the dose of total clindamycin.

Bromsulphthalein (BSP) is excreted both unchanged and as a glutathione conjugate in the bile.[182] Some compounds which are excreted in bile as glucuronide conjugates are listed in Table 18-11. This important conjugation reaction is catalyzed by the microsomal enzyme uridine diphosphate (UDP) glucuronyl transferase. Glucuronides are more water-soluble than the parent compounds because of the large hydrophilic carbohydrate moiety, and consequently are poorly absorbed from the intestine. They may, however, be hydrolyzed, a metabolic reaction catalyzed by β-glucuronidase which is present in the intestine, and the active compound may be released. It may be absorbed into portal venous blood or excreted in the feces, or it may be reduced, a further metabolic reaction which will inactivate the compound. When the

Table 18-11. Compounds excreted as glucuronide conjugates in the bile

Foreign Compounds	Endogenous Substances
Chloramphenicol	Bilirubin
Trimethoprim	Thyroxine
Sulfadimethoxine (N'−)	Stilbestrol
Morphine	
Iodopanoic acid (ester glucuronide)	

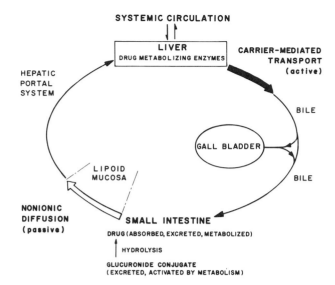

Figure 18–13. The enterohepatic circulation of a lipid-soluble foreign or endogenous compound. Glucuronide conjugates, formed in the liver and excreted in the bile, may be hydrolyzed in the small intestine and the liberated parent compound be reabsorbed. (Modified from Baggot: *Principles of Drug Disposition in Domestic Animals.* Philadelphia, W. B. Saunders Co., 1977.)

physicochemical properties of the compound in the intestine are favorable for absorption by passive diffusion, an enterohepatic cycle will be established (Fig. 18–13). This term implies the passage of a compound from hepatocytes into the bile and then into the intestine, from which it is absorbed and returned to hepatic sinusoids. The compound will gradually be removed from this cycle and the body by renal excretion. Ampicillin attains high concentrations in the bile;[183] some of the antibiotic is reabsorbed in the small intestine. The biliary concentration of ampicillin is markedly dependent on the integrity of the gallbladder and its ducts.[184] The pharmacologic significance of enterohepatic circulation for a drug depends on the fraction of the dose which enters the bile. When the amount is substantial, the effects of a single dose will be prolonged (e.g., digitoxin in the human) and reflected in the rate of elimination.

Generally, with compounds of molecular weight less than 300, there is little variation among species in the extent of their biliary excretion, even though different metabolites may be formed.[185] When the molecular weight of a polar compound is between 300 and 500, there is likely to be a species variation in extent of biliary excretion.[186]

Recycling processes, such as enterohepatic circulation, diffusion of amines into acidic gastric contents and reabsorption from small intestine, passage

of weak organic electrolytes into and reabsorption from ruminal fluid, may complicate the assessment of bioavailability. In monogastric animals, it is unlikely that enterogastric recycling would be of quantitative significance as, in the dog, the stomach receives only 1.2[187] to 4%[188] of the cardiac output. Enterohepatic circulation of a drug that is extensively cleared by the liver into bile may produce secondary peaks in the plasma level-time profile. One may discount erratic absorption when a relationship exists between the ingestion of food and the appearance of the secondary peak, especially when the drug is given intravenously or orally in solution.[189]

REFERENCES

1. Alexander, F.: An Introduction to Veterinary Pharmacology, 3rd ed. Edinburgh, Churchill Livingstone, 1976, p. 162.
2. Amend, J. F., and Klavano, P. A.: Xylazine, a new sedative-analgesic with predictable emetic properties in the cat. V.M./S.A.C. 68:741, 1973.
3. Yeary, R. A.: Syrup of ipecac as an emetic in the cat. J.A.V.M.A. 161:1677, 1972.
4. Sadusk, J. F., and Palmisano, P. A.: Teratogenic effect of meclizine, cyclizine and chlorcyclizine. J.A.M.A. 194:139, 1965.
5. Brand, E. D., Harris, T. D., Borison, H. L., and Goodman, L. S.: The antemetic activity of 10-(dimethylaminopropyl)-2-chlorophenothiazine (chlorpromazine) in the dog and cat. J. Pharmacol. Exp. Ther. 110:86, 1954.
6. Bank, S., Saunders, S. J., Marks, I. N., Novis, B. H., and Barbezat, G. O.: Gastrointestinal and hepatic diseases. In Drug Treatment. Principles and Practice of Clinical Pharmacology and Therapeutics. Edited by G. S. Avery. Acton, MA, Publishing Sciences Group, 1976, p. 519.
7. Kutt, H., and McDowell, F. H.: Drug-induced neurological diseases. In Drug Treatment. Principles and Practice of Clinical Pharmacology and Therapeutics. Edited by G. S. Avery. Acton, MA, Publishing Sciences Group, 1976, p. 793.
8. Davenport, H. W.: Physiology of the Digestive Tract, 3rd ed. Chicago, Year Book Medical Publishers, 1971, p. 29.
9. Daniel, E. E.: The effects of drugs on the gastrointestinal tract. In Gastroenterology. Edited by A. Bogoch. New York, McGraw-Hill Book Co., 1973, p. 103.
10. Molitor, H.: A comparative study of the effects of five choline compounds used in therapeutics: acetylcholine chloride, acetyl-beta-methylcholine chloride, carbaminoyl choline, ethyl ether beta-methylcholine chloride, carbaminoyl beta-methylcholine chloride. J. Pharmacol. Exp. Ther. 58:337, 1936.
11. Alexander, F.: An Introduction to Veterinary Pharmacology, 3rd ed. Edinburgh, Churchill Livingstone, 1976, p. 165.
12. Cutting, W. C.: Handbook of Pharmacology, 4th ed. New York, Meredith, 1969, p. 535.
13. Ibid, p. 487.
14. Jenden, D. J.: Antimuscarinic agents. In Essentials of Pharmacology. Edited by J. A. Bevan. New York, Hoeber, 1969, p. 119.
15. Bülbring, E., and Crema, A.: Observations concerning the action of 5-hydroxytryptamine on the peristaltic reflex. Br. J. Pharmacol. 13:444, 1958.
16. Sollmann, T.: A Manual of Pharmacology, 8th ed. Philadelphia, W. B. Saunders Co., 1957, p. 544.
17. Short, C. R., and Davis, L. E.: Post-natal development of drug-metabolizing enzyme activity in swine. J. Pharmacol. Exp. Ther. 174:185, 1970.
18. Phillips, R. W., and Lewis, L. D.: Drugs affecting gastrointestinal motility and ingesta movement. In Veterinary Pharmacology and Therapeutics. Edited by L. M. Jones, N. H. Booth, and L. E. McDonald. Ames, Iowa State University Press, 1977, p. 726.
19. Seckington, I. M.: Treatment of colic from a practitioner's point of view. Equine Vet. J. 4:188, 1972.
20. Lish, P. M.: Some pharmacologic effects of dioctyl sodium sulfosuccinate on the gastrointestinal tract of the rat. Gastroenterology 41:580, 1961.

21. Alexander, B., Lorenzen, E., Hoffman, R., and Garfinkel, A.: The effect of ingested mineral oil on plasma carotene and vitamin A. Proc. Soc. Exp. Biol. Med. 65:275, 1947.
22. Stryker, W. A.: Absorption of liquid petrolatum ("mineral oil") from the intestine. A histologic and chemical study. Arch. Pathol. 31:670, 1941.
23. Davis, L. E.: Review of the clinical pharmacology of the equine digestive tract. J. Equine Med. Surg. 1:27, 1977.
24. Daniel, E. E.: The effects of drugs on the gastrointestinal tract. In Gastroenterology. Edited by A. Bogoch. New York, McGraw-Hill Book Co., 1973, p. 109.
25. Burks, T. F.: Mediation by 5-hydroxytryptamine of morphine stimulant actions in dog intestine. J. Pharmacol. Exp. Ther. 185:530, 1973.
26. Jaffe, J. H., and Martin, W. R.: Narcotic analgesics and antagonists. In The Pharmacological Basis of Therapeutics, 5th ed. Edited by L. S. Goodman and A. Gilman. New York, Macmillan Publishing Co., 1975, p. 274.
27. Coffman, J. R., and Garner, H. G.: Acute abdominal diseases of the horse. J.A.V.M.A. 161:1195, 1972.
28. Phillipson, A. T.: Ruminant digestion. In Dukes' Physiology of Domestic Animals. Edited by M. J. Swenson. Ithaca, Cornell University Press, 1970, p. 449.
29. Dougherty, R. W.: A study of drugs affecting the motility of the bovine rumen. Cornell Vet. 32:269, 1942.
30. Duncan, D. L.: Responses of the gastric musculature of the sheep to some humoral agents and related substances. J. Physiol. (Lond.) 125:475, 1954.
31. Amadon, R. S.: An experimental study of drugs stimulating the motility of the ruminant stomach. J.A.V.M.A. 76:65, 1930.
32. Stowe, C. M.: Cholinergic (parasympathomimetic) drugs. In Veterinary Pharmacology and Therapeutics, 3rd ed. Edited by L. M. Jones. Ames, Iowa State University Press, 1965, p. 313.
33. Alexander, F.: An Introduction to Veterinary Pharmacology, 3rd ed. New York, Churchill Livingstone, 1976, p. 165.
34. Rossoff, I. S.: Handbook of Veterinary Drugs. New York, Springer, 1974, p. 635.
35. Harvey, S. C.: Gastric antacids and digestants. In The Pharmacological Basis of Therapeutics, 5th ed. Edited by L. S. Goodman and A. Gilman. New York, Macmillan Publishing Co., 1975, p. 970.
36. Bevan, J. A.: Essentials of Pharmacology. New York, Hoeber, 1969, p. 94.
37. Emmelin, N.: Action of histamine upon salivary glands. In Histamine: Its Chemistry, Metabolism and Physiological and Pharmacological Actions Handb. exp. Pharmak. Edited by M. Rocha e Silva. Vol. 18, Part 1. Berlin, Springer-Verlag, 1966, p. 294.
38. Bailey, C. B.: Saliva secretion and its relation to feeding in cattle. III. The rate of secretion of mixed saliva in the cow during eating, with an estimate of the magnitude of the total daily secretion of mixed saliva. Br. J. Nutr. 15:443, 1961.
39. Kay, R. N. B.: Continuous and reflex secretion of the parotid gland in ruminants: the effects of stimulation of the sympathetic nerve and of adrenaline on the flow of parotid saliva in sheep. J. Physiol. 144:463, 1958.
40. Leeson, C. R., and Leeson, T. S.: Histology, 3rd ed. Philadelphia, W. B. Saunders Co., 1976, p. 350.
41. Black, J. W., Duncan, W. A. M., Durant, C. J., Ganellin, C. R., and Parsons, E. M.: Definition and antagonism of histamine H2-receptors. Nature 236:385, 1972.
42. Parsons, M. E.: The evidence that inhibition of histamine-stimulated gastric secretion is a result of the blockade of histamine H2-receptors. In International Symposium of Histamine H2-Receptor Antagonists. Edited by C. J. Wood and M. A. Simkins. Welwyn Garden City, England, Smith, Kline & French, 1973, p. 207.
43. Konturek, S. J., Dimitrescu, T., Radecki, T., and Dimbinski, A.: Effect of metiamide, a histamine H2-receptor antagonist on gastric and pancreatic secretion and peptic ulcers induced by histamine and pentagastrin in cats. In International Symposium on Histamine H2-Receptor Antagonists. Edited by C. J. Wood and M. A. Simkins. Welwyn Garden City, England, Smith, Kline & French, 1973, p. 247.
44. Menguy, R., and Desbaillets, L.: The gastric mucous barrier: influence of protein-bound carbohydrate in mucus on the rate of proteolysis of gastric mucus. Ann. Surg. 168:475, 1968.
45. Ewing, G. O.: Indomethacin associated gastrointestinal hemorrhage in a dog. J.A.V.M.A. 161:1665, 1972.
46. Bayliss, W. M., and Starling, E. H.: The mechanism of pancreatic secretion. J. Physiol. 28:323, 1902.
47. Harper, A. A., and Raper, H. S.: Pancreozymin, a stimulant of the secretion of pancreatic enzymes in extracts of small intestine. J. Physiol. 102:115, 1943.
48. Crittenden, P. J., and Ivy, A. C.: The nervous control of pancreatic secretion in the dog. Am. J. Physiol. 119:724, 1937.
49. Kostina, T. E.: The role of the sympathetic innervation in the humoral phase of pancreatic secretion. Sechov. Physiol. J. USSR 44:142, 1958.
50. Jerzy-Glass, G. B.: Introduction to Gastrointestinal Physiology. Englewood Cliffs, N.J., Prentice-Hall, 1968, p. 104.
51. Dyck, W. P., Rudick, J., Hoexter, B., and Janowitz, H. D.: Influence of glucagon on pancreatic exocrine secretion. Gastroenterology 56:531, 1969.
52. Javitt, N. B.: Hepatic bile formation. N. Engl. J. Med. 295:1464 and 1511, 1976.
53. Sperber, I.: Secretion of organic anions in the formation of urine and bile. Pharmacol. Rev. 11:109, 1959.
54. Vonk, R. J., Jekel, P., and Meijer, D. K. F.: Choleresis and hepatic transport mechanisms. II. Influence of bile salt choleresis and biliary micelle binding on biliary excretion of various organic anions. Naunyn. Schmiedebergs Arch. Pharmacol. 290:375, 1975.
55. Wheeler, H. O., Ross, E. D., and Bradley, S. E.: Canalicular bile production in dogs. Am. J. Physiol. 214:866, 1968.
56. Thistle, J. L., and Hoffman, A. F.: Efficacy and specificity of chenodeoxycholic acid therapy for dissolving gallstones. N. Engl. J. Med. 289:655, 1973.
57. Schultz, S. G., and Curran, P. F.: Coupled transport of sodium and organic solutes. Physiol. Rev. 50:637, 1970.
58. Graf, J., Korn, P., and Peterlik, M.: Choleretic effects of ouabain and ethacrynic acid in the isolated perfused rat liver. Naunyn Schmiedebergs Arch. Pharmacol. 272:230, 1972.
59. Shaw, H., Caple, I., and Heath, T.: Effect of ethacrynic acid on bile formation in sheep, dogs, rats, guinea pigs and rabbits. J. Pharmacol. Exp. Ther. 182:27, 1972.
60. Barnhart, J., and Combes, B.: Characteristics common to choleretic increments of bile induced by theophylline, glucagon and SQ-20009 in the dog. Proc. Soc. Exp. Biol. Med. 150:591, 1975.
61. Macarol, V., Morris, T. Q., Baker, K. J., and Bradley, S. E.: Hydrocortisone choleresis in the dog. J. Clin. Invest. 49:1714, 1970.
62. Berthelot, P., Erlinger, S., Dhumeaux, D., and Preaux, A.-M.: Mechanism of phenobarbital-induced hypercholeresis in the rat. Am. J. Physiol. 219:809, 1970.
63. Robins, R. E., Trueman, G. E., and Bogoch, A.: The gallbladder and extrahepatic bile ducts. In Gastroenterology. Edited by A. Bogoch. New York, McGraw-Hill Publishing Co., 1973, p. 852.
64. Eichhorn, E. P., Jr., and Boyden, E. A.: The choledochoduodenal junction in the dog—a restudy of Oddi's sphincter. Am. J. Anat. 97:431, 1955.
65. Crema, A., and Benzi, G.: In vitro behavior of the sphincter of Oddi in various animals. Arch. Fisiol. 60:374, 1961.
66. Robins, R. E., Trueman, G. E., and Bogoch, A.: The gallbladder and extrahepatic bile ducts. In Gastroenterology. Edited by A. Bogoch. New York, McGraw-Hill Publishing Co., 1973, p. 855.
67. Hendrix, T. R., and Bayless, T. M.: Digestion: intestinal secretion. Annu. Rev. Physiol. 32:139, 1970.
68. Hubel, K. A.: Effects of bethanechol on intestinal ion transport in the rat. Proc. Soc. Exp. Biol. Med. 154:41, 1977.
69. Sommers, H. M.: Infectious diarrhea. In The Biologic and Clinical Basis of Infectious Diseases. Edited by G. P. Youmans, P. Y. Paterson, and H. M. Sommers. Philadelphia, W. B. Saunders Co., 1975, p. 499.
70. Wilson, D. E.: Prostaglandins, their actions on the gastrointestinal tract. Arch. Intern. Med. 133:112, 1974.
71. McKenzie, A. D., and Palmer, R. A.: Diseases of the colon, rectum and anus. In Gastroenterology. Edited by A. Bogoch. New York, McGraw-Hill Publishing Co., 1973, p. 610.
72. Anand, B. K., and Brobeck, J. R.: Hypothalamic control of food intake in rats and cats. Yale J. Biol. Med. 24:123, 1951.
73. Janowitz, H. D.: Hunger and appetite: physiologic regulation of food intake. Am. J. Med. 25:327, 1958.
74. Paintal, A. S.: Study of gastric stretch receptors: their role in peripheral mechanism of satiation of hunger and thirst. J. Physiol. 126:255, 1954.
75. Herrin, R. C., and Meek, W. J.: Afferent nerves excited by intestinal distension. Am. J. Physiol. 144:720, 1945.
76. Jones, L. M.: Bitters, carminatives, antacids, bile salts, emetics and antemetics. In Veterinary Pharmacology and Therapeutics, 3rd ed. Edited by L. M. Jones. Ames, Iowa State University Press, 1965, p. 65.
77. Carroll, F. D., Goss, H., and Howell, C. E.: The synthesis of B vitamins in the horse. J. Anim. Sci. 8:290, 1949.
78. Steele, J. R.: Further observations on the use of B vitamins in standardbred horses. Vet. Med., 45:48, 1950.

79. Penfold, J. L.: Effect of cyproheptadine and a multivitamin preparation of appetite stimulation, weight gain and linear growth. Med. J. Aust. *1*:307, 1971.

80. Modell, W.: Status and prospect of drugs for overeating. J.A.M.A., *173*:1131, 1960.

81. Murray, M., Robinson, P. B., and McKeating, F. S.: Peptic ulceration in the dog: a clinical-pathological study. Vet. Rec. *91*:445, 1972.

82. McMillan, D. E., and Freeman, R. B.: The milk-alkali syndrome: a study of the acute disorder with comments on the development of the chronic condition. Medicine *44*:485, 1965.

83. Newberne, P. M., and Wilson, R. B.: Renal damage associated with silicon compounds in dogs. Proc. Natl. Acad. Sci. *65*:872, 1970.

84. Fordtran, J. S., Morawski, S. G., and Richardson, C. T.: *In vivo* and *in vitro* evaluation of liquid antacids. N. Engl. J. Med. *288*:923, 1973.

85. Dunlop, R. H.: Pathogenesis of ruminant lactic acidosis. Adv. Vet. Sci. Comp. Med. *16*:259, 1970.

86. Cocking, J. B., and MacCaig, J. N.: Effect of low dosage of carbenoxolone sodium on gastric ulcer healing and acid secretion. Gut *10*:219, 1969.

87. Turpie, A. G. G., Runcie, J., and Thompson, T. J.: Clinical trial of deglycyrrhizinized liquorice in gastric ulcer. Gut *10*:299, 1969.

88. Combes, B., and Stakelum, G. S.: Conjugation of sulfobromophthalein sodium with glutathione in thioether linkage by the rat. J. Clin. Invest. *39*:1214, 1960.

89. Bevan, J. A.: Essentials of Pharmacology. New York, Hoeber, 1969, p. 644.

90. Lim, R. K. S.: A revised concept of the mechanism of analgesia and pain. *In* Pain. Edited by R. S. Knighton and P. R. Dumke. Boston, Little, Brown and Co., 1966, p. 117.

91. Davis, L. E.: Pharmacology of anti-inflammatory drugs. Proc. Symposium on Equine Pharmacology and Therapeutics. A.A.E.P., Golden, Colo., 1969, pp. 61–74.

92. Modell, W., Schild, H. O., and Wilson, A.: Applied Pharmacology. Philadelphia, W. B. Saunders Co., 1976, p. 395.

93. Gray, G. W., and Yano, B. L.: A study of the actions of methampyrone and of a commercial intestinal extract preparation on intestinal motility. Am. J. Vet. Res. *36*:201, 1975.

94. Davis, L. E., and Jenkins, W. L.: Some considerations regarding drug therapy in ruminant animals. Bovine Pract. *9*:57, 1974.

95. Davis, L. E., and Donnelly, E. J.: Analgesic drugs in the cat. J.A.V.M.A. *153*:1161, 1968.

96. Hall, L. W.: Wright's Anesthesia and Analgesia, 7th ed. London, Bailliere Tindall, 1971, p. 153.

97. Hall, L. W.: Wright's Anesthesia and Analgesia, 7th ed. London, Bailliere Tindall, 1971, p. 155.

98. Anonymous: Conditions for the distribution and use of methadone. Code of Federal Regulations, Title 21, Sec. 130.44.

99. Lowe, J. E.: Pentazocine (Talwin-V) for the relief of abdominal pain in ponies—a comparative evaluation with description of a colic model for analgesia evaluation. Proceedings of the American Association of Equine Practitioners, 1969, p. 31.

100. Chase, Patricia E.: Personal communication.

101. Davis, L. E., and Sturm, B. L.: Drug effects and plasma concentration of pentazocine in domesticated animals. Am. J. Vet. Res. *31*:1631, 1970.

102. Paddleford, R. R., and Short, C. E.: An evaluation of naloxone as a narcotic antagonist in the dog. J.A.V.M.A. *163*:144, 1973.

103. Blevins, D., and Lowe, J. E.: Unpublished data.

104. Moye, R. J., Pailet, A., and Smith, M. W., Jr.: Clinical use of xylazine in dogs and cats. V.M./S.A.C. *68*:236, 1973.

105. McCashin, F. B., and Gabel, A. A.: Evaluation of xylazine as a sedative and preanesthetic agent in horses. Am. J. Vet. Res. *36*:1421, 1975.

106. Hopkins, T. J.: The clinical pharmacology of xylazine in cattle. Aust. Vet. J. *48*:109, 1972.

107. Hoffman, P. E.: Clinical evaluation of xylazine as a chemical restraining agent, sedative and analgesic in horses. J.A.V.M.A. *164*:42, 1974.

108. Newkirk, H. L., and Miles, D. G.: Xylazine as a sedative-analgesic for dogs and cats. Mod. Vet. Pract. *55*:677, 1974.

109. Clarke, K. W., and Hall, L. W.: "Xylazine"—a new sedative for horses and cattle. Vet. Rec. *85*:512, 1969.

110. Cabana, B. E.: Importance of biopharmaceutics and pharmacokinetics in clinical medicine. Arzneim. Forsch. *26*:151, 1976.

111. Siekevitz, P.: The organization of biologic membranes. N. Engl. J. Med. *283*:1035, 1970.

112. Singer, S. J., and Nicolson, G. L.: The fluid mosaic model of the structure of cell membranes. Science (N.Y.) *175*:720, 1972.

113. Schanker, L. S.: Passage of drugs across body membranes. Pharmacol. Rev. *14*:501, 1962.

114. Travell, J.: The influence of the hydrogen ion concentration on the absorption of alkaloids from the stomach. J. Pharmacol. Exp. Ther. *69*:21, 1940.

115. McGuigan, J. E.: On the distribution of gastrin release (editorial). Gastroenterology *64*:497, 1973.

116. Gregory, R. A.: The gastrointestinal hormones: a review of recent advances. J. Physiol. (Lond.) *241*:1, 1974.

117. Jacobs, M. H.: Some aspects of cell permeability to weak electrolytes. Cold Spring Harbor Symp. Quant. Biol. *8*:30, 1940.

118. Phillipson, A. T., and McAnally, R. A.: Studies on the fate of carbohydrates in the rumen of the sheep. J. Exp. Biol. *19*:199, 1942.

119. Masson, M. J., and Phillipson, A. T.: The absorption of acetate, propionate and butyrate from the rumen of sheep. J. Physiol. (Lond.) *113*:189, 1951.

120. Gingerich, D. A., Baggot, J. D., and Yeary, R. A.: Pharmacokinetics and dosage of aspirin in cattle. J.A.V.M.A. *167*:945, 1975.

121. Brodie, B. B., and Hogben, C. A. M.: Some physicochemical factors in drug action. J. Pharm. Pharmacol. *9*:345, 1957.

122. Hogben, C. A. M., Tocco, D. J., Brodie, B. B., and Schanker, L. S.: On the mechanism of the intestinal absorption of drugs. J. Pharmacol. Exp. Ther. *125*:275, 1959.

123. Wilbrandt, W., and Rosenberg, T.: The concept of carrier transport and its corollaries in pharmacology. Pharmacol. Rev. *13*:109, 1961.

124. Stein, W. D.: The Movement of Molecules Across Cell Membranes. New York, Academic Press, 1967, p. 1.

125. Lewis, W. H.: Pinocytosis. Johns Hopkins Hosp. Bull. *49*:17, 1931.

126. Fawcett, D. W.: Surface specializations of absorbing cells. J. Histochem. Cytochem. *13*:75, 1965.

127. Levy, G.: Kinetics and implications of dissolution rate limited gastrointestinal absorption of drugs. *In* Physicochemical Aspects of Drug Action. Proceedings of the Third International Pharmacological Meeting, Vol. 7. Edited by E. J. Ariens, Oxford. Pergamon Press, 1968, p. 330.

128. Cabana, B. E., Willhite, L. E., and Bierwagen, M. E.: Pharmacokinetic evaluation of the oral absorption of different ampicillin preparations in beagle dogs. Antimicrob. Agents Chemother. Suppl., p. 35, 1969.

129. Rowland, M., Riegelman, S., and Epstein, W. L.: Absorption kinetics of griseofulvin in man. J. Pharm. Sci. *57*:984, 1968.

130. Riegelman, S.: Clinical evaluation of the effect of formulation variables on therapeutic performance of drugs. Drug Inform. Bull. *3*:59, 1969.

131. Bates, T. R., Sequeira, J. A., and Tembo, A. V.: Effect of food on nitrofurantoin absorption. Clin. Pharmacol. Ther. *16*:63, 1974.

132. Kabasakabian, P., Katz, M., Rosenkrantz, B., and Townley, E.: Parameters affecting absorption of griseofulvin in a human subject using urinary metabolite excretion data. J. Pharm. Sci. *59*:595, 1970.

133. Welling, P. G., Lyons, L. L., Tse, F. L. S., and Craig, W. A.: Propoxyphene and norpropoxyphene: influence of diet and fluid on plasma levels. Clin. Pharmacol. Ther. *19*:559, 1976.

134. Waisbren, B. A., and Huechel, J. S.: Reduced absorption of aureomycin caused by aluminum hydroxide gel (Amphojel). Proc. Soc. Exp. Biol. Med. *73*:73, 1950.

135. Barr, W. H., Adir, J., and Garnetson, L.: Decrease of tetracycline absorption in man by sodium bicarbonate. Clin. Pharmacol. Ther. *12*:779, 1971.

136. Greenblatt, D. J., Shader, R. I. Harmatz, J. S., Franke, K., and Koch-Weser, J.: Influence of magnesium and aluminum hydroxide mixture on chlordiazepoxide absorption. Clin. Pharmacol. Ther. *19*:234, 1976.

137. Hurwitz, A.: The effects of antacids on the gastrointestinal drug absorption. II. Effect on sulfadiazine and quinine. J. Pharmacol. Exp. Ther. *179*:485, 1971.

138. Hurwitz, A., and Sheehan, M. B.: The effects of antacids on absorption of orally administered pentobarbital in the rat. J. Pharmacol. Exp. Ther. *179*:124, 1971.

139. Hurwitz, A., Robinson, R. G., Vats, T. S., Whittier, F. C., and Herrin, W. F.: Effects of antacids on gastric emptying. Gastroenterology *71*:268, 1976.

140. Wagner, J. G.: Biopharmaceutics: absorption aspects. J. Pharm. Sci. *50*:539, 1961.

141. Sacchetti, G., Nicholis, F. B., and Roncoroni, L.: Evaluation in man of the effects of an anticholinergic agent on the gastric emptying by a quantitative x-ray method. J. Pharmacol. Exp. Ther. *145*:393, 1964.

142. Burks, T. F.: Gastrointestinal pharmacology. Annu. Rev. Pharmacol. Toxicol *16*:15, 1976.

143. Consolo, S., and Garattini, S.: Effect of desipramine on intestinal absorption of phenylbutazone and other drugs. Eur. J. Pharmacol. *6*:322, 1969.

144. De Marco, T. J., and Levine, R. R.: Role of the lymphatics in the

intestinal absorption and distribution of drugs. J. Pharmacol. Exp. Ther. *169*:142, 1969.

145. Ther, L., and Winne, D.: Drug absorption. Annu. Rev. Pharmacol. *11*:57, 1971.

146. Rowland, M., Benet, L. Z., and Graham, G. G.: Clearance concepts in pharmacokinetics J. Pharmacokinet. Biopharm. *1*:123, 1973.

147. Robinson, J. W. L., Jequier, J. -Cl., Felber, J. -P., and Mirkowitch, V.: Amino acid absorption by the intestinal mucosa. J. Surg. Res. *5*:150, 1964.

148. Alexander, F.: Factors influencing motility of perfused horse intestine. Q. J. Exp. Physiol. *36*:1, 1950.

149. Annison, E. F., and Lewis, D.: Metabolism in the Rumen. London, Methuen, 1959, p. 124.

150. Balch, C. C., and Campling, R. C.: Physiology of Digestion in the Ruminant. London, Butterworths, 1965.

151. Masson, M. J., and Phillipson, A. T.: The composition of the digesta leaving the abomasum of sheep. J. Physiol. (Lond.) *116*:98, 1952.

152. Bailey, C. B.: Saliva secretion and its relation to feeding in cattle. III: The rate of secretion of mixed saliva in the cow during eating, with an estimate of the magnitude of the total daily secretion of mixed saliva. Br. J. Nutr. *15*:443, 1961.

153. Kay, R. N. B.: The rate of flow and composition of various salivary secretions in sheep and calves. J. Physiol. (Lond.) *150*:515, 1960.

154. Hungate, R. E.: The Rumen and its Microbes. New York, Academic Press, 1966.

155. Baggot, J. D., Davis, L. E., and Reuning, R. H.: The disposition kinetics of amphetamine in the ruminant animal. Arch. Int. Pharmacodyn. Ther. *202*:17, 1973.

156. Karjalainen, J., Ojala, K., and Reissell, P.: Tissue concentrations of digoxin in an autopsy material. Acta Pharmacol. Toxicol. *34*:385, 1974.

157. Vajda, F., Williams, F. M., Davidson, S., Falconer, M. A., and Breckenridge, A.: Human brain, cerebrospinal fluid, and plasma concentrations of diphenylhydantoin and phenobarbital. Clin. Pharmacol. Ther. *15*:597, 1974.

158. Houghton, G. W., Richens, A., Toseland, P. A., Davidson, S., and Falconer, M. A.: Brain concentrations of phenytoin, phenobarbitone and primidone in epileptic patients. Eur. J. Clin. Pharmacol. *9*:73, 1975.

159. Gibaldi, M., Nagashima, R., and Levy, G.: Relationship between drug concentrations in plasma or serum and amount of drug in the body. J. Pharm. Sci. *58*:193, 1969.

160. Riegelman, S., Loo, J. C. K., and Rowland, M.: Shortcomings in pharmacokinetic analysis by conceiving the body to exhibit properties of a single compartment. J. Pharm. Sci. *57*:117, 1968.

161. Davis, L. E., and Westfall, B. A.: Species differences in biotransformation and excretion of salicylate. Am. J. Vet. Res. *33*:1253, 1972.

162. Yeary, R. A., and Swanson, W.: Aspirin dosages for the cat. J.A.V.M.A. *163*:1177, 1973.

163. Notari, R. E.: Pharmacokinetics and molecular modification: implications in drug design and evaluation. J. Pharm. Sci. *62*:865, 1973.

164. Oehme, F. W.: A Comparative Study of the Biotransformation and Excretion of Phenol. Ph. D. Dissertation, Columbia, MO, University of Missouri, 1969.

165. Rowland, M.: Influence of route of administration on drug availability. J. Pharm. Sci. *61*:70, 1972.

166. Boniface, J., Picone, D., Schebalin, M., Zfass, A. M., and Makhlouf, G. M.: Clearance rate, half-life and secretory potency of human gastrin-17-I in different species. Gastroenterology *71*:291, 1976.

167. Baggot, J. D., Ludden, T. M., and Powers, T. E.: The bioavailability, disposition kinetics and dosage of sulphadimethoxine in dogs. Can. J. Comp. Med. *40*:310, 1976.

168. Sams, R. A., and Baggot, J. D.: Bioavailability, disposition kinetics, and dosage of sulphadimethoxine in dogs—a correction. Can. J. Comp. Med. *41*:479, 1977.

169. Loo, J. C. K., and Riegelman, S.: New method for calculating the intrinsic absorption rate of drugs. J. Pharm. Sci. *57*: 918, 1968.

170. Scheline, R. R.: Drug metabolism by intestinal microorganisms. J. Pharm. Sci. *57*:202, 1968.

171. Williams, R. T.: Toxicologic implications of biotransformation by intestinal microflora. Toxicol. Appl. Pharmacol. *23*:769, 1972.

172. Dutton, G. J.: Glucuronide conjugation. *In* Metabolic Factors Controlling Duration of Drug Action. Edited by B. Uvnas. Oxford, Pergamon Press, 1961, p. 39.

173. Gregory, J. D.: Sulfate conjugation. *In* Metabolic Factors Controlling Duration of Drug Action. Edited by B. Uvnas. Oxford, Pergamon Press, 1962, p. 53.

174. Fouts, J. R.: The metabolism of drugs by subfraction of hepatic microsomes. Biochem. Biophys. Res. Commun. *6*:373, 1961.

175. Boyes, R. N., Adams, H. J., and Duce, B. R.: Oral absorption and disposition kinetics of lidocaine hydrochloride in dogs. J. Pharmacol. Exp. Ther. *174*:1, 1970.

176. Dollery, C. T., Davies, D. S., and Conolly, M. E.: Differences in the metabolism of drugs, depending upon their routes of administration. Ann. N. Y. Acad. Sci. *179*:108, 1971.

177. Smith, R. L.: The biliary excretion and enterohepatic circulation of drugs and other organic compounds. Prog. Drug Res. *9*:299, 1966.

178. Dencker, H., Dencker, S. J., Green, A., and Nagy, A.: Intestinal absorption, demethylation, and enterohepatic circulation of imipramine. Clin. Pharmacol. Ther. *19*:584, 1976.

179. Bellamy, H. M., Bates, B. B., and Reinarz, J. A.: Lincomycin metabolism in patients with hepatic insufficiency: effect of liver disease on lincomycin serum concentrations. Antimicrob. Agents Chemother. p. 36, 1967.

180. Brandl, R., Arkenau, C., Simon, C., Malerczyk, V., and Eidelloth, G.: The pharmacokinetics of clindamycin in the presence of abnormal liver and renal function. Dtsch. Med. Wochenschr. *97*:1057, 1972.

181. Brown, R. B., Barza, M., Brusch, J. L., Hashimoto, Y., and Weinstein, L.: Pharmacokinetics of lincomycin and clindamycin phosphate in a canine model. J. Infect. Dis. *131*:252, 1975.

182. Grodsky, G. M., Carbone, J. V., and Fanska, R.: Identification of metabolites of sulfobromophthalein. J. Clin. Invest. *38*:1981, 1959.

183. Brown, D. M., and Acred, P.: "Penbritin"—a new broad-spectrum antibiotic. Preliminary pharmacology and chemotherapy. Br. Med. J. *2*:197, 1961.

184. Mortimer, P. R., Mackie, D. B., and Haynes, S.: Ampicillin levels in human bile in the presence of biliary tract disease. Br. Med. J. *3*:88, 1969.

185. Abou-El-Makarem, M. M., Millburn, P., Smith, R. L., and Williams, R. T.: Biliary excretion of foreign compounds. Biochem. J. *105*:1289, 1967.

186. Williams, R. T.: Species variations in drug biotransformations. *In* Fundamentals of Drug Metabolism and Drug Disposition. Edited by B. N. LaDu, H. G. Mandel, and E. L. Way. Baltimore, The Williams & Wilkins Co., 1971, p. 187.

187. Neff-Davis, C., Davis, L. E., and Powers, T. E.: Comparative body compositions of the dog and goat. Am. J. Vet. Res. *36*:309, 1975.

188. Grim, E.: Circulation. *In* Handbook of Physiology, Vol. II, Sec. 2. Baltimore, The Williams & Wilkins Co., 1963, p. 1439.

189. Jusko, W. J., and Levy, G.: Absorption, metabolism, and excretion of riboflavin-5'-phosphate in man. J. Pharm. Sci. *56*:58, 1967.

Chapter 19

ANTIMICROBIAL DRUGS

THOMAS E. POWERS and H. DWIGHT MERCER

Antimicrobial agents have had a tremendous influence upon the pattern of infectious diseases throughout the world. The benefits remain unquestionable, but as is the usual case, there is generally a rather substantial cost associated. In the process of treating infected patients with antimicrobial agents, many new problems have been created.

There are three major classes of antimicrobial agents employed for veterinary therapy, prophylaxis, and as low-level feed additives for growth promotion purposes. These are respectively: (1) the classic antibiotics, (2) the sulfonamides, and (3) the nitrofurans.

The number of individual compounds in each class is large. The situation is complicated by the fact that their use for a particular purpose is often determined as much by personal preference as it is by objective scientific considerations. These compounds are known to have great influence on the enteric flora following feeding use, prophylactic use, and therapeutic usage in human and veterinary medicine. It is now generally recognized and accepted that enteric microorganisms are not restricted to a single animal species nor to well-confined ecologic niches.

It is truly a short segment of modern history that man has had the benefits of antimicrobial agents. Following the introduction of sulfonamides in 1935, then came tyrothricin (1939), penicillin (1940), streptomycin (1944), bacitracin (1945), polymyxin (1947), chloramphenicol (1947), chlortetracycline (1948), neomycin (1949), oxytetracycline (1950), nystatin (1951), erythromycin (1952), isoniazid (1952), tetracycline (1953), novobiocin (1955), vancomycin (1956), kanamycin (1956), and gentamicin and the semi-synthetic penicillins in the 1960s.

The annual production and usage of antibiotics in the United States increased from a total of 4.2 million pounds in 1960 to a total of 16.9 million pounds by 1970 (Table 19–1). The amount utilized in human and veterinary pharmaceutical purposes was 9.6 million pounds and the other uses, which were predominantly as feed additives, totaled 7.3 million pounds by 1970.[1,2]

Table 19–1. Annual production of antibiotics in the United States[1]*

| | Year | | |
	1960	1965	1970
Medicinal	3.0	4.7	9.6
Feed additive	1.2	2.8	7.3
Total	4.2	7.5	16.9

* Production is in millions of pounds.

The antimicrobial agents have become the most commonly used drugs in the practice of veterinary medicine. In this chapter, we want to discuss their values and limitations as therapeutic agents and as feed additives, as these apply to gastroenterology. It is assumed that the reader has a thorough understanding of the mode of action, the spectrum, chemistry, pharmacology and toxicity of the various antimicrobial agents, or access to such information. Certain basic topics will be discussed as they apply to gastroenterology.

CHEMOTHERAPEUTIC TRIANGLE

The following, which has been designated the chemotherapeutic triangle, illustrates the relationship among the host, the parasite, and the therapeutic agent.

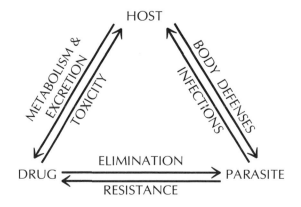

As we administer the drug to the host, we find that it cannot only act against the microorganism but also

311

affect the host directly or indirectly to produce an untoward effect. Direct untoward effects include nephrotoxicity and hepatotoxicity; indirect factors include alteration of the intestinal flora. Many antimicrobial agents may produce gastrointestinal signs such as anorexia, nausea, vomiting, diarrhea, and abdominal pain. These signs of disease may be due to irritation of the mucosa, to central action, or to alteration of the intestinal flora.

Some basic aspects emphasized by the chemotherapeutic triangle are (1) the potential value of even a single dose in reducing the severity of infection, (2) the importance of the host defenses in ultimately affecting a cure, (3) an inhibitory or bacteriostatic drug may effect a cure, possibly as well as a bactericidal drug, in the presence of adequate host defense mechanisms, (4) in the absence of adequate defense mechanisms, a preferred bactericidal agent may be ineffective, and (5) the host may overcome the infection in the absence of drugs.

Animals and man can and do recover from infections without antimicrobial therapy. The administration of an effective dose of the properly selected antibiotic may reduce the number of bacteria or slow their rate of multiplication adequately to permit the host defenses to overcome the infection more quickly. Even inhibitory agents as well as static agents can reduce the number of pathogens over time. Fortunately, many antimicrobial agents have relatively high therapeutic indices, such as the penicillins. It is hoped that untoward side effects are kept at a minimum. Not depicted in the diagram but acting at the level of the host are supportive therapy and environmental factors.

The gastrointestinal tracts of the various species of domestic animals possess a normal microbial flora which is part of the host defense barrier. The administration of antimicrobial agents in the intestinal tract will affect not only the pathogens but also the normal intestinal flora. The increased use of antibacterial chemotherapy has been reported to encourage commensal colonization by candida yeasts, particularly in the oropharyngeal cavity and the intestine.[3] This alteration of flora may result in a more dire outcome than the pathogen would cause. For this reason, it is considered extremely important to raise the question of the value of antimicrobial agents in the treatment of intestinal diseases. There appears to be little scientific evidence to prove that oral antimicrobials are effective in diarrhea of neonatal calves, for example.

Numerous studies have demonstrated that the routine prophylactic use of antimicrobial agents in simple surgical procedures is contraindicated. Increase in postoperative infection has been reported following the routine prophylactic use of antimicrobial agents.[4] On the other hand, in high-risk patients, it becomes necessary to employ antimicrobial agents, and several reports have shown a subsequent decrease in wound infections.[5,6] Others have reported equivocal results.[7,8]

The high risk cases requiring antimicrobial therapy are: (1) those that involve impaired natural defense mechanisms, (2) those in which the surgical procedure could result in massive bacterial contamination, and (3) those that involve prolonged and extensive surgery with unavoidable tissue damage. The best results are generally obtained when the antimicrobial agent is given before or close to the time of initial contamination. The longer the drug administration is delayed after the lesion has been established, the less its effectiveness.

Poorly absorbed drugs, such as the aminoglycosides and nonabsorbable sulfonamides such as sulfathalidine or sulfasuxidine, have been used to reduce bacterial flora prior to intestinal surgery. Neomycin or kanamycin sulfate at concentrations above 100 μg/g of feces is reported effective in eliminating bacteria from the gut.[9] Nystatin has been used currently to control fungi. In order to control anaerobic bacteria, especially bacteroides, a drug such as lincomycin,[10] clindamycin, or chloramphenicol would be needed.

The host eliminates the antimicrobial drug through metabolism, excretion, or a combination of the two. At the same time the host is reacting to the microorganism and attempting to rid itself of the infection. The antimicrobial agent should be capable of reducing the number of infectious organisms without interfering with defense mechanisms. On the other hand, the microorganism is also capable in many cases of responding to the antimicrobial agent and acquiring drug resistance through such mechanisms as mutation, transduction, transformation and/or conjugation.

SELECTION OF ANTIMICROBIAL AGENTS

The first premise in the treatment of infectious diseases is that specific infections are caused by one or more specific microorganisms. One then attempts to select that drug or drugs which will produce an inhibitory, bacteriostatic, or bactericidal effect on the microorganism(s) involved. This may not be a single drug or group of drugs for any given situation; instead, there may be several suitable treatments from which to choose. However, in most cases one drug or group of drugs would be preferred.

Some therapies are empirically based. For example, dosages of tylosin ranging from 11 to 200 mg/kg daily and lasting from 1 week to 5 years and 10 months were reported effective in a variety of long-standing spontaneous forms of canine inflammatory bowel disease. From this uncontrolled trial, it was suggested that the tylosin-vitamin combination had an effectiveness in canine enterocolitis far superior to that of salicylazosulfapyridine.[11]

Although clinical results are the only true measure of the value of therapy, one must be cautious in the interpretation of results. Even placebos have been credited with producing a wide variety of effects in veterinary medicine and human medicine.[12]

A list of suggested antimicrobial drugs of choice for different species of microorganisms is given in Tables 19–2 and 19–3. These tables are intended only as a guide to initiation of therapy. One must perform a sensitivity test to determine the true antimicrobial drug of choice.

Because bacteria become drug-resistant and new antimicrobial agents are developed, the drug or drugs of choice for particular diseases can and do change. However, the basic principles guiding therapy remain essentially unaltered.

The veterinarian, in determining the correct therapy for a suspected infectious disease, must

Table 19–2. Antimicrobial agents used in treatment of infections produced by gram-positive bacteria[13]

Antimicrobial Agent (Class)	Primary Agent in the Treatment of Infection Produced by:	Secondary Agent in the Treatment of Infection Produced by:
Cephalosporins		*Staphylococcus aureus, Staphylococcus epidermidis* *Streptococcus pneumoniae* *Streptococcus* Lancefield groups A-F Viridans group (alpha-hemolytic, non-Lancefield groupable streptococci) Peptostreptococcal species
Clindamycin, Lincomycin		Same as erythromycin Anaerobic bacteria
Erythromycin	*Corynebacterium diphtheriae*	*Staphylococcus aureus, Staphylococcus epidermidis* *Streptococcus pneumoniae* *Streptococcus* Lancefield groups A-F Viridans group (alpha-hemolytic, non-Lancefield groupable streptococci) Peptostreptococcal species Clostridia—all species
Penicillins Penicillin G	*Staphylococcus aureus, Staphylococcus epidermidis* (nonpenicillinase producing) *Streptococcus pneumoniae* *Streptococcus* Lancefield groups A-F Viridans groups (alpha-hemolytic, non-Lancefield groupable streptococci) Clostridia—all species *Corynebacterium diphtheriae* *Actinomyces israelii* Anaerobic bacteria	
Penicillinase-resistant penicillins	*Staphylococcus aureus, Staphylococcus epidermidis* (penicillinase-producing)	*Streptococcus pneumoniae* *Streptococcus* Lancefield groups A-F Viridans group (alpha-hemolytic, non-Lancefield groupable streptococci)
Vancomycin		*Staphylococcus aureus, Staphylococcus epidermidis* Enterococcal species (Lancefield group D streptococci) *Streptococcus faecalis*

Table 19–3. Antimicrobial agents used in treatment of infections produced by gram-negative bacteria[13]

Antimicrobial Agent (Class)	Primary Agent in the Treatment of Infection Produced by:	Secondary Agent in the Treatment of Infection Produced by:
Aminoglycosides Streptomycin	*Yersinia pestis, Francisella tularensis*	
Kanamycin	*Proteus morganii, Proteus rettgeri* (indol-positive species)	*Serratia marcescens*
	Klebsiella pneumoniae	*Providencia stuartii* and *Providencia alcalifaciens*
Gentamicin	*Pseudomonas aeruginosa* *Serratia marcescens* *Providencia stuartii* and *Providencia alcalifaciens*	Enterobacter sp. *Proteus rettgeri, Proteus morganii,* and *Proteus vulgaris* (indol-positive species)
Chloramphenicol	*Salmonella typhosa*	Shigella species *Haemophilus influenzae, Neisseria meningitidis, Bacteroides fragilis,* all subspecies
Cephalosporins	*Klebsiella pneumoniae*	*Escherichia coli* *Proteus mirabilis*
Clindamycin, Lincomycin	*Bacteroides fragilis*	Same as erythromycin Anaerobic bacteria
Penicillins Penicillin G	*Neisseria gonorrhoeae* *Neisseria meningitidis* *Bacteroides fragilis*	
Ampicillin- Amoxicillin	*Salmonella typhimurium* and *Salmonella enteritidis* Shigella sp., *Escherichia coli, Proteus mirabilis, Haemophilus influenzae*	
Carbenicillin	*Pseudomonas aeruginosa* *Proteus rettgeri, Proteus morganii,* and *Proteus vulgaris* (indol-positive species)	
Polymyxin B and E		*Escherichia coli* *Pseudomonas aeruginosa*
Sulfonamides	*Escherichia coli, Proteus mirabilis*	
Tetracyclines	*Vibrio cholerae* Moraxella sp.; Mima sp. Brucella sp.	Enterobacter species *Escherichia coli, Klebsiella pneumoniae,* Proteus sp.

assess the condition of the host, the characteristics of the infection, and the interactions between the two. One must find answers to the following: Is there definitely an infection present that warrants the use of antimicrobial agents? Does the animal possess adequate normal defense mechanisms and is the host responding in an adequate way to the infectious agent; i.e., are there normal inflammatory, immunologic and cellular-type responses? Are there available antimicrobial drugs that can be effective against the infection? Will the use of an antimicrobial drug be worth the risks as far as the alteration of the normal intestinal flora and the possible establishment of a flora that is resistant to the antimicrobial drug used?

INTERACTION OF ANTIMICROBIAL DRUGS IN COMBINATION

Some of the reasons proposed for use of combinations of antimicrobial drugs have been:

1. Prompt treatment of desperately ill patients
2. Treatment of a true mixed infection
3. Prevention of emergence of resistant strains
4. A synergistic action

The experienced veterinary clinician can, in many cases, make a presumptive diagnosis of the causative etiologic agent(s) prior to the return of the laboratory culture results. In such a case, one may correctly select the single antimicrobial drug or combinations thereof which may be effective against the microorganism. Quite often, however, the specific etiologic agent and its sensitivity spectrum to antimicrobial drugs are not known with certainty. One is then plagued with the fear of inadequate treatment of the patient. This uncertainty leads in too many cases to selecting for use two or more antibiotics in the hope of being more certain of having a drug active against the pathogens. This action neglects the risk that is taken by adding the second or third antimicrobial drug.

In addition to giving a false sense of security and increasing the cost of therapy, the chances for adverse drug reactions are increased. In most instances, a combination of antimicrobial drugs is no more effective than its single most effective member.[14]

A rational approach to the quantification and prediction of combined antibiotic action must be based on:[15]

1. Kinetics of the antimicrobial agents
2. Mechanism of action of each of the agents in question
3. Dose-response relationship over a wide concentration range for the separate antibiotics
4. The strain and species of the organism

In some life-threatening bacteremic infections in animals, the veterinarian may feel compelled to administer two or more antimicrobial drugs simultaneously. The selection of these two or more drugs should still be directed at the most probable causes of the infection. For example, if septicemia is a result of invasion of intestinal organisms, one should use drugs that are most active against the type of organism found in the intestinal tract. The drugs selected should usually consist of (1) an aminoglycoside other than the streptomycins, such as neomycin, spectinomycin, gentamicin, kanamycin, tobramycin, amikacin, netilmicin, sisomicin,[16,17,18,19] and (2) ampicillin, carbenicillin, or possibly one of the polymyxins. Because of the presence of Bacteroides in the intestinal flora, a drug active against anaerobes, such as carbenicillin, may also be used.[19,20,21]

Polymixins have been shown to be active against most species of gram-negative rods except Proteus and Providencia and many strains of Enterobacteriaceae. Ampicillin and amoxicillin usually have good activity against enterococci.[18]

A study of 610 strains of *Pseudomonas aeruginosa* isolates showed that the effectiveness of each drug ranked highest to lowest was: tobramycin, colistin, ticarcillin, carbenicillin, gentamicin, and kanamycin.[22] A high percentage of *E. coli* and *Klebsiella sp.* from dogs and cats are resistant to tetracycline and streptomycin while 30% of the *E. coli* and 50% of the *Klebsiella sp.* are resistant to chloramphenicol. Polymixin and gentamicin have good in vitro effect on pseudomonas.[23]

The presence of two or more microorganisms producing an infection in the intestinal tract or on a local mucous membrane may dictate the need for two antimicrobial agents. Such nonabsorbable drugs as neomycin, combined with bacitracin and/or polymixin, are an example of a combination of drugs providing a broader spectrum of activity.

Combinations of sulfonamides have been used, such as triple sulfonamides USP, in order to reduce the renal toxicity of same. This takes advantage of the principle of an additive antibacterial effect, but without additive effect as far as their tendency to crystallize in the nephron.

Drug Synergism

Certain combinations of drugs under certain conditions have been shown to exert a synergistic action. One of these is the combination of sulfonamide with a folic acid antagonist such as trimethoprim or pyrimethamine. By acting at two different sequential steps in the biosynthesis of tetrahydrofolic acid in the bacteria, these two bacteriostatic drugs may produce a bactericidal action,[24] and in certain species may require a considerably reduced amount of each to be effective in producing a cure. A combination of sulfamethoxazole, trimethroprim, and colistin is synergistic against several *Pseudomonas* strains.[25]

Antimicrobial synergism may be manifested by enhancement of bactericidal rate.[14] This type of synergism has been demonstrated with gram-negatives, rods, staphylococci, and other organisms. It has been studied the most with enterococci, *Streptococcus faecalis*. The utilization of an aminoglycoside such as streptomycin, kanamycin, or gentamicin in combination with penicillin results in an immediate striking increase in the rate of bactericidal action.[26] It is assumed that this type of synergism is related to an alteration of microbial permeability by one drug so the penetration of the second drug is enhanced; i.e., penicillin damages the cell membrane thereby permitting the streptomycin to penetrate intracellularly in greater concentrations to produce its bactericidal effect.

In enterococcal endocarditis in rabbits and also in vitro, synergism has been shown using penicillin plus gentamicin, streptomycin, or sisomicin.[27] Amoxicillin combined with streptomycin, kanamycin, or gentamicin showed synergy against enterococci homologous with that of combinations of penicillin or ampicillin with aminoglycoside antibiotics.[28]

Nafcillin and gentamicin were proved to be synergistic against eight strains of *Staphylococcus aureus* in broth culture and in rabbits with *S. aureus* endocarditis. Gentamicin was ineffective alone, but enhanced the bactericidal rate of nafcillin when in combination.[29] Combination of tobramycin and carbenicillin was shown to be synergistic against 7 of 35 isolates of *Pseudomonas aeruginosa* tested.[30]

In vitro experiments have shown either an additive or synergistic activity by combinations of penicillin with cephalothin, penicillin with rolitetracycline, and cephalothin with rolitetracycline in 40 to 50% of the *E. coli* and *S. aureus* strains tested.[31]

Synergism was demonstrated between aminoglycosides and tetracycline or chloramphenicol on urinary tract isolates of coliforms.[32] Ampicillin, plus aminoglycosides were synergistic against some *Proteus*, *Klebsiella*, and enterobacter.[33,34,35]

Michel demonstrated a synergistic bactericidal effect of a combination of chloramphenicol and penicillin G against 17 of 20 β-lactamase-producing strains of *S. aureus*. It was their interpretation that this synergism was due to the chloramphenicol-induced inhibition of a β-lactamase production by the bacteria. Synergism or antagonism could be obtained depending upon the concentration of chloramphenicol used. With some inhibitory (low) concentrations of chloramphenicol, a synergistic effect was obtained whereas higher concentrations produced an antagonism to the penicillin.[2]

Mixtures containing equipotent fractions of clindamycin and lincomycin showed equivalence or indifference of effects on *S. aureus*. On the other hand, combinations of clindamycin and lincomycin are less active than the a priori equipotent concentration of either drug alone in their action against *E. coli*, demonstrating unequivocally an antagonism of effects.[36]

It has been proposed that it is reasonable to use combinations of antibiotics for initial therapy when one suspects gram-negative infections, since a single antibiotic may not produce an antibacterial spectrum which is broad enough to act against the common pathogens encountered.[37] For instance, carbenicillin and gentamicin were synergistic against 70% of the strains of *Pseudomonas aeruginosa* tested. Cephalothin plus gentamicin appears to be the best combination against *Proteus* and *Klebsiella*

strains, inhibiting 81 and 73% of these strains, respectively.

Carbenicillin and cephalothin were also shown to have good activity against *Proteus* strains, inhibiting 76%. The carbenicillin and cephalothin combination showed the highest frequency of synergistic activity against the strains studied.[37]

To explain the synergy seen between certain penicillins, it is proposed that the poorly hydrolyzed compounds such as methicillin and cloxacillin, having markedly greater affinities for the active center of the enzyme penicillinase, interact with the penicillinase thereby acting as competitive inhibitors of the hydrolysis of other antibiotics such as ampicillin. In other words, the methicillin or cloxacillin acts as a penicillinase substrate, freeing the ampicillin to be active.

Disadvantages of Drug Combinations

There are several disadvantages to the combination of antimicrobial drugs. The first of these is the problem of dosage. Unless drugs have elimination kinetics that are very similar, it is difficult to predict when to give the second, third, and fourth dose of a combination product. For example, a combination of procaine penicillin G and dihydrostreptomycin, commonly used in veterinary medicine, has markedly different absorption and elimination kinetics in the dog. Procaine penicillin G, due to delayed absorption rate, may give an effective concentration for a period of 12 to 24 hours, when administered by the intramuscular or subcutaneous route. On the other hand, the effective concentration with dihydrostreptomycin may be as short as 4 to 8 hours. When does one repeat the second dose of such a combination product? If one does not maintain an adequate dihydrostreptomycin concentration, this can permit the emergence of resistant bacteria. In contrast, dihydrostreptomycin and procaine penicillin G have somewhat similar effective concentrations when given in combination to cattle and horses, and therefore, can be dosed at proper intervals.

A second disadvantage is that antagonism may occur between the drugs in combination. Just as two or more agents may be synergistic or additive to each other, they may also be antagonistic to each other; i.e., there may be less response with the combination than with either drug alone. Chlortetracycline, chloramphenicol, and macrolide antibiotics such as erythromycin are drugs that have been shown to antagonize penicillin and aminoglycosides.[38] The first group of drugs are all inhibitors of protein synthesis, whereas the penicillins are known to inhibit cell wall synthesis. The aminoglycosides interfere with ribosomal protein synthesis. Vancomycin and bacitracin inhibit cell wall synthesis and the polymixins act on the cell membrane, and have not been reported to antagonize the penicillins or aminoglycosides.

Antagonism between chloramphenicol and penicillin was shown in rabbits with *Streptococcus viridans* endocarditis. If the penicillin was administered before chloramphenicol, it was shown to eliminate the antagonism whereas if chloramphenicol was given before penicillin or with the penicillin, then there was an antagonism. In order to eliminate the antagonism, the chloramphenicol had to be injected 1 hour after the penicillin instead of 1 hour before penicillin.[39]

Eight strains of three genera isolated (*Proteus, Escherichia,* and *Pseudomonas*) showed antagonism of carbenicillin or ampicillin by cephaloridine, cloxacillin, or 6-aminophenicillinic acid.

Sulfonamides have also been shown to antagonize penicillin. It has been postulated that the antagonism is possibly due to a bacteriostatic drug slowing microbial metabolism in such a way that the maximal effect of a bactericidal agent cannot be manifested. The exact mechanism of this antagonism is not known. The combinations of solutions of sulfonamides, due to their high alkalinity, can react with and inactivate such drugs as penicillin G, an organic acid. This is an example of an antagonism that occurs when two or more chemically incompatible drugs are mixed in a bottle, vial, or syringe. This should always be avoided by the veterinarian.

BIOAVAILABILITY OF ANTIMICROBIAL DRUGS

The rate and extent to which a drug reaches the systemic circulation intact and in the active form is termed its bioavailability. Drugs, chemicals, food substances, and other factors may prevent the antimicrobial drug from reaching the systemic circulation following oral administration.

Substances may increase or decrease the absorption of drugs by the intestinal tract. The oral usage of chymotrypsin along with phenethicillin has been shown to enhance the absorption of the penicillin.[40] On the other hand, porcine gastric mucin has been shown to interfere with the bioavailability of tetracycline from the gastrointestinal tract of in vivo and in vitro preparations of rat intestines.[41] It is proposed that the drug may be bound in some way to the mucin macromolecule thereby preventing the tetracycline from being properly and adequately absorbed.

In addition to the antimicrobial interactions mentioned in the previous section, it is important to be aware that other drugs, chemicals, and factors may prevent the antimicrobial agent from reaching its site of activity following oral administration. Chemical and physical binding and interactions of drugs can and do occur in gastrointestinal lumen and may alter the rate of transport or rate of metabolism to inactive compounds.

Altered Motility

Disease itself can markedly influence absorption rate. The presence of bacterial enteritis reduced the percent of human patients with a detectable blood concentration following the administration of 25 mg/kg of meclocycline. This was associated with and may have been the result of increased movement of material through the intestinal tract and/or the increased number of bowel movements per day.[42]

On the other hand, it has been shown that drugs that reduce gut motility can also slow absorption of several drugs.[43] Chloramphenicol could have an effect on other drugs and their absorption since it has been shown to suppress the movement of smooth muscle of rabbit ileum and jejunum, rabbit aortic strips, and guinea pig trachea. It is 15 to 25 times more active than ephedrine in this respect.[44]

Reduced rumen motility can effectively reduce absorption of drugs.[45,46,47] The atropinized sheep rumen absorbed sulfanilamide much more slowly than that of normal sheep. Blood concentrations attained were four to five times greater in normal animals. Microorganisms of the rumen and gut may metabolize and inactivate certain antibiotics. Chloramphenicol is very well absorbed when given orally and produces effective blood concentration as well as does parenteral administration in the dog, cat, pony, and pig, but it produces no therapeutic activity in the ruminant due to ruminal organisms breaking it down.[48]

Adsorption and Chelation

Aluminum hydroxide gels have been shown to delay gastric emptying time from $t_{1/2}$ of 13 minutes to 48 minutes;[49] in addition, they have been shown to delay gastrointestinal absorption of sulfadiazine in animals.[50] Kaolin (hydrated aluminum silicate) is an adsorbent that also adsorbs drugs and limits activity and gastrointestinal absorption of antibiotics such as lincomycin,[51] neomycin,[52] and probably others.

Certain ions and anions have been shown to affect both absorption and biologic activity of antimicrobial agents. For example, the tetracyclines are chelating agents whose absorption from the gut is reduced when given simultaneously with substances containing multivalent cations (Ca^{++}, Mg^{++}, or Al^{++}).[53,54] Calcium ion also influences the biologic activity of several antibiotics. Calcium decreases the activity of neomycin, polymixin, dihydrostreptomycin, chlortetracycline, oxytetracycline, carbomycin, bacitracin, and oleandomycin against *Pseudomonas aeruginosa*.[55] Alkaline solutions are known to enhance activity of the aminoglycosides, whereas tetracycline are more active in an acidic environment.

The bioavailability of tetracycline was also significantly reduced when tetracycline was taken either with zinc sulfate or with zinc citrate complex.[56]

Studies on concentration time curves and urinary excretion of tetracycline showed the inhibition of tetracycline absorption by iron salts to decrease in the following order: Ferrous sulfate inhibiting greater than ferrous fumarate, followed by ferrous succinate, with ferrous gluconate greater than ferrous tartrate, which was greater than ferric sodium edetate. They concluded that not only the iron tablets or capsules, but also the type of iron salt used may significantly influence the absorption of simultaneously ingested tetracycline.[57]

Interactions with Foods

Foods such as milk products interfere with the absorption of several antibiotics including erythromycin, oleandomycin, and tetracyclines. Some oral penicillins such as phenoxymethyl penicillin (Pen V) and ampicillin are not significantly affected by food.[58]

Triolein actually had a negative effect on the bioavailability of griseofulvin in one study. This, of course, does not agree with the positive effect of lipid diets that had been reported in the literature previously. It is proposed that the differences in these results may be due to the strain of rat, or to the use of corn oil in earlier work rather than triolein, or to the volume of lipid administered by the previous workers, and to the particle size of the drug used in the other experiments. The lipids in this study did increase the bioavailability of a sulfasoxazole preparation. Their conclusion is that in general the extent of drug absorption from the lipids increased with the polarity of the lipid.[59]

Oral neomycin has been shown to reduce the absorption of phenoxymethyl penicillin[60] and vitamin B_{12} from the gastrointestinal tract.[61] Neomycin also adversely affects the intestinal absorption of fats.[62]

It has been proposed[63] that neomycin impairs fat absorption by precipitation of bile salts in the lumen of the small intestine and by changing the bacterial flora in favor of bacteroides, clostridia, and certain anaerobic lactobacilli. These produce amidases that can remove taurine and glycine from bile salts and also have a direct toxic effect on the intestinal mucosa. Polymixin, kanamycin, and bacitracin may cause malabsorption of fat, carbohydrates, and protein, but less so than neomycin.

Manufacturer

With the increase in number of generic products one becomes concerned as to the bioavailability of the various preparations from different manufacturers. The literature contains an increasing number of bioavailability studies, some of which may give conflicting results.

In a study of nine brands of tetracycline hydrochloride tablets, 250 mg size, the bioavailability was found to vary markedly from a 70 to 100% range to as low as 20 to 30% range.[64] Bioavailability of two preparations of penicillin V were studied and found to be identical.[65]

A bioavailability study of single lots of 250-mg ampicillin capsules available from 17 different distributors and/or manufacturers surprisingly showed no statistically significant difference between any of the 17 products tested as to their bioavailability. Several of these ampicillin products had been manufactured by the same company but distributed by different companies.[66]

Four ampicillin preparations were studied after four routes of administration in cats.[67] Following a dose of 10 mg/kg of body weight, the percentage of absorption calculated for each of these routes and preparations was 28% for anhydrous ampicillin (I.M.), 56% for ampicillin trihydrate (S.C.), 18% for anhydrous ampicillin (oral, suspension), and 42% for anhydrous ampicillin (oral, capsule).

Disintegration and Dissolution

Recently, several studies have been directed at attempting to correlate bioavailability and disintegration and dissolution. Studying the bioavailability of three different sulfadiazine tablets in vivo in man and in vitro, there was no correlation of disintegration and dissolution with bioavailability. The extent of bioavailability of the three products was 78, 73, and 100%, respectively. Although product 1 was superior in disintegration and product 2 was superior in dissolution, product 3 was obviously superior in in vivo bioavailability.[68] On the other hand, in another study, the dissolution time was found to be strongly associated with the bioavailability of tetracycline but not with chlortetracycline and oxytetracycline[69] and, therefore, was proposed as a tool in assessing tetracycline formulations as to their bioavailability.

In addition to disintegration and dissolution, many other factors such as physiologic state of the animal, method of administration (per os or stomach tube), and type of drug can affect results obtained in bioavailability studies. The limitations of kinetic studies themselves must be considered.[70] The traditional definition of bioavailability is the area under the time concentration curve by a nonintravenous route as compared to a comparable area by the intravenous route. A limitation of this parameter is that it is a function of the method used to estimate these areas. In addition to this limitation, it is important to estimate total area under the curve and not just the area to the end of the sampling period. Some authors use the terms bioavailability and percent absorbed synonymously even though the latter is not a ratio of areas. The Loo-Riegelman method of calculating percent absorbed is based on amount eliminated by the kidneys and amount in the "tissues"; both of these quantities are based on estimates derived from I.V. data which are subject to laboratory and estimation errors.

FAILURE OF ANTIMICROBIAL THERAPY

The most common cause of failure of antimicrobial therapy is inaccurate diagnosis. This often occurs when one depends too greatly on laboratory methods without knowing their limitations. In addition to normal human error, adequate facilities often are not available for anaerobic culture. For example, when E. coli is isolated from a deep lesion, one should suspect other enteric organisms, such as the anaerobes, e.g., Bacteroides.

A second factor is improper dosage schedule or route. The dosage of antimicrobials should be tailored to the patient if at all possible. The dosage given on the package may not be adequate if the infection is in a location not readily permeated by the drug and/or if the microorganism tends to be resistant at the usual blood concentration obtained. In such a case, one should increase the dose in order to increase blood concentration but also be aware of possibly increasing untoward side effects

and lengthening the required withdrawal time before marketing food animals. If septicemia is severe, one may have to use the intravenous route to attain high concentration quickly. Another factor is that proper dosage may have been prescribed, but the client may be failing to follow directions properly. Discontinuing therapy too early can and often does result in relapses. The importance of host defense in the ultimate cure cannot be overemphasized.

Interactions of drugs with other drugs, chemicals, and foods must be prevented. Whereas the simultaneous administration of food is of clinical value and should be done to prevent the emesis often seen with oral nitrofurantoin, the administration of foods (particularly milk) may interfere with the absorption of certain antibiotics such as tetracyclines, oxacillin, or penicillin G.

Another common reason for failure of antimicrobial therapy is bacterial resistance. This may be present before therapy or acquired during and after therapy. The acquisition of resistance may be correlated with some of the other reasons for failure with therapy, such as inadequate drug concentration at the site of infection.

It has recently been shown that the amount of aminoglycoside (gentamicin and tobramycin) required to inhibit bacterial growth of E. coli, P. mirabilis, and K. pneumoniae was increased by 4 to 20 times by anaerobiosis, in 20 of 25 strains tested.[71] Anaerobic conditions had no effect on the rate or extent of killing by the cephalosporins (cephalothin, cefazolin, and cefamandole). Since these organisms are facultative and if the infection is in an anaerobic area such as the gut or intra-abdominal abscess, the in vitro sensitivity tests should be done under anaerobic conditions.

The list of factors to recheck if antimicrobial therapy is not effective is:

1. Diagnosis
   a. Sensitivity of all pathogens producing the disease. The bacteria may be resistant to the drug.
   b. Superinfection. An improved definition of the problem requires that superinfection be suspected and the organism cultured.
   c. Possible presence of diseases additional to those already correctly diagnosed.
   d. Spectrum of antibiotic therapy is too narrow, e.g., multiple infections or gram-negative infection.
2. Dosage schedule
   a. Client compliance with directions.

   b. Inadequate dose prescribed.

   c. Improper dosage interval used.

3. Interaction and neutralization of activity by other drugs, solutions, or chemicals.

4. Interference with absorption from site of administration, e.g., oral administration in the presence of enteritis.

5. Adequacy of other components of therapy
   a. Debridement
   b. Drainage
   c. Supportive therapy
   d. Environmental factors

6. Possibility of cure of disease, but persistence of a drug-induced fever.

7. Inadequacy of host defense mechanisms.

8. Drug may be too toxic to dose and use effectively.

9. Organisms insensitive due to anaerobic environment.

DRUG RESISTANCE

The introduction of antimicrobial agents was not the cause of the development of drug resistance. Nevertheless, the selective pressure from using these agents allows for great increases in the numbers of resistant organisms in exposed microbial populations.

A bacterial strain is termed as resistant when a genetic modification allows it to tolerate a significant increase in concentration of an antibiotic. Resistance is the result of: (1) molecular change in the site of action of the antibiotic, (2) the production of an inactivating enzyme, or (3) modifications in the penetration of the antibiotic.[72]

Bacteria may acquire resistance by spontaneous chromosomal mutation and/or by transfer of a small independent extrachromosomal genetic element called a resistance plasmid or resistance factor (R-factor) from a resistant microorganism to a sensitive one.[73]

The consequences for health of these two mechanisms are different. Chromosomal mutation is specific for one group of related antibiotics. The selective pressure due to the use of one product of this group will lead only to the selection of bacteria that are resistant to this group. There is no evidence that transfer of chromosomal DNA frequently occurs under natural conditions. On the other hand, when one factor (R factor) is able to mediate resistances to several different groups of commercially available antimicrobial drugs, the consequences are of more concern. If an antibiotic belonging to one group is given for any purpose, it selects for resistance not only for its group but for several other groups as well. Such transfer of genetic factors may occur in natural conditions. Based upon these facts, it is generally accepted that a large majority of "resistance" in wild type bacteria is related to R factors, i.e., extrachromosomal DNA.

Plasmids—Extrachromosomal DNA

Plasmids are genetic elements which exist stably in the autonomous or extrachromosomal state. All bacterial plasmids described thus far are composed of double-stranded DNA. Like the chromosome they contain genes for the initiation of replication. Indeed, the single indispensable and therefore most important property of any plasmid is its ability to replicate autonomously in the cytoplasm of the host cell. Also, like the chromosome, plasmids have a site of attachment to a cell component, presumably the membrane, to ensure maintenance and distribution to daughter cells. Two characteristics distinguish plasmids from the chromosome. First, a plasmid is only a small fraction the size of the bacterial chromosome. The amount of DNA may be as little as 0.1 to 0.2% of that in the chromosome. Second, plasmids can be lost from the cell without affecting the cell's ability to grow; i.e., plasmids are not essential but are dispensable to a cell under ordinary conditions of growth.[74]

Two parts constitute an R factor: One part codes for resistance characters, while the other is necessary for transfer. These two parts may or may not be associated. Transfer in gram-negative rods can occur by direct contact (conjugation) between the resistant and the sensitive bacteria. This contact is related to special appendages called sex pili. In gram-negative rods and in gram-positive cocci, the transfer may occur through an intermediate host, a bacteriophage (transduction).[74]

The following mechanisms of resistance are mediated by R factors:

1. Resistance to penicillins and cephalosporins: R factors mediate the production of enzymes (penicillinase) able to split the β-lactam ring of these compounds, which is essential for their activity.

2. Resistance to aminoglycoside antibiotics, such as streptomycin, neomycin, kanamycin, and gentamicin: Eight different enzymes are able to adenylate, phosphorylate, or acetylate and thereby inactivate the antibiotics.

3. Resistance to chloramphenicol: R factors or R plasmids mediate the production of different acetyl transferases inactivating the antibiotic.

4. Resistance to tetracyclines.

5. Resistance to sulfonamides and trimethoprim.

6. Resistance to macrolides: In staphylococci

and streptococci, resistance is not transferred by R factors, but is linked to plasmids. These plasmids consequently mediate resistance to erythromycin, spiramycin, oleandomycin, lincomycin, and tylosin.[72]

R factors have been found in all species of enterobacteria, *Salmonella, Shigella, Escherichia coli, Klebsiella, Enterobacteriaceae, Proteus, Providencia, Pseudomonas, Vibrio cholerae, Pasteurella,* and in *Aeromonas* from fish. Some R factors have been transferred to soil bacteria, such as *Rhizobium* and *Agrobacterium.* Resistance plasmids are well known in staphylococci and have been recently observed in streptococci.[72,74]

Other cell characteristics are also mediated by plasmids. Plasmids in intestinal bacteria control the synthesis of a wide variety of bacterial products, many of which are significant in the survival of the bacteria and in their interrelationships with their host and with other microorganisms. These products include hemolysins, colicins, substances that confer resistance (R factors as already mentioned) to antimicrobial agents, as well as fimbrial antigens, enterotoxins, and certain surface antigens which are related to the pathogenic activity of enterobacteria. These plasmid-mediated characteristics may be of great practical importance if they are in any way associated with transferable drug resistance and are conjunctively transferred with R factors under the selective pressure of antibiotic usage.[75]

The Hemolysin Plasmid. Plasmid control of alpha hemolysin production in *Escherichia coli* was first reported in 1968. It was demonstrated that the hemolysin plasmid could be transferred by conjugation not only to other *E. coli* strains, but also to *Shigella* and *Salmonella.* The formation of alpha hemolysin by *E. coli* has been of particular interest to workers investigating the pathogenicity of *E. coli* for certain animal species. Most strains of *E. coli* that cause diarrhea in pigs are hemolytic; however, the hemolytic plasmid has not been implicated in the disease. Hemolytic *E. coli* have also been implicated in enteric and systemic disease in dogs and cats.

The Colicin Plasmid. The substance colicin is capable of killing strains of *E. coli* but is ineffective against the toxin-producing strains. This is clearly a potential asset to an *E. coli* strain trying to colonize the intestinal tract (in competition with a multitude of other strains), and therefore may be considered a virulence factor.[76]

The K-88 and K-99 Plasmids. The K-88 plasmid codes for the K-88 fimbrial antigen, which is found exclusively on *E. coli* strains enteropathogenic for swine. It has recently been shown that the K-88 fimbriae play an important role in the colonizing ability and, hence, the enteropathogenicity of *E. coli* strains in pigs. The K-99 plasmid, while not as well described, plays a similar role in calves.[76]

The Enterotoxin (Ent) Plasmid. It appears that enterotoxin is an essential factor in the enteropathogenicity of *E. coli* strains. *E. coli* strains implicated in infantile diarrhea, diarrhea in human adults, and diarrhea in pigs and calves have been shown to possess a plasmid that codes for enterotoxin production.[75]

Functional relationships between these different plasmids in intestinal bacteria are only now being identified. It is quite conceivable that a plasmid that codes for a virulence determinant, such as the enterotoxin plasmid, could become linked with an R factor. Such a linkage, combined with the continued indiscriminate use of an antibiotic agent, could provide the selection required to increase markedly the range of enteropathogenic types of *E. coli.* This may potentially be the most serious consequence of R factor-mediated resistance in Enterobacteriaceae.[74,77]

The Origin and Ecology of R Factors

The origin of R factor genes and the environmental pressures responsible for their selection remain poorly defined. Thirty strains of enteric bacteria isolated prior to the widespread usage of antibiotics (prior to 1950) have been screened for drug resistance and R factor infection. One strain was resistant only to sulfadiazine, two strains only to spectinomycin, and one *E. coli* was found to be multiply resistant to streptomycin, tetracycline, and bluensomycin. The other strains were sensitive to all inhibitory agents. This one strain that was multiply resistant did contain an R factor and was confirmed as being isolated prior to 1937. This is the earliest reported isolate infected with an R factor. These findings indicate that R factors are not a recent phenomenon, need not have been transferred (recently) to the United States from the Far East or Europe, and may not have originally carried multiple genes mediating resistance to antibacterial agents.[78]

A study of a "preantibiotic" community in Borneo to trace the evolution of R factor was concluded in 1970. Penicillin was used in the population on one occasion in 1941. Out of 1017 viable isolates, 50 were found to be multiply resistant to any two of the following antibiotics: ampicillin, tetracycline, chloramphenicol, and streptomycin. Only six strains were found capable of transferring resistance and were thus considered to be R factor-bearing strains. Only 0.5% of the flora from this community contained R factors.[79] Other studies have confirmed the virtual absence of R factors in antibiotic-free communities.[78]

The most likely explanation of the source of these R factors is generally believed to be naturally occurring antibiotics produced by soil microorganisms. If this source of antibiotics is responsible for the development in Enterobacteriaceae of genes mediating resistance to antibiotics, it is also reasonable to assume that these genes evolved and survived in the free-living members of this group. Therefore, these bacteria, *E. coli, Aerobacter, Proteus*, and the *Providencia* group, would receive a selective advantage from the possession of such genetic information, while the obligate enteropathogen in the preantibiotic period would not have been exposed to antibiotics in its natural habitat and would not have profited from such genetic material.[74] The members of the enteropathogens that fortuitously receive R factors by conjugation possess a selective advantage after the introduction of therapeutic antibiotics and have since emerged as the predominant members of their populations.[72]

Such a process of development of R factors would support the theory that there is a limit or threshold of acceptable antibiotic pressure. Otherwise, given the ability of these enterobacteria to adapt to their environment of inhibitory substances, man could potentially reach a point in time where antimicrobial agents become totally ineffective against enteropathogens that have received R factors by the conjugational process.

Regional Prevalence of R Factor

Illinois

In order to determine the current levels of resistance in farm animals in 1974, a survey was conducted on the antibacterial drugs used on farms in Illinois. All Illinois swine, beef cattle, calf, and poultry farms in the reported study used feed containing antibacterial drugs. The antibacterial agents used as feed supplements are presented in Table 19–4.[80]

The predominant antimicrobial agents used on these farms were tetracycline, penicillin, neomycin, and sulfonamides. While it was not possible to detail the occasional use of parenteral or oral therapeutic uses, it is fair to speculate that the same four classes of drugs are often used for therapeutic purposes.

Table 19–4. Antibacterial drugs used continuously in feeds of Illinois swine, poultry, and beef cattle and calves, 1974[80]

Antibacterial Drugs	Percent of Farms Using Each Antibacterial Drug		
	Swine	Poultry	Beef Cattle and Calves
Tetracyclines	76	100	80
Penicillin	52	50	0
Sulfonamides	68	50	20
Streptomycin	20	0	0
Neomycin	16	50	40
Tylosin	16	0	0
Furazolidone	8	0	0
No. of farms	25	2	5

The percentage of antibiotic-resistant, gram-negative enteric organisms was determined for the major categories of animals found in these farms.

The proportions of antibiotic-resistant organisms to total organisms in fecal specimens from Illinois swine are presented in Figure 19–1. Ninety-five percent of the swine samples examined contained between 10 and 100% oxytetracycline-resistant organisms, whereas 82% of the samples demonstrated 10 to 100% ampicillin-resistant organisms.

The proportions of antibiotic-resistant organisms to total organisms in fecal specimens from Illinois cattle are presented in Figure 19–2. Seventy-seven percent of the Illinois beef cattle samples contained from 10 to 100% oxytetracycline- or dihydrostreptomycin-resistant organisms. Forty-five percent of

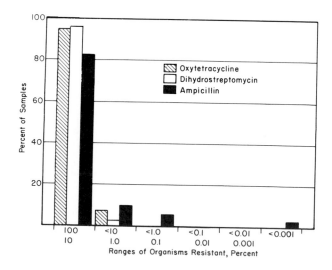

Figure 19–1. Quantitation of the proportions of antibiotic-resistant gram-negative enteric organisms in fecal specimens (n=133) from Illinois swine.[80]

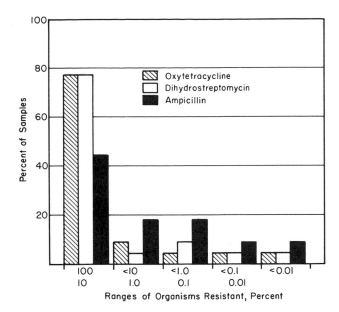

Figure 19-2. Quantitation of the proportions of antibiotic-resistant gram-negative enteric organisms in fecal specimens (n=22) from Illinois beef cattle and calves.[80]

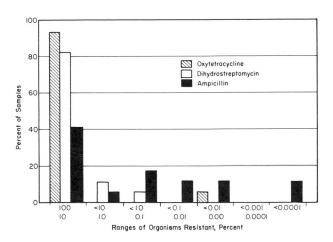

Figure 19-3. Quantitation of the proportions of antibiotic-resistant gram-negative enteric organisms in composite fecal specimens (n=18) of Illinois poultry.[80]

the samples were in the 10 to 100% range of ampicillin-resistant organisms.

The results obtained from quantitating proportions of resistant organisms in 18 composite poultry samples from 10 Illinois farms are presented in Figure 19-3. Again, high proportions of the samples examined were composed of largely antibiotic-resistant organisms. Ninety-four percent of the samples had between 10 and 100% oxytetracycline-resistant organisms. Eighty-two percent of the samples contained 10% or greater dihydrostrepto-

mycin-resistant organisms. Forty-one percent of the poultry samples fell into the 10 to 100% range of ampicillin-resistant organisms.

Montana

Providing a contrast to the Illinois farm animals and their resistance profiles is the percentage of antibiotic-resistant gram-negative organisms in fecal samples from Montana range cattle. The distribution of these samples according to ranges of antibiotic-resistant organisms is presented in Figure 19-4. Only one (1.4%) of the samples contained greater than 0.1% oxytetracycline-resistant organisms. Three (3%) of the samples contained approximately 0.1% dihydrostreptomycin-resistant organisms. One of 72 samples had 1% and 4 had 0.1% ampicillin-resistant organisms.

U.S. Cross-Section

Five hundred fifty-five (555) isolates of *E. coli* were obtained from fecal specimens of a representative number of animals from five farms in the United States. Antibiotic exposure of the selected herds was determined by an epidemiologic survey of these farms. The results of this study are presented in Table 19-5. The incidence of multiple resistance in the *E. coli* isolates was higher in herds exposed to continuous feeding of antimicrobial agents (84.8%) than in a herd not receiving antimicrobials (15.7%). The most frequent resistant pattern observed was the triple pattern of dihydrostreptomycin, sulfonamide, and tetracycline.[81]

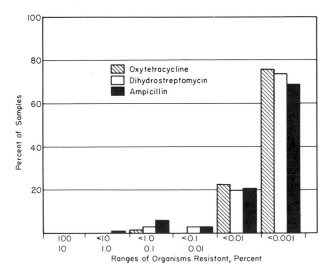

Figure 19-4. Quantitation of the proportions of antibiotic-resistant gram-negative enteric organisms in fecal specimens (n=72) from Montana range cattle.[80]

Table 19–5. Relationship between exposure to antimicrobials and frequency of resistances of E. coli[81]

			Percentage of Strains		
Exposed	Nature of Exposure	Total Strains	Multiply Sensitive	Singly Resistant	Multiply Resistant
Farm 1	Continuous	99	0.0	4.1	95.9
Farm 2	Intermittent	138	44.9	16.7	38.4
Farm 3	Continuous	131	10.7	22.2	67.2
Farm 4	Continuous	77	4.9	0.0	95.1
Farm 5					
(A) Swine	Continuous	25	8.0	16.0	76.0
(B) Calf	Intermittent (therapeutic at birth)	21	76.2	4.8	19.0
Subtotal		491	24.1	10.6	65.3
Not Exposed					
Farm 5					
(C) Dairy cows	None	64	78.1	6.2	15.7
Total		555	31.8	9.9	58.2

Nebraska

Fecal specimens were collected on 22 different Nebraska ranches and at the Department of Veterinary Science from young calves and pigs with neonatal diarrhea. Enterobacteriaceae isolated from these fecal specimens were screened for resistance to 8 antibiotics. The results indicate that of the 92 strains studied, 57 were resistant to one or more antimicrobial agents. Resistant strains were obtained from all herds involved in the study. The two most common resistance patterns were tetracycline/streptomycin/sulfamethazole (22 of 57) and tetracycline (13 of 57). Forty-three of the 57 resistant strains were positive for R factor (R^+).[82]

New York

In another study, a detailed one-year survey was conducted of fecal specimens from a herd of dairy cattle in Upper New York State. This herd received no antimicrobial agents in feed or water, but were treated intramammarily in a dry cow mastitis therapy program (Fig. 19–5). The baseline in this herd was less than 5% resistant organisms in feces. During peak treatment intervals with high doses of penicillin and dihydrostreptomycin, the incidence of resistant organisms would spike to about 10% multiply-resistant organisms. An interesting aspect of this study also involved an examination of environmental samples coincidental with fecal sampling from the dairy cattle. These environmental sources consisted of sampling from the manure spreader, barn cleaner, and lot area around water

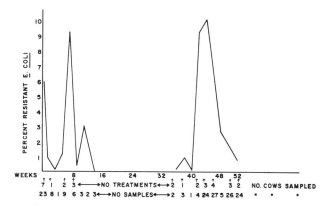

Figure 19–5. Influence of intramammary treatment of dry cows with penicillin and dihydrostreptomycin on drug resistance of E. coli isolates in feces from the herd.[83]

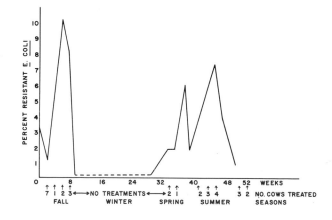

Figure 19–6. Influence of intramammary treatment of dry cows with penicillin and dihydrostreptomycin on drug resistance of E. coli isolates from the immediate environment of the herd.[83]

tanks. Figure 19–6 clearly demonstrates the interrelationships of resistant organisms from the animals and their immediate environment. The percentage of organisms manifesting resistance stimulated by this therapeutic use of drugs was considerably lower than those seen with continuous antibiotic usage in other studies.[83]

Other Studies

Beagle dogs were fed a diet containing 0, 2, or 10 μg/g (equivalent to 0, 2, or 10 ppm) of dihydrostreptomycin. In both treatment groups, the medicated feed resulted in a shift from a predominantly sensitive coliform fecal population to a fecal population resistant to dihydrostreptomycin, which peaked at 73% within 30 days from initiation of exposure (Table 19–6). Fifty-nine percent of the streptomycin-resistant strains were able to transfer, by conjugation, their resistance determinants.[84]

The most significant aspect in these studies was the very small dose of the drug and the significant response of the enteric flora to the antibiotic.

Salmonella cultures were obtained from outbreaks of animal disease from 37 states and 1 territory. They were screened for resistance to 11 antimicrobial drugs. Of the 1251 strains examined, 935 (75%) were resistant to one or more of these agents. The most common resistance pattern was ampicillin, dihydrostreptomycin, sulfonamide, and tetracycline. R factors and resistance transfer factors were commonly demonstrated in this study.[85,86]

In contrast to the relatively large number of studies with farm animals, very few studies have been reported in which isolates from dogs and cats have been examined. In those cases where they have been studied, multiple resistance and R factors have been demonstrated in organisms isolated from a variety of disease conditions.[87]

A high prevalence of multiple antibiotic resistance was observed in populations of E. coli isolated from two large groups of calves in a commercial veal rearing unit. Almost all of the organisms isolated were resistant to tetracycline, streptomycin, neomycin, and kanamycin after the calves had been given rations containing neomycin for 1 week. The number of cultures with resistance to ampicillin also increased during antibiotic feeding despite the fact that it was not utilized in the ration or for therapy. Sixty-five percent of these cultures contained transferable R factors.[88]

Feces of healthy adults and of children under the age of 5, none of whom were hospitalized or receiving antibiotics, were examined for the presence of antibiotic-resistant coliform bacilli. A higher proportion of children (62%) than of adults (46%) carried resistant strains, and this difference was observed in both rural and urban groups. Rural members of both age groups more often carried resistant organisms than did urban members. Among rural adults, the incidence of drug-resistant strains was 63% in those whose occupation involved close contact with farm animals, compared

Table 19–6. The incidence of lactose-fermenting bacteria resistant to specific antimicrobial drugs before, during, and after treatment with dihydrostreptomycin (DSM)[84]

Treatment Phase	DSM Treatment μg/g	Percent Isolates Resistant					Number Tested
		SM*	SU	TE	AM	Other†	
Pretreatment	0	7	5	0	2	10	100
	2	7	13	8	0	3	60
	10	5	3	2	2	3	59
During Treatment	0	2	2	2	2	1	125
	2	51	46	20	9	6	74
	10	73	52	25	6	11	85
After Treatment	0	18	12	8	0	2	50
	2	62	22	40	22	0	50
	10	58	42	25	0	2	48

* Streptomycin
Sulfamethoxypyridazine (SU)
Tetracycline (TE)
Ampicillin (AM)
† Isolates in this category were resistant to one of the following drugs:

cephalothin	chloramphenicol	polymyxin B
furazolidone	kanamycin	naladixic acid
gentamicin	neomycin	

with 29% in those with other occupations. Transmissible plasmids (R factors) were demonstrated in 61% of the resistant strains.[89]

Method of Exposure and Prevalence. Fecal samples were collected from five groups of people differing in the manner of their exposure to antibacterial drugs. The groups included (1) people working on farms who were continuously in contact with the predominantly resistant flora of farm animals that ate rations containing antibacterial drugs; (2) people residing on the same farms with no direct exposure to the farm animals; (3) people treated with antibacterial drugs; (4) untreated people residing with treated individuals; and (5) untreated people with no exposure to farm animals or treated individuals. The results indicated that the people in groups 1, 2, and 3 demonstrated a maximum of 62% of the samples resistant to oxytetracycline (resistance presented as 10,000 or more oxytetracycline-resistant organisms per 100,000 colony forming units); group 4 samples demonstrated 37% oxytetracycline-resistant organisms, while group 5 demonstrated only 13% resistant organisms. For dihydrostreptomycin, groups 1, 2, and 3 showed 59% resistant organisms, whereas group 5 infrequently contained high proportions of dihydrostreptomycin-resistant organisms. Statistically significant differences ($P<0.05$) in frequencies of ampicillin-resistant organisms occurred between group 5 and groups 1, 2, 3, and 4. It may be concluded that samples from persons recently treated with antibacterial drugs (group 3) and samples from persons working and/or living on farms (groups 1 and 2) contained the highest proportions of gram-negative enteric organisms resistant to oxytetracycline, dihydrostreptomycin, and ampicillin.[80]

Removal of Antibiotic Pressure and Persistence of Resistance. Given the fact that exposure to almost any level of most common antibacterial drugs will induce a resistance response, it becomes of interest to examine the persistence of resistant enteric flora when antibiotic pressure is removed. Female patients suffering from urinary tract infections were treated with various drugs and the resistance profile followed in their enteric flora. Therapeutic courses of ampicillin or sulfonamide had only a slight effect in selecting fecal *E. coli* resistant to the relevant drug. Tetracycline exerted strong selection, not only for tetracycline resistance, but also for multiple resistance, significantly increasing the frequency of resistance to ampicillin, streptomycin, chloramphenicol, and sulfonamides. The resistance effects had disappeared 5 weeks after the end of

treatment. A very critical point was that the change of the predominant fecal *E. coli* from sensitive to resistant, or back from resistant to sensitive, always resulted from a change of serotype, never from acquisition or loss of resistance in a resident strain.[90]

In contrast, six groups of swine (85 animals) were fed a combination of antimicrobial drugs (sulfamethazine, chlortetracycline, and penicillin) for 2 weeks. After 2 weeks, the drugs were removed from two groups of animals and these groups were isolated in their environment. The remaining groups remained on feed-additive antimicrobial drugs. Thirty-two weeks after cessation of dietary antibiotics, resistance to oxytetracycline and dihydrostreptomycin remained at 100% and 89%, respectively, which was the level of resistance observed at the outset of the experiment.[91]

When antibiotic usage is of a short duration, and the baseline of resistant organisms is low, it is often observed that the incidence of resistant bacteria will decrease in a relatively short time after antibiotic administration has ceased. Conversely, where antimicrobials are fed to all animals in each generation year after year, sufficient pressure is exerted to establish and maintain an enteric flora *and* an environmental flora that is mostly resistant. The key element in such circumstances may be the lack of availability of sensitive serotypes to recolonize the enteric tract. It is also feasible to consider that one may have selected resistant organisms which are well adapted to colonize specific species and persist even when the selective pressure is withdrawn.

Plasmid-Mediated Antibiotic Resistance

The available data would indicate that several general principles can be stated regarding plasmid-mediated antibiotic resistant characteristics.

Principle 1. R factors did not evolve with the availability and conventional use of commercial antibiotics; R factor plasmids were apparently a part of the microorganisms' survival capabilities at an earlier time, probably due to exposure to naturally occurring antibiotic substances.

Principle 2. The broad spectrum of usage of most antimicrobial agents, including therapeutic use in animals and man as well as feed and water usage, does cause R factor-mediated resistances to occur in enteric flora, often involving a high percentage of the enteric flora.

Principle 3. There is an interrelationship between the resistance spectrum in the enteric flora and the immediate environment, which may be referred to as a local enteric gene pool.

Principle 4. A higher correlation exists between duration of exposure to antimicrobial agents and percent resistance than exists with the dosage of a drug. Short term, high level therapeutic usage, while resulting in a resistant enteric flora, does not seem to affect the local pool of resistant plasmids nearly as adversely as does long term usage at a variety of dose levels.

Principle 5. Plasmid-mediated resistance has increased during the past decade in certain study populations and areas; in some species such as swine, in which antibiotics have been intensively used in feed and water, virtually the entire population of organisms in the immediate environment are multiply-resistant and contain R factors that are transferable.

Potential Consequences of R Factors

Four general consequences of R factors have been defined which attract scientific concern, and for which the likelihood of these occurrences have been partially or fully documented.

1. The pool of resistance in the bacteria themselves has been fully documented in a variety of animal species, and for a variety of antimicrobial drugs. This has direct implications to the clinical use of antimicrobials.

2. The ability of the bacterial plasmid (R factor) to promote its own transfer from a resistant non-pathogen to a sensitive pathogenic strain has been fully documented.

3. The interrelationships between the R factor plasmids and other plasmids that contribute to the pathogenicity of an organism, such as hemolysins, colicins, K-antigens, and enterotoxin plasmids, are only now being fully studied and understood.

4. There is evidence which suggests that animals and other environmental sources may serve as reservoirs for resistant enteric flora in humans and/or vice versa. This potential for an environmental pool or source of R factors warrants further discussion.

Studies were conducted in a large European city to determine the R factor content of sewage from different sources. Many strains of enteric bacteria in sewage carry R factors. About 2% of all coliforms obtained in sewage outflow from a domestic housing district carried R factors conferring resistance to tetracyclines and/or streptomycin. Comparison with the incidence of R factors in the coliforms in sewage from hospitals showed a number of interesting points:[92]

a. The proportion of coliforms resistant to tetracycline and/or streptomycin in hospital sewage was substantially higher (about 20%) than in sewage from domestic sources.

b. The resistance patterns exhibited by R factors in coliforms from hospital sources generally tended to be more complex than those strains from domestic sources. Many isolates from domestic sources carried only one resistance marker, while isolates from hospital sources carried multiple resistance markers.

c. However, if the comparison of absolute numbers of R factors is made between hospital and non-hospital subjects, the conclusion can be drawn that more than 95% of all R factors in this large European city are carried by bacteria inhabiting the population outside the hospitals.

Since the great majority of these subjects outside the hospital environment will not have received prescribed antibiotic treatment in the recent past, this observation seems to stress a vital point in the ecology of R factors. Expansion of the R factor pool in humans by person to person transfer is most likely to take place in people who are outside hospitals and who are, therefore, less likely to be undergoing purposive antibiotic treatment at the time. Under these circumstances, it becomes extremely important to identify the source of the selection pressure that maintains R factor-carrying (R^+) coliforms among the gut flora of the human population outside hospitals.

Certainly, the therapeutic use of antibiotics in outpatients and in domiciliary practice is likely to be one source, but it is highly dubious whether it is the only one. For example, several studies show that run-off from feedlots and downstream samples contain high numbers of R^+ microorganisms.[15,93,94]

As mentioned earlier, the production and use of antibiotics for both humans and animals increased considerably (over threefold) in the decade between 1960 and 1970, while the population increased only 11%. It should be clear that the increase in antibiotic production probably relates to the variety and extent of antimicrobial usage, and thus greatly potentiates the sources of R factors.[95]

While the Food and Drug Administration in the United States has been reviewing the hazards and benefits of sub-therapeutic feed additive usage of antimicrobials since 1970, they have been unable to reach any definitive conclusions or to recommend any actions to date. However, it is highly possible that a more restrictive policy will emerge regarding feed-additive antibiotics. The American Medical Association is now studying methods to control and reduce the apparent overuse and abuse of antimicrobial agents in the hospital environment. The issue of the therapeutic use of antimicrobials by the veterinary profession has yet to be addressed by any national body of experts.[95]

Transfer of Resistant Bacteria from Domestic Animals to Man

The potential interaction between the feed additive use of antimicrobial agents and humans has been clearly delineated in a recent study. An *E. coli*, in which a temperature-sensitive chloramphenicol-resistant gene was used as a marker to identify a particular plasmid, was introduced into a group of chickens maintained by a specific family and caretakers under controlled circumstances. The mobility of this specific plasmid, which conferred resistance to chloramphenicol, tetracycline, sulfonamides, and streptomycin, was followed over a 2-month period. On two occasions the plasmid was detected in human feces. The first occurred in the fecal sample from the 12-year-old son of a farm owner. Two days after he had cleaned the cage in which chickens harboring the *E. coli* with the marker plasmid in the intestine were housed, 78% of the coliforms in his fecal flora were resistant to chloramphenicol. The second human host was observed excreting *E. coli* with this plasmid 1 week after handling the chickens. The same plasmid was found in chickens in clean cages in the vicinity, thus confirming the transfer of a specific plasmid from enteric flora of poultry to man and from poultry to poultry.[96]

Escherichia coli from 14 Missouri farm families and their livestock were characterized as to their patterns of resistance to antibiotics. Identical antibiograms that were found in *E. coli* of members of the farm family and associated groups of animals were counted as matches, using three types of counting techniques. Statistical tests indicated a strong association between the resistance patterns of the *E. coli* isolated from people and those isolated from their livestock. A follow-up study in which correlations were made between those families that consumed home-grown pork or beef and those that lived on a farm but did not consume their own home-grown meat products firmly established that the food chain was a definite indirect source of resistant coliforms.[93]

While the direct route of transfer from animals to man is of interest, it should be recognized that under the current circumstances of today's livestock production and management, only a small segment of the population would be exposed directly to animal production units.[97] Several indirect routes may be of even more concern. Run-off water and environmental contamination originating from livestock operations where antibiotics are used in feeds has been found to contain R factor enteric organisms. The contribution this source might make to man's burden of R[+] enteric flora has yet to be defined.[94]

Another indirect, and probably the most important, source are the R[+] enteric flora which can be commonly found on foodstuffs originating from a variety of food animals. A number of studies have been conducted, and a wide variety of numbers and types of R[+] enteric flora have been found to be a stable part of the food chain. The real significance of this source of R[+] organisms to the human enteric flora has not been fully defined. There remains much controversy over the extent to which non-pathogenic *E. coli* in the animal community act as a source of R factor bearing strains for man. Most scientists agree that the most probable route by which transfer can occur is by ingestion of meat foods contaminated with R[+] *E. coli* of animal origin.[98,99,100]

A study in 1976 has shown the distribution of O-antigen types of *Escherichia coli* in calves over a 10-month period. Four hundred calves from separate farms located over a wide area were surveyed. Of the 148 O-types recognized, 93 were found in calves, compared with 107 in a previous survey in man. Forty-two of these O-types isolated were resistant to at least one antibiotic. Of these, 71% belonged to 10 O-types, 9 of which were also found in man. It was concluded that calves form a potential reservoir of R[+] plasmid-carrying *E. coli* for man.[101]

The one other potential mechanism by which the use of antimicrobial agents may play an important role on the enteric and environmental pool of R[+] microflora involves the occurrence of drug residues in animal tissues. These residues may result from therapeutic and/or feed-use antibiotics in food animals. The U.S. Department of Agriculture reports an annual rate of 1 to 2% incidence of antibiotic residues in red meat and poultry carcasses at slaughter time. For the past 2 or 3 years, the incidence of sulfonamide residues has been about 12 to 15%, with the larger percentage of sulfonamide residues occurring in swine and poultry. The data were presented in an earlier section of this chapter, which confirms that residues as low as 1 to 2 ppm can cause a distinct increase in the R[+] enteric flora of either man or animals. During 1976, the majority of residue violations could be attributed to the feed additive use of antimicrobial agents.

Therapeutic Use of Antibiotic and R Factor Resistance

The treatment with antibiotics to which R factor-linked resistance determinants exists leads to immediate conversion of the gut flora to one showing the appropriate resistance pattern mediated by one or more R factors. In practice, this response can be seen best by feeding a tetracycline. Within 36 hours of the start of a standard therapeutic course of 250 mg of tetracycline four times daily, the incidence of R factor-carrying, tetracycline resistant *E. coli* in the fecal flora starts to rise and frequently reaches more than 95% of the total *E. coli* count. Figure 19–7 shows the overall response to feeding tetracycline to a number of individuals on various occasions and the time course of return to sensitivity.[92,93,102]

Although in some cases the coliform flora had reverted to being predominantly susceptible within 5 days of the end of the course of therapy, in others substantial populations of resistant organisms were still detectable some weeks after the end of treat-

ment. In fact, in one case the resistant organisms could still be detected after more than 2 months.[97]

The introduction of antibiotics into clinical use is commonly followed by the appearance of resistant bacterial populations as was indicated previously. However, the fear that in time all gram-negative bacteria would become R factor carriers has not yet been realized. An end to antibiotic treatment often leads to a decrease in the resistant flora, albeit sometimes more slowly than is perhaps desirable. This observation supports the contention that resistant organisms must be at a growth disadvantage when compared with susceptible ones, and the limited amount of evidence available suggests that this is so. Several studies have indicated that carriage of R factor seems to confer some growth disadvantages to the host bacterium, when that bacterium is not in an environment where the plasmid(s) gives a competitive advantage.

Transfer of Resistance in the Hospital Environment

While it would be desirable to provide information on the nature and characteristics of resistance in microflora in the veterinary clinic and hospital, no data can be cited. There are, however, numerous studies in human hospitals from which reasonable comparisons can be drawn. The emergence of nosocomial pathogens highly resistant to available antimicrobial agents is a cause for concern in any hospital. Gram-negative organisms are being encountered as nosocomial pathogens with increasing frequency, and selective pressures of antimicrobial therapy favor the persistence of more resistant strains.[103] Furthermore, the ability of these organisms to cause disease is enhanced by the increasing prevalence in hospitals of patients with impaired host defenses. Seven large epidemics of urinary tract infection have been studied by the Center for Disease Control during the last 5 years. The seven outbreaks were caused by three different organisms: *Klebsiella pneumoniae, Serratia marcescens,* and *Proteus rettgeri.* In all seven epidemics, a major initial concern of hospital personnel was the lack of effective antimicrobial therapy or fear that, with selective pressure, resistance to the only effective agent would develop. The major reservoir for the *K. pneumoniae* infections was the gastrointestinal tract. The major reservoir for both *S. marcescens* and *P. rettgeri* appear to be the genitourinary tracts of catheterized patients.[103]

Epidemiologic investigation suggests that the epidemic organism was transmitted from patient to

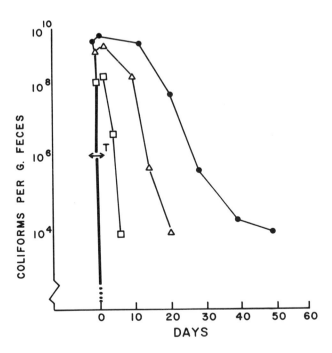

Figure 19–7. Response of gut coliforms in humans to ingestion of tetracycline. Duration of feeding (250 mg four times daily) is shown by the arrow with the T above. The curves show the longest (●), shortest (□), and average (△) survival of tetracycline-resistant coliforms in the feces. Data from 92, 93, 102.

patient on the hands of personnel in all seven outbreaks, contrary to common thought that hospital equipment and paraphernalia would be the most common vectors. The most frequently observed factors that predisposed patients to urinary infection with these multi-drug-resistant strains were urinary catheterization *and* prior exposure to broad-spectrum antimicrobial therapy.

Infants whose intestinal tracts were colonized by enteric organisms with R factor-mediated resistance to kanamycin during their stay in an intensive care nursery were cultured at intervals after discharge from the hospital. Forty-six percent of the infants remained carriers of R factors for 12 months or longer after discharge. Enteric organisms with R factor-mediated resistance to kanamycin were also found in the rectal flora of 33% of the infant's family members. A control group, consisting of infants who were discharged from a well-baby nursery, had an intestinal carriage rate of 5%. The results of this study indicate that R factors of nosocomial origin may persist in an antibiotic-free environment for a considerable period of time. It may also indicate that R factors obtained from a hospital are commonly disseminated in a community.[102]

An important aspect of the acquisition of R factors by pathogens is that the entire resistance spectrum, extending to as many as seven drugs, may be acquired in one or very few events. Since pathogens are invasive in their own right, and therefore need no selective support from the antibiotics to promote the infections they cause, a resistant pathogen with epidemic potentialities may spread widely in a susceptible human population in which it is disseminated by its normal epidemic routes. If one of the resistances it carries is directly against a drug that can be used in the treatment of the disease, the treatment then becomes ineffective.[104]

The disastrous outbreak of chloramphenicol-resistant typhoid in Mexico is an excellent illustration of these points. Only one strain of the typhoid bacillus was involved, and the R factor concerned, which had the resistance spectrum chloramphenicol, streptomycin, sulfonamide, and tetracycline (CSSuT), was transferred to it as a single linkage group, that is, in one event. The entire outbreak, involving some thousands of deaths, was thus caused by a single line of the typhoid bacillus, which needed only one R factor transfer and the opportunity of epidemic spread to cause the largest and most troublesome typhoid outbreak on record.[105] Many analogous examples can be cited, and

the appearance of plasmid-mediated drug resistance in genera such as *Vibrio, Haemophilus, Clostridium, Streptococcus,* and other organisms widely different from the enterobacteria, may be a hint that R factors have greater transfer potentialities than was previously thought.

Effects of Resistance upon Antimicrobial Therapy in Animals

Pneumonia is widely acknowledged to be the most important disease of feedlot cattle. In a recent report, it was stated that in a 13,000 head capacity feedlot in northern California, uncomplicated bacterial pneumonias were responsible for 42.5% of all deaths over an 18-month period. During an experiment in which chlortetracycline was used continuously in the feeding program, it was noted that an increasing proportion of sick cattle were not responding satisfactorily to treatment. This refractoriness was found to be correlated with a great increase in the occurrence of antimicrobial resistance. It was soon determined that it was not practical to attempt treatment of infections with antibiotics to which the causative organism was classified resistant.[106]

A series of studies was conducted in experimentally infected pigs with a multiply resistant *E. coli* which had been isolated from an outbreak of swine bacterial enteritis. Typical clinical signs of colibacillosis were reproduced in piglets. The *E. coli* involved contained an R factor which conferred resistance to seven antibiotics, one of which was chlortetracycline. The causative organism was susceptible to chloramphenicol. Following the production of frank clinical colibacillosis, pigs were treated with therapeutic levels of either chloramphenicol or chlortetracycline. Chloramphenicol was significantly more effective in terminating experimentally induced colibacillosis in piglets than no treatment, or treatment with chlortetracycline. Chlortetracycline was not significantly better than no treatment. This study provides clear evidence that a disease caused by a resistant *E. coli* will not respond as effectively to a therapeutic agent for which a resistance plasmid exists.[93]

R Factors and Plasmids Conferring Potential Pathogenic Characters

It has been known for a considerable time that *E. coli*, while being a normal inhabitant of the intestinal tract, can also be associated with a variety of pathologic conditions in man and animals. For many years this organism has been considered to be a major etiologic agent in diarrhea of the newly born of several species, particularly pigs, calves, and man. In fact, during 1974, examination of numerous cultures of *E. coli* isolated from cases of diarrhea and examined by a major veterinary diagnostic laboratory revealed that over 95% of these isolates were multiply resistant to antimicrobial agents.[107]

It is now well established that the intestines of a healthy pig are sterile at birth, and that the normal bacterial flora (lactobacilli, gram-positive cocci, *Clostridium perfringens, E. coli,* and Bacteroides) are established within the first 24 hours of life. Evidence already presented indicates that, in many instances, this flora may be 95 to 100% multiply resistant, particularly in swine populations that are raised in areas where pigs generally receive antibiotics in their feed. By the 48th hour of life, the production of acid in the stomach has increased, and with the fall of pH in the stomach contents the multiplication of most organisms except lactobacilli is suppressed. At this point in time the gut flora is composed mainly of lactobacilli, Bacteroides, Veillonellae, and yeasts. It has been shown that *E. coli* diarrhea is characterized by the proliferation of certain serotypes of *E. coli* anterior in the small intestines. Moreover, the evidence indicates that this colonization process in swine often requires the presence of K-88 antigens, which are mediated by plasmids, and in a majority of cases these pathogenic *E. coli* are capable of producing enterotoxin, which is mediated by the Ent plasmid. Most of these organisms are also hemolytic, the hemolysin factor being mediated by another plasmid.[108]

Thus, several key properties of pathogenic *E. coli* owe their pathogenicity to plasmid-mediated characters. These R factors are, however, simply another type of plasmid which conveys the antibiotic-resistance profile. Under the conditions of selective pressure, as is imposed by the use of antimicrobial agents in feeds, the R^+ plasmids are mobilized, and as has been shown, the process of conjugation and R^+ factor transfer can occur easily and readily. Under these circumstances where conjugation and R^+ plasmids are being consolidated and transferred, there is strong suspicion and reasonable scientific data to support the concept of transfer of these additional plasmids which confer pathogenic properties to *E. coli*. If this phenomenon can and does occur under normal husbandry conditions then it is easy to understand the concern for the potential danger implied; e.g., antimicrobial agents may provide a focal point for increasing the pathogenesis of enteric *E. coli* which are also multiply antibiotic resistant.[109]

Future Considerations

The World Health Organization (WHO) convened a group of public health experts in October 1973 to study two issues: (1) the control of harmful residues in food for human and animal consumption, and (2) the public health aspects of antibiotics in foodstuffs.[72] The WHO also convened a panel of experts in December, 1975 to discuss the public health aspects of antibiotic-resistant bacteria in the environment.[104]

This august body of experts was able to reach several conclusions which represent a sound and logical scientific basis for future considerations on the way physicians, veterinarians, and farmers should use antibiotics. It seems appropriate to close this chapter with a direct quote of their conclusions:

(1) Antibiotics are indispensable in human and veterinary therapy and have brought great progress in the treatment and control of human and animal disease.

(2) The widespread resistance among bacteria already poses difficulties in human and veterinary therapy and may, if the present trend continues, render antibiotics far less effective than at present, thus depriving mankind of a most valuable weapon against many diseases.

(3) The selection of bacterial strains resistant to antibiotics is closely related to problems of environmental hygiene, a situation exacerbated by the continuing interchange in ecological systems.

(4) All uses of antibiotics for human and veterinary purposes, including low-level additions to animal feed for growth promotion, are responsible for the selection of antibiotic-resistant strains in bacteria.

(5) Low levels of antibiotics in animal feed contribute to increased production of animal protein for human consumption.

(6) Certain antibiotics which are not generally used in medicine or veterinary therapy are as effective and economic for growth promotion as those which are now commonly used in therapy.

Thus, on the basis of available information, the WHO working group agreed on the following classification of antibiotics, arranged in categories of increasing risk with respect to the development of bacterial resistance and their value as therapeutic agents: (1) bacitracin, flavomycin, virginiamycin and related products, (2) polymyxins, furans, tylosin (and other macrolides), (3) penicillins, tetracyclines, (4) ampicillin, cephalosporins, (5) sulfonamides, trimethoprim and related compounds, aminoglycoside antibiotics (streptomycin and neomycin), and (6) chloramphenicol.

The important general recommendation to emerge from this group of specialists was that only antibiotics other than those of therapeutic value should be used for growth promotion in animals; i.e., category 1, above. Since such compounds are already available, certain restrictions of use would not appear to cause any great hardships or economic loss to the animal industries.

The potential benefit of adopting a definite restriction policy for antimicrobial drugs at this time could well mean the preservation of the effectiveness of these drugs. Moreover, adopting a restriction policy, combined with renewed educational efforts directed at physicians and veterinarians, could be a critical decision in the future evolution and control of disease in man and animals.

It should be added that only those antibiotics that do not cause resistance to antibiotics commonly used therapeutically should be used for growth promotion in animals.

REFERENCES

1. Mercer, H. D.: Antimicrobial drugs in food-producing animals. Vet. Clin. North Am. 5:3, 1975.
2. Reference deleted.
3. Muller, J.: Fungal infection after antibiotic therapy. Munch. Med. Wochenschr. 118:669, 1976.
4. Aronson, A. L.: The use, misuse and abuse of antibacterial agents. Mod. Vet. Pract. 56:383, 1975.
5. Stone, H. H., Hooper, A., Kolb, L. D., Geheber, C. E., and Dawkins, E. J.: Antibiotic prophylaxis in gastric, biliary and colonic surgery. Ann. Surg. 184:443, 1976.
6. Gunn, A. A.: Antibiotics in biliary surgery. Br. J. Surg. 63:627, 1976.
7. Brenner, E. J., and Tellman, W. H.: Pseudomembranous colitis as a sequel to oral lincomycin therapy. Am. J. Gastroenterol. 54:55, 1970.
8. Jensen, M. J., McKenzie, R. J., Hugh, T. B., and Lake, B.: Topical ampicillin-cloxacillin in the prevention of abdominal wound sepsis. Br. J. Clin. Pract. 29:115, 1975.
9. Hayes, N. R., van der Waaig, D., and Cohen, B. J.: Elimination of bacteria from dogs with antibiotics. J. Hyg. (Camb.) 73:205, 1974.
10. Leigh, D. A., Pease, R., Henderson, H., Simmons, K., and Russ, R.: Prophylactic lincomycin in the prevention of wound infection following appendectomy: a double blind study. Br. J. Surg. 63:973, 1976.
11. VanKruiningen, H. J.: Clinical efficacy of tylosin in canine inflammatory bowel disease. J.A.A.H.A. 12:498, 1976.
12. Hamlin, R. L., and Smith, C. R.: Placebo effects in veterinary medicine. Fed. Proc. 24:329, 1965.
13. Reisberg, B.: In The Biologic and Clinical Basis of Infectious Diseases. 2nd Ed. Edited by G. Youmans. Chapter 46. Philadelphia, W. B. Saunders Co., 1979.
14. Jawetz, E.: Synergism and antagonism among antimicrobial drugs. West. J. Med. 123:87, 1975.
15. Claudon, D. G., Thompson, D. I., Christenson, E. H., Lawton, G. W., and Dick, E. C.: Prolonged salmonella contamination of a recreational lake by runoff waters. Appl. Microbiol. 21:875, 1971.
16. Gerding, D. N., Kromhout, J. P., Sullivan, J. J., and Hall, H. W.: Antibiotic penetrance of ascitic fluid in dogs. Antimicrob. Agents Chemother. 10:850, 1976.
17. Meyer, R. D., Kraus, L. L., and Pasiecznik, K. A.: In vitro susceptibility of gentamicin-resistant Enterobacteriaceae and Pseudomonas aeruginosa to netilmicin and selected aminoglycoside antibiotics. Antimicrob. Agents Chemother. 10:677, 1976.
18. Finland, M., Garner, C., Wilcox, C., and Sabath, L. D.: Susceptibility of "enterobacteria" to aminoglycoside antibiotics: comparisons with tetracyclines, polymyxins, chloramphenicol and spectinomycin. J. Infect. Dis. 134:557, 1976.
19. Weinstein, A. J.: Newer Antibiotics. Guidelines for Use. Postgrad. Med. 60:75, 1976.
20. Meny, R., Webb, C. D., and Fiedelman, W.: Carbenicillin therapy of anaerobic infections. Curr. Ther. Res. 17:478, 1975.
21. Schoutens, E., and Yourassowsky, E.: Speed of bactericidal action of penicillin G, ampicillin and carbenicillin on Bacteroides fragilis. Antimicrob. Agents Chemother. 6:227, 1974.
22. Dulong de Rosnay, H. L. C., Grimont, P. A. D., Dessaut, B., and Lesgouarres, M.-T.: Comparative in vitro activity of tobramycin, gentamicin, kanamycin, colistin, carbenicillin and ticarcillin on clinical isolate of Pseudomonas aeruginosa: epidemiological and therapeutic implications. J. Infect. Dis. 134:S50, 1976.
23. Hariharan, H., and Barnum, D. A.: Antimicrobial drug susceptibility of certain bacterial pathogens from dogs and cats. Can. Vet. J. 15:108, 1974.
24. Bushby, S. R. M.: Combined antibacterial action in vitro of trimethoprim and sulfonamides. Postgrad. Med. J. (Suppl.) 45:10, 1969.
25. Nord, C.-E., Wadstrom, T., and Wretland, B.: Synergistic effect of combinations of sulfamethoxazole, trimethoprim, colistin against Pseudomonas maltophilia and Pseudomonas cepacia. Antimicrob. Agents Chemother. 6:521, 1974.
26. Miles, C. P., Coleman, V. R., Gunnison, J. B., and Jawetz, E.: Antibiotic synergism requires simultaneous presence of both members of a synergistic drug pair. Proc. Soc. Exp. Biol. Med. 78:738, 1951.
27. Carrizosa, J., and Kaye, D.: Antibiotic synergism in enterococcal endocarditis. J. Lab. Clin. Med. 88:132, 1976.
28. Russell, E. J., and Sutherland, R.: Activity of amoxycillin against enterococci and synergism with aminoglycoside antibiotics. J. Med. Microbiol. 8:1, 1975.
29. Sande, M. A., and Courtney, K. B.: Nafcillin-gentamicin synergism in experimental staphylococcal endocarditis. J. Lab. Clin. Med. 88:118, 1976.
30. Watanakunakorn, C., and Bannister, T.: In vitro activity of tobramycin and gentamicin against Enterobacteriaceae and gentamicin-resistant, carbenicillin-resistant Pseudomonas aeruginosa. Curr. Ther. Res. 17:488, 1975.
31. Daschner, F. D.: Combination of bacteriostatic and bactericidal drugs: lack of significant in vitro antagonism between penicillin, cephalothin, and rolitetracycline. Antimicrob. Agents Chemother. 10:802, 1976.
32. McCabe, W. R., and Jackson, G. G.: Treatment of pyelonephritis. Bacterial, drug and host factors in success or failure among 252 patients. N. Engl. J. Med. 272:1037, 1965.
33. Bulger, R. J., and Kirby, W. M.: Gentamicin and ampicillin: synergism with other antibiotics. Am. J. Med. Sci. 246:717, 1963.
34. Bulger, R. J., and Rossen-Runge, U.: Bactericidal activity of the ampicillin/kanamycin combination against Escherichia coli, Enterobacter-Klebsiella, and Proteus. Am. J. Med. Sci. 258:7, 1969.
35. Kaye, D., Koenig, M. G., and Hook, E. W.: The action of certain antibiotics and combinations against Proteus mirabilis. Am. J. Med. Sci. 242:320, 1961.
36. Heman-Ackah, S. M.: Microbial kinetics of drug action against gram-positive and gram-negative organisms. III. Effect of lincomycin and clindamycin combinations on Staphylococcus aureus and Escherichia coli. J. Pharm. Sci. 64:1621, 1975.
37. Klastersky, J.: Clinical Use of Combinations of Antibiotics. New York, John Wiley & Sons, 1975.
38. Jawetz, E., Gunnison, J. B., and Speck, R. S.: Studies on antibiotic synergism and antagonism: the interference of aurcomycin, chloramphenicol, and terramycin with the action of streptomycin. Am. J. Med. Sci. 222:404, 1951.
39. Carrizosa, J., Kobasa, W. B., and Kaye, D.: Antagonism between chloramphenicol and penicillin in streptococcal endocarditis in rabbits. J. Lab. Clin. Med. 85:307, 1975.
40. Avakian, S., and Kabacoff, B. L.: Enhancement of blood antibiotic levels through the combined oral administration of phenethicillin and chymotrypsin. Clin. Pharmacol. Ther. 5:716, 1964.

41. Braybrooks, M. P., Barry, B. W., and Abbs, E. T.: The effect of mucin on the bioavailability of tetracycline from the gastrointestinal tract: *in vivo, in vitro* correlations. J. Pharm. Pharmacol. *27*:508, 1975.
42. Zanini, A. C., Sertie, J. A., and Oga, S.: Gastrointestinal absorption of meclocycline in healthy volunteers and patients with enteric infections. Curr. Ther. Res. *18*:733, 1975.
43. Frey, H. H., and Kampmann, E.: Interaction of amphetamine with anticonvulsant drugs. II. Effect of amphetamine on the absorption of anticonvulsant drugs. Acta Pharmacol. Toxicol. *24*:310, 1966.
44. Banergee, S., and Mitra, C.: Muscle relaxant properties of chloramphenicol. J. Pharm. Sci. *64*:704, 1976.
45. Young, L. S., and Hewitt, W. L.: Activity of five aminoglycoside antibiotics *in vitro* against gram-negative bacilli and *Staphylococcus aureus*. Antimicrob. Agents Chemother. *4*:617, 1973.
46. Bischop, C. R., Janzen, R. E., Landals, D. C., Manns, B. D., McCortney, D. J., Morgan, G. A., Pawlyshyn, V. P., Schienbein, A. J., Scigliano, B. W., and Taylor, K. L.: Effects of rumen stasis on sulfamethazine blood levels after oral administration in sheep. Can. Vet. J. *14*:269, 1973.
47. Oyaert, W., Quin, J. E., and Clark, R.: Studies on the alimentary tract of the Merino sheep in South Africa. XIX. The influence of sulphanilamide on the activity of the ruminal flora of sheep and cattle. Onderstepoort J. Vet. Res. *25*:59, 1951.
48. Davis, L. E., Neff, C. A., Baggot, J. D., and Powers, T. E.: Pharmacokinetics of chloramphenicol in domesticated animals. Am. J. Vet. Res. *33*:2259, 1972.
49. Hurwitz, A., Robinson, R. G., Vats, T. S., Whittier, F. C., and Herrin, W. F.: Effects of antacids on gastric emptying. Gastroenterology *71*:258, 1976.
50. Hurwitz, A.: The effects of antacids on gastrointestinal drug absorption. II. Effect of sulfadiazine and quinine. J. Pharmacol. Exp. Ther. *179*:485, 1971.
51. Wagner, J. G.: Biopharmaceutics: absorption aspects. J. Pharm. Sci. *50*:359, 1961.
52. Danti, A. G., and Guth, E. P.: A study of the release of selected antibiotics from cation-saturated bentonites. J. Am. Pharm. Assoc. *44*:249, 1957.
53. Dearborn, E. H., Litchfield, J. T., Eisner, J. H., Corbett, J. J., and Dunnett, C. W.: The effects of various substances on the absorption of tetracycline in rats. Antibiot. Med. *4*:627, 1957.
54. Kunin, C. M., and Finland, M.: Clinical pharmacology of the tetracycline antibiotics. Clin. Pharmacol. Ther. *2*:51, 1961.
55. Price, K. E., Zolli, Z., Atkinson, J. C., and Luther, H. G.: Antibiotic inhibitors. II. Studies on the inhibitory action of selected divalent cations for oxytetracycline. Antibiot. Chemother. *42*:689, 1957.
56. Andersson, K.-E., Bratt, L., Dencker, H., Kamme, C., and Lanner, E.: Inhibition of tetracycline absorption by zinc. Eur. J. Clin. Pharmacol. *10*:59, 1976.
57. Neuvonen, J. P., and Turakka, H.: Inhibitory effect of various iron salts on the absorption of tetracycline in man. Eur. J. Clin. Pharmacol. *7*:357, 1974.
58. Krondl, A.: Present understanding of the interaction of drugs and food during absorption. Can. Med. Assoc. J. *103*:360, 1970.
59. Bloedow, D. C., and Hayton, W. L.: Effects of lipids on bioavailability of sulfisoxazole acetyl, dicumarol, and griseofulvin in rats. J. Pharm. Sci. *65*:328, 1976.
60. Cheng, S. H., and White, A.: Effect of orally administered neomycin on the absorption of penicillin V. N. Engl. J. Med. *267*:1296, 1962.
61. Jacobson, E. D., Chodos, R. B., and Faloon, W. W.: An experimental malabsorption syndrome induced by neomycin. Am. J. Med. *28*:524, 1960.
62. Dobbins, W. O.: Drug-induced steatorrhea. Gastroenterology *54*:1193, 1968.
63. Bartelink, A.: Clinical Drug Interactions in the G.I. Tract of Man. Clinical Effects of Interaction Between Drugs, New York, American Elsevier Publishing Co., 1974, p. 103.
64. Lovering, E. G., McGilveray, I. J., McMillan, J., Tostowaryk, W., Matula, T., and Marier, G.: The bioavailability and dissolution behavior of nine brands of tetracycline tablets. Can. J. Pharm. Sci. *10*:36, 1975.
65. Dimmling, T. H., Bredehorst, H. B., and VanderElst, E.: Bioavailability of various preparations and doses of penicillin V. Eur. J. Clin. Pharmacol. *10*:55, 1976.
66. Whyatt, P. L., Slywka, G. W. A., Melikian, A. P., and Meyer, M. C.: Bioavailability of 17 ampicillin products. J. Pharm. Sci. *65*:652, 1976.
67. Mercer, H. D., Garg, R. C., Powers, J. D., and Powers, T. E.: Bioavailability and pharmacokinetics of several dosage forms of ampicillin in the cat. J. Vet. Res. *38*:1353, 1977.
68. Ritschel, W. A., Ritschel, G., Buncher, C. R., and Rotmensch, J.: Study on bioavailability of sulfadiazine tablets in man. Drug Intelligence Clin. Pharm. *10*:402, 1976.
69. Mizazaki, S., Nakano, M., and Arita, T.: Effect of crystal forms on the dissolution behavior and bioavailability of tetracycline, chlortetracycline, and oxytetracycline bases. Chem. Pharm. Bull. *23*:552, 1975.
70. Powers, J. D., Powers, T. E., Baggot, J. D., Kowalski, J., and Kerr, K.: Automated processing of data from pharmacokinetic investigations. Comput. Biomed. Res. *9*:543, 1976.
71. Verklin, R. M., and Mandell, G. L.: Alteration of effectiveness of antibiotics by anaerobiosis. J. Lab. Clin. Med. *89*:65, 1977.
72. Long-Term Programs in Environmental Pollution Control in Europe: Report on a Working Group on Control of Harmful Residues in Food for Human Consumption and Public Health Aspects of Antibiotics in Foodstuffs. Regional Office for Europe, Copenhagen, World Health Organization, 1974.
73. Baldwin, R. A.: The development of transferrable drug resistance in salmonella and its public health implications. J.A.V.M.A. *157*:1841, 1970.
74. Falkow, S., Williams, L. P., Seaman, S. L., and Rollins, L. D.: Increased survival in calves of *Escherichia coli* K-12 carrying an Ent. plasmid. Infect. Immun. *13*:1005, 1976.
75. Gyles, C. L.: Plasmids in intestinal bacteria. Am. J. Clin. Nutr. *25*:1455, 1972.
76. Smith, D. H.: R-Factor infection of *Escherichia coli* lyophilized in 1946. J. Bacteriol. *94*:2071, 1967.
77. Ingram, L. C., Anderson, J. D., Arrand, J. E., and Richmond, M. H.: Probable example of R-factor recombination in the human gastrointestinal tract. J. Med. Microbiol. *7*:251, 1974.
78. Maré, I. J.: Incidence of R-factors among gram-negative bacteria in drug-free human and animal communities. Nature (Lond.) *220*:1046, 1968.
79. Davis, C. E., and Anandan, J.: The evolution of R-factor: a study of a "preantibiotic" community in Borneo. N. Engl. J. Med. *282*:117, 1970.
80. Siegel, D., Huber, W. G., and Enloe, F.: Continuous nontherapeutic use of antibacterial drugs in feed and drug resistance of gram-negative enteric flora of food-producing animals. Antimicrob. Agents Chemother. *6*:697, 1974.
81. Mercer, H. D., Pocurull, D., Gaines, S., Wilson, S., and Bennett, J. V.: Characteristics of antimicrobial resistances among fecal flora of animals: relationship to veterinary and management uses of antimicrobials. Appl. Microbiol. *22*:700, 1971.
82. Aden, D. P., Reed, N. D., Underdahl, N. R., and Mebus, C. A.: Transferable drug resistance among Enterobacteriaceae isolated from cases of neonatal diarrhea in calves and piglets. Appl. Microbiol. *18*:961, 1969.
83. Rollins, L. D., Pocurull, D. W., Mercer, H. D., Natzke, R. P., and Postle, D. S.: Use of antibiotics in a dairy herd and their effect on resistance determinants in enteric flora and environmental *Escherichia coli*. J. Dairy Sci. *57*:944, 1974.
84. Rollins, L. D., Gaines, S. A., Pocurull, D. W., and Mercer, H. D.: Animal model for determining no-effect level of an antimicrobial drug on drug resistance in lactose fermenting enteric flora. Antimicrob. Agents Chemother. *7*:661, 1975.
85. Polacek, M. A., and Sanfelippo, P.: Oral antibiotic bowel preparation and complications in colon surgery. Arch. Surg. *97*:412, 1968.
86. Neu, H. C., Cherubin, C. E., Longo, E. D., Flouton, B., and Winter, J.: Antimicrobial resistance and R-factor transfer among isolates of salmonella in the Northeastern United States: a comparison of human and animal isolates. J. Infect. Dis. *132*:617, 1975.
87. Roy, R. S.: Presence de facteurs R chez des souches d'enterobacteries, pathogenes isolées d'animaux domestiques, et plus particulièrement du chien. Can. J. Comp. Med. *36*:1, 1972.
88. Loken, K. I., Wagner, W. L., and Henke, C. L.: Transmissible drug resistance in Enterobacteriaceae isolated from calves given antibiotics. Am. J. Vet. Res. *32*:1207, 1971.
89. Linton, K. B., Lee, P. A., Richmond, M. H., Gillespie, W. A., Rowland, A. J., and Baker, V. N.: Antibiotic resistance and transmissible R-factors in the intestinal coliform flora of healthy adults and children in an urban and a rural community. J. Hyg. (Camb.) *70*:99, 1972.
90. Datta, N., Brumfitt, W., Saiers, M. C., Orskov, F., Reeves, D. S. and Orskov, I.: R-factors in *Escherichia coli* in feces after oral chemotherapy in general practice. Lancet, #7694, Feb. 13, 1971, pp. 312–315.
91. Rollins, D. E., and Moeller, D.: Acute migratory polyarthritis associated with antibiotic induced pseudomembranous colitis. Am. J. Gastroenterol. *65*:353, 1976.

92. Richmond, M.H.: R-factors in man and his environment. *In* Microbiology. Edited by D. Schlessinger. Washington, D.C., American Society for Microbiology, 1975, p. 27.

93. FDA Contracts 71-269, University of Illinois, July 1976, and 71-306, University of Missouri, October 1974: Ecological Effects of Antimicrobial Agents on the Enteric Flora of Animals and Man.

94. Miner, J. R., Fina, L. R., and Platt, C.: *Salmonella infantis* in cattle feedlot runoff. Appl. Microbiol. *15*:627, 1967.

95. Simmons, H. E., and Stolley, P. D.: This is medical progress? Trends and consequences of antibiotic use in the United States. J.A.M.A. *227*:1023, 1974.

96. Levy, S. B., Fitzgerald, G. B., and Malone, A. B.: Spread of antibiotic-resistant plasmids from chicken to chicken and from chicken to man. Nature *260*:40, 1976.

97. Richmond, M. H.: Antibiotics and bacterial resistance, R-factors in farm animals and their possible consequences for human health. Norden News, Spring, 1976, p. 19.

98. Shooter, R. A., Rousseau, S. A., Cooke, E. M., and Breaden, A. L.: Animal sources of common serotypes of *Escherichia coli* in the food of hospital patients: possible significance in urinary-tract infections. Lancet No. 7666:226, 1970.

99. Jones, A. M.: *Escherichia coli* in retail samples of milk and their resistance to antibiotics. Lancet No. 7720:347, 1971.

100. Walton, J. R.: Contamination of meat carcasses by antibiotic-resistant coliform bacteria. Lancet No. 7672:561, 1970.

101. Howe, K., and Linton, A. H.: The distribution of O-antigen types of *Escherichia coli* in normal calves compared with man, and their R-plasmid carriage. J. Appl. Bacteriol. *40*:317, 1976.

102. Damato, J. J., Eitzman, D. V., and Baer, H.: Persistence and dissemination in the community of R-factors of nosocomial origin. J. Infect. Dis. *129*:205, 1974.

103. Schaberg, D. R., Weinstein, R. A., and Stamm, W. E.: Epidemics of nosocomial urinary tract infection caused by multiple resistant gram-negative bacilli: epidemiology and control. J. Infect. Dis. *133*:363, 1976.

104. Public Health Aspects of Antibiotic-Resistant Bacteria in the Environment. Regional Office for Europe, Brussels, World Health Organization, 1975.

105. Datta, N., and Olarte, J.: R-factors in strains of *Salmonella typhi* and *Shigella dysenteriae* isolated during epidemics in Mexico: classification by compatibility. Antimicrob. Agents. Chemother. *5*:310, 1974.

106. Hjerpe, C.A., and Routen, T.A.: Practical and theoretical considerations concerning treatment of bacterial pneumonia in feedlot cattle, with special reference to antimicrobic therapy. Edited by E.I. Williams. Proceedings of 9th Annual Convention, American Association of Bovine Practitioners, Dec. 8–11, 1976, 97–140.

107. FDA Contract 72-39, Colorado State University, March 14, 1975: Study on the Relationship Between Drugs and Their Subsequent Effect on Therapy of Disease in Veal Calves.

108. Smith, H. W.: A search for transmissible pathogenic characters in invasive strains of *Escherichia coli:* the discovery of a plasmid-controlled toxin and a plasmid-controlled lethal character closely associated or identical with colicine V. J. Gen. Microbiol. *83*:95, 1974.

109. Smith, H. W., and Linggood, M. A.: Transfer factors in *Escherichia coli* with particular regard to their incidence in enteropathogenic strains. J. Gen. Microbiol. *62*:287, 1970.

Section Three

GASTROINTESTINAL DISEASES OF DOMESTIC ANIMALS

Chapter 20

THE MOUTH

JERRY H. JOHNSON, BRUCE L. HULL,
and ALBERT S. DORN

Diseases of the mouth and its associated structures constitute a substantial portion of gastrointestinal diagnoses in every species. Animals with oropharyngeal disease are likely to be poorly nourished animals, at least for the short term, resulting in loss of production and/or performance. The mouth is also a site at which may be found clues to the presence of disease in another part of the body.

The oropharyngeal, salivary, and dental diseases of horses, cattle, and dogs will be discussed in that order in this chapter, continuing the order of species that was generally followed in Section One. For each species, diseases are clustered according to cause, so that trauma, infection, congenital malformations, and neoplasia are recurring themes throughout the chapter. Special topics are included as appropriate to the segment; e.g., nutritional disorders as evidenced in the mouth, guttural pouch disease in horses, and sialoliths and sialoceles associated with salivary glands.

LIPS, TONGUE, AND SOFT PALATE

Horse

The upper lip, the main prehensile structure in the horse, is sensitive, strong, and mobile.[1] Severe damage to the lips, whether traumatic, infectious, or neurogenic, will affect the horse's ability to graze, since during grazing, the lips direct the forage between the incisor teeth.

The tongue is large and mobile and fills the mouth when closed. It provides the vacuum for suckling by the young horse and for the intake of solid and liquid food by the adult.

The soft palate is quite long in the horse and will not permit mouth breathing, because the epiglottis overlies the trailing edge of the palate. The soft palate can be partially visualized through the mouth, but endoscopy is required for complete visualization.

Trauma

Trauma to the lips may result in distortion of the facial features, as well as impairing the horse's grazing ability. If severe lacerations occur, surgical correction is suggested. Healing by primary union may be difficult to achieve due to constant movement of the lips. Cross tieing and muzzling, and feeding via nasogastric tube are aids in patient management.

Facial nerve paralysis due to direct trauma or neuritis (depending on the location of the nerve involvement) can result in a drooping of the lips on the affected side. This interferes with grazing as well as increasing the risk of the lips being lacerated by the teeth. The nostril on the affected side may be partially collapsed. The most serious consequence of facial nerve paralysis is that food may collect between the cheek and the molar teeth. The impacted food ferments, resulting in a fetid odor, and may cause erosion of the buccal mucosa. The mouth should be cleaned out at least once per day to minimize erosion. Reconstructive surgery of the lips (removal of one or more elliptical pieces of lip) is done primarily for the sake of a pleasing cosmetic effect but the lip trauma and food accumulation may also be reduced.[2]

Trauma to the tongue in the horse is primarily due to the use of improper bits or overzealous use of a rough bit during training. Transverse tongue lacerations slightly anterior to the frenulum are not uncommon. In some cases the laceration extends through as much as half of the thickness of the tongue. If the lesion is acute, surgical correction is indicated, but owing to continuous movement of the tongue some of the sutures may not hold. In rare cases, the laceration may extend through the entire tongue resulting in loss of the tip. These horses have some problems grazing but appear to thrive if fed hay and grain. Sharp teeth can also cause trauma to the lips and tongue, and this can be corrected by "floating" the sharp points down so there is no additional trauma. Direct visualization of the teeth, lips, and tongue will reveal the problem. The horse also may lose weight, taking a long time to eat and drooling food and saliva from the mouth, thereby effectively reducing its total daily intake.

Infection

Infections of the lips, tongue, and palate are rare. Viral pox lesions occur but these are generally of little consequence and persist for only a few days. Viral papillomas of the nose and lips are not uncommon, appear mostly in the spring, and cause little interference with eating. If the papillomas are numerous and become irritated while the horse grazes, food intake may decline. The horse should be removed from pasture and fed good-quality hay and grain. The papillomas are unsightly, but in some cases will disappear in 2 or 3 months. Crushing several of the lesions may hasten regression. Viral papillomas have also been observed on the lips and extremities of foals at birth. Surgical excision with scissors is effective in those instances. In severe cases an autogenous bacterin may be considered.

Palatitis

Palatitis or lampas is an inflammation and swelling of the palate immediately posterior to the upper incisors. This disorder occurs primarily among young horses during the eruption of the permanent incisors and is usually noticed when the horse fails to eat properly. The swelling may extend beyond the table surface of the incisors. Therapy consists of changing the ration to a soft mash and leafy hay. Rarely will this disorder need any specific treatment other than a change of diet. The outmoded practice of fulguration cautery of the palate is to be condemned.

Soft Palate Paresis

This condition may be seen in the acute stage with food being expelled from both nostrils because of inability to swallow or in a clinically normal horse that develops a respiratory noise after forced exercise. Guttural pouch infection and distention leading to a neuritis of cranial nerves IX and XII is the most logical explanation of the cause. A patent airway is the first consideration in an acute case. Catheterization and supportive therapy, such as flushing or draining the guttural pouches as needed and maintaining hydration and feeding via nasogastric tube, should also be considered.[3] In the chronic case that occurs with a respiratory "gurgle" after forced exercise and with a history of poor perfor-

mance, an endoscopic exam should be conducted at rest and immediately after exercise. If the endoscopic exam reveals the soft palate covering the epiglottis after several induced swallowing movements, a section of the posterior edge of the palate may need to be removed surgically to correct the disorder permanently.[4,5]

Congenital Malformations

Congenital malformations of the lips and tongue are seen rarely and in most cases the affected foal is stillborn. Cleft soft palate may be seen in foals that survive the immediate neonatal period.[6] The clinical sign of milk flowing from the nostril after nursing should alert one to its possible presence.[7] The appearance of milk at the nostril is not pathognomonic for cleft soft palate, since foals with an intact soft palate may have this sign for the first 1 to 3 days of life. Visual demonstration of the cleft soft palate is made either through the mouth or by endoscopy.[4,8] Surgical correction, although not highly successful, is the only method of treatment. In all cases recorded, the cleft in the live foal involves the soft palate only and not the hard palate.[9,10,11,12,13] These horses should not be used for breeding, even if a successful surgical repair permits survival.

Neoplasia

Sarcoid has the highest frequency of all tumors in the horse,[14] perhaps because it is transmissible from horse to horse. A virus is suspected as the causative agent. Surgical removal by excision or cryosurgery should be considered if the lesions are unsightly, interfere with lip motion, or enlarge rapidly. Sarcoid occurs more frequently about the face and ears and less frequently on the lips.

Papillomatosis is the most frequent tumor reported in the soft tissues of the lips and muzzle.[15] This tumor is also thought to be viral-induced.

Other tumors may be seen; these should be biopsied and then treated appropriately.

Cow

Examination of the bovine mouth can be performed with or without the aid of a speculum. Although the use of a speculum affords a superior visual examination, there is value in a digital examination. Digital examination is probably more helpful in detecting temperature changes, abnormal teeth, and foreign bodies. After the hand has been withdrawn from the mouth, abnormal odors can be detected at the fingertips. If necessary, one may also bring one's nose near the cow's mouth. When performing digital examination within the mouth, the pharyngeal area should be palpated for foreign bodies, lacerations, or swellings.

The bovine tongue is extremely strong. Therefore, in performing a digital examination due caution must be exercised to avoid being bitten or lacerated by the molar or premolar teeth. Visual examination is probably best for observing hemorrhages, pustules, ulcers, or lacerations. Whenever the oral cavity is examined, one must be cognizant of the potential of rabies and take necessary precautions by wearing gloves.

Trauma

Trauma to the bovine mouth is uncommon as compared to trauma to the equine mouth. Lacerations to the lips and tongue are rare. However, if such lacerations do occur, they should be treated as described for the horse.

Fracture of the mandible is usually due to sharp external trauma, and is usually bilateral. It may be self-inflicted by an extremely fractious animal when halter training is begun. Although these mandibular fractures are often compounded and contaminated, they usually heal surprisingly well. Treatment can be with plates or wires, but probably the most satisfactory procedure is with intramedullary pins. The pin is introduced just ventral to the first incisor (penetrating gingival mucosa rather than skin). Then the pin is directed caudally in the medullary cavity of the mandible. Usually these fractures are bilateral and may even involve the mandibular symphysis. After pinning one mandible, the procedure is repeated on the second. Then the most rostral ends of the two pins are joined in a stable fixation such as with a Kirschner apparatus.

Postoperatively, the animal should be fed a ration of milled grain. Hay should be gradually reintroduced after 7 to 14 days. Intramuscular injection of antibiotics for 5 to 7 days and local irrigation with saline solution daily is beneficial for compound fractures. The pins should be removed in 4 to 6 weeks. If they remain stable, the 6-week period is preferable; however, if the pins loosen, they may be removed after the fourth week.

Infection

Many infectious oral lesions in cattle have a similar appearance. Some of these diseases are localized to the mouth and are not serious. Others are visible evidence of highly contagious diseases that threaten great economic loss to herds and must be reported to government agencies. Therefore, correct diagnosis is extremely important. The following distinguishing features of the important oral infections in cattle are shown in Table 20–1.

Proliferative stomatitis is a common transmissible viral disease of young calves (2 to 8 weeks of age). Hyperkeratosis has been associated with this disease but does not appear to be an essential feature in the pathogenesis of the lesion. The disease is not serious in its own right.

The earliest clinical sign is a small (less than 1 cm), swollen, congested lesion which ulcerates within 2 to 5 days and may then proliferate. These lesions may be seen on the tongue, lips, palate, and buccal mucosa. The proliferative lesions persist for several weeks, but heal spontaneously and treatment is usually not indicated. There is little loss of condition or production as a result of proliferative stomatitis.

Papular stomatitis was first reported in cattle in the United States in 1960.[16] It is a viral disease causing little systemic disturbance. Its chief importance is its close resemblance to other, more devastating viral diseases of the bovine digestive tract.

Cattle up to 2 years of age are susceptible and often the morbidity approaches 100% in a herd, but without death loss. The lesions consist of raised reddish papules (0.5 to 1.0 cm in diameter) which occur on the muzzle, inside the nostrils, and on the buccal mucosa. Although the disease often goes unnoticed, it may cause transient anorexia and fever. Individual lesions heal quickly, but new lesions may continue to develop for several months. Treatment for papular stomatitis is neither indicated nor beneficial.

The bovine virus diarrhea-mucosal disease complex (BVD-MD) is probably the most prevalent oral problem of cattle in North America. It is a highly contagious viral disease of cattle and appears with a variety of clinical signs. The oral lesions are but one of many manifestations of the disease, and this discussion will focus on recognition of the oral lesions of BVD-MD.

Oral lesions initially start as reddened, congested areas, which erode into pinpoint ulcers within 24 hours. The ulcers gradually enlarge in diameter to 1 to 2 cm and may coalesce to form large denuded areas. The lesions, which typically remain shallow, can be found on the muzzle, gingiva, buccal mucosa, dental pad, tongue, palate, and pharynx as well as in the esophagus and in the abdominal segments of the digestive tract. Ulcers of BVD-MD should not be confused with the more linear erosions on the dental pad which are caused by trauma from the incisors. Chronic BVD-MD typically produces blunting and rounding of the buccal papillae.

Table 20–1. Oral lesions in cattle as evidence of local or systemic viral disease

Disease	Causative Agent	Age Affected	Oral Lesions	Location of Lesions	Associated Signs and Findings	Other Systemic Involvement	Morbidity	Mortality	Treatment	Diagnosis
1. Proliferative Stomatitis	Virus	Calves; 2–8 wk	Raised congested, ulcerated, proliferative 1 cm diam.	Tongue, lips, palate, buccal mucosa	Anorexia	Hyperkeratosis	High	None	None	Clinical history and physical examination
2. Papular Stomatitis	Virus	Birth to 2 yr	Raised reddish papules	Buccal mucosa, muzzle, inside nares	Transient anorexia and fever	—	Up to 100%	None	None	Histopathology, virus isolation
3. Bovine Virus Diarrhea-Mucosal Disease Complex (BVD-MD)	Virus	All ages	Reddened, erosions, pinpoint ulcers Blunting, rounding of buccal papillae at commissures of lips	Buccal mucosa, dental pad, tongue, palate, gingiva, pharynx, muzzle, esophagus, forestomachs, abomasum, small intestine, coronary band of hooves	Anorexia, persistent fever, leukopenia (1000–3000/cmm), neutropenia	Pneumonia, cough, inflammation at coronary band causes lameness	Variable to high (many asymptomatic infections)	Low	Supportive, fluid therapy	Virus isolation from nasal scrapings or bronchial lymph node. Increase in paired titers, fluorescent antibody test
4. Foot-and-Mouth Disease (FMD, all cloven-footed animals)	Virus	All ages	Vesicular and bullous eruptions, erosions	Buccal cavity, cleft and coronary band of hooves, teats	Transient fever, anorexia, ptyalism, dullness, reduced milk yield	Feet (vesicles at coronary band, and interdigital cleft). *Severe lameness.* Teats, vulva, perineum	Up to 100%	Low; 5–10% of affected animals	None	Virus isolation; neutralization by known antisera
5. Vesicular Stomatitis (cattle, horses, swine)	Virus	Adult cattle (calves more resistant)	Vesicular eruptions, erosions	Buccal cavity, coronary band	Fever, anorexia	None	High	Low	None	Virus isolation; fluorescent antibody test
6. Rinderpest	Virus	All ages	1–5 mm discrete ulcers (*no vesicles*)	Lower lip, adjacent gingival mucosa, ventral surface of tongue. Ulcers may coalescece	Fever, nasal and lacrimal discharge, thirst, depression	—	Up to 100%	Up to 90%	None	Virus isolation; fluorescent antibody test
7. Bluetongue (primarily sheep)	Virus	All ages	Ulcers	Tongue, dental pad, muzzle, coronary band (sloughing of hoof, ulcers on udder)	Fever, anorexia	None	Low	High	None	Serum neutralization, microagar gel diffusion, complement fixation
8. Photosensitization	Actinic rays of sun/photodynamic agent in skin	All ages	Ulceration	Lips, ventral surface of anterior 1/3 of tongue, nose	Depression	Hairless and white-skinned areas of body	Low to high	Low	Remove from sunlight	Identify agent

This is usually best observed at the commissure of the lips. Inflammation of the coronary band may occur, causing lameness. Separation of the sensitive and insensitive laminae may occur; in severe cases, the hoof wall may become detached. A fever of 104 to 105° F is typical; however, it may subside before other clinical signs become evident. Thus, fever may not be detected at the time of clinical examination.

Diagnosis can usually be made after a thorough physical examination and/or a postmortem. BVD-MD typically produces a severe leukopenia (1000 to 3000 per cubic mm) early in the clinical syndrome. The primary cell type remaining in the circulation is the lymphocyte, accounting for 75 to 100% of the cells in the differential count. The virus may be isolated from the blood during the febrile period, while virus isolation from nasal scrapings or bronchial lymph node is also diagnostic. Demonstrating a significant increase in antibody titer in paired serum samples taken 2 to 4 weeks apart indicates an active infection. The fluorescent antibody technique may be used on nasal scrapings or on tissues collected at necropsy to demonstrate the presence of BVD antigen.

A high percentage of the cattle in North America have a titer to BVD-MD. In calves and feedlot cattle, it seems to be associated with acute or chronic pneumonia as well as with digestive disease, especially in the midwestern United States.

Foot and mouth disease is an acute, highly contagious disease of cloven-footed animals. Morbidity often approaches 100% within a herd; however, mortality is usually low (5 to 10% of affected animals). The disease is characterized by vesicular eruption and subsequent erosion of the epithelium of the mouth and feet. In the acute stage of the disease a high fever (104 to 106°F) occurs, but this usually subsides before the appearance of lesions. The high fever is often accompanied by anorexia, dullness, and decreased milk yield in dairy cattle. Following the brief febrile period, vesicles of various sizes form on the buccal mucosa, dental pad, and tongue. These vesicles are filled with a clear fluid and are easily ruptured. During vesiculation, the animal may salivate profusely and open and close its mouth with a "characteristic smacking sound."[17] Concurrently, vesicles occur on the feet, especially in the interdigital cleft and the coronary band area. The teats, vulva, and perineum may also be affected with vesicles. As discussed in the previous section, BVD-MD also causes coronary band lesions and lameness, but BVD-MD does not cause the severe lameness that occurs with foot and mouth disease. The foot lesions and severe lameness of foot and mouth disease are the basis for culling of affected cattle in endemic areas.

Foot and mouth disease has not been diagnosed in the United States since 1929. Cattle in the United States and Canada are not vaccinated for foot and mouth disease and would be extremely susceptible should the disease be reintroduced. Considering the seriousness of foot and mouth disease and the fact it can be easily confused with several other vesicular diseases, one should report to the federal veterinarian any case that strongly resembles foot and mouth disease. At this point, the federal veterinarian can conduct the appropriate diagnostic tests and may quarantine the herd if necessary.

Vesicular stomatitis is a highly contagious, febrile viral disease which naturally affects cattle, horses, and swine. The mouth lesions of vesicular stomatitis in cattle are often indistinguishable from those of foot and mouth disease. While vesicular stomatitis is important in its own right, it is especially important because of its similarity to the oral manifestations of foot and mouth disease. Whenever vesicular stomatitis is suspected, it should be reported to the federal veterinarian so appropriate diagnostic tests can be performed.

Rinderpest is a highly contagious viral disease of cattle and buffalo. In susceptible cattle the morbidity approaches 100% and mortality may reach 90%. Although this disease is enzootic in many parts of the world, it is not presently found in North or South America.

Rinderpest is characterized by sudden onset after a variable incubation period of 3 to 15 days. The temperature rises quickly to above 104°F and is accompanied by nasal and lacrimal discharges, anorexia, thirst, and depression. Oral lesions appear 2 to 3 days after the onset of the fever. These small (1 to 5 mm) discrete ulcers appear initially on the inside of the lower lip and adjacent gingival mucosa as well as on the ventral surface of the tongue. Later these ulcers may coalesce and become generalized throughout the mouth. There is never any vesicle formation, but rather just a sloughing of the necrotic areas.

The signs and lesions of rinderpest are very difficult to distinguish from BVD-MD. However, the mortality is much greater in rinderpest. Since rinderpest is an exotic disease with potentially disastrous consequences to the cattle population of the United States, the federal veterinarian should be contacted in suspicious cases. Treatment is not effective and should not be undertaken.

Bluetongue has been reported in cattle, although

it is primarily a disease of sheep. Excessive salivation and edema of the lips as well as ulcerative lesions on the tongue, dental pad, and muzzle are seen in cattle. Bluetongue usually affects an individual animal or several animals, but is rarely epidemic in cattle. The clinical diagnosis must be confirmed by laboratory tests. Useful laboratory tests are serum neutralization, micro-agar-gel diffusion, or complement fixation. Treatment is ineffective and cannot be recommended at this time.

Photosensitization may be accompanied by oral lesions, which are easily confused with those of the previously described viral diseases. The ulcerations of photosensitized cattle characteristically involve the nose, lips, and ventral surface of the anterior one third of the tongue as well as the more classic lesions of the hairless and white-haired areas. The oral lesions are of the nature of complete yet very superficial sloughs, which could be confused with viral stomatitis in its more advanced form. The distribution of other lesions on the animal should help differentiate photosensitization from viral stomatitis.

Although treatment is not generally effective, removing the animals from direct sunlight will allow the lesions to regress.

Necrotic stomatitis and necrotic pharyngitis (laryngitis) are discussed as necrobacillosis since the lesions, causative agents, and treatment are similar.

Necrobacillosis, caused by infection with *Fusobacterium necrophorum,* is characterized by a fever of 103 to 106°F, increased salivation, painful swallowing, complete anorexia, severe depression, and a necrotic, foul-smelling breath. In classic necrotic stomatitis, the lesions are traditionally found in the mucosa of the cheek (giving the animal a puffy-cheeked appearance), while necrotic pharyngitis involves the pharyngeal and laryngeal mucosa.

Treatment is often unsatisfactory unless begun early in the course of the disease. Sulfapyridine, sulfamethazine (sulfadimidine), as well as penicillin, streptomycin, and tetracyclines have been successful in arresting the disease. Antihistamines and corticosteroids are useful adjuncts to relieve swelling and ease breathing.

Actinomycosis or "lumpy jaw" is a rarefying osteomyelitis of the mandible and maxilla, caused by *Actinomyces bovis.* Other organisms may be cultured from these lesions, especially if the lesions have ulcerated and developed fistulous tracts. *Actinomyces bovis* typically produces "sulfur granules," yellow concretions in the exudate which are a distinguishing feature helpful in diagnosis. Staining the crushed "sulfur granules" reveals gram-positive filaments, which are diagnostic.

The mode of infection with *A. bovis* is not definitively known. Since *A. bovis* is a normal inhabitant of the mucous membranes, upper respiratory tract, and digestive tract,[18] it may be introduced into the tissues as a result of mechanical lacerations from feedstuffs or foreign materials during mastication, as well as into open alveoli resulting from the loss of deciduous teeth. Once the organism penetrates the tissues, primary necrosis takes place and a tract is produced. Enlargement of the lesion and the development of osteomyelitis takes place after anaerobic conditions have been established.

The granulomatous mass may protrude into the oral cavity as well as outwardly from the jaws. After an abscess has developed, it will usually rupture. Exudate is thick, tenacious, light-green and purulent, containing the characteristic "sulfur granules." These are actually colonies (3 to 4 mm in diameter) of the organism. The draining tract heals, only to break out in another skin site over the lesion. A long-standing lesion will have numerous protrusions of granulomatous tissue. These granulomatous masses are quite characteristic of actinomycosis.

Clinically, actinomycosis may be well advanced before external signs are visible. Early signs include difficult mastication and a slight bulge over the maxilla or mandible. The enlargments are hard and immobile when palpated. Often, loose teeth can be noted in the area of the lesion.

Although the physical findings are fairly characteristic, the diagnosis can be confirmed only by: (1) culture (special media and conditions are required); (2) staining of the crushed "sulfur granules" with New Methylene Blue, or (3) radiography. Well-advanced lesions have a typical "sponge-like" radiographic appearance of the affected bone.

Once bony involvement has occurred, treatment will probably only arrest further development of the lesions rather than effect a cure. These arrested lesions may recrudesce later and again become an active infection requiring treatment.

Iodides, both organic and inorganic, are still the standard treatment for both actinomycosis and actinobacillosis. These can be given intravenously, orally or in combination. Iodides probably have little effect against *Actinomyces bovis*, but they are effective in reducing fibrous reaction and allowing other antimicrobials or the animal's defenses to function. The intravenous dose of sodium iodide is 9 g/100 kg as a 20% solution. If oral treatment is given, organic iodide salts are preferable, since they are more palatable than potassium iodide.

Penicillin has proven to be effective against actinomycosis when given locally (into and around the lesion) as well as parenterally. Streptomycin seems to be effective against both actinomycosis and actinobacillosis. Combining penicillin and streptomycin has given excellent results in actinobacillosis and good results in actinomycosis. Sulfonamides and erythromycin have each been reported to produce an excellent response in pigs.[19]

Radiation therapy does not produce good clinical response when used alone. However, it seems to potentiate sodium iodide therapy. Radiation therapy should not be used if iodides have been administered in the previous 30 days, as large sloughs can be produced. Therefore, radiation therapy should be used initially (500 R every other day for 10 days) and then followed by sodium iodide therapy.

Isoniazid has been used to treat a limited number of cases of actinomycosis and some improvement has been obtained.[20,21] The dosage rate is 12 to 22 mg/kg of body weight daily for 30 days. Isoniazid is excreted in milk; therefore, it should not be used in lactating dairy animals. Since the infection is acquired at contaminated troughs and waterers, animals with discharging lesions should be isolated or eliminated from the herd.

Actinobacillosis or "wooden tongue" affects the soft tissues of the mouth, usually the tongue and less commonly the pharyngeal lymph nodes. The abscesses of actinobacillosis may drain in a manner similar to those of actinomycosis. Again, the purulent exudate contains "sulfur granules," which are differentiated from those of actinomycosis by the same crush-and-stain preparation described for actinomycosis. The causative organisms appear as rather short gram-negative rods, in contrast to the gram-positive filaments of *A. bovis*. *Actinobacillus lignieresi* enters through lacerations of the buccal mucosa, as does *A. bovis*. Once entry is gained, granulomatous lesions with necrosis and suppuration develop.

The first clinical signs of actinobacillosis are inability to eat and ptyalism. The animal often manipulates the tongue as if a foreign body were caught in the mouth. Visual or digital examination may be necessary to differentiate between actinobacillosis and a foreign body. Examination often reveals a hard swollen tongue, especially at the base. The anterior third of the tongue is usually normal. Occasionally ulcers and granulomatous lesions are present on either side of the base of the tongue.

If infection involves the retropharyngeal lymph nodes, dysphagia occurs and stertorous, snoring respirations may be heard. Even if the animal has no food in its mouth, it may repeatedly attempt to swallow. As the disease progresses, the affected animal becomes emaciated or dehydrated due to interference with prehension of food and drinking of water.

Treatment is similar to the treatments discussed previously for actinomycosis. However, treatment for actinobacillosis is generally more successful than is treatment for actinomycosis.

Nutritional Disorders

Nutritional stomatitis can be produced experimentally, but is not recognized as a clinical entity in the bovine.

Cleft Palate

Cleft palate occurs in calves with a lesser frequency than in foals. Clinical signs in the suckling calf are as described earlier for foals. The Charolais breed was at a sixfold risk as compared with other cattle breeds, according to one epidemiologic study.[22]

Dogs

Infectious and Traumatic Diseases

Cheilitis or inflammation of the lips has a variety of causes in dogs. The lips may be injured as the result of chewing sharp or abrasive objects. The buccal surface of the lip may develop contact ulcers as a result of the abrasive action of dental tartar or malpositioned teeth. Inflammation and ulceration of the lip-fold occurs in breeds with a deep furrow, which entraps saliva and debris and enhances the development of local infection. Excessive salivation may occur which predisposes to infection of the lips. The lips also become affected in generalized diseases of the skin, such as acute pustular dermatitis, dermatomycosis, urticaria, and demodectic mange.

The signs of cheilitis vary depending upon the severity of the lesion. The most consistent physical findings are pawing at the mouth or rubbing the muzzle against surfaces and objects, ptyalism, persistent presence of moisture on the chin, foul odor, and loss of hair about the site. Infection of the lip fold is manifested by a brown stain on the surrounding hair and swelling of the skin. In heavy coated dogs, the exudate may be contained within the hair of the chin, and foul odor may be mistakenly attributed to diseases of the oral cavity or stomach.

Treatment of cheilitis involves removing the predisposing cause and treating the inflammation. Injuries to the lips should be repaired, foreign objects should be removed, and wounds should be sutured as soon as possible. With inflammatory lesions, hair is clipped from the involved area, the lesion is cleansed, and drugs are applied topically to relieve irritation. Astringents, antibacterial agents, and antibiotic or sulfonamide combinations containing corticosteroid are useful. When irritation is severe, topical anesthetics or an Elizabethan collar may be used to prevent self-trauma. Infections of the lip folds usually respond to cleansing and medical treatment, but if sustained response is not obtained, surgical removal of the lip fold is indicated.

Stomatitis or generalized inflammation of the mouth may extend to the gums (gingivitis) or the tongue (glossitis). Primary stomatitis most frequently results from extension of gingivitis which accompanies periodontal disease. Chemical, thermal, or mechanical irritation may also cause stomatitis. Specific infections may be involved, such as Vincent's stomatitis, caused by a spirochete and fusiform bacteria, and mycotic stomatitis due to *Candida albicans*. Stomatitis occurs as a secondary disorder in uremia, leptospirosis, infectious canine hepatitis, canine distemper, and niacin deficiency.

The signs of stomatitis are quite variable, and may range from slight ptyalism and drooling to complete anorexia and severe discomfort. Most affected animals eat carefully and slowly, and drool considerable amounts of saliva. They exhibit apparent thirst by spending considerable time at the water pan. The mouth is sensitive, and sedation or anesthesia may be required for examination. The regional lymph nodes may be enlarged and tender, and the breath malodorous.

After the primary cause of stomatitis is identified and removed, the oral lesions are cleansed, palliative agents are applied to relieve pain, and supportive medication is provided. It usually is necessary to anesthetize or sedate the patient to cleanse the mouth thoroughly, after which an antiseptic solution is applied. The subcutaneous administration of atropine sulfate reduces salivation, prolonging the effects of topical applications. Dogs with stomatitis should be given a systemic antibiotic. The bacteria associated with oral infections usually are sensitive to penicillin. Because stomatitis is often associated with periodontal disease, dental prophylaxis should

be included as part of both treatment and prevention.

A generalized stomatitis called "idiopathic necro-ulcerative stomatitis" has been described. It is characterized by sloughing of the oral mucosa with deep ulcers of the entire mouth. Salivation is profuse, and dermatitis frequently develops on the forelegs where the skin is moistened by saliva. A slight fever is present and the animal appears depressed. The disease may last for 3 to 8 weeks before spontaneous remission occurs. A specific cause has not been determined,[23] and antibiotic treatment is not effective in shortening the course of the disease.

Pemphigus vulgaris[24,25] is an autoimmune disease of dogs, characterized by chronic bullous eruptions of the mouth, nose, ears, and skin. The bullae initially appear as vesicles but the propensity of mouth and lip lesions to erode commonly yields the visual appearance of ulcerative stomatitis, glossitis, and cheilitis. Other clinical findings associated with these diseases include halitosis, ptyalism, gingivitis, dental deposits, difficulty in eating, sneezing and nasal discharge. Fever and lymphadenopathy are inconstant findings. Other mucocutaneous sites, e.g., anus, vulva, prepuce, and periorbital skin, may also be affected with bullous lesions. The skin manifestations may be so severe that toenails are sloughed. Bullous pemphigoid,[26] another bullous disease of dogs, produces similar skin lesions but without oral involvement. A variant form of pemphigus called pemphigus foliaceous, has been described in a dog, in which the lesions spread extensively over the skin "far distant from any mucocutaneous junction."[27] However, mucosal lesions were never noted in this dog.

Intercurrent bacterial infection may be present at the time of examination, and bullae may not be readily found on inflamed mucosae. Antibiotic therapy is of little or no benefit, and such negative evidence in the history will alert the veterinarian to the possibility of these bullous diseases. Biopsy and histopathologic examination of both mucosal and cutaneous lesions will provide support for the diagnosis. Acantholysis (separation of epidermal cells from one another) is evident, with clefts and bullae being formed within the epidermis in a suprabasilar location in pemphigus vulgaris, while cleft formation is below the epidermis in bullous pemphigoid.

Positive direct and indirect immunofluorescent findings are diagnostic.[24,25] Immunoglobulin G is demonstrable in the intercellular space cement substance (ICSS) of affected epidermis in cases of pemphigus vulgaris, while the indirect immunofluorescence technique can be used to demonstrate the presence of circulating antibodies to ICSS, using canine lip or esophagus as substrate. In bullous pemphigoid, direct immunofluoresence technique has been used to demonstrate immunoglobulin G and the third component of complement (C_3) at the basement membrane zone. Indirect immunofluorescence using canine esophagus as substrate tissue demonstrated that antibodies directed against basement membrane were present in the serum. In both diseases in dogs, the pathogenetic role of immunoglobulin autoantibodies has yet to be defined, although anti-ICSS serum from some humans with pemphigus vulgaris has been used to induce skin blisters in monkeys. These blisters have the histopathologic features of the original lesions in the patient whose serum was used for injection. Further studies in dogs are indicated.

Corticosteroid is the key to treatment, with antibiotic, local antiseptic, moist dressings, and fluids as adjunct therapy. In humans, pemphigus vulgaris requires high doses of corticosteroid to maintain adequate immunosuppression, while bullous pemphigoid in humans is controlled with lesser doses. Corticosteroid therapy must be maintained continuously in humans with pemphigus vulgaris, but the dose is tapered and later discontinued in bullous pemphigoid with anticipation of continued remission. Dogs with pemphigus vulgaris require high doses of corticosteroid (1.0 mg prednisolone/kg/day or greater to attain control). Although some affected dogs are later kept in remission by much reduced or alternate-day corticosteroid therapy, other canine patients with pemphigus vulgaris do not attain complete remission even with sustained high doses. Bullous pemphigoid in dogs may parallel the disorder in humans by being controllable with lower doses of corticosteroid, although more experience by veterinarians is needed to establish the point. One reported case continued in remission after corticosteroid was discontinued. Cyclophosphamide (2.2 mg/kg/day) has been used to treat pemphigus vulgaris, with the dose being tapered to 1 mg/kg every third day.[25]

With the dependence on corticosteroid in the management of these bullous diseases and the extensive use of corticosteroid in veterinary practice, one should be alert to any clues in the history that suggest that improvement or temporary remission of bullous or ulcerative mouth and/or skin lesions has previously been obtained with any type of immunosuppressive drug.

Stomatitis and gingivitis have been described in silver-gray Collies as part of a disorder called the "Gray Collie syndrome." This disease is characterized by cyclic neutropenia, thrombocytopenia, anemia, bilateral fundic ectasia, lameness, malabsorption, diarrhea, and severe gingivitis.[28] The oral lesions are unresponsive to symptomatic local treatment.

In the cat, feline rhinotracheitis virus (FRV) and feline calicivirus (FCV) may cause ulcerative stomatitis and glossitis. The ulcerative lesions produced by these viruses may cause inappetence. Treatment is usually directed against the systemic effects of these diseases, and parenteral feeding may be necessary to maintain adequate nutrition. Placement of pharyngostomy tube may facilitate feeding while the disease runs its course.

Glossitis or inflammation of the tongue is another common oral disease in dogs and cats. Glossitis may accompany stomatitis or the tongue alone may be affected. Injuries to the tongue are a common cause of glossitis. The tongue may be lacerated or injured by licking sharp surfaces, ingesting foreign bodies, and biting electrical cords. Clinical signs of laceration or foreign body penetration of the tongue are lingual swelling, drooling of blood-tinged saliva, and pawing at the mouth. A linear foreign body such as a string or thread may become caught at the frenulum of the tongue after both ends have been swallowed. The animal moves its tongue constantly trying to remove the offending object, causing the string to penetrate into the frenulum.

Other primary causes of glossitis include insect bites, dental tartar, and chemical burns. In the cat, feline rhinotracheitis virus (FRV) and feline calicivirus (FCV) cause glossitis. In most cases of primary glossitis, the cause will be evident during history-taking and physical examination. For example, bee stings occur when the animal is outside in the warm weather when flowers are blooming. Glossitis may also be associated with dental tartar when the margins of the tongue contact the teeth. Chemical burns affect the tip of the tongue and also the roof of the mouth. The feline respiratory viruses are associated with well-demarcated erosions of the epithelium at the margins and dorsum of the tongue. Electrical burns may cause coagulative necrosis across both lips and tongue.

Treatment for lesions of the tongue is symptomatic. Clean lacerations should be sutured with absorbable suture to control bleeding and appose cut edges. Jagged lacerations may require debridement. If a necrotic section of the tongue has sloughed, the tongue heals by granulation. Dogs manage well if the caudal two thirds of the tongue is intact, even though the rostral one third is lost. Lingual foreign bodies should be removed under sedation or general anesthesia. Administration of systemic broad-spectrum antibiotics and removal of dental calculus will facilitate healing of lesions on the tongue. A soft diet, such as canned food mixed with water, is indicated during the convalescent period. A pharyngostomy tube may be necessary to maintain a proper nutritional plane until healing progresses.

A specific type of inflammation affecting the anterior third or free end of the tongue is called "gangrenous glossitis." This characteristic lesion is caused by interference with the blood supply to the tongue and is commonly seen in chronic leptospirosis, end-stage kidney disease, and endocarditis with embolic nephritis. The usual clinical signs of gangrenous glossitis include anorexia, excessive salivation, and malodorous breath. A tenacious, necrotic exudate which may be blood-tinged is noted in the mouth. Pain is severe, and one cannot examine the tongue without anesthetizing the patient. The free end of the tongue is discolored, congested, and may become light gray as gangrene develops.[23]

A unique pathologic condition of the tongue of military working dogs in South Vietnam has been reported.[29] Names for this condition include acute glossitis, atrophic glossitis, and "red tongue." The tongue of affected animals is characterized by variable redness and loss of papillae on the anterodorsal third. The main clinical signs are ptyalism and inappetence. Symptomatic treatment is only partially effective. The most effective treatment includes withholding the dogs from duty and training and confining the dogs in the shade. Attempts were made to reproduce the tongue lesions in German Shepherd dogs.[30] Artificial sunlight, heat, and humidity, in combination with tetracycline, iodine solutions, and natural oral flora from the native Vietnamese dogs were used. The experiments suggested that chronic exposure to artificial and natural sunlight may produce irreversible changes in the lingual epithelium of the tongue.

Foreign bodies may involve any part of the oral cavity. The most common oral foreign body is a bone wedged between or over the teeth. Other foreign objects include porcupine quills, fishhooks, and sewing needles. The intensity of signs depends upon the type of foreign body. Dogs usually paw and scratch at the face and drool saliva. Treatment simply involves removing the offending object. Sedatives or a general anesthetic are required, depending on the nature of the dog and the type and location of the foreign body. Radiography is indicated when signs are typical but the object has penetrated beneath the mucous membrane.

Infectious oral papillomatosis is a contagious viral disease seen most frequently in young dogs, manifested by the development of benign papillomas. The common sites of involvement are the mucous membranes of the mouth, tongue, pharynx, and lips. Attempts to infect other tissues of the dog have been generally unsuccessful.[31] The exception has been the conjunctival epithelium where 8 of 17 dogs developed papillomas following inoculation with canine oral papilloma virus (COPV).

The disease tends to be self-limiting and usually within 3 months the dog develops resistance to the papillomas. Because of the unsightly appearance of the lesions, and the apparent discomfort associated with the problem, some dogs require treatment. The most effective method is surgical removal of the papillomas with electrocautery. Complete removal of all papillomas may not be possible, but the development of resistance causes regression of the remaining lesions. Cyclophosphamide (Cytoxan) has been effective in preventing the formation of new papillomas. Immunity following spontaneous recovery is life-long, but occasionally papillomas have reappeared. Autogenous vaccines have been recommended for treatment, but they are generally considered ineffective.

Congenital Anomalies

Congenital fissure of the lip (formerly called hairlip) is a developmental anomaly of the lips, anterior nasal septum, columella, and premaxilla. The preferred term for this anomaly is primary cleft palate. The primary palate includes all structures rostral to the incisive papilla. Secondary cleft palate (formerly called cleft palate) involves palate structures posterior to the incisive papilla. Primary and secondary cleft palates may occur simultaneously in the same animal.[32]

A variety of factors are thought to be involved in the development of primary and secondary cleft palates in dogs. These include mutant genes, chromosomal alterations, teratogens, multifocal inheritance, hormones, mechanical influences, and trauma.[33] Clefts of the primary palate are considered to be hereditary, whereas clefts of the secondary palate are not necessarily inherited. In man, only 10% of cleft palates are thought to be inherited.

The overall incidence of cleft palate in all domestic animals has been reported.[22] Of over 406,000 animals evaluated, 248 had primary and/or secondary cleft palates. Cats had one fourth the risk of dogs. Within the canine species, purebreds had three times the risk of mixed breeds. Canine breeds with especially high risks were Miniature

Schnauzer, Welsh Corgi, Boston Terrier, and Yorkshire Terrier. Altogether, small breeds had three times the risk of larger breeds. In the bovine species Charolais were at a sixfold risk. These epidemiologic findings support the genetic heterogeneity of spontaneous cleft palate in domestic animals.

Various surgical procedures have been described to correct primary and secondary cleft palates. These techniques have been described in detail.[32,33]

A lethal glossopharyngeal defect has been described in dogs.[34] All of the affected animals have unusually narrow tongues, and the name "bird tongue" has been applied. Puppies are alive at birth and the first indication of abnormality is a lack of interest in suckling. The tongues curl upward and inward at the fimbriated margins. Affected puppies are unable to swallow and die in a few days from starvation. Genetic analyses suggest that the defect is caused by a simple, recessive, autosomal gene in the homozygous condition. Treatment is not indicated.

Neoplasia

Neoplasia of the oral cavity in dogs and cats is common. One survey reported 20.4 cases of oral and pharyngeal cancer per 100,000 dogs.[35] Estimated rates were higher for males (26.5 per 100,000) as compared to females (14.6 per 100,000). The incidence for German Shepherds was significantly higher than for other breeds. The incidence rate of oral and pharyngeal cancer in cats was 11.6 per 100,000 cases. A recent survey of 361 cases of canine oral and pharyngeal tumors, summarizing the biologic behavior of these tumors, is seen in Table 20–2.[36,36a]

The most common malignant neoplasms of the mouth of the dogs are squamous cell carcinoma of both the tonsils and gums, malignant melanoma, and fibrosarcoma.[36a] Malignant melanoma (which may be amelanotic) occurs with greater frequency in Cocker Spaniels, while German Shepherds develop fibrosarcoma more frequently than other breeds. In general, malignant oropharyngeal neoplasms occur in old dogs. Fibrosarcoma occurs at a younger age than other types of oral tumors, 4.5 years in one series[35] and 7.9 years (mean) in another.[36a] An example of this type of tumor is seen in Figure 20–1.[37]

Neoplastic lesions are usually not recognized by clients until the tumor is well advanced. When seen, neoplastic lesions appear both proliferative and ulcerated, although destructive lesions with little tissue proliferation may be observed. Clinical signs of the disease include anorexia, weight loss, and dysphagia. Blood-tinged saliva and halitosis may also occur.

Biopsy and histopathologic examination are essential to confirm the correct diagnosis. Cytologic examination of a specimen scraped from the surface of the lesion may also be useful. Thoracic radiographs are necessary to prognose the case, particularly if malignant melanoma or squamous cell carcinoma is suspected, because pulmonary metastases may occur from these lesions. Fibrosarcoma is less likely to metastasize to the lungs.[36a]

After a histopathologic diagnosis of oropharyngeal neoplasia has been established, treatment and prognosis should be discussed with the owner. Surgical treatment is rarely rewarding because malignant melanoma, fibrosarcoma, and squamous cell carcinoma tend to invade surrounding tissue and have a high recurrence rate.

Table 20–2.   Summary of the biologic behavior of 361 cases of canine oral and pharyngeal cancer

Tumor type	No. of Cases	Site of Origin	Average Age (yr)	Male-Female Ratio	Breed Predilection	Percent of Regional Node Metastasis	Percent of Distant Metastasis	Prognosis
Malignant melanoma	121	Gum, cheek, lip, palate, tonsil, and tongue	11	4.2:1	None	81(n=54)	—	Very poor
Squamous cell carcinoma	80	Tonsil	9.6	1.5:1	None	77(n=48)	—	Very poor
Squamous cell carcinoma	84	Other than tonsil	8.8	1:1	None	82(n=11)	—	Fair to poor
Fibrosarcoma	76	Gum, lip, cheek, palate	7.6	1.8:1	None	35(n=26)	—	Usually poor

From R. S. Brodey,[36] and R. J. Todoroff and R. S. Brodey.[36a]

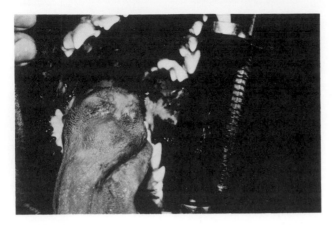

Figure 20–1. Lingual fibrosarcoma involving the tongue of a 5-year-old male Pit Bull Terrier. (From Dorn and Olmstead.[37])

Radiation therapy has been used to control many malignant oral neoplasms. The treatment and prognosis depend on the type of tumor, radiosensitivity, tissue dose of radiation, and the amount of tumor infiltration of adjacent tissues such as bone. A veterinary radiologist with experience in radiation therapy should supervise the treatment. Because relatively few cases are treated with radiation therapy in veterinary medicine, more information must be exchanged between veterinarians using this technique. Standard protocols should be established for each tumor type. Radiation therapy can be combined with other types of therapy for the most efficacious results.

Recently, cryosurgery has been recommended as the treatment of choice for oral and pharyngeal neoplasms of the dog.[38] Cryosurgery involves the use of profound cold to destroy accessible cancerous tissues. The extent of tissue destruction depends on the rate of freezing and thawing. The patient is anesthetized and surrounding normal tissues are protected. A large trephine biopsy is taken from the center mass for positive histopathologic diagnosis. The peripheral portions of lesion are immediately frozen with an appropriate cryosurgical instrument and the effect of freezing is measured with thermocouples. The patient is re-evaluated in 2 weeks and another biopsy and repeat freezing may be considered.

In many patients with oral malignancies, cryosurgery must be considered as being palliative. Beneficial results include relief of pain, improved appearance, decreased odor and improvement in eating, swallowing, and breathing. Specific tumor types which have been subjected to cryosurgery include fibrosarcoma, malignant melanoma, squamous cell carcinoma, and mast cell sarcoma.[39]

Cryosurgery has also been used in combination with chemotherapy for the treatment of specific cancerous lesions.[40] The rationale of this therapy is based on three assumptions:

1. A lack of success of chemotherapy alone relates to the excessive size and age of tumor cell population at the time of therapy.
2. Carcinoma usually flourishes in the face of a progressive local circulatory and hemodynamic disadvantage as compared to normal host tissues. This relationship is a major encumbrance to effective chemotherapy.
3. Cryosurgery is a relatively benign means of altering tumor cell mass and microcirculatory dynamics.

The prognosis for long-term survival (>1 yr) of dogs with oral malignancy is poor, based upon the results of surgery, cryosurgery, radiation therapy, chemotherapy, and immunotherapy.[36a]

Another type of oral neoplasm occasionally encountered is the adamantinoma. This tumor is also known as ameloblastoma and arises from the enamel organ, the embryonic predecessor of a tooth (Fig. 20–2). One survey of 205 canine oral neoplasms revealed 18 adamantinomas. These tumors lyse bone and are most common in the mandible. Microscopically, the adamantinoma consists of cords or nests of epithelium with intercellular bridges. Occasional small cysts are found. The stroma varies from dense fibrous to loose myxomatous connective tissue.[41]

In another study of 57 cases of primary oral adamantinomas and ameloblastic odontomas, radiation therapy was used to treat 16 selected cases with beneficial results.[42] The results suggested that radiation therapy may be effective for this type of tumor.

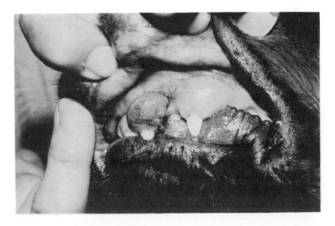

Figure 20–2. Ameloblastoma involving the third incisor in the mouth of a 6-month-old male Irish Setter.

PHARYNX

Horse

The pharynx of the horse is rarely involved in direct trauma owing to the length of the head. Foreign bodies are more apt to be trapped in the mouth and teeth before reaching the pharynx, which is partially protected by the long soft palate.

Infection

Pharyngitis is a clinical entity of major importance in performance horses. The exact cause and pathogenesis of this disorder have not been defined although viruses are suspected. Affected horses usually become dyspneic, breathe noisily, cough during exercise, tire easily, and have nasal or guttural pouch discharges. Pharyngitis in the horse sometimes produces gastrointestinal signs, in that acute cases may have reduced appetite for grain. Hay or grass will rarely be refused. Chronic pharyngitis produces little effect on swallowing or appetite. This contrasts sharply with pharyngitis in cattle, dogs, and cats, in which species anorexia may be severe and prolonged, accompanied by ptyalism, repeated swallowing, and aerophagia (dogs and cats).

Equine pharyngitis may have an acute or chronic course. The acute form usually appears in two phases. The initial phase, possibly of viral origin, is characterized by fever, pharyngeal hyperemia, and a serous to mucoid discharge. The subsequent phase, complicated by secondary bacterial infection, has lymphoid infiltration and follicular hyperplasia of the pharyngeal mucosa.

The chronic form is visualized endoscopically as a severe and persistent chronic lymphoid follicular hyperplasia (CLFH). The chronically affected equine pharynx has a "cobblestone" appearance as viewed endoscopically.

CLFH appears to be a nonspecific inflammatory response of the nasopharynx. Any noxious stimulus to the nasopharynx, or viral or bacterial infection of the upper respiratory tract, seems to cause the lymphoid tissue to proliferate. Lymphoid follicles may appear within 5 days following onset of clinical signs.[43] Some horses will cough excessively in both the acute and chronic phase when digital pressure is applied externally to the laryngeal area and when the cricotracheal space is manipulated.

The diagnosis of pharyngitis is confirmed by endoscopic examination. Severely affected horses will have lymphoid follicles and nodular lymphoid hyperplasia in the naso- and oropharynx, as well as in the dorsal pharyngeal recess and on the dorsum of the soft palate. A few small follicles are commonly seen in clinically normal young horses, although the number of follicles diminishes with age. Normal horses over 4 years of age will have few if any follicles on the pharyngeal wall.[5,43,44]

Treatment is symptomatic, including a broad-spectrum antibiotic if desired. Nasal sprays may be of some benefit. Electrocautery of the lymphoid follicles in the chronic case has also been advocated. Rest is essential during the convalescent period. Vaccination for rhinopneumonitis at a young age may be of some benefit in prevention.

Malformations and Tumors

Congenital malformations and primary tumors of the pharynx are rare in the horse. Congenital malformations of the larynx such as a small epiglottis, small arytenoid cartilages, and an extremely small rima glottis have all been observed.

Diseases of Guttural Pouches

The paired guttural pouches are large hollow pockets that are formed as outpouchings of the eustachian tubes. The horse, tapir, and hyrax are unique in that all have guttural pouches. Each guttural pouch is divided by the stylohyoid bone into a medial and lateral compartment. In the adult horse each pouch has an average capacity of 300 ml, of which the lateral compartment contains 100 ml. The guttural pouches are lined with ciliated epithelium and are supplied with mucous glands. Numerous lymph nodes are present in the guttural pouches of the young horse.

Specific viral infections of the guttural pouches are not recognized. The most common infection is bacterial in origin and is caused by *Streptococcus equi,* the agent of "strangles," of which empyema of the guttural pouches is a sequelae. The organism is introduced by way of the pharyngeal orifice of the eustachian tubes. The resulting infection causes inflammation and swelling of the guttural pouch openings, trapping the exudate in the guttural pouches. This exudate can develop into caseous or solid concrements called chondroids.

The clinical signs vary depending on the severity of the disorder. In mild cases of guttural pouch empyema, the only clinical sign may be a slight nasal discharge. It is usually unilateral, indicating that only one guttural pouch is involved. The exudate is usually without odor, somewhat mucoid, slightly milky and opaque. The exudate is discharged when the horse lowers the head because the pharyngeal opening of the guttural pouch is not located at the most ventral portion of the pouch.

Empyema may vary from no external change in the anatomy of the head and neck, to the severely distended guttural pouches that are visibly distended. The horse with the distended pouch(es) may be anorectic due to swelling in the pharyngeal region, which decreases air flow during respirations. The horse may not be able to move air rapidly enough to allow for eating or swallowing. Another reason for anorexia may be due to pressure of the exudate-filled pouch on the glossopharyngeal (IX) and hypoglossal (XII) nerves that course the lateral wall of the pouches. Such pressure can cause partial to complete paralysis of the soft palate, pharynx, and tongue. The paralysis is usually temporary, with the exception that the soft palate will interfere with respiration during forced exercise. The patient may be thought to be choked because of a partial or complete inability to swallow.

The client may complain that food is being expelled from both nostrils of the horse with empyema of the guttural pouches. This greenish exudate may be mistakenly thought to be the result of a pharyngeal abscess. Rather, it is exudate with particles of masticated food, which is not expelled from the mouth because of the long soft palate in the horse. Radiographic demonstration of a fluid line in the guttural pouches or direct visualization of the pharynx and guttural pouches via endoscopy are very useful diagnostic procedures. The classic endoscopic sign, other than exudate in the guttural pouch, is a displacement of the soft palate over the epiglottis that remains after repeated swallowing movements.[4,45]

Initial therapy consists of life-saving measures (i.e., tracheostomy) and specific antibiotic therapy. Supportive measures include tube feeding and draining the exudate from the pouch. The latter is done by catheterization of the pouch(es) with a Chambers mare catheter and installing a self-retaining catheter in the pouch, or by surgical drainage.[3] The guttural pouch may be opened surgically by one of three approaches. The approach at Viborg's triangle, a midline approach (Whitehouse's method), or the hyovertebrotomy technique (Chabert's method) have been described.

Mycosis or "Guttural Pouch Diphtheria" may show a variety of clinical signs. The clinical signs in order of frequency are: epistaxis, dysphagia, abnormal head posture, nasal catarrh, head shyness, abnormal respiratory noises, sweating and shivering, Horner's syndrome and other ocular defects, colic and facial paralysis.[46] These signs are explained on the basis of erosion of blood vessels, local pain, paralysis of cranial nerves, and paralysis

or stimulation of the sympathetic nervous system. Evidence of "parotid pain" may be detected by palpation. The spurious evidence of pain in the parotid gland occurs because of its proximity to the diseased guttural pouches.

Aspergillus nidulans is the most frequently isolated causative agent, with concurrent bacterial infection. A positive diagnosis is made by isolating the organism from the mucosal lesion, which is generally located in the dorsum of the medial compartment of the pouch.[47-49] The internal carotid artery, the vagus, accessory, and sympathetic nerves, the cranial cervical ganglion and ventral cerebral vein are situated in a fold in this area, and erosions into these structures produce the clinical signs.

If epistaxis is a part of the clinical history, diagnostic workup is needed to establish whether the hemorrhage is originating in the guttural pouches or elsewhere. Generally if the expistaxis is spontaneous and not associated with forced exercise, the guttural pouch is the prime suspect. Endoscopy and angiography may help localize the lesion. If the epistaxis is observed during or immediately after forced exercise, the lung is the most likely source of the hemorrhage.[50-52] Ligation of the internal carotid surgically or placing a balloon catheter proximal to the lesion may be indicated if the lesion is located in the guttural pouch.

Other therapy to consider is daily irrigation of the pouch with a 1:4 dilution of povidone-iodine solution (Betadine Solution Veterinary) for 7 to 10 days, or until there is no endoscopic evidence of a severe diffuse inflammatory reaction upon chemical debridement of the mucous membrane. Consideration has been given to trichloracetic acid or formalin for use in chemical debridement of the guttural pouch.[53]

Tympanites (emphysema) of the guttural pouch(es) is seen in young horses and is thought to be caused by a congenital malformation. The clinical signs are distention of one or both guttural pouches in the region of Viborg's triangle.[4] Percussion reveals an air-filled cavity, and firm digital pressure may result in expulsion of the air so that the contour of the neck appears normal. After a few breaths, the pouch(es) will refill. Radiographs will reveal an abnormally large guttural pouch(es) with no fluid line.

The size and involvement (unilateral or bilateral) will dictate the severity of clinical signs. Nursing foals are susceptible to aspiration pneumonia. Regurgitation of milk may be observed at the external nares as occurs with cleft soft palate.

The cause apparently is related to hyperplasia of

the mucous membrane at the pharyngeal orifice of the guttural pouch. Air is allowed to enter but the membrane acts as a one-way valve preventing escape of air. Correction is through a lateral surgical approach, in which a section of the mucous membrane is removed and the pharyngeal orifice dilated in a retrograde manner.[54,55] If both pouches are affected, the foregoing procedure is done on one pouch and a section of the medial wall of the pouch is removed to allow access to the opposite pouch and the same procedure conducted on the pharyngeal orifice. Only one lateral skin incision is necessary.

Tumors of the guttural pouch occur and the clinical signs vary with the size and location of the lesion. Similar clinical signs as mentioned with guttural pouch mycosis could be observed. Cases of facial paralysis with ptosis of the upper eyelid and drooping of the ear on the same side warrant a guttural pouch examination via endoscopy and radiography of the head. The types of tumors reported and observed are fibroma, squamous cell carcinoma, and melanoma.[15,56] The prognosis is dependent on whether the tumor is benign or malignant, and whether it is accessible to surgical removal.

Cow

Trauma and Obstruction

The most common form of pharyngeal obstruction is probably swelling secondary to trauma. Swelling and cellulitis can actually progress to abscess or fistula formation. Most cases of pharyngeal trauma are iatrogenic and due to improper use of the balling gun, dose syringe, or stomach tube. These instruments, if kept free of rough edges or burrs at the tip, usually cause no problem when used carefully. However, injudicious use or even proper use with an extremely fractious animal can lead to pharyngeal trauma, secondary swelling, and phlegmon.

Pharyngeal trauma can usually be diagnosed by visual examination with a speculum or by digital palpation. Occasionally, radiographs are needed to identify foreign bodies in the pharyngeal area.

Treatment consists of antibiotic to combat secondary bacterial infection. Steroid and antihistamine are sometimes indicated because of severe edema and swelling. A stomach tube passed through the nose and left in place for 2 weeks may provide a route for alimentation and fluid intake while the pharyngeal area heals. If foreign bodies (i.e., bolus or food material) are involved, they must be extracted by hand or surgically removed. In severe cases, a tracheotomy (to maintain an airway) and a rumen fistula (for decompression of the rumen and for feeding) are indicated for temporary relief until the pharyngeal area heals.

Pharyngeal paralysis is evidenced by inability to swallow, with retention of food in the mouth. Ptyalism occurs, with saliva hanging from the mouth in ropey strings. In these cases, a careful oral examination (visual and digital) is indicated as the signs of pharyngeal paralysis are similar to those of pharyngeal foreign body or obstruction. Caution is essential since rabies is a possibility whenever pharyngeal paralysis is present.

If foreign body, obstruction, and trauma can be ruled out after examination, a diagnosis of pharyngeal paralysis is probably justified. There is no known treatment for pharyngeal paralysis although some cases improve with time.

Dog

The pharynx is continuous with both the alimentary and respiratory systems and may be involved in diseases of both systems. The pharynx is somewhat difficult to examine in the conscious dog, and it may be advantageous to anesthetize or sedate the dog to perform a complete examination. Use of an artificial light source and retraction of the soft palate will permit visualization of the ventral, lateral, and posterior walls. The nasopharynx can be examined with a dental mirror or a pharyngeal mirror and light.

Infectious and Traumatic Diseases

Pharyngitis usually results from extension of infection from adjacent areas, such as the mouth, tonsils, or nasal cavities, or may occur as an acute primary infection associated with a foreign body or a systemic disease. Chronic pharyngitis may be observed in animals with elongation of the soft palate, pharyngeal cysts, disturbed pharyngeal innervation, tonsillitis, megaesophagus, and cricopharyngeal achalasia.

Animals with acute pharyngitis usually have a history of anorexia and gagging which lead to expectoration of white, foamy phlegm. The client may comment that the animal acts hungry, but stops eating because of the discomfort associated with swallowing. A rise in temperature corresponds with the severity of the infection. After a few days, a cough may develop. In severe cases, submandibular edema, complete anorexia, severe coughing, and impaired breathing may be observed.

Examination of the pharynx reveals thick foamy

mucus and secondary tonsillitis. The pharynx may be hyperemic and ulcerated, and a pseudomembrane may be seen. Diagnosis of pharyngitis is based on history and clinical signs of anorexia, gagging, and expectoration of white, tenacious, foamy exudate.

Successful treatment depends on removing the primary cause of the pharyngitis. Bacteria associated with pharyngitis generally respond to penicillin, sulfonamide, or broad-spectrum antibiotic. These drugs may be combined with low doses of corticosteroid to provide symptomatic relief. Removal of pseudomembranes and local treatment with antiseptics or antibiotics may be beneficial. Food should be bland and easy to swallow. In severe cases, parenteral feeding or placement of a pharyngostomy tube may be necessary to provide nutrients until the inflammation subsides.

Perforating foreign bodies such as plant awns and seeds, needles, wood splinters, and bone chips may be found in the pharynx of dogs. Large nonperforating foreign bodies seldom lodge in the pharynx because the dog can usually expel them quickly. The tonsillar crypts, posterior pillars of the mouth, and the posterolateral aspect of the pharynx are the usual locations of small perforating objects. The clinical signs of pharyngeal foreign body include coughing and retching. Swallowing is difficult and painful, and anorexia is common. Mucus or blood may be evident in expectorated material, and dysphagia may accompany increased salivation. External palpation of the pharyngeal region may elicit pain. Pharyngeal examination may not be possible unless the animal is anesthetized. Radiographs are indicated and will confirm the presence of radiopaque foreign bodies.

Small foreign bodies may enter the posterior pillar of the mouth or tonsillar region, and migrate dorsally producing a temporal or postorbital abscess. Heavier foreign bodies enter the posterosuperior aspect of the pharynx and migrate caudally causing an abscess in the cervical area. The pharyngitis resulting from the foreign body should be treated as previously described following removal of the inciting cause. The most frequent sequel to a foreign body which penetrates the pharynx is a retropharyngeal abscess.

The tonsils are closely associated with the pharynx, located in crypts at the lateral pharyngeal wall. The tonsils form part of a ring of lymphoid tissue in the orpharynx. Exposure to a variety of irritants and infectious agents makes tonsillitis relatively common in dogs. Small-breed dogs are most frequently affected with primary tonsillitis. Dogs

retch, cough, expectorate mucus, and have malaise, fever, and inappetence. The clinical signs may be caused by inflammation of the pharyngeal mucosa with or without tonsillar swelling. The appearance of the tonsils in the dog varies considerably and may have little correlation with the condition of the animal. Color is the most accurate indication of disease, as acutely inflamed tonsils appear bright red. Inflammation of the surrounding mucosa may be obvious and punctate hemorrhages may be seen. Localized abscesses may be visible as white specks on the surface of the tonsil. The acutely inflamed tonsil is friable and bleeds easily if touched.

The diagnosis of tonsillitis is based on direct inspection and clinical signs. Treatment with antibiotics usually results in clinical improvement, although tonsillar swelling may persist for weeks or months. Low doses of corticosteroid in combination with antibiotic may provide symptomatic relief while the cause of the infection is being treated. Tonsillectomy is not indicated for acute tonsillitis.

An important cause of chronic tonsillitis, seemingly more so in small breeds of dogs, is chronic anal sac disease. The anal sac duct becomes obstructed, the anal sac becomes inflamed, and the dog grooms the anal region, ingesting contaminated material. Regular medical treatment of diseased anal sacs or removal of the sacs will improve the anal problem as well as the tonsillitis. Tonsillectomy is seldom indicated in such cases.

Occasionally tonsillitis and pharyngitis may be recurrent in young dogs. Tonsillectomy provides permanent relief from clinical signs caused by chronic, primary tonsillitis but is rarely necessary. This disease usually runs its course as the animal matures.

When performing a tonsillectomy, general anesthesia and endotracheal intubation are essential. To prevent aspiration of blood, a moist gauze sponge should be placed in the pharynx around the endotracheal tube prior to removal of the tonsillar tissue by electrocautery. Tonsillectomy is occasionally indicated in mature animals when the enlarged tonsils stand out of their crypts, causing mechanical interference with swallowing or with airflow. This is usually seen in brachycephalic dogs with upper airway disease and a superimposed mechanical obstruction.[57]

Neoplasia

Tonsillitis may be confused with neoplastic diseases of the tonsil. These neoplasms are squamous cell carcinoma and lymphosarcoma. Table 20–3 describes the differential diagnosis of three common

Table 20–3. Differential diagnosis of inflammatory and neoplastic lesions of the tonsils

Item	Tonsillitis	Squamous Cell Carcinoma	Lymphosarcoma
Age incidence	Usually young animals.	Usually old animals (average age 9 years).	Usually middle-aged or old animals (average age lower than for carcinoma).
Size of tonsils	Uniform enlargement—may be 2–3 times normal size. Usually bilateral.	Nodular enlargement; may form huge irregular mass, or tonsil may be replaced by a plaque-like ulcer. Usually unilateral.	Uniform enlargement may become quite large. Usually bilateral.
Color of tonsils	Reddened—may be tiny foci of necrosis or suppuration.	Gray, pinkish-gray, or red.	Pink or red.
Consistency of tonsils	Slightly increased.	Very firm to hard.	Much softer than carcinoma.
Surrounding tissues	Normal or hyperemic.	Often diffusely infiltrated with gray, granular, tumor tissue.	Usually normal.
Regional lymph nodes (mandibular and retropharyngeal)	Slight uniform enlargement; may be hot and painful. Usually bilateral.	Moderate to massive enlargement, irregularly lobulated. Node is very firm but not hot or painful. Usually unilateral involvement, but may be bilateral.	Moderate to massive, often irregularly lobulated. Node is not as firm as with carcinoma, no heat or pain. Usually bilateral involvement.
Superficial body lymph nodes	Negative.	May have prescapular adenopathy; rest of nodes negative.	Usually greatly enlarged (also internal nodes, liver, and spleen often involved).
Signs	Fever, gagging, cough, depression, anorexia.	Dysphagia, dyspnea, choking, lateral cervical mass, pain, ptyalism, anorexia.	Very variable; depends on the involvement in body cavities or cervical nodes and not on tonsillar lesions.
Blood findings	Leukopenia or leukocytosis.	Negative.	Leukocytosis with neutrophilia, usually; a few have lymphatic leukemia.
Radiograph of thorax	Negative.	May have metastatic lung nodules.	Often have hilar or anterior mediastinal lymphadenopathy.

From R. S. Brodey.[58]

tonsillar lesions in the dog.[58] The most common tonsillar tumor of the dog and cat is squamous cell carcinoma.[58] It is the opinion of some authors that carcinoma of the tonsil occurs with greater frequency in urban dogs.[59] Another neoplasm of the tonsil is lymphosarcoma, which occurs in middle-aged or older dogs (Table 20–3).

Presenting signs in dogs and cats with tonsillar neoplasia are similar to other types of oral neoplasms. These signs include anorexia, weight loss, and dysphagia. Tonsillar carcinomas often appear as unilateral, irregular, firm, ulcerated masses. Enlargement of regional lymph nodes may also occur. Conversely, tonsillar lymphosarcoma is usually bilaterally symmetrical with smooth surfaced enlargements.

The prognosis for tonsillar neoplasia must be guarded. Biopsy of all lesions is essential to confirm the diagnosis. Treatment plans used for other types of oral neoplasms have been recommended for tonsillar neoplasia with variable results. Lymphosarcoma of the tonsil may be treated with chemotherapeutic drugs, as part of the treatment of what is probably multicentric lymphosarcoma, with the tonsils being the most easily found of many lesions.

SALIVARY GLANDS

Horse

The salivary glands of the horse have received little attention either owing to lack of problems or the inability of veterinarians to diagnose the problem(s). In a study conducted on function of the horse's parotid gland, it was found that saliva flowed only during mastication. Local anesthesia of the oral mucous membrane inhibited salivary secretion, and secretion was stimulated by pilocarpine and inhibited by atropine. The ponies used in this study secreted approximately 8 liters of saliva from one parotid salivary gland in a 24-hour period. The weight of the ponies was not recorded. Electrolyte concentrations of the saliva were highest during periods of high flow rate. Horse parotid saliva contained a high concentration of calcium and, in the absence of a dietary supplement of sodium bicarbonate, the sodium concentration of the saliva fell after about 21 days. The addition of a sodium supplement restored the sodium concentration of the saliva within 24 hours. Lactic acid is produced by fermentation in the horse's stomach and its neutralization would be facilitated by the addition of a bicarbonate buffer such as saliva. The buffering properties of the horse parotid saliva, however, fall far short of that of sheep, which contains twice as much bicarbonate per liter as horse parotid saliva does, as well as a substantial amount of phosphate.[60]

Inflammation of the Parotid Salivary Gland

This condition can occur as a separate entity in the horse and must be differentiated from "parotid pain," as seen in some guttural pouch disorders in which pain is exhibited in the hyoid region. Specific infections of the salivary glands have not been recorded, leading one to think that salivary infections are rare.

Sialoliths (Calculi)

These do occur in the horse although they are not seen as frequently as in cattle. They occur most frequently in the parotid duct (Stenson's duct). The calculi are usually smooth on the surface and gray or yellowish-gray. In the usual case, the calculus is thought to be a foreign body. The composition of sialoliths in horses is not recorded. The clinical signs are pain and swelling along the course of the parotid duct.[61]

Therapy consists of removing the calculi by enlarging the parotid papilla and evacuating the calculi into the mouth, or by surgically opening the duct. Closure of the duct must be complete at the time of surgery, and food and water should be withheld for 3 or 4 days and the horse isolated from other animals at feeding time. If healing does not occur by first intention, a fistula usually develops and healing is delayed.[61] The same would apply to an injury or laceration involving the parotid duct.

Sialocele

This condition of the parotid salivary gland, presumably a congenital malformation, has been observed by the author. Surgical correction included careful dissection of the entire parotid gland on the affected side. The parotid gland was not functioning

prior to the surgery; therefore, no adverse effect on mastication and swallowing was expected nor observed. There are reports of similar extirpation of the parotid salivary gland because of fistula.[61,62] Formerly, therapy consisted of injecting an irritant into the gland to destroy the parenchyma. Ten ml of Lugol's iodine solution were injected into the parotid duct and the duct was ligated to contain the solution within the gland. Subsequent injections were made if the entire gland was not destroyed. If the parotid duct cannot be located, the Lugol's solution can be injected into the gland proper, using no more than 2 ml at 2- to 3-cm intervals, for a total volume of approximately 15 ml. This technique will result in fever and a stiff carriage of the neck for a few days. Also, the horse should be held off feed for 2 to 3 days post injection.[61]

Neoplasms

These tumors of the salivary glands are rare and would probably be extensions from another primary site. Malignant melanomas in grey horses have been observed in the region of the parotid salivary gland.

Cow

Salivary diseases are extremely rare in the bovine. When they occur, the appearance is similar to and should be treated as described for the horse.

Dog

There are four major pairs of salivary glands in the dog; the parotid, mandibular, sublingual, and zygomatic. The most important disorders that affect these glands are infections and cysts or mucoceles.

Infectious and Traumatic Diseases

Sialadenitis or inflammation of the salivary glands is uncommon, but when seen, the zygomatic or parotid glands are usually involved. Infected bite wounds and trauma are the most common causes for infection of the parotid gland. Both glands may be infected by bloodborne organisms, mouth organisms which ascend through the ducts, or migrating foreign bodies. Clinical signs include swelling or abscessation in the region of the gland. The rectal temperature is elevated. Pain is manifested when the mouth is opened. Infected parotid glands become swollen, and edema occurs at the base of the ear. Zygomatic salivary gland infection results in swelling of the eyelids and protrusion of the eyeball. Inflammation of this gland is a common form of retrobulbar abscess.

Early parenteral treatment with antibiotic causes regression of the infection and limits development of abscesses. Parotid salivary gland abscess should be incised at the most superficial point. Zygomatic salivary gland abscesses should be drained behind the last upper molar in the oral cavity. After making a small stab incision with a scalpel, the opening is enlarged with a forceps. Occasionally, a zygomatic salivary gland abscess ruptures and drains near the lateral canthus. Irrigation of the abscess with an antiseptic solution and concurrent parenteral administration of antibiotic result in prompt healing in most cases.[23]

Sialocele or salivary mucocele is the most common clinical problem of salivary glands in the dog. Salivary mucocele is a collection of salivary secretion in a nonepithelial-lined swelling. After damage to the salivary gland or duct, saliva leaks into the tissues and follows the path of least resistance. The sublingual gland is most frequently involved. Frequent sites for collection of the extravasated saliva are the sublingual tissues on the floor of the mouth on one side of the tongue, and the superficial connective tissues of the intermandibular or cranial cervical area. The lesion may be unilateral or bilateral. The cause of the gland or duct damage is rarely found.

The incidence of salivary cysts has been reported.[63] Of 4688 dogs examined, 16 had salivary cysts. The highest incidence was seen in Toy and Miniature Poodles, and the age range of 2 to 4 years was most frequently represented. There was no difference in incidence between males and females.

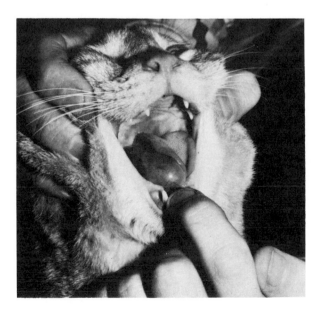

Figure 20–3. Ranula in the oral cavity of an adult cat.

Another report suggests a higher incidence in German Shepherds.[64]

Clinical signs of sialocele depend on the location. A large sublingual swelling, commonly known as a ranula, is likely to push the tongue to the opposite side, causing reluctance to eat and the flow of blood-tinged saliva (Fig. 20–3). Usually the owner will observe the lesion in the mouth. Intermandibular salivary mucocele may have an acute onset when the swelling is firm, but gradual enlargement of a soft nonpainful mass is the most common presenting complaint.

Diagnosis of a sialocele is based on palpation and aspiration biopsy of the mass. The material obtained by aspiration is clear or blood-tinged. Occasionally the aspirate is brown-colored from the lysis of red blood cells within the cyst. Some chronic cervical mucoceles contain nodules which are free within the swelling and which resemble calculi. These nodules are folds of inflammatory lining sloughed into the cavity. Tests other than aspiration biopsy are rarely needed to confirm a diagnosis of salivary mucocele. Although sialography confirms the affected side of salivary gland or duct leakage, this radiographic technique is necessary only when the involved side cannot be identified by inspection and palpation.

Intermandibular salivary mucocele usually causes little problem to the dog after the initial inflammatory reaction has subsided, but occasionally mucoceles become large enough to cause physical discomfort. Mucoceles usually recur after aspiration but periodic aspiration may be sufficient treatment. Surgical drainage of the mucocele and removal of the affected sublingual and mandibular salivary glands is the preferred treatment. Results of the operation are excellent if all of the affected glandular tissue is removed. The wall of the cyst or mucocele does not have to be excised. If the affected side cannot be determined by sialography, the glands of both sides can be removed.

Ranula can be treated by marsupialization, which is the creation of a fistula from the mucocele into the oral cavity. A section of the mucocele wall is removed with a scalpel or scissors. The inner lining of the mucocele is sutured to the oral mucous membrane with nonabsorbable suture such as silk. Stainless steel wire has been suggested as an alternate suture material to maintain patency of the fistula.[65] Ranula can also be treated satisfactorily by mandibular and sublingual gland removal on the affected side.

Neoplasia of the salivary glands of the dog and cat is extremely rare. When a methodical workup of submandibular and anterior cervical masses is done, the diagnosis will usually be obtained by examination of biopsy material.

TEETH AND GUMS

Horse

The teeth are hard, white or yellowish-white structures implanted in the alveoli of the bones of the jaw. Functionally, they are organs of prehension and mastication and may serve as weapons. Horses have two sets of teeth. The first set which appears during early life is known as deciduous or temporary teeth. These are replaced by the permanent teeth during the period of growth (1 to 5 years). The incisor teeth are situated in front (rostrally) and are implanted in the premaxilla and mandible. The canine teeth are situated further back in the interalveolar space. The canine teeth are prominent in the male and may be small or absent in the female.

In the adult horse, the dental arcade is made up of six teeth. The premolars form the anterior part of the arcade and the molars form the posterior part. The premolars appear in both the deciduous and the permanent series, but the molars appear only in the permanent dentition. The term cheek teeth is used to include both premolars and molars.[66]

In the upper arcade the first premolar may be vestigial or absent. When present, it is seen medial to the anterior margin of the dental arcade and is known as the "wolf tooth." The first and sixth upper teeth are triangular with the apex rostral in the first tooth and caudal in the sixth. The central four are almost square and the complete arcade presents a slight convex curve to the cheek.

All cheek teeth have a buccal, lingual, and two contact surfaces. The contact surfaces between adjacent teeth are close, and there is normally only a very narrow interproximal area at the gum margin. This intimate contact along the arcade is maintained throughout life as the tooth erupts and as the crown is worn away.

The six mandibular teeth are rectangular with the long axis rostrocaudal and a straight arcade. In all horses the distance between the left and right mandible, measured at any tooth, is 30% narrower than in the upper jaw. Consequently, the teeth in the lower arcades become more eroded on the buccal aspect and those of the upper arcades on the lingual aspect, with the formation of sharp enamel edges.[67]

The upper cheek teeth differ from the lower teeth in that the enamel is formed from an enamel organ which is folded vertically across the tooth as well as longitudinally. As these folds erupt and are worn away, an upper tooth is produced with its distinctive enamel lakes filled with cement and a central canal, the infundibulum, or "cup."

Each tooth is composed of four tissues; pulp, dentine, enamel, and cement. The pulp is a soft, gelatinous tissue which occupies the central part of the tooth, i.e., the pulp cavity. In the upper teeth the pulp cavity has five main divisions within the folds of the enamel and in the lower teeth there are two main divisions. Dentine forms the bulk of the tooth and progressively encroaches on the pulp cavity with age. The enamel is very hard and bluish-white in appearance. The cement is the peripheral tooth substance and progressive cementation of the peripheral enamel irregularities takes place, thus leveling up the surface. It is similar in structure to bone. The embedded part of the tooth is united to the alveolus by a vascular layer of connective tissue, the alveolar periosteum.[66]

The position of the embedded crowns and roots of the last four upper cheek teeth varies at different ages and in different types of horse. All of these teeth are developed in the posterior part of the body of the maxilla and are related to the maxillary sinuses. Commonly the third and fourth teeth project upward into the anterior maxillary sinus and the fifth and sixth into the posterior maxillary sinus. This relationship is clinically important in that periapical infection of these four teeth may lead to maxillary sinus empyema.

The gums are composed of dense fibrous tissue which is intimately connected with the periosteum of the alveolar processes and blends at the edges of the alveoli with the alveolar periosteum. They are covered by a smooth stratified epithelium and have few glands and are relatively insensitive.

Trauma

Cracked, broken, or split teeth are not uncommon in the horse. All of the teeth may be involved but the incisors are more prone to trauma due to location. A minor crack or break in the tooth may cause no discomfort, but the tooth may be extremely painful if the crack or split extends below the gum level. The incisors may be cracked because the horse nibbles on hard objects, and may get the teeth caught between two boards; cracking is also due to direct trauma such as a kick or falling on a hard surface. A small hard stone in hay or grain could cause the cheek tooth to break if the horse bites down very hard.

Trauma may also cause a fractured jaw as well as broken teeth. The location of the fracture and the number of teeth involved and the age of the horse must all be considered in rendering a prognosis and choosing an approach to therapy. For example, if only the central incisors are fractured and displaced anteriorly in a 1-year-old horse, the therapy may simply consist of extraction since the permanent teeth are not involved. In the most severe fractures and more so in older horses, heavy-gauge stainless steel wire, bone pins, and/or plates may be required to maintain reduction of the fracture.

The severity and location of the fracture will dictate the type of postoperative care and feeding practice. In severe cases, a nasogastric tube is placed and secured to the halter. Feed and water are then provided as needed. The horse is muzzled to prevent displacement of the fracture. The mucosa around the fracture may be lacerated and, if so, is usually friable and may not hold sutures. An open wound may develop at the fracture site and, if so, should be flushed at least twice daily with an antiseptic, and a broad-spectrum antibiotic should be administered parenterally. Healing of the mucosa and the bone is usually quite rapid unless complications develop. If a draining tract develops and persists, plain and contrast radiographs may be helpful in localizing the problem. Periostitis, irritation from the wire or plate, or development of a sequestrum are all possible complications. Establishment of drainage, treatment with specific chemotherapy, and removal of the cause such as embedded wire, or removal and curettage of a sequestrum, should allow second intention healing.

Infundibular Necrosis (Dental Caries)

The maxillary cheek teeth are the most common site of infundibular necrosis. The lesion may start in one infundibulum and expand centrifugally, forming a deep central valley of necrosis if there is coalescence of several lesions within anterior and posterior cement lakes of the same tooth. Pulpitis may develop in the pulp cavity of the tooth, leading to a periapical granuloma and localized apical osteitis. In severe cases, the tooth may split along the cavity.[68]

Early cases may be difficult to diagnose in that the primary complaint may be slobbering, taking a prolonged period of time to eat, or holding the head to one side while chewing. On the initial examination, the sharp enamel points should be removed by floating, and retained deciduous teeth "caps" removed in young horses. If the clinical signs persist, a more thorough examination of the teeth is indicated, paying particular attention to the infundibulum. An infundibular pick can be fashioned so that the shank is long enough to reach the third

molar. This pick is used to check the infundibulum of all of the teeth. The point on the pick should be about the diameter of a 20-gauge needle and approximately ½ inch in length. If an infundibular pick is not available, a 20-gauge needle or straightened paper clip can be held in long needle holder and used for this purpose. If the infundibular pick can be inserted into the infundibulum over 3 mm, coupled with a foul odor and the clinical signs described previously, a patent infundibulum should be suspected. Radiographic evaluation of the teeth and sinuses will help the examiner to arrive at the correct diagnosis. Sinusitis frequently accompanies this lesion, and if left untreated, the sinus will swell externally distorting the face and may open and drain. Removal of the infected tooth, followed by sinus curettage, is the effective method of treatment. The severity of the lesion increases with age of onset and the fourth upper cheek tooth is most frequently diseased.[67–69]

Periodontal Diseases

These diseases of the horse are inflammatory— the initial lesion being a marginal gingivitis with hyperemia and edema. The gingival sulcus becomes eroded and a triangular pocket is formed usually on the buccal aspect. The cavity harbors food material and bacteria, establishing a cycle of irritation, inflammation, and erosion. This destructive process extends around the tooth to the lingual aspect and deeper into the periodontium resulting in gross alveolar sepsis. Affected teeth are lost through spontaneous extrusion or by dental extraction. Clinical signs are similar to infundibular necrosis, with the end point being an abscessed tooth.

The teeth most commonly diseased are the first and fifth in the upper jaw and the first, second, and fifth in the lower jaw. The incidence increases with age, and 60% of horses over 15 years of age have some degree of periodontal erosion. Immature horses (40%) also have periodontal inflammation associated with eruption of the permanent dentition. When eruption is completed and the occlusal plane has been established, the incidence decreases and the disease process may reverse.[67,69]

The most severe form of periodontal disease is found in association with extreme abnormalities of wear. These changes are most frequently observed in older horses and can cause a chronic unthriftiness and a premature end to an otherwise useful horse.

Dental Prophylaxis

Horses use their teeth to grind food; therefore, the lower jaw (approximately 30% narrower than the upper jaw) traverses laterally to one side or the other as the jaws are closed. This causes the teeth in the lower arcades to be worn more on the buccal aspect and those of the upper arcades on the lingual aspect, forming sharp enamel edges on the upper buccal and the lower lingual aspect. These sharp points should be rasped down using an instrument called a "float." It is important that the teeth are floated properly—only the sharp points should be removed and not too much of the tooth. Young horses (between the ages of 18 months and 4 years) have more dental disease than any other age group except the very old horse.[70]

Since horses wear a bit in their mouth while working, teeth conditions such as enamel points cutting their cheek or tongue can be a real problem. Young horses (2½ to 4 years of age) that have a first premolar "wolf tooth" can develop a head-shaking problem. These horses may have a problem in chewing owing to soreness until the deciduous tooth is removed.

The first step in the treatment of any dental case is a thorough systematic examination. The head should be visually examined for the presence of any obvious swellings of the face or jaws. The presence of any nasal discharge or draining tract or foul odor that could originate from fermented food packed in the mouth or from an abscessed tooth will be detected on initial examination of the head. Next, the head should be palpated for swelling, the sinuses percussed and the buccal side of the upper arcade palpated through the cheeks. By grasping the bridge of the nose and the mandible close to the lips, and moving the jaws from side to side, an indication as to the roughness of the teeth will be obtained. This initial check gives the examiner a general indication as to what might be expected in the mouth and also it gives the two of them a chance to get acquainted.

The inside of the mouth and teeth are examined next, but first the mouth should be rinsed thoroughly using a bulb or dose syringe. This procedure also gives the examiner a clue as to the horse's disposition before trying to insert a hand into the mouth.

The incisors are most readily accessible and should not be overlooked. The incisors can be examined by raising the upper lip. If the horse opens its mouth during this maneuver, be sure to examine the teeth closely to check the horse's bite. The age of the horse should be determined at this stage and this should help in determining what dental care is needed. Brachygnathism or "parrot mouth" or "overshot" is a disorder in which the

upper incisors extend beyond the lower ones. With this condition, and depending on the severity, the horse would experience difficulty in grazing and since this condition is thought to be an inherited trait, these horses should not be considered for breeding purposes.

The opposite disorder, in which the lower jaw is longer than the upper jaw, is termed prognathia of the mandible or "undershot" or "sow mouth." This also is an undesirable trait and these horses will have difficulty in grazing and should not be considered for breeding purposes.

To examine the premolars and molars, the tongue is grasped by slipping the hand in the interdental space with the palm down and the thumb pointing in the direction of the incisor teeth. After grasping the tongue, the hand is rotated so that the thumb is against the palate; with thumb pressure, most horses will open their mouth wide enough for a visual inspection of one side. This technique is then repeated for inspection of the opposite side. In examining a horse's mouth, the tongue should never be grasped and held alone because if the horse jumps or pulls back suddenly, the frenulum could be torn or the tongue may be lacerated by the teeth. To prevent damage to the tongue and a possible bite to the hand, the horse's head should be well restrained by an assistant and the hand that is not introduced into the mouth can be used to hold onto the halter or placed over the bridge of the nose to prevent a sudden upward movement of the head. If the horse refuses to open the mouth, a mouth wedge or gag may be used to force it open. A mouth speculum can also be used to hold the mouth open, but generally the horse that tolerates a speculum can be examined without its use. A mouth speculum can be a dangerous instrument to both the examiner and the conscious patient. A mouth speculum should be used only on an anesthetized horse, unless the horse is extremely cooperative and the examiner has previous experience with this speculum and can remove it quickly. Good assistants who will stick with you in time of need, such as when a horse strikes, are to be highly prized!

A dental pick that is long enough to check the back teeth is helpful in checking for a patent infundibulum or caries. Digital palpation of the teeth can be conducted with the hand placed in the horse's mouth. This must be conducted with extreme care. The right hand is used to check the left side of the mouth and vice versa. The technique consists of grasping the tongue with one hand and pulling the tip of the tongue out of the side of the mouth. The other hand is inserted into the mouth forcing the tongue, with the back of the hand, between the arcades on the opposite side of the one being examined. It is important that considerable pressure be applied with the back of the hand, for carelessness at this point could be disastrous. This procedure should be conducted quickly since most horses will tolerate this for only a short time. Some horses have little respect for their tongue and many bite down during this procedure; therefore, the examiner must exercise extreme caution.

If the temperament of the horse is such that the examiner feels that the examination is incomplete or proper visualization of the teeth is not obtained, general anesthesia should be considered and the examination then done with the speculum in place. The examiner should be prepared to treat the disorder if possible while the horse is under general anesthesia. Time spent in initial preparation will save time in the end and additional anesthesia may well be avoided.

Sharp Enamel Points are the most common problem related to the horse's dental health. These points develop due to the anatomic shape of the head and the grinding motion of premolar and molar teeth. Clinical signs related to enamel points vary from severe cases, in which there is such discomfort that the horse reduces food consumption and loses weight, to milder cases that are characterized by prolonged chewing time to consume the grain ration. Lacerations of the buccal surface and tongue are common findings with sharp enamel points. In older horses the anterior edge of the second superior premolar may be elongate owing to lack of wear. The opposing lower premolar is frequently slightly caudal to the superior premolar. If this point on the superior premolar is excessively long and the other teeth are wearing down, the point can injure the lower gum causing a gingivitis that may become infected. Also in older horses, the last cheek tooth (third molar), either superior or inferior, may wear with a sharp point on the most posterior edge that may injure the opposing gum; therefore, it is important when floating teeth that the last cheek teeth be checked carefully.

Elongation of individual teeth indicates absence or excessive wear of the opposing teeth. An undulating table surface may result, and this abnormality predisposes to excessive wear of some teeth and possibly to alveolar periostitis. The client should be informed of the problem and encouraged to watch their horses carefully so that re-evaluation could be done when signs indicate worsening of the problem.

Frequently, veterinarians are asked how often a horse's teeth should be examined or "floated." This question is difficult to answer in that young horses (2 to 4 years) probable need to have their mouth examined twice per year whereas older horses that do not have any obvious problems need only yearly examinations. I am sure many horses have lived a long useful life without anyone ever looking into their mouth, but for the best use of their teeth for masticating their food (and since false teeth are not practical!), it would be best to have their teeth examined yearly. If the teeth continue to wear evenly, the client is reassured; if tooth wear is abnormal, prompt treatment will minimize further damage.

Congenital Malformations

Brachygnathism and prognathism of the lower jaw have been mentioned previously and are considered inherited traits. Parvignathism ("scissor mouth" or "shear mouth") is another congenital deformity in which the upper and lower teeth fail to meet properly. This deformity occurs when the difference in width between the upper and lower arcade is excessive, preventing the lateral movement of the teeth and interfering with mastication of food. The problem occurs most frequently in older horses after the teeth have grown in length and have not worn properly. The teeth are treated by cutting or rasping to create the desired level, but the end result is frequently less than optimal in that the horse will probably continue to have problems eating.

Neoplasia

Adamantinomas presumably of tooth germ origin may be more common in the horse than in other species. These tumors are firm, possibly cystic, masses usually affecting the mandible. They are usually found in young horses and may be present at birth.[15] These tumors present themselves as an enlargement of the jaw with the overlying mucosa and skin being intact. Radiography and biopsy are beneficial in definitively diagnosing this condition.

Ameloblastic odontoma has been reported in young and older horses. Because of the amount of bone present, such tumors may mistakenly be called osteosarcomas,[15] because of radiographic and gross pathologic appearance.

Squamous cell carcinoma appears to arise from the epithelium of the upper gum or hard palate. These tumors have an ulcerated area in the center from which emanates a foul fetid odor. A squamous cell carcinoma may also originate in the sinuses, resulting in a visible facial swelling along with a mucopurulent or hemorrhagic nasal discharge. Progressive hematomas of the ethmoid region may also result in mucopurulent or hemorrhagic nasal discharge.[71]

Epidermoid cyst in the premaxilla causing stertorous respiration due to the size of the mass has been reported and may be confused with a dental tumor.[72] Surgical extirpation of any neoplasm of tooth germ origin is likely to be attended by problems of postsurgical infection and/or recurrence of the tumor.

Cow

Porphyria is a rare congenital metabolic disease of cattle and swine. It has been recorded in Shorthorn, Holstein, Black and White Danish, and Jamaica Red and Black cattle.[73,74] This disease is characterized by a red-brown discoloration of the teeth as well as discoloration of bones, photosensitization, and red-brown urine. Teeth in affected animals fluoresce when irradiated with ultraviolet light. The dental lesions do not adversely affect these animals. However, to avoid the skin lesions of photosensitization requires special management effort, since affected animals must never be exposed to direct sunlight.

Fluorosis is first evident as changes in the teeth, the result of chronic fluorine toxicity. Only permanent teeth, exposed to fluorine before eruption, have been found to be affected. The observable change is mottling, which appears as horizontal lines of light yellow to brown or black discoloration. The mottled areas are prone to wear and are brittle. This leads to uneven wear of teeth, inadequate mastication, and subsequent poor nutrition. Affected animals are often noted to avoid cold water and prefer to lap at water rather than to drink normally. Lameness is also associated with fluorosis, but at higher concentrations of fluorine or with longer duration of exposure. Sudden severe lameness may appear and is usually due to a transverse fracture of the third phalanx.[75]

Tooth Capping (Bovine Crowns)

In the early 1960s, tooth capping became a popular conservation technique for cows on sandy or short pastures. These grazing conditions contribute to abnormally rapid wear of incisors because of the abrasive effect of sand and soil which is ingested with forage.

Stainless steel caps are used as a long-term salvage procedure for this problem. The stainless steel caps must be applied while there is still a good tooth root to support the cap. Nine different sizes are available to provide a properly sized cap for each tooth (depending on shape and degree of wear). All eight incisors should be capped at the same time to prevent uneven wear.

When the proper caps have been selected, they should be placed in order on a clean surface and thoroughly dried. The cement is then mixed and the teeth are dried and sterilized with thymol solution. The caps are then filled with the cement and placed on the appropriate teeth. Excess cement is removed and the caps are allowed to dry for 5 to 10 minutes. A mouth block is used to prevent chewing while applying the caps and while they are drying.

The use of dental crowns in range cattle is influenced by potential profit-margins, as are most elective therapies in food animal practice. Application of dental crowns is likely to be limited to genetically valuable breeding stock.

Prognathism and Brachygnathism

Prognathism or projection of the lower jaw is one of the more common congenital defects in cattle. Often the degree of prognathism is mild enough to go unnoticed. However, in the more extreme case, prognathism can interfere with prehension of food. In ruminants, there is good evidence that mandibular length is inherited. The defect is more common in beef breeds than in dairy breeds.[76]

Brachygnathism or short lower jaw has been reported in cattle as well as sheep. However, this defect is rare. As both prognathism and brachygnathism are proven genetic defects, correction should not be attempted.

Neoplasia

Adamantinomas, odontomas, and epuli, all of rare occurrence, make up the majority of the oral tumors of cattle.

Adamantinoma is an epithelial tumor arising from the embryonic precursor of the tooth. Although derived from enamel-forming tissue, the adamantinoma is a soft tissue tumor. The tumor may become locally invasive, but metastasis rarely occurs. Adamantinomas usually involve the incisor area in the bovine.

Odontomas may be found on the mandible or maxilla. They often will become cystic and contain tooth-like structures.

Epulis is a neoplasm involving the gingiva at its junction with the teeth. These neoplasms are usually fibromas and show no evidence of malignancy.

Each of these three types of tumors can be dissected out under general anesthesia; however, the results are not always successful. Since they are usually benign, there is little value in surgical treatment.

Dog

Dentistry once again became an important part of veterinary practice in the 1960s, with the dramatic increase in numbers of horses in North America and the willingness of clients to pay for more sophisticated dental procedures in horses, dogs, and cats.[77]

The adaptation of the ultrasonic scaler to veterinary dentistry has enabled the veterinarian to remove stubborn supragingival dental deposits more effectively and more efficiently. The collaboration of veterinarians with dentists has introduced new techniques to veterinary dentistry. Examples include repositioning of maloccluded teeth, restoration of teeth with enamel hypoplasia, the application of endodontic therapy to broken canine teeth in dogs, root canal procedures, and the development of artificial tooth implants. Growing interest in dentistry is reflected in the change from extraction as a first resort solution toward preservation of

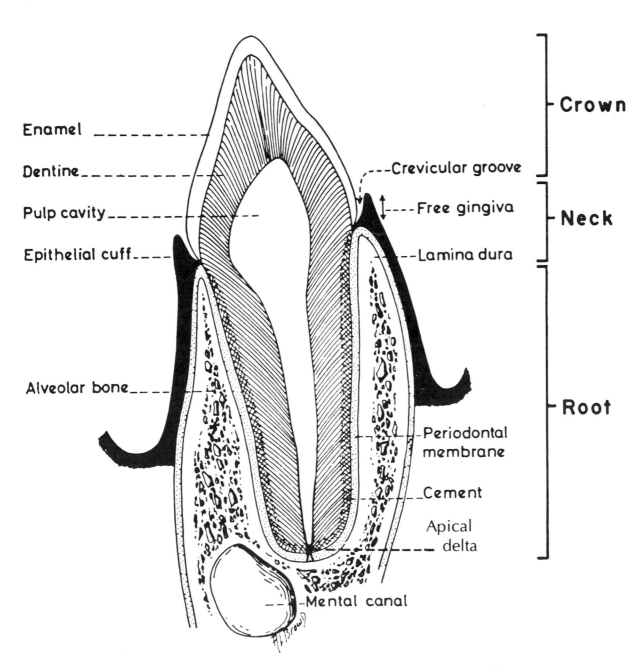

Figure 20–4.   Cross section of the lower first molar tooth. (Modified from Bell.[79])

teeth with a variety of these techniques.[78] The organization of the American Veterinary Dentistry Society and the growing number of papers at meetings on veterinary dentistry verify the increasing importance of this specialty in veterinary medicine.

Dental Terminology

A recent report has described the acceptable dental terms used by veterinary anatomists.[78] Previous terminology had been confusing and was not always anatomically correct. The new terms describe the directions within the mouth:

Rostral = toward the nose
Caudal = toward the tail
Labial = toward the lips = facing the lips
Lingual = toward the tongue = facing the tongue
Mesial = toward the center line of the
            dental arch
Distal = away from the center line of the
            dental arch
Contact = where a tooth touches an adjacent
            tooth
Occlusal (or masticatory) = biting surface

Incidence of Dental Disease in Dogs

The incidence of dental disease in dogs has been reported in a survey of over 600 cases.[79] A classification of occurrence reveals that periodontal disease is diagnosed in almost 75% of the cases. Diagnoses made less frequently are maxillary dentoalveolar abscess (malar abscess), epulis, caries,

persistent temporary dentition, enamel hypoplasia, neoplasms, and injury. Attrition and pigmentation of teeth were observed but not included in the survey. The percentages represented by various types of canine dental disease are represented in Figure 20–5.[79]

Periodontal Disease in Dogs

Periodontal disease is defined as any pathologic process involving the periodontium. Several structures may be involved, including the gingiva, cementum, alveolar bone, or periodontal membrane. The origin of periodontal disease is in the crevicular groove, formed by a cuff of epithelium surrounding the tooth (Fig. 20–6).[79] The periodontal membrane is the most important structure of this area and is necessary for the preservation and maintenance of dental health.

The periodontal membrane is composed of white fibrous connective tissue and consists of principal fibers and indefinite fibers. Six bundles of principal fibers extend from the cementum on one side to the bone on the other, except in the areas of the gums.

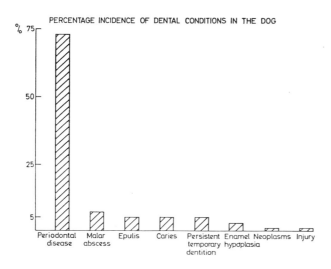

Figure 20–5. Percentage incidence of dental conditions in the dog. (From Bell.[79]) The proportion of dental injuries shown here would be typical of confined house pets; working dogs or free-ranging dogs might have a greater proportion of injuries because of greater environmental exposure.

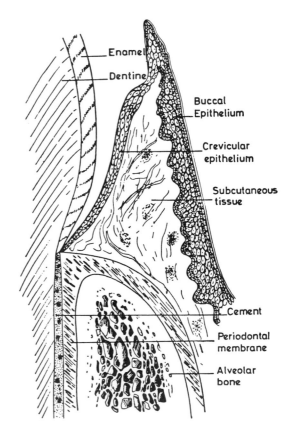

Figure 20–6. Microscopic section of the crevicular groove formed by the cuff of epithelium surrounding the tooth. (From Bell.[79])

The free-gingival group extends from the cementum to the gums and functions to firm the gums. The transseptal group extends from the cementum of one tooth to the cementum of the adjacent tooth and binds two adjacent teeth together. The alveolar crest group extends from the cementum of the root to the crest of the alveolar process. The horizontal, oblique, and apical groups are attached to cementum and bone. The last three groups along with the alveolar crest group suspend the tooth in the socket. The indefinite fibers of the periodontal membrane fill the spaces between the bundles of principal fibers and are supporting tissues. The minute capillaries and nerves which supply the tooth pass through the indefinite fibers.

The functions of the periodontal membrane are to: (1) act as a shock absorber and diminish trauma both on biting and during the course of a blow to the tooth; (2) afford a fibrous attachment to the tooth; (3) provide a layer of soft material through which blood vessels and nerves may pass from the bone to the tooth without undue risk of damage or injury by mechanical shock; and (4) maintain a proper relation between the gums and the teeth. The tooth is dependent on the existence and proper functioning of the fibers of the periodontal membrane for physical support, nutrition, and sensitivity. If the periodontal membrane is damaged, the tooth will suffer.[80,81]

Periodontal disease is responsible for the loss of more teeth in the small animal population than any other factor. The effects of periodontal disease on the tissues of the mouth are well documented, but the relationship between periodontal disease and total body health is unclear.

The onset of periodontal disease in animals is rarely acute. Occasionally, severe symptoms may be seen in 2- to 4-year-old dogs. However, a periodontal disease is often seen in middle-aged dogs, and signs are quite common in the geriatric age group (Fig. 20–7). Although the disorder may be quite advanced before being noted, there is often a 3- to 5-year period of subclinical disease preceding the onset of obvious signs.

The oral cavity can never be completely sterilized in the normal animal and it exists under a continuous insult of microorganisms. In healthy gingiva, a delicate balance exists between destruction and repair of the epithelial lining of the crevicular groove. Periodontal disease begins as an infiltration of the crevicular groove by bacteria and their toxins. These microorganisms produce microscopic ulcers in the crevicular epithelium. The process begins with the collection of dental plaque, which

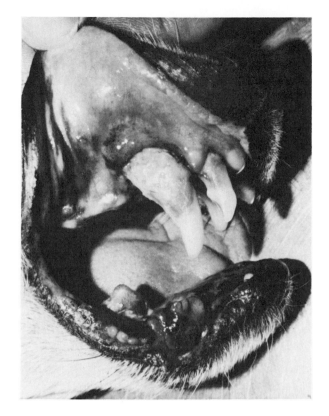

Figure 20–7. Severe periodontal disease in a 12-year-old male Terrier. Note the calculus deposits and gingival retraction of the mandibular canine tooth and incisors. Extraction of the affected teeth will relieve the disorder but will cause an oronasal fistula to persist.

consists of organic matrix, dead epithelial cells, food debris, and microorganisms. The plaque causes a deepened crevicular groove which disrupts the enamel cuticle. The result is a periodontal pocket, which is defined as a crevicular groove deeper than 3 mm. Once initiated, the disruption continues into the principal fibers of the periodontal membrane. The newly formed periodontal pocket is a route for oral bacterial to invade and produce an inflammation of the surrounding gingivae.[81]

The invasion of bacteria is accompanied by swelling, which inhibits the ability of gingival tissue to contain the infection. Swelling eliminates the normal knife-like margin of the gingiva and increases the tendency of food debris to be trapped within the periodontal pocket. As bacteria grow, epithelial ulceration and destruction of gingival tissue increase. The gums then recede from the crown of the tooth. Eventually, the process involves the alveolar bone, unprotected cementum and dentin of the tooth root. The end result is massive infection, destruction of bone, and loss of the tooth. Once the tooth is lost, the infection is contained and the alveolus heals. In the terminal stages, the tooth acts less like a normal body constituent and more like a foreign body, producing an abscess.[81]

The main clinical features of periodontal disease are: (1) halitosis or fetid breath, (2) gingival inflammation and ulceration, (3) gingival recession, (4) pus in the periodontal pocket, and (5) loosened teeth. The severity of the disease will determine the intensity of clinical signs. Dental deposits (dental plaque or calculus) may or may not be present on the affected teeth.

Dental Deposits

Deposits on teeth may accompany periodontal disease in small animals. Dental deposits are classified as uncalcified (dental plaque) and calcified (calculus). Uncalcified or dental plaque is composed of food debris, dead epithelial cells, organic matrix, and bacteria. Calculus is an adherent calcified mass which forms on tooth surfaces and is classified on the basis of location on the tooth and relation to the gingival margin. Supragingival calculus (supramarginal, salivary) consists of calcium phosphate and calcium carbonate held together by an agglutinin formed after attachment to teeth. It is located above the gum margin and is most commonly found on teeth near the orifice of salivary ducts. Calculus is grayish-white to clear white. Subgingival calculus develops below the gum margin and is distributed on all teeth.[82]

Dental deposits have been historically incriminated as a primary predisposing cause of periodontal disease. However, it is now generally accepted that bacterial invasion is basic to the process. However, effective dental prophylaxis must include meticulous removal of all deposits on teeth.

Although the cause of calculus deposit is unknown, two theories on calculus formation have been advanced. The first is based on the precipitation of calcium salts from saliva by a physico-chemical process initiated by a phosphatase enzyme. Phosphatase is liberated by desquamated epithelial cells and acts on the organic phosphates of saliva to form inorganic salts which enter into calculus formation. Another theory incriminates bacteria which precipitate calcium salts from saliva in the same manner as does phosphatase.[80]

The sequence of events in the epidemiology of periodontal disease and calculus formation in Beagle dogs has been described.[83] The observations were based on careful clinical examinations supported by objective recording and assessment.

Calculus deposition on the teeth of the Beagles was observed as early as 9 months of age on the surfaces of the teeth that are in close proximity to the opening of the ducts of the parotid glands. Calcified deposits were preceded by an accumulation of stain and soft debris which indicated that teeth were no longer self-cleansing (Fig. 20–8).[83]

During the period from 16 months to 26 months, calculus formation increased in surface area, became thicker, more textured in appearance, and more difficult to separate from the teeth. During this period, free-margin gingival inflammation increased. After 26 months of age, 95% of the observed animals had heavy calculus deposits. The teeth of the maxillary arch were subject to earlier deposition of calculus than those of the mandibular arch, suggesting a greater self-cleansing action in the mandibular arch (Fig. 20–9).[83] This cleansing was probably due to the large tongue and method of mastication of the Beagle. After 26 months of age, the gingival inflammation became severe with suppuration and acute abscess formation. The calculus had overcome the defensive resistance of the gingi-

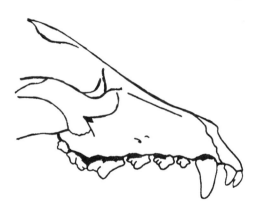

Figure 20–8. Dark shaded area indicates calculus deposition at 14 to 15 months of age. (Modified from Rosenberg et al.[83])

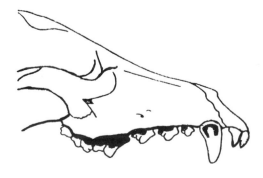

Figure 20–9. Dark shaded area indicates calculus deposition at 19 to 20 months of age. (Modified from Rosenberg et al.[83])

val tissue and the accompanying periodontal disease was irreversible.

The occurrence of calculus and gingival inflammation did not parallel the chronologic ages of the Beagles. This suggested an individual predisposing factor toward calculus formation and gingival inflammation. Physical consistency of the diet apparently is a factor in the development of periodontal disease and calculus formation. The feeding of bone, sinew, and tendon may be necessary for physical cleansing to control calculus accumulation and gingival inflammation.[83]

Factors Related to Periodontal Disease

Numerous factors have been incriminated in the development of periodontal disease in dogs. The role of dental deposits has been discussed. These deposits and persistent gingival infection are common denominators for the development of periodontal disease. The role of gingivitis accompanying periodontal disease has undergone considerable investigation. Periodontal lesions developing over an 18-month period in Beagles occurred in three stages: (1) subclinical gingivitis, (2) clinical gingivitis, and (3) periodontal breakdown. Subclinical gingivitis was characterized by increasing gingival exudation and migration of leukocytes into the crevicular groove. Clinical gingivitis was characterized by alterations of gingival color and texture, the presence of hemorrhage, but only minor alterations in the number of crevicular leukocytes. Periodontal breakdown was associated with clinical gingivitis and loss of attachment.[84,85]

Another report has described the conversion of chronic gingivitis into destructive periodontitis in 4-year-old Beagles. Cotton-floss ligatures were placed supragingivally around the crown of teeth, resulting in enhanced plaque accumulation, increased gingival exudation, and rapid formation of periodontal pockets. There was also an overt loss of alveolar bone and apical displacement of gingival tissue. The chronic inflammatory infiltrate around ligated teeth contained a plasma-cell dominated chronic lesion.[86]

Numerous other factors may be involved in the development of periodontal disease. Uneven wear, trauma, and malfunction due to loss of other teeth may predispose to gingivitis. Furthermore, these dogs may not be able to self-clean the teeth properly, resulting in accumulation of dental deposits. Fusospirochetal disease, which is similar to "trench mouth" in man, may also be involved. This infection is caused by *Spirochaeta vincenti* or *Fusiformis bacillus*, which are anaerobic microorganisms. The crevicular epithelium becomes swollen, and these microorganisms proliferate deep within the crevicular groove. Dental prophylaxis and extractions may have to accompany appropriate topical and systemic antibacterial treatment.

The diet may also affect the development of periodontal disease. Physically soft rations may not permit adequate self-cleansing of the teeth. Many veterinarians feel that the practice of leaving food in front of dogs at all times increases the risk of periodontal disease, because food substrate is constantly in the mouth. Specific vitamin deficiencies (A, B_2, C, D) may also play a role.

Dental Prophylaxis

Dental prophylaxis is the term used for the combination of treatment and prevention of periodontal disease. All small animals patients should be placed on a regular dental prophylaxis program by the veterinarian. Dental prophylaxis ensures that the teeth will remain healthy throughout most of the life of the animal.

Dental prophylaxis is a four-step program. The first step is scaling of teeth and removal of calculus. Certain precautions should be followed when scaling teeth. In most cases the dog should be anesthetized. Endotracheal intubation with inflation of the cuff should be done whenever general anesthesia is used for dental procedures. This prevents the aspiration of blood or mucus and ensures a patent airway. Keeping the dog tilted with the head lower than the rest of the body also prevents aspiration.

Dental deposits may be removed manually or by using ultrasonic scaling equipment. This equipment has reduced the time required to clean teeth with dental deposits, but the use of this equipment does present problems. Considerable heat can be generated by the tip of the scaling probe. Excessive force on the probe can damage the crevicular and buccal epithelium and the periodontal pocket. Therefore, all scaling below gingival margins should be performed with hand instruments of appropriate size. The standard-sized dental scalers (tartar scrapers) used in many practices are too large for most small animal patients. Their use results in excessive trauma and hemorrhage. Rather, one should use small curettes.

Ultrasonic dental cleaning can also lead to contamination of the local environment. Aerosol spread of microorganisms occurs at least 48 inches from the mouth of the patient, and the heaviest zone of contamination occurs within a 15-inch radius immediately in front of the mouth. The resulting mist

Table 20–4. Tooth disclosing solution

3.3 g iodine crystals
1 g potassium iodide
1 g zinc iodide
16.0 ml glycerine
16.0 ml distilled water

is a potential hazard to the operator. A surgical mask may lessen the danger to the operator and should be worn by individuals using ultrasonic scalers. It is also inadvisable to use dental ultrasonic equipment in an aseptic area such as a surgery room.[87]

A disclosing solution may be used to stain the calculus to facilitate its identification and aid in removal. A formula for this solution is listed in Table 20–4. This solution is also available from dental drug supply companies.

Removal of subgingival calculus should be performed manually, since ultrasonic devices may traumatize the crevicular groove or periodontal pocket. Hand scaling removes bacteria-laden calculus and plaque from the surface of the tooth and from within the periodontal pockets. Scaling toward the gum margins may disrupt the enamel cuticle or cause penetration of gums. The removal of embedded stains should be avoided, since it damages the enamel and may predispose to cavities. If subgingival calculus is allowed to remain, the periodontal pocket will continue to deepen.[81]

The second step of the dental prophylaxis is subgingival curettage and root planing. These techniques are indicated in cases of deepened periodontal pockets or root exposure or both. Subgingival curettage and root planing are often accomplished simultaneously when dental curettes are passed to the bottom of the periodontal pocket and withdrawn. The cutting edges of the curettes are directed alternately against the root surface and soft tissue wall of the pocket. Necrotic tissue debris and epithelium are removed from the soft tissue side and the irregular, cementum-dentin wall is planed smooth.[81]

The use of systemic antibiotic is advisable prior to the therapy and should be continued for at least 48 hours postoperatively to reduce intragingival bacteria populations. If dental prophylaxis does not return the gingiva to a healthy functional state within 10 to 14 days, surgery is indicated to eliminate gingival or osseous periodontal pockets. Teeth can usually be salvaged and returned to a functional state if one third of the root structure is within

healthy alveolar bone and an oral hygiene program is started.

The third step of the dental prophylaxis is polishing of the teeth. "The professional prophylaxis should be completed by polishing all exposed tooth surfaces to remove microscopic surface irregularities. Polishing presents the smoothest possible surfaces to the oral environment which helps retard accumulation of plaque for as long as possible."[81] The equipment for polishing is a dental hand piece and motor available at any dental supply house. A handpiece with adapted dental-type chuck and rheostat, to control speed, is very useful. Rubber polishing cups are used to apply a paste which consists of flour of pumice, and hydrogen peroxide and glycerin in equal parts. When polishing, the paste is applied by the rubber rotary polishing cup below the gum line in the gingival crevice. The enamel cuticle must not be damaged. Polishing in one place too long will cause heat from friction and damage the tooth. After some practice, one will be able to determine the amount of pressure to apply without wearing away too much enamel.[81]

The fourth and final step of any periodontal therapy is to encourage the owner to provide an effective measure of oral hygiene care for the animal at home. The oral hygiene techniques applicable to the dog and cat are rather basic. A small, soft toothbrush may be used to remove accumulations of soft debris from the surfaces of the teeth. The most common dentifrices used for animals are hydrogen peroxide, baking soda and water, although their continued use alters the oral flora. Human dentifrices cannot be recommended for pets because of their detergent-base formulations. A digestible dentifrice for dogs is available. When animals will not tolerate toothbrushes, the owner may be able to wrap a soft cloth around a forefinger and wipe the debris from the tooth surfaces. Milk bones, vinyl chew toys, and dry foods also provide valuable chewing exercise and reduce plaque.[81]

Methods of preventing the formation of dental deposits have been evaluated. The daily application of gel containing 0.5% chlorhexidine gluconate has been shown to reduce the formation of bacterial plaque and calculus on clean tooth surfaces in the Beagle dog. The gel had no effect on established calculus. Plaque and calculus formed rapidly when treatment was discontinued. However, an undesirable side effect was brown discoloration of tooth surfaces.[88] Another report suggested that 8-hydroxyquinoline sulfate inhibited formation of dental plaque in dogs.[89]

Treatment of Periodontal Disease

Treatment and control of periodontal disease require the four-step program previously described. Veterinarians should initiate a program of regular dental care in small animal patients. Calculus removal accompanied by subgingival curettage, root planing, and polishing are indicated for early cases of periodontal disease. Later, gingivectomy may be necessary to slow the process. In some cases, the gum may reattach to the teeth, decreasing the size of the pocket. If the teeth are quite loose, they must be extracted in an attempt to eradicate the infection.

Systemic antibiotic should always be administered when teeth are scaled. Penicillin or broad-spectrum antibiotic is usually indicated to reduce the extension of localized infections.

Mandibular frenectomy is indicated when recession of the gingiva around the mandibular teeth produces deep pockets and traps food. Simple excision of the frenuli next to the gingiva opens the pockets and may slow periodontal recession. The mandibular frenulum is one wall of the periodontal pocket and contributes to the retention of food debris, calculus accumulation, and periodontal disease. The detachment of the frenulum from its insertion on the buccal surface allows removal of debris from the area. Mandibular frenectomy combined with gingivectomy, root planing, and subgingival curettage reduces the progress of periodontal disease.[90]

Severe periodontal disease involving mandibular canine and incisor teeth may lead to oronasal fistula. Extraction of the involved teeth may be necessary and compounds the problem. The fistula is usually established prior to the loss of the tooth. The treatment of choice is a mucoperiosteal flap covering the healed alveolus of the extracted tooth. Prior to preparing the flap, the underlying bone is curetted. This technique is contraindicated when insufficient soft tissue is available for closure. If the suture line opens and the fistula is re-established, attempted reclosure should be delayed 3 to 6 months.[91]

Recent studies have shown the value of technetium-99m-tin diphosphonate radiopharmaceutical for determining the severity of periodontal disease in dogs. Scan images of soft tissue and vascular pools were normal for all dogs. Densitometric data from bone scans were compared. Radionuclide uptake in bone of dogs with chronic destructive periodontal disease was six times greater than corresponding values for control dogs.[92] This technique may be useful in determining whether corrective surgery or extraction is the treatment of choice.

Injuries to the Teeth and Endodontics

Fractures occur at all levels of the teeth. If the pulp is not exposed by the injury, the tooth needs no further attention. When the pulp is exposed, stimulation of afferent nerves produce an acutely painful condition especially when the dog drinks water. Pulp necrosis will develop as a sequela to pulp exposure. The pulp tissues are exposed to bacteria in the mouth when the teeth are worn or broken. Infection fills the pulp chamber and bacteria gain access to periapical tissues. Abscess formation at the apical delta occurs within a few weeks. Death of the pulp can also occur without bacterial exposure. The tooth is usually discolored because of traumatic injury and pulpal hemorrhage. Untreated pulpal death eventually results in loss of the tooth. Between pulpal death and tooth loss, there may be some time of body stress. Loss of pulp vitality is an indication for endodontic therapy or immediate extraction.[93]

The diagnosis and treatment of problems associated with diseased pulp tissues is called endodontics. Endodontic therapy consists of exposing the pulp chamber and removing pulp contents. An endodontic file is used to clean the walls of the pulp chamber, removing the cellular debris. Flushing with sodium hypochlorite, hydrogen peroxide, or saline solution aids in the cleaning process. The canal is then dried and filled.[93]

Various techniques for the repair of fractured teeth have been reported. Fractures of the canine teeth without exposure of the pulp cavity have been repaired with calcium hydroxydatum fastened to the injured surface by a crown of chrome-cobalt alloy. When the pulp cavity is exposed, it may be restored by removing all contents of the cavity and sealing by insertion of several gutta percha cones into the cleaned cavity. After 5 months one case had no difficulty with mastication or prehension and the teeth remained white. Failure from this method occurs because capping does not eliminate the bacteria within the canal or relieve the periapical abscess. A 20 to 25% failure rate was observed after 18 to 24 months when zinc oxide and eugenol paste was used to fill the canal. Failures occurred because of percolation of body fluids around the periapical delta, dissolution of the apical seal, and bacteria thereby gaining access to the pulp canal.[94]

The preferred method of restoring pulpal injuries is through apicoectomy and retrograde amalgam filling, done aseptically. Removal of maxillary bone is begun over the apex of the root through a mucosal flap. Exposure is continued until the outline of the root is seen and the apical foramen is visualized. Hemorrhage is controlled around the apical foramen and the seat of the apex is packaged with amalgam. The area is swabbed and the dental flap resutured. Zinc oxide and eugenol paste are forced into the filed pulp canal and the crown sealed with amalgam. Success depends on a double hermetic apical seal. The retrograde amalgam technique satisfies this requirement. Over 200 procedures have been performed with no technique failures.[94]

Recent work has suggested that root canal filling with calcium hydroxide paste is superior to other widely used materials. Calcium hydroxide-containing materials appeared to be particularly useful in an infected environment.[95]

Numerous reports have recently appeared in the veterinary literature describing restoration of broken teeth. Gold alloy crowns filled with crown and bridge cement have been attached to tooth remnants with pins, posts, and dental fixatives. The crowns have lasted for months following restoration.[96-99]

A new innovation in veterinary dentistry may be the use of prosthetic dental implants in man and laboratory animals including the dog. A variety of materials have been used as abutments for prostheses or for mandibular and maxillary reconstructions. These materials include metals, plastics, and ceramics. Endosteal titanium implants have been placed in dogs up to 12 months with some success.[100] Another report described varying degrees of inflammation accompanying endosteal metal implants of 8 months' duration. No epithelial or fibrous connective tissue adherence or attachment to the blades was evident.[101] Studies with ceramic tooth implants have suggested that they may be the best implantable substitutes for hard tissues. Ceramics are well-tolerated by tissues and are resistant to chemical action and corrosion. When ceramics are fabricated with controlled porosity, soft and mineralized tissue with the appearance of haversian bone will readily penetrate into porous spaces. The least desirable property of ceramics is the time and difficulty required to fabricate the material in the desired form.[102]

The criteria for successful tooth implantation should include: (1) stable physiologic retention, (2) nontoxicity, (3) durability and sound function in the oral cavity, (4) noncarcinogenicity, and (5) esthetic satisfaction. Other complex factors such as healing of the periodontal membrane, viability of the periodontal membrane in tooth implants, microbial flora, health of the implant recipient, nontraumatic occlusion, and physical and chemical properties of artificial implant material will influence the success of tooth implants.[103] It would appear that additional investigation is necessary before these techniques can be applied to clinical patients.

Maxillary Dento-Alveolar Abscess

Maxillary dento-alveolar abscess is a soft fluctuant swelling or draining sinus on the side of the head just below the medial canthus of the eye. This condition is also known as carnassial abscess, dental fistula, or malar abscess. It is a common dental disorder in dogs and may occur in the cat. The cause is thought to be damage to the lateral alveolar plate of the rostral lateral root of the upper carnassial tooth, caused by fracture of the tooth or intermittent concussion. Bacteria enter the alveolus and establish an abscess. The abscess may erode the maxillary bone, break through the skin, and give rise to a chronic fistula. The swelling of the abscess or draining fistula may regress and reappear. The carnassial tooth may show no apparent clinical relation to the abscess. In approximately one half of the involved cases, the rostral root of the first molar is also affected.

Treatment usually consists of extracting the upper carnassial tooth on the affected side. The first molar on that side should also be removed. Antibiotic therapy should be given for 3 to 5 days following the extraction.

Epulis

Epulis is a non-neoplastic fibrous proliferation of tissue surrounding the teeth, and may originate from the supporting structures of the teeth or from chronic inflammation (Fig. 20–10). Most epuli are found on the labial aspect of the dental arcade of dogs 6 years of age or older. Boxers, Spaniels, Labradors, and German Shepherds are most commonly affected. The canine teeth and premolars are usually involved.

The epulis should be allowed to remain until it interferes with normal mastication. The treatment consists of removing the affected tissue with electrocautery, including all of the tumor base. When multiple epuli are involved, gingivectomy, including the alveolar periosteum, has been useful. Occasionally removal of the affected tooth is indicated, with curettage of the alveolus.

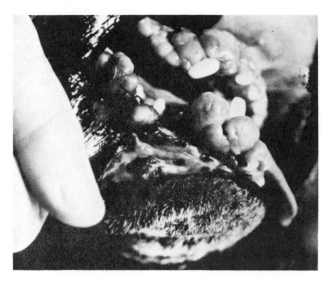

Figure 20–10. Multiple epuli on an 8-year-old male Boxer. Note the envelopment of many teeth with proliferative tissue growth.

Caries

Caries are a pathologic process involving the destruction of the enamel layer of teeth with subsequent invasion of the dentin by bacteria. It was formerly believed that caries did not occur in the dog, but caries have been documented.[104–106] One study reported the incidence of dental caries in 2113 dogs over a 15-year period to be 5.8%.[107] Another survey of 209 dogs suggested that dental caries do not occur spontaneously in dogs.[108] Both authors concluded that trauma is generally responsible for carious lesions.

Canine caries occur with the highest incidence on the occlusal surfaces. The upper first molar has the highest incidence of caries because the occlusal surface is subjected to trauma by the distobuccal cusp of the lower first molar. The mechanical destruction of enamel permits bacteria to be pressed into the tooth, giving rise to fissure or pit caries. Premolar teeth have a low incidence of caries. Brachycephalic dogs have irregular occlusion of upper and lower teeth and caries are rare in this group.[104]

The lower incidence in dogs as compared to man is attributed to a greater natural resistance in the canine mouth. Experimentally implanted carious human teeth became sterile after 4 or 5 months in a canine mouth. Cavities cut in teeth and left open 18 months did not become carious. Other techniques have been used in an attempt to induce caries in the dog. These techniques are: (1) completely removing the salivary gland, (2) feeding a highly refined carbohydrate diet, (3) producing traumatic spots on the dentinoenamel junction with a burr, and (4) applying lactobacillus culture in broth. During one 24-month study, none of these techniques produced carious lesions.[109] This resistance is attributed to: (1) strong bactericidal action of saliva with an alkaline pH of 7.5 to 8.3, (2) absence of ptyalin, a starch reducing enzyme in the saliva, (3) abundance of phosphates in diet, (4) anatomic form of the teeth with pointed crowns and few fissures, and (5) higher urea content of saliva which neutralizes the oral acids that assist in enamel breakdown.

Caries are manifested by halitosis, difficult chewing, refusal of hard food, salivation, rubbing of the mouth on the floor, and the finding of a cavity in a tooth filled with brown necrotic debris.[104] If the disorder can be detected early, an amalgam filling may be placed in the cavity. The cavity may be enlarged with a dental burr to about 3 mm depth and lined with zinc oxide and oil of cloves paste prior to inserting the amalgam. Results with amalgam fillings in dogs have been variable. Carious teeth not repaired in the early stages should be extracted if decay has become quite extensive.

Enamel Hypoplasia

Enamel hypoplasia is the failure of enamel to form before the eruption of the tooth. Enamel erosion, a posteruptive damage, may be confused with hypoplasia. The primary cause of enamel hypoplasia in dogs is canine distemper. The distemper virus causes a dull, chalky, or discolored tooth surface in the mildly affected cases. Excavations, grooves, and furrows of the dentin occur in the more severe cases. The dark-brown staining of the pitted areas is protective secondary dentin. The distemper virus alters the desmolytic action of the enamel epithelium preventing resorption of the connective tissue between the crown and the oral epithelium. The roots of retained teeth showed normal development with normal length. Distemper virus exerts an influence on the regulating mechanism of the hard tissues of the teeth. These changes have been demonstrated by histopathologic investigation of young canine jaws examined after death from distemper. A section of permanent tooth showed the inner enamel epithelium (ganoblast layer) detached from the underlying dentin resulting in a cavity filled with fibrinous exudate.[110]

Hypoplastic enamel has also been produced in puppies from bitches fed diets deficient in the fat-soluble vitamins. Destructive enzymes, chemical deficiencies, and bacterial invasion have also been recognized as playing a role in enamel hypoplasia. High fever and tetracycline drugs have been incriminated for enamel hypoplasia but no scientific data have been found to substantiate these theories.

Teeth with hypoplastic enamel are predisposed to fracture, and attempts have been made to restore the affected teeth. Maxillary canine teeth with hypoplastic enamel have been successfully restored with gold alloy crowns and composite resins.[111,112]

REFERENCES

1. Talukdar, A. H., Calhoun, M. L., and Stinson, A. W.: Sensory end organs in the upper lip of the horse. Am. J. Vet. Res. 31:1751, 1970.
2. Frank, E. R.: Veterinary Surgery, 7th ed. Minneapolis, Burgess Publishing Co., 1964.
3. Tritschler, L. G., and Morrow, L. L.: Guttural pouch catheter. V.M./S.A.C. 67:532, 1972.
4. Johnson, J. H., and Merriam, J. G.: Equine endoscopy. Vet. Scope 19:2, 1975.
5. Raker, C. W.: Diseases of the pharynx: paresis, paralysis, and/or elongation of the soft palate. Mod. Vet. Pract. 57:471, 1976.
6. Huston, R., Saperstein, G., and Leipold, H. W.: Congenital defects in foals. J. Equine Med. Surg. 1:146, 1977.
7. Johnson, J. H.: Infections of the upper respiratory tract. Vet. Clin. North Am. 3:255, 1973.
8. Johnson, J. H.: Selection, care and maintenance of endoscopic equipment for use in horses. J.A.V.M.A. 172:374, 1978.
9. Jones, R. S., Maiselo, D. O., Geus, J. J., and Lovius, B. B. J.: Surgical repair of cleft palate in the horse. Equine Vet. J. 7:86, 1975.
10. Mason, T. A., Speirs, V. C., Maclean, A. A., and Smyth, G. B.: Surgical repair of cleft soft palate in the horse. Vet. Rec. 100:6, 1977.
11. Nelson, A. W., Curley, B. M., and Kainer, R. A.: Mandibular symphysiotomy to provide adequate exposure for intraoral surgery in the horse. J.A.V.M.A. 159:1025, 1971.
12. Stickle, R. L., Goble, D. O., and Braden, T. D.: Surgical repair of cleft soft palate in a foal. V.M./S.A.C. 68:159, 1973.
13. Tolksdorff, E.: Surgical Approach to Cleft Palate. Proceedings of the American Association of Equine Practitioners 12:41, 1966.
14. Sundberg, J. P., Burnstein, T., Page, E. H., Kirkham, W. W., and Robinson, F. R.: Neoplasms of equidae. J.A.V.M.A. 170:150, 1977.
15. Cotchin, E.: A general survey of tumours in the horse. Equine Vet. J. 9:16, 1977.
16. Griesemer, R. A., and Cole, C. R.: Bovine papular stomatitis. J.A.V.M.A. 137:404, 1960.
17. Blood, D. C., Henderson, J. A., and Radostits, O. M.: Veterinary Medicine, 5th ed. Baltimore, The Williams & Wilkins Co., 1974.
18. Merchant, I. A., and Packer, R. A.: Veterinary Bacteriology and Virology, 7th ed. Ames, Iowa State University Press, 1967.
19. Buschman, G., and Dupree, C.: Oral treatment of actinomycosis in sows. D.T.W. 138:14, 1976.
20. Brodie, B., and Manning, J. P.: Isoniazid treatment of actinomycosis. Mod. Vet. Pract. 48:70, 1967.
21. Watts, T. C., Olson, S. M., and Rhodes, C. S.: Treatment of bovine actinomycosis with isoniazid. Can. Vet. J. 14:223, 1973.
22. Mulvihill, J. J., Mulvihill, C. G., and Priester, W. A.: Epidemiologic features of cleft lip and/or cleft palate in domestic animals. Teratology 13:31A, 1976.
23. Severin, G. A.: Diseases of the Digestive System. Canine Medicine. Santa Barbara, CA, American Veterinary Publications, 1968, p. 279.
24. Stannard, A. A., Gribble, D. H., and Baker, B. B.: A mucocutaneous disease in the dog resembling pemphigus vulgaris in man. J.A.V.M.A. 166:575, 1975.
25. Hurvitz, A. I., and Feldman, E.: A disease in dogs resembling human pemphigus vulgaris: case reports. J.A.V.M.A. 166:585, 1975.
26. Kunkle, G., Goldschmidt, M. H., and Halliwell, R. E. W.: Bullous pemphigoid in a dog: a case report with immunofluorescent findings. J.A.A.H.A. 14:52, 1978.
27. Halliwell, R. E. W., and Goldschmidt, M. H.: Pemphigus foliaceus in the canine: a case report and discussion. J.A.A.H.A. 13:431, 1977.
28. Cheville, N. F.: The Gray Collie syndrome, J.A.V.M.A. 152:620, 1968.
29. Stedham, M. A., Jennings, P. B., Moe, J. B., Elwell, P. A., Perry, L. R., and Montgomery, C. A.: Glossitis of military working dogs in South Vietnam: history and clinical characteristics. J.A.V.M.A. 162:272, 1973.
30. Jennings, P. B., Lewis Jr., G. E., Crumrine, M. H., Coppinger, T. S., and Stedham, M. A.: Glossitis of military working dogs in Vietnam: experimental production of tongue lesions. Am. J. Vet. Res. 35:1295, 1974.
31. Tokita, H., and Konishi, S.: Studies of canine oral papillomatosis, II. Oncogenicity of canine oral papilloma virus to various tissues of dogs with special reference to eye tumor. Jpn. J. Vet. Sci. 37:109, 1975.
32. Hammer, D. L., and Sachs, M.: Clefts of the primary and secondary palate. In Current Techniques in Small Animal Surgery. Edited by M. J. Bojrab. Philadelphia, Lea & Febiger, 1975, p. 75.
33. Howard, D. R., Merkley, D. F., Lammerding, J. J., Ford, R. B., Bloomberg, M. S., and Davis, D. G.: Primary cleft palate (harelip) and closure repair in puppies. J.A.A.H.A. 12:636, 1976.
34. Hutt, F. B., and deLahunta, A.: A lethal glossopharyngeal defect in the dog. J. Hered. 62:291, 1971.
35. Dorn, C. R., Taylor, D. O. N., Schneider, R., Hibbard, H. H., and Klauber, M. R.: Survey of animal neoplasms in Alameda and Contra Costa Counties, California. II Cancer morbidity in dogs and cats from Alameda County. J. Natl. Cancer Inst. 40:307, 1968.
36. Brodey, R. S.: The biological behaviour of canine oral and pharyngeal neoplasms. J. Small Anim. Pract. 11:45, 1970.
36a. Todoroff, R. J., and Brodey, R. S.: Oral and pharyngeal neoplasia in the dog: a retrospective survey of 361 cases. J.A.V.M.A. 175:567, 1979.
37. Dorn, A. S., and Olmstead, M. L.: Surgical excision of a lingual fibrosarcoma in a dog. Canine Pract. 6:41, 1977.
38. Withrow, S. J., Greiner, T. R., and Liska, W. D.: Cryosurgery. Veterinary considerations. J.A.A.H.A. 11:271, 1975.
39. Goldstein, R. S., and Hess, P. W.: Cryosurgery of canine and feline tumors. J.A.A.H.A. 12:340, 1976.
40. Benson, J. W.: Regional chemotherapy and local cryotherapy for cancer. Oncology 26:134, 1972.
41. Langham, R. F., Keahey, K. K., Mostosky, U. V., and Schirmer, R. G.: Oral adamantinomas in the dog. J.A.V.M.A. 146:474, 1965.
42. Langham, R. F., Mostosky, U. V., and Schirmer, R. G.: X-ray therapy of selected odontogenic neoplasms in the dog. J.A.V.M.A. 170:820, 1977.
43. McAllister, E. S., and Blakeslee, J. R.: Clinical observations of pharyngitis in the horse. J.A.V.M.A. 170:739, 1977.
44. Raker, C. W.: Diseases of the pharynx. Mod. Vet. Pract. 57:396, 1976.
45. Johnson, J. H.: Endoscopy of the pharynx, larynx and guttural pouch in the horse. V.M./S.A.C. 66:47, 1971.
46. Cook, W. R.: The clinical features of guttural pouch mycosis in the horse. Vet. Rec. 83:336, 1968.
47. Cook, W. R.: Observations on the aetiology of epistaxis and cranial nerve paralysis in the horse. Vet. Rec. 78:396, 1966.
48. Cook, W. R., Campbell, R. S. F., and Dawson, C.: The pathology and aetiology of guttural pouch mycosis in the horse. Vet. Rec. 83:422, 1968.
49. Johnson, J. H., Merriam, J. G., and Attleberger, M.: A case of guttural pouch mycosis caused by Aspergillus nidulans. V.M./S.A.C. 68:771, 1973.
50. Cook, W. R.: Epistaxis in the racehorse. Equine Vet. J. 6:1, 1974.
51. Johnson, J. H., Garner, H. E., Hutcheson, P. P., and Merriam, J. G.: Epistaxis. Proceedings of the American Association of Equine Practitioners 19:115, 1973.
52. Johnson, J. H., Garner, H. E., and Hutcheson, D. P.: Some Coagulation Aspects of Epistaxis in the Conditioned Thoroughbred. 1st International Symposium on Equine Hematology, 1975, p. 560.
53. Raker, C. W.: Diseases of the guttural pouch. Mod. Vet. Pract. 57:549, 1976.
54. Lokai, M. D., Hardenbrook, H. J., and Benson, G. J.: Guttural pouch tympanites in a foal. V.M./S.A.C. 71:1625, 1976.
55. Wheat, J. D.: Tympanites of the guttural pouch of the horse. J.A.V.M.A. 140:453, 1962.
56. Merriam, J. G.: Guttural pouch fibroma in a mare. J.A.V.M.A. 161:487, 1972.
57. Harvey, C. E., and O'Brien, J. A.: Disorders of the oropharynx and salivary glands. In Textbook of Veterinary Internal Medicine, Vol. 2. Edited by S. J. Ettinger. Philadelphia, W. B. Saunders Co., 1975, p. 1068.
58. Brodey, R. S.: A clinical and pathologic study of 130 neoplasms of the mouth and pharynx in the dog. Am. J. Vet. Res. 21:787, 1960.
59. Ragland, W. L., and Gorham, J. R.: Tonsillar carcinoma in rural dogs. Nature 214:925, 1967.
60. Alexander, B. F.: A study of parotid salivation in the horse. J. Physiol. 184:646, 1966.
61. Bracegirdle, J. R.: Removal of the parotid and mandibular salivary glands from a pony mare. Vet. Rec. 98:507, 1976.

62. Peddie, J. F., Tobler, E. E., and Walker, E. J.: Extirpation of the parotid gland in a mare. V.M./S.A.C. 66:605, 1971.
63. Knecht, C. D., and Phares, J.: Characterization of dogs with salivary cyst. J.A.V.M.A. 158:612, 1971.
64. Harvey, C. E.: Canine salivary mucocele. J.A.A.H.A. 5:155, 1969.
65. Prescott, C. W.: Ranula in the dog—a surgical treatment. Aust. Vet. J. 44:382, 1968.
66. Getty, R.: Sisson & Grossman's Anatomy of the Domestic Animals, 5th ed. Philadelphia, W. B. Saunders Co., 1975.
67. Baker, G. L.: Some aspects of equine dental radiology. Equine Vet. J. 3:46, 1971.
68. Baker, G. J.: Incidence of caries and periodontal disease in horses. J. Bone Joint Surg. 51:384, 1969.
69. Baker, G. J.: Some aspects of equine dental decay. Equine Vet. J. 6:127, 1974.
70. Beeman, G. M.: Equine Dentistry. Proceedings of the American Association of Equine Practitioners 8:235, 1962.
71. Cook, W. R., and Littlewort, M. C. G.: Progressive haematoma of the ethmoid region in the horse. Equine Vet. J. 6:101, 1974.
72. Wagner, P. G., Grant, B. D., Farrell, R. K., and Miller, R. A.: Epidermoid cyst in the premaxilla of the horse: a case report. J. Equine Med. Surg. 1:53, 1977.
73. Jorgensen, S. K.: Studies on congenital porphyria in cattle in Denmark. Br. Vet. J. 117:61, 1961.
74. Nestel, B. L.: Bovine congenital porphyria (pink tooth) with a note on five cases observed in Jamaica. Cornell Vet. 48:430, 1958.
75. Burns, K. N.: Report of 3rd International Meeting, Diseases of Dairy Cattle, Copenhagen, 1964, p. 292.
76. Wiener, G., and Gardiner, W. J. F.: Dental occlusion in young bulls of different breeds. Anim. Prod. 12:7, 1970.
77. Freeman, A.: Editorial—veterinary dentistry. J.A.V.M.A. 150:634, 1967.
78. Zontine, W. J.: Canine dental radiology: radiographic technique, development and anatomy of the teeth. J. Am. Vet. Radiol. Soc. 16:75, 1975.
79. Bell, A. F.: Dental disease in the dog. J. Small Anim. Pract. 6:421, 1967.
80. Boulton, G.: Animal dentistry. I. Diseases of the teeth and their supporting structures. Can. Vet. J. 1:162, 1960.
81. Ross, D. L.: Chapter 38, Veterinary dentistry. In Textbook of Veterinary Internal Medicine, Vol. 2. Edited by S. J. Ettinger. Philadelphia, W. B. Saunders Co., 1975, p. 1047.
82. Hofmeyer, C. F. B.: Comparative dental pathology (with particular references to caries and periodontal disease in the horse and the dog). J. S. Afr. Vet. Med. Assoc. 31:471, 1960.
83. Rosenberg, H. M., Rehfeld, C. E., and Emmering, T. E.: A method for the epidemiologic assessment of periodontal health-disease state in a Beagle hound colony. J. Periodontol. 37:208, 1966.
84. Lindhe, J., Hamp, S., and Loe, H.: Experimental periodontitis in the Beagle dog. Int. Dent. J., 23:432, 1973.
85. Lindhe, J., Hamp, S., and Loe, H.: Experimental periodontitis in the Beagle dog. J. Periodont. Res. 8:1, 1973.
86. Schroeder, H. E., and Lindhe, J.: Conversion of stable established gingivitis in the dog into destructive periodontitis. Arch. Oral Biol. 20:775, 1975.
87. Zontine, W. J., Sims, S., and Donovan, M. L.: Bacterial environmental contamination associated with ultrasonic dental procedures in dogs. J.A.A.H.A. 5:150, 1969.
88. Hull, P. S., and Davies, R. M.: The effect of a chlorhexidine gel on tooth deposits in Beagle dogs. J. Small Anim. Pract. 13:207, 1972.
89. DePalma, P. D., Loux, J. J., Hutchman, J., Dolan, M. M., and Yankell, S. L.: Anticalculus and antiplaque activity of 8-hydroxyquinoline sulfate. J. Dent. Res. 55:292, 1976.
90. Ross, D. L.: Therapeutics of Veterinary Dentistry. A.A.H.A. Proceedings, 1973, p. 128.
91. Hess, J. L., and Lowe, J. W.: A simple surgical treatment for acute periodontitis in the dog. V.M./S.A.C. 70:837, 1975.
92. Kaplan, M. L., Garcia, D. A., Goldhaber, P., Davis, M. A., and Adelstein, S. J.: Uptake of 99 mTc-Sn. EHDP in Beagles with advanced periodontal disease. Calcif. Tissue Res. 19:91, 1975.
93. Ross, D. L., and Myers, J. W.: Endodontic therapy for canine teeth in the dog. J.A.V.M.A. 157:1713, 1970.
94. Ramy, C. T., and Segreto, V. A.: Apicoectomy and root canal therapy for exposed pulp canal in the dog. J.A.V.M.A. 150:977, 1967.
95. Binnie, W. H., and Rowe, A. H. R.: A histological study of periapical tissues of incompletely formed pulpless teeth filled with calcium hydroxide. J. Dent. Res. 52:1110, 1973.
96. Wynne, W. P. D., Themaine, L. M., and Matthews, J. R.: Restoration of fractured canine tooth in a dog. J.A.V.M.A. 162:396, 1973.
97. Hamilton, C. J., and Ridgway, R. L.: Dowel and core preparation and full gold coverage of maxillary canine teeth in a German Shepherd. V.M./S.A.C. 71:176, 1976.
98. McIntosh, D. K., Wilson, J. B., and Adams, N. C.: Restoration of a mandibular canine tooth. Southwest. Vet. 22:235, 1969.
99. Wiest, L. M., and Sweeney, E. J.: Restoration of a fractured canine tooth in a dog. J.A.V.M.A. 164:601, 1974.
100. Richards, L. W., Gourley, I. M., and Cordy, D. R.: Titanium endosteal dental implants in the mandibles of dogs: preliminary studies. J. Prosthet. Dent. 31:198, 1974.
101. Piliero, S. J., Schnitman, P., Pentel, L. Cranin, A. N., and Dennison, T. A.: Histopathology of oral endosteal metallic implants in dogs. J. Dent. Res. 52:1117, 1973.
102. Garrington, G. E., and Lightbody, P. M.: Bioceramics and dentistry. J. Biomed. Mater. Res.—Symp. 6(2):333, 1972.
103. Hamner, J. E., and Reed, O. M.: The complex factors in tooth implantation. J. Biomed. Mater. Res.—Symp. 6(2):297, 1972.
104. Schneck, G. W.: Caries in the dog. J.A.V.M.A. 150:1142, 1967.
105. Spink, R. R.: Dental cavities in a dog. V.M./S.A.C. 71:466, 1976.
106. Gardner, A. F., Darke, B. H., and Keary, G. T.: Dental caries in domesticated dogs. J.A.V.M.A. 140:433, 1962.
107. Bodingbauer, J.: Comparative observations on the occurrences of caries in man and the dog. Z. Stomatol. 44:333, 1947. Abst. Vet. Rec. 60:40, 1948.
108. Rudinu, I.: Spontaneous dental caries in animals. Dent. Abst. (Chicago) 4:38, 1959.
109. Lewis, T. L.: Resistance of dogs to dental caries: a two-year study. J. Dent. Res. 44:1354, 1965.
110. Bodingbauer, J.: Retention of teeth in dogs as a sequel to distemper infection. Vet. Rec. 72:636, 1960.
111. Marvich, J. M.: Repair of enamel hypoplasia in the dog. V.M./S.A.C. 70:697, 1975.
112. Kaplan, B., and Marx, S. G.: Restorations of the maxillary canine teeth of a dog with enamel and dentin hypoplasia. J.A.V.M.A. 150:603, 1967.

Chapter 21

THE ESOPHAGUS

JOAN A. O'BRIEN
COLIN E. HARVEY
ROBERT S. BRODEY

The esophagus is a prosaic organ. Although essential for a normal quality of life, it was never exalted in Shakespearian metaphor or enshrined in culinary history by Escoffier.

The esophagus begins at the pharynx, passes through the neck and thorax, and enters the abdomen to end at the gastroesophageal junction. Commencing dorsal to the larynx and trachea, it inclines to the left in the mid- and caudal cervical region, and passes dorsal to the trachea at or caudal to the thoracic inlet. In the thorax it lies dorsal and to the left of the tracheal bifurcation and to the right of the aortic arch; it passes ventral to the aorta through the esophageal hiatus of the diaphragm, terminating at the cardia of the stomach. In the horse, dog, and cat, the esophagus has a short intra-abdominal component which is not present in the pig or cow.[1,2]

The esophagus is fixed cranially by the attachment of fascia and muscle to the cricoid cartilage of the larynx and vertebral fascia of the neck. It is movable where it passes through the neck and thorax, and is covered by deep cervical fascia, and mediastinal fascia and adventitia of adjacent organs. It is fixed caudally by the phrenico-esophageal membrane and stomach. This arrangement allows considerable normal movement of the esophagus along a cranial-caudal and transverse axis during respiration and swallowing.[3]

Histology

The esophagus consists of four layers: mucosa, submucosa, muscularis, and adventitia. The mucosal layer of the collapsed esophagus lies in longitudinal folds and consists of cornified, stratified squamous epithelium. This epithelium is very strong and is considered the "holding" layer for surgical sutures.

The esophageal epithelium has duct openings from the submucosal mucus-secreting glands. Areas of mucosal pigmentation are seen in some heavily pigmented animals such as Chow dogs. Cardiac (mucosal) glands occur in the distal esophagus in all species. In the cat, the mucosa of the distal thoracic esophagus has a scale-like surface, and the muscularis mucosa smooth muscle extends the entire length of the esophagus.[4] The muscularis mucosa is found only in the distal third of the esophagus in the dog and bovine.

The submucosal layer contains many elastic fibers and allows the mucosa to lie in longitudinal folds when the esophagus is empty. Submucosal (mucus-secreting) glands are present throughout the entire length of the canine esophagus but are found only in the pharyngoesophageal region of the feline and bovine esophagus and in the cranial half of the porcine esophagus.

The third layer of the esophagus is the muscularis. It consists of two layers of muscle usually described as inner circular (spiral) and outer longitudinal (oblique). The two layers interdigitate, particularly in the cow and dog where the ventral outer layer of muscle may pierce the dorsal muscle layer becoming the inner layer. In the cow, pig, and dog the muscle layer is striated throughout its length except for a small area of smooth muscle in the inner circular layer near the cardia. In the horse and cat, the muscle changes from striated to smooth at approximately the level of the heart base; all layers are smooth muscle in the caudal one to two thirds of the esophagus.

The myenteric plexuses (Auerbach plexus) are present between the inner and outer muscle layers. They are distributed evenly along the length of the esophagus in the ox and cat but are more concentrated in the caudal portion of the esophagus of the dog.

The fourth layer of the esophagus is the adventitia. It is variably made up of deep cervical fascia, adventitia of contiguous structures, pleura, and in those species with an abdominal component, peritoneum.

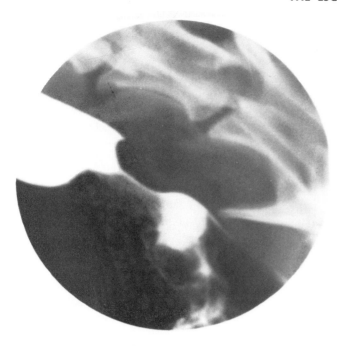

Figure 21–1. Lateral spot film of cricopharyngeal area in a normal dog during barium contrast esophagram.

Table 21–1. Factors influencing the caudal esophageal sphincter (High Pressure Zone)

Increase Pressure	Decrease Pressure
Gastric distention	Hiatal hernia (±)
Gastrin (±)	Secretin
Motilin (±)	Cholecystokinin-pancreozymin
Antacids	Increased gastric acidity
Methacholine (Bethanechol)	Vagotomy
Metoclopramide	Cardiomyotomy
Protein ingestion	Primary muscle disease
	Hypoglycemia

Cranial Esophageal Sphincter

In all species there is a cranial esophageal sphincter; it is composed mainly of the cricopharyngeus muscle, which blends imperceptibly with the caudal fibers of the thyropharyngeus muscle (a constrictor of the pharynx). The caudal aspect of the cricopharyngeus muscle blends with the cranial fibers of the longitudinal esophageal muscle layer. The innervation of this cranial esophageal sphincter is the pharyngoesophageal nerve, a branch of the vagus. In the dog the cricopharyngeus muscle is well developed and can often be recognized radiographically in both survey radiographs and contrast studies (Fig. 21–1): innervation in the dog is by the pharyngeal nerve, which leaves the vagus separately from the pharyngoesophageal nerve.

Caudal Esophageal Sphincter

The existence of a physiologic caudal esophageal sphincter is well recognized in species that have been studied carefully. Confusion arises from the variable terminology used to describe the caudal end of the esophagus. The endoscopist recognizes the area where the squamous epithelium changes to the columnar epithelium of the gastroesophageal junction. The surgeon sees the external landmark, the cardiac incisura, and insertion of the phrenicoesophageal ligaments. The physiologist recognizes the high pressure zone area in the caudal

esophagus: this pressure has been reported as 46 ± 2.5 cm H_2O in the dog and 32.6 to 38.6 mm Hg in the cat.[5,6,7,8]

The high pressure zone of the caudal esophageal sphincter is altered by certain hormones, gastric pH, esophageal and gastric distention, neurogenic influences, surgical interference, and anatomic abnormalities such as hiatal hernia (Table 21–1).[6,7,9,10,11,12,13]

The function of the esophagus in all species is to transport food, liquid, and saliva to the stomach. In the ruminant, function also includes bolus regurgitation for further mastication and eructation of ruminal gases. Regurgitation of food may occur in the bitch and queen in weaning their young.

The esophagus is quiet at rest and contracts during swallowing. Swallowing is a combined reflex-voluntary mechanism. In the normal pattern of events an ingested bolus is propelled by the tongue and muscles of the pharynx to the caudal pharynx and cricopharyngeus muscle, which relaxes to allow bolus passage. A swallowed bolus initiates a primary peristaltic wave, propagated throughout the length of the esophagus. Esophageal distention may elicit a secondary peristaltic wave that can commence at the area of distention anywhere along the length of the esophagus. The peristaltic wave is an annular contraction that moves aborally along the esophagus and is closely coordinated with upper and lower esophageal sphincter relaxation. Reverse peristaltic movements (except in the ruminant) and a large number of tertiary waves, or spontaneous contractions, are abnormal. Tertiary waves increase in frequency with age in man; it is not known whether this occurs in other species.

SIGNS OF ESOPHAGEAL DISEASE

Signs of esophageal disease are related to loss of function and include dysphagia, ptyalism, oral or nasal regurgitation, and bloat. Bloating is usual in the ruminant but is an uncommon sign of esophageal disease in other species. Pharyngeal and tonsillar inflammation are often seen secondary to repetitive regurgitation; the irritation of regurgitated material in the nasopharynx may lead to nasal discharge. The owner may notice a transient swelling in the neck following eating. Complaints of noisy eating and breathing may be due to mucus and air in an enlarged esophagus. Weight loss is common, although careful husbandry by the owner can minimize this loss. The animal may be anorectic if the esophageal disease causes pain, but in many cases the animal is very hungry and will reingest regurgitated material.

Regurgitation may occur with signs of dysphagia as the animal eats, or it may be delayed many hours. Regurgitation tends to be more passive with neurologic defects affecting the esophagus. Regurgitation is more active and may be accompanied by dysphagia in diseases such as foreign body obstructions, benign strictures, or tumors. Regurgitated material characteristically consists of mucus and undigested food; it may have a tubular shape as a result of compaction in the esophagus.

The veterinarian should inquire about the opportunity for access to caustics or previous medication, surgical procedure prior to onset, and the age of onset of dysphagia to determine the probability of a congenital abnormality.

The rate of onset of the disease is important, with acute onset more compatible with foreign body or caustic burn, while a gradually developing dysphagia is more typical of stricture or tumor. The type of dysphagia is important; e.g., liquids and semisolid foods are better tolerated when the esophagus is narrowed by organic disease.

Other signs of systemic illness should be investigated to rule out more generalized diseases such as myasthenia gravis, heavy metal poisoning, myositis, and neuromuscular disease.

FINDINGS IN ESOPHAGEAL DISEASE

The findings at physical examination may be non-contributory. However, pharyngitis, rhinitis, and nasal discharge are common in animals that repeatedly regurgitate decaying food. The animal's physical condition may vary from extreme cachexia to normal depending on the actual amount of nourishment the animal obtains. Dehydration may be severe with repeated regurgitation. High fever is unusual unless there has been perforation of the esophagus, although aspiration pneumonia may induce fever. Dyspnea may result from aspiration

pneumonia or encroachment on lung inflation by a greatly dilated esophagus. Repetitive swelling of a dilated cervical esophagus may occur spontaneously with expiration, or it may be induced by compressing the thorax during breath-holding. Abnormal auscultatory findings over the thorax may be rales associated with aspiration pneumonia or splashing sounds caused by a fluid/air mixture in the esophagus moving with changes in intrapleural pressure. Moving the stethoscope to auscultate the cervical esophagus will often document an esophageal origin of sound. Investigation of dysphagia should include observing the animal eat and drink.

Survey radiographs of animals with suspected esophageal disease should include the entire length of the esophagus from pharynx to stomach. These are useful in the diagnosis of radiopaque foreign bodies or a dilated, air-filled megaesophagus. Both survey radiographs and contrast studies should be made in the conscious animal to evaluate function and avoid pharmacologic dilation of the esophagus caused by anesthesia or sedation. Single radiograph contrast studies following administration of barium sulfate (or Gastrografin in suspected perforations) will outline a non-radiopaque foreign body or a perforation; fluoroscopy is needed to evaluate function and, in many instances, to localize areas of stricture.

Esophagoscopy is usually indicated in the diagnosis and treatment of esophageal diseases other than obvious megaesophagus and vascular ring obstruction. Esophageal biopsy and cytology are helpful when mucosal abnormalities may be due to infection, parasites, or neoplasia.

Examination of the regurgitated material should include both gross characteristics and measurement of pH. Regurgitated material is typically undigested food and may assume the tubular form of the esophagus. The pH of a freshly regurgitated sample may range from 7.5 to 8.3. Esophageal secretions have been measured in the dog and found to contain total solids of 1.25 to 1.48 g/dl with chloride concentrations approaching those in the stomach.[15]

Esophageal manometry (measurement of the pressure characteristics of peristaltic waves and changes in pressure in the lower esophageal sphincter) is reported for experimental animals, but these studies have rarely been used in clinical veterinary medicine to date. Abnormal manometric findings have been observed in naturally occurring canine megaesophagus, and a lowered distal esophageal sphincter pressure has been reported after experimentally induced esophagitis in the cat.[7,16]

DISEASES AFFECTING THE CRANIAL ESOPHAGEAL SPHINCTER

Dysphagia is seen frequently in domestic animals. In most instances, an obvious cause is found at physical examination. Oropharyngeal tumors, abscesses, and lacerations or tonsillitis and acute or chronic pharyngitis can all be manifested by difficulty in prehension, sialorrhea (ptyalism), and awkward gulping movements often followed by a nasal discharge or dropping of the food bolus from the mouth. Those animals having dysphagia but without directly visible, palpable, or radiographically demonstrable organic disease in the mouth, pharynx, or neck are a challenge to the clinician. In such animals, careful observation of the feeding pattern and functional studies such as contrast esophagrams are necessary.

The pattern of deglutition consists of a series of coordinated contractions and relaxations of the tongue and pharyngeal and laryngeal muscles in a careful balance of relative muscular effort.[17]

Derangement of deglutition can result from a single muscle abnormality or slight malfunction of more than one element. The usual result in a dysphagic animal is failure of the food bolus to enter the esophagus. The obvious inference is that the cricopharyngeus muscle (cranial esophageal sphincter) has failed to relax in sequence. It should be noted, however, that the same result would occur from incoordinated pharyngeal constrictor muscle activity failing to push the food bolus through the relaxed cricopharyngeus sphincter. Subtle differences such as this require careful evaluation of pharyngeal contrast radiographs and histopathologic examination of muscle to determine a true diagnosis. In contrast, surgical management directed at impairing the function of the cricopharyngeus muscle and allowing easier passage of food boluses into the esophagus is likely to be of benefit to any animal with pharyngeal or cricopharyngeal malfunction. The response to surgery, therefore, cannot be used as a confirmation of diagnosis.

Cricopharyngeal Achalasia

Cricopharyngeal achalasia has been described by several authors[18,19,20] as occurring in the dog. The diagnoses were based on a history of dysphagia and radiographic evidence of failure of food to enter the esophagus normally. Muscle disease or abnormal electromyograph tracings have not been reported, but we have observed EMG tracings compatible with myotonia in one dog. The six dogs described ranged from 13 weeks to 15 months old, and were of different breeds. Nasal exudation was reported as occurring in several of the dogs. Dysphagia in otherwise healthy young dogs has been seen on several occasions in our practice.* As with the case histories reported, physical examination was normal except for evidence of pharyngitis presumed to be secondary to the dysphagia. At operation, hypertrophy of the cricopharyngeus muscle was not observed; muscle fibers were histologically normal. It is our clinical impression that Cocker Spaniels, which have a high, narrow pharynx, may be more prone to dysphagia than other breeds. Gagging and retching superimposed on eating may mimic dysphagia in brachycephalic dogs.

When presented with a dysphagic dog, a complete physical examination and careful neurologic examination should be performed. If no neuromotor abnormalities are observed, and if cinefluorography demonstrates repeated failure of contrast material to enter the esophagus, a presumptive diagnosis of cricopharyngeal achalasia may be made.

In examining cinefluorographs of dogs during swallowing, relaxation of the cricopharyngeus muscle is seen for a short period only. For this reason, random single radiographs made during swallowing are unlikely to record cricopharyngeal relaxation, particularly if made without the benefit of fluoroscopy. (See Fig. 21–1) Pharyngeal contrast cinefluorography is not an easy procedure in the dog; allowance must be made for the gulping and squirming associated with forcible swallowing of contrast material by an untrained dog.

Treatment is manipulation of the diet to avoid all large particle or rough food, or cricopharyngomyotomy. Cricopharyngomyotomy is generally considered to be a procedure with few complications; postoperative aerophagia does not usually occur. The cricopharyngeus muscle does not remain in a "resting" state of tonic contraction except during deglutition as was previously thought, but rather contracts only during inspiration, breathholding, straining, or during pharyngeal stimulation.[21]

Pharyngeal Paralysis

In the horse, pharyngeal paralysis may be caused by central nervous system disease. Swallowing incoordination, muscle spasms, or blindness may be present. Guttural pouch mycosis may also cause pharyngeal paralysis.[22] Toxic factors (moldy corn poisoning, Yellow Star thistle poisoning and

---

*University of Pennsylvania, School of Veterinary Medicine, Philadelphia, Pennsylvania 19104.

botulism), metabolic disturbances such as eclampsia, and mechanical factors such an enlargement of pharyngeal and cervical lymph nodes secondary to strangles and pharyngeal polyps can cause dysphagia.[23] Nasal regurgitation of food or water is the principal clinical sign of dysphagia in the horse.

In the dog, dysphagia may be one clinical sign of more generalized neural disease. Specifically, a syndrome known as multiple cranial neuropathies (pharyngeal paralysis) is recognized. There is atrophy of the muscles of mastication, a weak or absent gag reflex, dysphagia, and regurgitation. The clinical course is the progression of neuropathy to include other cranial, or peripheral nerves. The cause of the neuropathy usually cannot be established. In man, the differential diagnoses include muscular dystrophy, thyrotoxicosis, myasthenia gravis, cerebrovascular disease, bulbar poliomyelitis, trauma (including surgical trauma) and idiopathic neuropathy.[24]

DISEASES OF THE BODY OF THE ESOPHAGUS

Vascular Ring Stricture

Partial occlusion of the esophagus by aberrant blood vessels in the heart base area is a common cause of esophageal obstruction in the dog and cat and has been described in a bull.[25] The embryonic patterns of these abnormalities have been reviewed in detail.[26] These vascular abnormalities have been seen in many breeds of dogs and in cats, with the highest incidence in the Irish Setter and German Shepherd dog. Persistent regurgitation present from the time of weaning is the most common presenting sign. Because of the high incidence of generalized

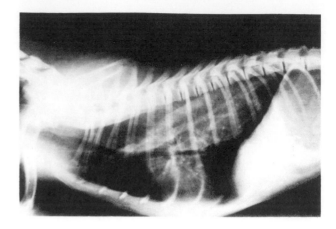

Figure 21–3. Lateral survey radiograph of a dog showing the generalized dilatation of megaesophagus.

megaesophagus and occluding vascular ring anomalies in the German Shepherd dog, confirmation of the diagnosis by esophageal contrast radiography must be obtained prior to surgical treatment. Esophageal dilatation, which may be very large cranial to the heart base, is seen with occluding vascular ring anomalies (Fig. 21–2), whereas dilatation of the entire thoracic and (sometimes) cervical esophagus is seen with generalized megaesophagus (Fig. 21–3). Both disorders can exist in the same dog. Esophageal motility may be abnormal cranial to an occluding vascular ring if the esophageal dilatation is very large. Esophageal motility and diameter are usually normal caudal to the vascular ring.

Endoscopic Appearance. The dilated esophagus is frequently filled with ingesta and saliva. The mucosa usually appears inflamed and has a velvet-like appearance. At the level of the occluding vascular ring, the mucosa may appear more inflamed and have small ulcerations, or it may be almost normal but extremely compressed. Abnormal pulsations may be seen if the constricting vessel is patent. Fibrous scarring of the mucosa is not present. The wall of the esophagus often appears paper-thin; care should be used when passing a sound at surgery or advancing an endoscope.

Treatment. Treatment consists of transecting the aberrant vessel to release the esophagus from the stricturing effect. Prior to surgery the esophageal contents should be evacuated by suction to reduce the likelihood of pre- or postoperative aspiration of esophageal contents. The surgical approach is made through a left fourth interspace thoracotomy. The cause of the stricture is determined by inspection,

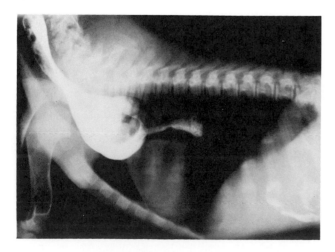

Figure 21–2. Lateral radiograph of a dog during barium contrast esophagram showing dilatation of the esophagus cranial to constriction by persistent right aortic arch.

using an esophageal sound if necessary. It is prudent to consider the constricting vessel patent, even though the most common vascular anomaly, persistent right aortic arch, has a closed ligamentum arteriosum rather than a patent ductus arteriosus. The vessel is gently dissected away from the underlying esophagus, ligated or clamped, and divided. An esophageal sound is then pushed cautiously across the area of stricture, and any remaining constricting fibrous bands are undermined and sectioned until the sound can pass easily caudal to the stricture level. Esophagoplasty following transection of the constricting vessel has been suggested.[27]

The prognosis following operation for vascular ring stricture is fair-to-good. The clinical impression is that the more dilated the esophagus is preoperatively, the poorer the functional result. One report describes a reduction in the number of myenteric ganglial cells (particularly in mid-esophagus) in two dogs with a persistent right aortic arch when they were compared with normal dogs and dogs with generalized megaesophagus.[28] Resection of part of the dilatation could prove beneficial in dogs with gross dilatation but has not been described clinically. Because of the inherited nature of vascular ring strictures, neutering affected animals is recommended. The presentation, treatment, and results of treatment in the cat are the same as for the dog.

Esophageal deviation caused by aberrant left subclavian and brachiocephalic arteries has been reported in English Bulldogs:[29] surgical redirection of the left subclavian artery resulted in remission of clinical signs.

Other Congenital Anomalies Causing Esophageal Obstruction

Congenital anomalies which are well recognized in man, such as esophageal atresia with or without tracheoesophageal fistula,[30] have been reported rarely in domestic species,[31] probably because death occurs very soon after birth. Immediate, radical surgical treatment would be required. Esophageal stenosis in a Norfolk Terrier,[19] and congenital esophageal diverticulum in a Miniature Schnauzer[32] have been briefly described with accompanying contrast radiographs; both lesions were at the thoracic inlet. Neither treatment nor prognosis was described.

Congenital anomalies of the esophagus have been mentioned as occurring in other species, although usually with insufficient documentation. The surgical excision of an esophageal intramural cyst or teratoma has been reported in the horse.[33]

DISEASES RESULTING IN MOTILITY ABNORMALITIES

Abnormalities of esophageal motility result in a reduction in the rate of flow of material through the affected part of the esophagus. If severe enough, this causes retention of food, dilatation of the esophagus, and subsequent regurgitation.

For many years, it was assumed that gross dilatation of the esophagus in the dog was caused by failure of the lower esophageal sphincter to relax ("achalasia"), a condition that is well documented in man (see below under Diseases of the Distal Esophagus and Lower Esophageal Sphincter). Treatment was based on this assumption. It has now been shown that in the dog generalized megaesophagus rarely if ever is caused by achalasia; indeed, there are no adequately documented reports of true achalasia in the dog. Based on esophageal manometry studies in dogs with generalized megaesophagus, lower esophageal sphincter function is normal, peristaltic motor activity is absent or poor in the mid- and cervical esophagus and swallowing frequently fails to produce a primary peristaltic wave (body motor response).[34] Neuromuscular function examined by nerve stimulation and gross observation and electromyography of affected dogs is somewhat confusing; one report states that complete tetanic contractions occurred along the entire esophageal length when vagal fibers were stimulated,[35] while in another report, only feeble, isolated, localized contractions resulted from vagal stimulation.[36]

Both reports suggested that abnormalities existed in the afferent nerve supply of the esophagus, which could eliminate secondary peristaltic waves. One possible reason for the difference in the observed results was the effect of age and maturation on esophageal motor units of affected dogs.[37] Histologic examination of the esophagus of affected animals confirms that megaesophagus in both dogs and cats is not associated with absence or reduction in myenteric ganglial cells; in humans with achalasia, myenteric ganglial cells are much reduced in number.[35,38,39] A condition similar to megaesophagus has been reported in the horse, although with no documentation.[40]

Megaesophagus—Clinical Features

The dog is the most commonly affected domestic animal. The German Shepherd dog is more likely to be affected than other breeds.[41] An autosomal pattern of inheritance has been suggested.[42] An hereditary basis in Miniature Schnauzers and Great Danes is suggested. Megaesophagus in the dog is most frequently congenital. In occasional instances, megaesophagus in the dog has been associated with myasthenia gravis (esophageal dilatation was present in 8 of 10 dogs),[43] and chronic lead or thallium poisoning, trypanosomiasis (Chagas' Disease), or glycogen storage-like disease in the dog.

Dogs with generalized megaesophagus have regurgitation and variable cervical esophageal enlargement, coughing or wheezing associated with aspiration pneumonia and varying degrees of emaciation. While most affected dogs commence regurgitating at, or soon after weaning, up to 25% of dogs may not have clinical signs until they are more than 2 years old.[41] Affected dogs eat with no difficulty, and often reingest the regurgitated food multiple times until it is retained. There is no correlation between the time of eating and regurgitation.

Diagnosis. The diagnosis is confirmed by radiographs. In many dogs, food or air within the esophagus provides sufficient contrast to determine that esophageal enlargement extends from the diaphragm cranially. Where doubt exists in differentiation between megaesophagus and vascular ring stricture or acquired esophageal stricture, an esophageal contrast study should be performed, preferably using fluoroscopy so the rate and extent of peristalsis can be assessed, particularly for dogs showing segmental rather than generalized megaesophagus.[44] With generalized megaesophagus, the contrast medium moves slowly to the area of maximum dilatation and moves synchronously in this area with respiration, with no or only very occasional weak, peristaltic contractions. Hypersensitivity of the esophageal muscle to parenterally administered methacholine does not occur in dogs with generalized megaesophagus as it does in man with achalasia.[34]

Endoscopic examination is generally not a helpful diagnostic aid except for the rare occurrence of a tumor of the cardia of the stomach causing generalized esophageal dilatation. The dilated esophagus is usually filled with secretions and partially broken down food. The mucosa is irritated, appears more velvety than normal, and is friable. The lumen is grossly enlarged and difficult to follow owing to the sacculations and redundancy of the esophageal wall. It is easy to lose sight of the lumen and to end up in blind sacs; to proceed further is to risk perforation. The most successful way to reach the stomach is to clear secretions continually and to keep the endoscope pressed against the dorsal wall of the esophagus as it is advanced to the cardia.

Treatment. Present treatment consists of reducing the esophageal contents to the minimum, commencing as young as possible to allow esophageal maturation without gross dilatation. Frequent small meals are the most important factor. Feeding the dog from a height, so that the esophagus is elevated, assists in esophageal emptying.[45] The use of rough-surfaced food to stimulate secondary peristaltic activity may be beneficial.[46]

Surgical treatment, either cardiomyotomy or cardioplasty, is no longer considered beneficial in dogs with megaesophagus. The clinical impression exists that the prognosis is dependent on the age of the dog and the degree of dilatation. Older dogs with gross dilatation will frequently continue to regurgitate and often die of aspiration pneumonia in spite of dietary therapy.

The treatment of cats with megaesophagus has been less successful than in the dog; in one report of four cats, all died.[47] Another report described 15 cats with pyloric obstruction, 5 of which had severe generalized esophageal dilatation. Four of the 5 cats with esophageal dilatation died or were euthanatized, and one cat became normal except for occasional regurgitation following pyloromyotomy.[48]

Acquired Esophageal Dilatation

Diseases that produce esophageal obstruction, such as vascular ring stricture, acquired esophageal stricture, and esophageal neoplasia, will usually produce some degree of prestenotic dilatation. Such diseases are easily diagnosed by radiographic contrast studies or esophagoscopy, and the esophageal dilatation may revert to normal if the cause of the obstruction can be corrected.

Segmental megaesophagus resulting from denervation is occasionally seen following esophageal surgery, particularly where resection and anastomosis were performed and where the esophagus was separated from its attachments to mobilize sufficient length. The effects of denervation on esophageal function have been extensively studied. Unilateral vagectomy produces no clinically observable abnormalities, but does cause slight delays in esophageal emptying. Bilateral vagectomy produces grossly reduced or absent peristalsis and variable degrees of esophageal dilatation, which occasionally persist and cause regurgitation. However, most bilaterally vagectomized cats show restoration of esophageal motility by 9 months after surgery.[49] The effects of denervation may be more obvious clinically following extensive surgical dissection because scar tissue may limit normal esophageal distensibility.

Regurgitation may be seen 1 to 2 months after esophageal anastomosis. Contrast radiography and esophagoscopy are used to rule out secondary stricture. Treatment is directed at prevention of enlargement of the dilatated esophageal area. Small meals given several times per day should be continued for 6 months or longer if regurgitation persists.

Esophageal dilatation may be seen caudal to areas of mediastinitis in dogs with perforation due to foreign bodies; such dilatation is transient and presumably due to interference with vagal function by the mediastinal cellulitis. Esophageal dilatation is common in upper airway obstruction with aerophagia and may be commonly seen in thoracic radiographs of anesthetized animals.

Acquired Esophageal Obstruction

Obstruction of the esophagus by ingested material occurs in most domestic species. Because the clinical signs differ for each species, they are described separately.

Esophageal Foreign Bodies in the Dog

The dog bolts its food with little attempt at mastication. Esophageal foreign bodies are seen in the dog with some frequency. The most common foreign body is a steak or pork chop bone which becomes lodged between the heart and diaphragm.[50] Sharp objects such as pins, fishhooks, chicken bones, or pieces of wood can become lodged anywhere in the esophagus.[51]

Once lodged, the foreign body may cause complete esophageal obstruction, e.g., by a steak bone with meat attached; partial esophageal obstruction, e.g., a thinner foreign body, or one with projections that stretch the esophageal wall creating spaces through which fluid can pass; or no obstruction.

Clinical signs result from the obstruction and esophageal stretching, esophagitis, ulceration, and perforation and mediastinitis. In dogs with partial esophageal obstruction, a delay of several days and occasionally a week or more may occur before veterinary advice is sought. If the esophagus remains intact, clinical signs are restricted to regurgitation of food and fluid, or food only. If esophageal erosion or perforation occurs, anorexia, pyrexia, and lethargy are seen. Gagging or retching is seen only when the foreign body is lodged close to the pharynx, or has injured the pharynx in passing. Foreign bodies with lines attached, such as sewing needles or fishhooks, may be suspended in the esophagus if the thread or line is caught around the tongue. The animal will show rapid awkward tongue

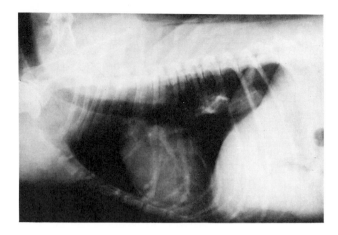

Figure 21–4. Lateral survey radiograph of a dog showing a piece of bone lodged in the esophagus just caudal to the heart base.

movements with the head held tucked in and the string may saw its way through the lingual frenulum, and be missed on casual inspection of the mouth. Elevating the base of the tongue by pressing a fingertip dorsally in the intermandibular space is helpful in demonstrating lesions of the lingual frenulum.

The presence of an esophageal foreign body is confirmed and its exact position determined by radiographs (Fig. 21–4). Occasionally, contrast radiography will be necessary to demonstrate a foreign body not otherwise visible because of an associated mediastinitis, or lack of radiographic contrast.

Treatment. To prevent further damage to the esophagus, foreign bodies should be removed without delay.

If appropriate equipment is available, esophagoscopy and forceps removal of the foreign body should be attempted. Advantages of esophagoscopy and forceps removal of the foreign body are the rapidity of the procedure, avoidance of thoracotomy and associated complications, and avoidance of esophageal incision and closure with associated complications. The esophagus is suctioned to remove food or fluid cranial to the obstructing foreign body, and the foreign body and surrounding esophagus and mucosa are examined. For bones and other bulky objects, the largest diameter esophagoscope available and a long-handled forceps matched to the length of the esophagoscope are used. The foreign body is grasped, carefully excluding the esophageal wall, and gently pulled cranially. If the foreign body does not move, the forceps is reapplied to the foreign body and gently twisted prior to pulling. If the foreign body becomes disengaged from the esophageal wall, the esophagoscope, forceps, and foreign body are removed as one unit. The most useful forceps for foreign bodies in the dog are alligator forceps and ring forceps, particularly for grasping bony projections of steak or chop bones. The esophagus is examined following removal of the foreign body. Clean mucosal lacerations or esophageal ulceration and abrasions can be left untreated. Severely damaged esophageal tissue or areas of obvious penetration into the mediastinum are indications for thoracotomy.

Sharp foreign bodies can also be removed by esophagoscope and forceps. The foreign body must be disengaged from the esophageal wall by pulling it directly opposite from its direction of penetration. Once disengaged, the foreign body is pulled into the esophagoscope (if small enough) or held parallel to the long axis of the esophagus as the esophagoscope, forceps, and foreign body are removed.

Used judiciously, forceps removal of esophageal foreign bodies is safe and effective.[51] An alternative conservative treatment method for bony foreign bodies is to push the foreign body into the stomach. Gastrotomy to remove the bone is not necessary.[50,51]

Should attempted forceps removal fail or equipment be unavailable, surgical removal of the foreign body is indicated. The surgical approach is determined from the radiographs. Foreign bodies located in the cervical and cranial mediastinal esophagus are approached through a midventral cervical incision, splitting the sternohyoid-thyroid muscles. Foreign bodies in the mid-thorax are approached through a right fifth or sixth intercostal incision, and foreign bodies in the caudal thorax are approached through seventh or eighth right or left intercostal incision or via laparotomy and gastrotomy. The foreign body is identified and the esophagus examined after packing off the immediate area. The esophagus is incised longitudinally close to or over the foreign body and the foreign body is removed. The esophagotomy incision is closed by placing sutures in the mucosa, with a separate layer in the muscularis layer. If the esophagus is ruptured or necrotic necessitating resection, sufficient length of the esophagus is gently dissected from the pleura, the esophagus is incised with a scalpel to provide clean edges for suturing, and the esophagus is sutured by end-to-end anastomosis in two layers. The pleura is not sutured. The packing sponges are removed and the esophagus is gently irrigated prior to closure of the thoracic incision.

Where esophageal perforation and mediastinitis exist, the area of disease must be drained. For cervical or cranial mediastinal foreign bodies where the pleura has not been penetrated during surgery, Penrose drains may be placed in the damaged tissue, exiting through the skin in the cervical area. Drainage of the esophagus in the mid or caudal thoracic area can only be achieved into the pleural cavity. The perforated esophagus is debrided and sutured closed; the mediastinum is debrided as necessary and no attempt is made to cover the damaged area with healthy pleura. A thoracentesis tube is placed to allow removal of fluid and air for 24 hours, or longer if fluid continues to accumulate.

The list of potential surgical and post-surgical complications is long and ominous, including intraoperative hemorrhage (aorta, azygos vein, bronchoesophageal and intercostal vessels), lung rupture and pneumothorax, chylothorax, mediastinal abscessation, breakdown of esophageal suture line, abscessation of the thoracotomy incision, vagal denervation causing esophageal motility abnormalities, and cardiac or respiratory failure associated with the pathophysiology of thoracotomy or aspiration of regurgitated esophageal contents.

Esophageal Foreign Bodies in the Cat

The cat is regarded as a more fastidious eater than the dog, and esophageal obstruction by food items is uncommon. Sharp objects such as sewing needles and fish and chicken bones are more commonly encountered. Removal by forceps should be attempted as in the dog. Such items, however, are often more difficult to remove with forceps than objects such as bone as they may have passed partially or completely through the esophageal wall. Surgical removal is indicated and the prognosis is favorable.

Esophageal Foreign Body in the Horse–"Choke"

The most common foreign bodies in the horse are compacted dry feed and medicinal boluses. Obstruction occurs most often in horses with pre-existing esophageal disease, in older horses with defective teeth in greedy eaters, and in Shetland ponies.

Clinical Signs. The horse initially shows distress, arches the neck and pulls its chin towards the sternum or extends the neck toward the ground. Drooling is often seen from the mouth or nose and may be tinged with food material or blood. Coughing, retching and regurgitation of food, or inability to swallow are also seen. The agitated or distressed condition often subsides in 18 to 36 hours following the onset of obstruction.

Diagnosis. Cervical obstructions are usually palpable. Attempts to pass a stomach tube will be unsuccessful. Contrast radiographs are being used more frequently to diagnose and locate esophageal obstructions in the horse.[52]

Treatment. Esophageal obstructions caused by compacted feed are the easiest to manage; spontaneous recovery often occurs within 2 days. Attempting to pass a stomach tube periodically helps saliva to penetrate and lubricate the mass. Smooth muscle relaxants or medications such as pilocarpine or arecoline, which increase salivation, have been suggested. Forcing water through a stomach tube placed at the obstruction may help to break up and flush out the compacted materials; the horse should be held with the head tied low to avoid aspiration. If conservative management is unsuccessful after 2 days, more aggressive measures are necessary. For thoracic obstructions, the horse is anesthetized and the cervical esophagus is exposed. A stomach tube is passed and water is pumped in while the esophagus is held firmly against the tube. The esophagus can be suctioned and the process repeated as often as necessary.

For cervical obstructions, the esophagus is exposed and the obstruction manipulated to break up the compacted material. If this is unsuccessful, esophagotomy is performed, the obstruction is cleared, and the esophageal incision is sutured. Where possible, esophagotomy is avoided, as stricture, fistula, and aspiration pneumonia may occur.

Following relief of the obstruction, the horse should be confined to a bare stall and fed soft, soaked feed for several days. Soaking the food thoroughly may be successful in preventing choke in horses which are prone to obstruction.

Esophageal obstruction in the horse can occur secondary to esophageal stenosis, esophageal dilatation, esophageal diverticulum, and esophageal spasm, each of which is noted as occurring in the horse, although poorly documented.[23]

Esophageal Obstruction in Cattle—"Choke"

With few exceptions, choke in cattle is caused by the rapid ingestion and/or incomplete mastication of food material such as apples, potatoes, cabbage, beets, turnips, corn ears, and compacted dry sugar beet pulp.

Clinical Signs. Bloat and sialorrhea are the principal clinical signs. Variable degrees of distress, frequent chewing movements, and extension, raising and lowering of the head with protrusion of the tongue may be seen. Coughing and, infrequently, retching can occur.

Diagnosis. Diagnosis is based on the clinical signs and availability of obstructing material. Most obstructions are cervical and can be palpated. Failure of normal passage of a stomach tube confirms the presence of esophageal obstruction. The tube must be passed slowly and carefully to avoid damaging the esophageal epithelium.

Treatment. If bloat is severe, a rumen trocar should be placed. Cervical obstructions are cleared by manipulating the foreign body cranially until it is at the esophageal opening, then reaching into the mouth through a speculum to grasp the foreign body as it is forced into the pharynx by one final external push.

If manipulation is unsuccessful, removal with a loop of steel wire can be attempted, or a large-diameter (Kingman) stomach tube can be used to push the offending object into the rumen. Esophagotomy is performed infrequently. If the foreign body is in the thoracic esophagus, rumenotomy and manual, wire loop, or forceps removal via the cardia can be attempted, or a rumen trocar is placed while awaiting maceration and passage of the object.[53] Transthoracic esophagotomy with successful recovery was reported for a distal esophageal compacted hay mass in a 5-year-old cow.[54]

INFECTIOUS AND INFLAMMATORY DISEASES OF THE ESOPHAGUS

The mucous membrane of the esophagus is exposed continually to pathogenic and opportunistic bacteria and fungi in all species. Specific antibacterial activity has not been described in the activity of the mucous glands of the esophagus, but the antibacterial activity of the vast amounts of swallowed saliva probably contributes a protective effect.

Bacterial Infections

There is no reported primary bacterial infection of the esophagus. Prior damage to the mucous membrane by corrosive substances or perforation allows bacterial invasion, but the emphasis in therapy is directed against the precipitating event or subsequent stricture.

Viral Infections

Many of the epitheliotropic viruses cause esophagitis, although the dominant clinical findings are skin and oral ulcerations. Salivation may be in part due to esophageal lesions.

Ulcerative esophagitis due to bovine papular stomatitis virus has been reported in one group of five sick calves: typical oral lesions were not seen.[55] Congestion of the esophagus is seen in cattle and sheep with rinderpest.[56]

Shallow esophageal ulcers have been recognized in cats with calicivirus respiratory disease although the signs have been dominated by respiratory disease.[57]

Fungal Infections

Candida is seen rarely as a cause of esophagitis in debilitated dogs which have been on long-term antibiotic treatment. Signs consisted of ptyalism, and inappetence and regurgitation with blood-tinged regurgitus. The esophagus appears partially or diffusely covered with gray or yellow pseudo-membrane which, when removed, exposes a slowly bleeding surface. Diagnosis is by cytology of the yeast organisms on wet-mounts of the pseudomembrane and by culture. Successful treatment has been reported in man with nystatin (Mycostatin) orally, as well as intravenous amphotericin B (Fungizone). It is important to stop antibiotic or steroid therapy. Candidial esophagitis is a growing cause of concern in immunosuppressed humans and it may prove to be a concern to veterinarians involved in cancer chemotherapy.

Corrosive Esophagitis

The incidence of corrosive esophagitis is much lower in domesticated animals than in man. The inadvertent ingestion of a caustic substance or administration of an improper drenching material or potentially caustic material in a pill or bolus can result in corrosive esophagitis. Administration of potentially caustic medications is particularly hazardous in weakened, or semi-anesthetized animals with depressed swallowing function. Over-zealous use of a concentrated solution of potassium permanganate or other oral antiseptics in the treatment of stomatitis can also cause caustic burns. Esophagitis and stomatitis have been maliciously induced by the forced ingestion of oven-cleaner and other strong alkalies.

The list of substances that can cause a chemical burn of the esophagus includes acids and alkalies, methylene blue, potassium permanganate, copper sulfate, phenol, iodine, and chlorine solutions.

Clinical Signs. Signs of esophagitis are similar in all species and include dysphagia and ptyalism. Regurgitation may occur if there is considerable esophageal edema and spasm.

Endoscopic Appearance. The esophageal mucosa may vary from inflamed and edematous to severely ulcerated and hemorrhagic depending upon the degree of the chemical burn. It is important that any endoscopic observations be performed extremely gently. Some endoscopists recommend that the esophagoscope be inserted only to the first lesion seen, while others suggest that it is important to recognize the extent of the damage. In veterinary medicine where prognosis and economics of treatment are vital, the latter view is usually held.

Radiography. Survey radiographs are useful in prognosis. If there is already evidence of mediastinitis from a full thickness burn, the prognosis must be extremely unfavorable. Barium studies and fluoroscopy are not usually indicated at this time unless there is suspicion of a stricture. If fluoroscopy is performed and corrosive esophagitis is present, there will be evidence of esophageal spasm, reverse peristalsis and tertiary waves. In the cat, the herringbone pattern of the caudal esophagus will be accentuated. Areas of mucosal ulceration may be seen in all species.

Treatment. The aim in treatment of esophagitis is to prevent stricture. In mild esophagitis, oral antibiotics and parenteral steroids (prednisolone, 2 mg/kg for 3 to 4 days) are given. Bouginage is indicated if stricture is present. Esophageal flushing is not helpful since the action of the chemical is usually immediate. Flushing with saline solution is useful if there is a disintegrating pill or bolus lodged in the esophagus.

The duration of therapy with steroids and the need for repeated bouginage depend on the response of the individual. Careful follow-up is important since it is common for the initial signs of dysphagia and ptyalism to lessen, only to reappear approximately 1 week later.

Prognosis. In massive chemical burns of the esophagus, mediastinitis and shock are common within hours, and there is every expectation of severe stricture development if the patient survives. Since the long-term prognosis is very unfavorable, euthanasia is indicated. In less massive burns and particularly in those associated with inadvertent swallowing of antiseptic solutions, prednisolone therapy should be started at the first onset of signs and continued for a week or two after signs abate.

Acquired Esophageal Stricture

Acquired esophageal stricture has been reported in many species, and is most common and best documented in the dog and cat. The causes of esophageal stricture are many; obvious causes include foreign body impaction, esophageal trauma associated with the passage of irritant materials or from esophageal manipulations (esophagoscopy or esophageal tube passage) or surgical procedures. Ingestion of caustics, common as a cause of stricture in children, is a rare cause in animals. Any cause of esophagitis can potentially cause esophageal ulceration and stricture formation; upper respiratory viral diseases in the cat, and viral stomatides in ungulates can cause sufficient damage to result in stricture. The most common strictures in the dog and cat are associated with an anesthetic or surgical episode 1 day to 6 weeks previously.[58,59,59a] It is postulated that the esophageal epithelial erosion is caused by reflux of gastric contents.[60] The incidence of acquired post-anesthetic ("reflux") esophageal stricture cannot be correlated with particular factors such as the use of atropine preoperatively, position of animal or manipulation of abdomen during anesthesia, use of endoesophageal stethoscope, or use of endotracheal tube. The majority of such idiopathic "reflux" strictures occur in the area of the thoracic inlet. It should be noted that reflux is common in the anesthetized or sedated, recumbent dog or cat.

Clinical Signs. Acquired esophageal stricture causes a gradual diminution of esophageal distensibility. Unless the stricture is high in the cervical area, the predominant clinical sign is regurgitation. An astute owner may notice that the animal suffers from a gradual reduction in the size of food particles that it can successfully swallow. Often finely blended food or fluids are all that will be tolerated. Aspiration pneumonia may be obvious, and progressive emaciation is seen.

Diagnosis. In the dog and cat, diagnosis is based on esophagoscopy and esophageal contrast radiography (Fig. 21–5). Mixing of contrast medium with food is necessary to visualize some strictures. In the horse or cow, the disorder may be initially difficult to distinguish from esophageal impaction as the usual initial presentation of a stricture is obstruction by impacted food: if obstruction recurs rapidly, a stricture or other esophageal lesion should be suspected. Contrast radiographs are the simplest way of confirming the diagnosis in the horse or cow.

Treatment. Two basic methods, dilatation or resection, are available for treatment. Dilatation is frequently used in man, and is gaining increased acceptance in the dog and cat. The stricture is examined through an endoscope after suctioning the accumulated debris cranial to the stricture. Fresh strictures appear as areas of ulcerated esophagus, often with a bright red, easily damaged surface; older, healed strictures have obvious loss of lumen, ranging from a single linear or circumferential scar to multiple scars, or continuous reduction of lumen extending over several centimeters. A well-lubricated esophageal bougie smaller than the visible lumen is introduced and gently manipulated across the stricture. Progressively larger diameter bougies are used until the stricture is stretched tight around the bougie. By a gentle twisting movement, the bougie is inserted a little further to dilate the lumen. The animal is given oral antibiotics and 1 mg/kg prednisolone for 3 to 4 weeks. Commencing with finely blended material, the food is gradually changed to a coarser consistency to establish what diameter bolus the animal can swallow. If necessary, the dilatation-bouginage procedure is repeated until, for a dog or cat, the animal can manage canned food. The owner should be alerted to the hazard of the dog or cat swallowing bones and chew toys.

The advantage of dilatation is the technical simplicity of the procedure and the ability to treat long strictures. The disadvantage of requiring multiple procedures has been much reduced since the advent of prolonged steroid treatment following dilatation. As an alternative to systemic prednisolone, triamcinolone (40 mg/ml) can be injected intralesionally through the esophagoscope using an esophageal varices needle. Treatment by bouginage with or without steroids has produced satisfactory results in approximately 75% of 30 strictures seen in our practice in the last several years. The use of lathyrogenic substances such as beta-aminoproprionitrile has been shown to be as effective without bouginage as steroids and bouginage in preventing esophageal stenosis following experimental esophageal corrosive injury in the dog;[61] however, its use in an established stricture has not been reported.

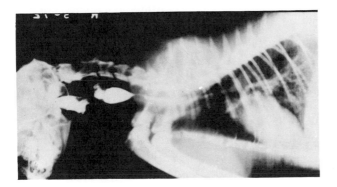

Figure 21–5. Lateral radiograph of a cat during barium contrast esophagram showing a stricture in the caudal cervical esophagus.

Esophageal Resection. Resection of a narrow stricture in the cervical esophagus is a technically simple procedure. The esophagus is exposed, avoiding the recurrent laryngeal nerve and vagosympathetic trunk, the stricture is identified either externally or by use of an esophageal sound, the esophagus is gently dissected, transected to eliminate the stricture, and closed with one of several recommended suture patterns. Restricturing, anastomotic leak with resultant cellulitis or fistula formation, or infection and breakdown of the incision approach are possible complications.

Surgical treatment of strictures longer than approximately 2 to 3 cm or those located in the thorax of the dog and cat presents more of a challenge, but is feasible.

Alternatives to resection include esophagoplasty (Heineke-Mikulicz), or use of an onlay graft to expand the lumen.

The use of esophagomyotomy,[52] dilatation via esophagotomy,[62] and muscle onlay grafting[63] have been reported for treatment of esophageal stricture in the horse. Satisfactory results were infrequent. Surgical treatment of a cervical esophageal stenosis and diverticulum in a 9-month-old calf was unsuccessful.[64] A distal esophageal stricture and prestenotic dilatation associated with a periesophageal abscess were diagnosed in a yearling Hereford heifer; treatment was not attempted.[65]

PARASITIC DISEASES OF THE ESOPHAGUS

Gongylonema Pulchrum

This nematode parasite is transmitted by an intermediate host, the dung beetle. It is found in the esophagus of cattle, sheep, goats, and occasionally swine. The parasite is of widespread distribution, but is not regarded as pathogenic or of economic importance.[66]

Spirocerca Lupi

This nematode parasite of dogs is endemic to Africa, Asia, and the warmer areas of the Americas and Southern Europe.[67] The incidence is higher in village and country animals than in city dogs, probably because of access to the dung beetle intermediate host and to transport hosts such as reptiles, mammals, and birds. The life cycle and oncogenic potential of this parasite are discussed under esophageal neoplasms.

Clinical Signs. In many infested dogs no signs are obvious and the disease is seen at necropsy. In other dogs the dominant signs may be related to sudden death due to rupture of an aortic aneurysm.

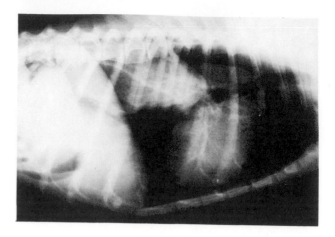

Figure 21–6. Lateral survey radiograph of a dog with *Spirocerca lupi* showing a mass lesion in the caudal esophagus and caudal thoracic vertebrae with bridging spondylosis.

Hypertrophic osteoarthropathy and lameness are common. Signs of esophageal involvement include anorexia, dysphagia, and bloodstained regurgitus.

The diagnosis may be made by fecal examination, radiographs, or endoscopy. Fecal flotation will demonstrate small elongated eggs, if a saturated solution of sodium nitrate, magnesium sulfate, or sodium dichromate is used.

Radiographic Findings. A mass lesion is seen in the caudal esophagus. Ventral spondylosis of the caudal thoracic vertebra may be present (Fig. 21–6).

Endoscopic Findings. Since most of the damage is in the esophageal wall, a relatively normal mucosa is seen with one or two (usually less than eight) 3 × 4 cm raised nodules with an umbilicated center. Occasionally the caudal end of a worm may be seen protruding through the crater-like opening. Esophageal washings from these areas will demonstrate eggs and worms.

Treatment. Disophenol (DNP) given at 7.7 mg/kg subcutaneously at 1-week intervals for two doses will kill adult parasites but has no effect on migrating immature worms in the aorta. Nodules in the esophagus can be removed surgically.[68]

A combination of surgical removal of esophageal lesions with repetitive DNP injections might prove worthwhile in the isolated dog that is to be removed from the continued source of infection. However, the possibility of malignant transformation of the lesions to sarcoma must be considered.

Trypanosoma Cruzi

This protozoan in natural and experimental infection of dogs has led to the development of megaesophagus and megacolon as well as the typical cardiac lesions of Chagas' disease.[69] Several species of triatomid insects serve as vectors and the disease is often associated with poor sanitation. The disease is prevalent in Central and South America and reservoirs have been found in many small mammals in the Southwestern United States. No effective treatment is known.

ESOPHAGEAL NEOPLASMS

Neoplasms of the esophagus are rare in all species of domestic animals.

Epithelial Neoplasms

Bovine: Single or multiple papillomas have been observed in the thoracic esophagus and esophageal groove of cattle, presumably caused by the virus causing cutaneous papillomatosis and transmissible genital fibropapillomatosis. The larger papillomas may become pedunculated by the actions of swallowing and result in stenosis with proximal dilatation.[70] In a remote valley of Kenya, papillomatous lesions along the length of the esophagus in three cattle were thought to represent an early phase in the development of multifocal esophageal and ruminal carcinoma.[71]

Canine: Multiple papillomas approximately 1 cm in size have been observed along the longitudinal mucosal folds of the esophagus in dogs with oral papillomatosis. These esophageal lesions are incidental findings and are not clinically important.[70]

Feline: Papillomas have occasionally been observed in British cats but appear to be very rare in North American cats.[70,72]

Squamous Cell Carcinoma

Equine: This uncommon neoplasm usually affects older horses and arises from the distal thoracic esophagus as well as the squamous component of the gastric esophageal mucosa of the stomach. It is usually an ulcerating crater-like lesion and may extend as far as 16 cm cranially along the distal esophageal wall. Although the tumor may result in stenosis of the esophagus, most horses die from inanition before there is a serious neoplastic penetration of the muscular wall.[70]

Canine: Four esophageal carcinomas have been reported in European dogs. One carcinoma that involved the proximal and distal esophagus of a 7-year-old Schnauzer also metastasized to the gastric wall, trachea, and middle cervical nodes. The second tumor occupied the entire thoracic esophagus in a 13-year-old male terrier and appeared to originate just cranial to the cardia: there was stenosis of the esophageal lumen and metastasis to the bronchial nodes and spleen. The third patient was an 11-year-old male spaniel and the fourth a 14-year-old male spaniel. In the latter, the lesions involved the proximal cervical esophagus and infiltrated the adjacent trachea and cervical muscles and tonsils. Smaller tumor nodules were found in the regional and bronchial nodes and lungs.[73]

Although not recorded in the literature, a few esophageal carcinomas have been observed in North American dogs. Such lesions should be considered in a middle-aged or older dog that exhibits intractable progressive regurgitation immediately following ingestion of solid food. Further diagnostic studies should include survey radiographs of the neck and chest. Irregular filling defects, various degrees of obstruction and segmental loss of normal esophageal motility seen on contrast fluoroscopy suggest an infiltrative lesion. Esophagoscopy and/or esophagotomy followed by biopsy would help differentiate an invasive carcinoma, which is rare, from fibrosis secondary to trauma or ingestion of a caustic.

Feline: Nineteen of 133 alimentary tract neoplasms in British cats were found to be esophageal carcinoma.[74] This unusually high frequency of esophageal neoplasia has not been reported elsewhere. A survey of 395 neoplasms in North American cats failed to reveal a single instance of this disease.[72] Further studies are needed to determine whether this neoplasm is still as common in Britain since environmental pollutants have been significantly reduced. The carcinoma characteristically produces an annular constricting lesion of the cranial thoracic portion, usually opposite to the first and second ribs. Most cats were middle-aged or older, and males were far more commonly affected. In three instances the tumors affected the cervical esophagus; two were cranial and the third involved most of the cervical esophagus.[74]

The major clinical sign was regurgitation, usually immediately after ingestion of solid foods. Because of the early onset of clinical signs, it was speculated that metastases had less time to develop. Metastasis to the mediastinal lymph nodes occurred in two cats, and in a third cat the esophageal tumor eroded into the adjacent tracheal wall.[74]

Mesenchymal Neoplasms

Almost all of these tumors are in dogs, and are malignant.

Leiomyoma

Canine: Although only three dogs with esophageal leiomyoma were reported in the literature prior to 1966, esophageal leiomyoma is not as rare as the literature might suggest. The three tumors reported involved the caudal thoracic esophagus of dogs from 10 to 13 years old. Two of the three were male and all were large-breed dogs (Boxer, Irish Setter, and Doberman Pinscher). At least two dogs had clinical signs of obstruction. Radiographically, the lesions were smooth-surfaced and ranged in size from 3.7 to 7.5 cm in their widest diameters.[73]

Leiomyomas are occasionally observed as incidental necropsy findings on one or both sides of the esophagogastric junction. Usually they appear as small, firm sessile submucosal nodules. In one instance the authors observed a 5-cm leiomyoma of the distal esophagus at necropsy. There had been no clinical signs referrable to the lesion. Radiographically, leiomyoma should be considered when one observes a smooth, rounded lesion at the distal esophagus of an older dog exhibiting gradual onset of obstructive signs. Definitive treatment involves transthoracic or abdominal esophagotomy and excision of the lesion: the prognosis is favorable.

Osteosarcoma and Fibrosarcoma

These two neoplasms are usually related to infection with *Spirocerca lupi*, the esophageal nematode, and constitute the best example in veterinary oncology of a malignant neoplasm that is closely related to a specific concomitant parasitic infection.[75,76] Clinicians in areas enzootic for *S. lupi* must always consider the possibility of esophageal granuloma or sarcoma in any dogs with signs of progressive esophageal disease, as in these areas sarcomas of the esophagus are by far the most common neoplastic entity of the esophagus.

Major *S. lupi* enzootic areas in North America are the Southeastern United States and, to a lesser extent, Oklahoma and Texas. In general this parasite occupies much of the subtropical and tropical regions of the world. Many dogs with *S. lupi* have been from Africa, India, and the Philippines. It is also seen in many temperate areas of Eurasia.[75,76] Because of the mobility of human populations, dogs with *S. lupi* related to esophageal sarcomas are occasionally observed in non-enzootic areas. In one reported instance, a Boxer which lived for 7 years in Kenya and later was moved to England developed clinical evidence of an esophageal sarcoma when it was 10 years old.

The life cycle of *S. lupi* is complex. Dung beetles act as intermediate hosts. Chickens act as paratenic transport hosts; i.e., they ingest infected beetles and the *S. lupi* larvae migrate to and encyst in the crop submucosa. If the dog eats infected dung beetles and/or the crop of infected chickens, the *S. lupi* larvae rapidly invade the gastric wall and migrate through the wall of the gastric arteries, usually reaching the abdominal aorta within a week. They then migrate cranially through the aortic adventitia and spend 2.5 to 4 months in the caudal thoracic aorta producing areas of necrosis, inflammation, and scarring that may result in aneurysms. The presence of *S. lupi* larvae in the ventral thoracic vertebral area is thought to be related to the thoracic spondylosis often seen in this disease. Finally the larvae migrate through the mediastinum and penetrate into the lumen of the caudal thoracic esophagus, and then re-enter the submucosa where they give rise to purulent granulomas. Eggs laid into the granuloma cavity escape into the lumen and then into the feces, from which dung beetles can ingest the eggs. Rural areas with large populations of cattle, chickens, and dung beetles are ideal for maximal canine infection.[74,78]

The clinical and radiographic features seen in dogs with these neoplasms are quite distinctive, and providing a high index of suspicion is maintained, the differential diagnosis is not difficult. In 58 affected dogs from the Southeastern United States, the median age was 6 years with a range of 2 to 11 years. The breed distribution primarily consisted of hounds (31 dogs), pointers (11 dogs), and setters (7 dogs). Whether this unusually high occurrence in hounds represents a specific genetic predisposition for these sarcomas and/or is related to unusual exposure factors to *S. lupi* is not clear.[75,76] In other parts of the world the German Shepherd dog breed is most commonly affected; however, without baseline population data, no breed predilection can be ascribed with certainty.

The clinical syndrome is usually characterized by rapidly progressive esophageal obstruction leading to inanition, weakness, and dehydration. Hypertrophic osteopathy is exceedingly common in dogs with esophageal sarcomas, being observed in 34 of 55 affected dogs in the Alabama area.[75,76] Indeed, in an area enzootic for *S. lupi* any dog with hypertrophic osteopathy should be suspected of having an esophageal sarcoma or rarely an esophageal granuloma.[77]

Radiographic examination is essential. Survey radiographs of the chest will usually reveal a mass in the distal thoracic esophagus and a characteristic deforming ventral spondylosis involving the fifth to tenth thoracic vertebrae (Fig. 21–6). The latter lesion, although very characteristic of *S. lupi* infection, is not always present. Many dogs will also have well-defined, often very radiopaque pulmonary metastases. When contrast radiography is performed, large irregular filling defects associated with obstruction are visible in the distal thoracic esophagus. A further diagnostic test includes fecal examination for *S. lupi* eggs. Artificial gastric juice is much better than sodium hydroxide as a fecal diluent as it facilitates visualization of the eggs by digesting fecal food particles.[78] A negative test, however, does not exclude the diagnosis of spirocercosis.

Hypertrophic osteopathy is readily diagnosed radiographically as it affects all four extremities. The characteristic diaphyseal osteophytes develop distally and may involve the pelvis.[77] This syndrome appears commonly in dogs with and without pulmonary metastases. Neoplastic invasion of the esophageal branches of the vagi may play a role in its development.[75,76]

Further diagnostic tests include esophagoscopy with biopsy, cytologic examination of esophageal washings, and exploratory thoracotomy and esophagotomy. Treatment is rarely satisfactory, as metastasis to lungs, regional nodes, and other distant sites is common. Furthermore, sarcomas are often large and locally invasive, making excision difficult and creating a large defect that must be surgically repaired.

The esophageal granuloma that forms as a reaction to the adult worms is histologically characterized by a loose, highly vascular granulation tissue containing many embryonal-appearing fibroblasts. The tissue is considered by many to be precancerous.[75,76] Transformation of the esophageal granulomas to osteo- or fibrosarcomas occurs in only a very small percentage of *S. lupi* infected dogs. The causes of the sarcomas are unclear but may include an oncogenic virus carried by the parasite, various metabolites of the worms, and genetic or immunologic host factors.

MISCELLANEOUS ESOPHAGEAL DISEASES

Esophageal Diverticulum

Esophageal diverticulum in the dog is very rare but has been described;[19,79,80,81] curiously, of the five dogs in the reports, two were Chihuahuas and two were Cairn Terriers. The disorder is mentioned as occurring in the horse.[23] A large diverticulum of the distal esophagus in a cow was detected by palpation via a rumenotomy: treatment was not attempted.[82] Whether these lesions are congenital, or result from esophageal muscle damage following esophageal foreign body lodgment or impaction has not been determined. In the dog, they may be unilateral or bilateral, occurring in the caudal thorax between the heart and diaphragm which is the most common site for large bone impactions to occur. Clinical signs in the dog are regurgitation and retching, which may be persistent.[19] Diagnosis is by contrast radiography or esophagoscopy. Treatment is surgical resection of the diverticulum. The prognosis is favorable in the dog.

Esophageal Perforation and Fistula

The most common cause of esophageal perforation is esophageal foreign body or choke, and the manipulations associated with treatment of same. Other causes include injection in the neck, esophageal surgery or surgery of adjacent structures such as tracheotomy, esophagoscopy or esophageal intubation, spike wounds from fences or railings, and bite wounds.

Perforation and leakage of esophageal contents cause cellulitis and abscess formation, which may be palpable in the neck as a hot, painful, crepitant area, and may cause edema of one or both sides of the ventral neck and head. If occurring in the chest, the lesion will not be palpable and signs such as pyrexia, anorexia, and listlessness may be the only indications of disease. Subcutaneous emphysema may be present, and in cattle, ventral cervical cellulitis may extend rostral to the mandible. In most animals, the tentative diagnosis is simple because of the history of the causative agent, or an external wound may be apparent. In the dog and cat, thoracic radiographs confirm the diagnosis; either a radiodense thickening of the mediastinum or pleural effusion will be noted. Where mediastinitis is obvious on survey radiographs following forceps or surgical removal of a foreign body, the existence of a perforation should be established prior to subjecting the animal to anesthesia and surgery. In such circumstances, contrast radiography carries with it the risk of leakage into the mediastinum. Contrast medium such as Gastrografin causes no significant histologic reaction whereas barium causes granuloma formation; the recommended sequence is to use Gastrografin first, followed by barium if the superior physical properties of barium are necessary.[83] If no perforation is obvious, the animal should be treated medically with antibiotics, and supported with intravenous fluids as necessary. Further radiographs should be taken at 12- or 24-hour intervals. If the mediastinal lesion increases in size, the chest should be explored and the mediastinum drained.

Treatment depends on the cause of perforation. In general, the perforated area should be explored, debrided, the esophagus sutured, and drains placed in the adjacent contaminated tissues. Drainage for mediastinitis or mediastinal abscess in the dog or cat associated with esophageal perforation was described previously. Surgical closure of esophageal perforation in the horse is usually unsuccessful, although it may close spontaneously over a period of several weeks.[52] Successful treatment with antibiotic is described for cervical esophageal lacerations in cattle caused by use of a probang to dislodge foreign bodies.[53]

Three dogs with esophagobronchial or esophagotracheal fistula have been reported,[84,85,86] and one cat was seen in our practice. All four lesions were believed to have been caused by foreign body penetration. Three animals died during or immediately following treatment.

DISEASES OF THE DISTAL ESOPHAGUS AND DISTAL ESOPHAGEAL SPHINCTER

Achalasia

Achalasia is defined as the failure of a gastrointestinal tract sphincter to relax, in this instance the distal esophageal sphincter. The condition is well documented in man where the resting lower esophageal sphincter pressure of an affected individual is twice that of normal, and the distal esophageal sphincter does not relax to the level of gastric pressure during swallowing.[86a] Treatment with dilatation of the cardia, or cardiomyotomy or cardioplasty, provides relief in the majority of patients.

As was discussed under Diseases Resulting in Abnormalities of Motility, the term achalasia has often been abused in veterinary medicine. In spite of much searching, true functional achalasia has yet to be documented in animals of veterinary interest.

Hiatal Hernia, Gastroesophageal Intussusception and Reflux Esophagitis

Abnormalities of anatomy or function of the esophageal diaphragmatic hiatus and/or distal esophageal sphincter have been reported on several occasions in the dog.

The abnormalities can be grouped into three categories: gastroesophageal intussusception, hiatal herniation of stomach into the thorax, and gastroesophageal reflux. Dogs with hiatal herniation of the stomach often have reflux visible at fluoroscopy, although not all dogs with reflux have hiatal herniation.

Gastroesophageal intussusception has been described frequently.[87-93] Of the 16 intussusceptions reported, 12 occurred in German Shepherd dogs; the other breeds reported were Afghan Hounds, Irish Setter, and Collie. With the exception of one dog of unknown age, all of the affected dogs were less than 6 months old, including a dog admitted for diagnosis at 2 days of age.

Clinical signs are regurgitation, vomiting, and distress. "Coffee-ground" vomitus is common because gastric acid and gastric mucosal hemorrhage pool in the distal esophagus prior to expulsion, allowing acid hematin to form. Differentiation of gastroesophageal intussusception from megaesophagus may be difficult. The absence of a gastric gas bubble should suggest the need for a contrast esophagram. One dog was unsuccessfully treated by gastropexy following reduction of the intussusception.[87]

Gastroesophageal reflux, with or without hiatal hernia, has been reported or seen by the present authors in Irish Setter, Chow, Poodle, Boxer, Labrador, and Welsh Terrier dogs.[19,94-97]

The age at presentation ranged from 2 months to 5 years. The clinical signs included frequent regurgitation or vomition of mucus which may be blood-tinged, drooling of saliva, and prolonged or "picky" eating. The diagnosis is based on contrast fluorography; several swallows should be observed followed by a period of time to observe the regurgitation or herniation. The extent of reflux or herniation is variable and may not correlate well with the clinical signs.

The extent of the disease is best assessed by esophagoscopy. The distal esophagus and cardia may have discrete linear or circular ulcerations, or more often a diffuse inflammation. The appearance of the distal esophagus may prevent accurate delineation of the gastric verge, partly because the cardia may be patulous.

Treatment is either medical or surgical. Frequent small meals with antacid preparations ameliorate the signs in some dogs; closure of the esophageal hiatus by fundoplication has also been attempted successfully.[95] Treatment with cimetidine (Tagamet) may also be beneficial in controlling the clinical signs in these dogs.

Papillomatous esophagitis has been described in a 1-year-old cat.[98] The lesion was most severe at the cardia. Treatment was not attempted.

Peptic esophagitis may be seen in the pig; it is

similar to that seen in the dog with gastroesophageal reflux.[70]

Esophageal hiatal hernia has been described in a 5-year-old Hereford bull showing signs of dysphagia and abnormal regurgitation. The diagnosis was made by rumenotomy: conservative management by restricting roughage was followed by satisfactory recovery.[99]

DISEASES OF OTHER SYSTEMS AFFECTING THE ESOPHAGUS

Hyperkeratosis and Parakeratosis

Hyperkeratosis of cattle is caused by ingestion of feed contaminated with penta- or hexachloronaphthalene. Esophageal lesions include hyperkeratosis and occasionally papillary projections up to 2 cm in diameter. However, the esophageal lesions are rarely of significance in the clinical syndrome.[100] Parakeratosis of swine, caused by zinc deficiency, may occasionally cause esophageal lesions, also of little clinical significance.

Central Nervous System Disease

Diseases of the brain and cranial nerves causing specific pharyngeal or esophageal derangement have been discussed previously. Esophageal dysfunction rarely occurs as part of the clinical picture associated with generalized central nervous system disease, although pharyngeal dysfunction does.

DISORDERS OBTUNDING ESOPHAGEAL FUNCTION

The esophagus runs a long course through which it is juxtaposed with many different structures. Because there are few fixed points (esophageal opening, thoracic inlet, esophageal hiatus) and because the esophagus is such a grossly distensible organ, obtundation of esophageal function rarely occurs. Structures that may cause interference at the pharyngeal or upper cervical level are discussed in this chapter under Dysphagia.

Thyroid carcinoma may distort the position of the esophagus, may invade the esophageal wall causing impaired peristalsis or stricture, or may interfere with normal vagal nerve function causing signs of esophageal dysfunction. In such circumstances, an externally palpable mass will be obvious, although thyrotoxicosis is rare.

Cranial mediastinal neoplasms such as lymphosarcoma or thymoma may deflect the esophagus sufficiently to cause a degree of obstruction and subsequent regurgitation in the dog. In the cat, lymphosarcoma may virtually fill the cranial mediastinum without causing clinically observable esophageal deficits. Caudal mediastinal lymph nodes which are enlarged due to lymphosarcoma or tuberculosis may cause sufficient interference with esophageal function to result in stenosis or a predisposition to esophageal food impaction and bloat in cattle.

REFERENCES

1. Getty, R.: Sisson and Grossman's Anatomy of the Domestic Animals, 5th ed. Philadelphia, W. B. Saunders Co., 1975, pp. 475 and 881.
2. Miller, M. (Ed.): Anatomy of the Dog. Philadelphia, W. B. Saunders Co., 1964, p. 662.
3. Dodds, W. J., Stewart, E. T., Hodges, D., and Zboralske, F. F.: Movement of the feline esophagus associated with respiration and peristalsis: an evaluation using tantalum markers. J. Clin. Invest. 51:1, 1973.
4. Bremner, C. G., Shorter, R. G., and Ellis, F. H., Jr.: Anatomy of feline esophagus with special reference to its muscular wall and phrenoesophageal membrane. J. Surg. Res. 10:327, 1970.
5. Rayl, J. E., Balison, J. R., Thomas, H. F., and Woodward, E. R.: Combined radiographic, manometric, and histologic localization of the canine lower esophageal sphincter. J. Surg. Res. 13:307, 1972.
6. Hollenbeck, J. I., Maher, J. W., Wickbom, G., Bushkin, F. L., McGuigan, J. E., and Woodward, E. R.: The effect of feeding on the canine lower esophageal sphincter. J. Surg. Res. 18:497, 1975.
7. Eastwood, G. L., Castell, D. O., and Higgs, R. H.: Experimental esophagitis in cats impairs lower esophageal sphincter pressure. Gastroenterology 69:146, 1975.
8. Rinaldo, J. A., Jr., Levey, J. F., Smathers, H. M., Gardner, L. W., and McGinnis, K. D.: An integrated anatomic, physiologic and cineradiologic study of the canine gastroesophageal sphincter. Dig. Dis. 16:556, 1971.
9. McCallum, R. W., Kline, M. M., Curry, N., and Sturdevant, R. A. L.: Comparative effects of metoclopramide and bethanechol on lower esophageal sphincter pressure in reflux patients. Gastroenterology 68:1114, 1975.
10. Castell, D. O., and Harris, L. D.: Hormonal control of gastroesophageal sphincter strength. N. Engl. J. Med. 282:886, 1970.
11. Castell, D. O.: Changes in lower esophageal sphincter pressure during insulin-induced hypoglycemia. Gastroenterology 61:10, 1971.
12. Watson, L. C., Reeder, D. D., and Thompson, J. C.: Hydrocortisone administration and gastrin and gastric secretion in dogs. Arch. Surg. 109:547, 1974.
13. Hogan, W. J., Dodds, W. J., Hoke, S. E., Reid, D. P., Kalkhoff, R. K., and Arndorfer, R. C.: Effect of glucagon on esophageal motor function. Gastroenterology 69:160, 1975.
14. Reference omitted.
15. Brooks, F.: The esophagus. In Gastroenterology. 2nd ed. Vol. 1. Edited by H. L. Bockus. Philadelphia, W. B. Saunders Co., 1964.
16. Hoffer, R. E., Valdes-Dapena, A., and Baue, A. E.: A comparative study of naturally occuring canine achalasia. Arch. Surg. 95:83, 1967.
17. Suzuki, M., Nomura, S.: Electromyographic studies on the deglutition movement in the dog. Jpn. J. Vet. Sci. 34:253, 1973.
17a. Watrous, B. J., and Suter, P. F.: Normal swallowing in the dog: a cineradiographic study. Vet. Rad. In press.
18. Sokolovsky, V.: Cricopharyngeal achalasia in a dog. J.A.V.M.A. 150:281, 1967.
19. Pearson, H.: The differential diagnosis of persistent vomiting in the young dog. J. Small Anim. Pract. 11:403, 1970.
20. Rosin, E., and Hanlon, G. F.: Canine cricopharyngeal achalasia. J.A.V.M.A. 160:1496, 1972.
21. Levitt, M. N., Dedo, H. H., and Ogura, J. H.: The cricopharyngeus muscle, an electromyographic study in the dog. Laryngoscope 75:122, 1965.
22. Cook, W. R.: Etiology of epistaxis and pharyngeal paralysis. Mod. Vet. Pract. 47:41, 1966.
23. Kingrey, B. W., and Lundvall, R. L.: Oral and esophageal conditions. In Equine Medicine and Surgery, 2nd ed. Edited by Catcott and Smithcors. Wheaton, IL, American Veterinary Publishing Co., 1972.
24. Bechara, F. A., and Blakeley, W. R.: Late assessment of results of cricopharyngeal myotomy for cervical dysphagia. Am. J. Surg. 128:818, 1974.

25. Roberts, S. J., Kennedy, P. C., and Delahanty, D. D.: Persistent right aortic arch in a Guernsey bull. Cornell Vet. *43*:537, 1953.
26. Buchanan, J. W., and Lawson, D. D.: Chapter 10, Cardiovascular surgery. *In* Canine Surgery, 2nd ed. Edited by J. Archibald. Santa Barbara, CA, American Veterinary Publications, 1974, p. 430.
27. Funkquist, B.: Oesophago-plasty as a supporting measure in the operation for oesophageal constriction following vascular malformation. J. Small Anim. Pract. *11*:421, 1970.
28. Clifford, D. H., Ross, J. N., Waddell, E. D., and Wilson, C. F.: Effect of persistent aortic arch on the ganglial cells of the canine esophagus. J.A.V.M.A. *158*:1401, 1971.
29. Woods, C. B., Rawlings, C., Barber, D., and Walker, M.: Esophageal deviation in four English Bulldogs. J.A.V.M.A. *172*:934, 1978.
30. Ashcraft, K. W., and Holder, T. M.: The story of esophageal atresia and tracheoesophageal fistula. Surgery *65*:332, 1969.
31. Clifford, D. H., and Malek, R.: Diseases of the canine esophagus due to prenatal influence. Am. J. Dig. Dis. *14*:578, 1969.
32. Bone, W. J.: What is your diagnosis? J.A.V.M.A. *155*:549, 1969.
33. Scott, E. A., Snoy, P., Prasse, K. W., Hoffman, P. E., and Thrall, D. E.: Intramural esophageal cyst in a horse. J.A.V.M.A. *171*:652, 1977.
34. Diamant, N., Szczepanski, M., and Mui, H.: Manometric characteristics of idiopathic megaesophagus in the dog: an unsuitable animal model for achalasia in man. Gastroenterology *65*:216, 1973.
35. Strombeck, D. R., and Troya, L.: Evaluation of lower motor neuron function in two dogs with megaesophagus. J.A.V.M.A. *169*:411, 1976.
36. Gray, G. W.: Acute experiments on neuroeffector function in canine esophageal achalasia. Am. J. Vet. Res. *35*:1075, 1974.
37. Diamant, N., Szczepanski, M., and Mui, H.: Idiopathic megaesophagus in the dog: reasons for spontaneous improvement and a possible method of medical therapy. Can. Vet. J. *15*:66, 1974.
38. Clifford, D. H.: Myenteric ganglial cells of the esophagus in cats with achalasia of the esophagus. Am. J. Vet. Res. *34*:1333, 1973.
39. Clifford, D. H., and Gyorkey, F.: Myenteric ganglial cells in dogs with and without achalasia of the esophagus. J.A.V.M.A. *150*:205, 1967.
40. Hofmyer, C. F. B.: The digestive system. *In* Textbook of Large Animal Surgery. Edited by F. W. Oehme and J. E. Prier. Baltimore, The Williams & Wilkins Co., 1974.
41. Harvey, C. E., O'Brien, J. A., Durie, V. R., Miller, D. J., and Veenema, R.: Megaesophagus in the dog: a clinical survey of 79 cases. J.A.V.M.A. *165*:443, 1974.
42. Osborne, C. A., Clifford, D. H., and Jessen, C.: Hereditary esophageal achalasia in dogs. J.A.V.M.A. *151*:572, 1967.
43. Palmer, A. C., and Barker, J.: Myasthenia in the dog. Vet. Rec. *95*:452, 1974.
44. Schwartz, A., Ravin, C. E., Greenspan, R. H., Schoemann, R. S., and Burt, J. K.: Congenital neuromuscular esophageal disease in a litter of Newfoundland puppies. J. Am. Vet. Radiol. Soc. *17*:101, 1976.
45. Sokolovsky, V.: Achalasia and paralysis of the canine esophagus. J.A.V.M.A. *160*:943, 1972.
46. Guffy, M. M.: Esophageal disorders. *In* Textbook of Veterinary Internal Medicine, Vol II. Edited by S. J. Ettinger. Philadelphia, W. B. Saunders Co., 1975, p. 1098.
47. Clifford, D. H., Soifer, F. K., Wilson, C. F., Waddell, E. D., and Guilloud, G. L.: Congenital achalasia of the esophagus in four cats of common ancestry. J.A.V.M.A. *158*:1554, 1971.
48. Pearson, H., Gaskell, C. J., Gibbs, C., and Waterman, A.: Pyloric and oesophageal dysfunction in the cat. J. Small Anim. Pract. *15*:487, 1974.
49. Burgess, J. N., Schlegel, J. F., and Ellis, F. H., Jr.: The effect of denervation on feline esophageal function and morphology. J. Surg. Res. *12*:24, 1972.
50. Pearson, H.: Symposium on conditions of the canine oesophagus—I. Foreign bodies in the oesophagus. J. Small Anim. Pract. *7*:107, 1966.
51. Ryan, W. W., and Greene, R. W.: The conservative management of esophageal foreign bodies and their complications: a review of 66 cases in dogs and cats. J.A.A.H.A. *11*:243, 1975.
52. Kerr, B. J., and Evans, L.: Clinico-Pathological Conference. University of Pennsylvania, New Bolton Center, 1972.
53. Fox, F. H.: The esophagus, stomach, intestines, and peritoneum. *In* Bovine Medicine and Surgery. Edited by W. J. Gibbons, E. J. Catcott, and J. F. Smithcors. Wheaton, IL, American Veterinary Publications, 1970.
54. Morgan, J. P.: What is your diagnosis? J.A.V.M.A. *147*:412, 1965.
55. Crandell, R. A., and Gosser, H. S.: Ulcerative esophagitis associated with poxvirus infection in a calf. J.A.V.M.A. *165*:282, 1974.
56. Newsom's Sheep Diseases. Edited by H. Marsh. Baltimore, The Williams & Wilkins Co., 1958, p. 123.
57. Wardley, R. C.: Personal communications.
58. Grier, R. L.: Esophageal disease as a result of improper patient positioning. Arch. J. Am. Coll. Vet. Surg. *4*:4, 1975.
59. Harvey, H. J.: Iatrogenic esophageal stricture in the dog. J.A.V.M.A. *166*:1100, 1975.
59a. Pearson, H., Darke, P. G. C., Gibbs, C., Kelly, D. F., and Orr, C. M.: Reflux esophagitis and stricture formation after anesthesia: a review of seven cases in dogs and cats. J. Small Anim. Pract. *19*:507, 1978.
60. Wilson, G. P.: Ulcerative esophagitis and esophageal stricture. J.A.A.H.A. *13*:180, 1977.
61. Davis, W. M. Madden, J. W., and Peacock, E. E., Jr.: A new approach to the control of esophageal stenosis. Ann. Surg. *176*:469, 1972.
62. Fretz, P. B.: Repair of esophageal stricture in a horse. Mod. Vet. Pract. *53*:31, 1972.
63. Hoffer, R. E., Barber, S. M., Kallfelz, F. A., and Petro, S. P.: Esophageal patch grafting as a treatment for esophageal stricture in a horse. J.A.V.M.A. *171*:350, 1977.
64. Thrall, D. E., and Brown, M. D.: What is your diagnosis? J.A.V.M.A. *159*:1040, 1971.
65. Alexander, J. E.: What is your diagnosis? J.A.V.M.A. *145*:699, 1964.
66. Dunn, A. M.: Veterinary Helminthology. Philadelphia, Lea & Febiger, 1969, p. 145.
67. Dunn, A. M.: Veterinary Helminthology, Philadelphia, Lea & Febiger, 1969, p. 221.
68. Colgrove, D. J.: Transthoracic esophageal surgery for obstructive lesions caused by Spirocerca lupi in dogs. J.A.V.M.A. *158*:2073, 1971.
69. Marsden, P. D., and Hagstrom, J. W. C.: Experimental Trypanosoma Cruzi Infection in Beagle Puppies. The Effect of Variations in the Dose and Source of Infecting Trypanosomes and the Route in Inoculation on the Course of the Infection. Trans. R. Soc. Trop. Med. Hyg. *62*:816, 1968.
70. Jubb, K. V. F., and Kennedy, P. C.: The Pathology of Domestic Animals, Vol. 2. New York and London, Academic Press, 1971, p. 43.
71. Plowright, W.: Malignant neoplasia of the oesophagus and rumen of cattle in Kenya. J. Comp. Pathol. Ther. *65*:108, 1955.
72. Engle, C. G., and Brodey, R. S.: A retrospective study of 395 feline neoplasms. J.A.A.H.A. *5*:21, 1969.
73. Lawson, D. D., and Pirie, H. M.: Conditions of the canine oesophagus. II. Vascular rings, achalasia, tumours and perioesophageal lesions. J. Small Anim. Pract. *7*:117, 1966.
74. Cotchin, E.: Neoplasia in the cat. Vet. Rec. *69*:425, 1957.
75. Bailey, W. S.: Parasites and cancer: sarcoma in dogs associated with *Spirocerca lupi*. Ann. N.Y. Acad. Sci. *108*(art. 3):890, 1963.
76. Bailey, W. S. *Spirocerca lupi*: a continuing inquiry. J. Parasitol. *58*:3, 1972.
77. Brodey, R. S.: Hypertrophic osteoarthropathy in the dog: a clinicopathologic survey of 60 cases. J.A.V.M.A. *159*:1242, 1971.
78. Cabera, D. J., and Bailey, W. S.: A modified Stoll Technique for detecting eggs of *Spirocerca lupi*. J.A.V.M.A. *145*:573, 1964.
79. Knecht, C. F., Small, E., Slusher, R., and Reynolds, H. A.: Epiphrenic diverticula of the esophagus in a dog. J.A.V.M.A. *152*:268, 1968.
80. Reed, J. H., and Cobb, L. M.: Diagnosis, radiographic study and surgical relief of a case of esophageal diverticulum. Can. Vet. J. *1*:323, 1960.
81. Noel, R. J.: What is your diagnosis? J.A.V.M.A. *157*:352, 1970.
82. McGavin, M. D., and Anderson, N. J.: Projectile expectoration associated with an esophageal diverticulum in a cow. J.A.V.M.A. *166*:247, 1975.
83. James, A. E., Jr., Montali, R. J., Chaffee, V. Strecker, E-P, and Vessal, K.: Barium or gastrografin: which contrast media for diagnosis of esophageal tears? Gastroenterology *68*:1103, 1975.
84. Thrall, D. E.: Esophagobronchial fistula in a dog. J. Am. Vet. Radiol. Soc. *14*:22, 1973.
85. Dodman, N. H., and Baker, G. J.: Tracheo-esophageal fistula as a complication of an esophageal foreign body in the dog—a case report. J. Small Anim. Pract. *19*:291, 1978.
86. Cohen, S., and Lipshutz, W.: Lower esophageal sphincter dysfunction in achalasia. Gastroenterology *61*:814, 1971.
86a. Schebitz, H.: Röntgenbefund einer oesophago-tracheal fistil nach freundkörperperforation beim hund. Tierarztl. Wnsch. *15*:87, 1960.
87. Tufvesson, G., and Viriden, P.: Surgical treatment of a case of invaginatio gastro-oesophagea in the dog. Nord. Vet. Med. *5*:435, 1953.

88. Carlson, W. D., and Lumb, W. V.: Esophageal invagination of the stomach in a dog. Mod. Vet. Pract. *39*:65, 1958.
89. McFadden, W. R.: What is Your Diagnosis? J.A.V.M.A. *160*:462, 1972.
90. Pollock, S., and Rhodes, W. H.: Gastroesophageal intussusception in an Afghan Hound: a case report. J. Am. Vet. Radiol. Soc. *11*:5, 1970.
91. Rice, D. F.: Esophageal intussusception in a dog. J.A.V.M.A. *151*:1055, 1967.
92. Schwab, L. M.: What is Your Diagnosis? J.A.V.M.A. *160*:1654, 1972.
93. Singer, A.: What is Your Diagnosis? J.A.V.M.A. *167*:951, 1975.
94. Kluth, G. A., and Kenna, T. L.: Hiatus hernia in a dog. Vet. Rec. *76*:501, 1964.
95. Gaskell, C. J., Gibbs, C., and Pearson, H.: Sliding hiatus hernia with reflux oesophagitis in two dogs. J. Small Anim. Pract. *15*:503, 1974.
96. Alexander, J. W., Hoffer, R. E., MacDonald, J. M., Bolton, G. R., and O'Neil, J. W.: Hiatal hernia in the dog: a case report and review of the literature. J.A.A.H.A. *11*:793, 1975.
97. Rogers, W. A., and Donovan, E. F.: Peptic esophagitis in a dog. J.A.V.M.A. *163*:462, 1973.
98. Wilkinson, G. T.: Chronic papillomatous oesophagitis in a young cat. Vet. Rec. *87*:355, 1970.
99. Kirkbride, C. A., and Noordsy, J. L.: An esophageal hiatus hernia in a bull. J.A.V.M.A. *152*:996, 1968.
100. McEntee, K., and Olafson, P.: Hyperkeratosis. *In* Bovine Medicine and Surgery. Edited by W. J. Gibbons, E. J. Catcott, and J. F. Smithcors. Wheaton, IL, American Veterinary Publications, 1970.

Chapter 22

THE STOMACH AND FORESTOMACHS

Part I. Equine Stomach Diseases

ROBERT H. WHITLOCK

_____

GASTRITIS

Gastritis is uncommon in the horse and is a very difficult diagnosis to make antemortem. At necropsy a reddish color of the stomach is not adequate for a diagnosis of gastritis, but true gastritis is characterized by excessive mucus production, severe hyperemia, and petechiation.[1] Trichostrongyles may cause such a lesion.

Chronic gastritis is characterized by patchy reddening, an increased cobblestone appearance and/or nodular formations. *Draschia megastoma* may cause large nodules (3 to 4 cm) with pores on the mucosal surface. Habronema infestation may on occasion cause chronic gastritis.

GASTRIC ULCERS

Gastric ulcers in horses are rarely reported. In eight cases of fatal perforating gastric ulcers in foals, two types of ulcers were seen.[2] One involved only the esophageal region and the other involved only the pyloric portion. The latter type seemed to be related to stress and prolonged antibiotic therapy. Fungal elements were not found in any of the cases. Five of the eight cases had multiple erosions and ulcerations of the esophageal region, most of which were adjacent to the margo plicatus.

Erosions, ulcers, and irregular cornification of the esophageal portion of the stomach are common postmortem findings, particularly adjacent to the margo plicatus.[2] The lesions vary from small focal erosions to confluent areas of ulceration. They may be related to bot infestation (*Gastrophilus intestinalis*) but their precise pathogenesis is unclear.

Perforated gastric ulcers are rarely reported in the adult horse. One horse with a chronic debilitating disease had a perforating ulcer in the nonglandular part leading to abdominal abscesses. The cause of the ulcer was unclear.[3]

GASTRIC NEOPLASIA

The primary neoplasm involving the equine stomach is squamous cell carcinoma. Lymphosarcoma and other neoplasms such as leiomyoma only rarely affect the stomach.[1,5] Only 3% of carcinomas in horses are of gastric origin,[6] while gastric carcinoma in man comprises a greater proportion of the total.

History

The chief complaints most often registered by the owner are gradual weight loss, anorexia, and lethargy.[7] Abdominal pain and difficulty in eating or swallowing are not features of gastric carcinoma. Most horses range in age from 6 to 10 years but the neoplasm is not restricted to this age group. Often, affected horses have been treated with a variety of medicaments with no response. The weight loss continues over a period of 2 to 6 months and most horses are killed for humane reasons.

Physical Examination

Emaciation and lethargy are the clinical hallmarks but are nonspecific signs. Rectal examination may determine the presence of nodules or masses in the cranial abdomen. Pallor of the membranes suggesting anemia occurs in some horses.[7] The vital signs are usually normal in the early stages but as the lesions develop, one or more become elevated. The pulse increases in response to the anemia, the respiratory rate increases in response to metastatic masses in the thorax, and a fever to 40°C is a result of necrosis in the neoplasm. Ascites and ventral edema may be the primary sign in a few horses and despite weight loss, the abdomen appears distended.[8] The presence of ascitic fluid can be confirmed by abdominocentesis or by rectal examination.

Fiberendoscopy and gastroscopy offer the possibility of direct visualization of the stomach and are of value in determining the presence of foreign bodies and neoplastic masses. Today a variety of sizes and types of fiberendoscopes are available as noninvasive techniques for gastric evaluation.

Laboratory Evaluation

Variable anemia (PCV range 12 to 28%) often accompanies squamous cell carcinomas.[7] The anemia can result from blood loss in the stomach and/or depressed erythrogenesis. Those horses losing blood from the stomach will have a positive fecal occult blood. Since occult blood rarely occurs in the horse, its presence should signal a possible gastric tumor.

Histologic evaluation of a biopsy specimen provides the definitive answer. The biopsy specimen can be obtained during an exploratory laparotomy or a percutaneous biopsy through the left seventh intercostal space. Additionally, evaluation of the peritoneal or thoracic fluid may demonstrate neoplastic cells. Rarely are samples of gastric washings diagnostic.

Diagnosis

Although gastric squamous cell carcinoma is not common in horses, it should be considered in any middle-aged horse with evidence of weight loss and anemia. A thorough physical examination, rectal examination for masses and peritoneocentesis to determine the presence of neoplastic cells should be done to assist in the diagnosis. A definitive diagnosis is virtually impossible short of histopathologic examination.

Treatment

No effective therapeutic agents are available to treat this neoplasm.

Prognosis

The prognosis for all cases of squamous cell carcinoma is grave. Most horses continue to lose weight and are destroyed for humane considerations within a few weeks of onset of clinical signs.[7]

GASTRIC PARASITISM

Gastric habronemiasis is relatively common in horses, but rarely causes clinical signs.[9] Three species of spirurids (*Habronema muscae*, *Habronema majus*, and *Draschia megastoma*) can infect the equine stomach. *Habronema* become embedded in the mucus normally covering the glandular areas. *Draschia megastoma* is the most pathogenic of the three and can produce mural abscesses and granulomatous lesions perforated by sinus tracts.[10] Rarely, ulceration is followed by perforation.

The major clinical significance of these parasites is not in the damage they can do to the stomach, but the damage they produce by infecting skin wounds causing exuberant granulation tissue.

The stomach "bots" of horses include the larva of: *Gastrophilus nasalis*, *G. intestinalis*, *G. hemorrhoidalis*, *G. pecorum*, and *G. inermis*. These parasites exist wherever horses are kept and may cause a mild gastritis, but rarely cause perforated ulcers.[10]

The adults live for only a short time (few days to two weeks) and lay eggs on the horse's coat. The *G. intestinalis* eggs are laid on the hair of the front legs, hatch after being licked and penetrate the buccal mucosa to migrate toward the stomach. In the stomach the *G. intestinalis* larva are found in clusters in the nonglandular cardia, while the *G. nasalis* larva are located in the glandular area. The extent of the larval-associated lesions are minimal and the larvae do not suck blood.

Neither gastric habronemiasis nor *Gastrophilus* infestation produce any characteristic signs. The presence of "bot" eggs on the horse's coat is good evidence of gastric infestation. Gastric habronemiasis is difficult to diagnose definitively. Direct visualization of either parasite by a gastroscope is possible using modern flexible fiberendoscopes.

Carbon disulfide continues to be one of the most effective vermifuges for gastric habronemiasis and *Gastrophilus sp*. The treatment efficacy is enhanced by pretreatment with 4 to 6 liters of 2% sodium bicarbonate to remove the excess mucus, followed by carbon disulfide (2.5 ml/45 kg body weight). Thiabendazole (50 mg/kg body weight) is also effective as are other anthelmintics.

GASTRIC DILATATION

Equine gastric distention occurs more frequently than reported in the literature.[11] A high proportion of horses with serious colic have gastric dilatation secondary to ileus. However, primary gastric dilatation (GD) occurs less commonly but sporadically when horses have accidental access to grains or concentrate feed. Less serious gastric dilatation may result from excessive consumption of water following a period of deprivation or following excessive swallowing of air (cribbing).

History

Primary GD most often occurs when the horse overeats on concentrate or grain. In previous eras this seemed to occur at harvest time, when a horse would overeat on wheat or another grain being harvested. The owner may note greenish ingesta at the nostrils and seek veterinary assistance, but the majority of cases have abdominal pain as the chief complaint.

Physical Examination

Ingesta at the nostrils is most striking when it occurs, and it should warrant consideration of GD if swallowing is normal. The "dog-sitting" posture is classically associated with GD but, in my experience, rarely occurs. The severity of the pain is highly variable depending on the nature of the primary lesion. Retching is an uncommon sign in the horse and seems to occur in the more chronic cases of GD.[12]

Laminitis may occur concurrently, especially in cases where GD is associated with overeating of concentrate. Borborygmus is usually decreased and a prominent metallic "ping" is often present over the cecal base. Rectal examination, when coupled with the use of sedatives and motility-modifying drugs, e.g., Pro-Banthine, may render the stomach palpable. Palpation of the spleen per rectum does not indicate gastric distention. The spleen can be palpated in most horses and on occasion it may rest just forward of the pelvic inlet without the stomach being distended.

If the stomach ruptures, vomiting ceases and the animal assumes a quiet reluctant-to-move stance. The pulse is weak and severely elevated (> 100/ min). The temperature is often subnormal. The mucous membranes become cyanotic and the capillary refill time is prolonged (> 3 seconds).

Laboratory Evaluation

Acidosis commonly accompanies most equine abdominal crises and that seems true of GD. However, in some cases of GD, metabolic alkalosis may occur, presumably as a sequela to chloride loss. Most animals will have variable hemoconcentration and mild hypokalemia, hyponatremia, and hypochloremia. The pH of the gastric contents most often approximates 7.0, and measurement of the pH does not give much information about the site of the obstruction.

Pathophysiology

Primary GD follows excessive consumption of feed grains or concentrate, whereas secondary GD occurs as a result of intestinal obstruction. GD is more prone to occur with small intestinal obstruction but can occur with ileus or physical obstruction

in any region of the intestinal tract. The reflux of intestinal secretions into the stomach occurs more quickly and is more severe following the higher (duodenal) obstructions.

Primary GD occurring with excessive grain consumption is further complicated by the increased osmotic pressure in the stomach. This "draws" in more fluid, which further contributes to the distention and leads to hypovolemic shock. Severe laminitis can be a sequel to toxin absorption. Some affected horses are ultimately euthanatized because of complications of pedal bone rotation.

Diagnosis

If fluid flows spontaneously after a nasogastric tube is placed in the stomach, a diagnosis of GD is apparent. However, the difficulty arises in differentiating primary from secondary GD. Complete removal and subsequent evaluation of the contents may indicate whether the condition was due to overeating. Occasionally, surgical intervention (gastrotomy) is necessary for both a definitive diagnosis and treatment. Recently, radiographic contrast medium was used to confirm a diagnosis of gastric stenosis.[12]

Treatment

Initial treatment, whether for primary or for secondary GD, is gastric decompression. It is recommended to pass the largest nasogastric tube possible. If difficulty is encountered passing the tube through the cardia, several milliliters of local anesthetic may facilitate passage. Once in place, fluid may flow spontaneously or a siphon may be started to initiate flow. Sedation with xylazine (Rompun) facilitates the procedure and minimizes the attendant risk of inhalation pneumonia, as the horse's head invariably hangs very low following sedation. If the tube was difficult to pass or if one expects continued reflux, the tube should be fixed in place to allow continual decompression. If fluid does not readily flow, a small amount of water may be pumped in and an attempt made to siphon the contents. This procedure should be repeated several times in cases of primary GD to soften and liquefy the mass of feed present. Occasionally it is necessary to perform a gastrotomy to remove the contents, which has been done successfully.[11] Secondary GD responds when the primary lesion is corrected.

Prognosis

Most horses with secondary GD have a fair to good prognosis. Gastric drainage can continue for

10 days due to ileus and then stop as normal intestinal function returns. Primary GD has a variable prognosis dependent on the amount and type of concentrate consumed. Those horses overeating on wheat often die acutely of gastric rupture. One horse with gastric stenosis died of surgical complications.[12]

DIAPHRAGMATIC AND HIATAL HERNIA

Ruptured diaphragm or hiatal hernia occurs rarely. An incidence of 304 diaphragmatic ruptures occurred in a series of 71,532 colic cases in Prussian army horses during the period 1892 to 1908.[13] Congenital diaphragmatic defects are apparently very rare.[14] Successful surgical repair has been reported in only two cases.[14,15]

History

Colic signs or a recent traumatic episode are the major facts reported by the owners of horses with diaphragmatic hernia (DH). Respiratory distress with exercise intolerance is less often the chief complaint.

Clinical Signs

The clinical signs of DH are extremely variable. Some horses show no clinical signs[16] while some horses die suddenly.[13] Respiratory embarrassment is reported less commonly than colic, which occurs in approximately 90% of the cases. The degree of pain is also highly variable, depending on the portion of bowel incarcerated and the severity of the incarceration.

Pathophysiology

Diaphragmatic defects can be congenital or acquired. The congenital type usually results from incomplete fusion of the pleuroperitoneal folds, with the resultant defect in the dorsal tendinous portion of the diaphragm, and represents an enlarged esophageal hiatus.[17] The acquired defect is produced by compression of the thorax or abdomen. External trauma is the primary cause but advanced pregnancy may be a predisposing cause.[18] Once the defect is present, abdominal viscera pass through and give rise to signs of respiratory embarrassment or to abdominal pain (colic). With large defects enough viscera enters the thorax to cause respiratory distress, while smaller defects usually result in intestinal incarceration and colic.

Diagnosis

As most horses with DH are admitted with colic, a carefully done physical examination is necessary even to be aware of the possibility of DH. Borborygmal sounds can be heard over the lung fields of any horse.[19] However, the absence of respiratory sounds in the ventral thorax should make one consider DH. Percussion of the chest with ventral dullness should evoke a consideration of DH. Further evidence can be obtained during the rectal examination as the abdomen may seem empty. This impression of emptiness in a horse with colic should make one consider DH.

Radiographic examination of the thorax will give a definitive diagnosis if intestinal loops can be visualized.

The frequency of thoracic wall injuries, in published accounts of this disorder, suggests that DH should be considered in any horse with colic and recent or healed thoracic wounds.

Treatment and Prognosis

Surgical intervention is the only rational approach to correction of the problem. However, the mechanical problems are enormous and only two cases have been successfully corrected.[14,15]

The anesthesia of horses with DH presents a challenge and necessitates mechanical intermittent positive pressure ventilation.[14]

The prognosis for life is poor to grave in cases of DH. Occasionally a horse will respond to symptomatic therapy only to have a recurrence and die later.

Part II. Bovine Stomach Diseases

ROBERT H. WHITLOCK

INDIGESTION

A diagnosis of simple indigestion is made when a cow is anorectic and has decreased milk production. It is a symptomatic diagnosis, treated as such, but also is indistinguishable from earlier phases of other more serious, progressive digestive disorders that bear a less favorable prognosis and greater risk of death loss. The more serious digestive disturbances may be ruled out with increasing confidence if the laboratory findings are in the normal range and/or if prompt, favorable response to treatment is obtained. However, worsening of the patient's condition or a static course in the face of symptomatic treatment dictates re-evaluation of both diagnosis and treatment.

History

Acute indigestion is usually precipitated by a change in the feeding program or a drastic change in environmental conditions so that cattle voluntarily and substantially alter their feed intake. The change in feed might range from a spoiled moldy feed to frozen feed or a feed contaminated with a pollutant, i.e., a herbicide. Certain cattle seem much more susceptible to bouts of indigestion than do others. Cattle in advanced gestation and so-called "greedy eaters" are more prone to indigestion as they are less discriminating in their feed preference and the expanding uterine size in later pregnancy decreases the available space for the rumen, which may slow its motility. Acute indigestion may occur as a single cow problem or in herd outbreaks depending on the cause and predisposing factors.

Physical Examination

The characteristic signs are partial anorexia, normal vital signs, a moderate hypolactia (if lactating), and most often a decreased rate and strength of ruminal contractions. Ballottement of the rumen reveals a "doughyness" in the dorsal aspects and gives the impression of more fluid ventrally. The general attitude of the patient is one of slight to moderate dullness and listlessness.

Laboratory Evaluation

The documented laboratory studies on bovine indigestion are sparse. One would typically expect to find a mild hemoconcentration as detected by a moderate elevation in the PCV and total plasma protein.

Etiologic Factors

Indigestion in ruminants can be subdivided into several different categories.

1. Consumption of indigestible feed material such as soil or sand by cattle with perverted appetites (pica) or the ingestion of the placenta by the cow after parturition.

2. The "eager eater" type of cow which, when fed with a group of animals, consumes more fermentable roughage and concentrate than she is accustomed to, predisposing to a mild rumenitis.

3. Damaged feed, i.e., spoiled from freezing and molding, or poor quality roughage, which may predispose to indigestion. Other factors include fatigue or stress of animals held off feed or not having feed available to them for 12 to 18 hours or longer and then being offered concentrate and roughage when they have a ravenous appetite.[10] A sudden change in feed formula or ingredients or a change in the character of the roughage could predispose to indigestion. Management factors such as lack of an appropriate water supply or lack of water due to drought, or environmental factors, e.g., the water might be frozen, could also predispose to irregular feed and water intake, which might lead to indigestion. Cattle in advanced pregnancy seem to be more predisposed to indigestion, presumably because the enlarging fetus in the uterus compresses the forestomachs against the diaphragm. These in turn may predispose to relative atony of the forestomachs.

Pathophysiology

The common factor seems to be that the ruminant microflora is poorly adaptable to sudden changes in the nature of the diet. Dairy cows consuming in excess of 3% of the body weight per day on a dry matter basis and producing large quantities of milk, or feedlot beef cattle that are being fed high quantities of concentrate are most predisposed to indigestion.

Diagnosis

One of the most important aspects of making diagnoses of indigestion is the history obtained from the observant owner or farm manager. There will often be an indication of a change in feed, a period of stress such as a severe change in the weather, transportation, vaccination, or advanced pregnancy. The lack of specific evidence of abdominal pain is a major factor in ruling out traumatic reticulitis or localized peritonitis. Other diagnostic rule-outs would include primary ketosis and abomasal displacement, which are quite common but usually limited to the early postpartum period. Abomasal displacements to the left or right could closely mimic indigestion and cause the cow to go off feed. Abomasal displacements include similar clinical signs in cattle. These cattle will have a mild ketonuria and ketolactia with a gas-filled viscus on the left or right side of the animal's body. In the absence of a gas-filled viscus and lack of ketonuria one would have a difficult time in differentiating abomasal displacement from indigestion. One word of caution: if a cow is examined immediately after transport, even when moved only a few miles, one must wait for 24 to 48 hours to pass before ruling out LDA/RDA with assurance. Early cases of so-called vagal indigestion also resemble simple indigestion.

Treatment

The symptomatic therapy of simple indigestion is designed to reestablish normal rumen motility and rumen microbiologic activity by correction of any defects in management or environmental conditions that may have predisposed to the indigestion. The administration of the so-called ruminatoric drugs may promote a mild catharsis and cause an emptying of the rumen, but is unlikely to enhance normal rumen motility.

The rational treatment of indigestion depends on the severity and the specificity of the clinical signs. Those animals with mild cases of indigestion may require little treatment other than the time for the rumen to reestablish normal function. Most cases of mild indigestion will respond to oral ruminatorics which contain a high proportion of magnesium hydroxide with added so-called stomachics, such as nux vomica, tartar emetic, ginger and capsicum. An average initial dose of 340 g (¾ lb) of a commercial ruminatoric (Carmilax) will promote a mild cathar-

sis and seemingly result in clinical recovery. The mode of action and actual efficacy of most ruminatorics are open for debate.

One drug specifically indicated in acute simple indigestion is calcium gluconate parenterally, to correct the mild hypocalcemia (6 to 9 mg/dl) that is often present. The pathogenesis of the hypocalcemia may be related to acute cessation of calcium absorption from the duodenum owing to diminished abomasal emptying and flow of ingesta. The calcium is best administered subcutaneously, from which site a prolonged absorptive phase promotes a mild hypercalcemia for several hours. If calcium is given intravenously, the animal will reestablish normocalcemia within a period of minutes and hypocalcemia may recur in 1 to 3 hours.

Prognosis

The prognosis of most cases of simple indigestion is quite favorable. These patients gradually come back on feed, reestablish milk production, and become productive members of the herd. It would be rare indeed that a cow with simple indigestion would have clinical signs for longer than several days without other complications. Thus, failure to respond within 48 to 72 hours of the onset of indigestion is prima facie evidence that a more serious disorder is present. In fact, many practitioners treat various undiagnosed digestive disorders initially as simple indigestion. Those that relapse or are slow to respond are reevaluated to ascertain the presence of a more deep-seated problem such as vagal indigestion or chronic liver abscesses. Economics often dictates this approach, and since most cows respond to symptomatic therapy, this approach may be justified.

LACTIC ACIDOSIS—RUMINAL ACIDOSIS

This form of acute indigestion develops in ruminants ingesting highly fermentable carbohydrate, usually in the form of grains rich in starch.[20,21] Other synonyms for this disease include: acute grain overload, acute rumen overload, overeating, grain engorgement, D-lactic acidosis, and indigestion with toxemia. Most of the numerous papers on ruminal acidosis deal primarily with the peracute or severe form of rumen acidosis.[22-28] Several recent observations suggest that other forms of ruminal hyperacidity exist, i.e., indigestion, chronic compensated acidosis and low milk-fat syndrome. Therefore, the clinical designation "rumen acidosis" should be considered a collective term for several digestive disturbances, each with a nonphysiologic depression of rumen pH.[29] Additional information on lactic acidosis can be found in literature reviews.[30-34]

History

This disease usually affects ruminants with accidental access to highly fermentable feed to which they are unaccustomed or to rations where the concentrate is increased too rapidly. Such accidents may occur when wheat or barley has been spilled from a bin or when cattle break out of their holding area and obtain access to grain. Other accidents usually occur at the time of harvest when cattle manage to obtain access to the grain in bags or piles around the area where the grain is being processed, or when cattle break into a field of corn. Offending feeds include apples, wheat, corn, pears, sprouted oats, potatoes, barley, bakery products, rye, sorghum, fodder beets, mangels, grapes, whey, molasses and brewers grains, among others.

In addition to accidental access to grain, other management factors also predispose to acidosis. One of the most common situations is where cattle are re-fed within 8 to 12 hours after their feed supply has been exhausted or when the roughage content of the ratio is decreased suddenly.[28] Even changes in the physical form of the grain may predispose to acidosis, i.e., a change from whole shelled corn to steamed flaked corn.

Clinical Signs

The clinical signs of lactic acidosis depend upon the amount of grain consumed, the time period since eating, and the severity of ruminal acidosis that has developed. The most acute dramatic form is associated with the sudden ingestion of massive amounts of concentrate and usually results in ruminal distention. Occasionally mild bloat, recumbency, and death occur within 12 to 14 hours after overeating. The first clinical signs occur 6 to 8 hours after overeating and precede the metabolic effects.[28] The signs include: complete anorexia, acute hypolactia (if lactating), dullness, muscular tremors, groaning, odontoprisis, and occasionally signs of colic. Soon after the onset of digestive disturbances, the feces become soft, yellow-green, and foamy; and occasionally they contain blood.[29] The eyes become sunken, appear glassy, and scleral injection becomes more prominent with the development of toxemia. Ruminal contractions are diminished and become absent as the pH decreases to less than 5.0.[35] The acid ingesta has a similar effect on cecal motility but a more erratic effect on the abomasum and small intestine. The decreased rumen motility may be a protective mechanism by

reducing lactic acid absorption in the rumen and small intestine and reducing fermentation by not mixing substrate with bacteria. The animals often show an unsteady staggering gait due to metabolic aberrations and lameness due to laminitis.[36-38]

The temperature and pulse are elevated, proportional to the severity of the disease; a pulse of 120 to 140 per minute is indicative of a severe case and a guarded prognosis. Urine flow is usually profuse for the first 8 to 12 hours after overeating, but then is decreased sharply as systemic dehydration occurs.[39] Terminally, most animals are recumbent and cannot be forced to rise. Their eyes are fixed in a staring gaze and they have intensely reddened mucous membranes. Some animals salivate and most will have a serous to mucopurulent nasal discharge. CNS signs consist of depression to the point of coma, while opisthotonus, head pressing, and extensor tonus are occasionally observed.[40]

In subacute cases, the clinical signs vary tremendously, dependent on which body system is affected, i.e., low milk fat or chronic lameness from laminitis. Laminitis or founder often occurs in the acute or subacute form with increased vascular supply to the feet resulting in a pounding digital pulse, warm hooves, and a stiff, stilted gait. Abortion, premature parturition, or birth of dead or weak calves, retained placenta, and reduced milk production all have been associated with subacute rumenitis.[37,41] The sudden death syndrome in which cattle die suddenly without premonitory signs has also been attributed to this syndrome.[42,43]

Sequelae to acute rumenitis include liver abscesses, which are present in a variety of syndromes including: (1) no clinical signs (occult abscesses), (2) acute death due to an abscess rupturing into the posterior vena cava and showering the lungs with septic emboli, (3) thrombosis of the posterior vena cava and resultant chronic diarrhea, (4) massive hepatic abscesses that may cause poor weight gains, and (5) epistaxis due to a metastatic pulmonary abscess from a hepatic abscess.

The subacute or chronic form of rumenitis may be associated with a mild ruminal acidosis which results in the clinical syndromes of low-fat milk, the "off-feed" syndrome, mild laminitis or the abomasal displacements and chemical rumenitis. The clinical signs may be transient: partial anorexia, decreased ruminal motility, and decreased fat content of the milk.

Laboratory Evaluation

Laboratory findings most commonly include: (1) hemoconcentration with the PCV elevated up to

55%; total serum protein increased from a normal of approximately 7.5 to 9.5 or 10 g/dl; (2) metabolic acidosis with a life-threatening blood pH of 7.0 or less with a decrease in plasma bicarbonate to less than 10 mEq/L; (3) elevated blood lactate to greater than 100 mg of L-lactate or a total lactate of 200 mg/dl; and (4) prerenal azotemia with the BUN up to 150 mg/dl and comparable elevations in plasma creatinine.[21,28,35,44] The rumen contents become more acid, with a pH as low as 4.0 or 5.0. Microscopic examination of rumen contents will indicate the loss of normal protozoa and bacteria. The gram-negative bacteria and protozoa are killed and the rumen population becomes predominately gram-positive.

Serum calcium and magnesium are both decreased which may contribute to the myasthenia. The serum phosphorus is likely elevated as a result of both increased phosphate absorption and decreased renal loss. The urine will be decreased in volume and have an increased specific gravity up to 1.060 with prominent aciduria and glucosuria. The blood glucose will increase to several times normal (> 200 mg/dl) and there may be an increase in blood pyruvate concentration.

Pathophysiology

Lactic acidosis is associated with inadequate ruminal microbial adaptation to an increased dietary concentrate to forage ratio. Increasing the daily concentrate intake does not invariably lead to severe clinical signs of ruminal acidosis, but perhaps only to reduced or irregular appetite (indigestion). It must be stressed that the amount of roughage in relation to concentrate is of importance in maintaining a normal rumen pH. The rumen may become acidotic when the dietary roughage content is decreased, even though the concentrate intake is stable. With a sudden increase in the quantity of concentrate, or with partial or complete anorexia for several days and then a return to concentrate feed, the animal may suddenly be predisposed to ruminal acidosis.[34] No predictable relationship seems to exist between the amount of concentrate ingested and the degree of clinical disease that results.[10]

The microbiologic changes are summarized as follows: Normally, gram-negative bacteria predominate in the rumen microflora with moderate numbers of protozoa. The rumen fermentation products are approximately 65% acetic acid, 25% propionic acid, and 10% butyric acid. As the amount of fermentable concentrate increases, gram-positive cocci (*Streptococcus bovis*) multiply rapidly utilizing starch or glucose as their substrate to produce lactic acid. As the rumen pH decreases to less than 4.5, their growth (*Str. bovis*) is inhibited, while most protozoa are killed at pH 5.0 or less.[45] As the rumen pH falls, *Streptococci* are rapidly overgrown by gram-positive rods (*Lactobacilli*) whose optimum pH is below 5.0 and by 24 hours represent the most numerous organisms in the rumen and cecum.[46] Some of the many (at least 265) strains of *Lactobacilli* isolated from the rumen contents of overfed animals are capable of forming histamine by decarboxylation of histidine.[47] Parenteral histamine causes cessation of ruminal contractions which can be prevented by H1 receptor antagonists; whereas endotoxin also causes rumen stasis, but cannot be blocked with H1 receptor antagonists.[48] Both toxins may be present in ruminal acidosis. In addition to producing lactic acid, *Streptococci* also consume thiamine, which may be a factor in the development of subsequent neurologic signs. Rumen thiamine concentration is normally maintained by a balance of thiamine-producing and thiamine-consuming bacteria.[49] Additional important microbic changes include the increased proportion of coliforms and *Clostridium perfringens* in the rumen and cecum.[46] These organisms are capable of elaborating an enterotoxin which could lead to a further compromise of the homeostatic mechanisms.

Organic acids formed by these organisms (strep) include formic, valeric, and succinic with a concomitant decrease in acetic, propionic and butyric acids.[50,51] The animal will become anorectic at this time.

The cessation of rumen motility is not due to the accumulation of lactic acid, but is rather due to the increased concentration of unassociated volatile fatty acids (VFA).[52] Butyric acid is more potent than propionic or acetic in this regard while lactic acid has almost no effect on rumen motility. As the rumen pH drops to 5.0 or less, *Lactobacilli* proliferate with formation of equal mixtures of the D and L-isomers of lactic acid. Once produced, one isomer may be changed to the other by isomerase. The decrease in rumen pH during the first 8 hours of acidosis is not caused by lactic acid but by an increased production of other organic acids, the proportion of which varies.[29] The lactic acid concentration usually reaches its peak within 7 to 24 hours after acute overeating and then decreases rapidly as the L-isomer is metabolized and the D-isomer is excreted.[29] However, the rumen pH may be low for several days. Additionally, the rumen concentrations of phosphate, chloride, and potassium are increased during the acute stages of acidosis.

The increased lactic acid and breakdown products of starch increase the rumen fluid osmolality, resulting in additional sequestration of fluid in the rumen as a compensatory mechanism tending to decrease the rumen osmolality. Approximately 60% of the increase in rumen osmolality to 400 milliosmoles is due to lactic acid.[53] This causes systemic dehydration with an increased PCV and total plasma protein. Clinically, the fluid influx in the rumen is determined by rumen ballottement and the "splashy" consistency which characterizes rumen acidosis. The increased PCV occurs in association with an increase in blood lactate and pyruvate.

The increased blood lactate concentrations are mainly due to increased D-lactate. In acute acidosis, the blood L-lactate may reach 100 mg/dl and the total lactate a maximum of 240 mg/dl.[20] The decreased extracellular fluid volume, increased lactic acid, and resultant poor peripheral perfusion lead to a metabolic acidosis, often to a life-threatening pH of 7.0 or less. The blood glucose and pyruvate concentrations in ruminal acidosis often increase to more than 200 mg/dl and 5.5 mg/dl, respectively.[53]

Rumenitis of varying forms is the common denominator of most aspects of the disease. The initial chemical rumenitis that results from the acidosis can heal without complication or can develop more extensive lesions. The production of lactic acid and decrease in rumen pH results in swollen edematous rumen papillae with the development of hyperemia and hemorrhage. Rumenitis begins with the development of microvesicles of the stratum lucidum, hyperemia, and then epithelial desquamation and detachment of areas of mucosa.[54] As this occurs, bacteria (notably *Fusobacterium necrophorum*) and fungi invade the rumen papillae. The hyphae of mycotic agents are highly invasive, spread rapidly, and have a specific affinity to invade blood vessels causing thrombosis.[20] These acute hemorrhagic lesions in the rumen, reticulum, and omasum are the hallmark of mycotic infections. It is virtually impossible to treat mycotic rumenitis effectively once it develops. With a less severe ruminal acidosis, a localized rumenitis with a localized abscess formation may result. These abscesses may metastasize to the liver causing liver abscesses, and develop one of several sequelae.

The changes in rumen microflora are also associated with production of toxins, specifically histamine, tyramine, tryptamine,[23,24,46,54,55] alcohol, and endotoxins, all of which may result in further cardiac damage, hepatic damage, renal damage, and development of azotemia and laminitis. However, since histamine is poorly absorbed and rapidly metabolized, and since large oral doses of histamine do not produce laminitis, it is unlikely that rumen-derived histamine causes laminitis.[56] The concurrent damage to rumen epithelium may allow toxin absorption that normally would not occur from the rumen.[53] Endotoxin has been demonstrated in the blood of animals experimentally overfed and in the rumen contents of cattle with so-called "sudden death syndrome."[35]

Polioencephalomalacia may result from alterations in the normal rumen microflora where microorganisms such as *Clostridium sporogenes* or *Bacillus thiaminolyticus* are capable of producing thiaminase.[57] Two types of thiaminases are produced by these organisms. Thiaminase I produces a thiamine analog while thiaminase II breaks down thiamine. Rumen environments associated with lactic acidosis are also conducive to the production of thiaminases.

Following death from ruminal acidosis, degenerative changes commonly occur in the heart, liver, muscle, and kidney.[29,58] Myocarditis may be a consistent feature of ovine acidosis.[25] Histologic changes in the brain include perivascular and perineuronal edema which resemble the early changes in polioencephalomalacia.[25] Additionally, neurologic lesions ranging from nonspecific gliosis to demyelination have been described in fatal cases of indigestion.

Diagnosis

Acute ruminal acidosis is best determined by a history of increased consumption of concentrate, the characteristic clinical signs, and the change in rumen pH. The macroscopic alterations in ruminal fluid characteristic of acidosis include a milky-grey color, a watery consistency, plant particles that do not float, and few gas bubbles. The fine particles sediment rapidly and a sour smell is very apparent.

Diagnostic rule-outs would include septic mastitis or metritis, which may also be associated with a "splashy" rumen, increased pulse rate, and diarrhea. Diffuse peritonitis would produce similar clinical signs, but could easily be ruled out by abdominocentesis. Poisoning by salt, cyanide, or nitrate might give similar clinical signs to those of a recumbent "downer" cow with acute grain overload. The diagnosis is best confirmed by a history of overeating or an abrupt change in diet with a development of a splashy rumen. The splashy rumen may occur in vagal indigestion but a simple clinical evaluation will differentiate the two symptom-complexes. In the final analysis, the low rumen pH is specific for lactic acidosis and would not be expected in cases of vagal indigestion.

Treatment

The therapy for lactic acidosis should include rumenotomy where the rumen is emptied of all ingesta, rinsed, reemptied, and inoculated with rumen liquor from a normal cow. An easier approach, but perhaps not as efficacious, is the use of gastric lavage where water is infused or siphoned from the rumen.[59] This has to be done with a marine bilge pump and not a regular stomach pump, which clogs easily due to the coarse ingesta. The pumping and siphoning have to be repeated several times and are fraught with such problems as clogging of the stomach tube and a greater risk of inhalation pneumonia, all of which makes it a cumbersome technique at best. If rumen contents cannot be emptied, another alternative is to administer several gallons of water to decrease the rumen hypertonicity and to treat with oral antibiotic (penicillin, 20 to 50 million units; neomycin, 1 to 2 g; chloramphenical, 2 to 5 g; or chlortetracycline, 5 to 10 g).[10] Intraruminal antibiotic has been shown to prevent the onset of lactic acid formation, but is ineffective once lactic acid formation has occurred. An organic iodine disinfectant (Weladol, Dow Chemical) has been effectively used in treatment of acute grain overload. Four ounces are given in mineral oil or water. If the rumen motility has ceased at the time, efforts are made to mix the disinfectant with the rumen contents by external ballottement and kneading of the rumen.[60] The mode of action is apparently the destruction of *Lactobacilli* and works best when given 4 to 8 hours postingestion. Other commercially available agents would be oral alkalinizing agents to correct the rumen pH such as magnesium hydroxide or sodium bicarbonate. Although sound in theory (i.e., to restore the rumen pH), the efficiency of oral alkalinizing agents such as sodium bicarbonate is questionable, at best. Ammonium hydroxide may help by increasing the numbers of lactate-utilizing bacteria.

Other supportive parenteral therapy would include use of antihistamine, 300 to 400 mg subcutaneously, 3 to 4 times per day; thiamine ½ to 1 g intramuscularly or intravenously; and calcium borogluconate subcutaneously to correct the hypocalcemia that often occurs in acute indigestion.

Sheep given parenteral thiamine were able to tolerate severe ruminal acidosis for 7 days compared to sheep not given thiamine. Intravenous fluids may be needed to correct the dehydration. Adequate amounts of intravenous bicarbonate are needed to correct the acidosis accompanying the dehydration. The fluid lost in ruminal acidosis is derived from both intracellular and extracellular fluid compartments. Plasma sodium, potassium, and chloride concentrations decrease in approximately isotonic proportions, which suggests a polyionic isotonic fluid with bicarbonate to be well justified.[11]

Prognosis

The eventual outcome of each case of ruminal acidosis is difficult to predict, but a serious condition is present with any of the following signs: (1) rumen atony, (2) rapid pulse (> 120/min), (3) ataxic or drunken gait, (4) severely sunken eyes, and (5) decreased skin temperature. If any of these signs are present within 10 to 12 hours following overeating, the prognosis is unfavorable.

Additionally, some animals temporarily respond to therapy only to relapse, become recumbent, and die 5 to 8 days later due to mycotic rumenitis.

Prevention

Nonadapted lambs and heifers, inoculated intraruminally with rumen fluid from sheep and steers adapted to a high-energy ration, did not have digestive problems when fed high-energy rations.[61,62] Inoculation did not increase average daily gain but did increase feed efficiency compared to unadapted animals. Lactate utilizing bacteria (*Megasphaeran elsdenii, Peptococcus asaccharolyticus,* and *Selenomonas ruminantium*) increase with increased concentrate feeding.[61] Gradual adaptation to increased concentrate feeding is best to prevent ruminal acidosis.[63,64] The crude fiber in the ration should be 14% of the TDN for fattening cattle and 18% of the TDN for milking cattle. Alkalinizing agents in the ration are of minor importance in the prevention of acidosis.

BLOAT

Bloat (rumen tympanites) can be subdivided into two major types: (1) acute bloat, which is life threatening and most often a frothy bloat, and (2) chronic bloat, which is usually a free-gas bloat.

Acute or chronic bloat is a disease of major importance to both the veterinarian and the livestock producer. Losses attributed to this disease occur due to death in acute frothy bloat or to production losses (failure to gain weight and produce milk) in chronic bloat.

History

Acute Bloat

These animals often have a history of change from a poorer pasture to a lush stand of alfalfa, clover or, less commonly, Bird's-foot trefoil. The new growth is often moist with dew and has been eaten early in the morning. Several animals (10 to 30%) are usually affected out of a group on the same feeding regime. The incidence is lower, but bloat often occurs in multiple animals in feedlots as well. Affected feedlot animals are usually on full feed and consuming more than 50% of their ration as concentrate. Acute or chronic frothy bloat can also occur in cattle fed primarily alfalfa hay, particularly when fed in combination with grain concentrate.

Chronic Bloat

This is usually a single animal disease and the owner may first notice a general increase in ruminal or abdominal size. Coincident with this are a gradual weight loss and decreased production. Chronic bloat has a variable course and therefore a variable history. Some animals may have a gradual onset of increased severity of ruminal distention and others have exacerbations of bloat with normal interictal periods.

Clinical Signs

Acute Bloat

The vital signs are elevated in proportion to the severity of the ruminal distention. Cattle in immediate danger of dying will have a pulse rate of 140 to 160 per minute. The respiratory effort becomes more labored with gasping efforts in the terminal stages. Milk production ceases abruptly as the intraruminal pressure increases, often up to 70 mm Hg. This severe distention mechanically interferes with respiration, which is further embarrassed by the absorption of CO_2 from the rumen and can result in death within 1 hour of commencing to feed.[65] The key finding on physical examination is the type of gas in the rumen (simple free-gas accumulation or a frothy mixture of ingesta and gas) which is determined when the stomach tube is passed. If simple gas accumulation has occurred, the problem is immediately relieved. If foam is present in the tube, a diagnosis of frothy bloat is made.

Chronic Free-Gas Bloat

The outstanding clinical sign of chronic bloat is the mild to moderate ruminal tympany which is easily relieved by passing a stomach tube. Occasionally the distention may be severe enough to cause discomfort. Some cases of frothy bloat will have a gas cap on the rumen froth leading to confusion of the two types of bloat. Examination of rumen contents offers the best method of differentiating the two forms of bloat. The term feedlot bloat should not be associated with either specific form of bloat, as both free-gas and frothy bloat occurs in feedlot animals.[66] Further description of chronic bloat will be covered in Vagal Indigestion.

Pathophysiology

Frothy or Legume Bloat

The cause of legume bloat is not excessive gas production but that the gas produced is contained by small bubbles (1 mm diameter), producing a foam or froth. This foam cannot be eructated; thus, it accumulates and leads to ruminal distention.

Many factors (plant, mineral and animal) contribute to the foam production in the rumen. Foaming agents include two broad categories: (1) the detergents and silicones which become concentrated on the surface of the solution and lower surface tension, permitting bubbles to form readily but have little persistence; (2) the proteins and polyuronides form monomolecular films on the surface, reducing surface tension but increasing surface viscosity (surface resistance to shearing force). Foams so formed have great strength, but are broken by the addition of detergents, which rupture the monomolecular layer (by further lowering surface tension and viscosity). Stable foam production is the optimal point in lowered surface tension and increased surface viscosity.[67,68]

The solubility of protein is vital to foam formation since plants with high protein content but a low concentration of soluble protein will not cause bloat, but those which have a high concentration of soluble proteins will do so.[67] Bird's-foot trefoil is a legume but, because of its low soluble protein content, seldom causes bloat; whereas red clover quite readily produces bloat and has a high level of soluble protein. This soluble protein of legumes (molecular weight 555,000) is a cytoplasmic protein (18-S) from chloroplasts. It has been identified as the enzyme ribulose diphosphate carboxylase and is the main plant factor in frothy bloat.[66,69] Forages that induce bloat contain about 4.5% of this protein, while nonbloatogenic forages contain less than 1%. Approximately 65% of the soluble protein in feed is released into the rumen fluid during mastication.[70] If the released protein is then mixed with the bubbles of gas from the ongoing fermentation process, frothy bloat may result.

The cow's capacity to eructate is about three times the normal amount of gas produced (2 liters/minute),[71,72] providing the vagus is intact and no esophageal obstruction exists nor is stable foam covering the esophageal orifice. It is difficult to overload the rumen or to elevate the hindquarters sufficiently to prevent eructation of gas.[71] Thus the basic problem is a stable foam and not excess gas production. However, the site of gas production in the rumen may be important. Legumes and concentrates sink to the floor of the rumen, so gas bubbles are forced to rise through the rumen fluid contributing to foam production.[73] Legumes are rich in citric, malonic, and succinic acids, which quickly react with the bicarbonate in the rumen to release large quantities of carbon dioxide giving rise to 40 to 70% of the total gas produced,[74] while methane accounts for 20 to 30%, and N_2, O_2, H_2 and H_2S are minor components.[70,75] Differences in fermentation rates between animals of differing susceptibility to bloat have not been demonstrated.

The stability or cohesiveness of the foam once produced is dependent upon two other major factors: (1) divalent cations—calcium and magnesium, and (2) rumen pH. The divalent cations bind together the 18-S protein at the isoelectric point—pH 5.4.[76] The isoelectric point (pH 5.4) is critical to the development of a stable foam as the cohesion between protein molecules is maximum and therefore surface viscosity and resistance to shear are maximum. Unless the rumen pH is near 5.4, the foam is less stable and serious bloat is not likely to occur.[66]

Once the soluble protein is whipped into a froth, the protein at the gas-water interface becomes denatured and stiffens, similar to the beaten egg white in a meringue pie. The smaller and more numerous the bubbles, the more stable the foam. The denatured protein is more resistant to bacterial degradation than is soluble protein, thus slowing bacterial destruction of the foam.[75] However, plants with higher concentrations of soluble protein do not invariably produce bloat. Many of these plants have antifoam factors which counteract the foam-stabilizing chemical. Plant fats have been shown to reduce foam and are found in the chloroplasts of many plants.[77] This explains why mineral oil is an effective treatment for frothy bloat. Rough, scabrous material stimulates rumen motility and the frequency of eructations.[78] Soft plant growth, such as young or prebloom plants, tends not to stimulate rumen motility as much and thus depresses the frequency of eructation. It has been observed that when a bloated animal is fed coarse roughage, foam production often decreases. This has often been used for treatment of frothy bloat. Thus, the response to roughage may be partially due to its stimulating effect on the rumen motility. Agitation also influences the foam stability in a negative way. The 18-S protein can be completely precipitated in vitro by agitation.[67] In the bloating animal the protein is denatured in the surface film of the foam bubble by agitation, which may explain why vigorous exercise sometimes relieves frothy bloat.

Saliva has components which both enhance and inhibit foaming. The HCO_3^- breaks down, with the release of CO_2 and aids in bubble formation. Mucin, however, has antifoaming properties. Saliva may also reduce the surface tension of the rumen contents by the action of other components. The HCO_3^- and mucin concentration depends on which gland the saliva is coming from, and whether bloat occurs depends not only on the amount of saliva but also on the glandular origin. The parotid and submaxillary glands have high concentrations of mucin and these are released when eating and when the rumen pressure is high. The parotid saliva also has a surface tension low enough to make foam less stable. Thus, release of the parotid and submaxillary saliva is a good defense mechanism when the animal bloats. The saliva, as a buffer, may also bring the pH into a range where the froth is less stable. Rumen bacteria (mucinolytic) are more numerous in bloated animals and in rumen ingesta of animals fed freshly cut alfalfa hay or a feedlot bloatogenic ration, compared to those fed alfalfa hay. Thus, salivary mucin normally inhibits bloat formation, but in the presence of aerobic or anaerobic mucinolytic rumen bacteria it may not be as effective as an antifoaming agent.[69] Salivary secretion is very likely inherited, which may be one of the reasons bloat seems to have a hereditary basis.[79]

In summary, primary frothy bloat occurs when the rumen ingesta contains foaming substances (primarily 18-S soluble protein), when the lowered pH of the rumen (~5) is suitable for the growth of encapsulated bacteria which produce extracellular polysaccharides (slime) and mucinolytic bacteria which destroy salivary mucin, or when salivation is insufficient. In some circumstances one or more of these factors may be in the critical range which triggers rumen distention by the accumulation of foam.

Acute Free-Gas Boat

Acute free-gas bloat is most often associated with esophageal obstruction due to foreign bodies (apples, pears, tubers, beets, carrots, or green corn). Bloat is seldom fatal if the object is irregular so gas can escape. Extra-esophageal obstructions such as inflammatory mediastinal masses or neoplasia, especially lymphosarcoma, may cause acute free-gas bloat. Passage of a stomach tube and palpation of the esophagus will help determine whether the obstruction is intra- or extraluminal.

Less common causes of extraluminal esophageal obstruction would include persistent right aortic arch, tuberculosis due to enlargement of the thoracic lymph nodes, or esophageal spasm due to tetanus. Chronic respiratory disease, especially shipping fever, has been implicated in chronic free-gas bloat by the inflammatory process extending to the vagus nerve, thus interfering with normal eructation.[80] Acute or chronic free-gas bloat is, with rare exception, due to failure of eructation and not to excessive gas production in the rumen. This is contrary to popular belief by many practicing veterinarians.

Normal eructation occurs following the second reticular contraction and the ruminoreticular fold remains contracted to act as a dam retaining fluid ingesta in the rumen and allowing gas accumulation in the relaxed reticulum.[81] Even when the back feet of the animal are elevated and water is introduced into the cardia, eructation is still possible as it is following the administration of drugs to stop rumen motility.

The majority of cattle with chronic free-gas bloat have evidence of chronic respiratory disease or chronic reticulitis when explored surgically. The adhesions seem to fix the reticulum in such a way as to prevent normal eructation. The prerequisite event prior to eructation is clearing the cardia. If the cardia is unable to be cleared of ingesta and to be filled with gas, then chronic bloat may result.

Certain anatomic factors must also be considered, such as the position of the cow's reticulum in reference to the normal standing position. For example: (1) cattle with milk fever may become recumbent and the cardia becomes flooded preventing eructation, (2) cows cast in dorsal recumbency for surgical purposes are very prone to bloat, (3) overfed veal calves at 12 to 14 weeks of age are very

prone to free-gas bloat owing to mechanical interference with eructation by the milk-flooded cardia, and (4) dwarf cattle are also prone to free-gas bloat, as it is the major cause of death in such animals. Free-gas bloat is considered the third most important disease complex of veal calves following diarrhea and pneumonia.[82] The sudden-onset free-gas bloat is primarily due to overfilling of the rumen as the calves are "pushed" on whole milk or milk replacer at 12 to 14 weeks of age. Calves with a short stocky conformation are more predisposed than are other calves. Chronic intermittent bloating in veal calves is more likely due to chronic localized peritonitis or is a sequela to chronic enzootic calf pneumonia. Both diseases interfere with the eructation mechanism.

Diagnosis

Simple passage of the stomach tube is a valid means of making a definite diagnosis of bloat, be it free-gas or frothy.

Chronic free-gas bloat may occur as a primary entity by itself or it may be associated with other forms of chronic indigestion, failure of omasal transport, or abomasal impaction. As a specific entity, chronic free-gas bloat or failure of eructation may be determined by passing a stomach tube. If the gas is removed and the rumen is relatively empty, or at least does not contain more than the normal amount of ingesta, the diagnosis is simply failure of eructation. If the rumen is full of ingesta (usually more fluid than normal; "splashy") then the chronic free-gas bloat is associated with another problem, such as chronic traumatic reticulitis.

Additional diagnostic rule-outs would include any cause of abdominal distention such as ascites, hydrops, or vagal indigestion.

Necropsy diagnosis of ruminal tympany is based on the findings of (1) compressed lungs, (2) congestion and hemorrhage in the cervical esophagus with a blanched, pale, thoracic esophagus, (3) pale muscles and lymph nodes in the caudal part of the cadaver while red and congested in the cranial half, and (4) frothiness of the rumen ingesta.[83]

Treatment

The principal therapeutic aim in the treatment of frothy bloat is to reduce the stability of the foam. Passage of a stomach tube may allow for some free gas to escape and bring a little relief. Then, one of many types of oil can be given: mineral oil, pine oil, creolin, fish and animal oils, turpentine or poloxalene in a ½ liter or less dosage. The surface tension is lowered and the gas bubbles break up

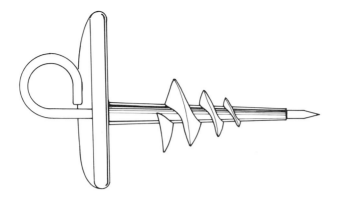

Figure 22–1. Buff's screw trocar used in the treatment of chronic free-gas bloat. The trocar will promote an adhesion of the rumen to the body wall and facilitates the development of a rumen fistula.

permitting eructation. Once the oil is administered, its distribution in the rumen is hastened by exercise or massaging the rumen but this may not be necessary. Emergency treatment by the owner is often required. In acute frothy bloat, the owner may resort to rumen trocarization with the attentant risks of peritonitis in an effort to prevent death from asphyxiation. Bloat of more gradual onset will often respond to placing a "gag" in the mouth. The gag in the form of a stick or broom-handle placed transversely across the mouth at the commissures will stimulate increased salivation. The increased salivary mucin, HCO_3^- and volume will all aid in the antifoaming activity of the rumen.

Free-gas bloat or failure of eructation that is not associated with another primary form of indigestion is treated most easily by the establishment of a rumen fistula. This can be done surgically, after the completion of a rumenotomy or by using a "screw" trocar (Fig. 22–1).[84] The treatment of chronic bloat associated with other forms of indigestion will be covered later in this chapter.

One new device (Rutickulator) was developed to stimulate rumen function mechanically. This plastic "spoke-like" instrument is given orally, and when in the rumen, the surrounding paper separates and the spokes expand. The device floats on the surface and serves to scratch or stimulate the inner surface of the rumen (in a manner similar to coarse roughage). In this way, it is advocated as an aid in the control of chronic bloat and other rumen dysfunctions.

Prognosis

The prognosis in most cases of bloat is favorable, especially if the animal is treated early. The outcome of most cases of failure of eructation (free-gas

bloat) is good to excellent. Usually these cows will regain their ability to eructate and the fistula will heal closed in a matter of weeks. Once cattle have become accustomed to leguminous forage, the incidence of bloat is reduced.

Prevention

Four major methods have been used for the prevention of frothy bloat: (1) pasture management, (2) feeding of roughage supplements, (3) administration of antibacterials, and (4) antifoaming materials. Currently frothy bloat is prevented almost entirely by pasture management and antifoaming agents, primarily poloxalene.[66]

Frothy bloat can be prevented by feeding 1 to 2 g poloxalene per 50 kg of body weight per day. However, it may not be possible to have the cattle eat a supplement containing poloxalene when grazing an immature stand of alfalfa. The animals should be given the grain supplement prior to being turned out. Another alternative is poloxalene in a molasses lick-wheel. One lick-wheel is needed for every 25 cattle and should be kept near drinking areas and within 400 meters of the cattle. A poloxalene block can be used at the rate of five blocks per 25 cattle.[85] Poloxalene is poorly absorbed from the gastrointestinal tract with 94% of recovery in the feces in 9 days, with only 4% appearing in the urine.[86] Detergent in an ethyl cellulose gel is slowly released into the rumen fluid and is effective in the prevention of chronic frothy feedlot bloat, which commonly occurs when concentrates comprise more than 50% of the ration.[87] A larger particle size of ration will decrease the incidence of bloat. Additional benefits of a larger particle size are the maintenance of a more stable rumen pH and decreased numbers of slime-producing bacteria.[88,89] The addition of water to feedlot rations also decreases the incidence of bloat by decreasing rumen viscosity.[66] Mineral oil given as 4 to 8% of the ration reduces bloat by 40%, but animal fats are not effective.[90]

Chronic free-gas bloat is very difficult to prevent, but the incidence can be reduced by minimizing the predisposing conditions, specifically chronic respiratory disease and localized traumatic reticulitis.

TRAUMATIC RETICULOPERITONITIS

Synonyms for traumatic reticuloperitonitis (TRP) include "hardware disease," traumatic gastritis, and traumatic reticulitis. This very common disease of adult cattle is more prevalent in dairy cattle compared to beef cattle, not because of their eating habits, but because of the environmental conditions where dairy cattle are kept, i.e., smaller pastures which are associated with a greater possibility for ingestion of metallic foreign bodies from old fences, silage, choppers, and other instruments, compared to the beef cow on the open range. Goats seem to have a low incidence of TRP, but under poor management conditions the incidence is significant.[91] The economic importance of traumatic reticuloperitonitis is high (2% of all cattle annually)[92] and is one of the most common diseases involving the gastrointestinal tract. Certainly, the economic losses are much greater with TRP than with the other common gastrointestinal diseases, especially abomasal displacements. One study reported 21% of 2184 cattle had lesions of traumatic reticulitis; another found 79% incidence in dairy cattle and 20.9% incidence in beef cattle of reticular adhesions in 34,000 carcasses examined.[92,93]

History

The typical patient with acute TRP has an abrupt decrease (typically 50%) in milk production and reduced appetite for grain, but not necessarily hay, from one milking to the next. For example, a cow producing 30 lb of milk twice daily would decrease to 15 lb twice daily and then to 5 or 10 lb twice daily over a 2- to 4-day period. Additionally, the farmer may recognize that the cow is reluctant to walk (like wearing a tight pair of shoes), may have an arched back and a capricious appetite. Eating, even greedily, then suddenly ceasing to eat followed by grunting, is characteristic of TRP.[94] The reluctance to walk may be manifested by a slow return to the barn when she previously was the second or third cow back from pasture. This point can be brought out in the history by asking the farmer when the cow came to the barn. The farmer may reply, "I had to send the dog after the cow" or "She would not come to the barn today."

Vomiting is occasionally one of the first signs noted by the herdsman, but probably occurs in less than 20% of the cases.[95] The clinical signs of vomiting are uncommon and should be regarded as a specific sign, probably due to a penetration of the anterior reticulum adjacent to the esophageal opening.

Occasionally, vomiting is so violent that ingesta splashes against the wall, which may be noted by the farmer. Mild free-gas bloat occurs in about 50% of TRP cases and may alert the owner to a problem.[96]

Physical Examination

The typical cow with TRP may have a slightly arched back (kyphosis) and have a dull, depressed attitude.[97] She may stand up all of the time or lie down most of the time, which is variable from cow to cow, but immobility is relatively constant. The cow may have a contracted ("tucked-up," gaunt) appearance of the abdomen. Occasionally one can hear a grunt emitted by the cow.[98] Closer inspection of the head will indicate an anxious expression and a glassy appearance to the eyes. Stiffness of the forelegs with abduction of the forelegs is occasionally seen. This may be an effort to "fix" the diaphragm and use the intercostal muscles for respiration. Trembling of the triceps muscles and abduction of the elbow has been associated with TRP, but neither sign was observed in 10 experimental cases of TRP.[99]

A mildly elevated temperature, 103.5°F to 104.5°F, often occurs in the early stages, but by 4 days only 58% had a temperature over 102°F.[100] The pulse rate is in the high normal range, 75 to 85. The fever and elevated pulse usually return to normal in 3 to 5 days. The rumen contractions are usually decreased in frequency and amplitude.[100] In both natural and experimental TRP, the reticular contraction interval was prolonged but was observed only in the acute stages. Prolongation of the second phase of the reticular contraction was most apparent 2 to 7 days post injury.[101] The reticular pressure was decreased in both groups of cattle with TRP and substantiates our clinical impressions of the decreased ruminal strength. Experimentally, rumen atony occurs within 2 hours of perforation. The rumen consistency as determined by ballottement is usually more firm than normal.

The recumbent cow with TRP will arise with her hind feet first and exert pressure against the reticulum and diaphragm and at this time may show pain or evoke a grunt. The manifestation of pain is

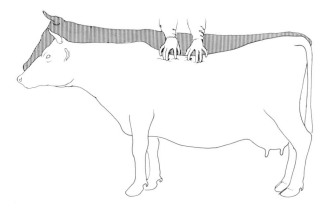

Figure 22–2. Digital pressure is exerted over the withers by pinching the muscles. The normal response is ventroflexion to become lordotic.

indicated by the tightness of the sternocephalicus muscle, often with an obvious groan. Grunting while walking is a good indication of peritonitis, but only occurs in 20% of the cases. Muscle trembling may occur in 15% of the early cases. Auscultation adjacent to the thoracic inlet may indicate a "catchy" respiration at the height of inspiration (30% of the cases). Pressure over the withers (Fig. 22–2) will indicate a failure to ventroflex the spine, which may be an indication of pain in the upper thorax area or in the anterior abdomen (positive in approximately 50% of TRP cases). It is not a specific test for reticulitis, but does indicate pain; and since TRP is one of the most common causes of abdominal disease, it must be considered.

The grunt test or Williams' reticular grunt test is done by determining the primary ruminal contraction and listening for a grunt 2 to 3 seconds before the primary ruminal contraction is palpated in the flank. The primary ruminal contraction is initiated by a reticular contraction, but is not associated with eructation.[97,102] Another method of detection of reticular pain is accomplished by gently lifting the fist in the area of the xiphoid at the height of inspiration. It is important to simultaneously auscult the trachea at the thoracic inlet. This should be done during several respiratory cycles in order not to miss a spontaneous grunt. Suddenly the fist, which is on one's knee, is forced upward in the area of the reticulum on the left side of the xiphoid (Fig. 22–3).[103] If pain is present, this will cause a pause or a grunt or an obvious groan. Occasionally, it is loud enough to be heard without a stethoscope but is best determined by auscultation. This test is not specific for traumatic reticulitis but suggests the presence of pain on the left side of the ventral abdomen and was positive in about 50% of cows with TRP.[96] The test

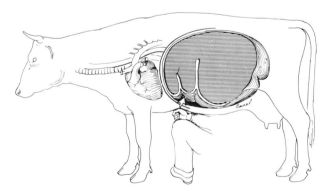

Figure 22–3. Pressure is exerted in the area of the xiphoid by elevating the fist on one's knee. The normal response is minimal discomfort. An audible grunt or tightening of the cervical muscles suggests pain, perhaps from traumatic reticuloperitonitis.

should be repeated on the right side, and if more intense, suggests localized peritonitis associated with perforated abomasal ulcer. In beef cattle or in a large dairy bull, which may be more stoic, a greater force may be needed to elicit the pain, i.e., a bar lifted against the abdomen or a kick with the foot. It is best to determine the response of the normal animal, and then the sick animal. The most valuable diagnostic aids are the history of an abrupt decrease in appetite and milk production, then the temperature elevation (>102°F), pain in the xiphoid region, decreased rumen motility, and decreased defecation.

The subacute or chronic form of TRP represents a diagnostic challenge. The clinical signs of weight loss, dehydration, rough haircoat, arched back, variable rumen motility, accompanied by less obvious localized abdominal pain, present a more nebulous clinical picture.[95] As more dairymen are now treating their own animals, this presents a more difficult problem when asked to offer a diagnosis on a cow sick with TRP for 10 days. In such cases, the temperature and pulse are often normal. The ability to localize the pain in the xiphoid region of such an animal is a diagnostic challenge to even the most astute veterinarian.

Laboratory Evaluation

A leukogram may show a neutrophilia with a total leukocyte count in excess of 13,000 by 24 hours after the onset of signs.[103] Simultaneously, band cells appeared in excess of 5% in 67 cases of TRP.[103] Absolute neutrophil counts greater than 8000/cmm are associated with a poorer prognosis.[104] The relative percentage of lymphocytes decreases, which alters the neutrophil to lymphocyte (N/L) ratio. An N/L ratio of 1:1 or greater is often the only hematologic abnormality in chronic TRP.

The fibrinogen often increases from a value of 300 to 400 mg/dl to 1000 mg/dl or greater, over a period of several days. Concurrently, but more gradually, the globulin increases from a normal of 3.5 to 4.0 g/dl to 5.0 or even 7.0 g/dl in chronic TRP. The hyperglobulinemia is a nonspecific response to antigenic stimulation.

The acid-base balance may be normal if the forestomachs continue to discharge contents into the small intestine. Occasionally there will be relative abomasal atony with the development of mild hypochloremia and a compensated metabolic alkalosis. The serum calcium may be lowered by 2 to 3 mg/dl down to 7 or 8 mg/dl. This is presumably associated with the decreased ingesta in the duodenal area (the site of calcium absorption).

Cattle with TRP often develop mild hypoglycemia but urinary ketones are rarely of sufficient concentration to reflect even secondary acetonemia.[104]

The diagnostic acumen regarding TRP can be confirmed by radiographic techniques.[105] Radiologic equipment is available in most group practices today. This affords a specific approach to the definitive diagnosis, which is most difficult in chronic cases. A radiograph of the reticulum may give other valuable information about the size, shape, and location of the foreign body, which, on occasion, one cannot detect even during the rumenotomy procedure since it may be too deeply embedded. Peritoneocentesis and cytologic evaluation of the cells are aids in the determination of inflammatory processes such as TRP within the peritoneal cavity. The normal peritoneal fluid contains approximately equal numbers of neutrophils and lymphocytes, while in inflammatory disease such as TRP, the percentage of neutrophils and band neutrophils increases.[106]

Etiologic Factors

TRP is most often caused by sharp pointed metallic objects (90%) consumed by the nondiscriminating ruminant. These foreign bodies are most commonly wires (76%), or nails (30%), and 96% were ferromagnetic in one study of 2140 foreign bodies.[107] Occasionally other metallic objects, slices of steel, and stones (usually less than 5% of the total) penetrate the reticulum and cause a localized peritonitis. The length of most penetrating foreign bodies exceeds 4 cm, while shorter objects are either free or wedged into the honeycomb. Only 4 or 5% of the objects exceeded 7 cm in one study of 2140 foreign bodies.[107]

This disease seems to be much more common in dairy cattle compared to beef cattle and rarely occurs in goats or sheep, which have more fastidious habits of eating roughage. Advanced pregnancy seems to predispose to TRP by virtue of a normally voluminous uterus compressing the reticulum,[108] increasing the risk of perforation by foreign bodies which may be present.

Pathophysiology

The ingestion of the foreign body and subsequent penetration of the reticular wall lead to the development of an acute localized inflammatory reaction (peritonitis). Sharpened foreign bodies administered to cows resulted in TRP within 48 hours.[99] If the penetration occurs only in the reticular folds, the course of the disease will be mild with temporary inappetence and reduced milk yield. Penetration of the anterior wall usually results in a localized peritonitis, but if it advances further forward (5 cm), substantial complications may result (pericarditis). Penetration of the posterior wall is potentially more serious and may result in severe peritonitis.

Migration is more apt to occur if the foreign body is straight, whereas wires with kinks or hooks more often remain embedded in the reticular wall and cause serious complications (abscess between the reticular wall and the diaphragm).

The sequelae of traumatic perforation of the reticulum and the development of the localized peritonitis are as follows: (1) complete resolution, once the foreign body has returned to the reticulum; (2) local peritonitis with abscess formation which may result in splenic, hepatic, and/or diaphragmatic abscesses; (3) penetration through the diaphragm to cause local pleuritis and/or pneumonitis: (4) penetration of pericardium to cause pericarditis; (5) rupture of the gastroepiploic artery causing fatal hemorrhage; or (6) localized abscess formation, which may be clinically silent or result in (7) chronic infection causing endocarditis and embolic nephritis.[10] Thus, the sequelae to traumatic perforation of reticulum are many and varied, and the clinical signs associated with each of these syndromes may be extremely variable.

Diagnosis

Few diseases of cattle are associated with such abrupt decreases in milk production and appetite from one feeding to the next as in TRP. Diagnosis is most easily made early (1 to 3 days) following penetration of the reticulum by the foreign body. The acute pain is associated with an acute inflammatory reaction; as the inflammatory reaction subsides, the pain is less apparent and not as easily localized. Thus, if called to evaluate a cow for a possible reticulitis, the pain and clinical signs associated with the acute inflammatory response are most apparent and easily detected in the first 24 to 72 hours. Following this there should be gradual diminution in the intensity of clinical signs, thus greater difficulty in making a definite diagnosis of TRP.

Other diseases that should be considered in the diagnostic rule-outs for reticulitis include acute indigestion, often with a history of more gradual decrease in milk production, and the feeding of spoiled feed.

Pyelonephritis will cause many of the same signs as reticulitis, but the acute inflammatory process is localized to the kidney and ureters. The cows will have an arched back, go abruptly off feed, have mild hyperthermia (103°F), and if a urine sample is collected, it should contain frank blood clots which characterize acute but not chronic pyelonephritis. There is also an absence of localized pain in the xiphoid area; however, such cows will have a positive (pain) withers test. Abomasal displacements may be considered in any diagnostic work-up for digestive diseases in cattle, but high correlation with parturition and the presence of a gas-filled viscus on the right or left side of the abdomen easily identifies an abomasal displacement.

Abomasal ulcers (type III) with perforation will cause a local peritonitis and many of the same clinical signs as will traumatic reticuloperitonitis. The only way to differentiate TRP from a perforated ulcer is the site of localized pain, which is more to the right of the xiphoid, compared to reticulitis with a pain to the left of the xiphoid. Occasionally, a cow with abomasal displacement will develop an abomasal ulcer and a localized peritonitis on either the right abdominal wall or left abdominal wall, depending upon which side the abomasum is displaced. Local pain at the rib cage dorsolateral to the xiphoid will help differentiate this type of abomasal ulcer from the localized peritonitis of the ventral abdomen associated with TRP.

Cattle with acute hepatic abscesses occasionally exhibit pain similar to reticulitis. The pain is usually manifest clinically as a reluctance to become lordotic when squeezing over the withers, but there will be no evidence of localized pain in the xiphoid area. Additionally, pain may be detected by percussion over the right side of the thorax.

Treatment

The conservative treatment of traumatic reticulitis is immobilization by confinement in a stall or stanchion. Exercise will cause shifting of the abdominal organs predisposing to a greater spread of inflammation, resulting in a greater area of peritonitis or even diffuse peritonitis. Along with stall rest, antibacterial drugs are indicated to control the infection. Penicillin (10 to 20,000 units per kg per day by parenteral injection) or oral sulfas (2 grains per kg body weight for 3 to 5 days) are efficacious, as are tetracycline and sulfa drugs given intravenously. This form of therapy usually results in 80 to 90% recovery.[109,110]

Most cattle will benefit from a bar magnet (1.5 × 6 cm) administered via a "balling" gun. Depending upon the rate of rumen contraction it will take 1 to 4 days for the magnet to move from the anterior ventral sac of the rumen into the reticulum. Withdrawing the foreign body to the magnet will take another 1 to 3 days. An inclined platform (a door or several planks) is used to elevate the front feet 15 to 20 cm and reduce the pressure of the reticulum against the diaphragm, thus decreasing pain and facilitating walling-off of the infection.

In one study, cows were kept inside on a raised platform and given antibiotics daily; this treatment resulted in 89% recovery.[110] If the cows were ill less than 24 hours, 95% recovered, emphasizing early diagnosis and treatment.[104,110]

Many animals are treated with oral cathartics which may act as a ruminatoric. Most of these drugs will promote a mild catharsis but their utility and effectiveness as a true ruminatoric must be questioned.

Another approach in the treatment and prevention of the disease is the use of a magnetic metal retriever (Fig. 22–4).[111–113] The retriever consists of a large magnet on the end of a wire cable, passed through a stiff plastic stomach tube. This is passed through a metal mouth speculum into the anterior dorsal sac of the rumen. The distal end of the stomach tube is bent in a "U" shape by a separate nylon cord so that the magnet can be placed in the reticulum. The metal cable is extended and retracted several times to sweep the surface of the reticulum. Here the more powerful magnet will attach to ferrous foreign bodies and remove them from the reticulum as the magnet and wire cable are withdrawn. The best results are obtained following a 12- to 18-hour fast from roughage, which facilitates easier entrance and mobility of the magnet in the reticulum.[114] When this instrument came into use, much concern was expressed about the potential damage to the esophageal mucosa by the foreign bodies during removal. This has not been a deterrent to the use of the instrument. Many veterinarians have become very adept in the use of the

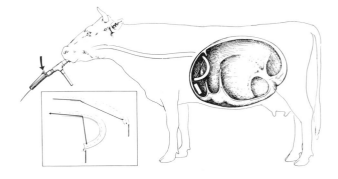

Figure 22–4. The "Muffley" magnetic metal retriever. Note the magnet in the reticulum and its proximity to penetrating foreign objects.

retriever in conjunction with an electromagnetic metal detector. The detector is a sensitive aid in the detection of ferrous foreign objects and provides further evidence that the offending nail has been removed by the retriever. The retriever has been used both as a treatment for TRP and as a preventative aid on all cows in "problem" herds on an annual or semiannual basis.

Prevention

Magnets are very efficacious in preventing TRP, and all dairy animals of breeding age should be given a bar magnet along with routine vaccination.[115–117] One author reported a 52% reduction in the incidence of TRP over a 6-month period in 100 heifers.[118] Further, the continued presence of the magnet in the reticulum should be determined annually with a compass or a "studfinder." Studfinders are cheap bar magnets on a swivel used to detect the studs in house walls. When the studfinder is held against the reticulum, it will detect the presence of a bar magnet and indicate the polarity. The compass or studfinder should always be used prior to giving a magnet. Two magnets depolarize each other and therefore diminish their effectiveness in withdrawing the foreign body.[119] The cage magnet is a recent German development which allows greater "pulling power" as the magnet is held 1 to 1½ cm from the reticular lining (Fig. 22–5). The cage magnet has a greater capacity for ferrous material, but the increased cost must be weighed against the use of the retriever to remove the simple bar magnet and clean it of foreign bodies.

Animals that do not respond to nonsurgical therapy should be considered for surgical removal of the foreign body via an exploratory rumenotomy. This procedure is very safe, usually done in the field quickly and effectively by most practicing veterinarians. The foreign body is removed and the animal is usually treated with an antibiotic after surgery because of possible contamination of the surgical site with rumen content.

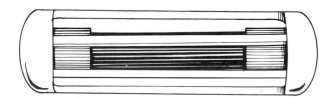

Figure 22–5. A "cage" magnet. It is designed to attract the foreign objects next to the bar magnet, which may provide greater "pulling power."

Prognosis

The prognosis for life and for return to milk production is good in most cases of traumatic reticuloperitonitis. Occasionally, pericarditis, vagal indigestion, abscesses, and hepatic thrombosis may result in unfavorable sequelae. The heart rate at the time of initial examination has served as a prognostic aid. If over 88 per minute, up to 30% may not recover.[110] Additionally, when TRP occurs in advanced pregnancy, the prognosis is diminished for two reasons: (1) The increasing size of the gravid uterus seems to impair forestomach function, and (2) most important, the farmer does not recognize illness in these dry cows as early as in lactating cows, so their lesions are more advanced when first treated.

VAGAL INDIGESTION

Chronic indigestion, Hoflund's syndrome, chronic localized peritonitis, or vagal indigestion all may be a part of a syndrome associated with gradual abdominal enlargement due to ruminal distention with fluid and/or gas.[119] Vagal indigestion is not one disease entity, but a collection of diseases that result in ruminal distention and abdominal distention. The site of functional disturbance within the forestomachs allows classification into four distinct types: type I, failure of eructation or free-gas bloat; type II, omasal transport failure; type III, abomasal impaction; and type IV, partial obstruction of the forestomachs. The term "vagus indigestion" was introduced in 1940 to describe a disorder of ruminants associated with a functional disturbance of the stomach.[119] By sectioning various branches of the vagus nerve, Hoflund was able to produce four types of functional disturbances, which were classified as follows:

1. Functional stenosis between the reticulum and omasum with atony of the rumen and reticulum.
2. Functional stenosis between the reticulum and omasum with normal or hyperactive ruminal and reticular motility.
3. Permanent functional stenosis of the pylorus with atony or retained activity of the reticulum.
4. Incomplete pyloric stenosis.

The symptoms produced in experimental animals were essentially the same as those recorded in spontaneous cases, and vagus nerve lesions were demonstrated at postmortem examination in spontaneous cases.

The classification outlined first includes a broader range of disease processes in the term "vagal indigestion," and differentiation should be based on clinical and clinicopathologic examinations. Additionally, it is doubtful that pyloric stenosis is the cause of abomasal impaction except in rare instances. The functional stenosis between the reticulum and omasum is equivalent to omasal transport failure. The motility of the reticulum and rumen associated with this syndrome varies with time in the same animal, depending on the degree of rumen distention. A more detailed discussion is presented under pathophysiology.

History

The history is often characterized by earlier bouts of indigestion, periods of anorexia, decreased milk production, and weight loss. The presenting signs are most often anorexia and constipation. The weight loss is more gradual than in lactating cows with ketosis. Occasionally this syndrome affects cattle in late gestation and the enlarging fetus may mask initial signs of weight loss, but the continuing loss of muscle mass becomes apparent as the abdomen increases in circumference. Vomiting and/or regurgitation may, on occasion, be the chief complaint noted by the owner. When several animals in a herd are vomiting, spoiled forage should be suspected. Other causes of vomiting in individual cows include: (1) frothy bloat, (2) reticulitis, and (3) toxic plants such as rhododendron and laurel.[120]

Acute or intermittent free-gas bloat may be another sign the owner may register as the chief complaint. This form of bloat is rarely life threatening, but may cause mild abdominal distress and require emergency treatment if only to alleviate the owner's apprehensions about the cow's problem. Interestingly, when the gas is removed from the rumen, these animals are hungry and may eat vigorously; but as the rumen distends, the feeding ceases because of the discomfort. Typically, animals with vagal indigestion have a capricious appetite early in the disease, but as the disease progresses, the inappetence becomes complete. Yet despite nearly complete inappetence, these cattle will often drink water normally or even excessively, further contributing to the rumen distention.

Clinical Signs

The clinical signs are usually gradual in onset, with a mild to gradual decrease in milk production (if lactating), gradual abdominal distention despite a poor appetite, and decreased fecal output compared to herdmates on a similar ration. The nature and character of the feces typify vagal indigestion. The amount passed is decreased in proportion to what the cow eats and, on close inspection, often contains 2 to 4 cm hay particles suggesting poor digestion. Actually, the omasal canal determines the particle size admitted to the abomasum and, if it is not properly functioning, allows larger particles of hay into the lower tract which can be evaluated by close inspection of the feces. The fecal consistency is thicker and more sticky (pasty) than normal. This is a reflection of prolonged transit time and mucous secretion in the colon.

Abdominal distention is one of the most important clinical signs of vagal indigestion.[121] Typically, when a cow becomes partially anorectic, the abdominal size decreases and appears contracted (gaunt or "tucked-up") (Fig. 22–6). However, if a cow retains the normal fullness or becomes distended following anorexia, then vagal indigestion should be considered in the rule-out process. The accumulation of gas and fluid in the rumen is the major factor for the distention. Frequently a small amount of gas accumulates on top of the rumen ingesta, giving the left side of the abdomen a very rotund appearance, i.e., "apple-shaped." In advanced abomasal impaction, the lower right abdominal quadrant may appear distended, giving a pear-shaped appearance to the right side when viewed from behind. Together these two shapes form the so-called "papple" (*apple* on the left "rumen" and *pear* on the right "abomasum"), which characterizes the abdominal contour in cattle with abomasal impaction (Fig. 22–7). As the abdominal distention becomes more severe, the animal becomes weak and has difficulty rising to its feet,

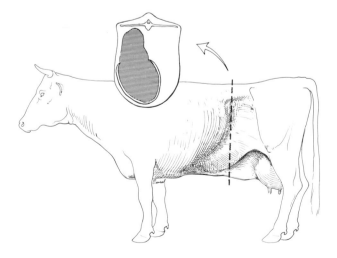

Figure 22–6. A gaunt, "tucked-up" cow suggestive of decreased rumen fill with an open gastrointestinal tract (contracted abdomen).

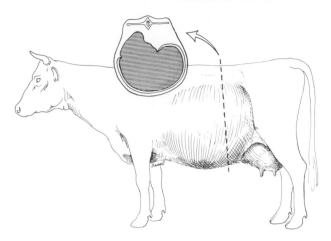

Figure 22–7. A distended abdomen due to excessive rumen contents. The ventral sac of the rumen often enlarges to form an "L" shape, as defined during the rectal examination. The external contour suggests the "papple" shape typical of abomasal impaction.

leading to the "downer-cow" syndrome. This can be further complicated by hypocalcemia, hypokalemia, and severe dehydration. The temperature and respiratory rates are often within normal ranges. The pulse is more variable and ranges from 34 to 80 per minute. Approximately 25 to 40% of the cows will have bradycardia (less than 60 per minute).[122] However, in the later stage of the disease the heart rate will increase to more than 100 per minute as the cow becomes terminal. The eyes lose their normal sparkle and become sunken as dehydration progresses. The haircoat is often rough, suggesting a chronic disease such as traumatic reticulitis. Diminished skin elasticity (most obvious on the lateral cervical area) parallels the sunken eyes. The longer the skin "tent" takes to return to normal, the more severe the dehydration and the more serious the forestomach problem.

Ballottement of the upper left paralumbar fossa is an important aid in the evaluation of any cow suspected of vagal indigestion. Typically, the rumen becomes firm or doughy as the contents become stratified following anorexia. However, with vagal indigestion, obstruction to ingesta flow results in the accumulation of saliva and possibly abomasal secretions in the forestomachs, giving the impression of a fluid or "splashy" consistency when the rumen is ballotted. Thus, the determination of rumen consistency is a key point in the physical examination of a patient suspected of vagal indigestion. Determination of rumen consistency and the assessment of rumen size will also assist in the evaluation of the acid-base and electrolyte status (Table 22–1).

Palpation of the rumen in the upper left paralumbar fossa may reveal a mild to moderate accumulation of gas. The free-gas bloat is easily removed by the passage of a stomach tube, but recurs within several hours. The presence of the free-gas bloat for several days easily differentiates it from frothy bloat.[121] The degree and severity of bloat do not seem to be related to the type of vagal indigestion with one exception. If the rumen and abdomen are distended primarily owing to gas accumulation in the rumen without retention of fluid ingesta, then type I vagal indigestion, "failure of eructation," should be suspected. The other forms of vagal indigestion are accompanied with excessive fluid, with or without gas, in the rumen. Occasionally, deep palpation in the anterior to mid-lower right quadrant will reveal a heavy mass (abomasum).

Table 22–1. Clinical guide for predicting the acid-base status of a bovine patient, 500 kg (1100 lb). The guide is based on the slightest detectable change in hydration, 1+, and the most severe, 4+

Clinical Signs*	Skin Turgor Dehydration†	Base Excess (mEq/L)*	Estimated Serum Bicarbonate (mEq/L)	Liters of Fluid to Correct Deficit‡
Fluid distended rumen—very sparse feces	4+	+20	50	60
"Splashy" rumen—sparse feces	3+	+15	45	45
Moderate distention—sparse feces	2+	+10	40	35
Doughy rumen—firm feces	1+	+ 5	35	25
NORMAL	NORMAL	± 3	25±5	0
Slight diarrhea	1+	− 5	20	25
Mild diarrhea	2+	−10	15	35
Moderate diarrhea—acute	3+	−15	10	45
Severe diarrhea—profuse, acute	4+	−20	5	60

*The correlating clinical sign for the prediction of alkalosis is abdominal distention; and for acidosis, it is the appearance of a dehydrated cow with a contracted ("tucked-up," gaunt) abdomen.
†The hydration status is based on the combination of lack of skin turgor in the mid-neck area and the retraction of the eye in the socket.
‡The estimated amount of fluid to correct the immediate deficit, not the amount necessary for maintenance.

Experience in this part of the physical examination is necessary to detect a massively distended, heavy abomasum. The tense body wall or gravid uterus makes this subjective evaluation difficult. However, if the abomasum can be palpated, then type III vagal indigestion is confirmed.

Auscultation of the rumen may detect no rumen contractions or excessive contractions (4 per minute). Extreme care must be used to assess rumen motility in those cattle with a distended rumen, where the liquid nature of the rumen contents produces little sound during a ruminal contraction. Palpation of the rumen may be a better technique to detect rumen motility in these cases. The absence of rumen motility often signifies a poor prognosis, as it is usually associated with more extensive reticular adhesions to the point of diffuse peritonitis. Simultaneous auscultation-percussion of the rumen will occasionally detect a ping or "tinkle" sound typical of a left abomasal displacement (LDA). However, if the size of the gas-filled viscus is critically evaluated, it will be too large for an LDA and the size and shape is more compatible with a rumen "ping." Rumen pings occur most often when associated with excessive fluid in the rumen or with minimal distention resulting from gas. Obvious cases of bloat rarely are associated with a ping or "tinkle" sound. Rectal examination is an important adjunct to any physical examination and, in animals with suspected vagal indigestion, the ventral sac of the rumen becomes disproportionately distended compared to the dorsal sac, and forms an "L" shape (Fig. 22–7). In advanced vagal indigestion the ventral sac may occupy 75% of the abdominal cavity (gas may then accumulate in the right side of the ventral sac to produce a ping sound), detected by simultaneous auscultation-percussion of the right abdominal wall.

In cases of advanced pregnancy, rectal examination is of little value as an aid in diagnosis as the enlarged uterus precludes accurate assessment of the rumen size. Only rarely can the distended impacted abomasum or omasum be palpated during a rectal examination, but if detected will confirm a diagnosis of abomasal impaction. If the omasum is palpated during a rectal exam, then liver disease should be suspected such as hepatic abscess or fibrosis.[123] The enlarged liver displaces the omasum caudally in the abdomen enabling palpation. Evidence of abdominal pain in cases of vagal indigestion is often difficult to assess as the cow may be depressed.[124] A carefully done Williams' reticular grunt test may occasionally give evidence of localized pain in the xiphoid region. The withers pinch test may also indicate pain in the anterior abdomen, but neither test will be strongly positive. Acute pain may be best elicited during the initial phase of foreign body penetration, whereas a dull diffuse pain or no detectable pain is likely to prevail during the later stages when the signs of vagal indigestion are obvious.

Laboratory Evaluation

The single most rewarding laboratory determination is the serum or plasma chloride determination. Cattle with a distended rumen and normal plasma chloride do not have abomasal reflux (Fig. 22–8), which implies the lesion is in the omasal canal or reticulum; whereas hypochloremia (< 85 mEq/L) is evidence of abomasal reflux from an abomasal impaction or stasis of the forestomachs. Cattle with abomasal impaction occasionally have a severe metabolic alkalosis with a plasma chloride of 50 mEq/L or less. Although very low plasma chloride values (> 50 mEq/L) suggest a grave prognosis, cattle may survive if treated vigorously.

Hypokalemia commonly accompanies the hypochloremia.[125] The normal plasma potassium is 4.0 to 5.0 mEq/L, which decreases to 2.0 mEq/L or less and necessitates vigorous potassium supplementation. Hypokalemia results from anorexia and a decreased intake of forage rich in potassium (a typical adult herbivore ingests 3000 to 6000 mEq/K^+/day), coupled with continued renal loss of potassium. The renal excretion decreases, but not in proportion to the decreased potassium intake. Some potassium is shifted intracellularly as a result of the alkalosis with a further net decrease in the plasma K^+ concentration. Concurrent with the hypokalemia, paradoxic aciduria is often present. The sodium reabsorption in the proximal convo-

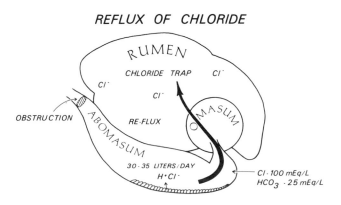

Figure 22–8. Diagram of abomasal reflux of chloride-rich fluid into the rumen. During most obstructive diseases the rumen acts as a chloride trap.

luted tubule must be balanced electrically and, as a result, H^+ is exchanged for the Na^+ resulting in aciduria in the face of a metabolic alkalosis.[126,127]

An assessment of abomasal reflux can also be established by determining rumen chloride concentration, as reflux causes the rumen chloride concentration to increase above 50 to 70 mEq/L.

Dehydration often results in prerenal azotemia with increased concentration of BUN and creatinine. The BUN rarely exceeds 80 mg/dl and the creatinine rarely exceeds 8 or 9 mg/dl in prerenal azotemia. Similarly, the packed cell volume (PCV) and total plasma proteins (TPP) are elevated as a reflection of dehydration. If vagal indigestion is associated with a chronic inflammatory process, such as an abscess, the TPP may be disproportionately elevated as a reflection of chronic antigenic stimulation and hypergammaglobulinemia. The PCV may be decreased ($< 30\%$) as a reflection of bone marrow depression-anemia of chronic disease.

The leukogram in cattle with vagal indigestion will reflect the lesions causing the problem. A lymphocytosis suggests lymphosarcoma; a reversal of the neutrophil/lymphocyte ratio suggests chronic inflammation; a leukocytosis suggests a subacute response to inflammation; and a leukopenia may herald the development of an overwhelming peritonitis.

A moderate hypocalcemia (6 to 8 mg/dl) often accompanies any type of indigestion. It may occasionally be sufficiently low to result in recumbency resembling milk fever. The blood glucose is variable, tending to be decreased (< 50 mg/dl) in mild, early cases while in advanced cases it may be greatly elevated to over 200 mg/dl. The hyperglycemic response is characteristic of ruminants with any severe, life-threatening disease and is commonly present in vagal indigestion.[124]

Pathophysiology

The pathophysiology of chronic indigestion represents a collection of several distinct disease entities in cattle, all characterized by disturbances of ingesta transit. The specific site of the lesion will determine the type of clinical signs exhibited. Most commonly, chronic indigestion is a sequel to traumatic reticuloperitonitis. Extensive controversy exists in the literature about the role of the vagus nerve in the pathogenesis of "vagal" indigestion. The question remains unanswered today, but evidence is accumulating to suggest that vagal neuritis or injury to the vagal nerve is a minor factor in the development of vagal indigestion.

The cause of chronic free-gas bloat may be associated with esophageal obstruction due to foreign bodies such as potatoes, tubers, apples or pears. Less commonly, extraesophageal compression such as lymphosarcoma, thyroid tumors or, rarely, chronic mediastinal inflammatory process, tuberculosis or lung abscess will be the cause of bloat.[128]

The cause of simple failure of eructation is most often associated with an inflammatory lesion around the vagus nerve (i.e., chronic pneumonia) or localized peritonitis in the left ventral wall of the reticulum which results in adhesions and pain interfering with cardia clearing. Normally, eructation occurs during the secondary ruminal contraction; but if the cardia is partially flooded with fluid, eructation proceeds more slowly and chronic free-gas bloat may develop.

Omasal transport failure may result from a number of causes, all of which prevent or inhibit the transport of ingesta from the reticulum through the omasal canal into the abomasum. The disease processes which impair this normal function lead to an organic or functional obstruction. A postparturient cow may eat the placenta and obstruct the omasal canal. Space-occupying lesions include lymphosarcoma, papilloma, squamous cell carcinoma, or a large ulcer (infarct) in the area.[129] Adhesions between the reticulum and diaphragm anterior to the omasum are the most common cause of omasal transport failure. Adhesions interfere with normal omasal function and cause omasal atony and the failure of omasal transport. These adhesions may include abscesses up to 35 cm in diameter. Abscesses can usually be palpated across the wall of the reticulum through a rumenotomy incision. Omasal canal atony is documented by palpation during a rumenotomy and by finding the omasal orifice atonic and easily distensible.

Abomasal impaction may be subdivided into two major categories. Primary impaction is associated with restricted access to water and/or may appear where cattle are fed very dry, coarse roughage such as wheat or oat straw. These disorders may occur on a herd basis, especially in western areas of Canada or the United States where beef cattle are pastured on straw and the water supply is frozen due to cold weather. The relative lack of water and coarse roughage can cause high mortality rates in beef cattle.

Secondary abomasal impactions occur as a result of decreased motility and are often a sequel to traumatic reticuloperitonitis. Often an abscess or an area of local adhesion interferes with the normal effective abomasal motility, leading to an impaction. It may appear that the pylorus is restricting the outflow of ingesta, but documented cases of pyloric stenosis in cattle are extremely rare. Occasionally, foreign bodies may obstruct the pylorus, such as hair balls in calves and the placenta in adult cattle.

The question of vagal neuritis as a cause of failure of omasal transport or abomasal impaction is still unclear, but evidence is accumulating that vagal nerve injury is not always involved in vagal indigestion. It is the opinion of the author that failure of omasal transport and abomasal impaction are often associated with mechanically impaired motility, due to adhesions or abscesses, which are sequelae to chronic traumatic reticuloperitonitis or abomasal ulceration with localized peritonitis. When the contents of the abscess are removed, cows with failure of omasal transport often recover, suggesting pressure to be an important factor.

The vagus nerve was histologically evaluated in 29 cases of vagal indigestion and degenerative changes were demonstrated in nine.[129] Two cases had infiltrated neoplastic cells (lymphosarcoma) in the thoracic vagus, three cases resulted from damage during the twisting associated with abomasal volvulus, two cases involved adhesions, and in another two no cause for the neuritis was found. Abomasal impaction has occurred as a sequela to abomasal volvulus (torsion).[124] The impaction seems to result from the loss of normal motility following surgical correction of the volvulus. Adhesions may develop occasionally between the abomasum and omasum (the site of the twist) which mechanically interferes with motility.[124] At necropsy the abomasum is severely distended with firm, dry, coarse ingesta. The pylorus invariably appears within normal limits.

The site of the adhesions or abscess formation is consistently in the right lateral wall of the reticulum, often with minimal involvement of the diaphragm.[129] The abscesses associated with failure of omasal transport are more dorsal but still predominately involve the right wall of the reticulum and more often involve the diaphragm.

Abomasal impaction has been reported in adult sheep with parasitic lesions about the vagus nerve.[130] The abomasums were firmly distended with fibrous ingesta and in some cases no lesions were found to account for the impaction.

Partial obstruction of the forestomachs is the most difficult type of vagal indigestion to define. It seems to be more common in dairy cattle in advanced pregnancy. As the gravid uterus enlarges, it forces the abomasum further forward interfering with normal motility, especially if adhesions are present. If abomasal motility has already diminished, then a partial impaction may result. Cattle with this form of vagal indigestion may represent a combination of omasal transport failure and abomasal impaction in the early stages. However, if prolonged and progressive, it often develops into one type or the other. Some cases even with advanced ruminal distention may have marginally low plasma chlorides (80 to 95 mEq/L), which makes definitive classification difficult.

The vagus supplying the abdominal viscera is composed of approximately 90% sensory and 10% motor fibers; hence from a numeric viewpoint it is primarily sensory. The gastric centers in the brain stem are dependent on the afferent input from these sensory receptors, principally the tension receptors in the reticulorumen.[131,132] The tension receptors are primarily located on the medial wall of the reticulum on either side of the reticular groove and the anterior dorsal sac of the rumen.[133] Reflex reticulorumen contractions occur when discharge of these low-threshold tension receptors is evoked by stretching the wall. By inference, any lesion in the medial wall of the reticulum or dorsal sac of the rumen would be expected to reduce tension receptor activity and then reduce input to the gastric centers, decreasing or abolishing primary cycle contractions of the reticulorumen.

The apparent increase in rumen motility in some cases of vagal indigestion may be due to increased secondary ruminal contractions with a possible decrease in primary contractions. Experimentally, if the rumen is insufflated with gas, the frequency of secondary contractions is independent of the primary contractions and the effective stimulus for the former is increased ruminal tension. As many cows with vagal indigestion have a mild chronic free-gas bloat, this is the most logical explanation for the observed increased rumen contraction rate.

Afferent vagal and splanchnic nerve input may also reflexly inhibit reticuloruminal movements by marked distention of the reticulorumen. The marked distention excites high-threshold tension receptors in contrast to the stimulation of low-threshold tension receptors, which stimulate contractions.[134]

A rise in the intraruminal pressure triggers the reflex opening of the cardia and other events involved in eructation. However, if the cardia is flooded with fluid or foam, the reflex cardial opening does not occur. Thus, if cattle are unable to clear the cardia because of frothy bloat, extensive reticular adhesions, or malpositions (recumbency), then more gas would accumulate to the point of respiratory embarrassment and/or death. Large increases in ruminal pressure stimulate the high-tension inhibitory receptors impairing rumen motility, which occurs in cases of severe bloat and is rarely seen in advanced vagal indigestion.

Diagnosis

Early cases of vagal indigestion may be confused with abomasal displacements or traumatic reticulitis.[124] The simultaneous auscultation-percussion technique should allow the detection of most abomasal displacements. The localized pain in the xiphoid region and lack of abdominal distention characterize the cow with traumatic reticulitis.

The diagnostic rule-outs for abdominal distention would include frothy bloat and uterine enlargement (hydrops allantois or hydrops amnii), which would be best determined by rectal examination or ballottement of the abdomen to determine the presence of the fetus. Cattle with prolonged gestation or with multiple feti should be considered in the diagnostic rule-outs. Ascites would cause abdominal distention and may be due to right heart failure, vena caval thrombosis, or abdominal neoplasia such as lymphosarcoma or mesothelioma. A ruptured bladder will also present as abdominal enlargement, but occurs much more commonly in feedlot steers than in dairy cattle. Occasionally, chronic diffuse peritonitis will cause abdominal distention but the clinical course is usually of shorter duration.

Intestinal obstruction such as a small intestinal intussusception, cecal volvulus, abomasal volvulus, inguinal hernia, or fat necrosis may cause intestinal distention, but with only a mild increase in abdominal size. Other physical findings (rectal examination and percussion) easily differentiate these syndromes from vagal indigestion. Bradycardia, if present, is an important diagnostic aid to suggest vagal indigestion. Since bradycardia is an unusual clinical sign (it may also occur with botulism, milk fever, Addisonian crisis, diaphragmatic hernia and pituitary abscess), a test was devised to differentiate conduction disturbances in the vagus nerve from abnormality within the conduction system of the heart. The atropine test consists of monitoring the heart rate every 5 minutes for 20 minutes following 30 mg atropine given subcutaneously. With a 5% or less increase in heart rate, the bradycardia is attributed to intracardial lesions; with a 7 to 16% increase, vagotonic bradycardia is considered; but a greater than 16% increase in heart rate is considered diagnostic for vagal indigestion in 95% of the cases.[135] The test is not reliable, according to the author's experience.

Treatment

The treatment for chronic free-gas bloat is relatively simple: the establishment of a rumen fistula. A rumenostomy can be performed by suturing the rumen to the body wall or by the use of a commercially available rumen trocar (Buff's screw trocar) (see Fig. 22–1). With a small 1- to 3-cm rumen fistula, the gases produced by fermentation can be expelled. The appetite returns, and as the omasal function is normal, ingesta will pass down the tract unimpeded, allowing return of the animal to the herd as a productive unit. In time (2 to 6 months), the fistula will granulate closed. Failure of eructation, be it due to adhesions of the reticulum or to an inflammatory lesion associated with a vagus nerve, is potentially reversible. If the lesion heals, the cow regains the ability to eructate normally in some cases. Contrary to popular opinion, antiferments such as turpentine or other noxious liquids containing turpentine are of no value in the prevention and/or treatment of free-gas bloat. The concentration of these materials necessary to inhibit gas formation by the rumen microflora is large and would cause death of most microflora prior to decreasing rumen gas production. Therefore, their use should not be encouraged in free-gas bloat but reserved for frothy bloat where they are effective as surface tension reducing agents.

The initial therapy in early cases of failure of omasal transport, abomasal impaction or partial obstruction would include ruminatorics and cathartics to promote gastrointestinal tract evacuation, calcium gluconate subcutaneously to maintain normocalcemia, and other supportive care. It is recognized that many so-called ruminatorics or parasympathomimetics do little to promote effective rumen contractions, but do promote catharsis, which is a desired effect. Some cattle will respond to this symptomatic therapy while others will require surgical intervention. Those cattle in advanced pregnancy will often benefit from a therapeutic abortion. Economics will dictate in what manner the cow will be treated, if at all. Especially important are the normal water supply, feed, and exercise. Exercise, even if forced, tends to enhance colonic evacuation and should be considered in vagal indigestion.

The treatment of failure of omasal transport is primarily surgical and usually includes a rumenotomy to remove any foreign bodies and to localize any foreign object which may be occluding the omasal canal, such as a placenta or papilloma. If a neoplasm is present, a needle biopsy may be obtained to make a definitive diagnosis, and then euthanasia recommended if confirmed. If a mass palpated between the reticulum and diaphragm is ascertained to be an abscess, it should be drained. The abscess can be drained via a needle suction apparatus where the pus is removed via a long tube through the rumenotomy incision. If the reticular wall is firmly adhered to the abscess, an incision can be made through the reticular wall directly into the abscess allowing purulent material to spew forth into the lumen of the reticulum. A certain degree of courage is needed to make the incision for fear of causing a diffuse peritonitis. It is occasionally advantageous to insert a 20 to 30 cm long, 8-gauge needle percutaneously through the body wall directly into the abscess and obtain drainage in this manner. On occasion, the abscess can be surgically extirpated via a paramedian incision if it is loosely attached to surrounding tissues.

Other supportive therapy considered of value for failure of omasal transport includes a stomach tube through the nasal passage down the esophageal groove and directly into the abomasum. In this way, gruel can be pumped through the nasogastric tube several times daily. As the abomasum and small intestine function normally, the gruel can be digested and help meet the metabolic requirements. If the tube is placed in the rumen, it would cause more ruminal distention and bloat adding to the severity of the problem. Other supportive therapy would include systemic antibiotic to control the localized peritonitis. The cathartics promote gastrointestinal evacuation, while subcutaneous calcium gluconate maintains normal plasma calcium concentrations.

Abomasal impaction requires vigorous therapy if it is to be treated at all. The owner should be made aware of the poor prognosis associated with this form of the disease. If the cow is not valuable, salvage is recommended. If the cow is valuable and worthy of therapy despite the poor prognosis, oral cathartics such as magnesium hydroxide and other commercially available laxatives are indicated in 0.5 to 1.0 kg amounts/day. Subcutaneous calcium gluconate to correct the mild hypocalcemia will help to increase the abomasal motility. Intravenous fluids are also very important to correct the metabolic alkalosis and hypokalemia that is usually present. Once the acid-base and electrolyte status is corrected, a rumenotomy may be indicated. If the abomasum is only partially impacted, dioctyl sodium sulfosuccinate (DDS) or magnesium sulfate may be infused directly into the abomasum. The abomasum is then massaged through the ruminal wall. In mild cases, this form of therapy seems to be effective. If an abscess is present between the rumen, reticulum, and diaphragm, and firmly adhered to the reticulum, it may be incised and the purulent contents drained into the reticulorumen. If not, it may be advantageous to drain the abscess percutaneously.

Abomasotomy is only used as a last alternative as it is usually not beneficial to the patient, in that most surgery will promote further adhesions in the fundic area and further diminish abomasal motility. It is best to enhance motility by extra-abomasal means, rather than directly removing the contents from the abomasum itself. It is possible to remove substantial abomasal contents through the omasal orifice during rumenotomy and not produce further adhesions.

Only rarely is there any evidence of a foreign body obstructing the pylorous. The use of the pyloromyotomy or the Heller-Paul procedure to correct pyloric stenosis in cattle is usually not effective.

Prognosis

The owner should be made aware that a rumen fistula will allow foul gas to escape from the rumen into the environment where cows are being milked and may cause "off-flavored" milk. Occasionally, spillage of rumen contents from the fistula may predispose to local peritonitis. However, adequate surgical technique carries a minimal risk of peritonitis. Overall, the success rate of rumenostomy for correction of simple failure of eructation is about 95% successful, i.e., an excellent prognosis. In feedlot cattle the prognosis is less favorable if a chronic respiratory disorder is the predisposing problem. Even with correction of the bloat, the animal may fail to thrive. Prognosis for life with omasal transport failure is guarded. A more definitive prognosis can be made at the time of surgical intervention. A neoplasm such as lymphosarcoma warrants a hopeless prognosis, whereas a pedunculated papilloma (wart) offers a good prognosis. An abscess between the omasum and diaphragm should warrant a fair prognosis, but a placenta causing the obstruction would bear a very good prognosis. In cases of abscesses or adhesions between the omasum, diaphragm, and reticulum, the prognosis is approximately 50 to 70% for survival depending on the size, extent of adhesions to the reticulum and, most important, whether its contents can be drained without causing diffuse peritonitis. The prognosis for life in this situation depends upon the stage of gestation. The closer to parturition, the better the prognosis. The loss of the fetus should allow improvement in abomasal motility and may improve the prognosis.

ABOMASAL DISPLACEMENTS: (LEFT, RIGHT OR VOLVULUS)

The abomasum of the average adult dairy cow is a sac-like elongated organ lying on the lower right quadrant of the abdominal cavity extending from its omasal attachment to the area of the tenth or eleventh rib where it is continued by the ascending duodenum.[136] Anteriorly it is firmly attached to the omasum, but the body of the abomasum is loosely suspended by the greater and lesser omenta which allow it to move to the left or distend to the right (displaced abomasum) or to rotate on its mesenteric axis to become incarcerated (abomasal volvulus, AV). The abomasum is truly a wandering organ and can move from its normal position to become a left-displaced abomasum (LDA), or transpose to the right, a right-displaced abomasum (RDA), in a matter of 2 to 3 hours. If the distention is severe and conditions allow, an abomasal volvulus (torsion) may result from an RDA.[137]

History

The clinical history is typical of cattle with ketosis. The appetite is capricious for grain and silage, but roughage consumption is variable to nearly normal. The milk production is moderately decreased (10 to 30%) and the owner asks for veterinary assistance since there does not seem to be an obvious reason for the decreased production. Approximately 40% of the cows with displaced abomasums (DA) have concurrent diseases such as retained placenta, metritis, or mastitis.[138]

Abomasal displacements occur at any time during the gestation period, including the dry period prior to calving; but approximately 80% of DA occur within 1 month of parturition and have been reported in bulls, calves, and sheep.[138,139,140] No breed predilection is apparent.[141] Older cattle (5 to 8 years) are more predisposed to LDA and RDA than young cattle (2 to 4 years).[141,142]

Abomasal disorders in general and DA in particular occur most commonly in high-producing dairy herds and in herds fed ad libitum corn silage and high moisture corn.[141]

Most cattle with abomasal displacements have a gradual decrease in milk production (3 to 7 lb per milking) in contrast to cattle with acute traumatic reticulitis (reticuloperitonitis), in which the milk

production drops approximately 50% from one milking to the next.[143] The course of the disease (LDA) is generally nonprogressive following the initial fall in milk production and decrease in appetite.[144] Occasionally recovery is spontaneous, as reflected in the return to normal appetite and milk production. This relapsing pattern is typical of many cows with recurrent DA. The history for RDA is identical to LDA except a higher percentage of RDA occurs postpartum, whereas LDA's more often occur prior to parturition.

Most cases of abomasal volvulus (AV) occur in the early postpartum period. They are characterized by an abrupt decrease (75% in 24 hours) in milk production, which contrasts to the gradual drop in milk production as occurs with LDA and RDA. The capricious appetite of LDA and RDA contrasts with the nearly complete anorexia in cattle with abomasal volvulus (torsion). The cow with AV will appear seriously ill to the owner, as evidenced by sunken eyes, mild diarrhea, abdominal distention, kicking at the abdomen, and a "slack" udder. Statistically, 25 clinical cases of LDA occur for every four or five RDA and one AV.[141,143]

Physical Examination

The temperature, pulse, and respiratory rate are usually in the normal range in the absence of concurrent diseases.

Palpation in the left paralumbar fossa may reveal a "nothingness" (void) between the body wall and the rumen, and occasionally (20% of cases), one may palpate the abomasum in the upper left paralumbar fossa immediately behind the last rib.[145]

Rumen contractions are often decreased in frequency and amplitude. Occasionally one can auscult the heartbeat over the rumen in the left paralumbar fossa. The heartbeat detected upon auscultation of the rumen is typically present with ketosis, but can be heard in many digestive diseases.

Mild abdominal pain or discomfort may be manifested by shifting weight from one leg to another (treading). The treading may occasionally be correlated with rumen contractions against a distended abomasum. The manifestations of abdominal discomfort are more fully appreciated by knowing the extent of rearrangement of abdominal viscera that may occur.[136]

The feces are sparse and different from those of herdmates on the same feed. The fecal consistency varies from diarrhea (20 to 40%), to constipation (25%), to normal (30%),[145] or putty-like or pasty in more chronic cases. Undigested hay fibers are often noted in the feces of cattle with chronic DA and diseases of the omasum.

Ketonuria (70%) and ketolactia are often present at moderate concentrations 2+/4.[145] If the owner or veterinarian has a good olfactory sense, the characteristic "ketotic" odor may be detected on the breath or from the milk.

Rectal palpation may reveal the rumen to be more medial than usual. Only rarely will an LDA be palpated during a rectal examination.

Auscultation over the upper left rib cage may reveal pinging sounds ("like a penny in a well"). These sounds are thought to be due to gas bubbling through the liquid ingesta of the displaced abomasum, and because of that are not a constant finding.

Simultaneous auscultation-percussion (snap-finger technique) to detect a gas-filled viscus is the most definitive clinical procedure for the diagnosis of abomasal displacement. If an LDA is suspected, one should percuss (snap-finger technique) from the sixth costochondral junction (point of elbow) to the upper portion of the paralumbar fossa, listening carefully for the pinging sounds (Fig. 22–9). These sounds are nearly diagnostic, but may occur with a fluid "splashy" rumen or with pneumoperitoneum. The "ping" area with DA is oval in outline and is smaller than the area of the rumen. Pneumoperitoneum will be associated with a ping on both sides of the body and extends caudally to the pelvic inlet area and may be detected dorsally over the lumbar region (Fig. 22–10).

The clinical signs of uncomplicated RDA are very similar to LDA except for the anatomic differences from the left to right sides. Rectal palpation may reveal a gas-distended viscus in the upper right quadrant. A cleft can be palpated on the medial

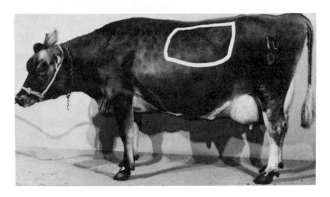

Figure 22–10. Outline of an area typically associated with pneumoperitoneum or rumen resonance. A rectal examination will differentiate between the two conditions.

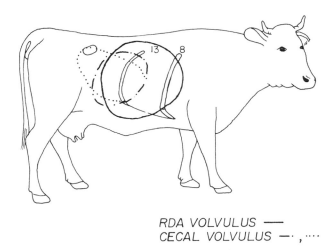

RDA VOLVULUS ———
CECAL VOLVULUS —·— , ·····

Figure 22–11. The encircled areas represent the sites of resonance associated with an abomasal volvulus or a cecal volvulus. Note the areas of overlap, although the cecum often extends more caudally than does the abomasum.

aspect of the abomasum during rectal examination. This cleft is formed by the pyloric portion folding over the abomasal fundus, as the pylorus is uppermost and folds forward toward the shoulder.

Auscultation over the last portion of the right rib cage will reveal pinging sounds (Fig. 22–11). The ping-pitch or resonance alone is not pathognomonic of RDA but, coupled with an outline of the anatomic location and rectal examinations, is diagnostic. Ballottement of the abdomen below the right costochondral junction (ventrolaterally) often elicits the splashing of gas and fluid in RDA. The Liptak test involves insertion of the needle through the body wall into a gas-filled viscus. The pH of the fluid thus obtained is measured by pH sensitive paper.* If the pH is 1 to 3, then an abomasal source

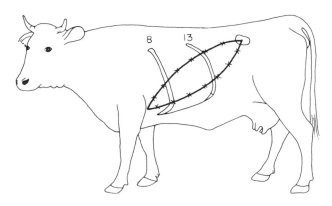

Figure 22–9. Outline of the area where one should use the snap-finger technique to determine the presence of a gas-filled viscus. Once a viscus is localized by noting a "ping," its size should be determined.

---

*EM Laboratories, Inc., 500 Executive Blvd., Elmsford, New York 10523.

should be suspected, but if it is 5 to 7, then rumen juice or blood has been aspirated. The procedure is relatively safe, but it is not always possible to obtain fluid.

Cows with abomasal volvulus (AV) appear more depressed in contrast to cattle with LDA or RDA where the attitude is brighter and the cows are more alert, except in long-standing cases. The cow with AV may grunt as if in pain, which rarely occurs with DA. Cows with AV usually have a fetid, watery diarrhea, presumably due to the toxic state of the animal and partial intestinal obstruction.

The upper right abdominal quadrant appears distended and the abomasum can be palpated through the flank behind the thirteenth rib.[146] It is nearly always possible to palpate the abomasum via rectal examination in these cases. In simple RDA the abomasum is palpated only occasionally per rectum.

The pulse rate is often above 100 per minute in cases of AV, while with RDA the pulse remains in the high normal range (75 to 80). The size of the gas-filled viscus in AV is characterically large and extends from the paralumbar fossa forward to the eighth rib (30 to 50 cm diameter) (Fig. 22–11).

In summary, the severity and acuteness of the onset of clinical signs, especially the rapid pulse and the acute decrease in milk production, help to differentiate AV from right abomasal displacement (in the absence of other diseases).

Laboratory Evaluation

Most cattle with abomasal disease (obstruction) typically develop a compensated metabolic hypochloremic, hypokalemic alkalosis (Table 22–2).[125] The severity of the hypochloremia varies proportionately with the degree of obstruction. The chloride continues to be secreted into the abomasum and, with obstructed pyloric flow, is refluxed through the omasal canal and sequestered in the rumen. The rumen then acts as a huge chloride trap which contributes to the plasma hypochloremia (see Fig. 22–8). The metabolic alkalosis results from compensation for the hypochloremia.

The hypokalemia with abomasal disease is associated with several factors: (1) decreased intake of potassium due to anorexia associated with the displacement, (2) potassium shift into the cell during alkalosis to permit hydrogen exchange, and (3) the renal excretion of potassium, which continues during a period of decreased oral intake and, thus, represents a net loss from the body.

Dehydration occurs simultaneously with the alkalosis. This is reflected in an elevated packed cell volume (normal is 30 to 33%; increased to 40 or 45%) and total plasma proteins (normal 6.5 to 7.5 g/dl; increased to 8.0 g/dl). The BUN may increase as a reflection of decreased glomerular filtration rate.

A mild to moderate hypoglycemia may occur and

Table 22–2. The plasma electrolytes of patients with obstructive gastrointestinal diseases compared to the composition of commonly available fluids for large animals

Patient	No. of Cases	Na$^+$*	K$^+$*	CL$^-$*	HCO$_3^-$*
Left abomasal displacement	75	137±0.6	3.5±0.1	86 ±4.0	27±0.7
Right abomasal displacement	18	133±1.0	2.9±0.2	81 ±3.0	34±2.5
Abomasal impaction	12	136±1.2	3.3±0.2	86 ±3.7	38±3.0
Intussusception	5	134±2.4	3.3±0.4	86.4±4.4	35±4.4
Cecal volvulus	4	134±2.1	3.1±0.2	91 ±3.0	32±2.4
Normal values	—	139±2	4.0±0.5	103 ±4.0	25±5.0
Abomasal volvulus	Typical case	140	2.0	65	55
Fluids					
Lactated Ringer's solution		130	4.0	111	27 (lactate)
Isotonic sodium chloride		154	—	154	—
(4 g potassium chloride and 5 g sodium chloride/L)		85	56	141	—
(4 g ammonium chloride and 5 g potassium chloride/L)		—	75	150	−(75)
1.3% (isotonic) sodium bicarbonate		156	—	—	156
5% sodium bicarbonate (50 g/L)		600	—	—	600
Lactated Ringer's and 5 g NaHCO$_3$/L		190	4.0	111	60+(27) lactate
6% dextrose (isotonic)		—	—	—	—

*Expressed as mEq/L

is often related to the severity of the ketosis. The normal plasma glucose in dairy cows is 60± 5 mg/dl. Many cows develop mild hypoglycemia (40 to 50 mg/dl), while some cows with AV develop hyperglycemia (> 100 mg/dl). The hyperglycemia is presumably due to stress reactions, i.e., epinephrine and corticosteroid release. A mild hypocalcemia (calcium 6.0 to 8.5 mg/dl) occurs with many digestive diseases, and abomasal disorders are no exception. See Indigestion for further discussion.

Paradoxical aciduria is a common finding with DA and occurs as a result of excretion of hydrogen ions (loss) and retention of sodium in the face of hypokalemia.[126,127] Aciduria is more common in chronic displacements compared to recent DA. This temporal difference may represent the catabolic state where the anorectic ruminant more closely represents the carnivore than the ruminant in the metabolic sense. The paradoxical aciduria is not constant and in some cases may not be dependent on hypokalemia; but in any event, the urine pH should not be used as an index of the animal's acid-base status.[126]

Pathophysiology

Abomasal displacements were reported as early as 1898[147] but not frequently until the middle of the 20th century.[148–152] Since that time they have been reported with increased frequency in countries with intensive dairy farming.

Abomasal displacements were first described in the United States in 1954[153] during standing laparotomies in dairy cattle. The DA were related to advanced pregnancy and to the extraomental position of the uterus.[153,154]

Strictures of the duodenum were associated with RDA[155,156] and sand (geosediment) with right abomasal displacements, but forced feeding of large amounts of sediment (sand) did not cause right abomasal displacements.[157] During parturition, the pregnant uterus may displace the rumen dorsally and allow the abomasum to move to the left.[150,158] Localized peritonitis,[159] ascites,[160] and inappropriate transportation of cattle[161] have all been suggested as etiologic factors in abomasal displacements.

Inappropriate transportation of cattle as a predisposing cause of LDA was noted when cattle were transported in a truck from a dry barn to a milking barn. At their destination, the cows jumped from the back end of the truck to the ground. Subsequently, there was a high incidence of LDA. Following this incident, cows were walked down a ramp from the back of a truck to the ground and the LDA incidence decreased remarkably.[161]

Thus, the pathogenesis of DA in dairy cows appears to be multifactorial.[142,162–167] Although LDA, RDA, and AV are usually regarded as separate clinical diseases, observations that spontaneous recovery from an LDA may lead to an RDA a few hours or days later supports the concept of a common etiology.[142,168]

Most authors believe abomasal atony with increased gas production are the prime requisites for abomasal displacements.[144,158] However, until recently the genesis of the abomasal atony was only speculative.

Abomasal hypomotility associated with high-concentrate, low-roughage rations is an important factor in genesis of DA.[142,162] Inherited predisposition,[152] positional changes of intra-abdominal organs, and concurrent disease are also contributing factors.[142] The abomasal hypomotility that accompanies high concentrate feeding is related to increased VFA in the abomasal ingesta.[169] The motility of the abomasum, normally 1.2 to 2.2 contractions per minute, seems to be related to the concentration of VFA in the abomasum.

Abomasal contractions are not continuous but are cyclic. The contractions are not peristaltic but occur in two regions: the fundus and the pylorus. These contractions are increased in rate and strength during the feeding of hay and concentrates to the cow, but following concentrate feeding the rate of contractions and the strength of contractions are diminished for 1 to 2 hours. The increased abomasal VFA concentration is associated with increased concentrate feeding. Gavage of high concentrate rumen contents from one cow into the abomasum of a second cow reduced abomasal contractions.[169]

Experiments in sheep showed that intra-abomasal infusion of a 300-mM solution of either acetic, propionic, or butyric acid was associated with a marked diminution of abomasal action-potential activity and of abomasal emptying rate. Butyric acid was the most potent in causing abomasal stasis, and the obvious association of increased concentration of volatile fatty acids in the abomasum and development of abomasal atony is further substantiated.[170] However, in another experiment cows were fed various rations: an increase in VFA was found in the rumen but not in the duodenum or abomasum following concentrate feeding.[171] Similarly, an earlier experiment failed to confirm the hypothesis of increased VFA in the abomasum following concentrate ingestion.[172] Explanation in part may be due to dilution of the omasal fluid by increased gastric secretion and the rapid absorption of VFA through the abomasal mucosa.[173]

The gas released by the normal abomasum when the cow is not eating approximates 500 ml per hour and, when fed hay, increases to 800 ml per hour. When 3 lb and then 15 lb of concentrate are given, gas production increases to 1100 and 2200 ml per hour, respectively. The gas consists primarily of variable amounts of carbon dioxide, methane, and nitrogen.[169] Thus, a linear relationship exists between the amount of gas produced and the amount of concentrate fed, and a partial explanation for the demonstrated association between concentrate feeding and DA is offered.

The relationship between concentrate feeding and the development of left abomasal displacement is well illustrated where four groups of 10 to 12 cows were each fed varying amounts of silage. As the percentage of dietary concentrate increased, the number of DA also increased significantly.[162]

Hypocalcemia may also contribute to the pathogenesis of DA, as hypocalcemia decreases abomasal motility.[168,174] In one experiment, 90 cows had serum calcium concentration evaluated at 1, 3, and 5 days postpartum. A cow was considered to have an abnormal calcium value if it was less than 6.5 mg/dl. LDA's occurred in seven of 26 cows with abnormally low calcium values, whereas only one of 64 normocalcemic cows had an LDA.[174]

The seasonal occurrence of DA must be influenced by factors other than parturition since the correlation between DA and parturition is high but the calving rate does not parallel the seasonal incidence.[142,152] One possible explanation is the seasonal fluctuation in acid-base balance (base-excess). Swedish cows tend to be more alkalotic during the late winter stabling season compared to the summer season. Further experiments have shown alkalosis to impair abomasal emptying, thus providing a plausible reason for the seasonal variation of DA incidence.[168]

Abomasal emptying time ($T_{1/2}$) using ^{51}Cr is normally 11 ± 3 minutes. Cattle given atropine or those with alkalosis (B.E. + 4 to 12 mEq/L) have an emptying time ($T_{1/2}$) of 27 and 19 minutes, respectively.[168] The average seasonal difference in base-excess was 3 to 4 mEq/L, suggesting the alkalosis during the stabling period may partially explain the higher incidence in DA in this season.

The interpretation of this data may be related to the gastrointestinal transit time, where cattle in the stabled environment tend to be fed less roughage, more concentrate, and may have prolonged (slowed) transit time. Cows on pasture with a high intake of grass will have rapid transit time and thus lose more base, producing a relative acidosis compared to the alkalosis in a stabling season.

Genetic factors may be linked to the occurrence of DA and may explain the variable incidence among herds. One study gave statistical evidence of an increased incidence (1.5 times) of LDA occurring if the cows were sired by relatives of one bull compared to other bulls.[152]

Thus, a combination of management factors may be altered to prevent or at least to decrease the incidence of DA. This would include the minimizing of lead feeding, the feeding of concentrate several times a day to prevent pulse increments of VFA in the abomasum, the feeding of at least 8 lb of hay each day, and the maintenance of a normocalcemia. This may be more difficult to achieve than one can easily appreciate. It is well known that cattle at parturition have a relative hypocalcemia, even though they may not develop clinical signs of milk fever. The diet should be adjusted appropriately to prevent hypocalcemia by feeding a low calcium diet prior to parturition. This will enhance bone calcium turnover and therefore increase calcium availability to maintain the plasma calcium pool. The metabolic alkalosis should be prevented by minimizing intestinal stasis. Concurrent diseases such as metritis, mastitis, and other diseases associated with parturition, especially ketosis, may be prevented, thus minimizing the hypocalcemia that can occur with inappetence.[175] A summary of factors responsible for abomasal atony and gas production is shown in Table 22–3.

Table 22–3. Predisposing factors for displaced abomasum

	Atony	Gas
Older cows	+	−
Larger cows	+	−
Higher producing cows	+	+
Parturition	+	−
Winter and spring months	+	−
Larger amounts of grain	+	+
Larger amounts of corn silage	+	+
Mastitis, metritis, milk fever	+	−
Lead feeding	+	+
Limited roughage	+	+
Hypocalcemia (6–8 mg/dl)	+	−
Lack of exercise	+	−
Metabolic alkalosis	+	−

Diagnosis

The most important aspect in the diagnosis of abomasal displacement (LDA, RDA, and AV) is simultaneous auscultation and percussion. Once a gas-filled viscus is detected, it must be defined anatomically to ascertain its size and shape. Other causes of a ping on the left side include a gas-filled rumen or pneumoperitoneum (see Fig. 22–10). It is fairly easy to differentiate either of these two from an LDA by anatomy and by the use of rectal examination. A most difficult task clinically is to diagnose an LDA when it is not possible to hear a ping. Many clinicians feel that cattle can have LDA's when a ping cannot be ausculted. In this situation, repeated percussion and auscultation may occasionally yield a ping sound. Also, increasing the intra-abdominal pressure by holding a knee or fist in the flank while using auscultation-percussion may elicit the ping if a displacement is present. Another technique is the use of the Liptak test. The measurement of abomasal pH or pepsin activity are indications of abomasal flow rate rather than an index of abomasal disease.[176]

Another technique would be the use of peritoneoscopy-endoscopy. A small incision is made in the flank and the endoscope is inserted with direct visualization of the abomasum.[145] This technique is more for academic use than of value to the practitioner. When the diagnosis is in question and the clinical signs are fully compatible with a displacement, surgical correction may be carried out in the absence of a diagnosis of another disease. If done with the cow in the standing position, the diagnosis will be confirmed by laparotomy.

A complete examination in all cows with acetonemia, where response to therapy is poor and marginal, may reveal other diseases such as retained placenta, metritis, mastitis, traumatic reticuloperitonitis, pyelonephritis, and fatty liver; but when these diagnostic rule-outs are eliminated, one must always examine and reexamine the cow for abomasal displacement.

The definitive diagnosis of RDA and AV is more complex and involves other organs that may yield a ping sound. An atonic coiled colon is the major diagnostic rule-out as it is the most common reason for a ping on the right side of a cow. Any reason for anorexia in a cow may cause a ping originating from the coiled colon (Fig. 22–12). A ping from an RDA is usually larger and extends forward to the tenth rib, while a ping from a cecal dislocation may encompass as large an area as an RDA ping but is

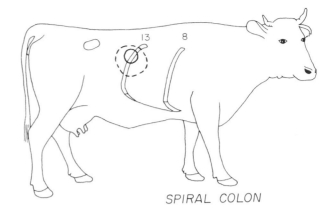

Figure 22–12. The encircled area deep to the last rib represents the site of a resonant sound ("ping") often associated with relative atony of the coiled colon.

located more caudally in the abdomen (see Fig. 22–11). Additionally, the cecum or dilated colon can be palpated during rectal examination.[177] The definite diagnosis of AV is fairly easy if the cow has the cardinal signs of an acute abdomen with a large gas-filled viscus on the right side of the abdomen (see Fig. 22–11).

Treatment

Principal approaches to therapy are either surgical or nonsurgical correction of the displaced abomasum. The major nonsurgical technique is to cast the cow on her left side, tie the feet together, and roll the cow from side to side in a 70° arc while the cow is in dorsal recumbency. This rolling motion causes the abomasum to slip over the ventral sac of the rumen to its normal position on the right side.[178] It is very important to allow the cow to recover to her feet from the left side. Some authors claim up to 70% success[179] but others feel that less than 30% respond permanently. Occasionally a cow may have an LDA and be asymptomatic, i.e., be displaced but not have decreased milk production nor inappetence; hence, all cows may not require therapy.[180,181]

Other medical therapy includes "supposed" gastrointestinal stimulants such as cascara sagrada, carbamylcholine, neostigmine, dipyrone, and oral laxatives. Most of these drugs do not have a direct effect on the abomasum, but may promote catharsis. Parasympathomimetics stimulate contractions, not normal rhythmic segmental contractions associated with normal peristalsis, but more spastic contractions of the entire organ. Cascara sagrada has minimal effect on the abomasum and its effect is directed primarily on the colon. Another therapeutic regime includes ½ kg of coffee in warm water given orally. Its mechanism of action is unknown.

Surgical correction may be carried out by at least five major approaches:[182]

1. When using the right flank omentopexy technique, the abomasal gas is removed, the abomasum is repositioned in its normal position, and is then anchored by suturing the omentum to the right abdominal wall.[183] The risk of peritonitis from puncturing the abomasum is minimal and the time spent in surgery (cow in standing position) is minimal (45 minutes).

2. The left flank abomasopexy is also done in the standing position. Suture material is anchored to the greater curvature of the abomasum or adjacent to the greater omentum and, via long needles, suture material is pulled through the abdominal wall to the right paramedian position. This requires a "long-armed" individual to push the abomasum back into its normal position and a second person to tie the sutures outside the cow.

3. Right paramedian abomasopexy provides the most secure fixation. It is more difficult as the cow is cast in a dorsal recumbent position and provides greater opportunity for inhalation pneumonia.

4. An alternative but less commonly used surgical procedure is the bilateral flank approach. One operator forces the abomasum ventrally, while the second surgeon (right flank) pulls on the omentum to return it to the normal position on the ventral abdomen.[136] An omentopexy is then utilized to fix the abomasum, preventing recurrence of the displacement.

5. The most recent surgical approach has been the percutaneous abomasopexy by the ventral paramedian approach.[182] This procedure does not require an open incision, can be done very quickly (15 to 20 minutes), and is less expensive for the owner. The cow is quickly cast in dorsal recumbency where it is extremely important to auscultate the abomasal ping to ascertain its normal position underneath the right xiphoid area. Once the abomasum has been located, a large (12 to 14 cm) ⅜-curved needle with nylon suture material is passed through the abdominal wall directly into the abomasal lumen and secured. The most critical part of this procedure is to make sure the abomasum is in the normal position. Some authors claim 95% success using this technique.[182]

Each surgical technique has a high rate of success ranging from 75% to 95% depending upon the report.[184-189] It is the impression of this author that whichever approach is utilized, one may achieve a high rate (> 90%) of success. The most important consideration is the use of one technique and its consistent use, so the surgeon is fully aware of all aspects of the approach.

The only satisfactory treatment for an abomasal volvulus is surgical intervention or immediate salvage at slaughter. These alternatives should be made known to the owner as soon as the diagnosis is confirmed. If the cow is valuable enough to justify surgical intervention, it must be done with dispatch. The choice of surgical approach, standing right flank laparotomy or right paramedian celiotomy, is left to the surgeon. Any approach may result in correction of the problem with an equal degree of success, provided the surgeon is experienced.

Most frequently, the direction of rotation in AV is counter clockwise viewed from behind the cow and involves both the omasum and abomasum. Some authors report greater success if an abomasotomy is not done prior to correction of the twist.[186] The gas is removed via a 13-gauge needle with tubing attached and then the twist is corrected. The sequestered chloride and electrolytes are then available for absorption from the small intestine. Fourteen of 20 cases (70%) recovered from surgery and were discharged following the right standing flank technique of surgical correction.[186]

A most important aspect of correction of AV is the correction of the massive fluid and electrolyte imbalance (usually a metabolic alkalosis and hypochloremia).[190] Table 22–2 indicates the severity of the problem. Several choices of fluid therapy may be utilized to correct abomasal volvulus. Enriched potassium solutions are indicated and are usually safe up to 40 mEq/L when given intravenously. Excessive potassium may be cardiotoxic. Potassium chloride orally (60 to 80 g two or three times daily) will also aid in the restoration of body potassium. Cattle should be provided free access to block salt. The extent of oral and intravenous therapy should be evaluated with each individual animal. Severely dehydrated animals may require 40 to 80 liters of intravenous fluids to correct the electrolyte and water imbalance.[191] Other supportive care such as subcutaneous calcium gluconate, multiple B-vitamins, repeated low doses (2 to 4 mg) of neostigmine, forced feeding of hay, and correction of any concurrent diseases should be carried out.

Prognosis

The prognosis for life and use following surgical correction for routine abomasal displacements is excellent, as 85 to 95% of these cows will respond if they do not have concurrent abdominal complications. With complications the prognosis may decrease to 40%.[192] Cattle with DA and concomitant diarrhea have a significantly poorer prognosis and a higher incidence of peritonitis.[193] The prognosis associated with AV decreases in proportion to the severity of the volvulus.[194] Those cases with a pulse > 100, chloride < 80 mEq/L, or fluid removed from the abomasum prior to untwisting the volvulus have a significantly poorer prognosis than cows without these changes.[194] Many cases of abomasal volvulus will die, not because of surgical mismanagement, but because of hemorrhagic infarction of the abomasal wall vis-a-vis thrombosis of the gastroepiploic veins. If thrombosis occurs as a sequela to the volvulus, no medical or surgical technique will correct it. Pyloromyotomy and abomasoduodenostomy have been attempted to correct the abomasal stasis that often develops in advanced cases, but to little avail.[194]

In order to prevent or minimize future occurrences the owner should be informed of all the factors involved in the pathogenesis of DA: minimizing lead feeding; feeding a complete ration instead of feeding grain in the parlor twice daily; if possible, feeding over 8 lb of hay per day; maintaining normocalcemia, if possible, by feeding a correct calcium-phosphorus amount; minimizing metabolic alkalosis (good in theory, difficult in practice); and minimizing concurrent diseases such as mastitis and metritis. These will all help decrease the incidence of DA, but will not prevent all cases.

ABOMASAL ULCERS

Four types or forms of abomasal ulcerations will be discussed, as the clinical signs are different, although the pathogenesis of the ulcer may be similar. Each of the four major types of abomasal ulcers will be discussed separately, except for pathophysiology.

Of 1535 slaughtered beef cattle, 28 (1.8%) had innocuous abomasal ulcers and in another study 1.9% had perforating lesions suggesting a prevalence of about 3.0 to 3.5% in fattened cattle.[195] Dairy cattle had an incidence of 9.1% of fatal bleeding ulcers in 141 cows sent to emergency slaughter and 1% in "normal cows" brought to slaughter.[196] Dairy calves may have a high incidence (97%) of ulcers when the abomasum is examined at slaughter.[197]

History: Type I Erosions and Ulcers

Retrospectively, this form of abomasal erosion and ulceration is easy to diagnose. Most cases are associated with or are believed to be secondary to septic diseases, such as coliform mastitis or septic metritis. The characteristic feature of the disease is the darkened, usually soft to fluid feces. However, the chief complaint by the owner is invariably the primary disease (sepsis) and the changes in the feces are of passing interest.

Clinical Signs: Type I Erosions and Ulcers

The first syndrome of abomasal ulceration is that associated with slight erosion or ulceration of the abomasum mucosa. This type of ulcer results in only mild to no clinical signs. These erosions or ulcers of the mucosa are usually multiple and manifested clinically by dark, fetid feces.[198] They usually respond to supportive therapy aimed at treatment of the primary disease associated with the abomasal ulceration. Other causes would be nitrate toxicosis, arsenic poisoning, or other caustic agents which may cause ulceration of the mucosa. Clinicians should consider abomasal ulcers in their clinical diagnosis or differential diagnosis when evaluating animals with septic diseases. The diagnosis can only be definitively made at necropsy.

History: Type II Bleeding Ulcers and Anemia

The history may vary from sudden death without clinical signs to a black tarry stool with resultant weakness due to anemia. Of 141 dairy cows with fatal bleeding abomasal ulcers, 109 did not have any illness more than 1 day prior to death.[196] One or more nonbleeding ulcers or scars from earlier healed ulcers were found in many cows suffering from bleeding ulcers. In the 141 cows with bleeding ulcers, 54 (38.3%) had only one ulcer.

In a study of 2700 cows, where the abomasums were inspected following slaughter, only a few cows had any evidence of localized peritonitis associated with perforation from a total of 250 cows with bleeding ulcers. Most of the bleeding ulcers were located in the greater curvature of the fundic area as opposed to the pyloric area. The ulcers bled from distal branches of the right or left gastroepiploic arteries. Bleeding ulcers were very uncommon in cows less than 2 years of age and significantly more common in cows over 3 years old.

Physical Examination: Type II Bleeding Ulcers and Anemia

The clinical signs in bleeding ulcers are related to the anemia, i.e., pallor of the mucous membranes, tachycardia, muscular weakness, and death if enough blood is lost. If enough time has elapsed, digested blood is present in the feces. This would be dark black pigment in contrast to hemorrhage lower in the intestinal tract, which would appear as bright red feces. Rarely a cow will "bleed out" prior to the appearance of melena, but sudden death and pale membranes may be the only sign noted by the owner or veterinarian.

Serum pepsinogen may be abnormally high or in high normal limits (normal 22.7 ± 7.4 μg/dl) in cattle with acute bleeding ulcers.[196] Leukocytosis and elevated lactic dehydrogenase may result but are very nonspecific compared to serum pepsinogen, which when elevated is indicative of damage to the gastric mucosa.[199]

Diagnosis: Type II Bleeding Ulcers and Anemia

The diagnostic rule-outs of bleeding abomasal ulcers would include blood in the digestive tract from other sources, such as a duodenal ulcer; or a neoplasm causing bleeding into the forestomachs, such as squamous cell carcinoma or, less commonly, lymphosarcoma. Another cause of blood in the digestive tract is a pulmonary abscess metastatic from a postcaval thrombosis. This type of pulmonary abscess often erodes blood vessels causing the cow to cough up blood, swallow it, and produce dark black feces and anemia in the same manner as a cow with an abomasal ulcer. Therefore, it is incumbent on the clinician in the examination of a cow with a tentative diagnosis of a bleeding abomasal ulcer to rule out a pulmonary abscess. Rarely, lesions of the larynx and oral cavity may also bleed sufficiently to cause the melena.

A major diagnostic rule-out for a bleeding abomasal ulcer would be lymphosarcoma, as it has a predilection for the uterus, heart, and abomasum. Many times, when lymphosarcoma primarily involves the abomasum, it will result in a bleeding ulcer and this may be, in fact, the chief complaint by the owner. Therefore, it is incumbent upon a veterinarian examining a cow with a bleeding ulcer to rule out lymphosarcoma as the cause of the ulcer. A hemogram may indicate an absolute lymphocytosis. Lactic dehydrogenase is of diagnostic value in cattle with leukemia or lymphosarcoma. A value of greater than 3500 bb units is diagnostic for lymphosarcoma. Other aspects of a physical examination, such as a rectal examination and palpation of the external lymph nodes (finding all of these normal), would lessen the possibility of lymphosarcoma. A bovine leukemia titer, if negative, should rule out the possibility of lymphosarcoma; but if positive, the cow may or may not have lymphosarcoma.

Treatment: Type II Bleeding Ulcers and Anemia

Bleeding abomasal ulcers are best treated by providing a nonstressful environment for the cow, with stall rest, good feed, and water. Supportive therapy may include the oral astringents, which would contain gum catechu and zinc phenylsulfate. Propantheline bromide (30 mg, 3 to 4 times per day) should dramatically decrease acid secretion and has been used successfully in cattle. If the packed cell volumes drop to 12%, blood transfusion may be in order, but the life span of transfused bovine red cells is extremely low (half-life about 48 hours on the first transfusion).[200] Thus, a blood transfusion in the treatment of any severe anemia in the cow should be regarded as emergency therapy in a life-threatening situation and not as supportive therapy only. The use of symptomatic hematinics such as oral iron and cobalt, although safe, are probably not efficacious, as these are blood-loss anemias and not iron-deficiency anemias. If the bleeding continues and there is reason to believe that lymphosarcoma is absent, exploratory laparotomy via a right paramedian incision may help in the localization of the ulcer and surgical extirpation of the defect.[201] Usually bleeding ulcers are single and not at multiple sites in the abomasum. However, in order to localize the lesion in the abomasal wall, the abomasum may have to be entered and viewed directly. Rarely can one localize the bleeding ulcer by evaluation of the serosal surface.

The prognosis for bleeding abomasal ulcers is guarded at best. Many of these may be associated with lymphosarcoma and are incurable; in many the blood loss will continue and the cows may die from exsanguination.[196]

Type III Abomasal Ulcers—Acute Circumscribed Peritonitis

In this syndrome there is a perforating abomasal ulcer with minimal bleeding which results in a localized peritonitis.

Clinical Signs: Type III Acute Circumscribed Peritonitis

The clinical signs closely resemble traumatic reticulitis (TRP). The primary differentiating feature between the acute peritonitis associated with abomasal perforation and TRP is the localization of pain. With abomasal perforation, it is on the right side of the xiphoid, in contrast to the typical case of TRP, where pain is localized on the left of the xiphoid.

Laboratory Evaluation: Type III Acute Circumscribed Peritonitis

The laboratory findings of acute circumscribed peritonitis would be very similar, if not identical, to those associated with TRP: a reversal of the neutrophil-lymphocyte ratio with a mild neutrophilia after 8 to 10 hours, increased fibrinogen, and gammaglobulin levels. If the lesion resolved with resolution toward normal, blood values would tend to return to baseline.

Diagnosis: Type III Acute Circumscribed Peritonitis

Diagnostic rule-outs would include TRP and other causes of localized peritonitis. One major differentiating feature would be the time of onset in relationship to parturition. Abomasal ulcers in general are most common in the early postpartum period;[202] however, this is not the typical time one would see an onset of traumatic reticuloperitonitis, which tends to be scattered throughout the gestation period and not closely correlated to parturition. These perforating abomasal ulcers that cause localized peritonitis rarely bleed enough to cause dark, tarry feces as is typically associated with a bleeding abomasal ulcer.

Treatment: Type III Acute Circumscribed Peritonitis

Treatment of this form of abomasal ulcer patient is similar to that for TRP.

Prognosis: Type III Acute Circumscribed Peritonitis

The prognosis for cases of perforated abomasal ulcer with local peritonitis is not good if the lesion is in the fundic portion of the abomasum, which it usually is. A perforating ulcer toward the pylorus will occasionally result in interference of normal motility of the abomasum and lead to the syndrome of abomasal impaction.

Type IV Abomasal Ulceration Resulting in Perforation with Diffuse Peritonitis

Of 1988 beef cattle necropsied, 31 (1.6%) had perforating or extensive bleeding ulcers. The incidence was higher during the winter than during other times and more often occurred during the first 45 days on full feed. They were located primarily in the pyloric region and invariably were single lesions.

Perhaps the most uncommon form of the abomasal ulceration results in a fulminant peritonitis, with death resulting 24 to 48 hours after the onset of clinical signs. The ulcer perforates the mucosa and abomasal wall spilling abomasal contents into the peritoneal cavity.[203] The diffuse peritonitis that results from ingesta spillage is impossible to treat and almost all of these cows or calves will die.[197] I am not aware of a cow surviving this form of the disease. Surgical attempts at repair have been made without success.[202] Again, if the diagnosis were made and prompt surgical correction instituted, the cow could be saved as these ulcers are usually single and could be oversewn quite easily.

Pathophysiology of Ulcers

The cause of abomasal ulcers in cattle has not been fully investigated. In man, increased gastric acid secretion is important in the pathogenesis of ulcer formation. Hyperacidity and physical stressors may operate in cattle, as in man. Lactic acidosis may be an additional factor in cattle, as the ruminal lactic acid concentration increases up to 320 mM/L and that of histamine up to 70 mg/ml of rumen ingesta.[204] Abomasal stasis facilitates histamine absorption, thus stimulating abomasal acid secretion. The excess HCl and pepsin gravitate to the greater curvature (ventral part) and the local concentration of HCl and pepsin may be ulcerogenic.

So-called "stress" factors have long been implicated in cattle as a cause of ulcers. A high stocking rate of dairy cattle per acre was shown to have a statistically significant, positive influence on incidence of ulcers.[196] Other stress factors such as recent parturition and the attainment of peak lactation may predispose to a higher incidence of ulcers in the early postpartum period.[202] One study reported 11 of 18 (60%) bleeding or perforating ulcers occurred within 1 month of parturition.[205]

Of all perforating ulcers, 58% occurred within 1 month of parturition and 25 of 30 (80%) postpartum ulcers occurred within the first 4 weeks after calving.[206,207] Additionally, transient hypocalcemia, which is more prevalent during the early postpartum period, has been associated with increased gastric acid secretion.

The volume and VFA content of the digesta reaching the abomasum have a great influence on the abomasal secretion.[208] The abomasal secretion is fairly constant in amount, as a result of continuous flow: the ingestion of low dry matter content forage (lush pastures) or high VFA feeds could damage the gastric mucosa by allowing diffusion of H^+ ions from the lumen to the tissue predisposing to ulcer formation.[196]

Under these circumstances, the stress effects could be mediated through increased ACTH and endogenous steroids which increase gastric acid secretion or through sympathetic discharge of epinephrine and norepinephrine.

Prednisone (10 mg/kg/day for 8 days) produced a significant increase in the volume and the acidity of gastric secretion in swine, but no change in pepsin secretion.[209] The peak changes occurred at 3 to 4 days with a gradual decrease to pretreatment values by the end of the treatment period.

The metabolic cellular enzymes of the gastric mucosa seem very sensitive to effects of hypovolemic shock, apparently resulting in part from the gastric mucosa's lack of glycogen and a relative inability to utilize anaerobic glycolysis as an alternate energy pathway.[210]

The major factors identified as requisites for ulcer formation in experimental animals are: (1) acid, (2) increased mucosal permeability to H^+ (induced by such agents as bile acids, aspirin, VFA), and (3) altered mucosal blood flow (secondary to shock), all necessary for the development of stress ulcers.[211] These factors may be similar to the ones which produce ulcers in cattle.

Classically, histamine effects include: (1) vasodilation, (2) hypotension, (3) stimulation of the smooth muscle of the gut and bronchi, (4) tachycardia, (5) gastric acid secretion, and (6) inhibition of uterine contraction. The first three responses are mediated through histamine H1 receptors. The last 3 effects may be antagonized by recently discovered H2 antagonists, metiamide and cimetidine, both of which significantly reduce basal acid and meal-stimulated secretion.[212]

Dairy calves tend to have a higher incidence of ulcers than any other type of animal. Similarly, calf ulcers usually have mucoraceous phycomycete hyphae present in the tissue adjacent to the defect.[213–215] The abomasal content also contained spores of mucoraceous fungi which probably were ingested by the calf and secondarily invaded the ulcer. Antibiotic treatment has been shown to enhance the growth of *Candida sp.* but the same is not true of phycomycetes. Considering the frequency of infectious bovine rhinotracheitis-associated rumenitis in calves, one might assume the erosive rumenitis as predisposing to the mycotic gastritis.[214,216,217] The disease could not be reproduced experimentally by feeding calves *Rhizopus* orally.[218]

GASTRIC ULCERS IN SWINE

Gastric ulcers occur frequently, often up to 50%, in swine[219,220] and normally occur in the higher regions of the stomach, i.e., nonacid-secreting quadrilateral area around the cardia and esophagus (nonglandular stratified squamous epithelium).

History

Sudden death with pale membranes is the most obvious form noted by the owner. Melena is next, with failure to thrive the least obvious finding noted. All breeds appear equally susceptible but barrows have a higher incidence than gilts.

The disease may be peracute, acute, subacute, chronic or subclinical. The peracute disease is often insidious, with unexpected death the result of massive hemorrhage into the stomach. This type can occur at anytime, but seemingly has a higher incidence during the last part of pregnancy or early postpartum. If pigs survive the massive hemorrhage, they become weak, dull, and depressed, refuse to eat or drink, become hypothermic, and have pallor of the mucous membranes.

Physical Examination

Swine with gastric ulcers have dyspnea and cold extremities. If forced to rise, they will have a staggering gait and then may collapse and die. Their pen may be blood covered as a result of hematemesis; if they defecate, melena should be obvious. These animals often die in 3 to 5 days following the first bleedout.

Those pigs with the subacute form have less severe hemorrhage characterized by the recurrence of melena, with intermittent periods of anorexia, constipation, decreased weight gain, and mild lethargy. Those that survive this stage may develop emaciation, become stunted, and have intermittent melena. If perforation of the stomach wall occurs, acute local or diffuse peritonitis results and death often follows.

The subclinical form of the disease occurs most commonly when the pigs do not manifest any clinical signs and the lesions are detected only at slaughter or by gastroscopy.

Laboratory Evaluation

Hematologic changes usually suggest a moderate progressive microcytic anemia. Plasma pepsinogen and plasma corticosteroid concentrations are found to be unrelated to the presence or severity of gastric lesions in swine.[209] This is unlike man, where high pepsinogen values are correlated with a higher incidence of duodenal ulcers[221] and in rats with gastric ulcers,[222,223] and abomasal ulcers in cattle.[196]

Diagnosis

The diagnosis may be difficult because of the multiplicity of clinical signs. The acute and subacute bleeding types are most easy to evaluate. A positive fecal occult blood should not be regarded as pathognomonic, as other intestinal diseases will also give positive results. Also, pigs can have massive hemorrhage from perforating ulcers, with negative fecal occult blood.

If the ulcers are not complicated by any acute infectious process, the body temperature is normal or subnormal. Hematemesis, although not common, is nearly pathognomonic of a bleeding gastric ulcer if present. Intermittent dark bowel movements with an afebrile course and evidence of anemia should elicit concern about gastric ulcers.

Treatment

Any therapy is symptomatic and should *not* be considered otherwise. A blood transfusion should be done as quickly as possible in valuable breeding animals. Fluid therapy with balanced electrolytes may be of value as adjunctive therapy to restore blood volume. Parenteral administration of iron and B-complex vitamins to promote optimal hematopoiesis is a rational approach.

Prevention

As ulceration is a stress-associated disease, all possible factors should be evaluated to minimize stress, including adequate ventilation, space, heating, humidity, and ammonia accumulation. Proper nutrition, especially vitamin E and selenium, the fiber content and particle size of the grain (smaller particles are more ulcerogenic) are all important. Added oat hulls with the diet (swine) and reduced animal density and outdoor rearing are measures which may reduce the incidence of ulcers.

PARASITIC DISEASES OF BOVINE STOMACHS

Stunted growth, weight loss, and decreased weight gain have long been the accepted classic picture associated with parasitism. However, overwhelming parasitic infestations can occur and present an entirely different picture such as anemia and severe debility and death.

Rumen Parasites

Flukes of the family Paramphistomidae are commonly found in the rumen. These parasites produce neither clinical signs nor lesions in the rumen. The immature flukes burrow into the mucosa of the small intestine and cause damage to the mucosa. Carbon tetrachloride may be effective (5 to 10 ml/500 kg) and the control is similar to fascioliasis.[10]

Abomasal Parasites

History

Most owners report weight loss, diarrhea, and generally unthrifty condition as the major complaints in cattle with parasitic gastritis. Seasonal occurrences are commonly expressed in the summer and fall months or early spring months.

Physical Examination

Anemia and bottlejaw (hypoproteinemia) are two of the outstanding findings in advanced gastric parasitism. The anemia is most severe in heavy *Haemonchus* infections. Diarrhea varies from pasty loose feces to a profuse watery consistency and is most often accompanied by heavy *Ostertagia* and *Trichostrongylus* infections. Cattle with primary *Haemonchus* infections have no diarrhea and may be constipated.

Less severe infections produce weight loss, decreased production, rough haircoats, partial anorexia, and dehydration.

Gastric *Ostertagia* infections have been divided into two phases. Type I corresponds to the classic description of parasitic gastritis, i.e., weight loss and diarrhea when young animals have recently been put out on grass. Pre-type II infections are clinically inapparent where more than 80% of the larvae are inhibited in the early fourth stage. These animals would have been first infected in late fall and have no clinical signs during the early winter months. This stage of arrested development may last from several weeks to several months.[224]

Type II infections result from the maturation, up to 6 months later, of sufficient numbers of previously inhibited larvae to cause clinical signs of parasitic gastritis. This often occurs during the time when the cattle are stabled or during the late winter months.[225]

Laboratory Evaluation

A quantitative fecal egg count is one of the most helpful aids in determining a diagnosis of parasitic gastritis. In type I, counts of over 1000 *Ostertagia* eggs per gram (epg) are found only in clinically affected animals. In type II, the fecal egg counts are of little value. Plasma pepsinogen concentration is of diagnostic value to evaluate the severity of the abomasal lesion and thus of the infection.[226]

Etiologic Factors

Haemonchus placei (large stomach worm), *Ostertagia ostertagi* (brown stomach worm) and *Trichostrongylus axei* (small stomach worm) are the most important stomach worms in cattle.[10] These parasites exist virtually wherever cattle are kept and the incidence of infection varies widely.

Although *Haemonchus* is called the large stomach worm, the adults are small (1.5 to 3.5 cm long) and not easy to see without careful inspection. Adult *Ostertagia* are about 0.75 cm long and adult *Trichostrongylus* about 0.5 cm long. The life cycles are similar with all three parasites. The first stage larvae hatch and develop to the third stage larvae within 5 days under favorable conditions. *Ostertagia* are more resistant to environmental influence than the others. Following ingestion of the infective larvae by the host, they will become adults within 21 to 25 days. *Ostertagia* burrow into the abomasal mucosa where they may stay for extended periods.[227]

Pathophysiology

These parasites are usually present as multiple infections, causing a debilitating syndrome often referred to as the "HOT" *(Haemonchus, Ostertagia, Trichostrongylus)* complex. Younger animals are seemingly more susceptible to the effects of the parasites than adult animals, but losses will occur at any age. Malnutrition, concurrent disease, and previous parasitic infections influence the host's response.

The number of parasites necessary to cause clinical disease varies, but often less than 10,000 *Haemonchus* are present. Some few animals may have upward of 300,000 in the abomasum. Approximately 40,000 to 60,000 *Ostertagia* or *Trichostrongylus* are present in clinically parasitized animals.[228] In massive infections, up to one million (usually immature) larvae may be present.

The *Haemonchus* parasites produce their clinical signs by utilizing protein and blood from the host. *Trichostrongylus* remove relatively little blood from the stomach and some blood loss may occur with *Ostertagia*. The major pathogenic effect of *Ostertagia* occurs with the emergence of the parasite from the abomasal mucosa. This process stimulates gastric hyperplasia with the formation of nodules. Simultaneously, the stomach pH increases and pepsinogen is not activated. During parasitic emergence, albumin and protein are lost into the lumen of the stomach, leading to a hypoproteinemia and bottlejaw if the loss is severe enough.

Immunity to gastric parasites exists but its effects are short lived in the case of *H. contortus*. IgA specific immunoglobulins have been detected in the abomasal mucus, but the concentration decreases rapidly when exposure to larvae ceases.[229,230]

Protective immunity develops in growing animals as a result of subclinical infections. Thus, if cattle are brought from an area of light infection to a moderately infected area, severe clinical parasitism may result since the immunity is low. The resistance in native cattle (continually exposed to parasite infection) is rarely sufficient to withstand a massive exposure.[231]

Diagnosis

Whenever a clinician is presented with an animal showing evidence of weight loss, rough haircoat, and soft, unformed feces, gastric parasitism must be considered at the top of the diagnostic rule-out list. This is especially true in young animals, as parasitism is the most common cause of these clinical signs. A presumptive diagnosis is based on the clinical signs and history concerning management and previous anthelmintic therapy. A definitive diagnosis is possible by repeated fecal egg counts or at necropsy.

Malnutrition is the major diagnostic rule-out in younger animals but can be ruled out by a good history and evaluation of the management and nutrition program. Rarely will primary malnutrition produce a severe hypoproteinemia as occurs with parasitic gastritis.

Johne's disease in adult cattle produces identical clinical signs, but most commonly only one or two animals in a group are involved with Johne's. Occasionally, Johne's and gastric parasitism may occur simultaneously.

Other diseases producing weight loss, loose feces, and a rough haircoat would include: (1) liver abscesses, (2) fat necrosis, (3) copper deficiency, (4) abdominal abscesses, (5) chronic localized peritonitis, and (6) toxicosis such as aflatoxins.

Treatment

Phenothiazine is one of the older anthelmintics and is being replaced by newer chemotherapeutic agents such as organophosphates. Thiabendazole at the rate of 50 to 100 mg/kg is one of the more widely used drugs today. It is effective against both stomach and intestinal parasites and has a wide margin of safety.[232] It is not effective for the *Ostertagia* buried in the submucosa, but at the higher dose (100 mg/kg) thiabendazole may be effective. Levamisole and tetramisole are both effective against these parasites at the rate of 8 and 15 mg/kg orally or subcutaneously.[233]

As most drugs are effective only against the adults, treatments should be repeated in 14- to 21-day intervals. All animals in a group should be treated to decrease exposure to other animals and to reduce pasture contamination.

Prevention

The most effective treatment for any disease is prevention and this is especially true for gastric parasitism. Each step in the development of parasitic gastritis must be prevented to control the problem effectively. These steps include: (1) initial exposure to a large number of infective larvae, (2) lowered resistance due to malnutrition or intercurrent disease, and (3) increased exposure to larvae to overcome the resistance developed during previous infections.

Decreased exposure to infective larvae is best accomplished by having the animals dispersed over a wide area to prevent ingestion. Increased concentration of animals under any circumstances may produce stress conditions and also predispose to concurrent diseases.

Wet areas (ponds, streams, and swamps) in the pasture should be fenced off, as these areas provide the environmental conditions conducive to larval viability. Adequate pasture forage should be available, since poor pasture growth is conducive to increased ingestion of infective larvae. Young animals develop a more severe parasitic gastritis than older animals exposed to a similar load of parasites. Separation of the two age groups is preferred. If possible, the younger animals should be placed in a relatively parasite-free area.

DIAPHRAGMATIC DEFECTS (HERNIA) IN CATTLE

Diaphragmatic defects (DD) in cattle are infrequently reported,[108,234-243] but probably occur more frequently in practice. When the disorder is encountered, surgical repair is usually unsatisfactory.[239,244]

History

Chronic free-gas bloat is the single most common sign noted by owners of cattle with diaphragmatic defects. A history of traumatic reticulitis may be present in some cattle with DD.[237] Recent parturition and subsequent weight loss with abnormal respiratory motions often precede the diagnosis of DD.[234,238] Unusual respiratory actions such as periodic breath-holding and mouth breathing occurs in some cattle. The clinical course of the disorder varies from a few weeks to a few months and is usually progressive to cachexia or to severe free-gas bloat.

Physical Examination

Chronic bloat is the dominant clinical finding (9 of 18 cases) in cattle with diaphragmatic defects (DD). Abdominal distention not related to bloat occurs in some cattle, making them resemble vagal indigestion. The appetite is at best capricious and seems related to the severity of the bloat rather than the diaphragmatic defect.

The respiratory rate may be elevated but the irregularity of the rate and change in respiratory effort are more striking than the hyperpnea. Bradycardia (pulse less than 60 per minute) occurs in approximately 50% of the animals with DD.[108] Respiratory involvement, as evidenced by the increased respiratory rate and reduced vesicular sounds over one side of the thorax (usually left), occurs in some cattle.

Auscultation over the thorax may reveal muffled heart sounds more commonly on the right side and borborygmal (peristaltic) sounds in the lower aspect of the chest. The recognition of borborygmal sounds on one side of the thorax is nearly pathognomonic for DD. A heart murmur has been detected in some cattle with DD and may be the result of cardiac compression by the reticulum. Rarely tinkling, gurgling sounds can be detected in the pericardial sac.[238] Percussion of the thorax may indicate a dullness on the affected side and a hyperresonance on the opposite side. Odontoprisis occurs commonly and is likely a nonspecific manifestation of pain.

In approximately half of the cattle, the rumen contractions are weak and slow. Increased rumen contractions ($>$ 2 per minute) occur in a minority of cases. Rumination is absent or occurs rarely. Vomition may occur in some cases.[236,243] The feces tend to be firm and dryer than normal. Elicited pain is difficult to assess at best, and most cases do not manifest positive xiphoid pain.

Laboratory Evaluation

Radiographic examination of the thorax is the most important aid in making a definitive diagnosis. Usually a defect in the outline of the diaphragmatic reflection can be demonstrated and a viscus visualized in the thorax. Exploratory laparotomy is another alternative to establish a definitive diagnosis, since it allows for both diagnosis and treatment in one procedure.

Pathophysiology

Diaphragmatic defects can occur as a result of traumatic injury, from congenital defects,[237] or as a sequel to traumatic reticulitis.[235] Cattle with congenital diaphragmatic defects usually show clinical signs prior to 1 year of age, while defects secondary to reticulitis or trauma occur in older animals (2 to 7 years). Trauma can occur at any age but pregnant animals seem to be more predisposed. Traumatic reticulitis has been the predisposing factor in the majority of the calves as evidenced by the abscesses and foreign bodies found at necropsy. The size of the diaphragmatic defect is variable but ranges from 10 to 25 cm, with the majority of the defects on the right side of the diaphragm.

The reticulum is the usual structure to pass through the diaphragm (usually to the right) and, as a result, dullness is often present on the lower right portion of the thorax.[240] The heart may be pushed to the left to an extent that its transverse diameter is decreased. The extent of reticular, abomasal, and omasal herniation through the defect not only determine the severity of signs but also the type of signs, i.e., bloat, failure of omasal transport, or a contracted abdomen (emaciation).

Diagnosis

Chronic, intermittently bloating patients should be evaluated for a diaphragmatic defect. A tentative diagnosis can be made on the basis of clinical signs but a thoracic radiograph or an exploratory laparotomy is needed to confirm the diagnosis. Laboratory procedures such as blood gases or examination of thoracic fluid may aid in the diagnosis but are rarely confirmatory.

Treatment

Surgical correction is the only effective treatment for DD. The surgical approach is difficult and the closure of the defect is nearly impossible; however, several cases have been successfully repaired both in practice[241] and in academic institutions.[237] The milder lesion of esophageal hiatal hernia may respond to conservative (nonsurgical) therapy.[237a]

Prognosis

The prognosis for recovery for diaphragmatic defects is guarded at best but must depend on the success of the surgical procedure. Defects can be repaired successfully but the congenital forms seem more prone to successful outcome than do other types.

NEOPLASIA OF THE BOVINE STOMACHS

Neoplasms of the bovine stomach occur with a wide range of clinical signs. A small benign papilloma of the esophageal groove may appear as severe free-gas bloat, while a massive involvement of the abomasum may show only mild or no clinical signs. Some tumors seem to be age related (mesothelioma in young calves), while others are not (lymphosarcoma).

History

As with neoplasia in any organ, the history and onset of clinical signs are extremely variable. Papillomas of the rumen and, specifically, of the esophageal groove will often appear as free-gas bloat. Lymphosarcoma of the forestomachs may occur in a variety of ways, including failure of omasal transport, if it occludes or blocks the omasal canal; abomasal impaction, if it interferes with motility of the abomasum; but perhaps the most common form is a bleeding abomasal ulcer. The history may include weight loss and on clinical examination melena, pale mucous membranes, lymphadenopathy, and exophthalmos.

Squamous cell carcinoma of the esophageal groove is uncommon, but when it occurs, it involves weight loss, anemia, and occasionally vagal indigestion. A high incidence of esophageal and forestomach squamous cell carcinoma has been reported in the Nosampolai Valley in Kenya.[245] Many of these cattle have bloat, dysphagia, regurgitation of food, sialosis, and polydipsia. Weight loss is gradual over the course of 6 to nine months.

Mesotheliomas are rare, but when they are present, they occur as ascites in the fetus or young calves up to 8 months of age.[246,247] The tumor arises from the mesothelial surface of the peritoneum and causes ascites by obstructing the lymphatic drainage of peritoneal fluid in the diaphragm.

Neurofibromas may cause disease of the forestomachs by interfering in normal abomasal emptying. The clinical signs are those of vagal indigestion.

Laboratory Evaluation

The most definitive means for assessment of the problem is a biopsy of the mass. A needle biopsy or excision of the mass can be taken during an exploratory laparotomy. In most instances, if a neoplasm is present, the biopsy is obtained for academic purposes rather than therapeutic reasons, as most tumors are not treated. In the case of a mesothelioma, a peritoneocentesis and cytologic evaluation will demonstrate the characteristic cells.

Pathophysiology

Neoplasms tend to produce their clinical signs by virtue of their size and mechanical interference in homeostatic processes. The esophageal papillomas interfere with eructation or with the normal flow of ingesta through the omasal canal. Mesotheliomas obstruct the normal reabsorption of peritoneal fluid in the diaphragm. Squamous cell carcinomas cause physical obstruction of ingesta flow or occasionally cause ascites in a manner similar to mesotheliomas. Lymphosarcoma often invades the abomasal wall and may interfere with the normal blood supply to the mucosa, predisposing to ulceration and bleeding. Some lymphosarcomas mechanically obstruct flow of ingesta; others remain clinically quiescent, but are found at necropsy.

Diagnosis and Prognosis

An accurate diagnosis is made only after biopsy of the mass. The differential diagnoses are variable and depend on the clinical signs presented.

The only neoplasm with a good prognosis is the papilloma which may be surgically extirpated. Malignant neoplasms are progressive and not amenable to treatment, at least on an economic basis.

Part III. Small Animal Gastric Diseases

WAYNE E. WINGFIELD

ACUTE GASTRITIS

The diagnosis of acute gastritis is often made by inference, unless made at the time of operation or necropsy. Endoscopy has provided a new dimension to the clinician's ability to view the stomach mucosa and to obtain biopsy specimens. In the absence of endoscopy or biopsy, one must rely on clinical history, a few objective physical and laboratory abnormalities, and often the patient's response to therapy.

History

The term "acute gastritis" usually refers to a short and self-limiting disorder accompanied by a history of sudden onset of vomiting. Eating of garbage, foreign material, spoiled foods, grass, toxins, bones, or iatrogenically administered drugs may cause an acute gastritis. The irritated gastric mucosa initiates the reflex act of vomiting via the medulla. Lethargy often accompanies the episode of acute gastritis. With an increased frequency of vomiting, the patient has polydypsia, which often leads to more frequent vomiting with subsequent losses of additional fluids and electrolytes.

Clinical Signs

Vomiting is the most frequent clinical sign associated with an acute gastritis, and leads to variable signs of dehydration and lethargy. Hematemesis may be seen with more severe mucosal erosions following ingestion of certain drugs, garbage, and foreign materials.

Physical Examination

Evidence of vomiting is usually seen with patients having acute gastritis. The animal may vomit during the examination which provides the best documentation. It is critical for the clinician to differentiate vomiting from regurgitation. The vomitus may be observed for its character, amount of mucus, bile, presence of foreign materials or tissue, blood, and may be cultured for the presence of infectious agents.

Dehydration of varying severity will be present depending upon the duration of the vomiting. Fluid depletion will be due to loss of gastric fluids or to reduced fluid intake. Normally, salivary and gastric secretions will be reabsorbed, but with vomiting the fluids will be lost.

With the loss of sodium, chloride, and potassium from gastric secretions in vomitus, an animal may show varying degrees of lethargy, weakness, and depression. If fever is associated with an acute vomiting syndrome, one should rule out an infectious or systemic disease. Abdominal palpation is usually unrewarding in terms of contacting the stomach because of its anatomic location; however, some discomfort may be observed when attempts are made at abdominal palpation. Abdominal splinting is often noted.

Laboratory Evaluation

When acute gastritis is suspected, only a few laboratory tests are usually evaluated. Evidence of dehydration is assessed in the light of the total plasma protein, packed cell volume, and hemoglobin values.

A complete blood count is usually normal but may show a stress leukogram. A significant alteration from normal necessitates consideration of systemic disease or a gastric disease of a more chronic nature.

A biochemical profile to include alanine amino transferase (formerly serum glutamic pyruvic transaminase—SGPT), blood urea nitrogen (BUN), glucose, serum alkaline phosphatase (SAP), total serum protein, amylase, electrolytes, and acid-base studies has been suggested.[248] This biochemical profile will provide data for its differentiation from systemic or metabolic diseases which may also present with sign of persistent vomiting.

The metabolic changes associated with acute gastritis depend upon the duration of vomiting. Hypochloremia, hyponatremia, and hypokalemia are associated with vomiting of gastric contents. The metabolic alkalosis associated with vomiting is usually mild (7.45 to 7.55) and may be complicated by acidosis secondary to dehydration and inadequate tissue perfusion,[249] which tends to lower the arterial blood pH.

The urinalysis will usually show a high specific gravity unless renal disease is present. Urine pH is often acid even in the presence of a metabolic alkalosis. Paradoxical aciduria results when the kidney tubules increase sodium reabsorption (increased aldosterone influence); increase excretion of anions such as phosphates, sulfates, and organic acids; and reabsorb bicarbonate ions to replace lost chloride ions.

In the presence of hematemesis, two urgent questions must be answered: what volume of blood has been lost to that point; and, more pertinent, what is the patient's physiologic response to the loss?[250]

Usually, the exact duration of bleeding is not known. The first laboratory reports may or may not reflect dilution from efforts at volume restoration. Additionally, anemia or polycythemia may have been present prior to the blood loss. Even with acute bleeding, it may require upward of 12 hours for significant changes in packed cell volume to be manifest. With hematemesis, serial hemoglobin or hematocrit determinations will be most useful.

Objective indirect recording of a patient's blood pressure through means of a Doppler Ultrasound, a noninvasive technique, is being more widely used in the practice of veterinary medicine. If the blood pressure, pulse rate, and respiratory rate are known, a patient's response to the loss of blood can be monitored. Serial examinations should be recorded. A drop in blood pressure and a rise in pulse and respiratory rate indicates a loss of large volumes of blood. The physiologic response a patient makes will depend upon the status of cardiovascular function, the excitement induced with handling, the amount of blood lost, and the rapidity of the loss.

Etiology

The inflammatory process involved in acute gastritis usually involves only the mucosa, but more severe abnormalities involve the submucosa, muscularis and serosal surfaces. Indeed, the inflammatory processes may not be limited to the stomach; at times, it may extend to the esophagus, as in the ingestion of caustic irritants or with reflux esophagitis. With some infectious processes it may extend to the small intestine. Systemic processes often may involve the entire digestive tract. In general, it is possible to classify the etiologic agents of acute gastritis into *exogenous* causes and *endogenous* causes.

Exogenous acute gastritis is most frequently encountered in the dog and cat following the ingestion of garbage or spoiled foods. This "garbage-can poisoning" has a complex etiology which involves bacterial toxins, mycotoxins, and putrefactive or decomposition by-products.[251] The cat is a more fastidious animal and therefore less likely to ingest garbage toxins than the dog; but owing to its curiosity and hunting instincts (ingesting dead or dying rodents already poisoned), acute gastritis does occur in cats.[252]

Voluntary ingestion of foreign material such as aluminum foil, stones, dirt, toys, and other similar material will cause an acute gastritis. The ingestion of grass may subsequently develop into gastritis, which is usually of a mild nature unless the grass has been contaminated with toxic herbicides, pesticides, or fertilizers.[253]

Chemical agents known to cause an acute gastritis in the dog and cat include arsenic, thallium, lead, ethylene glycol (antifreeze), agricultural chemicals (herbicides, fungicides), alpha-naphthyl thiourea (ANTU-rodenticide), and lawn fertilizers high in nitrogen.

Poisonous plants have been implicated as causes of acute gastritis. Also implicated are laurel, rhododendron, rose-bay, azalea, poinsettias, bulbs of daffodils, narcissus, jonquil, and hyacinth.[252] Other plants causing gastric signs are the yew, box, euonymus, daphne, wisteria seeds, lily of the valley, aconite, nightshades, castor bean seeds, precatory bean, and mushrooms of the genus *Amanita*.

Pharmaceutical agents implicated as the cause of acute gastritis include aspirin,[254-256] indomethacin,[257,258] phenylbutazone,[259] and corticosteroids.[260]

Endogenous infectious causes of acute gastritis include salmonellosis, canine distemper, infectious canine hepatitis, and leptospirosis. Mycotic infections have been associated with acute gastritis in the dog but without mention of genus.[261] Dogs have been shown to have a rising antibody titer to the virus of transmissible gastroenteritis in pigs (TGE), and it is believed this virus will produce a disease in dogs similar to that in pigs.[262] Internal parasites may also be associated with acute gastritis and vomiting.[263]

An acute hemorrhagic gastroenteritis has been described.[264] The cause of this syndrome is unknown, but aggressive symptomatic treatment is usually successful.

Pathophysiology

Morphologic signs of inflammation do occur with parasitism and ingestion of a number of irritant agents, but many of the lesions of the stomach referred to as "gastritis" are noninflammatory.[17]

True gastritis is characterized by an inflammation of the musosal lining of the stomach. Functionally, the mucosal resistance of the stomach to the movement of hydrogen and sodium ions is reduced,[265,266] and back-diffusion of acid (H[+]) from gastric lumen to blood occurs.

Certain drugs such as aspirin have been shown to increase the back-diffusion of hydrogen ions into the gastric mucosa.[266,267] At the same time, more sodium ions move into the lumen. The degree of damage to the mucosa is proportional to the amount of hydrogen ions moving back into the mucosa.[268] Table 22–4 lists the drugs known to alter the gastric mucosal barrier.

Table 22–4. Drugs known to alter the gastric mucosal barrier[268]

Bile salts
Short chain fatty acids (e.g., acetic, propionic)
Acetylsalicylic and salicylic acid
Aliphatic alcohols (e.g., ethanol, butanol)
Hypertonic solutions of glucose, sucrose, urea
Eugenol
Diethylaminoethyl
Acetazolamide
Sodium fluoride
Decyl sulphate
Lysolecithin
Phospholipase
Digitoxin
Oxethazaine
Promethazine hydrochloride
Mersalyl
Dithiothreital
N-ethyl maleimide iodoacetamide
Thiocyanate
2,3-Dimercaptopropanol (BAL)
p-chloromercuribenzoate
Indomethacin
Pancreatic juice

Corticosteroids may or may not alter the gastric mucosal barrier.[269] The pathogenesis of production of gastric erosions has been suggested to be due to a decrease in acid secretion. The decrease in acid secretion is the result of back-diffusion of hydrogen ions from the lumen of the stomach into the mucosa.[270] Another mechanism for the pathogenesis of steroid-induced gastric lesions is a reduction in the rate and renewal of gastric mucosal cells.[271] Other mechanisms suggested are altered pepsin secretion[272] and altered mucous secretion.[273]

Back-diffusion of acid frequently causes gastric bleeding. The hematocrit of the bloody fluid lost from erosions is frequently as low as 10%, suggesting plasma proteins are lost through the gastric barrier preferentially to erythrocytes.[274]

The clinical significance of this back-diffusion of hydrogen ions is to direct therapy at the complete neutralization of the intragastric contents; neutralization will allow restoration of the gastric mucosal barrier when the cause has been eliminated. Healing of the gastric lesions will then proceed.

A transient hypochlorhydria or achlorhydria may be observed during episodes of acute gastritis. This may be explained in part by the back-diffusion of hydrogen ions through the damaged mucosa. Isolated reports of achlorhydria in dogs seem to be self-resolving.[275] Perhaps one is dealing with gastritis and not a true, documented achlorhydria.

Diagnosis

The diagnosis of acute gastritis is usually made clinically. It is based upon a history of vomiting and/or anorexia and abdominal tenderness to palpation. There will be few consistent laboratory abnormalities, except in the presence of profuse vomiting.

Gastroscopy will reveal diffuse hyperemia, edema, patchy areas of mucus and petechial hemorrhage, and occasionally mucosal erosions. There may be little correlation between histopathologic changes and endoscopic appearance of the stomach, particularly if emphasis is placed on the variations in color of the mucosa which likely represent vasomotor phenomena.

Biopsy of the stomach may be made at the time of celiotomy or by peroral techniques. Peroral techniques involve the use of a fiberoptic endoscope with a biopsy channel or through the use of a biopsy capsule.[276]

Radiologic examination has not been found to be a reliable means for diagnosing acute gastritis. An experienced radiologist may deduce general information regarding localized, segmental, or diffuse gastric involvement. These mucosal abnormalities vary from an ill-defined, smudged appearance produced by blood, exudate, and secretions along the mucosal surface, to frank ulcer niches, craters, or fissures of varying size.[277]

With hematemesis, the initial problem is to define the site of bleeding within the digestive tract. Endoscopy affords the most accurate means of assessing gastric hemorrhage.[278] Passage of a gastric tube may afford some value in aspirating gastric fluids and examining them for evidence of erythrocytes. Contrast radiography of the stomach may show filling defects but will not differentiate blood from mucus, exudates, or food.

Treatment

Acute gastritis is usually self-limiting and will resolve spontaneously following withdrawal of the offending agent. The dog or cat should be confined and all water (12 hours) and food (24 hours) withheld. Providing ice cubes to lick will help relieve the thirst of vomiting and usually does not result in further vomiting. Following the initial 24 hours, small quantities of a bland food should be given. If this food is retained, a return to the normal diet can be accomplished after 2 to 3 days. If this empirical approach fails to produce a therapeutic response within 48 hours, a more aggressive diagnostic approach is warranted.

Antacids have been advocated for the treatment of gastritis.[279] The antacid reduces the concentration and total load of acid in the gastric contents. By this means the amount of acid available for back-diffusion through the mucosa is reduced. Raising the gastric pH will then permit neutralization to occur more quickly when the gastric juice comes into contact with pancreatic bicarbonate.

In addition to reducing the total amount of available hydrogen ion, antacids have the in vitro property of irreversibly inactivating pepsin if the gastric contents can be brought to a pH above 6.0. This is very difficult to achieve in vivo. The third effect of antacids on gastric juice is a diminution of peptic activity as the pH is raised above the optimal range for proteolysis.

Usefulness of antacid therapy will depend upon the rate of gastric emptying. Large, infrequent dosages are less likely to provide sustained buffering than a more frequent ingestion of the same quantity in smaller doses. Frequently, anticholinergic drugs are used to prolong the duration of action of antacids. Antacids themselves are known to delay gastric emptying.[280]

No antacid is free of hazard. Sodium bicarbonate presents a potential for sodium overload and systemic alkalosis; magnesium preparations may cause diarrheas and are dangerous to the patients with renal disease; and calcium carbonate carries the hazards of hypercalcemia, renal impairment, and gastric secretion. Aluminum hydroxide may lead to phosphate depletion, with consequent muscle weakness, bone resorption, and hypercalcemia.[279] These side effects are rarely encountered with the usual short-term usage in acute gastritis.

Antiemetics such as the phenothiazine tranquilizers are useful in the treatment of refractory vomiting, if obstruction and foreign body have been ruled-out. They must be used with caution in the presence of dehydration. Their α-adrenergic blocking action will cause arteriolar vasodilation and hypotension.

With dehydration, electrolyte losses and metabolic imbalances, fluid therapy should be initiated. In the absence of specific laboratory data about electrolyte and acid-base balance, an isotonic fluid that contains sodium, chloride, and potassium should be used. In fluid replacement one must administer not only the volume of deficit but also the maintenance requirement and contemporary loss. Intravenous fluid administration is preferred in the presence of gastric disease. A quantity of isotonic, polyionic solution equal to that of the blood volume can be administered over a 60-minute period, provided that cardiopulmonary and renal functions are not severely impaired. This rate of fluid administration is equal to 40 ml/lb in the dog and 35/lb in the cat.[281]

When gastric hemorrhage is identified, an ice-water lavage will provide the best noninvasive means for controlling bleeding.[250] Ice water or chilled saline solution may be used. The cold solution is added to the stomach via a gastric tube and allowed to flow out by gravity or with gentle syringe aspiration. The process is continued until all evidence of bleeding has stopped. With continued bleeding, a more aggressive therapeutic approach involving celiotomy may be required. Blood transfusion is indicated for the patient with severe blood loss, for continuing blood losses, or perhaps for the potential surgical patient.

Prognosis

The action of the causative factor is usually of short duration; the inflammatory response subsides and the gastric mucosa returns to normal. It is considered likely, however, that repeated episodes of acute gastritis or prolonged exposure to the causative factor may lead to permanent damage, a prolonged course, and possible chronic gastritis.

CHRONIC GASTRITIS

Chronic gastritis in the dog and cat is less common than acute gastritis. It is possible for acute and chronic gastritis to coexist.

History

In most instances, the causes of chronic gastritis are obscure and may be preceded by repeated attacks of acute gastritis. Owners often report that the animal has a poor haircoat, fails to gain weight or has lost weight, and shows other obscure clinical signs. Sporadic vomiting, which may or may not be associated with eating, may be noted.

Physical Examination

Significant findings associated with chronic gastritis are usually lacking. There may be signs of weight loss but this is not always the case. Depending upon the intensity or frequency of chronic vomiting, dehydration may be noted. One may be fortunate enough to palpate a gastric foreign body. Generally, the physical examination should be utilized to rule out other causes of vomiting and the presence of systemic disease.

Laboratory Evaluation

Evaluation of blood and serum has been unrewarding in the diagnosis of chronic gastritis. Evidence of chronic disease may be reflected in an absolute monocytosis. Signs of dehydration may or may not be supported by a finding of hemoconcentration.

Radiography will provide little assistance in the diagnosis of chronic gastritis. The radiographic appearance is described under Acute Gastritis. The presence of a radiopaque foreign body is occasionally noted. Subjective assessment of the gastric folds as appearing hypertrophic may be made. Delayed gastric emptying time associated with the administration of barium is occasionally seen with chronic gastritis.

Gastroscopic evaluation of the stomach will detect a thickening of the gastric mucosa over the entire surface or in localized areas. The mucosal surface has often been noted to have a tenacious, thickened layer of mucus. Occasionally, small areas of erosions may be noted on the mucosa with or without associated hemorrhage.

Biopsy of the gastric mucosa is the only way to confirm the existence of chronic disease. These biopsies may be taken at the time of gastroscopy or perhaps during celiotomy. The histopathologic findings of chronic gastritis include occlusion of the pyloric glands which results in tiny retention cysts and infiltration with chronic inflammatory cells, largely plasma cells, lymphocytes and eosinophils. As with any chronically irritated mucosa, the lymphocytic nodules are hypertrophic.[17]

Etiologic Factors

The cause of chronic gastritis is usually obscure. Prolonged exposure to any of the agents causing acute disease may lead to a chronic gastritis. Chronic uremia has been found to cause a diffuse chronic, follicular, hypertrophic-hyperplastic gastritis in the dog.[282] In cats, especially those with long hair, licking and swallowing of hair in the grooming process sometimes lead to hair-ball-induced chronic gastritis.[253]

A chronic hypertrophic gastritis resembling Menetrier's disease in man has been reported in a Boxer dog.[283] This disease is characterized by giant hypertrophic gastric rugae, hypoproteinemia, and edema of the extremities of man. Two variants are seen: one has protein-losing gastropathy and hypochlorhydria, and the other has hypersecretion of gastric acid but does not waste protein through the gastrointestinal tract.[284]

Diagnosis

A good clinical history and the absence of significant findings suggestive of systemic disease is important in establishing a diagnosis of chronic gastritis. It is especially important to question the client regarding the animal's eating habits and diet.

Gastroscopic examination with mucosal biopsy or full-thickness biopsy at the time of abdominal celiotomy is the only conclusive means for making the diagnosis.

Treatment

As with acute gastritis, removal of the offending agent is the prime prerequisite in the successful treatment of chronic gastritis. With foreign-body-induced gastritis, this is most easily accomplished via endoscopy or gastrotomy. Hair balls will often be passed if small amounts of petrolatum are administered orally for several days.

Should the chronic disease produce substantial hypertrophy of the gastric mucosa, surgical resection of that area is indicated. If there is delay in gastric emptying, either a pyloromyotomy or pyloroplasty may be indicated.

Prognosis

With the elimination of the causative agent, the prognosis is good. With continued exposure or persistence of the lesion, the animal may develop gastric ulcers or pyloric stenosis.

GASTRIC ULCERS

Gastric ulcers are not commonly seen in dogs or cats. When present, they are usually peptic ulcers: benign, acute, or chronic circumscribed mucosal defects which extend through the muscularis mucosae and have a firm, raised margin. They can be located in any portion of the alimentary tract exposed to the acid from gastric secretions. Ulcers are known to be caused by exogenous agents, occur as a sequela to gastritis, or appear in association with mastocytomas.

History

Peptic ulcers have been reported in adult dogs ranging from 2½ to 12 years of age.[285] Females had a higher incidence than males and there was no breed predilection.

Gastrointestinal ulcerations of dogs with mastocytomas were found in 20 of 24 animals. The most frequent site of ulceration was in the stomach.[286] Mast cell tumors are one of the most common skin tumors of the dog, occur most frequently in older dogs, have no sex predisposition, and have been shown to be more frequently encountered in Boxer and Boston Terrier breeds.[287] Peptic ulcers secondary to mast cell tumors have also been reported in the cat.[288]

Chronic vomiting is the most frequently encountered complaint associated with gastric ulcers. The vomitus may have a "coffee-grounds" appearance when partially digested blood is present. Other signs of gastric ulcers are the occasional presence of melena, variable appetite, and weight loss. With blood loss, anemia may be present. Dehydration is noted with chronic vomiting. Polydipsia is seen as the patient's response to dehydration.

Gastric, duodenal, and colonic ulcerations have been reported in dogs during the postoperative recovery period following spinal decompressive surgery. These animals had received low dosages of corticosteroids.[289]

Some animals with gastric ulcers are asymptomatic, while sudden death due to perforation may also be encountered.

Physical Examination

Abdominal pain represents the most frequently encountered finding upon palpation. Depending upon the depth of the ulceration, signs referable to peritonitis may be noted.

Vomitus around the muzzle occasionally is seen. Hematemesis and melena may be associated with anemia, as suggested by pale mucous membranes.

A previous history of mastocytomas, or evidence of these skin tumors, should include a careful evaluation for gastrointestinal ulceration.

Laboratory Evaluation

Objective evidence of anemia, usually regenerative, affords one of the few clinical laboratory findings associated with gastric ulcers. Generally, peptic ulceration in dogs is in association with, or secondary to, other diseases such as mast cell tumors. In 16 of 22 cases of peptic ulceration in dogs, evidence of liver disease was also noted. Pathologic changes in liver ranged from severe disease to fatty and degenerative changes.[285] Lead poisoning has also been reported to cause gastric ulcers in the dog.[290] Clinical laboratory tests should therefore be associated with defining primary disease entities which may cause hepatic disease or gastritis.

Endoscopic evaluation of the canine stomach

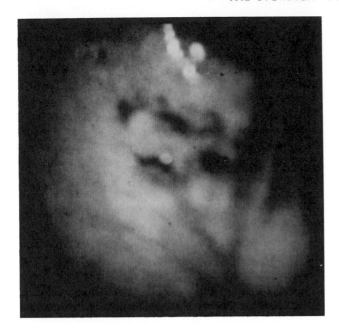

Figure 22–13. Endoscopic view of a dog with bleeding gastric ulcers. (Courtesy of Dr. Brent Jones, University of Missouri, Columbia.)

affords objective evidence of gastric ulcers. With acute ulcers, the mucosal lesions may be bleeding, have an inflammatory appearance around their periphery, and usually have no evidence of fibrin in the ulcer crater (Fig. 22–13). Chronic ulcers may show little inflammatory response and have a fibrin-filled crater and wrinkled mucosa peripheral to the ulcer.

Radiography with contrast materials will show frank ulcer, niches, craters, or fissures of varying sizes. Depending upon the chronicity of the disease and the location of the lesion, i.e., pylorus, gastric emptying may be slowed with gastric ulceration. With severe ulcers, evidence of stenosis is noted.

Exploratory gastrotomy can be a useful diagnostic tool in the diagnosis of gastric ulcers.

Etiologic Factors

Gastric ulcers may result from any of the agents causing acute or chronic gastritis. The relationship between liver disease and gastric ulcers is not known.

In mastocytoma-related peptic ulcers, histamine is probably responsible for the ulceration. The mast cell contains histidine decarboxylase and is capable of converting histidine to histamine.[291] The histamine is stored in association with heparin in the metachromatic cytoplasmic granules which characterize the mast cell. Heparin has been shown to prevent mucosal ulceration in the stomachs of the guinea pig[292] and the dog[286] following exogenous histamine administration. This would suggest that dogs with mastocytomas have a pronounced histamine intoxication without a concomitant heparinemia. Either the heparin in the mast cells is not being released or it is being rapidly bound or metabolized following its release. Additionally, many canine mastocytomas are anaplastic and contain little cytoplasmic metachromasia, suggesting a lack of heparin.

Pathophysiology

The principal sites of peptic ulcers are the proximal duodenum and the non-acid producing areas of the stomach (pyloric antrum and lesser curvature). The ulcers are usually solitary and may range from small mucosal fissures to as large as 4 cm in diameter. The depth of the ulcers ranges from erosions of the mucosa to perforation of the serosal surface.

Gastritis occurs in most human patients with gastric ulcers.[293] There has been some debate as to whether the gastritis produces or is due to the gastric ulcer. Experimentally, mucosa affected by gastritis is more susceptible to ulcer formation from peptic digestion.[294] In man, it has been noted that gastritis persists even after the gastric ulcer has healed.[295]

The gastric mucosal barrier is important in ulcer formation. Gastric ulcer patients (human) have been shown to have significantly higher back-diffusion of hydrogen ions than controls or patients with duodenal ulcers.[296]

Bile is known to produce a gastritis when refluxed into the stomach. This gastritis is due to a breaking of the gastric mucosal barrier. In the pathogenesis of gastric ulcer, human patients have been shown to have a higher than normal concentration of bile acids in the stomach.[297] Whether this bile reflux is due to pyloric sphincter incompetence or reversed peristalsis is not known. With experimental exposure of the dog's stomach to bile, the serum gastrin levels rise, there is an increase in parietal cell density, and the acid secretion increases.[298]

In animals, gastric ulceration can be produced by creation of a pyloric stenosis or obstruction.[294] If gastric emptying is impaired, the pyloric antrum becomes distended, gastrin is released, and hyperacidity results. The hyperacidity produced by obstruction of the pylorus is not borne out in human gastric ulcer patients and most ulcer patients do not have delayed gastric emptying times.[293]

The specific site of gastric ulcer formation is

probably determined by local factors such as blood flow, mucosal cell turnover, and mucus production.[293] With an alteration of blood flow, the viability of the underlying cells will be impaired. In fact, bile salts, aspirin, and other causes of gastritis do decrease mucosal blood flow in the experimental dog.[299]

Gastric epithelial cells serve a protective function in gastric ulcer formation. These cells have a short life span, averaging 4 days and are continually undergoing replication, shedding, and renewal.[293] In rats undergoing restraint stress, epithelial cell replication is depressed and gastric erosions occur.[300]

Mucus of gastric epithelial cells serves to help neutralize acid. Many of the anti-inflammatory drugs such as aspirin, cortisone, and indomethacin decrease mucous secretion and may subsequently lead to gastritis and ulcer formation with their chronic usage.[300]

Diagnosis

The diagnosis of gastric ulcers may be difficult. A history of chronic vomiting, especially with evidence of hematemesis, is useful. Endoscopic visualization of the ulcer will afford conclusive evidence but visualization of the lesser curvature, where many of the ulcers are located, is difficult. Barium contrast studies may be useful in chronic, deep ulceration but are nearly useless in mucosal erosions. Abdominal celiotomy may afford the best opportunity to diagnose gastric ulcers; but here again, unless the ulcer is actively bleeding or is invasive of deeper gastric layers, many will be overlooked.

Treatment

Successful treatment of gastric ulcers may involve medical, surgical, or combination therapy. If the cause of the gastritis-induced ulcer is known, elimination of this factor will hasten recovery. Antacid therapy has been shown to be efficacious in treating gastric ulcers in man.[279] Antiemetic drugs such as the promazine tranquilizers may be useful in cases not associated with anemia or dehydration. Intragastric lavage with ice water is indicated with acute gastric hemorrhage. Levarterenol (norepinephrine) is a potent alpha-adrenergic vasoconstrictive agent. It is almost completely destroyed in one passage through the normal liver. This product may be instilled into the stomach (8 mg in 100 ml saline), left in the stomach for 30 minutes, and lavage used to determine whether gastric bleeding has stopped. Multiple usages are usually required.[301]

A new approach to upper gastrointestinal bleed-

ing involves the use of specific H2-antagonist drugs. These agents act to increase gastric pH by antagonizing the action of many stimuli to acid production. The site of action is presumed to be at a final step involving histamine. Cimetidine is the drug currently in clinical use for control of gastric acid secretion.[301]

Dietary management of gastric ulcers is similar to that described under Acute Gastritis.

Surgical treatment for gastric ulcers may involve partial gastrectomy for removal of the ulcer. This technique, along with pyloromyotomy and vagotomy, has been used successfully in the dog.[282] In man, no one operation has emerged as one which is used for all patients requiring surgery. At present, truncal vagotomy with antrectomy appears to be the current favorite.[302] With perforated gastric ulcer, immediate surgical intervention is indicated.

Prognosis

Sufficient data are unavailable to provide a prognosis for dogs and cats with gastric ulcers. Sudden death due to perforation may occur. If the primary cause recurs (e.g., mastocytoma) further clinical episodes are to be expected.

FOREIGN BODIES IN THE STOMACH

Gastric foreign bodies are commonly seen in the practice of small animal medicine. The type of foreign body encountered is usually a swallowed object or a bezoar. Swallowed objects are of almost innumerable variety: pins and needles, rocks, children's toys, keys, sticks, bones, and other more bizarre objects such as ice cream spatulas, sharp knives, and coins (Fig. 22–14).

A bezoar is defined as a "concretion of various character sometimes found in the stomach or intestines of man or other animals." They may belong to

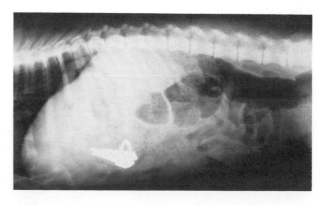

Figure 22–14. Lateral radiograph of a 9-month-old dog with a gastric foreign body.

one of four types: trichobezoar (hair), phytobezoar (fruit and vegetable fibers), trichophytobezoar (a mixture of hair, fruit, and vegetable fibers), or concretions of shellac.[303]

Bezoars were formerly supposed to have remarkable medicinal properties. The word "bezoar" is derived from the Persian word "badzahi" or "pad-zahr," "pad" meaning protecting (against) and "zahr" meaning poison; thus, bezoar originally meant a counter poison or antidote.[304]

History

Clinical signs of gastric foreign body are variable and inconstant. They may be so subtle that the patient is essentially asymptomatic, or so severe as to present signs of pyloric obstruction. Periodic episodes of vomiting, with associated signs of anorexia and discomfort, are most commonly observed. An abrupt increase in the frequency and intensity of vomiting sometimes provides the impetus to present the patient to the veterinarian. Gastric perforation may have occurred, followed by peritonitis, or the foreign body may have become lodged in the pyloric antrum.

Clients will occasionally report seeing the patient swallow the foreign object or, more commonly, will report a missing toy or other object with which the animal plays. Young dogs and cats are more likely to swallow foreign objects than are adults.

Physical Examination

Due to the variety of foreign materials swallowed, and their variable periods of residence in the stomach, diagnosis of a gastric foreign body on physical examination is not common. Palpation of the abdomen may elicit signs of discomfort, but actual grasping of a gastric foreign body is rather unlikely.

Pyrexia, abdominal fluid, pain upon palpation of the abdomen, and other findings consistent with peritonitis may be noted with perforation. However, it is more usual that the findings are consistent with an acute or chronic gastritis. Hematemesis and/or melena may be observed or reported.

Special Physical Examinations

Roentgenologic examination is an important aid to the diagnosis of a gastric foreign body. Although radiopaque lesions are visible on plain radiographs, contrast medium is often required to visualize the object clearly. Ingestion of large quantities of hair, fiber, or string produces filling defects on positive contrast radiography. Use of air or carbon dioxide in conjunction with the positive contrast agents may at times be useful in delineating gastric foreign bodies.

Endoscopic visualization of the stomach is often helpful in finding the foreign material.

Laboratory Evaluation

Complete blood counts are rarely abnormal in the presence of an uncomplicated gastric foreign body. With increased frequency of vomiting, the microhematocrit value will increase, and electrolyte imbalances may be evident.

Diagnosis

The history is often the initial clue to the presence of gastric foreign bodies. Radiology affords the greatest assistance in confirming the diagnosis.

Treatment

Treatment for the ingestion of foreign material depends upon the condition of the patient, the duration and intensity of vomiting, and the nature and type of the object. The presence of complications (fever, leukocytosis) should be assessed in planning therapy. Surgical removal of the foreign body is curative and seldom contraindicated. However, pins, needles, and other sharp, pointed objects will often pass spontaneously. A policy of watchful waiting is justifiable, particularly from the economic viewpoint. Hospital observation is advisable; methylcellulose, high-fiber moist food, and vigorous fluid therapy are given. This regime enhances normal bowel motility, lubricates the object, and fills the bowel around the object. The client must understand that surgery will likely be indicated if the object does not pass through the digestive tract, and that the ultimate fee may be greatly increased by prolonged hospitalization and medical treatment. Radiographs taken each day should show continued movement of the object. If the object remains stationary in the bowel for 24 hours, it may be engaged in the tissue with danger of perforation. Immediate surgical intervention is then indicated.

Emetics and purgatives should be avoided. The dangers associated with laceration, perforation, or obstruction do not warrant their risk.

Endoscopic retrieval of foreign materials may be rewarding. Additionally, removal of the object with forceps under fluoroscopy or by use of magnets has proven feasible.

Vaseline or other petrolatum products of a gelatinous consistency may be given in the presence of trichobezoars. These bezoars are most commonly encountered in the long-haired dog or cat and are associated with the self-grooming habits of these animals. Use of orally administered mineral oil is to be discouraged, due to the ease of inhalation and concomitant foreign body pneumonias produced by this product.

Surgical intervention is indicated when there is evidence of gastric impaction, failure of an object to move out of the stomach within 24 to 72 hours, failure of nonsurgical attempts at retrieval, accumulation of large numbers of foreign bodies, abnormally large or sharp-edged foreign bodies, more than minimal hematemesis or evidence of perforation. Gastrotomy is usually an uncomplicated procedure, and postoperative complications are minimal with aseptic technique and gentle handling of tissues. Prior to removal of the foreign body, it is imperative that the abdominal contents be protected from accidental gastric spillage. With trichobezoars and other radiolucent foreign bodies, the entire gastrointestinal tract should be explored for additional foreign bodies. Should a gastric ulcer be encountered, it is likely to be traumatically induced and, in the absence of impending perforation or excessive hemorrhage, will heal spontaneously.

Postoperatively, the dog or cat may be given water after 12 hours and placed on a highly digestible, low-fiber diet after 24 hours. A normal diet can be resumed within 3 or 4 days. It is advisable to feed the animal several times daily in smaller quantities for 2 to 3 weeks, in order to allow the gastric tissues to heal.

Prognosis

Removal of the gastric foreign body should afford a good prognosis. Gastritis or gastric erosions will heal spontaneously with removal of the offending object.

GASTRIC NEOPLASIA

Benign and malignant tumors of the stomach occur in the dog and cat. A review of available literature revealed 100 adenocarcinomas, 12 sarcomas, and 25 benign gastric neoplasms in the dog. Additionally, five surveys involving 20,529 total neoplasms included only 39 gastric adenocarcinomas, which accounted for fewer than 1% of the canine neoplasms identified. Only four gastric neoplasms, all sarcomas, were reported from six surveys of 1708 tumor-bearing cats.[305] The annual incidence rate for malignant tumor of the stomach and intestine of man is approximately 16 times the canine rate and 11 times the feline rate.[306]

The domestic cat apparently has predominantly sarcomas in the stomach. One report of 46 alimen-

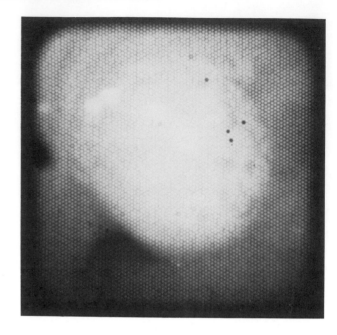

Figure 22–15. Gastric polyp as seen via endoscopy of the dog stomach. (Courtesy of Dr. Brent Jones, University of Missouri, Columbia.)

tary tract neoplasms in cats did not include any gastric carcinomas.[307] Gastric adenocarcinoma has been reported and reviewed for wild Felidae.[308]

Adenocarcinomas are the most frequent canine gastric neoplasms, with fibrosarcomas, leiomyosarcomas, and reticulum cell sarcomas (lymphosarcomas) also being reported.[309–321]

Leiomyomas are reported to be the second most frequent gastric neoplasm.[321] Other benign tumors are generally adenomatous polyps.[315,317] These polyps are nodules of tissue that protrude above the level of the gastric mucosa and are often pedunculated (Fig. 22–15). An unresolved problem in human medicine is the malignant potential for these polyps. There is circumstantial evidence that malignant transformation may occur, but this has not been proven.

History

Animals affected with gastric neoplasms range in age from 3 to 13 years. The average age in dogs is 9.3 years. Males have about a 2:1 incidence of gastric tumors over the female. No specific breeds nor geographic predispositions have been identified.

Vomiting is the most frequent clinical sign associated with gastric neoplasia. The frequency of vomiting increases with time, paralleling the weight loss that often occurs. Hematemesis and melena result when there is mucosal erosion or ulcer formation.

Other nonspecific findings include weight loss, anorexia, and possible anemia. Ascites, jaundice, diarrhea, coughing, and dyspnea are less common signs.

Physical Examination

There are no specific physical findings to suggest the presence of gastric neoplasia. The animal is usually anorectic and may show varying degrees of dehydration associated with chronic vomiting. In that many ulcer craters and mucosal erosions are often found in association with the neoplasm, anemia may be suggested by the presence of pale mucous membranes.

Abdominal pain occasionally is elicited upon palpation. Rarely is the primary neoplasm palpated. Dyspnea, hyperpnea, and coughing may be observed with metastasis to the lung.

Special Physical Examinations

Radiography affords objective diagnostic evidence of possible gastric neoplasia. Usually plain films are unremarkable, but barium contrast studies are useful in delineating gastric malignancy. Most changes are located in the pyloric antrum and along the lesser curvature. Characteristic features are the demonstration of a space-occupying lesion near the pyloric antrum, a lack of normal motility (fluoroscopy), and delayed emptying of the stomach.[322] A thickening of the gastric wall, distortion of the gastric lumen, and derangement of mucosal folds are occasionally noted. With small lesions it is possible to have an absence of radiographic abnormalities.[276,323] Lack of evidence for metastasis has not been rewarding in ruling out the existence of neoplasia. The tumors spread primarily to the hepatic lymph nodes and liver, although occasionally there is lung metastasis.

Endoscopy is associated with a low morbidity and mortality rate, yet will permit good documentation of disease. It is difficult to distinguish inflammatory lesions from neoplasia, and thus multiple biopsies are indicated with gastroscopy[324] (Fig. 22–16). A special nylon brush attached to a flexible spiral wire has been used successfully in preoperatively diagnosing leiomyosarcomas under fiberoptic visualization.[325]

Exfoliative cytology has been useful in the preoperative diagnosis of gastric cancer of man. Two techniques have been described: (1) saline gastric lavage and (2) chymotrypsin gastric lavage. With chymotrypsin lavage, accuracy in the diagnosis of gastric malignancy is greater than 90%.[326]

Abdominal celiotomy has been most frequently

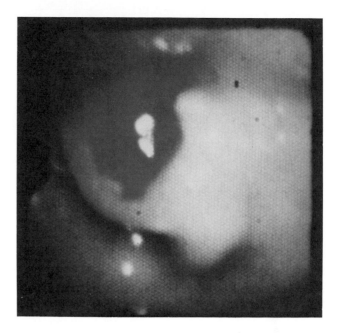

Figure 22–16. Pyloric leiomyoma after a biopsy has been taken via gastroscopy. (Courtesy of Dr. Brent Jones, University of Missouri, Columbia.)

used in the diagnosis of gastric neoplasia in the dog and cat. Unfortunately, the disease is usually so far advanced prior to surgery that total extirpation of cancerous tissue is not possible.

Laboratory Evaluation

The hemogram usually reflects nonspecific changes. Anemia may be reflected in a low packed cell volume, hemoglobin, and total red blood cell count. Biochemical profiles have been unrewarding.

Etiologic Factors

The cause of gastric neoplasms is unknown. Ingestion of carcinogenic chemicals would be one possible cause for gastric tumors, but no spontaneous cases have been proven in the dog and cat. Chronic gastritis is often seen in association with adenomatous gastric polyps, but neither cause nor effect has been established.

Diagnosis

Gastric neoplasms should be considered as a diagnostic rule-out for dogs admitted with a clinical history of chronic vomiting, weight loss, and hematemesis.

Preoperative confirmation of the diagnosis awaits cytologic evidence of neoplastic cells. Radiography often demonstrates a thickened gastric wall in the pyloric antrum or along the lesser curvature,

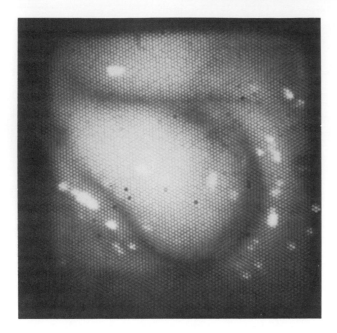

Figure 22–17. Pyloric obstruction extending from the lesser curvature. Biopsy and histopathology revealed the presence of an adenocarcinoma. (Courtesy of Dr. Brent Jones, University of Missouri, Columbia.)

space-occupying masses with contrast studies, and delayed gastric emptying; these are strong but not incontrovertible evidences of gastric neoplasia. Endoscopy should always be accompanied by gastric biopsy procedures (Fig. 22–17). Abdominal celiotomy affords the best opportunity for assessing the stomach, as well as for searching for evidence of metastasis.

Treatment

Wide surgical excision of gastric adenocarcinomas, in which lung or widespread metastasis has not occurred, will often prolong an animal's life. Occasionally, the surgeon is advised to consider partial gastrectomy procedures, which include bypass of certain parts of the gastrointestinal tract, e.g., gastrojejunostomy. With metastasis commonly extending to regional lymph nodes, surgical excision of the hepatic nodes is indicated to provide therapeutic as well as prognostic assessment. Lung metastasis does occur, but seems to be less frequent than to regional nodes draining the stomach and the liver.

Prognosis

Wide excision can provide a fair prognosis in dogs with gastric adenocarcinomas. Careful attention must be focused on surgical ablation of the

lesion *and* the adjacent lymph nodes. Survival rate for dogs and cats with gastric cancer, which have undergone surgical treatment, is not available; but all too often is limited to several weeks or months. In man, surgical cure rate for patients with lymph node involvement is 20%, in contrast to 50% for those who did not have lymph node involvement.[327]

GASTRIC PARASITISM

Internal parasites in the stomach of the dog and cat do not commonly produce clinical signs except in severe infestations. The overall incidence of these parasites is low.

History

Young animals are more likely to be infected with gastric parasites; wild carnivores are more likely infected than domestic. With severe infestations, the animal may show signs of an acute gastritis, perhaps complicated by bloody feces and anemia. With a loss of appetite, weight loss is common.

Physical Examination

Specific signs of gastric parasitism are lacking. Evidence of vomiting, weight loss, poor haircoat, and perhaps dehydration may be noted. With large numbers of parasites the animal may have hematemesis, melena, and a secondary anemia.

Special Physical Examinations

Gastroscopy may afford a view of the parasite, as well as confirming acute gastritis with mucosal erosions.

Laboratory Evaluation

Fecal flotation and identification of the characteristic eggs afford the best means for identification. Gastric parasites may be found in vomitus.

The hemogram may reflect the presence of an anemia.

Etiologic Factors

Several nematodes have been identified in the stomach of dogs, cats, and wild carnivora. *Physaloptera praeputialis, P. canis, P. felidis,* and *P. rara* are the most frequently encountered stomach parasites.[328] These are thick worms, about 3 to 6 cm long, and are usually attached to the gastric or duodenal mucosa. The life cycle of these parasites is indirect, with cockroaches, beetles, and crickets serving as intermediate hosts. Diagnosis of *Physaloptera* may be difficult, as the eggs do not float well on commonly used media. At necropsy *Physaloptera* may, at first glance, be mistaken for an ascarid, but closer examination will distinguish the adults. There will be a characteristic collar surrounding the parasite's head with a pair of trilobed lips.

Gnathostoma spinigerum has been reported from the gastric tumor-like nodules of domestic and wild cats, dogs, lions, leopards, mink, and raccoon.[329] They are 1 to 3 cm in length and have a large head with four "ballonets" or cavities. The cuticle has six to eleven transverse rows of hooks. Eggs of *Gnathostoma* hatch after about 4 days in the water, and the indirect life cycle is initiated when the ova are ingested by the water flea *(Cyclops)*. When the *Cyclops* is eaten by a fresh-water fish, frog, or reptile, the parasites become encysted and are infective when ingested. When the young worms are ingested, they may wander through several organs in the peritoneal and pleural cavities. The adult worms penetrate into the wall of the stomach via the serosal surface and produce cavities in which several worms live. The cavities may provide a channel for gastric contents to leak into the peritoneal cavity, causing peritonitis and possibly death.

Spirocerca lupi granulomas are occasionally found in the stomach of the dog. Small intestinal parasites such as *Toxacara canis*, *T. cati*, and *Toxascaris leonina* are on rare occasions found in the stomach of a dog or cat.

Diagnosis

The finding of characteristic eggs in the feces will provide the diagnosis of gastric parasites of *Physaloptera* or *Gnathostoma*. These eggs do not float well and it would be advisable to use saturated solutions of sodium nitrate, magnesium sulfate, or sodium dichromate, since saturated sodium chloride or dextrose solution will not float these eggs.

Endoscopy or necropsy will occasionally find these parasites in association with acute gastritis and mucosal erosions.

Treatment

Specific therapeutic measures for gastric parasites are lacking. Carbon disulfide has been used in the treatment of *Physaloptera* infestation in a badger,[330] and dichlorvos has partial efficacy in dogs and cats.

Control of intermediate hosts of both *Physaloptera* and *Gnathostoma* probably affords the best means for preventing reinfection.

PYLORIC DISEASES

As a motor unit, the stomach classically is considered to have two functional areas: a proximal *receptacle*—the fundus and body; and a distal *pump*—the antrum. At the end of the antrum is the pylorus, the function of which is not clear. The pylorus may have a sphincteric function to impede emptying of the stomach, or may act to prevent reflux of small intestinal contents.

Diseases of the pylorus in small animals can be classified as obstructive diseases or functional diseases. The obstructive diseases usually have mechanical impairment of the pylorus, whereas the functional diseases are usually manifestations of other organ systems on the stomach's ability to empty normally.

Obstructive Diseases

Stenosis of the pyloric canal may result from hypertrophy of the circular muscle fibers of the pyloric sphincter; intrinsic pyloric neoplasia; extrinsic pyloric lesions such as pancreatic abscesses, neoplasia, inflammatory lesions, or histoplasmosis; and obturation obstructions such as foreign bodies, gastric ulcers, or prolapses of the gastric mucosa through the pyloric canal.

There appear to be two distinct groups of animals associated with pyloric obstruction: (1) neonates, many times manifesting signs as the puppy or kitten is placed on solid foods, or (2) older animals which may have swallowed a foreign body, are recovering from a bout of gastritis, or perhaps have impingement of a gastric neoplasm upon the pyloric canal.

History

In the congenital form of pyloric obstruction, the most frequent client complaint is vomiting at fairly regular intervals after the ingestion of solid foods. The vomitus is usually undigested food and is almost never bile stained. Repeated episodes of vomiting may cause dehydration, loss of weight, and death.

The term "projectile vomiting" has been associated with pyloric diseases. The meaning of "projectile" is broadly inclusive. Some use the term to mean very forceful vomiting, which throws the vomitus for a considerable distance and usually empties the stomach in a single event. Others consider it to mean that the vomiting arrives as a projectile does, i.e., abruptly and without the warning of increased salivation and retching.[331] Both definitions are met in most patients.

Brachiocephalic breeds seem to be most commonly affected, with the predominance of reported cases in the Boston Terrier and Boxer breeds. A high proportion of cats reported with pyloric diseases are of the Siamese breed.[332] From previous reports in the dog and cat, no specific sex incidence could be determined. In man, where the congenital hypertrophic form of pyloric stenosis is so common, males predominate over females at a ratio of nearly 4:1.[333] With the congenital nature of the disease, inheritance is considered a factor. Literature citations in veterinary medicine are lacking, but two female kittens from the same litter with pyloric stenosis have been reported.[334] In man, the risk of pyloric stenosis is four times greater in children if the mother had pyloric stenosis than if the father had it.[335]

Dogs of any age and breed may have anatomic alterations in, on, or about the pyloric canal, which will result in an acquired, mechanical, pyloric obstruction. These alterations are usually the result of chronic gastritis, gastric ulcers, or neoplasms.

Physical Examination

The classic clinical signs of congenital hypertrophic pyloric stenosis in man include a palpable pyloric enlargement ("olive") in 92% of the cases, projectile vomiting in 91% of the cases, and visible gastric peristalsis in all cases.[336] Due to the conformation of the canine and feline abdomen, palpation of the pylorus is difficult and visualization of gastric peristalsis nearly impossible.

Observation of emesis is helpful in making the diagnosis. With vomiting of a chronic nature, signs of weight loss and dehydration are usually evident. After vomiting, the animal usually readily resumes feeding, only to vomit again at variable intervals.

Special Physical Examinations

Radiography affords the most definitive method of diagnosing pyloric obstruction. Obstruction results in distention of the stomach with food, fluid and/or air, long after ingesta would normally have entered the small intestine.[337] In the cat, a consistent finding was an increase in gastric volume, with the fundus and body becoming elongated craniocaudally but remaining on the left side of the midline. The mucosal folds became stretched and had a smooth appearance.[332] The pyloric antrum was often enlarged in size and the pyloric canal narrow and elongated.

Contrast radiography may be helpful to assess the rate of gastric emptying. The term "gastric emptying time," in radiology, is usually regarded as the

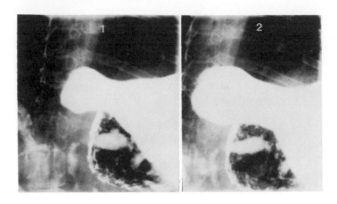

Figure 22–18. Pyloric stenosis as viewed in sequential radiographs taken at the time of fluoroscopy. Note how the barium pools in the pyloric antrum but does not proceed through the obstructed pylorus.

time required for the stomach to begin to empty—but not empty completely. Gastric emptying time has been reported to be 60 minutes.[337] In the cat, the onset of gastric emptying is variable. Even with pyloric dysfunction, barium has been noted in the duodenum within 5 to 10 minutes after administration.[332] The presence of barium within the stomach for greater than 12 to 24 hours is abnormal and should be considered a sign of delayed gastric emptying. The stress of chemical[338] and manual restraint may falsely delay emptying of the stomach.

Fluoroscopy enables the demonstration of gastric peristaltic waves. Many times these waves are of normal rate and intensity, but there is usually an enlargement of the pyloric antrum and a diminution in the quantity of barium passing through the pyloric canal (Fig. 22–18).

Gastroscopy in the canine patient with pyloric stenosis due to muscular hypertrophy may reveal the pyloric orifice to be fixed and narrowed. Peristaltic waves passing down the antrum may result in a slight narrowing but incomplete closure of the orifice.[339] Gastroscopy may also reveal the presence of a foreign body, ulcer, gastritis, or neoplasm within the pyloric antrum or canal.

Laboratory Evaluation

Hematologic changes with pyloric obstruction are usually associated with dehydration and, occasionally, a metabolic alkalosis. A transient trace of protein and increased white cells are occasionally seen in the urinalysis, but are readily cleared with rehydration. Urine pH is usually acid even in the presence of metabolic alkalosis.[340]

Etiologic Factors

The cause of the congenital form of hypertrophic pyloric stenosis is unknown. Heredity may play an important role. Many theories have been offered but none have been entirely acceptable. Some of the theories are: (1) pylorospasm as the primary lesion, followed by muscle hypertrophy; (2) muscle hypertrophy as the primary lesion, followed by pylorospasm; (3) imbalance of the autonomic nervous system with hypertonia of the vagi; (4) gastrointestinal allergy; (5) vitamin B deficiency in the mother during gestation; (6) pituitary lesions; (7) injury to the central nervous system during birth; (8) myenteric ganglion cell degeneration or lack, analogous to Hirschsprung's disease; (9) neoplasm; (10) glycogen storage disease; (11) adrenal cortical deficiency or dysfunction; (12) mother that elaborates a hormone which is "pylorotropic" in males, leading to hypertrophy of pylorus; in females, to hypertrophy of the uterus; (13) maternal emotional disturbances; and (14) anomalous blood supply to the pylorus.[331]

Pentagastrin is a synthetic substance of which the terminal tetrapeptide is identical to natural gastrin and has physiologic effects that resemble those of the natural substance.[341] Chronic stimulation of the parietal cells, of puppies and adult dogs, with pentagastrin produced duodenal ulceration. Moreover, pyloric hypertrophy was also produced in young puppies and, in at least one case, seems to have occurred as a result of prenatal administration of pentagastrin to the bitch.[342] Whether native gastrin from the bitch has an influence on the development of the pylorus of the pups is not known.

Transient mucosal edema or comparatively mild forms of gastritis in the pyloric region may compromise the passage of food into the duodenum. It remains unclear whether the increased work required to pass this ingesta results in muscle hypertrophy, or whether the hypertrophy was the cause of the initial gastritis or edema.[343]

Pathophysiology

The muscular coat of the stomach has two layers: an outer longitudinal layer, and an inner circular layer of smooth muscle fibers. Additionally, there is a weak inner oblique or longitudinal layer which is usually incomplete in the pyloric region. At the pylorus, the circular muscle layer is several times thicker than the outer longitudinal layer. The circular muscle is continuous with that of the antrum and is completely separated from the circular muscle of the duodenum by a thin fibrous septum.[344] Many of the longitudinal fibers continue into the duodenum.

The circular muscle fibers of the pyloric canal form two distinct loops: a right (oral or proximal) loop, and a left (aboral or distal) loop. At the lesser curvature, both loops are united in a muscle torus and usually cover ½ to 1½ cm of the gastric wall at the lesser curvature and are spread over 2 to 5 cm near the greater curvature. Both loops have an equal claim upon the name "pyloric sphincter."[345]

In all forms of pyloric hypertrophy, it is the circular muscle that becomes affected. The hypertrophy may be focal or circular and may involve the pylorus or pyloric antral areas.[343]

The muscle hypertrophy ultimately leads to a delay in gastric emptying. The delay in food passage causes hyperplasia of the gastric mucosa and seems to result in the retention of food and secretions.[346] The increase in gastric parietal cells leads to greater acid secretion and more acid is delivered to the duodenum, further retarding gastric emptying.[347] Thus, with food retention and gastric stasis, a "pylorospasm" and antiperistalsis result.[348]

Diagnosis

The congenital form of pyloric stenosis is common in the brachiocephalic breeds and a clinical picture which includes projectile vomiting is useful to render a tentative diagnosis. Obstruction of the pylorus in either the congenital or acquired form is most commonly diagnosed with radiographic techniques. The demonstration of a delay in gastric emptying, gastric distention, and ineffectual gastric peristalsis is sufficient evidence for consideration of a pyloric lesion. With contrast studies of the stomach, space-occupying lesions are occasionally identified.

Treatment

Surgery is the preferred treatment for obstructive lesions of the pylorus. Pyloromyotomy and pyloroplasty have been used successfully in the treatment of pyloric stenosis in the dog and cat.[334,349–352] Occasionally, complications have resulted, such as stricture of a previous myotomy incision, and have necessitated more elaborate surgical dismemberment of the pylorus, such as a gastroduodenostomy.[353]

In acquired pyloric stenosis the treatment is directed at the cause. Medical therapy is many times sufficient, but surgery is indicated for mechanical obstruction impeding ingesta passing into the duodenum.

Medical management of pyloric stenosis in human infants has been reported to be successful in Europe. Methscopolamine nitrate given orally, in combination with good supportive therapy plus a period of gastric lavage and discontinuation of oral feeding, was as effective as surgical therapy in some cases.[354,355] There are no comparable reports of medical therapy in dogs or cats with pyloric obstructive stenosis.

Prognosis

The congenital form of pyloric stenosis responds to a pyloromyotomy with few complications. The complications are due to insufficient length or depth of myotomy incision, or leakage from accidental and unrecognized perforation of the mucosa. The prognosis for acquired pyloric stenosis, of course, depends upon the cause.

Postoperative vomiting is not unusual following pyloric surgery and should not be considered as evidence of an inadequate operation. There is usually mucosal edema and gastritis present which requires resolution before cessation of vomiting can be expected.

Functional Diseases

Intermittent, projectile, postprandial vomiting in toy or miniature breeds, and especially in very nervous dogs, has been attributed to an undocumented entity entitled "pylorospasm." The general impression is that pylorospasm results from nervousness or through viscero-visceral or somato-visceral reflexes, initiated by irritation of any portion of the body. It is also believed that the delay in gastric evacuation which results from such irritation is largely or entirely due to this pylorospasm. Additionally, spasm of the pylorus has been identified and associated with antral gastritis, organic lesions elsewhere in the stomach or in the duodenum and secondary to pyloric ulcer.[356]

History

Toy or miniature breeds or nervous dogs are usually the ones associated with intermittent, postprandial, projectile vomiting. It affects dogs of all ages but is more common in animals less than 3 years of age.[357] The interval of emesis is variable during the postprandial period.

Physical Examination

Usually the animal with a functional pyloric disease is normal in all aspects of the physical examination. Witnessing of the projectile vomiting is often useful.

Special Physical Examinations

Radiography with contrast material affords the best opportunity for objectively documenting pyloric disease. A delay in the gastric emptying time with no other apparent abnormalities is usually noted. In a functional impairment of the pylorus, peristaltic waves in the stomach will vary in intensity from weak to vigorous. Little or no barium may pass through the pyloric canal.[358] Caution must be applied in making this diagnosis, as chemical or physical restraint may provide false positive findings of a delay in gastric emptying.

Etiologic Factors

Retention of gastric contents without organic obstruction has been reported to occur in the following ways: (1) psychogenic: fear or excitement; (2) neurogenic: autonomic nervous system abnormalities with histologically identifiable lesions, both central and peripheral; and (3) receptor-induced: gastric stasis induced by pH, fat, or amino acid stimulation of duodenal receptors.[359]

Diagnosis

Radiographic evidence of a delay in gastric evacuation in the absence of organic obstruction, coupled with a clinical history of postprandial, projectile vomiting in a nervous dog, usually affords the diagnosis of a functional pyloric disease or pylorospasm.

Treatment

Animals with a functional disorder of the pylorus have classically been treated by feeding small meals three to four times daily which helps diminish the gastric distention usually seen with this condition. Centrally arising emetic stimuli can be controlled through the use of phenothiazine tranquilizers. These will also have a calming effect on the animal, which will allow a return of gastric motility. In the past, anticholinergic drugs such as propantheline bromide have been advocated.[253,357] If gastric motility is slowed with gastric retention and pylorospasm, the use of parasympathomimetic drugs such as bethanechol has been found to be efficacious.[359]

Dietary management should be initiated through the use of more liquid solutions to facilitate passage. By diluting the food in water, the osmolar concentration is lessened and will increase gastric evacuation.

Correction of alterations in other organ systems which may be affecting gastric motility will often alleviate symptoms. Surgical treatment of a functional pyloric stenosis should be undertaken with caution.

ACUTE GASTRIC DILATATION

There are two types of acute gastric dilatation within small animal practice: (1) acute gastric dilatation of the young dog where overengorgement of food is the predominant etiologic factor, and (2) acute gastric dilatation of the older dog where gas and fluids accumulate within the stomach for reasons not yet clearly defined.

History

Acute dilatation occurs in all breeds at any age. The animal is usually noted to have a distended, painful abdomen. Nonproductive vomiting and excessive salivation may accompany the abdominal distention. Listlessness becomes more apparent as the duration of symptoms persists. Most of these animals have been noted to be greedy eaters, and to belch and pass flatus postprandially. The owner may report the dog to have overengorged by eating his own food and the food of littermates, or that the animal was fed some 6 to 8 hours previously and signs of gastric dilatation have only recently appeared. The importance of gastric dilatation in small animal practice is to differentiate it from the more rapidly fatal condition of gastric volvulus.

Physical Examination

Cranial abdominal distention is most commonly noted by observing the patient. This distention may protrude to either the left, right, or both sides, depending upon the degree of dilatation and the displacement of abdominal organs. Percussion of the cranial abdomen may reveal a resonant, tympanic sound if the stomach has a predominance of air, or may be dull to percussion with large volumes of fluid or food. Succussion may result in audible fluid and gas sounds in the stomach.

A very taut abdomen will be noted and many times the animal will make a grunting sound as it is manipulated. Deep palpation of the caudal abdomen may reveal a firm, thickened spleen as well as gas-filled intestines. Borborygmal sounds vary in their frequency and intensity according to the duration of distention and excitability of the patient. Some polypnea as well as tachycardia will be noted, but this again must be assessed in accordance with the disposition of the animal and the duration of gastric dilatation. Progression of the disease may

give clinical signs of impending hypovolemic, hypotensive shock.

Special Physical Examinations

The diagnosis of gastric dilatation can best be confirmed by radiographs of the abdomen. Air, fluid, and/or food will massively dilate the stomach. Other abdominal organs will be displaced caudally and slightly dorsally until nearly reaching the pelvis. The spleen will occasionally be enlarged and displaced from its normal position. The position of the spleen and pylorus will provide the distinguishing features between simple dilatation and gastric dilatation complicated by volvulus of the stomach. In dilatation, the pylorus will be forced caudally and slightly dorsally as a result of expansion of the greater curvature of the stomach. The spleen is displaced passively by the gastrosplenic ligament from the left toward the right.[360] Contrast studies of the stomach are usually not rewarding and the stress of handling could be detrimental to the animal.[361]

Laboratory Evaluation

Clinical laboratory studies usually reflect the consequences of vomiting, sequestration of large volumes of gastrointestinal secretions, and organ changes associated with dehydration and shock. The most consistent findings in experimentally induced gastric dilatation are elevations in the blood urea nitrogen (BUN), inorganic phosphorus, serum creatinine phosphokinase (SCPK), potassium, and creatinine. After release of the experimentally induced gastric dilatation, the serum potassium, alanine transaminase (formerly serum glutamic pyruvic transaminase—SGPT), aspartate transaminase (formerly serum glutamic oxaloacetic transaminase—SGOT), SCPK, BUN, creatinine, and inorganic phosphorus made significant increases.[360,362]

Etiologic Factors

Simple acute gastric dilatation seen in young animals is usually due to overeating. The stomach is filled with food; gastric distention results in excessive secretion; vomiting may be associated with aerophagia; and the stomach becomes massively enlarged.

Acute gastric dilatation is more commonly seen in the large, deep-chested breeds of dogs.[363] In these animals, it is of primary importance to differentiate simple dilatation from gastric dilatation with volvulus.

Many factors have been implicated as causes for gastric dilatation. Emesis, parturition, trauma, gastric neoplasms, overeating, pica, and abdominal surgery are most commonly associated with gastric dilatation.[364] Other factors mentioned are aerophagia,[365,366] and neurogenic stimulation of the vagus with splanchnic inhibition.[365] Other causes have been suggested in a review of acute gastric dilatation of animals.[367]

The question of bacteria producing gas from a suitable food substrate is not resolved. In a series of dogs dead for 1 to 24 hours, *Clostridium perfringens* was found.[367] Attempts at isolation of this gas-producing bacteria in most clinical cases has been fruitless. In fact, the only stomachs yielding *C. perfringens* are the black, discolored, chronic, necrotic stomachs of the moribund patient described in the review of necropsy patients.

The role of diet in the production of gastric dilatation is unresolved. Animals being fed, free-choice or selectively, meat or cereal, soybean-containing or soybean-free, small quantities or large quantities have all been identified as having gastric dilatation. Of greater consequence than the type of food are the management of the animal and hereditary factors. Postprandial exercise or excitement may elicit aerophagia as well as stretch the gastric wall and its supportive ligaments, which may lead to gastric retention and atony. Hereditary factors are probably important in predisposing some animals to acute gastric dilatation. Some family lines with high incidence of acute gastric dilatation are known to have a higher prevalence of the disease than others.

In summary, except in the case of the overeating puppy or kitten, the etiology of gastric dilatation is unknown. In all likelihood, it is a multifactorial disease involving aerophagia, feeding and management practices, hereditary factors, and other as yet unidentified causes.

Pathophysiology

Two conditions are necessary for gastric dilatation to occur: (1) a source for the distending gas, fluid, or food; and (2) an obstruction which prevents relief of distention either through eructation, emesis, absorption, or passage of the gastric contents into the small bowel.[368] As has been noted, the source of gas is unknown. Aerophagia is the most obvious means for allowing atmospheric air to enter the gastrointestinal tract.[369]

Many of the animals presented with acute gastric dilatation have a history of gulping their food rapidly. Postprandially, the animal frequently belches excessively and experiences excessive flatus. The source of this gas has been conclusively shown in man to be associated with abnormal swallowing of air.[370,371]

As the stomach dilates, it undergoes anatomic changes which, if allowed to progress, will lead to obstruction of both the pylorus and esophagus. This dilatation will involve the twisting of the fundus, allowing the duodenum to move dorsally and cranially and the greater curvature to rotate ventrally and eventually become aligned in a craniocaudal direction.

As these physical and anatomic changes occur, the venous drainage from the stomach becomes impaired leading to a localized hypoxemia and acidosis. The continued increase in the intragastric pressure causes the pyloric region to undergo abnormal excitation resulting in antiperistaltic waves[348] and later the stomach wall becomes atonic.

Gastric distention produces several cardiopulmonary effects which may culminate in the death of the patient if not rapidly reversed. The tremendous enlargement of the stomach encroaches upon the thoracic space producing an initial decreased tidal volume and increased respiratory rate. The inability to expand the thoracic cavity severely decreases lung compliance.[365] Decreased lung compliance and restricted respiratory excursion hamper effective alveolar ventilation, resulting in abnormal ventilation-perfusion ratios (V/Q) and lesions compatible with congestive atelectasis or shock lung.[372]

With acute gastric dilatation, shock is initiated by decreasing venous return to the heart. Arterial hypotension develops as central venous pressure decreases and caudal vena caval pressure increases. Experimentally, cardiac output has been shown to decrease 50% with gastric dilatation.[373]

The hemodynamic affects of caudal vena caval compression result in a decreased venous return to the heart.[374-377] Further sequestration of blood is produced, as the portal vein is also obstructed with increasing intragastric pressure.[378,379]

In summary, with acute gastric dilatation, the motility of the stomach is altered leading to atony and gastric retention. This enlarged stomach affects pulmonary and cardiovascular function resulting in hypovolemic shock.

Diagnosis

A history of overeating or having a bloated appearance is usually obtained from the pet owner. Many times the owner reports that the animal rapidly consumes its food and is affected with postprandial belching and/or flatus.

Examination of the dog will reveal a cranial

abdominal distention, usually with tympany upon percussion. The dog many times will be noted to retch with a nonproductive emesis.

Radiography affords the best means for confirmation of gastric dilatation and its differentiation from gastric volvulus. Extreme caution should be used in order to minimize additional stress to a patient already in shock.

Passage of a stomach tube has been advocated in the past as a diagnostic tool in differentiating simple dilatation from gastric volvulus.[364,380] This has not been found to be without error and many of the large breed, deep-chested dogs with gastric dilatation have had their stomach decompressed via gastric tube, only to have their stomach later noted to be in volvulus at radiography or at surgical exploration. One's ability to pass the gastric tube depends not only upon the cooperativeness of the patient, but also on the stiffness of the tube and degree of esophagogastric obstruction.

If radiography and passage of a gastric tube fail in terms of conclusively defining the problem as either simple dilatation or volvulus of the stomach, assume the stomach is in volvulus if it is a middle-aged or older, large, deep-chested dog.

Treatment

Prompt, vigorous treatment should be initiated in all cases of acute gastric dilatation. Initially, two factors deserve attention: (1) gastric dilatation and (2) shock produced by the gastric dilatation.

Early decompression of the stomach is mandatory. If a gastric tube cannot be passed, decompression may be achieved via gastric trocarization or gastrostomy.[381] Relief of distention will allow a partial return of circulating blood volume. Problems may arise at this point by the sudden, rapid release of a hypoxemic, acidotic fluid. The most likely source of the problems will be associated with the metabolic acidosis of shock and marked rise in the serum potassium concentration after gastric decompression.[360,362]

Fluid therapy at rapid rates have been advocated. The choice of fluids probably makes little difference, but lactated Ringer's or 2.5% dextrose in 0.45% sodium chloride are most frequently chosen.[381,382]

Corticosteroids are administered after the circulating fluid volume has been partially restored. Their usage will provide some protection from septic shock by decreasing either complement or complement fixation, thus preventing the production of anaphylatoxin and other shock factors. Additionally, corticosteroids afford assistance in protecting against microvascular and subcellular results of shock.[383–386]

Antibiotics have been shown to be effective in the treatment of patients with septic shock.[387]

Gastric lavage with warm saline or Ringer's solution should be instituted in cases of gastric dilatation. This lavage will remove foreign debris or excessive food which might be a source for recurrence of gastric dilatation. Lavaging is continued until contents returned are nearly clear, indicating removal of all gastric material.

Post-treatment monitoring of the patient is extremely important especially in the large breed, deep-chested dog. Gastric dilatation may recur within hours. With recurring gastric dilatation, consideration should be made to further diagnostic tests either to determine the cause of the dilatation or to note the appearance or progression of gastric dilatation to gastric volvulus.

Prognosis

Early, prompt, vigorous therapy is usually associated with a good prognosis. The animal must be closely observed for the first 3 or 4 days for signs of recurring gastric dilatation, vomiting, or signs of shock. Gastric dilatations do frequently recur and, in the susceptible animals, may progress to gastric volvulus.[363,388]

GASTRIC VOLVULUS

Gastric volvulus is a life-threatening condition most commonly seen in the large breed, deep-chested dog. Associated with the volvulus is a gastric dilatation of varying degrees. Dilatation of the stomach of moderate to severe proportions will lead to interference with the blood supply to the stomach and pathophysiologic changes affecting nearly every organ system of the animal. Additionally, a more chronic form of gastric volvulus is now being clinically recognized. In the chronic form, the stomach has rotated about its mesenteric axis but there is no significant gas accumulation and, thus, clinical signs of shock experienced by the animal with gastric dilatation and volvulus are lacking. Chronic vomiting and a history of recurrent gastric dilatation, belching, and flatulence are often noted by the client whose dog has chronic gastric volvulus.

History

Gastric dilatation complicated with volvulus is most frequently seen in the large, deep-chested breeds of dogs.[363,389,390] Rotation of the stomach about its mesenteric axis has also been reported in the Dachshund, Pekingese, and the domestic cat.[364,391-393] Gastric volvulus is more common in the male than the female[362] and in the older animal.[363,389]

A history of feeding the dog from a few hours to as many as 24 hours previously is usually obtained from the owner. Postprandial exercise or excitement also seem to precipitate the onset of gastric dilatation and volvulus.

The appearance of a gastric dilatation usually characterizes the animal with gastric volvulus. Marked cranial abdominal distention with tympany upon percussion, retching with inability to vomit, and clinical appearance of epigastric pain is usually exhibited. With pain the animal will salivate profusely, become restless, and as the duration of dilatation-volvulus increases, lethargy and shock become more apparent.

In both the acute and chronic forms of gastric volvulus, the owner often reports the dog to be a ravenous eater with frequent episodes of belching and flatulence during the postprandial interval.

Physical Examination

Acute volvulus with interference of the blood supply is an emergency. Cranial abdominal distention with tympany and retching with nonproductive emesis characterize the condition of gastric volvulus with dilatation. The appearance of the animal upon presentation varies with the interval of time elapsed since the onset of the symptoms. The animal which walks into the hospital of its own accord usually has not been affected very long. Conversely, the patient which has to be carried into the examination area, has extreme lethargy and injected mucous membranes, bears a poor prognosis.

Polypnea and tachycardia are frequently noted. These signs are considered to represent compensatory attempts at overcoming the encroachment upon the thoracic cavity and impeded venous return resulting from the gastric dilatation.

Passage of a gastric tube has been advocated in differentiating gastric dilatation from gastric volvulus. Depending upon the cooperativeness of the patient, skill of the operator, degree of gastroesophageal obstruction, and stiffness of the tube, the tube may or may not pass in the face of gastric volvulus. Passage of the gastric tube into the stomach does *not* eliminate gastric volvulus from further consideration.

When emesis occurs, it has varying appearances. With early postprandial vomiting, the food is usually undigested and rarely bile-stained. More fre-

quently, when gastric lavage is administered, the fluid is foul-smelling, coffee-colored, and may contain foreign debris such as bones, feathers, or garbage.

The body temperature can vary from hyperthermic to normothermic and even hypothermic with the onset of a septic shock. The mucous membranes may be variable in appearance from pale to normal or markedly congested. Scleral congestion is usually most pronounced in the dog with significant clinical signs of shock.

Abdominal palpation is not readily accomplished, due to the extreme distention of the stomach and associated epigastric pain. Occasionally, splenomegaly is noted, as is a displacement of the spleen either caudally or occasionally to the right side. Gas-filled intestines are usually palpated in the caudal aspect of the abdomen.

Animals with the chronic form of gastric volvulus

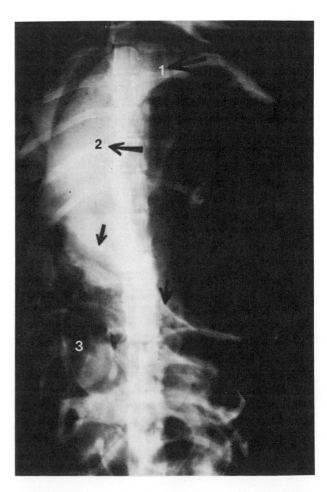

Figure 22–19. Ventrodorsal radiograph of a dog with gastric dilatation-volvulus. Note the position of the pylorus (1), spleen (2), and adynamic ileus (3).

are usually noted to have no apparent abnormalities upon physical examination.

Special Physical Examinations

Roentgenographic evaluation should be undertaken with extreme caution since the animal incurs additional stress during positioning. Frequently, it is advantageous to consider gastric decompression and therapy for shock before taking plain film or contrast radiographs.

Gastric dilatation-volvulus results in the distinguishing features of gas accumulation in the stomach, displacement of the pylorus, frequently the appearance of sacculation of the gastric fundus, and occasionally visualization of enlargement and displacement of the spleen.[361] The pylorus and duodenum are displaced cranially, dorsally, and to the left of the midline in the presence of gastric volvulus (Figs. 22–19 and 22–20).

In the chronic form of gastric volvulus, the cardia is noted to be on the right, the pylorus displaced dorsally and towards the left, and some gas noted in the stomach.[394]

Rarely, a pneumoperitoneum is noted on plain film roentgenography. If this is seen, it usually represents either an iatrogenic laceration of the stomach following gastric intubation, or gastric rupture.[395]

Adynamic ileus is frequently noted upon plain film roentgenography. The presence of air in the intestines is usually associated with swallowed air and not bacterial gas production.

Laboratory Evaluation

Clinical laboratory findings from spontaneous cases of gastric dilatation-volvulus are not currently available in the veterinary literature. Expected findings in acute volvulus should parallel those of acute dilatation with increases in blood urea nitrogen (BUN), inorganic phosphorus, alanine transaminase (SGPT), serum creatinine phosphokinase (SCPK), and aspartate transaminase (SGOT). A stress leukogram with increased packed cell volume and total protein can be expected.

Disseminated intravascular coagulation (DIC) is noted in dogs with gastric volvulus of prolonged duration. With DIC, a decrease in total platelet count (< 75,000/cu mm), prolonged prothrombin time (PT), prolonged partial thromboplastin time (PTT) and the presence of fibrin degradation products (FDP) at less than the ratio of 1:50 is expected.

Etiologic Factors

Gastric dilatation is generally conceded to precede gastric volvulus; thus, the causes of gastric dilatation must also be incriminated in gastric volvulus. One factor that most agree upon as being essential for the development of gastric volvulus is a

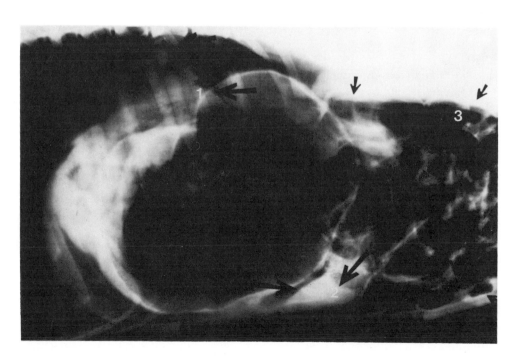

Figure 22–20. Lateral radiograph of a dog with gastric dilatation-volvulus. Note the position of the pylorus and duodenum (1), the spleen (2), and the presence of an adynamic ileus (3).

relaxation of the ligamentous supports of the stomach.[396] This relaxation is probably most notable in the gastrohepatic ligament of the dog. The cause for this ligamentous relaxation remains obscure; but recurrent gastric dilatation, overfeeding, postprandial exercise, and hereditary factors are likely involved. An atonic stomach, especially when partially fluid-filled, will twist quite readily with an absence of gastric supportive ligaments, whereas it is nearly impossible to rotate the empty stomach with intact supports.

Other anatomic features which have been implicated as causes of gastric volvulus include large, deep chests; splenic rotation;[396,397] pyloric sphincter dysfunction;[389,398] and gastric atony.[380,399] Hereditary factors also are suggested to be associated with a predisposition toward gastric volvulus.[389,390]

The etiologic factor associated with chronic gastric volvulus seems to be recurrences of gastric dilatation. These animals seem to experience episodes of gastric dilatation, each causing ligamentous lengthening, enlarging the gastric fundus, and predisposing to atony. Eventually, the stomach undergoes a twisting, but it is insufficient to cause obstruction at both the gastroesophageal and gastroduodenal segments, and accumulated gas and/or fluid is vomited or passed into the duodenum. With atony of the muscles and no supportive structures to the stomach, it remains in its position of volvulus; but little compromise of cardiovascular function results in the absence of distention or shock.

Pathophysiology

Acute gastric volvulus patients undergo the same pathophysiologic changes as patients with acute gastric dilatation. The only difference is the additional ischemia, disruption of venous return via the portal vein (Fig. 22–21) and caudal vena cava, and potential gastric necrosis resulting from the hypoxia and ischemia.[368]

The importance of hypovolemic, hypotensive shock is manifest in microvascular and subcellular organelle changes. With occlusion of the splenic vasculature, the production of factors VIII and IX is decreased.[100] A decreased circulating concentration of these clotting factors, plus many other inciting causes, may result in a disseminated intravascular coagulopathy (DIC).[401,402]

The exact cause for the high mortality seen with gastric volvulus is still disputed, but recently the failure of the reticuloendothelial system's capacity to neutralize endotoxins has been shown to contribute to the shock syndrome associated with portal

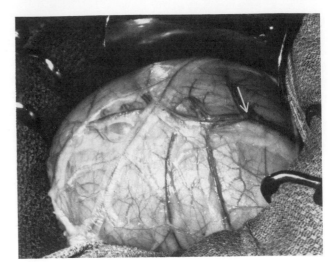

Figure 22–21. Venous congestion in the stomach of a dog with gastric dilatation-volvulus.

venous occlusion.[403,404] Endotoxin has not been identified in gastric volvulus, but cardiovascular and pathologic findings are consistent with a septic shock.

Diagnosis

A clinical history of gaseous problems after eating in a large breed, deep-chested dog suggests gastric dilatation with volvulus. These animals are admitted to the hospital usually in the acute condition where cranial abdominal distention with tympany is easily noted. The client usually reports that the animal's abdomen dilated quite rapidly and this was followed by retching with nonproductive emesis.

Radiographic evidence of gastric dilatation, with pylorus and duodenum rotated to a cranial, dorsal and leftward position over the stomach, is diagnostic for gastric volvulus. Soft tissue lines suggesting a sacculation of the stomach also confirm the radiographic diagnosis.

An inability to pass a gastric tube will suggest the diagnosis of gastric volvulus, but just because the tube passes the gastroesophageal area does not rule out gastric volvulus.

Chronic vomiting and a malpositioning of the pylorus and duodenum are suggestive of chronic gastric volvulus. This is especially true if the animal has had recurring bouts of gastric dilatation.

Treatment

As with acute dilatation, early recognition and prompt vigorous therapy are mandatory. Decompression of the stomach via gastric tube, trocariza-

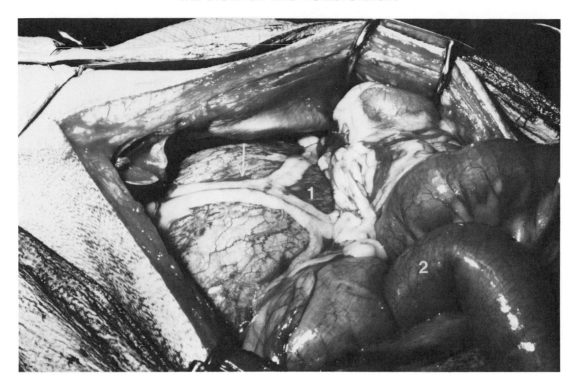

Figure 22–22. Surgical appearance following a cranial midventral abdominal incision into a dog with gastric dilatation-volvulus. Note how the greater omentum (arrow) has been pulled cranially to cover the stomach (1). An adynamic ileus is also noted with the many gas-filled loops of bowel (2).

tion, or gastrostomy is extremely important in stabilizing the patient in preparation for surgery.

Shock therapy with fluid administration, corticosteroids, and antibiotics is required in all cases of gastric volvulus with interference to the gastric blood supply. Patient monitoring during this stabilization period is a necessity.[382]

After the patient has been stabilized, anesthesia should be administered[382] and surgical correction of the volvulus undertaken. Repositioning of the stomach to its normal anatomic alignment should first be undertaken (Fig. 22–22). After the stomach has been repositioned, the gross appearance is evaluated. With areas of marked discoloration, bruising, or necrosis, a partial gastrectomy is indicated for removal of these areas.[405] Splenectomy will not prevent recurrence.[388]

Several authors have advocated the use of pyloric surgery, either pyloromyotomy or pyloroplasty, in the treatment of gastric volvulus,[364,405] to prevent its recurrence.

Gastropexy also has been advocated in the prevention of recurrence of gastric volvulus. The routine gastropexy[405] is probably effective in preventing gastric volvulus only in the immediate postoperative period.

The technique of using a tube gastrostomy[406] has many advantages. These advantages include an ease of placement at the time of the original surgery; a means for keeping the stomach decompressed; a route for administration of medication, fluids, and food, and a rigid gastropexy following removal of the tube.

Other methods to prevent a recurrence of gastric volvulus include a gastrocolopexy[407] and a "permanent" gastropexy.[408]

Prognosis

The mortality rate of dogs with gastric volvulus has been reported to be 26.8%[363] to 33%.[381] In all cases, the earlier in the course of the disease that vigorous medical and surgical therapy is initiated, the lower the mortality. Deaths associated with gastric volvulus are usually associated with necrotic areas of the stomach not removed at the time of surgery, cardiac abnormalities of an unknown etiology,[381a] peritonitis, and other unknown causes.[381]

Recurrence of gastric volvulus following surgery has been reported.[409] Close control of feeding and exercise at home may minimize that risk.

REFERENCES

1. Rooney, J. R.: Autopsy of the Horse: Technique and Interpretation. Baltimore, The Williams & Wilkins Co., 1970.
2. Rooney, J. R.: Gastric ulceration in foals. Pathol. Vet. *1*:497, 1964.
3. O'Brien, J. J.: Observations on debility and extensive hair loss in a filly. Equine Vet. J. *4*:227, 1972.
4. Neufeld, J. L.: Lymphosarcoma in the horse: a review. Can. Vet. J., *14*:129, 1973.
5. Neufeld, J. L.: Lymphosarcoma in a mare and a review of cases at the Ontario Veterinary College. Can. Vet. J. *14*:149, 1973.
6. Feldman, W. H.: Neoplasms of Domesticated Animals. Philadelphia, W. B. Saunders Co., 1932.
7. Meagher, D. M., Wheat, J. D., Tennant, B., and Osburn, B. I.: Squamous cell carcinoma of the equine stomach. J.A.V.M.A. *164*:81, 1974.
8. Kraus, E. E.: Carcinoma causing portal obstruction in the horse. North Am. Vet. *13*:25, 1932.
9. Soulsby, E. J. L.: Helminths, Arthropods and Protozoa of Domesticated Animals. Philadelphia, Lea & Febiger, 1968.
10. Blood, D. C., Henderson, J. A., and Radostits, O. M.: Veterinary Medicine, 5th ed. Philadelphia, Lea & Febiger, 1978.
11. Jones, D. G. C., Greatorex, J. C., Stockman, M. J. R., and Harris, C. P. J.: Gastric impaction in a pony: relief via laparotomy. Equine Vet. J. *4*:98, 1972.
12. Peterson, F. B., Donawick, W. J., Merritt, A. M., Raker, C. W., Reid, C. F., and Rooney, J. R.: Gastric stenosis in a horse. J.A.V.M.A. *160*:328, 1972.
13. Hutyra, F., and Marek, J.: Special Pathology and Therapeutics of the Diseases of Domestic Animals, 3rd ed. Vol. II. London, Bailliere, Tindall and Cox, 1926.
14. Speirs, V. C., and Reynolds, W. T.: Successful repair of a diaphragmatic hernia in a foal. Equine Vet. J. *8*:170, 1976.
15. Scott, E. A., and Fishback, W. A.: Surgical repair of diaphragmatic hernia in a horse. J.A.V.M.A. *168*:45, 1976.
16. McCunn, J.: Rupture of the diaphragm. Vet. Rec. *5*:556, 1925.
17. Jubb, K. V. F. and Kennedy, P. C.: Pathology of Domestic Animals, 2nd ed. New York, Academic Press, 1970.
18. Firth, E. C.: Diaphragmatic hernia in horses. Cornell Vet. *66*:353, 1976.
19. Coffman, J. R., and Kintner, L. D.: Strangulated diaphragmatic hernia in a horse. V.M./S.A.C. *67*:423, 1972.
20. Dunlop, R. H., and Hammond, P. B.: D-lactic acidosis of ruminants. Ann. N.Y. Acad. Sci. *119*:1109, 1965.
21. Dunlop, R. H.: Pathogenesis of ruminant lactic acidosis. Adv. Vet. Sci. Comp. Med. *16*:259, 1972.
22. Hungate, R. E., Dougherty, R. W., Bryant, M. P., and Cello, R. M.: Microbiological and physiological changes associated with acute indigestion in sheep. Cornell Vet. *42*:432, 1952.
23. Dain, J. A., Neal, A. L., and Dougherty, R. W.: The occurrence of histamine and tyramine in rumen ingesta of experimentally overfed sheep. J. Anim. Sci. *14*:930, 1955.
24. Irwin, L. N., Tucker, R. E., Mitchell, G. E., Jr., and Shelling, G. T.: Amine production by sheep with glucose-induced lactic acidosis. J. Anim. Sci. *35*:267, 1972.
25. Vestweber, J. G. E., and Leipold, H. W.: Experimentally induced ovine ruminal acidosis: pathologic changes. Am. J. Vet. Res. *35*:1537, 1974.
26. Dougherty, R. W., Coburn, K. S., Cook, H. M., and Allison, M. J.: Preliminary study of appearance of endotoxin in circulatory system of sheep and cattle after grain engorgement. Am. J. Vet. Res. *36*:831, 1975.
27. Dougherty, R. W., Riley, J. L., and Cook, H. M.: Changes in motility and pH in the digestive tract of experimentally overfed sheep. Am. J. Vet. Res. *36*:827, 1975.
28. Mullen, P. A.: Overfeeding in cattle: clinical, biochemical and therapeutic aspects. Vet. Rec. *98*:439, 1976.
29. Dirksen, G. A.: Acidosis. *In* Physiology of Digestion and Metabolism of Ruminant. Edited by A. T. Phillipson. Newcastle, England, Oriel Press, 1970, p. 612.
30. Gordon, E. E.: Etiology of lactic acidosis. Am. J. Med. Sci. *265*:463, 1973.
31. Morrow, L. L., Tumbleson, M. E., Kintner, L. D., Pfander, W. H., and Preston, R. L.: Laminitis in lambs injected with lactic acid. Am. J. Vet. Res. *34*:1305, 1973.
32. Telle, P. P., and Preston, R. L.: Ovine lactic acidosis: intraruminal and systemic. J. Anim. Sci. *33*:698, 1971.
33. Slyter, L. L.: Influence of acidosis on rumen function. J. Anim. Sci. *43*:910, 1976.
34. Elam, C. J.: Acidosis in feedlot cattle: practical observations. J. Anim. Sci. *43*:898, 1976.
35. Dougherty, R. W., Riley, J. L., Baetz, A. L., Cook, H. M., and Coburn, K. S.: Physiologic studies of experimentally grain engorged cattle and sheep. Am. J. Vet. Res. *36*:833, 1975.
36. Nilsson, S. A.: Clinical, morphological, and experimental studies of laminitis in cattle. Acta Vet. Scand. *4*(Suppl. 1):1, 1963.
37. MacLean, C. W.: Observations of laminitis in intensive beef units. Vet. Rec. *78*:223, 1966.
38. MacLean, C. W.: A post-mortem x-ray study of laminitis in barley beef animals. Vet. Rec. *86*:457, 1970.
39. Huber, T. L.: Lactic acidosis and renal function of sheep. J. Anim. Sci. *29*:612, 1969.
40. Vestweber, J. G. E., Leipold, H. W., and Smith, J. E.: Ovine ruminal acidosis: clinical studies. Am. J. Vet. Res. *35*:1587, 1974.
41. Nicholson, J. W. G., and Cunningham, H. M.: Retained placenta, abortion and abnormal calves from beef cows fed all-barley rations. Can. Vet. J. *6*:275, 1965.
42. Nilo, L., Dorward, W. J., and Avery, R. J.: A note on an investigation of mortality in feedlot cattle. Can. Vet. J. *8*:101, 1967.
43. Wilson, J. R., Bartley, E. E., Anthony, H. D., Brent, B. E., Sapienza, D. A., Chapman, T. E., Dayton, A. D., Milleret, R. J., Frey, R. A., and Meyer, R. M.: Analysis of rumen fluid from "sudden death" lactic acidotic and healthy cattle fed high concentrate ration. J. Anim. Sci. *41*:1249, 1975.
44. Huber, T. L.: Effect of acute indigestion on compartmental water volumes and osmolality in sheep. Am. J. Vet. Res. *32*:887, 1971.
45. Krogh, N.: Studies on alterations in the rumen fluid of sheep, especially concerning the microbial composition when readily available carbohydrates are added to the food. III. Starch. Acta Vet. Scand. *2*:103, 1961.
46. Allison, M. J., Robinson, I. M., Dougherty, R. W., and Bucklin, J. A.: Grain overload in cattle and sheep: changes in microbial populations in the cecum and rumen. Am. J. Vet. Res. *36*:181, 1975.
47. Rodwell, A. A.: The occurrence and distribution of amino-acid decarboxylases within the genus *Lactobacillus*. J. Gen. Microbiol. *8*:224, 1953.
48. Van Miert, A. S. J. P. A., Van Duin, C. Th. M., and Veenendall, G. H.: Role of histamine in the genesis of pyrogen (endotoxin)-induced reticuloruminal stasis in goats. Zentralbl. Veterinaermed[A] *23*:819, 1976.
49. Phillipson, A. T., and Reid, R. S.: Thiamine in the contents of the alimentary tract of sheep. Br. J. Nutr. *11*:27, 1957.
50. Ryan, R. K.: A study of the phenomenon of adaptation by sheep to gradual increase in grain intake as an approach to an understanding of the pathogenesis of grain engorgements in sheep. Ph.D. Thesis, Ithaca, NY, Cornell University, 1963.
51. Ryan, K. K.: Concentrations of glucose and low-molecular-weight acids in the rumen of sheep following the addition of large amounts of wheat to the rumen. Am. J. Vet. Res. *25*:646, 1964.
52. Svendsen, P.: The effect of volatile fatty acids and lactic acid on rumen motility in sheep. Nord. Vet. Med. *25*:226, 1973.
53. Huber, T. L.: Physiological effects of acidosis on feedlot cattle. J. Anim. Sci. *43*:902, 1976.
54. Ahrens, F. A.: Histamine, lactic acid, and hypertonicity as factors in the development of ruminitis in cattle. Am. J. Vet. Res. *28*:1335, 1967.
55. Sandford, J.: Formation of histamine in ruminal fluid. Nature *199*:829, 1963.
56. Brent, B. E.: Relationship of acidosis to other feedlot ailments. J. Anim. Sci. *43*:930, 1976.
57. Streeve, J. E., and Edwin, E. E.: Thiaminase producing strains of *Cl. sporogenes* associated with outbreaks of cerebrocortical necrosis. Vet. Rec. *94*:330, 1974.
58. Thomson, R. G.: Rumenitis in cattle. Can. Vet. J. *8*:189, 1967.
59. Radostits, O. M., and Magnusson, R. A.: A modification of an old method for emptying the rumen of cattle. Can. Vet. J. *12*:150, 1971.
60. Muri, P.: Post-ingestion prevention of rumen overload syndrome in cattle. Can. Vet. J. *15*:54, 1974.
61. Huber, T. L.: Effect of intraruminal inoculation on adaptation of lambs and heifers to a high energy ration. Am. J. Vet. Res. *35*:639, 1974.
62. Huber, T. L., Cooley, J. H., Goetsch, D. D., and Das, N. K.: Lactic acid-utilizing bacteria in ruminal fluid of a steer adapted from hay feeding to a high-grain ration. Am. J. Vet. Res. *37*:611, 1976.
63. Cook, M. K., Cooley, J. H., Edens, J. D., Goetsch, D. D., Das, N. K., and Huber, T. L.: Effect of ruminal lactic acid-utilizing bacteria on adaptation of cattle to high energy rations. Am. J. Vet. Res. *38*:1015, 1977.
64. Tremere, A. W., Merrill, W. G., and Loosli, J. K.: Adaptation to high concentrate feeding as related to acidosis in digestive disturbances in dairy heifers. J. Dairy Sci. *51*:1065, 1968.
65. Boda, J. M., Cupps, P. T., Colvin, H., and Cole, H. H.: The

sequence of events preceding death in a cow in acute experimental bloat on fresh alfalfa tops. J.A.V.M.A. *128*:531, 1956.

66. Howarth, R. E.: A review of bloat in cattle. Can. Vet. J. *16*:281, 1975.

67. McArthur, J. M., Miltimore, J. E., and Pratt, M. J.: Bloat investigations. The foam stabilizing protein of alfalfa. Can. J. Anim. Sci. *44*:200, 1964.

68. McArthur, J. M., and Miltimore, J. E.: Bloat investigations. The pH of rumen contents and its role on bloat. Can. J. Anim. Sci. *49*:69, 1969.

69. Bartley, E. E.: An analysis of the bloat complex and progress towards its prevention. J.A.V.M.A. *147*:1397, 1965.

70. Reid, C. S. W., Lyttleton, J. W., and Mangan, J. L.: Bloat in cattle XXIV. A method for measuring the effectiveness of chewing in the release of plant cell contents from ingested feed. N.Z. J. Agric. Res. *5*:237, 1962.

71. Dougherty, R. W.: The continuing quest for the cause of bloat in ruminants. J.A.V.M.A. *122*:345, 1953.

72. Kintner, L. D.: Bloat. Proc. Annu. Conf. Am. Assoc. Bovine Pract. *7*:163, 1974.

73. Nichols, R. E.: Frothy tympanities—its causes and control. North Am. Vet. *38*:168, 1957.

74. Rosen, W. G., Hester, F., and Nichols, R. E.: Etiology of legume bloat—non-volatile fatty acids. Am. J. Vet. Res. *22*:117, 1961.

75. Clarke, R. T. J., and Hungate, R. E.: Bloating in cattle. Microbial activities in the reticulo-rumens of cows differently susceptible to legume bloat. N. Z. J. Agric. Res. *14*:108, 1971.

76. Stifel, F. B., Vetter, R. L., and Allen, R. S.: Relationship between calcium and magnesium binding to fraction I chloroplasts protein and bloat. J. Agric. Food Chem. *16*:500, 1968.

77. Stifel, F. B., and Vetter, R. L.: Effects of feed intake upon bloating patterns in lambs fed alfalfa silage. J. Anim. Sci. *26*:385, 1967.

78. Colvin, H. W., and Daniels, L. B.: Rumen motility as influenced by physical form of oat hay. J. Dairy Sci. *48*:935, 1965.

79. Medel, V. E., and Boda, J. M.: Physiological studies of the rumen with emphasis on the animal factors associated with bloat. J. Dairy Sci. *64*:1881, 1961.

80. Pounden, W. D., Frank, N. A., Sanger, V. L., and King, N. B.: Feedlot bloat. J.A.V.M.A. *137*:503, 1960.

81. Dougherty, R. W.: Cinefluorographic studies of the ruminant stomach and of eructation. Am. J. Vet. Res. *16*:96, 1955.

82. Whitlock, R. H., and Ley, H.: Bloat in veal calves. Veal Grower *8*:12. 1976.

83. Mills, J. H. L., and Christian, R. G.: Lesions of bovine tympany. J.A.V.M.A. *157*:947, 1970.

84. Buff, B.: Die behandlung chronisch—rezidivierender tympanien bein rind. mit einem schraubtrokor. D.T.W. *76*:601, 1969.

85. Miller, C. R.: Prevention and management of frothy bloat in cattle. Bovine Pract. *5*:20, 1970.

86. Meyer, R. M., Helmer, L. G., and Bartley, E. E.: Bloat in cattle. VIII. Extent of elimination in milk and body tissues of C^{14}-labeled poloxalene used to prevent legume bloat. J. Dairy Sci. *48*:503, 1965.

87. Jacobsen, D. R., Lindahl, I. L., McNeill, J. J., Shaw, J. C., Doetsch, R. N., and Davis, R. E.: Feedlot bloat studies. Two physical factors involved in the etiology of frothy bloat. J. Anim. Sci. *16*:515, 1957.

88. Bryant, M. P., Barrentine, B. F., Sykes, J. F., Robinson, I. M., Shawver, D. V., and Williams, L. W.: Predominant bacteria in the rumen of cattle on bloat-provoking ladino clover pasture. J. Dairy Sci. *43*:1435, 1960.

89. Grosskopf, J. F. W.: Advances in research on acute frothy bloat in ruminants. J. S. Afr. Vet. Med. Assoc. *35*:169, 1964.

90. Elam, C. J., and Davis, R. E.: Ruminal characteristics and feedlot bloat incidence in cattle as influenced by vegetable oil, mineral oil and animal fat. J. Anim. Sci. *21*:568, 1962.

91. Roztocil, V., Chaudhari, A. Q., and El Mouty, I. A.: Induced traumatic reticuloperitonitis in goats. Vet. Rec. *83*:667, 1968.

92. Poulsen, J. S. D.: Prevention of traumatic indigestion in cattle. Vet. Rec. *98*:149, 1976.

93. Maddy, K. T.: Incidence of perforation of the bovine reticulum. J.A.V.M.A. *124*:113, 1954.

94. Hofmeyr, C. F. B.: The diagnosis and differential diagnosis of traumatic reticulitis in the cow. J.A.V.M.A. *130*:183, 1957.

95. Hughes, J. P., and Kennedy, P. C.: Traumatic reticulitis—an outbreak in a large dairy. J.A.V.M.A. *134*:383, 1958.

96. Hjerpe, C. A.: Studies of acute bovine traumatic reticuloperitonitis. II. Signs of traumatic reticuloperitonitis. J.A.V.M.A. *139*:230, 1961.

97. Kingrey, B. W.: Experimental bovine traumatic gastritis. J.A.V.M.A. *127*:477, 1955.

98. Hansen, A. G.: Traumatic reticulitis. J.A.V.M.A. *122*:290, 1953.

99. Churchill, E. A.: Diagnosis and surgical treatment of traumatic gastritis. J.A.V.M.A. *116*:196, 1950.

100. Holtenius, P., Jacobson, S. O., and Jonson, G.: Recording of the reticular motility in cattle with experimental and spontaneous traumatic reticuloperitonitis. Acta Vet. Scand. *12*:325, 1971.

101. Williams, E. I.: A study on reticuloruminal motility in adult cattle in relation to bloat and traumatic reticulitis with an account of the latter condition as seen in a general practice. Vet. Rec. *67*:922, 1955.

102. Williams, E. I.: Further observations on traumatic reticulitis and bloat in cattle. Vet. Rec. *68*:835, 1956.

103. Hjerpe, C. A.: Studies on acute bovine traumatic reticuloperitonitis. III. Haematology. J.A.V.M.A. *139*:233, 1961.

104. Blood, D. C., and Hutchins, D. R.: Traumatic reticular perforation of cattle with particular reference to the efficiency of conservative treatment. Aust. Vet. J. *31*:113, 1955.

105. Spurrell, F. A., and Kernkamp, H. C. H.: Radiological localization in diagnosis of foreign bodies in cattle. Proc. Annu. Meet. Am. Vet. Med. Assoc. *90*:79, 1952.

106. Oehme, F. W.: Cytological examination of the peritoneal fluid in the diagnosis of cattle disease. J.A.V.M.A. *155*:1923, 1969.

107. Jagos, P.: The characteristics of foreign bodies in traumatic inflammation of cattle. Acta Vet. (Brno) *38*:545, 1969.

108. Hutchins, D. R., Blood, D. C., and Hyne, R.: Residual defects in stomach motility after traumatic reticuloperitonitis of cattle. Pyloric obstruction, diaphragmatic hernia and indigestion due to reticular adhesions. Aust. Vet. J. *33*:77, 1957.

109. Fraser, C. M.: Conservative treatment of traumatic reticulitis. Can. Vet. J. *2*:65, 1961.

110. Hjerpe, C. A.: Studies on acute bovine traumatic reticuloperitonitis. I. Platform method of treatment. J.A.V.M.A. *139*:227, 1961.

111. Nusbaum, S. R.: A technique for treatment of bovine reticulitis. J.A.V.M.A. *126*:473, 1955.

112. Muffly, J. A., and Pint, L. H.: Nonsurgical removal of foreign bodies with a magnet. Proc. Ann. Meet. Am. Vet. Med. Assoc. *92*:48, 1955.

113. Kettle, E. W., and Snook, M. D.: Prevention of so-called "hardware disease" in cattle using a magnetic metal retriever. J.A.V.M.A. *130*:285, 1957.

114. Carroll, R. E.: Magnets in the control of traumatic gastritis. J.A.V.M.A. *127*:311, 1955.

115. Dunn, H. O., Roberts, S. J., McEntee, K., and Wagner, W. C.: Prevention of traumatic gastritis in bulls by use of magnets. Cornell Vet. *55*:204, 1965.

116. Rosenberger, G., and Stober, M.: Consideration of the treatment and prevention of foreign body diseases in cattle using magnetic instruments. D.T.W. *65*:57, 1958.

117. Albright, J. L., Briggs, J. L., and Jessup, R. V.: Long term effects of magnets and management in the control of traumatic reticulitis (hardware disease) in large commercial dairy herds. J. Dairy Sci. *45*:547, 1962.

118. Carroll, R. E.: Use of magnets in the control of traumatic gastritis of cattle. J.A.V.M.A. *129*:376, 1956.

119. Hoflund, S.: Investigations in functional disorders of the bovine stomach caused by lesions of the nervus vagus. Svensk. Vet. Tidskr. *45*(Suppl.), 1940.

120. Begg, H.: Diseases of the stomach of the adult ruminant. Vet. Rec. *62*:797, 1950.

121. Clark, C. H.: Clinical signs of vagal nerve injuries in ruminants. Vet. Med. *48*:389, 1953.

122. Dirksen, G., and Stober, M.: Beitrag zu den durch schadigungen des nervus vagus bedigten funktionsstorungen des rindermagens—hoflundsches syndrom. D.T.W. *69*:1, 1962.

123. Whitlock, R. H., and Brown, W. R.: Chronic cholangiohepatitis in a dairy cow. Cornell Vet. *59*:515, 1969.

124. Pope, D. C.: Abomasal impaction of adult cattle. Vet. Rec. *73*:1174, 1961.

125. Whitlock, R. H., Tasker, J. B., and Tennant, B. C.: Hypochloremic metabolic alkalosis and hypokalemia in cattle with upper gastrointestinal tract obstruction. Am. J. Dig. Dis. *20*:595, 1975.

126. Gingerich, D. A., and Murdick, P. W.: Paradoxic aciduria in bovine metabolic alkalosis. J.A.V.M.A. *166*:227, 1975.

127. Gingerich, D. A., and Murdick, P. W.: Experimentally induced intestinal obstruction in sheep: paradoxical aciduria and metabolic alkalosis. Am. J. Vet. Res. *36*:663, 1975.

128. Norrdin, R. W.: Thymoma and pulmonary metastasis in a 12-year-old bull with chronic bloat. Cornell Vet. *60*:617, 1970.

129. Neal, P. A. and Edwards, G. B.: "Vagus indigestion" in cattle. Vet. Rec. *82*:396, 1968.

130. Naerland, G., and Helle, O.: Functional pyloric stenosis in sheep. Vet. Rec. *74*:85, 1962.

131. Leek, B. F.: Vagus indigestion in cattle. Vet. Rec. *82*:498, 1968.

132. Titchen, D. A.: Reflex stimulation and inhibition of reticulum contractions in the ruminant stomach. J. Physiol. *141*:1, 1958.

133. Leek, B. F.: Reticulo-ruminal function and dysfunction. Vet. Rec. *84*:238, 1969.

134. Sellers, A. F., and Stevens, C. E.: Motor function of the ruminant forestomach. Physiol. Rev. *46*:643, 1966.

135. Dirksen, G., and Rantze, H.: Untersuchungen über die brauchbarkeit der atropinprobe fur die differential-diagnose de bradykardie beim rind. Berl. Munch. Tierarztl. Wochenschr. *81*:171, 1968.

136. Sack, W. O.: Abdominal topography of a cow with left abomasal displacement. Am. J. Vet. Res. *29*:1567, 1968.

137. Steere, J. H.: The wandering abomasum. Mod. Vet. Pract. *42*:29, 1961.

138. Mather, M. F., and Dedrick, R. S.: Displacement of the abomasum. Cornell Vet. *56*:323, 1966.

139. Martin, J. A.: Dilation with torsion of the abomasum in a six-week-old calf. Vet. Rec. *76*:297, 1964.

140. Fraser, J. A., Imlah, P., and McPherson, E. A.: Displacement of the abomasum in the ewe. Vet. Rec. *71*:858, 1959.

141. Whitlock, R. H.: Diseases of the abomasum associated with current feeding practices. J.A.V.M.A. *154*:1203,1969.

142. Robertson, J. M., and Boucher, W. B.: Left displacement of the bovine abomasum: epizootiologic factors. Am. J. Vet. Res. *29*:421, 1966.

143. Fox, F. H.: Abomasal disorders. J.A.V.M.A. *147*:383, 1965.

144. Pinsent, P. J. N., Neal, P. A., and Ritchie, H. E.: Displacement of the bovine abomasum. A review of 80 clinical cases. Vet. Rec. *73*:729, 1961.

145. Robertson, J. M.: Left displacement of the bovine abomasum: clinical findings. Vet. Rec. *79*:530, 1966.

146. Boucher, W. B., and Abt, D.: Right sided dilation of the bovine abomasum with torsion. J.A.V.M.A. *153*:76, 1968.

147. Corougeau and Prestat: Torsion de la caillette chez un veau. J. Med. Vet. *2*:340, 1898.

148. Jones, W.: Abomasal displacement in cattle. Cornell Vet. *42*:53, 1954.

149. Neal, P. A., and Pinsent, P. J. N.: Dilatation and torsion of the bovine abomasum. Vet. Rec. *72*:175, 1960.

150. Pinsent, P. J. N.: The differential diagnosis of abdominal disorders of the bovine animal. Vet. Rec. *74*:1282, 1962.

151. Neal, P. A.: Some clinical observations on the etiology of displacement of the abomasum in the dairy cow. Nord. Vet. Med. *16*:361, 1964.

152. Martin, W.: Left abomasal displacement: an epidemiological study. Can. Vet. J. *13*:61, 1972.

153. Moore, G. R., Riley, W. F., Westcott, R. W., and Conner, G. H.: Displacement of the bovine abomasum. Vet. Med. *49*:49, 1954.

154. Hansen, A. G., Elefson, E. P., Warsinske, H. E., Hjort, O., and Schornberg, R.: Displaced abomasum: a relatively common bovine syndrome. North Am. Vet. *38*:129, 1957.

155. Esperson, G.: Dilatatio et dislocatio ad dextram abomasi bovis. Nord. Vet. Med. *13*(Suppl. 1):1, 1961.

156. Bischoff, P.: Torsio abomasi bovis with special reference to etiology and pathogenesis. Stockholm, 15th World Veterinary Congress, 1953, p. 1040.

157. Svendsen, P.: Geosedimentum abomasi bovis. Nord. Vet. Med. *17*:500, 1965.

158. Dirksen, G.: Vorkommen, ursachen und entwicklung der linksseitigen labmagenverlagerung. (Dislocatio abomasi sinistra des Rinder.) (Occurrences, cause and development of left-side abomasal displacement in cattle.) D.T.W. *68*:8, 1961.

159. Marr, A., and Jarrett, W. F.: Displacement of the abomasum associated with peptic ulceration in a cow. Vet. Rec. *67*:332, 1955.

160. Albert, T. F., and Ramey, D. B.: Abomasal displacement associated with ingestion of gasoline. J.A.V.M.A. *145*:460, 1964.

161. Nilsson, L. S., Jr.: Etiology of abomasal displacement. Mod. Vet. Pract. *43*:68, 1962.

162. Coppock, C. E., Noller, C. H., Wolfe, S. A., Callahan, C. J., and Baker, J. S.: Effect of forage-concentrate ratio in complete feeds fed *ad libitum* on feed intake prepartum and the occurrence of abomasal displacement in dairy cows. J. Dairy Sci. *55*:783, 1972.

163. Hull, B. L., and Wass, W. M.: Causative factors in abomasal displacement. I. Literature review. V. M./S. A. C. *68*:283, 1973.

164. Dirksen, G.: Die erweiterung, verlagerung und drehung des labmagens beim rind. Berlin and Hamburg, Paul Parey, 1962.

165. Ide, P., and Henry, J. H.: Abomasal abnormalities in dairy cattle: a review of 90 clinical cases. Can. Vet. J. *5*:46, 1964.

166. Svendsen, P.: Abomasal displacement in cattle. Nord. Vet. Med. *22*:571, 1970.

167. Poulsen, J. S. D.: Aetiology and pathogenesis of abomasal displacement in dairy cattle. Nord. Vet. Med. *28*:299, 1976.

168. Poulsen, J. S. D.: Abomasal displacements in dairy cows: clinical chemistry and studies on the aetiology. Thesis. Stockholm, Royal Veterinary College, 1973.

169. Svendsen, P.: Etiology and pathogenesis of abomasal displacement in cattle. Nord. Vet. Med. *21*:1, 1969.

170. Bolton, J. R., Merritt, A. M., Carlson, G. M., and Donawick, W. J.: Normal abomasal electromyography and emptying in sheep and the effects of intra-abomasal volatile fatty acid infusion. Am. J. Vet. Res. *37*:1387, 1976.

171. Breukink, H. J., and de Ruyter, T.: Abomasal displacement in cattle: influence of concentrates in the ration on fatty acid concentrations in ruminal, abomasal and duodenal contents. Am. J. Vet. Res. *37*:1181, 1976.

172. Twisselman, K. L.: The role of fatty acids in the etiology of abomasal displacement. M. S. Thesis. Ithaca, NY, Cornell University, 1972.

173. Ash, R. W.: Stimuli influencing the secretion of acid by the abomasum of sheep. J. Physiol. *157*:185, 1961.

174. Hull, B. L., and Wass, W. M.: Abomasal displacement. II. Hypocalcemia as a contributing causative factor. V. M./S. A. C. *68*:412, 1973.

175. Gakala, S. Z., Rakalska, A., Albrycht, J., Staniszewska-Barkouska, K., Bienick, S., and Barkowski, T.: Effects of starvation on some clinical and biochemical parameters in cattle. Milano, 8th International Congress Diseases of Cattle, *8*:111, 1974.

176. Breukink, H. J.: Het verLoop van pH en popsinogeholte van de Lebmaginhoud. bij het volwassen rund. Tijdschr. Diergeneeskd. *98*:1051, 1973.

177. Whitlock, R. H.: Cecal volvulus in dairy cattle. Paris, Proceedings 9th International Congress on Diseases of Cattle. *9*:68, 1976.

178. Cote, J. F.: Displaced abomasum—a method of correction. Can. Vet. J. *1*:58, 1960.

179. Braun, R. K.: Non-surgical correction of left abomasal displacement in the cow. Cornell Vet. *58*:111, 1968.

180. Albert, T. F., and Ramey, D. B.: Apparent asymptomatic left abomasal displacement in a cow. J.A.V.M.A. *152*:1125, 1968.

181. Ingling, A. L., Albert, T. F., and Schueler, R. L.: Left abomasal displacement in a clinically normal cow. J.A.V.M.A. *166*:601, 1975.

182. Hull, B. L.: Surgical procedures for correction of abomasal displacement. Paris, Proceedings 9th International Congress on Cattle Diseases, *9*:47, 1976.

183. Hoffsis, G. F.: Right paralumbar omentopexy for the correction of left displaced abomasum. Proc. Am. Assoc. Bovine Pract. *4*:179, 1970.

184. Ames, S.: Repositioning the displaced abomasum in the cow. J.A.V.M.A. *153*:1470, 1968.

185. Baker, J. S.: Right displacement of the abomasum in the bovine—a modified procedure for treatment. Bovine Pract. *11*:58, 1976.

186. Gabel, A. G., and Heath, R. B.: Treatment of right-sided torsion of the abomasum in cattle. J.A.V.M.A. *155*:642, 1969.

187. Gabel, A. G., and Heath, R. B.: Correction and right sided omentopexy in treatment of left sided displacement of the abomasum in dairy cattle. J.A.V.M.A. *155*:632, 1969.

188. Lowe, J. E., Loomis, W. K., and Kramer, L. L.: Abomasopexy for repair of left abomasal displacement in dairy cattle. J.A.V.M.A. *147*:389, 1965.

189. Robertson, J. M., and Boucher, W. B.: Treatment of left displacement of bovine abomasum. J.A.V.M.A. *149*:1423, 1966.

190. Poulson, J. S. D.: Right-sided abomasal displacement in dairy cows: pre- and postoperative clinical chemical findings. Nord. Vet. Med. *26*:65, 1974.

191. Whitlock, R. H.: Non-infectious abdominal diseases of cattle. Abstracts 64th Annual Conference for Veterinarians, Ithaca, N.Y., NY State Veterinary College, 1972.

192. Weaver, A. D.: A postmortem survey of some features of the bovine abomasum. Br. Vet. J. *120*:539, 1964.

193. Wallace, C. E.: Prognostic significance of diarrhea in cows with left displacement of the abomasum. Bovine Pract. *11*:62, 1976.

194. Smith, D. F.: Right sided torsion of the abomasum in dairy cows: retrospective analysis and proposed classification of severity. J.A.V.M.A. *173* (1):108, 1978.

195. Jensen, R., Person, R. E., Braddy, D. A., Snari, D. A., Benitez, A., Laverman, L. H., Horton, D. P., and McChesney, A. E.: Fatal abomasal ulcers in yearling feedlot cattle. J.A.V.M.A. *169*:524, 1976.

196. Aukema, J. J., and Breukink, H. J.: Abomasal ulcer in adult cattle with fatal hemorrhage. Cornell Vet., *64*:303, 1974.

197. Rooney, J. R., Watson, D. F., and Hoag, W. G.: Abomasal ulceration and perforation. North Am. Vet. 37:750, 1956.
198. Whitlock, R. H.: What's new in the lower digestive tract? Proc. Amer. Assoc. Bovine Pract. 4:32, 1971.
199. Schotman, A. J. H., and Staver, C. J. M.: The determination of serum pepsinogen in clinically healthy cows. Tijdschr. Diergeneeskd. 94:653, 1969.
200. Kallfelz, F. A., and Whitlock, R. H.: Survival of ^{59}Fe-labeled erythrocytes in cross-transfused bovine blood. Am. J. Vet. Res. 34:1041, 1973.
201. Tasker, J. B., Roberts, S. J., Fox, F. H., and Hall, C. E.: Abomasal ulcers in cattle. Recovery of one cow after surgery. J.A.V.M.A. 133:365, 1958.
202. Whitlock, R. H.: Personal communication.
203. Pope, D. C., and Bennett, J. B.: Abomasal ulceration in a Jersey cow. Can. Vet. J. 2:189, 1961.
204. Hungate, R. E.: The Rumen and its Microbes. New York, Academic Press. 1966.
205. King, J. M.: Personal communication. Ithaca, NY, New York State College of Veterinary Medicine, 1975.
206. Hemmingsen, I.: Erosiones et ulcera abomasal bovis. Nord. Vet. Med., 18:354, 1966.
207. Hemmingsen, I.: Ulcus perforans abomasi bovis. Nord. Vet. Med., 19:17, 1967.
208. Hill, H. J.: Abomasal secretion in sheep. J. Physiol. 154:115, 1960.
209. Hirschowitz, B. I.: The physiology of pepsinogen. In Pathophysiology of Peptic Ulcer. Edited by S. C. Skoryna. Philadelphia, J. B. Lippincott Co., 1963.
210. Menguy, R., Desbaillets, L., and Masters, Y. F.: Mechanism of stress ulcer: influence of hypovolemic shock on energy metabolism in the gastric mucosa. Gastroentrology 66:46, 1974.
211. Safaie-Shirazi, S., Foster, L. D., and Hardy, B. M.: The effect of metiamide, an H_2-receptor antagonist in the prevention of experimental stress ulcers. Gastroenterol. 71:421, 1976.
212. Henn, R. M., Isenberg, J. I., Maxwell, V., and Sturdevant, R. A. L.: Inhibition of gastric acid secretion by cimetidine in patient with duodenal ulcer. N. Engl. J. Med. 293:371, 1975.
213. Gitter, M., and Austwick, P. K. C.: The presence of fungi in abomasal ulcers of young calves: a report of seven cases. Vet. Rec. 69:924, 1957.
214. Neitzke, J. P., and Schiefer, B.: Incidence of mycotic gastritis in calves up to 30 days of age. Can. Vet. J. 15:139, 1974.
215. Ohshima, K., Miura, S., Selmiya, Y., and Chihaya, Y.: Pathological studies on mucormyosis of the forestomach and abomasum in ruminants: a report on six cases complicated with candidiasis or pulmonary aspergillosis. Jpn. J. Vet. Sci. 38:269, 1976.
216. Mills, J. H., and Hirth, R. S.: Systemic candidiasis in calves on prolonged antibiotic therapy. J.A.V.M.A. 150:862, 1967.
217. Gleiser, C. A.: Mucormycosis in animals. J.A.V.M.A. 123:441, 1953.
218. Kharole, M. U., Gupta, P. P., Singh, B., Mandal, P. C., and Hothl, D. S.: Phycomycotic gastritis in buffalo calves (Bubalis bubalis). Vet. Pathol. 13:409, 1976.
219. Perry, T. W., Jimenez, A. A., Shively, J. E., Curtin, T. M., Pickett, R. A., and Beeson, W. M.: Incidence of gastric ulcers in swine. Science 139:349, 1963.
220. Muggenberg, B. A., Reese, N., Kowalczyk, T., Grummer, R. H., and Hoekstra, W. G.: Survey of the prevalence of gastric ulcers in swine. Am. J. Vet.Res. 25:1673, 1964.
221. Niederman, J. C., Spiro, H. M., and Sheldon, W. H.: Blood pepsin as a marker of susceptibility to duodenal ulcer disease. Arch. Environ. Health, 8:540, 1964.
222. Ader, R., Beels, C. C., and Tatum, R.: Blood pepsinogen and gastric erosions in the rat. Psychosom. Med. 22:1, 1960.
223. Ader, R.: Plasma pepsinogen level as a predictor of susceptibility to gastric erosions in the rat. Psychosom. Med. 25:221, 1963.
224. Armour, J., and Bruce, R. G.: Inhibited development in Ostertagia ostertagi infections—a diapause phenomenon in a nematode. Parasitology 69:161, 1974.
225. Michel, J. F., Lancaster, M. B., and Hong, C.: Observations on the resumed development of arrested Ostertagia ostertagi in naturally infected yearling cattle. J. Comp. Pathol. 86:73, 1976.
226. Anderson, N., Armour, J., Jarrett, W. F. H., Jennings, F. W., Ritchie, J. S. D., and Urquhart, G. M.: A field study of parasitic gastritis in cattle. Vet. Rec. 77:1196, 1965.
227. Murray, M., Jennings, F. W., and Armour, J.: Bovine ostertagiasis: structure, function and mode of differentiation of the bovine gastric mucosa and kinetics of the worm loss. Res. Vet. Sci. 11:417, 1970.
228. Doran, D. J.: The course of infection and pathogenic effect of Trichostronglyus axei in calves. Am. J. Vet. Res. 16:401, 1955.
229. Smith, W. P.: Anti-larval antibodies in the serum and abomasal mucus of sheep hyperinfected with Haemonchus contortus. Res. Vet. Sci. 22:334, 1977.
230. Soulsby, E. J. L.: Mechanism of immunity of helminths. J.A.V.M.A. 38:335, 1961.
231. Michel, J. F., Lancaster, M. B., and Hong, C.: Ostertagia ostertagi: protective immunity in calves. The development in calves of a protective immunity to infection with Ostertagia ostertagi. Exp. Pathol. 33:179, 1973.
232. Smith, H. J., and Archibald, R. M.: Critical trials on the efficiency of thiabendazole against Ostertagia, Cooperia and Nematodirus. Can. Vet. J. 9:57, 1968.
233. Robertson, E. L.: Chapter 52. Antinematodal drugs. In Veterinary Pharmacology and Therapeutics. Edited by L. M. Jones, N. H. Booth, and L. E. McDonald. Ames, Iowa State University Press, 1977.
234. Robinson, R. W.: Diaphragmatic hernia in a heifer. North Am. Vet. 37:375, 1956.
235. Milne, F. J.: Diaphragmatic hernia in the cow. J.A.V.M.A. 118:374, 1951.
236. Danks, A. G.: Rupture of the diaphragm. Cornell Vet. 29:420, 1939.
237. Troutt, H. F., Fessler, J. F., Page, E. H., and Amstutz, H. E.: Diaphragmatic defects in cattle. J.A.V.M.A. 151:1421, 1967.
237a.Kirkbride, C. A., and Noordsy, J. L.: An esophageal hiatus hernia in a bull. J.A.V.M.A. 152:996, 1968.
238. Roberts, S. J.: Diaphragmatic hernia in the bovine. Cornell Vet. 36:92, 1946.
239. Horney, F. D., and Cote, J.: Congenital diaphragmatic hernia in a calf. Can. Vet. J. 2:422, 1961.
240. Diesem, C. D., Mauger, H. M., and Tharp, V. L.: A bovine diaphragmatic hernia with extensive involvement of the thorax. J.A.V.M.A. 124:93, 1954.
241. Hall, R. F.: Repair of diaphragmatic hernia in a cow. Vet. Med. 58:328, 1963.
242. Tubbs, C. R.: Diaphragmatic hernia in two calves. J.A.V.M.A. 122:371, 1953.
243. Frost, J. N., and Danks, A. G.: Atypical indigestion in the bovine. Cornell Vet. 29:70, 1939.
244. Dietz, O.: Differential diagnosis of traumatic reticulo-peritonitis. J. S. Afr. Vet. Med. Assoc. 32:3, 1961.
245. Plowright, W., Linsell, C. A., and Peers, F. G.: A focus of ruminal cancer in Kenyan cattle. Br. J. Cancer 25:72, 1971.
246. Baskerville, A.: Mesothelioma in the calf. Pathol. Vet. 4:149, 1967.
247. Grant, C. A.: Congenital tumors of calves: report of two cases of "mesothelioma" and a tumor apparently of reticuloendothelial origin. Zentralbl. Veterinaermed. 5:231, 1958.
248. Lorenz, M. D.: Laboratory diagnosis of gastrointestinal disease and pancreatic insufficiency. Vet. Clin. North Am. 6:663, 1976.
249. Haskins, S. C.: An overview of acid-base physiology. J.A.M.A. 170:423, 1977.
250. Palmer, E. D.: Upper gastrointestinal hemorrhage. J.A.M.A. 231:853, 1975.
251. Harris, W. F.: Clinical toxicities in dogs. Vet. Clin. North Am. 5:605, 1975.
252. Atkins, C. E., and Johnson, R. K.: Clinical toxicities of cats. Vet. Clin. North Am. 5:623, 1975.
253. Cornelius, L. M., and Wingfield, W. E.: Diseases of the stomach. In Textbook of Veterinary Internal Medicine. Edited by S. J. Ettinger. Philadelphia, W. B. Saunders Co., 1975.
254. Herrgessel, J. D.: Aspirin poisoning in the cat. J.A.V.M.A. 151:452, 1967.
255. Taylor, L. A., and Crawford, L. M.: Aspirin-induced gastrointestinal lesions in the dog. J.A.V.M.A. 152:617, 1968.
256. Bonneau, N. H., Reed, J. H., Pennock, P. Q., and Little, P. B.: Comparison of gastro-photography and contrast radiography for diagnosis of aspirin-induced gastritis in the dog. J.A.V.M.A. 161:190, 1972.
257. Nicoloff, D. M.: Indomethacin: effect on gastric secretion, parietal cell population and ulcer provocation in the dog. Arch. Surg. 97:809, 1968.
258. Ewing, G. O.: Indomethacin-associated gastrointestinal hemorrhage in a dog. J.A.V.M.A. 161:1665, 1972.
259. Max, M., and Menguy, R.: Influence of aspirin and phenylbutazone on rate of turnover of gastric mucosal cells. Digestion 2:67, 1969.
260. Nicoloff, D. M.: Effect of cortisone and corticotropin on gastric secretion and peptic ulceration in the dog. Arch. Surg. 98:640, 1969.
261. Osborne, A. D., and Wilson, M. R.: Mycotic gastritis in a dog. Vet. Rec. 85:487, 1969.

262. Cartwright, S., and Lucas, M.: Vomiting and diarrhea in dogs. Vet. Rec. 88:571, 1972.
263. Schnelle, G. B.: Acute gastritis. In Current Veterinary Therapy, Vol. IV. Edited by R. W. Kirk, Philadelphia, W. B. Saunders Co., 1971.
264. Bernstein, M.: Hemorrhagic gastroenteritis. In Current Veterinary Therapy, Vol. VI. Edited by R. W. Kirk. Philadelphia, W. B. Saunders Co., 1977.
265. Davenport, H. W.: The gastric mucosal barrier. Mayo Clin. Proc. 50:507, 1975.
266. Ivey, K. J.: Gastric mucosal barrier—recent advances. Acta Hepatogastroenterol. 20:517, 1973.
267. Davenport, H. W.: Salicylate damage to the gastric mucosal barrier. N. Engl. J. Med. 276:1307, 1967.
268. Ivey, K. J.: Gastritis. Med. Clin. North Am. 58:1289, 1974.
269. Chvasta, T. E., and Cooke, A. R.: The effect of several ulcerogenic drugs on the canine gastric mucosal barrier. J. Lab. Clin. Med. 79:302, 1972.
270. Davenport, H. W.: Back Diffusion of Acid Through the Gastric Mucosa and Its Physiological Consequences. Progress in Gastroenterology, Vol. II. Edited by G. B. J. Glass. New York, Grune and Stratton, 1970.
271. Max, M., and Menguy, R.: Influence of adrenocorticotropin, cortisone, aspirin and phenylbutazone on the rate of exfoliation and the rate of renewal of gastric mucosal cells. Gastroenterology 58:329, 1970.
272. Bremen, J., Ley, R., Woussen-Colle, M. C., Verbeustel, S., and DeGraef, J.: Effects of cortisone on acid, pepsin, sulfated polysaccharides, and glycoprotein secretion by the mucosa of denervated fundic pouches of dogs. Digestion 4:81, 1971.
273. Zamora, C. S., Kowlczyk, T., Hoekstra, W. G., Grummer, R. H., and Will, J. A.: Effects of prednisone on gastric secretion and development of stomach lesions in swine. Am. J. Vet. Res. 36:33, 1975.
274. Davenport, H. W.: Fluid produced by the gastric mucosa during damage by acetic and salicylic acids. Gastroenterology 50:487, 1966.
275. Ditchfield, J., and Phillipson, M. H.: Achlorhydria in dogs, with report of a case complicated by avitaminosis C. Can. Vet. J. 1:396, 1960.
276. Anderson, N. V.: Biopsy of the gastrointestinal system. Vet. Clin. North Am. 4:317, 1974.
277. Gomez, J. A.: The gastrointestinal contrast study. Vet. Clin. North Am. 4:805, 1974.
278. Hedberg, S. E.: Endoscopy in gastrointestinal bleeding. A systematic approach to diagnosis. Surg. Clin. North Am. 54:549, 1974.
279. Morrissey, J. F., and Barreras, R. F.: Antacid therapy. N. Engl. J. Med. 290:550, 1974.
280. Hurwitz, A., Robinson, R. G., Vats, T. S., Whittier, F. C., and Herrin, W. F.: Effects of antacids on gastric emptying. Gastroenterology 71:268, 1976.
281. Finco, D. R., and Osborne, C. A.: Practical application and principles of fluid and electrolyte therapy. Proc. Am. Anim. Hosp. Assoc. 39th Annu. Meet., Las Vegas, 1972.
282. Damiano, S.: Chronic follicular hypertrophic-hyperplastic gastritis in a dog. Acta Med. Vet. 13:363, 1967.
283. Van Der Gaag, II, Happé, R. P., and Wovekamp, W. T. C.: A Boxer dog with chronic hypertrophic gastritis resembling Menetrier's disease in man. Vet. Pathol. 13:172, 1976.
284. Russell, I. J., Smith, J., Dozors, R. R., Wahner, H. W., and Bartholomew, L. G.: Menetrier's disease: effect of medical and surgical vagotomy. Mayo Clin. Proc. 52:91, 1977.
285. Murray, M., McKeating, F. J., and Lauder, I. M.: Peptic ulceration in the dog: a clinico-pathological study. Vet. Rec. 91:441, 1972.
286. Howard, E. B., Sarva, T. R., Nielsen, S. W., and Kenyon, A. J.: Mastocytoma and gastroduodenal ulceration. Pathol. Vet. 6:146, 1969.
287. Hess, P. W.: Canine mast cell tumors. Vet. Clin. North Am. 7:133, 1977.
288. Seawright, A. A., and Grono, L. R.: Malignant mast cell tumors in a cat with perforating duodenal ulcer. J. Pathol. Bacteriol. 87:107, 1964.
289. Hoerlein, B. F., and Spano, J. S.: Non-neurological complications following decompressive spinal cord surgery. Arch. Am. Coll. Vet. Surg. 4:11, 1975.
290. Sass, B.: Perforating gastric ulcer associated with lead poisoning in a dog. J.A.V.M.A. 157:76, 1970.
291. Schayer, R. W.: Formation and binding of histamine by free mast cells of rat peritoneal fluid. Am. J. Physiol. 186:199, 1956.
292. Watt, J., Eagleton, G. B., and Marcus, R.: The effect of heparin on gastric secretion stimulated by histamine or ametazole hydrochloride. J. Pharm. Pharmacol. 18:615, 1966.

293. Ippoliti, A., and Walsh, J.: Newer concepts in the pathogenesis of peptic ulcer disease. Surg. Clin. North Am. 56:1479, 1976.
294. Rhodes, J.: Etiology of gastric ulcer. Gastroenterology 63:171, 1972.
295. Gear, M., Truelove, S., and Whitehead, R.: Gastric ulcer and gastritis. Gut 12:639, 1971.
296. Overbolt, B., and Pollard, H.: Acid diffusion into the human gastric mucosa. Gastroenterology 54:182, 1968.
297. DePlessis, D.: Pathogenesis of gastric ulceration. Lancet 1:974, 1965.
298. Robbins, P. L., Boradie, R. A., Sosin, H., and Delaney, J. P.: Reflux gastritis: the consequences of intestinal juice in the stomach. Am. J. Surg. 131:23, 1976.
299. O'Brien, P., and Silen, W.: Effect of bile salts and aspirin on the mucosal blood flow. Gastroenterology 64:246, 1973.
300. Lipkin, M.: In defense of the gastric mucosa. Gut 12:599, 1971.
301. Fleshler, B.: Medical management of bleeding duodenal ulcers. Surg. Clin. North Am. 56:1375, 1976.
302. Hoerr, S. O.: A review and evaluation of operative procedures used for chronic duodenal ulcer. Surg. Clin. North Am. 56:1289, 1976.
303. Dorland's Illustrated Medical Dictionary, 25th ed., Philadelphia and London, W. B. Saunders Co., 1974.
304. Siffert, G.: Foreign bodies in the stomach. In Gastroenterology. Edited by H. L. Bockus. Philadelphia, W. B. Saunders Co., 1974.
305. Tyler, D. E.: Gastric neoplasia in the dog and cat. Arch. Am. Coll. Vet. Surg. 6:47, 1977. (Abst.)
306. Dorn, C. R.: Epidemiology of canine and feline tumors. J.A.A.H.A. 12:307, 1976.
307. Brodey, R. S.: Alimentary tract neoplasms in the cat: a clinicopathologic survey of 46 cases. Am. J. Vet. Res. 27:74, 1966.
308. Sagartz, J. W., Garner, F. M., and Sauer, R. M.: Multiple neoplasia in a captive jungle cat (Felis chaus)—thyroid adenocarcinoma, gastric adenocarcinoma, renal adenoma and Sertoli cell tumor. J. Wildl. Dis. 8:375, 1972.
309. Drake, J. C., and Hime, J. M.: Gastric carcinoma in the dog, two further cases. J. Small Anim. Pract. 6:313, 1965.
310. Ewing, G. O.: Gastric carcinoma in the dog: report of two cases. Calif. Vet. 21:28, 1967.
311. Jacquier, P. C.: Adenocarcinome du pylore chez le chien. Schweiz. Arch. Tierheilkd. 110:95, 1968.
312. Nomura, Y., Tsuchiya, T., Saito, Y., and Sawaya, H.: Pathological observations and classification of tumors found in domestic animals: III. Sixty-four cases examined in 1969. Bull. Azabu. Vet. Coll. 22:51, 1971.
313. Lingeman, C. H., Garner, F. M., and Taylor, D. O. N.: Spontaneous gastric adenocarcinomas of dogs: a review. J. Natl. Cancer Inst. 47:137, 1971.
314. Nomura, Y., Saito, Y., Tsuchiya, T., Kotani, Y., and Yagi, H.: Gastric cancer (scirrhous adenocarcinoma) with adrenocortical adenoma in a dog. Bull. Azabu. Vet. Coll. 24:17, 1972.
315. Murray, M., McKeating, F. J., Baker, G. J., and Lauder, I. M.: Primary gastric neoplasia in the dog: a clinico-pathological study. Vet. Rec. 91:474, 1972.
316. Pollock, S., and Wagner, B. M.: Gastric adenocarcinoma of linitis plastica in a dog. V. M./S. A. C. 68:139, 1973.
317. Hayden, D. W., and Nielsen, S. W.: Canine alimentary neoplasia. Zentralbl. Veterinaermed. 20:1, 1973.
318. Pass, M. A., Bengis, R. G., and Allen, H. L.: Clinico-pathologic conference. J.A.V.M.A. 163:1384, 1973.
319. Sautter, J. H., and Hanlon, G. F.: Gastric neoplasms in the dog: a report of 20 cases. J.A.V.M.A. 166:691, 1975.
320. Dorn, A. S., Anderson, N. V., Guffy, M. M., Cho, D. Y., and Leipold, H. W.: Gastric carcinoma in a dog. J. Small Anim. Pract. 17:109, 1976.
321. Patnaik, A. K., and Hurvitz, A. I.: Neoplasms of the digestive tract in the dog. In Current Veterinary Therapy, Vol. VI. Edited by R. W. Kirk. Philadelphia, W. B. Saunders Co., 1977.
322. Weaver, A. D.: Radiological diagnosis and prognosis of primary abdominal neoplasia in the dog. J. Small Anim. Pract. 17:357, 1976.
323. Berg, P., Rhodes, W. H., and O'Brien, J. B.: Radiographic diagnosis of gastric adenocarcinoma in a dog. J. Am. Vet. Radiol. Soc. 5:47, 1964.
324. Johnson, G. F., and Twedt, D. C.: Endoscopy and laparoscopy in the diagnosis and management of neoplasia in small animals. Vet. Clin. North Am. 7:77, 1977.
325. Cabre-Fiol, V., Vilardell, F., Sala-Cladera, E., and Perez-Mota, A.: Preoperative cytological diagnosis of gastric leiomyosarcoma. Gastroenterology 68:563, 1975.
326. Brandborg, L. L.: Polyps, tumors and cancer of the stomach. In Gastrointestinal Disease. Edited by M. H. Sleisenger and J. S. Fordtran. Philadelphia, W. B. Saunders Co., 1973.

327. ReMine, W. H., and Priestley, J. T.: Trends in prognosis and surgical treatment of cancer of the stomach. Ann. Surg. *163*:736, 1966.

328. Lapage, G.: Veterinary Helminthology and Entomology. Baltimore, The Williams & Wilkins Co., 1962.

329. Nayak, B. C., and Rao, A. T.: Pathology of gastric lesions in *Gnathostoma spinigerum* infection in a dog. Indian Vet. J. *49*:750, 1972.

330. Ehlers, G. H.: The anthelmintic treatment of infestations of the badger with spirurids *(Physaloptera)*. J.A.V.M.A. *78*:79, 1931.

331. Pollock, W. F., and Norris, W. J.: The management of hypertrophic pyloric stenosis at the Los Angeles Childrens Hospital. Am. J. Surg. *94*:335, 1957.

332. Pearson, H., Gaskell, C. J., Gibbs, C., and Waterman, A.: Pyloric and oesophageal dysfunction in the cat. J. Small Anim. Pract. *15*:487, 1974.

333. Benson, C. D., and Lloyd, J. R.: Infantile pyloric stenosis: a review of 1,120 cases. Am. J. Surg. *107*,429, 1964.

334. Twaddle, A. A.: Congenital pyloric stenosis in two kittens corrected by pyloroplasty. N. Z. Vet. J. *19*:26, 1971.

335. McKeoun, T., and MacMahon, B.: Infantile hypertrophic pyloric stenosis in parent and child. Arch. Dis. Child. *30*:497, 1955.

336. Gibbs, M. K., VanHeerden, H. A., and Lynn, H. B.: Congenital hypertrophic pyloric stenosis. Mayo Clin. Proc. *50*:312, 1975.

337. Gibbs, C., and Pearson, H.: The radiological diagnosis of gastrointestinal obstruction in the dog. J. Small Anim. Pract. *14*:61, 1973.

338. Zontine, W. J.: Effect of chemical restraint drugs on the passage of barium sulfate through the stomach and duodenum of dogs. J.A.V.M.A. *162*:878, 1973.

339. Zimmer, J. F.: Gastrointestinal fiberoptic endoscopy. *In* Current Veterinary Therapy, Vol. VI. Edited by R. W. Kirk. Philadelphia, W. B. Saunders Co., 1977.

340. Gardham, J. R. C.: Pyloric stenosis: an experimental study of alkalosis and the paradox of acid urine in dogs. Br. J. Surg. *56*:628, 1969 (Abst.).

341. Walsh, J. H., and Grossman, M. I.: Gastrin. N. Engl. J. Med. *292*:1324, 1975.

342. Dodge, J. A.: Production of duodenal ulcers and hypertrophic pyloric stenosis by administration of pentagastrin to pregnant and newborn dogs. Nature *225*:284, 1970.

343. Wellman, K. F., Kagan, A., and Fang, H.: Hypertrophic pyloric stenosis in adults. Gastroenterology *46*:601, 1964.

344. Belding, H. H., III, and Kernohan, J. W.: A morphologic study of the myenteric plexus and musculature of the pylorus with special reference to the changes in hypertrophic pyloric stenosis. Surg. Gynecol. Obstet. *97*:322, 1953.

345. Torgersen, J.: The muscular build and movements of the stomach and duodenal bulb, especially with regard to the problem of segmental divisions of the stomach in the light of comparative anatomy and embryology. Acta Radiol. (Stockh.) Suppl. *45*:80, 1942.

346. Crean, G. P., Hogg, D. F., and Rumsey, R. D. E.: Hyperplasia of the gastric mucosa produced by duodenal obstruction. Gastroenterology *56*:193, 1969.

347. Cooke, A. R.: Control of gastric emptying and motility. Gastroenterology *68*:804, 1975.

348. Nagoaka, K.: Electromyography study on the mechanism of delayed gastric emptying after vagotomy in dogs. Tohoku J. Exp. Med. *95*:1, 1968.

349. Archibald, R. McG., and Milton, A. R.: Surgical relief of pyloric stenosis in the dog. Can. J. Comp. Med. *18*:394, 1954.

350. Archibald, J. A., Cawley, A. J., and Reed, J. H.: Surgical technic for correcting pyloric stenosis. Mod. Vet. Pract. *41*:28, 1960.

351. Lawther, W. A.: Pyloric stenosis in a puppy. Aust. Vet. J. *37*:317, 1961.

352. Twaddle, A. A.: Pyloric stenosis in three cats and its correction by pyloroplasty. N. Z. Vet. J. *18*:15, 1970.

353. Butler, H. C.: Gastroduodenostomy in the dog. J.A.V.M.A. *155*:1347, 1969.

354. Corner, B. D.: Hypertrophic pyloric stenosis in infancy treated with methyl scopolamine nitrate. Arch. Dis. Child. *30*:377, 1955.

355. Day, L. R.: Medical management of pyloric stenosis. J.A.M.A. *207*:948, 1969.

356. Keet, A. D., Jr.: The prepyloric contractions in certain abnormal conditions. Acta Radiol. *50*:413, 1958.

357. Ewing, G. O.: Pyloric stenosis. *In* Current Veterinary Therapy, Vol. IV. Edited by R. W. Kirk. Philadelphia, W. B. Saunders Co., 1971.

358. Rhodes, W. H., and Brodey, R. S.: The differential diagnosis of pyloric obstructions in the dog. J. Am. Vet. Radiol. Soc. *6*:65, 1965.

359. Bolt, R. J.: Gastric evacuation and clinical syndromes. Med. Clin. North Am. *53*:1403, 1969.

360. Wingfield, W. E., Cornelius, L. M., and DeYoung, D. W.: Experimental gastric dilatation and torsion in the dog. I. Changes in biochemical and acid-base parameters. J. Small Anim. Pract. *15*:41, 1974.

361. Kneller, S. K.: Radiographic interpretation of the gastric dilatation-volvulus complex in the dog. J.A.A.H.A. *12*:154, 1976.

362. Merkley, D. F., Howard, D. R., Krehbiel, J. D., Eyster, G. E., Krahwinkel, D. J., and Sawyer, D. C.: Experimentally induced acute gastric dilatation in the dog. Clinico-pathologic findings. J.A.A.H.A. *12*:149, 1976.

363. Betts, C. W., Wingfield, W. E., and Greene, R. W.: A retrospective study of gastric dilation-torsion in the dog. J. Small Anim. Pract. *15*:727, 1974.

364. DeHoff, W. D., and Greene, R. W.: Gastric dilatation and the gastric torsion complex. Vet. Clin. North Am. *2*:141, 1972.

365. Morris, C. R., Ivy, A. C., and Maddock, W. G.: Mechanism of acute abdominal distension. Arch. Surg. *55*:101, 1947.

366. Caywood, D., Teague, H. D., Jackson, D. A., Levitt, M. D., and Bond, J. H., Jr.: Gastric gas analysis in the canine gastric dilatation-volvulus syndrome. J.A.A.H.A. *13*:459, 1977.

367. VanKruiningen, H. J., Gregoire, K., and Meuten, D. J.: Acute gastric dilatation: a review of comparative aspects, by species, and a study in dogs and monkeys. J.A.A.H.A. *10*:294, 1974.

368. Wingfield, W. E., Betts, C. W., and Rawlings, C. A.: Pathophysiology associated with gastric dilatation-volvulus in the dog. J.A.A.H.A. *12*:136, 1976.

369. Roth, J. L. A.: The symptom patterns of gaseousness. Ann. N. Y. Acad. Sci. *150*:109, 1968.

370. Anderson, K., and Ringsted, A.: Clinical and experimental investigations of ileus with particular reference to the genesis of intestinal gas. Acta. Chir. Scand. *88*:475, 1943.

371. Maddock, W. G., Bell, J. L., and Tremaine, M. J.: Gastrointestinal gas. Observations on belching during anesthesia, operations and pyelography; and rapid passage of gas. Ann. Surg. *130*:512, 1949.

372. Proctor, H. J., Ballantine, T. V. N., and Broussard, N. D.: An analysis of pulmonary function following non-thoracic trauma, with recommendations for therapy. Ann. Surg. *172*:180, 1970.

373. Merkley, D. F., Howard, D. R., Eyster, G. E., Krahwinkel, D. J., Sawyer, D. C., and Krehbiel, J. D.: Experimentally induced acute gastric dilatation in the dog. Cardiopulmonary effects. J.A.A.H.A. *12*:143, 1976.

374. Doppman, J. L., and Johnson, R. H.: The mechanism of shock in acute gastric dilatation: an angiographic study in monkeys. Br. J. Radiol. *42*:613, 1969.

375. Jakhanwal, D. P., Bhardwaj, G. P., Dalta, A. K., and Mohanty, P.: Obstruction of inferior vena cava as a factor for reduced blood pressure on distension of stomach in dogs. Indian J. Physiol. Pharmacol. *14*:19, 1970.

376. Passi, R. B., Kraft, A. R., and Vasko, J. S.: Pathophysiologic mechanisms of shock in acute gastric dilatation. Surgery *65*:298, 1969.

377. Wingfield, W. E., Cornelius, L. M., Ackerman, N., and DeYoung, D. W.: Experimental acute gastric dilation and torsion in the dog. 2. Venous angiographic alterations seen in gastric dilation. J. Small Anim. Pract. *16*:55, 1975.

378. Berman, J. K., Opsahl, T., Moore, W., Bakemeier, R. E., and Chen, T.: The relationship of intragastric and portal venous pressures. Surgery *51*:486, 1962.

379. Mooney, C. S., Bryant, W. M., and Griffen, W. O., Jr.: Metabolic and portal venous changes in acute gastric dilatation. Surg. Forum *20*:352, 1969.

380. Berg, P.: Gastric torsion. *In* Current Veterinary Therapy, Vol. IV. Edited by R. W. Kirk. Philadelphia, W. B. Saunders Co., 1971.

381. Walshaw, R., and Johnston, D. E.: Treatment of gastric dilatation-volvulus by gastric decompression and patient stabilization before major surgery. J.A.A.H.A. *12*:162, 1976.

381a. Muir, W. W., and Lipowitz, A. J.: Cardiac dysrhythmias associated with gastric dilatation-volvulus in the dog. J.A.V.M.A. *172*:683, 1978.

382. Rawlings, C. A., Wingfield, W. E., and Betts, C. W.: Shock therapy and anesthetic management in gastric dilation-volvulus. J.A.A.H.A. *12*:158, 1976.

383. Schumer, W., Erve, P. R., and Obernolte, R. P.: Mechanisms of steroid protection in septic shock. Surgery *72*:119, 1972.

384. Hassen, A.: Gram-negative bacteremic shock. Med. Clin. North Am. *54*:1403, 1973.

385. Reichgott, M. J., and Melmon, K. L.: Should corticosteroids be used in shock? Med. Clin. North Am. *57*:1211, 1973.

386. Rai, D. K., Gupta, L. P., Singh, R. H., and Udupa, K. N.: A study of microcirculation in endotoxin shock. Surg. Gynecol. Obstet. *139*:11, 1974.

387. Condon, R. E.: Rational use of prophylactic antibiotics in gastrointestinal surgery. Surg. Clin. North Am. *6*:1309, 1975.

388. Wingfield, W. E., Betts, C. W., and Greene, R. W.: Operative techniques and recurrence rates associated with gastric volvulus in the dog. J. Small Anim. Pract. *16*:427, 1976.

389. Funkquist, B., and Garmer, L.: Pathogenetic and therapeutic aspects of torsion of the canine stomach. J. Small Anim. Pract. *8*:523, 1967.

390. Andrews, A. H.: A study of ten cases of gastric torsion in the Bloodhound. Vet. Rec. *86*:689, 1970.

391. Turner, T.: A case of torsion of the stomach in an 11-year-old Dachshund bitch. Vet. Rec. *76*:243, 1964.

392. Turner, T.: Clinical communication: a case of torsion of the stomach in a five-year-old cat. J. Small Anim. Pract. *9*:231, 1968.

393. Herr, D. M., Thompson, P. L., and Cunningham, J. H.: What is your diagnosis? J.A.V.M.A. *162*:491, 1973.

394. Boothe, H. W., and Ackerman, N.: Partial gastric torsion in two dogs. J.A.A.H.A. *12*:27, 1976.

395. Dingwall, J. S., and Eger, C. E.: Management of acute gastric dilatation with torsion and rupture: a case report. J.A.A.H.A. *12*:23, 1976.

396. Blackburn, P. S., and McFarlane, D.: Acute fatal dilatation of the stomach in the dog. J. Comp. Pathol. *54*:89, 1944.

397. Maxie, M. G., Reed, J. H., Pennock, P. W., and Hoff, B.: Splenic torsion in three Great Danes. Can. Vet. J. *11*:249, 1970.

398. Funkquist, B.: Gastric torsion in the dog. Non-surgical reposition. J. Small Anim. Pract. *10*:507, 1969.

399. Fink, D. W.: Gastric volvulus: the angiographic appearance. Am. J. Roentgenol. *115*:268, 1972.

400. Tsapagas, M. J., Peabody, R. A., Karmody, A. M., Chuntrasakul, C., Goussous, H., and Eckert, C.: Pathophysiological changes following ischemia of the spleen. Ann. Surg. *178*:179, 1973.

401. Roberts, H. R., and Cedarbaum, A. I.: The liver and blood coagulation: physiology and pathology. Gastroenterology *63*:297, 1972.

402. Greene, C. E.: Disseminated intravascular coagulation in the dog: a review. J.A.A.H.A. *11*:674, 1975.

403. Greene, R., Wiznitzer, T., Ruttenburg, S., Frank, E., and Fine, J.: Hepatic clearance of endotoxin absorbed from the intestine. Proc. Soc. Exp. Biol. Med. *108*:261, 1961.

404. Olkay, I., Kitahama, A., Miller, R. H., Drapanas, T., Trejo, R. A., and Diluzio, N. R.: Reticuloendothelial dysfunction and endotoxemia following portal vein occlusion. Surgery *75*:64, 1974.

405. Wingfield, W. E., and Hoffer, R. E.: Gastric dilatation-torsion complex in the dog: etiology, treatment and surgical techniques. *In* Current Techniques in Small Animal Surgery. Edited by M. J. Bojrab. Philadelphia, Lea & Febiger, 1975.

406. Parks, J. L., and Greene, R. W.: Tube gastrostomy for the treatment of gastric volvulus. J.A.A.H.A. *12*:168, 1976.

407. Christie, T. R., and Smith, C. W.: Gastrocolopexy for prevention of recurrent gastric volvulus. J.A.A.H.A. *12*:173, 1976.

408. Betts, C. W., Wingfield, W. E., and Rosin, E.: "Permanent" gastropexy—as a prophylactic measure against gastric volvulus. J.A.A.H.A. *12*:177, 1976.

409. Betts, C. W., Kneller, S. K., and Rosin, E.: Recurring gastric volvulus in the dog. J. Small Anim. Pract. *16*:433, 1975.

Chapter 23

SMALL INTESTINAL DISEASES

ALFRED M. MERRITT

This chapter is divided into two major sections. Part I deals with small intestinal diseases of neonates and is organized in the traditional fashion—by causative agent. Part II is concerned with those diseases that occur, in the main, after weaning and throughout adulthood. The discussion of Part II is divided according to presenting patterns of clinical signs; the rationale for this approach is outlined in the special introduction to this part.

Small intestinal diseases are often difficult to diagnose because of the relative inaccessibility of the organ and the tendency for numerous types of disorders to be manifested by very similar signs (Table 23–1). This statement is particularly true for the neonatal diarrheas. The need before us as veterinarians is to develop a more orderly approach to enteric disease, first to decide *which* part of the bowel is malfunctioning and then *why*. Certain initial diagnostic procedures and tests should be routine (Table 23–2), the results of which dictate the formulation of an additional list of procedures (Table 23–3).

Therefore, it is the aim of this chapter to discuss the well-documented small intestinal diseases of domestic animals and provide guidelines for: (1) important epidemiologic considerations; (2) initial clinical categorization, (3) recognition of key signs and laboratory or necropsy findings that indicate a definite diagnosis, (4) understanding of pathogenetic and pathophysiologic mechanisms; and (5) formulation of therapeutic and prophylactic measures.

Table 23–1. Initial Impact—General History/Signs Signaling Potential Small Intestinal Disease

1. Abnormal feces
2. Weight loss
3. Edema
4. Vomiting
5. Colic
6. Hyperphagia
7. Dermatosis
8. Abdominal distention

Table 23–2. Minimum Data Base for All Cases of Suspected Small Intestinal Disease

1. Examination of feces for presence of parasite ova.
2. Complete blood count.
3. Serum albumin and globulin concentrations.
4. Serum Na, K, Cl, Ca, Mg, P concentrations.
5. Fecal culture
6. Fecal leukocytes
7. Peritoneal fluid analysis (horses)
8. Blood gas analysis (if marked dehydration and/or shock present)

Table 23–3. Procedures Specifically Applicable to Assessment of Small Intestinal Function

Procedure	Assessment
1. D-glucose absorption	General small intestinal absorptive function
2. D-xylose absorption	General small intestinal absorptive function
3. Fecal fat analysis	Fat assimilation
4. Serum carotene concentration	General small intestinal absorptive function
5. Prothrombin time	Fat soluble vitamin assimilation
6. Lactose tolerance	Specific lactose digestion
7. Intestinal biopsy	Pathologic classification of dysfunction
8. Radiography	Location and character of gross lesions
9. ^{51}Cr albumin excretion	Protein-losing enteropathy?
10. Fecal pH	Hypersecretion of $NaHCO_3$ (alkaline) or a malabsorption (acid)?

Part I. Small Intestinal Diseases of Neonates

ACUTE BACTERIAL INFECTIONS OF NEONATES

Acute bacterial infections of the small intestine in neonates of any species cause diarrhea either by invading into the gut wall to cause inflammation and destruction, or by elaborating a toxin that causes the gut to hypersecrete electrolytes and water, or by both mechanisms. If one has a general understanding of these mechanisms, the basis for certain epidemiologic features, clinical signs, and laboratory findings becomes much more obvious, thus helping the clinician to decide initially whether he is dealing with "invasive" or "toxigenic" disease.

Escherichia coli ("Colibacillosis")

Epidemiology

Much has been written on the subject of *E. coli* diseases of neonatal animals over the years. From the present perspective one thing becomes quite clear, however. Many of the diarrheas attributed to "colibacillosis" in the past probably were caused by viruses or salmonellae. There is no question that enteropathogenic *E. coli* exist and cause disease but it is doubtful that their incidence as primary pathogens is as high as previously suspected.

E. coli is part of the normal flora of the gastrointestinal tract of all species. Their highest concentrations are in the lower ileum and large bowel.[1] The population kinetics are quite dynamic; there are "resident" (autochthonous) and "transient" (allochthonous) strains.[2] The transient serotypes appear and disappear within the span of a few days. The resident serotypes predominate in number and turn over every few months or less. The factors that govern this population turnover are not well understood, but diet seems to play a part.[3,4,5]

At present well over 100 serotypes of *E. coli* have been found to be pathogenic. This figure cannot be precise because it is under constant modification. *E. coli* are typed according to their somatic (O), flagellar (H), and capsular (K) antigenic makeup. A serotype is designated as pathogenic if it is found to produce enterotoxin or have invasive properties.

All neonatal animals can contract "colibacillosis." In terms of incidence and economic considerations, calves and piglets predominate. The single most important factor regarding incidence is husbandry. If the premises, particularly where dams are confined for parturition and the young stock are housed, are cleaned and disinfected routinely, the neonates ingest or are force-fed colostrum within the first few hours after birth, and all young stock are fed properly from clean equipment, diarrhea due to enteropathogenic *E. coli* can be kept to a minimum. In addition, exposure of the dams to the area of infant housing for at least 2 weeks prior to parturition will increase the probability that antibodies against any indigenous enteropathogenic *E. coli* will appear in their colostrum.[6] Some workers maintain that ingestion of adequate colostrum within the first 4 to 5 hours after birth is the single most important deterrent to the development of colibacillosis;[7,8,9] this assumes, of course, that the appropriate K antibodies are there and that the animals can absorb them normally.[10]

Colibacillosis has its highest incidence within the first 2 weeks of life and, in contrast to most neonatal viral enteropathies, it spreads slowly and is sporadic among individuals (e.g., calves) or litters (e.g., piglets).[11]

Clinical Signs

The progression of signs from initial diarrhea to severe dehydration, acidosis, and collapse can vary even among animals within the same environment. Reasons for this variability are no doubt numerous, including amount of colostrum ingested, infecting dose, nutritional status, degree of general stress, and *E. coli* serotype involved. In some, only transient diarrhea will be seen. There are no definitive signs.

Pathophysiology

The septicemic form of *E. coli* infection usually manifests itself as shock, collapse, and death within the first 24 hours after birth. Our interest is primarily in the intestinal form of the disease. As mentioned earlier, most enteropathogenic *E. coli* are strictly toxigenic. In other words, they produce an enterotoxin that can attach to receptors in the small intestinal mucosa and thus activate adenyl cyclase, which increases the production of cyclic-AMP within the crypt cells. This results in the hypersecretion of electrolytes, primarily Na and Cl, and associated water.[5,12,13] While this is occurring, absorptive function at the villous tip is normal, an important point to remember when considering therapeutic principles discussed later.[14] The net effect, however, is that more water and electrolytes are dumped into the large intestine than it can absorb and a profuse saline diarrhea is manifested. Studies in calves suggest that the electrolytes and water are preferentially removed from the plasma space so that hypovolemic shock and metabolic acidosis are major consequences.[15,16,17]

We now also recognize the existence, at present only in humans and laboratory animals, of some serotypes of invasive *E. coli* which physically disrupt the mucosal cells causing malabsorption and gross leakage of plasma proteins (perhaps even blood) along with water and electrolytes into the intestine.[18] In contrast to the enterotoxigenic forms, these invasive *E. coli* have the potential for affecting the colon as well as the small intestines. The resulting diarrhea is a true "dysentery"; that is, the feces may contain shreds of mucosa, frank blood, and leukocytes (see Table 23–7).

Some recent work has shown that both enterotoxigenic and invasive forms of *E. coli* also disrupt small intestinal motility. Basically they cause the normal rhythmic contractions to cease. These are replaced by periods of quiescence that are interrupted frequently by single abnormally long peristaltic sweeps which essentially "strip" the fluid en masse into the colon.[19] The mechanism of elaboration of these effects remains to be elucidated, but cyclic-AMP is probably involved.[20]

Diagnostic Criteria

Laboratory Findings. In calves the most significant changes are found in the blood where indications of dehydration and metabolic acidosis are present to varying degrees. The hematocrit is invariably increased. Total serum protein concentration is an unreliable indicator of hydration unless colostral intake status is known. Serum sodium concentration is usually near normal, which goes along with a saline-type diarrhea, rather than a primary water loss, which would cause hypernatremia. In advanced cases, hyperkalemia is commonly seen[21,22] which reflects both the acidosis and preferential fluid loss from the plasma space.[16] If blood gas analyses are done, base deficits up to 20 mEq/L may be recorded.[15] Fecal cultures should be done to rule out other enteropathogens, but without further testing, the isolation of *E. coli* from such cultures is not diagnostic.

The most definitive way to indicate the presence of an enterotoxigenic form of *E. coli* is through inoculation of intestinal loops of young mice (heat-stable toxin) or adrenocortical tissue cultures (heat-labile toxin) with organisms cultured from the feces or, better still, from the small intestine of freshly killed sick animals.[23,24] This is much more reliable for demonstrating enteropathogenicity than serotyping.

Invasive *E. coli* are identified by their ability to cause conjunctivitis within 24 hours after application to the eye of a guinea pig.[25]

Necropsy Findings. With the enterotoxigenic form of the disease, lesions of the small intestinal mucosa are minimal. Some plasma cell infiltration or minor changes in villous architecture have been described,[26,27,28] but these may reflect the consequences of the infection rather than the effects of the organism. The invasive serotypes cause the usual necrosis and inflammation typical of any acute enteritis. As mentioned, such enteritis due to *E. coli* may prospectively be found in both small and large intestine. Objective proof of the presence of enteritis due to invasive *E. coli* in domestic animals remains to be documented.

Therapy

Treatment should be primarily directed at restoring normal hydration and acid/base balance, with secondary consideration of reducing coliforms in the gut with antibiotics. This philosophy applies most practically to those species whose veins are relatively accessible, as intravenous fluid administration is most desirable. Subcutaneous and intraperitoneal administration will suffice if the intravenous route is impractical or impossible.

Antibiotic Therapy. Heated arguments persist regarding the use of antibiotics for treating bacterial enteric infections. The consensus in human medicine is to use no antibiotics unless there is good evidence of sepsis, and then to use them systemically rather than topically; that is, do not use nonabsorbable antibiotics given orally. This would apply to either enterotoxigenic or invasive infections. Proponents of this approach say that giving antibiotics does nothing to hasten recovery and enhances the chances of carrier states of resistant organisms[29] or, on occasion, may provoke a carrier state into a systemic infection.[30] These remarks apply particularly to Shigella and Salmonella infections. Practical experiences in both veterinary and human medicine suggest that adjunct antibiotic therapy may be helpful in some instances in controlling the incidence of enterotoxigenic coliform infection throughout a barn or nursery and may increase chances of survival of neonates that are already sick.[11,31,32,33] Others find no help from antibiotics.[34,35] Many pathogenic *E. coli* cultured from premises where antibiotics are not used prophylactically are sensitive to numerous antibacterial agents, particularly the aminoglycosides, nitrofurans, and certain sulfas. One of the more effective sulfas that has been produced for specific use against colibacillosis infections in calves and pigs is sulfachlorpyridazine. Many of the aminoglycosides are not approved for use in food producing animals in the United States. Nitrofurans should be used with caution since they have been reported to cause central nervous disturbances[36] and blood clotting dyscrasia[37] in calves.

There is no doubt that antibiotics are grossly misused, particularly by laymen and food companies, in an attempt to treat and control neonatal diarrhea. They are not a panacea for poor husbandry practices and their abuse has often been needlessly expensive for farmers and caused a proliferation of resistant organisms.

Fluid Therapy. The base fluid of choice is one that is isotonic and contains either bicarbonate or a bicarbonate precursor such as acetate or pyruvate. It may be necessary to add extra $NaHCO_3$ to this solution, depending upon the clinical signs. The amount of fluid to replace depends upon the clinician's assessment of degree of dehydration. Table 23–4 summarizes the guidelines that I use for fluid replacement in young calves or foals suffering from an enterotoxigenic form of diarrhea. These guidelines were developed based upon clinical cases where arterial blood gas analyses were performed.

The rate of administration of intravenous fluid to calves and foals depends somewhat upon the condition of the patient but should be 30 to 40 ml per kilogram body weight per hour for the first hour.[17] Even though one estimates that a 50-kg calf has lost

10% of its body weight (5 L) in water, 1.5 to 2 liters of fluid, including the extra bicarbonate, will be all that is needed intravenously to help the animal through the crisis.

Some differences of opinion do exist regarding the composition of fluid for therapy of calves with colibacillosis. Some workers prefer to add extra potassium rather than bicarbonate to their solution.[38] They have developed this after extensive studies of fluid and electrolyte movement in sick calves. Their rationale is based upon observations that the cells of a severely sick calf are depleted in potassium because of the metabolic acidosis which has shifted the potassium to the plasma space. They feel the intercellular hypokalemia is what may be most immediately fatal, thus the need to drive K^+ back into the cells by extra-loading the plasma with the cation. They have given this type of solution both intravenously and subcutaneously. Others, and I am among this group, feel that large amounts of potassium are not necessary.[17]

It is highly recommended that fluids given either subcutaneously or intraperitoneally be isotonic. If hypertonic, they will cause pooling at the site of injection and further exacerbate the dehydration; if hypotonic, serious undesirable shifts in electrolyte distribution may result. Fluid therapy for neonates such as piglets or puppies must for all practical purposes usually be given extravascularly because of their small size. The formulation suggested for piglets with TGE (see p. 477) should suffice.

If the patient is relatively alert and is suckling, either upon initial examination or after stabilization with intravenous fluids, oral replacement of further water and electrolyte needs is the most practical and efficient method of therapy for enterotoxigenic forms of diarrhea. This takes advantage of the observation that the sodium/glucose absorptive

Table 23–4. Field Approximations—Acid/Base Status Foals and Calves with Severe Acute Diarrhea

Example: 45 kg. (100 lb.) Calf

Estimated Degree of Dehydration	Total Fluid Loss (liters)	Approximate Base Deficit (mEq/L)	Immediate HCO_3^- Needs (as $NaHCO_3$)			
			mEq	g	oz	Tbsp
10% Body Weight (depressed, sunken eyes, dry skin, ambulatory or sternal)	4.5	15–20	270–360	25–30	1	2
15% Body Weight (comatose)	6.75	25–30	455–545	40–45	1.5	3

1. HCO_3^- need (mEq) = base deficit (mEq/L) × body weight (kg) × 0.4.
2. 50 g of $NaHCO_3$ yields approximately 600 mEq of HCO_3^-.

2 tsp. NaCl
2 tsp. KCl (Lites salt)   q.s. to 1 gallon
1 TBL NaHCO₃ (baking soda)
   ½# sugar or ½ pt. Karo

Table 23–5. Oral Replacement Fluid for Calves with Severe Scours[39]

Mix thoroughly:	NaCl	117 g (4 oz)
	KCl	150 g (5 oz)
	NaHCO₃	168 g (5.5 oz)
	K₂HPO₄	135 g (4.5 oz)
Formula:	30 g (1 oz)	Electrolyte mixture
	250 g (½ lb)	Dextrose
	q.s. 4 liters	(1 gallon) Water

Feed as sole nutriment for 1–2 days. Estimate maintenance needs at 100 ml/kg/d plus losses in feces; administer in 4–5 doses. Allow access to fresh water on a free choice basis. Return to replacer or milk gradually, using above mixture as diluent. Exactly when and how fast to return the calf to original diet depends upon one's judgement of the case.

mechanism is intact. Sodium absorption is enhanced if small amounts of glucose or α-amino acid are present and vice versa. The absorption of these solutes "pulls" water and electrolytes into the plasma.[14] These principles were first applied successfully to people suffering from *Vibrio cholerae* infection and have subsequently been used in calves with colibacillosis. Multielectrolyte preparations containing dextrose of about 5% concentrations work best. The recipe for a preparation that has been designed for calves,[39] and that they drink readily, is given in Table 23–5. It may be used as the sole source of water, electrolytes, and energy for calves for 2 to 3 days, gradually being replaced by whole or artificial milk. The minimal daily water need of 80 ml/kg//day was established by studies done at Colorado State University.[40] Remember that estimates of excess water lost in the form of diarrhea must be added to the previously mentioned maintenance needs.

Other Therapy. There are recent studies indicating that bismuth subsalicylate, a major ingredient of Pepto-Bismol, inhibits the activity of *E. coli* enterotoxin so long as the toxin is still free within the intestinal lumen.[41] It has no effect on toxin already bound to mucosal cells and thus may be most helpful therapeutically in controlling further exacerbation of a case of colibacillosis. In addition, the salicylate component of Pepto-Bismol probably has local anti-prostaglandin synthetase activity to directly counteract the effects of the enterotoxin.[42]

In my opinion, anticholinergic agents are contraindicated in the treatment of colibacillosis. As indicated, intestinal motility is already reduced in this disease, and that which is manifested may be necessary to strip the bowel of the infective agent. There is no evidence to show that anticholinergics

are efficacious in reducing enterotoxin-induced intestinal hypersecretion.

Prophylaxis

As has already been suggested, the basic foundation of a good prophylactic program is making sure the newborn animals receive sufficient colostrum within the first few hours of birth, that the nursery areas have decent drainage and are routinely cleaned and disinfected, and that youngsters on artificial feeding programs are fed according to directions. Exposure of the dams to the nursery area for at least 2 weeks prior to parturition may also help reduce the incidence of disease since the adults will produce antibodies to pathogens present, which they will secrete into their colostrum.

Two systems developed for quantitative assessment of colostral intake can be very helpful in the evaluation of a herd diarrhea problem. One system involves the precipitation of the globulins in a serum sample by a dilute solution of zinc sulfate.[43] There is a good correlation between degree of turbidity and total IgG/IgM, but without the appropriate electronic equipment the degree of turbidity cannot be easily quantitated. Thus the practitioner is left to decide the response by "eyeballing" it, which is not very accurate. Recently, results of measurement of total serum protein in young calves, using a Goldberg refractometer, were compared with quantitated zinc sulfate turbidity tests, and the correlation was highly significant.[44] Therefore, the refractometer reading for total protein can be used as an index of susceptibility to diarrheal disease in young calves. A reading of less than 6 g/dl suggests that the chances for a calf to contract an infectious diarrhea are high.[45]

With regard to cattle, numerous attempts have been made to establish successful immunization programs whereby dams are vaccinated against pathogenic serotypes. There have been some problems with this approach, not because of failure to induce sufficient antibody titers, but because the pathogenic bacteria on a particular premises may change from one year to another.[46,47] Nonserotype-specific immunization of the bovine fetus, in utero, has met with some success.[48]

Immunization against colibacillosis has been more consistently successful in swine. Subcutaneous, intramammary, and oral vaccination of sows against certain strains, especially K-88 serotypes, caused protection in their piglets via colostrum.[49,50,51,52] Orally applied bacterins to young pigs have also been successful in conferring protection against serotypes used in the preparation of the bacterin,[53] perhaps by a "mucosal blockade" phenomenon.[54] The problem of changing pathogenic serotypes and its effect on a continually successful immunization program applies to swine as it does to cattle, however.

Salmonellosis

Epidemiology

All Salmonella serotypes with the exception of *S. typhi* should be considered enteropathogenic for all lower animals (and humans). Serotypes commonly encountered in veterinary medicine are *S. typhimurium, S. newport,* and *S. dublin.* When one is dealing with an outbreak of salmonellosis, the serotype is more important in helping to identify the source of the infection; the clinical signs are not serotype-specific.

Salmonella organisms are no doubt ubiquitous in the environment. Disease is produced when a susceptible animal ingests an appropriate dose of organisms (judged to be about 100,000 as a minimal infective dose in healthy humans).[13] Any stressful event,[55-58] any situation such as oral antibiotic therapy which can upset the normal enteric flora,[59] or diseases which disrupt the immune system, will increase the susceptibility of the animal to clinically apparent infection.[60]

The most insidious aspect of salmonellosis is the carrier state where the host is clinically normal but organisms are intermittently shed in the feces, usually when the host suffers a stress of some sort, such as shipping, pregnancy, drug treatment, exhaustion, general anesthesia, surgery, and even a change in weather. The incidence of fecal excretion of salmonella by swine, for example, is greatly altered by transportation. In one study, salmonella was isolated from one of 491 pen-adapted pigs but after 4 hours of transportation salmonellae were isolated from 72% of 491 pigs.[56] Increased warmth and humidity (i.e., summer) increases the incidence of salmonellosis.[60]

Pathogenesis

At least four distinct forms of salmonellosis occur, with one being the peracute form, which may be rapidly fatal.[61] After ingestion of the organism, invasion of the lymphoid tissue of the pharynx and possibly the small intestine and colon occurs. The organism invades the bloodstream via the lymphatics. Thus, a bacteremia and possibly a rapidly fatal septicemia may develop. This form of the disease is more common in young animals, e.g., suckling foals, 1 to 6 months of age and calves usually older than 2 weeks.[62-65] The disease usually occurs in pigs at 2 to 4 months of age and is either the septicemic or enteric form, but not both. Puppies that pass through holding points (brokers, retail pet outlets) after weaning are susceptible to either the septicemic or enteric form.

If the animal survives the peracute phase, an acute enteritis may develop. The organisms localize in extravascular sites such as mesenteric lymph nodes, liver, spleen and gallbladder and continue to proliferate. The organism can gain entrance to the intestine via the bile and it is in this stage that enteric localization occurs.[66] In the calf, distal ileum, cecum, and colon are primarily involved.[67] In severe cases, mucofibrinous casts are present in the lumen.

Electron microscopic studies have shown the microvillus border of intestinal mucosal cells to be the principal site of invasion.[68] Degeneration of the microvilli and the apical cytoplasm occurs when the organism is in critical proximity to the cell. Occasionally the organism penetrates the tight junction. However, as soon as the organism penetrates the intercellular space, the tight junction closes. The bacterium then fuses with the lateral membrane of the cell and is delivered into the cytoplasm. Thus, gross damage of the tight junction and intercellular space is not demonstrated and this may be why permeability characteristics do not seem to be changed in this disease. However, as the organism penetrates across the mucosal membrane into the cell, there is an interval when the cell is open to communication with the gut lumen. As the organism advances, the microvillus border is reconstituted. The bacteria then penetrate the basal laminae and multiply in the lamina propria, where a dense infiltrate of polymorphonuclear and mononuclear cells appears. Capillaries are engorged and subserous edema is present.

During this stage, the signs of acute enterocolitis develop, with an acute profuse, watery diarrhea, dehydration, and debilitation. Salmonellae also produce an effect which will cause functional crypt cells to hypersecrete water and electrolyte, by activation of adenyl cyclase.[69] If the animal survives this stage, a chronic enteritis with diarrhea may develop. These animals represent a commercial loss even if they do not die, and are also a continued source of contamination of the environment. The fourth type is the clinically silent salmonella shedder.

Pathophysiology

The enteric lesions suggest that the fluid loss associated with salmonellosis is due to increased permeability of the mucosa with the inflammatory edema providing the driving force for net secretion. However, this is not the case in experimental animals which have been studied. The blood to lumen permeability of the intestinal mucosa is unchanged and jejunal permeability is even decreased.[70] This is not to say that the lumen-to-blood permeability is not decreased owing to loss of the microvilli. However, the net secretion which is present cannot be due to altered permeability.

In monkeys experimentally infected with *S. typhimurium*, an acute inflammatory reaction is present which is more severe in the ileum and colon than in the jejunum.[71] The histologic alterations and water transport abnormalities correlate with the number of organisms which are present in the lumen. This correlation implies that rapid transit, which is characteristic of the upper small bowel, participates in removal of organisms from this region. This emphasizes once again that rapid transit rate (hypermotility?), if present, may be beneficial in certain instances. In fact, when animals are pretreated with opium, which stimulates segmental contractions of the jejunum thus slowing transit rate, the infection rate is greater.[68]

Ion transport changes in the jejunum are the least severe. Only a modest decrease in Na^+ absorption in detected and even in severe cases, significant net secretion is not elicited.[72] However, glucose-stimulated Na^+ absorption is absent[71] and this may reflect the decrease in jejunal permeability. Severe salmonella enteritis in the ileum results in net Na^+, Cl^-, and water secretion.[72] The normal $Cl^- -HCO_3^-$ exchange process is reversed and HCO_3^- is absorbed. However, HCO_3^- absorption appears to be mediated by H^+ secretion, which may be a manifestation of anaerobic metabolism by the inflamed, injured bowel. The net result is that HCl and Na^+ are delivered into the lumen. The glucose-stimulated Na^+ absorption in the ileum is at least partially intact and addition of glucose can reverse net Na^+ secretion to net absorption.

In vitro studies of ion transport by salmonella-infected rabbit ileum[69] have now shown that active Cl^- secretion is elicited and active Na^+ absorption (non-glucose mediated) is abolished although net Na^+ secretion may follow Cl^- passively in vivo. These transport changes are characteristic of the fluid secretion resulting from *E. coli* enterotoxin, mediated by cyclic AMP. Further studies have shown an activation of adenyl cyclase and an increase in mucosal cAMP in infected rabbit ileum. The Na^+-K^+ ATPase at the serosal border is unchanged despite the invasion of these cells by the pathogen. Pretreatment or post-treatment with indomethacin inhibits net fluid secretion which strongly suggests that activation of adenyl cyclase is mediated via prostaglandins (indomethacin inhibits prostaglandin synthesis).[73] Further studies indicate that the inflammatory reaction is in fact necessary for net fluid secretion[74] which further supports the hypothesis that prostaglandins or some other mediator are involved. (*Caution:* Indomethacin is absolutely contraindicated for use in dogs because it is associated with gastrointestinal hemorrhages.)

Although mechanisms of altered ion transport in the colon have not yet been investigated, it is clear that the colon participates in the net fluid loss. Not only is net colonic absorption abolished, but in severe cases, net secretion of Na^+, Cl^-, and water by the colon occurs.[72] In all likelihood these changes also are mediated by cAMP and prostaglandins.

Clinical Signs

Outstanding clinical signs of salmonellosis in neonates can include fever, fluid diarrhea often containing frank blood, anorexia, severe depression, and eventual collapse. Dehydration is usually not as precipitous in onset or as severe as that seen with *E. coli* infections. In calves it is not uncommon to find pneumonia associated with salmonellosis.[75] The question arises whether the stress caused by the pneumonia predisposes the animals to secondary *Salmonella* infection, or vice versa.

In calves, the acute form of salmonellosis resembles enterotoxigenic colibacillosis, with anorexia, dullness, and listlessness. Feces are bright yellow and contain necrotic shreds of tissue and small blood clots. However, *E. coli* infections are more common in the first week of life, while salmonellosis usually occurs after the second to third week. Coccidiosis must also be considered as a diagnostic rule-out. The rectal temperature is usually normal or subnormal and tenesmus is particularly prominent in coccidiosis. A profound anemia is usually a feature of coccidiosis, associated with the prominent necrotizing colitis. A positive diagnosis of coccidiosis may be obtained by detection of large numbers of oocysts in the feces. Bovine virus diarrhea (BVD) may mimic salmonellosis in young stock or adults but rarely causes profuse diarrhea in calves 2 to 10 weeks old. Mucosal erosions and ulcers in the mouth, so common with BVD, rarely occur in salmonellosis. BVD often is of slower onset with slower progression of signs than salmonellosis. Both may be associated with a leukopenia but it often persists longer in BVD.

Calves that recover from salmonellosis may develop a dry gangrene of the extremities which resembles ergotism.[76]

Following an outbreak of salmonellosis in a group of calves, the carrier rate may reach 50% or more.[77] During the active outbreak persons working with the calves or drinking raw milk of shedder cows can contact and develop enteric disease due to salmonellosis.[78,79] The carrier rate in swine may be high and some surveys have a similar number of isolations from visceral organs (mesenteric lymph nodes) as from the feces.[80]

Pigs with the acute enteric form of salmonellosis have signs and physical findings that are similar to those of swine dysentery and hog cholera. They demonstrate a profuse, watery diarrhea as early as 36 to 44 hours after experimental infection with *S. typhimurium*.[81] The diarrhea may be constant for 3 weeks unless the pigs die earlier. Dehydration, inanition, and progressive emaciation are prominent clinical features. Death may occur within 72 hours. In some field cases, diarrhea is not present.

The acute diarrheal phase of swine dysentery resembles that of salmonellosis. The animals are febrile initially, but with the onset of diarrhea, the fever subsides. No skin discoloration is present in swine dysentery and the internal lesions are confined to the large intestine. A positive diagnosis of swine dysentery can be obtained by identification of many small spirochetes in the feces.

If the animals are older than 6 months, the possibility of hog cholera must be considered even though eradication seems complete in certain areas of the Western Hemisphere. In pigs that die acutely of hog cholera, it is common to find an absence of macroscopic lesions while in salmonellosis, purple discoloration of the skin is present even in peracute deaths. In hog cholera there is an early pronounced leukopenia and then a leukocytosis associated with intercurrent bacterial invasion. The internal petechial hemorrhages of hog cholera are remarkably similar in distribution to those of salmonellosis. Since the disease affects the vascular system, infarcts, which are manifested as "button ulcers," are present in the colon and these resemble the discrete ulcers of salmonellosis. A non-suppurative encephalitis is usually present and is sufficient for a presumptive diagnosis of hog cholera.[66] Tests for the presence of the virus are necessary to establish the diagnosis with certainty. Appropriate regulatory officials should be consulted.

Diagnostic Criteria

Laboratory Findings. Outstanding findings consistent with salmonellosis are degenerative, followed in a day or two by regenerative, left shift, hypoalbuminemia, and fecal leukocytosis. These all result from the intense enteritis and are thus entirely distinct from effects of pure enterotoxigenic disease (see Table 23–7).[18] Unfortunately this whole spectrum of findings does not occur in every case, but depends upon severity of infection, stage of disease, concurrent infections. and previous therapy.

Culture of Salmonella organisms from the feces of animals showing signs of acute enteritis virtually confirms the diagnosis. This may be easier said than done. Unless fecal samples of adequate volume are submitted and appropriate media used, the organisms may be missed. Ideally, the fecal specimens submitted to the lab should be fresh and should be collected every other day until at least three samples have been cultured.

If a whole nursery is involved, environmental samples should also be gathered for culture. This may involve wiping cracks and surfaces with sterile swabs or actual collection and culture of water, feeds, cake collected on feeding buckets, soil around pens or stalls, material caught in drains or left in liquid manure systems, or any other substances that seem suspicious. This can help identify the original source of the infection and will most certainly emphasize the need to institute strong sanitation procedures immediately and to maintain strict adherence to good husbandry practices.

The diagnosis can be missed not only where sampling methods are inadequate but also when improper culturing techniques are employed. The best recourse for the practitioner is to submit the material to a nearby state or institutional laboratory which is set up to culture Salmonellae.

Necropsy Findings. Because Salmonellae are invasive, they evoke a true inflammatory response in affected portions of the bowel; small intestine or colon, or both. This may be indicated grossly by hyperemic intestinal mucosa and/or the presence of blood and tissue debris within the intestinal lumen. It has been my experience, on occasion, that gross indications of enteritis may not be very severe in calves or piglets with salmonellosis. Histologically, however, polymorphonuclear infiltration of the lamina propria and destruction of the mucosal lining are consistently found when the disease is active.

Therapy

When dealing with an outbreak of salmonellosis in a group of young animals, the most appropriate therapy is directed toward providing adequate fluids, electrolytes, and nutrition. Antibiotic therapy is inappropriate and a needless expense in most situations in that it is usually ineffective and has the potential of inducing a prolonged carrier state in survivors.[29,30] If particularly valuable individual animals show signs of severe, possibly septic, infection (high fever, shock, diffuse intravascular coagulation), systemic antibiotics are indicated. Intravenous chloramphenicol, 12 mg/kg q.i.d., is my antibiotic of choice for foals and calves since it has, to date, been found to be consistently effective against salmonellae in vitro. It is not licensed for such use in animals in the United States. Some of the newer, very expensive aminoglycosides such as gentamicin should also be effective.

Fluid therapy of any sort for small helpless newborn animals such as kittens or puppies and piglets requires a controlled environment (e.g., incubator) and involves frequent tube feedings and intraperitoneal or subcutaneous injections. Calves are somewhat easier to deal with, especially if they are still drinking. The oral replacement fluid (see Table 23–5) can be used with very satisfactory effects, particularly for calves that are pail or nipple fed, if the small intestine is not too badly damaged. In commercial operations, this is the only practical approach to take; any animals which are so sick that they will not drink should be removed from the premises and destroyed in an attempt to cut down on sources of infection. In fact, the commercial producer may find it more economical to remove all the existing young stock, completely clean the premises, disinfect, and repopulate.

More valuable large animal neonates, and this usually includes most foals, may require treatment on an individual basis. Their larger size, relative tractability, and value justify an individual-animal approach to therapy. Intravenous fluid therapy may be used with an isotonic replacement solution containing bicarbonate precursors (acetate, pyruvate) as the fluid of choice. (See under Salmonella Infection, Part II.)

Prophylaxis

The most effective prophylaxis is good management. If salmonellosis has been definitely established as existing on a premises, strict sanitation procedures should be instituted immediately. The area involved should be isolated from general traffic with foot baths containing a phenol-based product at its entrances and special clothing and equipment for use inside. Vacated stalls, pens, and all exposed spaces should be disinfected with phenol-base antiseptic, steam-cleaned and left vacant until the problem is resolved. Do not overlook rafters and other areas where dust collects. Dirt in stable stall floors should be removed to a depth of at least 15 cm.

Any new animals brought into these premises should be confined to areas known to be free of infection, and these areas ideally should be capable of serving as isolation units.

Fecal cultures should be taken of selected adult animals, particularly those that have recently given birth or who were known to be near the source of the outbreak. This may identify carrier animals which have perpetuated or will perpetuate the infection.

It is often virtually impossible to meet the conditions described previously because of one of a number of factors, including physical arrangement of the buildings, continued movement of animals, and reluctance of clients to cooperate. An advantage in dealing with neonates, when faced with these problems, in contrast to adults, is that immunization of the pregnant dam with type-specific antigen may be very effective in reducing the incidence of disease in the newborn. This, at least, has been my experience and that of others in dealing with outbreaks in groups of calves[82] and foals. In calves, some protection is afforded by high serum IgM but very little by IgA.[83] In these large animals with a long gestation period, the dams should be given a bacterin subcutaneously 6 weeks and again 2 weeks prior to projected parturition date. Owners should be warned that horses will develop quite a local reaction at the site of the injection. The bacterin used may be autogenous, made especially in the lab doing the culturing, especially if the serotype encountered is one of the more rare varieties. An *S. typhimurium/dublin* product is available commercially, made by Cutter Laboratories, (Paratyphol). Though developed for use in cattle, it is effective in horses as well.

Clostridium Perfringens Type C (or B)

Epidemiology

This is primarily a disease of large animal offspring, seen within the first 2 weeks postpartum. Its incidence is not widespread, but it can become endemic in certain areas or on particular farms. Calves, lambs, and piglets are more likely to be affected than foals or kids.[11,84] As with other clostridial diseases of intestinal origin, infection is often precipitated by a situation that disrupts the routine of a young stock, whereby a period of diminished availability of feed or milk is followed by a period of overconsumption. The alpha and beta toxins produced by type C are responsible for the clinical manifestation.[84]

Clinical Signs

Affected animals may simply be found dead; this is often the case with lambs. Signs, when seen, are colic and hematochezia. In addition, there is often evidence of toxemia, with bizarre behavior, aimless running, opisthotonus, or just severe depression, as possible signs.[11,84] In contrast to salmonellosis, however, there is no fever, affected animals usually die within a few hours, and central nervous system disturbance is a prominent feature.

Pathophysiology

The activated exotoxins cause severe necrosis of the intestinal mucosa. The rapid mucosal sloughing results in severe bleeding. Affected animals die of toxemia rather than exsanguination, however. The beta toxin is inactivated by trypsin;[85] thus pancreatic secretions must be abnormal if this toxin is to cause disease.

Diagnostic Criteria

Laboratory Findings. The only definitive help the laboratory could give is to demonstrate the presence of *C. perfringens type C* or its toxins in significant quantities within affected intestine. This is very difficult because (1) the toxins break down very rapidly, so the intestinal tract contents must be collected and frozen as soon as possible after death; (2) culture of organisms requires rapid collection into an anaerobic environment and maintenance of that environment during media and culture. A mouse neutralization test may be used, however, to detect toxin in very fresh intestinal contents.[86] Once the organisms have been cultured, they must be specifically identified through biochemical and serologic methods.[87]

Necropsy Findings. Classically, there is a severe hemorrhagic enteritis which, grossly, is impossible to distinguish from salmonellosis. Large ulcers may be present and the whole small intestine, especially the jejunum and ileum, may have a bluish-red tinge.[84] In contrast to salmonellosis, however, the large intestine is rarely affected. Histologically, in early lesions there is a preferential necrosis of the villous tips with clostridia present in the epithelial debris. The crypt epithelium is intact.[88]

Therapy

There is no reliably effective treatment for this disease. Hyperimmune serum has reportedly been successful in calves,[85] but most affected animals are usually beyond the treatment stage when examined.

Prophylaxis

As with salmonellosis, clostridial enteritis in neonates is best controlled by vaccination of the dams early enough before the expected parturition date that there will be effective titers of antitoxin in their colostrum.[86] A toxoid is used, therefore, instead of a bacterin. Youngsters born of unvaccinated dams can be given antitoxin immediately after birth and should probably receive a booster at 2 weeks of age to get them through the most susceptible age range.[84]

Acute Viral Infections of Neonates

In recent years it has become increasingly more apparent that enteric viruses are responsible for many cases of infant diarrhea in humans and domestic animals. The rota (reo) and corona types *seem* to be most important. One suggestion is that these viruses do not produce their typical clinical signs solely on their own but in concert with resident pathogenic enterobacteria.[89] The details regarding this interaction need to be elucidated.

Rota (Reo) Virus Enteropathy

Epidemiology

Calf rotavirus infection was formerly referred to as reovirus infection. Reo is the acronym for ''respiratory-enteric-orphan'' since, for many years, this type of virus was found in respiratory secretions and feces but could not be associated with any particular disease; thus, it was an orphan. The virus was first definitively implicated as a cause of enteric disease in calves by workers at the University of Nebraska,[90] and it is more properly referred to as a ''reovirus-like'' agent or rotavirus. This agent has also been shown to cause enteropathy in foals,[91,92] piglets,[93] and lambs.[94] Serologically there are cross-reactions between agents isolated from the various species.[95]

Epidemiologically, the incidence of the disease is endemic, usually to individual farms, although the organism appears to be ''ubiquitous.'' This implies that management may have a strong influence on whether the infection becomes apparent. Conditions of overcrowding, poor sanitation, improper feeding of calves, deficient colostrum intake, or failure to isolate newly acquired animals will favor an outbreak. In addition, adverse weather conditions seem to trigger outbreaks of disease.

As has been suggested, it is probable that rotavirus agents often interact with resident bacterial enteropathogens to produce clinical signs of severe diarrhea. For instance, in a recent study of a small beef herd in Canada,[96] 80% of the calves developed diarrhea before 10 days of age. Enteropathogenic *E. coli* were isolated from the feces of 30% of these calves, reovirus-like particles from 50%, and both agents from 20% of cases.

Clinical Signs

The clinical signs of enteric disease induced by the rotavirus agent, namely profuse diarrhea and dehydration, are virtually impossible to distinguish from those caused by enterotoxigenic *E. coli*. Infected calves usually show signs within the first week of life. Morbidity in severe outbreaks can reach 100% with mortality varying from 0 to 50% depending upon environmental factors.[89] Age limits for other species have not been so well delineated since outbreaks in them are rare.

Pathophysiology

The virus replicates within the mucosal cells lining the villi of the small intestines. As the infection continues, migration of infected cells to villus tips and their subsequent sloughing are accelerated. Replacement cells developing within the crypts move up while still immature so that the villi are eventually covered with cuboidal rather than mature functional columnar epithelium.[5,89] What this does, in effect, is produce an acute transient small intestinal malabsorption. In germ-free calves, for instance, the outstanding clinical signs are rapid onset of depression, salivation, and nonprofuse diarrhea with return to normal within 24 hours. Calves monocontaminated with pathogenic *E. coli* not present in large enough numbers to cause disease by themselves or, possessing the usual mix of neonatal flora containing some enteropathogens, become much sicker than the germ-free subjects when fed rotavirus.[89]

Diagnostic Criteria

Laboratory Findings. The only definitive laboratory finding is the demonstration of the rotavirus agent in the feces by a fluorescent antibody technique, immunoelectron microscopy, or culture.[89,97-99] The first is by far the most common and many regional laboratories are equipped to set it up, at least for calves. The earlier in the illness the fecal sample is collected, the better. Samples from as many animals as possible should be checked, and they should be frozen before shipment to the laboratory to prevent autolysis of antigen-bearing (infected) epithelial cells in the feces. Infected epithelial cells contain the antigen which reacts with the fluorescent antibody. Immunofluorescent technique can also be applied to small intestinal mucosa from *fresh* necropsy specimens.

Immunoelectron microscopy is much more precise in that it can demonstrate antibody attachment to individual virions, causing their clumping (Fig. 23–1), but most clinical laboratories do not have the expensive equipment needed. This technique has provided much insight into rotavirus infections, however, by sensitively demonstrating cross-reactivity between rotavirus agents isolated from different animal species and from children.

Necropsy Findings. Grossly, very little if any intestinal damage is seen at necropsy. Some disruption of normal villous architecture might be appreciated upon examination of fresh specimens of small intestinal mucosa under the dissecting microscope, if the carcass is very fresh. Histologically, the predominance of cuboidal epithelium covering the villi of the small intestine is quite characteristic; again, this will be seen only if the animal has been dead less than 1 hour before necropsy.[89]

Therapy

There is no specific antiviral therapy. Treatment is aimed at supporting the sick animal's water and electrolyte balance, either intravenously or orally. The intensity of treatment is determined by the degree of the illness and the animal's stated worth to the client.

Orally administered fluids will be less effective here than in animals with pure enterotoxigenic *E. coli* infection since the small intestinal epithelium is damaged. If a mixed bacterial-viral infection is suspected, oral antibiotics with known effectiveness against *E. coli* such as sulfachlorpyridazine, nitrofuran, or chloramphenicol (in non-food-producing animals) may reduce the severity of signs and thus mortality;[100] but these should be used only therapeutically, not prophylactically.

Prophylaxis

A very effective modified-live-virus vaccine has been developed for control of rotavirus-induced diarrhea in calves. In herds where rotavirus has been definitively implicated, all calves should be vaccinated via the oral route as soon after birth as possible. Once this is introduced into a particular

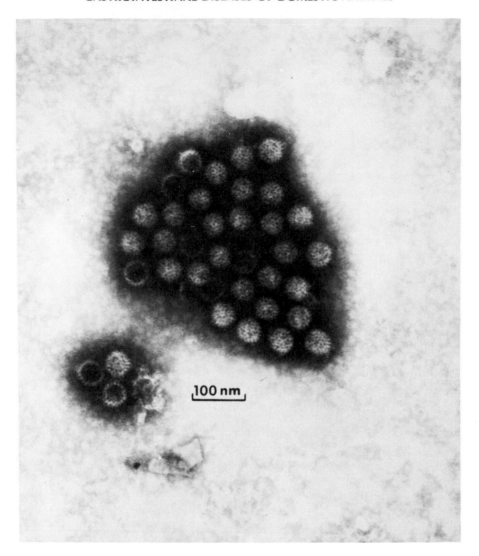

Figure 23–1. Immunoelectron micrograph (130,500×) of porcine rotavirus collected from the intestinal contents of a naturally infected 4-week-old piglet. Agglutination was created by incubation with electron-dense antiporcine rotavirus serum. (Photograph courtesy of Dr. Linda Saif, Ohio Agricultural Research and Development Center, Wooster, OH.)

operation, it may be necessary to continue it indefinitely unless the area can be totally depopulated and disinfected or husbandry and isolated procedures can be changed (see previous section on *E. coli* infections.)

One may rightly ask how a modified-live-virus vaccine could possibly provide protection against a disease the highest incidence of which is within the first 7 days of life. This rapid development of protection is due to the attachment of modified viral particles to the mucosal surface of the gastrointestinal tract, which block the reception of the wild virus particles and prevent their intracellular penetration.[101]

Vaccines are not yet available against rotavirus enteropathogens in species other than the bovine.

Coronavirus Enteropathy

Epidemiology

Coronavirus enteropathy is presently recognized in calves,[101] puppies,[102] and foals,[103] and in piglets in which it is called transmissible gastroenteritis (TGE). The conditions controlling its incidence and persistence are generally the same as those discussed under the rotavirus section. Its prevalence in calves is as yet not as great as rotavirus. In piglets, transmissible gastroenteritis is seen more commonly during the winter months and is widespread in hog raising areas.[104]

The virus gets its name from its morphology. Under the electron microscope it appears as a round body surrounded by numerous small projections resem-

Table 23–6. Infectious Diarrheal Diseases of Calves

Etiology	Age	Fever	Dehydration	Character of Feces	Other Clinical Features	Definitive Diagnosis	Specific Prophylaxis
Toxigenic Escherichia coli	<2 wk	No	Moderate to severe	—Profuse, watery —Fetid, yellow in color —Alkaline pH	—Hyperkalemia —No leukocytosis in CBC —Severe metabolic acidosis —Minimal gut pathology	—Demonstrate toxin production in infant mouse intestine (ST) or adrenal cell culture (LT) or gut loop	—Expose dam to environment >2 wk before calving —Improve husbandry —Vaccinate dam and/or calf
Salmonella	All	Yes	Mild to moderate	—Soft to watery —Shreds of mucosa and frank blood may be seen (dysentery)	—Degenerative left shift in CBC —Gross enterocolitis —Fecal leukocytosis	—Fecal culture	—Vaccinate dam —Depopulate and sanitize —Strict sanitation on premises —Eliminate known carriers
Clostridium perfringens Type C	<2 wk	No	Mild to moderate	—Marked hematochezia	—CNS disturbance —Rapid onset —Stress associated? —Gross hemorrhagic enteritis	—Histopathology shows necrotizing enteritis, clostridia in cellular debris —Anaerobic culture	—Vaccinate dams
Rotavirus	<1 wk	No or mild	Moderate to severe	—Profuse, watery —Acid pH	—Rapid spread, 100% morbidity	—Fecal fluorescent antibody —Fecal culture —Fecal immunoelectron microscopy	—Oral vaccine (MLV) at birth —Vaccinate dam (MLV) last trimester
Coronavirus	5–21 d	No or mild	Severe, develops rapidly	—Profuse, watery —Acid pH	—Rapid spread, 100% morbidity —Very resistant to fluid therapy	—Fecal culture —Fecal immunoelectron microscopy —Colon fluorescent antibody	—Oral vaccine (MLV) at birth —Vaccinate dam (MLV) last trimester
Virus Diarrhea (BVD)	>3 wk	Biphasic	Mild	—Watery, not profuse	—Sporadic morbidity and mortality —Lesions of buccal mucosa —Leukopenia	—Fecal, or intestinal contents/ lymph node culture —Pathognomonic GI erosions	—Vaccinate dams (while not pregnant) —MLV vaccine and hyperimmune serum to calves
Adenovirus	>10 d	?	Mild to moderate	—Watery	—Respiratory disease —Colic	—Culture pharynx	—None

bling a crown. As with the rotavirus, it replicates in small intestinal mucosal cells but causes a more severe and longer-lasting lesion.[105] The highest incidence of disease in calves is between 5 and 21 days of age. Infected pigs up to young adulthood may show clinical signs but those less than 3 weeks old are the more severely affected. Although resident bacterial enteropathogens may contribute to the severity of clinical signs, coronavirus infection can, in contrast to rotavirus, cause death in gnotobiotic calves.[106]

Clinical Signs

In calves, severe depression, non-bloody diarrhea, and dehydration progressing over a 4- to 5-day period to a moribund state and death are the usual signs. Supportive therapy often does little to alter the course of the disease. As mentioned, the highest incidence is between 5 and 21 days, although calves 2 or 3 days old can be affected. Features of differentiation from other calfhood diarrheas are outlined in Table 23–6.

Piglets with coronavirus infection (TGE) also have severe diarrhea, which is impossible to distinguish grossly from that caused by *E. coli*. A cardinal sign of TGE infection in pigs is vomiting.[104] All ages of animals in the herd can be affected, with piglets less than 10 days old having the highest mortality. Diarrheic feces in TGE outbreaks may be more acid, as a result of metabolic products from bacterial digestion of unabsorbed nutrients, than in colibacillosis where bicarbonate hypersecretion is a feature of the disease.[104] Most piglets less than 10 days old die in 2 to 7 days; most over 3 weeks old survive.[107] Other differentiating aspects of colibacillosis versus TGE in piglets are listed in Table 23–7. *Clostridium perfringens* type C causes hemorrhagic enteritis with bloody diarrhea which is uncharacteristic of TGE.

Table 23–7. Clinical, Epidemiologic, and Pathologic Findings Useful in Differentiating Colibacillosis from TGE in Piglets[104]

Characteristics	Colibacillosis	TGE
Incubation	4–24 hr	16–72 hr
Vomition	Seldom	Usually
Age	Only piglets	All ages
Morbidity	Variable	About 100%
Mortality (newborn)	Variable	About 100%
Seasonal	No	Yes, winter
pH (cecum)	Usually alkaline	Usually acid
Villous atrophy	Very seldom, patchy	Yes, extensive
Lactase (jejunum)	Present	Reduced or absent
Fat in chyle	Variable	Usually absent

Coronavirus infection in dogs can manifest itself at any age, but like TGE in pigs, the infant animals are most susceptible.[108] The most prominent sign in puppies is diarrhea and all members of the litter are affected in rapid succession. Villous atrophy occurs in piglets, so that malabsorption is the basic cause of the diarrhea; thus the feces should be acidic rather than basic. See Table 23–11 for comparison to parvovirus infection.

Pathophysiology

Coronavirus invades mature absorptive cells along the sides and tips of small intestinal villi. The early effect is a sodium and water hypersecretion.[109] Severe villous atrophy persists until cells can be replaced by regeneration from the crypts.[105,110] During this period of villous atrophy, absorptive function is severely impaired; unabsorbed nutrients hold water within the intestinal lumen and this osmotic activity is exacerbated through intraluminal digestion of these nutrients by intestinal flora. Undigested carbohydrates are easily hydrolyzed to organic acids by intestinal bacteria. This tends to give the feces a low pH.

Diagnostic Criteria

Laboratory Findings. Coronavirus infections in calves and piglets are substantiated at a diagnostic laboratory by immunofluorescent detection of the virus in infected gut tissue.[107] For calves, the middle of the spiral colon is the tissue of choice. For piglets with suspected TGE, the mid-jejunum is preferred; duodenal mucosa is rarely affected.[111] These tissues should be collected as soon after death as possible and frozen before delivery to the laboratory. Feces from calves may also be submitted if they have been collected very soon after clinical signs develop, but these should not be relied upon solely to provide a diagnosis, since if not handled carefully, the exfoliated epithelial cells containing virus particles are autolyzed.

Other systems to detect TGE infection, such as serum neutralization testing using cytopathogenic effect (CPE) suppression as the indicator, and acid bentonite agglutination, have been used, with the former proving to be more satisfactory.[104] Again, however, more equipment is necessary to do these tests than is required for immunofluorescence.

The highly sensitive technique of immunoelectronmicroscopy is now being used to detect the presence of agglutination of corona virions in the feces by specific antibodies.[112]

Techniques have been described for qualitatively assessing disaccharidase activity in intestinal mucosa of piglets suspected of having TGE (see Chapter 16), where activity should be diminished. Absolutely *fresh* tissue must be used for this test.

Necropsy Findings. At necropsy there are no definitive gross diagnostic findings of coronavirus infection. The absence of visible lymphatic channels within the mesentery in spite of plenty of digesta within the intestines suggests a malabsorptive state but this is certainly not definitive.

As mentioned, the findings of villous atrophy upon examination of a piece of the small intestinal mucosa through a dissecting microscope is highly indicative of coronavirus infection. Pieces of jejunum and ileum should be examined since the damage usually begins high in the tract and progresses aborad.[111] The examination again should be done on very fresh tissue which is floated in a Petri dish containing 0.9% saline solution.

Microscopically, the outstanding lesion suggesting coronavirus infection is marked villous atrophy of jejunal or ileal mucosa. Any indications of inflammation that may be present are probably due to effects of intestinal bacterial flora rather than to the virus. Indications of colonic mucosal damage have been found in calves;[113] this has not been seen in pigs or puppies.

Therapy

No decent trials concerning the effectiveness of antibiotics in suppressing the ravages of enteric viral infection have been done.

As with rotaviral-induced enteropathy, therapy should be directed first at reestablishing and maintaining fluid, electrolyte, and acid-base balance. Clinically, my experience with calves suggests this is more difficult in coronavirus infections for reasons that are not well understood. Perhaps it is because the effects of this infection upon the intestinal tract are more persistent. A methodology for subcutaneous fluid replacement for piglets infected with TGE has been developed[114] and is as follows:

1. Prepare 1.2% $NaHCO_3$/5% dextrose solution.
2. Inject 15 to 20 ml amounts in 4 sites subcutaneously, twice a day.
3. Do not give until second day of disease or it will cause alkalosis.

This therapy needs further clinical trial to assess its practicality as well as its effectiveness.

Prophylaxis

A vaccine has recently been developed for use against coronavirus infections in calves. This modified-live-virus preparation (Scourvax II) is combined with the rotavirus vaccine to be given orally within a few hours of birth.

The experimental evaluation of the effectiveness of the coronavirus immunizing product proved to be exceedingly difficult since both double-blind and odd-even techniques in groups of calves suggested that the vaccine was no better than the placebo in affecting morbidity but that both were better than nothing in reducing mortality. Only when an alternate-interval system of evaluation was employed—where efficacy when all calves born within a 1-month period of time were vaccinated was compared with results where all calves born the next month were not vaccinated—did both morbidity and mortality drop convincingly.[115]

Prophylactic procedures against TGE in swine are more complicated. It is well established that sows which have recovered from TGE, or been experimentally challenged, can pass immunity to their piglets through colostrum.[116] The duration of this immunity seems to vary between 9 and 12 months. So long as the sow's titer is high, any pigs suckling her will receive TGE neutralizing antibodies, which gets the piglets through the period of highest mortality. The practice then developed among swine producers to freeze intestines and their contents from piglets that died from TGE and feed some of these to sows about 3 to 4 weeks prior to farrowing. This practice is dangerous, however, for a number of reasons: (1) the existence of the virus on a given property is perpetuated rather than eliminated, (2) the disease can be spread to susceptible neighboring TGE-free herds, and (3) other pathogens, such as Salmonella, can be spread and maintained in the herd. The rational alternative is the use of a modified-live or inactivated virus for immunization of the sows or piglets, some of which are available commercially in certain regions of the United States.

The management practices in any herd ravaged by coronavirus infection should naturally be evaluated and changed where indicated. The role of colostrum and the circulating antibodies derived from its absorption, in protecting against the mucosal damage caused by coronavirus, is debatable. Evidence has been presented which suggests that circulating antibodies even if specific are ineffective in neutralizing intraluminal virus, in contrast to their effect on organisms which invade into the bloodstream.[117] This does not mean that colostrum is unimportant, since colostrum-deprived animals seem to stay sick longer and die in greater numbers.

Transmission of TGE virus within and between production units can occur not only due to human carelessness but by birds, particularly starlings, and perhaps even dogs.[107] It has been postulated that the prevalence of the disease in the winter months may be because this is when flocks of starlings and blackbirds travel from farm to farm feeding on the grain that has been set out for the pigs. This factor must be taken into account when attempting to control this disease.

Bovine Virus Diarrhea (BVD) in Calves

Epidemiology

Virus diarrhea (BVD) is common in young calves and must be considered in a complete differential diagnosis of neonatal diarrhea in this species. It is seen most commonly in intense production situations, such as vealing and feedlot operations, where the main source of animals is from auctions or similar type sales and reliability of colostral intake by calves is questionable. Calves of any age may be affected; some may even be infected in utero.[118] There is a suggestion that BVD virus may interact with other infectious agents of calves to exacerbate the enteric disease.[96,119] BVD virus is isolated from lung and bronchial lymph nodes in calves and feedlot cattle that have died of pneumonia.

Clinical Signs

Calves with BVD usually, but not always, have diarrhea. The feces are often more fluid but less voluminous than in other neonatal diarrheal diseases. The author's clinical impression is that the calf is depressed and anorectic more because it feels sick rather than because it is very dehydrated. Severe dehydration is not a particular feature of this disease. Some animals die within a few days; others may have diarrhea for weeks.[120,121]

Other findings that are compatible with BVD are a biphasic fever spike (if the animal lives that long) and nasal discharge. Erosions of the buccal mucosa along the hard palate, inside the lower lip, and under the tongue are also highly pathognomonic but do not occur consistently. Blunting of papillae at the commissures of the mouth may be seen.

Pathophysiology

The pathogenesis of gastrointestinal lesions and pathophysiology of the diarrhea in BVD is not well understood. Nor is it clear whether resident or pathogenic enteric bacterial flora influence the severity of disease.

Diagnostic Criteria

Laboratory Findings. A profound leukopenia (often to less than 1000 WBC/mm³) is consistently found and is very diagnostic. Both viral isolation and serology can be done on a herd basis to establish the presence of the virus. For isolation, nasal swabs and feces can be used. These should be frozen unless they can be transported immediately to the laboratory. Mesenteric lymph nodes also contain virus for weeks after exposure.[120] Serology is most helpful if a rising titer can be demonstrated in blood samples taken 2 weeks apart. Not all animals infected with BVD will show a rise in titer.[121]

Necropsy Findings. Pathognomonic gross lesions are erosions in any or all parts of the gastrointestinal tract, most commonly esophagus and small intestine. The lesions are characteristically linear in the esophagus while in the small intestine they tend to involve the Peyer's patches.[121] It must be emphasized, however, that gross lesions may not be seen but histologically there will be extensive lymphoid infiltration into the submucosa and possibly necrosis of the center of definitive lymphoid nodules.

Therapy

There is no specific treatment for BVD infection. Therapy, whether intravenous or oral, is directed toward support of potential fluid and electrolyte imbalance and may be helpful in some cases. There is anecdotal support for the intramuscular injection of 50 to 100 ml of whole blood from the dam, but this certainly is not consistently effective. Some patients die in spite of all treatments.

Prophylaxis

Since BVD virus is so ubiquitous within the adult cattle population, if a calf ingests sufficient colostrum at birth, there is a good chance that it will be passively protected until 2 to 3 months of age. Calves coming into a feeder or replacement operation via auction or sale where colostral intake status is unknown may be vaccinated and given a commercial hyperimmune serum preparation. Some feel that it reduces, but does not eliminate, signs of BVD infection and mortality in young calves.[122]

If the BVD is a persistent and widespread herd problem, vaccination of the cows with the modified live virus 3 to 4 weeks prior to breeding should protect at least *their* progeny from neonatal infection, via colostral antibody transfer. Once herd vaccination is started, the whole herd should be done as soon as possible. Since the modified virus can cause abortion, pregnant cows should not be vaccinated.

Finally, the management factors should be considered, as in all the other neonatal diarrheal problems. Particular attention should be paid to feeding practices. Is replacer rather than whole milk used? Is replacer being mixed properly? Are feed buckets properly sanitized between feedings? While in well-run operations it is economically more feasible to feed replacers, there are protective factors in the form of secretory globulins in whole milk, even beyond the colostrum phase, that would no doubt reduce the incidence of disease on a farm where husbandry is marginal.

Adenoviral Infection in Calves

Epidemiology

There are, to date, eight different serotypes of adenovirus recognized to be present in cattle. Types 2, 3, and 4 appear to be the most virulent with respect to causing disease in calves.[123] We do not yet recognize adenoviral infection to be a widespread major cause of diarrhea in calves, either because it is not, or because no one has looked carefully enough for it. However, economically important outbreaks have been described in Hungary and in the state of Oregon. The organism causes disease in both enteric and respiratory tracts, thus producing a so-called "pneumoenteritis complex." The incidence of disease is highest in calves of first-calf heifers, suggesting that continued exposure of older dams keeps antibody titers high enough to be secreted in sufficient amounts into the milk.[123]

Clinical Signs

Calves showing clinical signs of adenoviral infection are usually over 10 days old. Provisional signs are excessive lacrimation and increased nasal discharge. These discharges are serous at first but become mucopurulent and last 3 to 5 days. Signs of enteropathy begin a day or two after seeing the discharges. Gaseous distention of the bowel and colic along with the diarrhea are seen quite frequently, which is usually not the case with other causes of calfhood enteropathy.[124] The degree of polypnea and coughing indicative of pulmonary disease will vary although most infected calves will show signs of respiratory embarrassment if forced to exercise.

Pathophysiology

The way in which adenoviruses cause malfunction of the intestinal tract is not known.

Diagnostic Criteria

Laboratory Findings. There is nothing pathognomonic for adenoviral infection that can be seen in the results of the usual laboratory procedures. Nasal and lacrimal secretions, fresh feces and swabs of the posterior pharynx should be submitted for viral cultures. These samples should be frozen immediately unless they can be transferred to the laboratory directly. The positive culture of adenovirus to the exclusion of other enteropathogenic agents, along with signs of pneumoenteritis complex, should be quite conclusive. Failure to isolate adenovirus, however, does not discount the diagnosis completely.[123]

Necropsy Findings. The various serotypes of adenovirus appear to have varying tissue specific tropism with regard to severity of lesions. Type 3 is primarily pneumotropic, type 2 more enterotropic.[123] Gross pulmonary lesions consist of scattered areas of lobular consolidation, more prominent with ventral and hilar lobes. Mild to moderate interlobular edema is also seen. Histologically there is evidence of proliferation and necrosis of bronchiolar epithelial cells, bronchiolar occlusion and subsequent alveolar collapse. Large intranuclear inclusion bodies can be found in bronchiolar and alveolar epithelial cells and in the reticulum cells of regional lymph nodes.

Gross lesions in the intestinal tract are few and nonspecific. Histologically there seems to be particular tropism for endothelial cells, at least with type 2 infection, not only locally but throughout the body.

Therapy

There is no specific therapy. The viral infection appears to be rather short—7 to 8 days in most cases. Systemic broad spectrum antibiotics, particularly those known to be effective against respiratory tract infections in calves, such as tetracycline or tylosin, are indicated to control intercurrent bacterial infection.

Prophylaxis

Vaccines against adenoviral infection are not available. As with rota- and coronavirus, it has been shown experimentally that adenovirus can cause disease even though serum antibodies against it, derived from sufficient colostral ingestion, are high.[124] This suggests, therefore, that immune dams can confer protection to the very young calf only so long as their milk is being continually ingested. After 2 weeks of age, exposed calves ought to have a high enough titer in their secretory antibodies (intestinal and respiratory IgA) to protect them.

Chlamydial Enteritis in Calves

Chlamydia are members of the psittacosis-lymphogranuloma group of organisms. Those which cause enteritis in calves are antigenically distinct from other chlamydial agents of bovine origin.[125] At present, it is not clear whether chlamydia alone can cause natural outbreaks of diarrhea in calves or whether this is a laboratory phenomenon. These agents have been cultured, usually mixed with other organisms known to cause diarrhea, from feces of calves where diarrhea is endemic.[126] Experimentally, low and high virulence strains are recognized with those of high virulence causing enteritis in both colostrum-replete and colostrum-deprived animals. Critical studies testing the severity of disease in gnotobiotic calves have not been published. These would be necessary to gain a more accurate indication of importance of interaction with other intestinal flora.

The fact remains that experimental infection with pure chlamydial cultures causes calves to become depressed, be feverish, and have diarrhea. Those animals given large doses of virulent organisms have become moribund and died. Grossly, the small intestine was edematous and there were small ulcers of the mucosa. Microscopically, chlamydia could be found within enterocytes primarily along the sides of the villi in the intervillus zone and in the endothelial cells lining the lacteals.[127] Neutrophils were present in significant numbers; thus these, along with the edema, caused the reaction to be classified as a true enteritis. It has been found that the E. coli population density increased significantly in the small intestinal lumen of calves infected with chlamydia.[126] Thus, it was suggested that changes in the ecology of the resident enteric bacterial flora may be induced by the invasion of chlamydial agents and that this may exacerbate the enteritis.

Parvovirus Enteropathy in Calves

Parvovirus is known to cause diarrhea in humans; the infection spreads rapidly among both adults and children. Recently a number of bovine parvoviruses have been discovered which are antigenically related among themselves but antigenically distinct from the human strains.[128] The bovine types have been isolated from calves affected with enteric disease. Surviving animals developed antibodies but continued to shed the virus in their feces.

When bovine parvoviruses were fed to normal, colostrum-fed calves, they caused diarrhea, at first mucoid and then fluid in consistency.[128] By numerous immunofluorescence studies, the virions were found in highest numbers within the mucosal cells of the jejunum and ileum. There was accompanying evidence of enterocyte destruction.

At present, the seriousness of parvovirus as a primary pathogen in outbreaks of calf diarrhea still needs to be elucidated. We do not, as yet, routinely consider it in the list of differential diagnoses; perhaps we should.

PARASITIC INFECTIONS OF NEONATES

Coccidiosis

Epidemiology

Both *Eimeria* and *Isospora* genuses of coccidia can infect domestic animals, although the former are more common and more pathogenic. Details regarding species-specific infections and life cycles can be found in many textbooks of veterinary parasitology. In general, coccidiosis is *not* a problem in animals less than 1 month of age, but occasionally, particularly when there is crowding and poor sanitary procedures, outbreaks in 2- to 4-week-old neonates can occur. Calves, lambs, piglets, or puppies are susceptible.[129]

Clinical Signs

Tenesmus and bloody diarrhea are hallmarks of the disease. Degrees of depression, dehydration, and anemia are variable resulting in signs ranging from very little evidence of systemic disturbance, to rapid onset of collapse and death. Fever is not part of the syndrome. In chronic cases, signs of unthriftiness soon occur.

Diagnostic Criteria

Laboratory Findings. The demonstration of large numbers of oocysts in the fecal material is definitive. The problem is that severe signs of disease can be seen before the oocysts are passed in significant numbers. Usually the WBC count is within normal limits and the hematocrit is low, in contrast to what would be found with bacterial causes of dysentery. In the more chronic cases total serum protein concentration will be low as well.

It should be cautioned that the finding of a few bodies that look like oocytes in the feces of an animal showing signs consistent with coccidiosis is *not* definitive, however. If, in fact, it is an oocyst, it must be determined to be of a species known to cause disease in the host in question. If other phases of the life cycle of the coccidia can be seen in the feces, such as merozoites, trophozoites, or gametocytes, there is probable active disease present since such forms could come only from sloughed mucosal tissue.[129]

Necropsy Findings. Typically, there is a catarrhal enteritis with varying degrees of mucosal hemorrhage and sloughing, seen most prominently in terminal ileum and proximal colon. There may be clots of whole blood within the intestinal lumen. Tissues are often very pale due to the blood-loss anemia. Various stages of the life cycle of the organism can be found in smears of infected intestinal mucosa.

Therapy

Most of the sulfa preparations given orally in therapeutic doses will markedly reduce oocyte excretion in the feces and cause an amelioration of the signs. This class of drugs is used most frequently in domestic animals. Amprolium has been used extensively in poultry with good success, and has been cleared for use in food-producing animals. Clinicians' experience concerning which sulfa works best seems to vary; some find sulfamethazine is satisfactory while others like sulfaquinoxaline. In severely dehydrated patients, the nonabsorbable varieties may be preferred to avoid possible secondary renal problems. The mechanisms by which sulfas inhibit coccidia is not known.

Intravenous, subcutaneous, or oral fluid therapy is indicated for those very dehydrated animals in order to speed their recovery.

Prophylaxis

If the premises are kept clean, of fecal material in particular, and animals are not too densely housed, coccidiosis should not be a problem.

Cryptosporidiosis in Calves

Cryptosporidium is a small coccidioid that has traditionally been incidentally found in mice (*C. muris*), rabbits and chickens (*C. parvum*) and foxes (*C. vulpis*) where no signs of intestinal disease are present.

Recently cryptosporidia have been found in young calves that have diarrhea.[130,131] The disease is not fulminant but is persistent. Enteric infections with cryptosporidia in neonatal calves with diarrhea is common throughout North America.[131] It remains to be demonstrated whether cryptosporidia have a pathogenic or commensal role in small bowel disease of calves.

A thorough cleaning of the pens in which affected calves are kept and an effort to keep fecally contaminated bedding from piling up stop the disease from occurring.

Ascariasis in Puppies

Epidemiology

Pregnant bitches have the unfortunate ability to infect their young with both ascarids (*Toxocara canis*) and hookworms (*Ancylostoma caninum*) in utero.[132] As a result puppies may show signs of parasitosis, with either of these agents or both, by the time they are 2 weeks old. In contrast, ascarid larvae which are ingested by puppies after their birth and reach the intestinal tract via the respiratory system do *not* cause clinically apparent disease within the first month of the host's life. Details of the life cycles can be found in most textbooks of veterinary parasitology and will not be discussed here.

Clinical Signs

An early, and sometimes the only, sign of ascariasis in infant puppies is reduction in growth rate and chronic abdominal distention. Additional compatible signs include vomiting, diarrhea, and excessive crying. Large numbers of adult and immature worms may be seen in the vomitus or feces. Some infected pups develop a peculiar straddle-posture of the hind limbs when standing or walking.

Diagnostic Criteria

The presence of ascarid ova in the feces, along with the clinical signs just described, is as definitive as can be achieved ante mortem.

Therapy

The piperazine-containing preparations, such as a piperazine-HCl, are highly effective against the ascarids within the intestine. Thiabendazole paste fed daily at a dose rate of 150 mg/kg body weight for 5 to 20 days postpartum is also effective in clearing prepatent infection.[133]

Prophylaxis

The basic aim in reducing transplacental infection is to keep the bitch away from surfaces that are, or have been, contaminated with dog feces. The ova of ascarids are extremely resistant to environmental factors and can survive in soil for years. Even when all these precautions are taken, owners should be warned that the bitch may not be free of encysted larvae, which she can transfer during subsequent pregnancies over the next few years.[134]

Finally, pups born of dams known to transfer infection transplacentally should be given piperazine at least 2 times within the first month of life. This is not only to give the pups protection but also to reduce reinfection of the dam by their fecal material.[135]

Hookworm Infection of Puppies and Kittens

Epidemiology

As with ascariasis, the main reason that hookworms can cause a clinically significant parasitosis in infant carnivores is because infected larvae can be transmitted transplacentally and to an even greater degree via the colostrum.[132] *Ancylostoma caninum* is the most common and virulent organism, followed by *A. braziliense* and *Uncinaria stenocephala*. Infective larvae develop optimally where the temperature is moderate, the soil moist but not waterlogged, and sunlight is not continuous or direct. Thus both eggs and larvae are more susceptible to harsh environmental conditions than are those of *Toxocara*.

Since newborn puppies do not develop immunity to hookworms when they are exposed in utero, they are most susceptible to the parasite's ravages. Larvae attained either transplacentally or through colostrum can be patent adults in the intestine within 2 weeks.

Clinical Signs

Ancylostoma caninum is most dangerous to neonatal puppies or kittens because of hematophagy. Sleek, healthy looking animals can lose their condition and weaken in a matter of days owing to blood-loss anemia. They will become sluggish and cry continually. Mucous membranes become very pale. Unless the infection is extremely severe, intestinal secretion, digestion, absorption and motility continue quite normally. Thus, signs of gastrointestinal disturbance in this peracute form are usually minimal and there may be few, if any, hookworm ova in the feces. With slightly less peracute forms, melena, hematochezia, mild diarrhea, and dehydration may be seen. With this form, many ova are usually present in the feces.[134]

A. braziliense and *U. stenocephala* will, if in sufficient numbers, cause a mild indigestion with diarrhea.

Laboratory Findings

Even the finding of one hookworm ovum in the feces of a sick 2- to 3-week-old puppy should alert the clinician to consider this form of parasitosis in the differential diagnosis. If *A. caninum* is involved, normocytic normochromic anemia will prevail in the CBC. With *A. braziliense* or *U. stenocephala*, hypoproteinemia will be more prominent than anemia.

Therapy

With the peracute form of ancylostomosis, treatment of any kind may be to no avail. Blood transfusions and direct anthelmintic therapy are essential components of initial therapy. An orally administered anthelmintic such as dichlorvos or mebendazole is preferred, if the pup can retain it, over parenteral disophenol, since it will be brought into contact with the parasite sooner.[136] Transfusions may need to be repeated until the pup's hematocrit stabilizes above 20%. Since these animals are usually hypothermic, warmth in the form of heating pads or infrared lamps is indicated.

Pups with the less peracute form of the disease may also need a transfusion. The clinician will decide this after examining the color of the mucous membranes and the hematocrit. The amount of additional fluid therapy including electrolytes, vitamins, and nutrients will also depend upon the clinician's evaluation of the patient. All affected pups will need some following supportive care of this kind.

Prophylaxis

Prophylactic measures must be directed at destruction of infective larvae, and reduction of environmental contamination. These measures are directed at stopping reinfection of the dam.

Destruction of the larvae can be affected by spreading sodium borate (10 lb/100 sq ft) over gravel or loam surfaced runs.[137] More impervious surfaces such as concrete, steel, or tile should be washed thoroughly and sprayed with dilute sodium hypochlorite.[134]

Destruction of larvae is of short-term benefit unless measures are also taken to reduce recontamination. Resident adult bitches should be routinely treated with appropriate anthelmintics until no ova can be found in 3 to 4 serial fecal samples examined a few weeks apart.[136] If possible, housing of animals should be modified to reduce crowding. Ideally, soil or gravel bottom runs that have been used for many years should be dug out and replaced with new soil or concrete.

Part II. Small Intestinal Disease in Other Than Neonates

This section will deal with small intestinal diseases in other than neonates. The general plan is to categorize disease entities on the basis of possible presenting history and clinical signs. This most closely complies with the way in which a case is worked up; i.e., the clinician is first presented with the general complaint and makes some observations during the initial physical examination. At this point he constructs a broad list of rule-outs (differential diagnoses) which is gradually narrowed as particulars regarding history, results of laboratory tests and special examinations, and daily observation of clinical progression are collected.

The lists of compatible history and clinical signs that head each major subsection of this section are intended to aid the clinician in making the initial general categorization. *It must be emphasized* that it is virtually impossible to find a patient whose features of disease will match any given list completely. In fact, many of the same items appear in a number of subsection lists. The point is, if facts regarding the patient are consistent with 40 to 50% of the items on a given list, that group of diseases in that subsection must be considered in the initial broad group of differential diagnoses.

Details concerning diseases included within a subdivision are discussed according to a more traditional format. Species peculiarities will be emphasized where necessary; if these are not mentioned, assume the discussion is referring to all species. Some diseases are unique to a given species and this will be clearly pointed out. When discussing diseases that affect *all* animals, pertinent comparative information will be presented in the following species order: horse, cow, sheep, goat, pig, dog, cat. Accordingly, species-specific diseases within a subsection category (e.g., "Infections") will be discussed after those that affect all animals, and in the same species order.

ACUTE (FULMINATING) ENTERITIDES

History and Signs Compatible

1. Fever
2. Explosive Fluid Diarrhea (Dysentery)
   —may contain frank blood
   —may contain shreds of mucosa
3. Tenesmus during defecation
4. Colic
5. Vomiting
6. Hyperemic mucous membranes
7. Increased borborygmi
8. Mild to severe dehydration.

Bacterial Infections

Bacterial infections of the gastrointestinal tract which cause dysentery are due to invasive organisms which penetrate and eventually destroy mucosal cells. The local reaction is classic inflammation with erythema, edema, and neutrophil infiltration. Malabsorption and leakage of plasma or blood components can occur at the site of infiltration, the degree dependent upon the amount of damage. Often both large and small intestines are involved and many of the signs may be more related to colonic than small intestinal dysfunction. At present, recognized enteric bacterial pathogens in animals are few. With further sophistication of bacteriologic techniques, more organisms will no doubt be implicated.

Salmonellosis

Salmonellosis has been discussed in the first section of this chapter. Only the highlights of the epidemiology, clinical signs, therapy, and prophylaxis as they relate to older animals will be reviewed here. Salmonellosis in horses is discussed with large bowel problems in Chapter 24.

Epidemiology. In adult domestic animals *S. typhimurium*, *S. dublin*, and *S. enteritidis* are the serotypes commonly cultured where outbreaks occur. It is most important to remember that humans are also susceptible. The insidious aspect of salmonellosis is that asymptomatic carrier states exist and are probably responsible for many outbreaks. Fecal culturing to detect carriers is often futile since the organisms may not be shed until the carrier is exposed to a stressful event, at which time the animal may or may not show signs of infection. It is estimated that a normal healthy human must ingest in excess of 100,000 organisms to become sick,[13] with proportionately less being necessary if the patient's resistance has been lowered by oral antibiotics,[59] some illness, or other stressful event.[56,64,65] Minimal infective doses have not been established for all domestic animals. In one study in calves, the LD_{50} was 100,000 organisms.[138] In healthy swine, 10^8 organisms may be necessary to cause disease.[64]

Faulty management practices, most especially improper disposal of fecal material, and failure to provide proper isolation for animals with signs suggestive of infectious enteritis, are responsible for many cases of salmonellosis. Infected feedstuffs, especially those of animal origin such as bone meal, may be implicated as the source of an outbreak.[62,139]

Rodents and bats must be considered as potential vectors for salmonellae.[64] Up to 8% of rats caught on a dairy farm in England where an outbreak of *S. dublin* infection had recently occurred were found to be shedding the same serotype in their feces.[57]

Because of their close contact with humans, special attention should be given to salmonella infection in dogs. It has been estimated that up to 15% of the canine population in the United States may be carriers, with even higher percentages in younger dogs.[64] Dogs may also harbor and shed more than one serotype at a time. As carriers and fecal shedders, dogs and pigs may well be the most notorious.

Finally, human-to-animal transmission should not be overlooked. There are documented incidents of infections in farm animals from human carriers.[57,140]

Clinical Signs. *Horses.* Salmonellosis in horses is discussed with large bowel problems in Chapter 24.

Cattle. Diarrhea, dysentery, severe hematochezia, colic, and tenesmus are common clinical features of acute salmonellosis in cattle. Clots of whole blood may be voided in feces. Sloughing of the bowel mucosa also occurs and is associated with mild abdominal pain.[67,141] Variable anorexia and weakness, even recumbency, which is responsive to calcium injection, can occur.[142] There is a fever of 105 to 106° C, but the surface of the body is cold.[143] Abortion may follow the diarrhea, especially if *S. dublin* is present.[144]

In spite of fever and depression as well as the preceding signs, the rumen usually continues to move quite normally and appetite remains fair. Pregnant animals may abort. As with horses, a few cows with severe salmonellosis die within a few days, most recover within 7 to 14 days, and a few continue with less severe signs of intermittent fever and diarrhea, and progressive weight loss for many months.[60]

All cattle that have recovered clinically from a salmonella infection should be considered carriers whether the organism can be cultured from the feces or not. Some studies done in England suggest that carriers may spread the infection transplacentally or through the colostrum to their young.[65]

Swine. Occasionally pigs may die of sepsis before much diarrhea is seen and salmonellosis must be distinguished from vitamin E-selenium deficiency or bacterial endocarditis which can also cause sudden death in pigs. A chronic enterocolitis with diarrhea and wasting is more common in swine over 1 month of age than is the acute fulminating disease. This condition is covered in more detail under Chronic Enteritides or Neoplasia.

Dogs. Along with the usual fever and dysentery, dogs with salmonellosis may also show signs of upper respiratory disease, incoordination, partial posterior paralysis, blindness, or other neurologic disturbance such as running fits or persistent barking.[145,146] Abortions or persistent vaginal discharge may also occur. The finding of small punctate erosions or ulcers in the colon mucosa upon colonoscopic examination is consistent with the diagnosis, but these lesions can also be seen with other causes of colitis.

Salmonella organisms may be cultured from many organs other than the intestines of infected dogs.[147]

Laboratory Findings. Initial neutropenia followed by neutrophilia and leukocytosis, hypoalbuminemia, and hyponatremia are all consistent with acute salmonellosis. The definitive diagnosis is contingent upon culture of salmonella organisms from the feces, however. A single negative fecal culture is meaningless; at least three cultures from feces collected at 48-hour intervals should be made. Preferably the animal should not be given antibiotic during this time, certainly not oral antibiotic, but this depends upon the clinician's judgment of the severity of sepsis. Collect feces from the rectum whenever possible; avoid depending upon rectal swabs. If after three or more cultures the organism is still not isolated from the feces but the clinical signs and other laboratory data are consistent with salmonellosis, persistent diagnostic effort is encouraged.

Necropsy Findings. Salmonella infection causes a severe enterocolitis. Grossly, the mucosa is thickened and may be covered with a layer of serosanguineous fluid or fibrin. Sometimes frank clots of blood are found within the lumen. Upon close examination, the affected mucosa has a greyish granular appearance with what look like small pustules within the inflamed mucosal tissue.

Histologically, affected small intestine has marked disruption of the villous pattern, discontinuities along the mucosa through which red and white cells are exuding, and severe polymorphonuclear infiltration of mucosa and submucosa. There is nothing characteristic about a salmonella enteritis that is definitively pathognomonic, however.

Therapy. There is considerable controversy concerning whether antibiotics should be used in the treatment of acute salmonellosis. There is evidence that oral antibiotic therapy in humans induces a more persistent carrier state.[29,148,149] Other studies in experimental animals have shown that disruption of

page 487

nonabsorbable antibiotics means that fewer salmonella organisms are needed to cause disease.[59] These observations suggest that orally administered nonabsorbable antibacterial drugs should be avoided.

If there is clinical or laboratory evidence of septicemia, parenteral antibiotic is definitely indicated. Unfortunately the most expensive drugs, such as chloramphenicol, ampicillin, and gentamicin are the most effective, but may be cost-prohibitive when dealing with large animals. In food animals, the choice is restricted to ampicillin in the United States because of FDA regulations. If septicemia is not a problem, avoid using antibiotic altogether.

A combination of oral and intravenous fluid therapy may be necessary to support animals with salmonellosis through the acute stages of the disease. Oral electrolyte solutions should be offered on a *free choice* basis and not force-fed (Table 23–8). Fresh water should always be available as well. If fluid ingestion provokes vomiting, the intravenous route may have to be used exclusively.

The intravenous fluid of choice is an isotonic multielectrolyte replacement solution that contains bicarbonate precursors. Unless an animal is tending toward a shock state, it is not necessary to add extra bicarbonate to this solution or to infuse large

Table 23–8. Oral electrolyte replacement solutions for adult cattle or horses with severe diarrhea (should be provided on a free choice basis along with fresh water sources)

A. *For Cattle*
    2 oz (60 g) NaCl
    1 oz (30 g) KCl or KHCO$_3$
    q.s. 5 gallons (20 L) fresh water

B. *For Horses*
  1. Make up a supply of powder containing the following proportions of electrolytes
    NaCl 4 oz (117 g)
    KCl 5 oz (150 g)
    NaHCO$_3$ 5.5 oz (168 g)
    K$_2$HPO$_4$ 4.5 oz (135 g)
  2. Add 3 oz (90 g) of above mixture to 12 qt (12 L) pail of fresh water.

amounts of NaHCO$_3$. In fact, doing so may provoke a state of metabolic alkalosis.

It has been the testimonial clinical experience of some veterinarians, including the author, that orally administered activated charcoal has reduced both the severity and duration of signs. The rationale is that toxic substances, including any salmonella toxins, in the gut lumen are absorbed and thus deactivated. This therapy would be most indicated in non-ruminants and in monogastrics where orally applied medication does not induce vomiting. For dogs, charcoal pills are available.

Prophylaxis. In situations where salmonellosis occurs, effective sanitary measures and consideration of immunization procedures are in order. This is particularly true of outbreaks in groups of food-producing animals where individual animal therapy is often uneconomical and not in the public interest, and in any situation where neonates are involved. The specific procedures have been discussed in Part I of this chapter.

Invasive Escherichia coli

It has become clear over the last few years that there are strains of *E. coli* that are invasive and cause clinical signs that are difficult to distinguish from salmonellosis—namely fever, dysentery, abdominal pain, and sometimes vomiting. This is one of the causes of "traveler's diarrhea" in humans.[18] In domestic animals, it has only been documented to date in dogs,[150] and even in this report invasive properties of the organism were not substantiated. Therefore, veterinary experience with invasive *E. coli* is extremely limited, perhaps in part because techniques for making positive diagnoses are not known.

Suffice to say, if an outbreak of enteritis occurs in which all attempts to isolate salmonella, from either feces or autopsy material, fail, one should consider invasive *E. coli.* Documentation of invasiveness is by injection of approximately 10^8 organisms into the conjunctival sac of adult guinea pigs;[18,25] if the organism is invasive, a keratoconjunctivitis will result.

As with salmonellosis, antibiotic therapy may be indicated for treating individual animals that have signs of bacteremia but, in general, invasive coliform infection is a management problem where the usual principles of sanitation and isolation apply.

Yersiniosis

Yersinia (Pasteurella) *enterocolitica* is being found with greater frequency worldwide as a cause of enteritis in humans[151] and dogs.[152] Initially, signs are similar to salmonellosis, but the disease is not easily diagnosed or controlled and commonly becomes chronic,[151,153] where signs and pathology resemble those of other chronic inflammatory bowel disease (see Chronic Enteritides or Neoplasia).

"Winter Dysentery" in Cattle (WD)

Epidemiology. Traditionally, winter dysentery in cattle and a specific dysentery syndrome in swine were regarded as infections by *Vibrio jejuni* and *Vibrio coli,* respectively. It is now clear that the inciting cause of either disease is *not a Vibrio.*[154] A spirochete interacting with some normal gut flora is the probable cause of the porcine disease; the cause of winter dysentery remains to be elucidated.

True to its name, the greatest incidence of winter dysentery is in adult dairy cattle during the winter months (November 30–April 1) when the animals are usually more confined. There is an explosive herd outbreak of acute projectile diarrhea. Many cows will have a cough. Animals in early lactation seem to be most susceptible but the disease spreads rapidly to affect virtually all of the adults. Young stock may show mild signs. The disease is transient and feces usually return to normal in 5 to 7 days. Infected cows are immune for about 6 months after an attack, but the usual cycle of the disease through a given herd is 2 to 3 years. The incidence of this disease seems to be declining in regions where loose housing and milking parlors have replaced the stanchion barn.[155] The explanation for this is not clear.

Clinical Signs. The outstanding clinical signs are the projectile defecation of copious amounts of dark, fluid feces. The consistency of the fecal material is quite uniform although some very small shreds of epithelial tissue may be seen. There is no gross hematochezia. Affected animals often have signs of a mild upper respiratory disease, and the coughing that results often exacerbates the projectile character of the defecation.

Fever up to 103 to 104° F accompanied by mild depression and anorexia precedes the outbreak of diarrhea. Once the signs of enteritis are apparent, the animal's temperature and appetite are usually normal. Milk production is not markedly affected.[155] Mortality is uncommon.

Laboratory Findings. Many vibrios are seen in a fresh smear of fecal material. Otherwise, there are no indicative laboratory findings.

Therapy. A therapeutic procedure that will do most to hasten recovery of normal hydration and milk production is to provide free choice electrolyte water (see Table 23–8A). This can be made up in bulk in a container in the exercise yard or some other convenient spot. Make sure fresh water is also available at all times.

Prophylaxis. A specific immunizing product is not available. Some protection may be afforded by controlling traffic of both humans and animals onto the farm premises known to be infected. Once the disease is established, however, virtually nothing can be done to stop its spread.[155]

Viral Infections

In contrast to bacteria, viruses that cause lesions in the intestinal tract seem to have an affinity for certain cell types. Damage to those cells leads to a cascade of secondary effects that result in more complex dysfunction involving the resident enteric bacterial flora. The equine arteritis virus, for instance, damages only the small vessels within the submucosa, and any mucosal damage (it is usually minimal) is due to resultant circulatory dysfunction.[156] Feline panleukopenia virus, however, has a predilection for mucosal crypt cells which eventually causes villous atrophy and breakdown of the intestinal mucosal barrier because a generation of mature absorptive cells has been destroyed at its source in the crypts.[157] With the mucosal barrier broken, the enteric bacteria can penetrate into the submucosa and cause inflammation. Bovine virus diarrhea (BVD) virus preferentially invades lymphoid tissue within the intestinal wall as well as the vessels in the submucosa. Less frequently, BVD virus destroys mucosal tissue directly having, as does panleukopenia, a predilection for crypt cells.[158]

As suggested here and in the discussions of neonatal viral-induced enteropathies, contributions to the severity and duration of disease by the resident enteric bacterial flora need to be understood more fully. For example, the enteric component of panleukopenia in a germ-free cat is a fairly mild disorder, but a serious problem in conventionally raised cats.[159]

There is no one virus that, like salmonella, causes enteritis in all species of domestic animals. Diseases discussed here will be for the most part species-specified.

Equine Viral Arteritis (EVA)

Epidemiology. EVA is infrequent in its occurrence but has a worldwide distribution.[160] Method of transmission is most likely through animal to animal contact. Mortality is low but abortions can cause severe economic damage on a breeding farm.

Clinical Signs. The classic signs of this disease, high fever, severe depression, ventral edema, keratitis, petechial hemorrhages in the mucous membranes, and dyspnea should help distinguish EVA from other causes of acute equine diarrhea.

Laboratory Findings. A definitive diagnosis may be made by culture of the virus from the patient and the demonstration of a rising antibody titer in the serum.

Necropsy Findings. Equine viral arteritis virus can cause submucosal vascular damage within all portions of the small and large intestinal tract as part of its endotheliotropism. Lesions in the small intestine tend to be segmental, causing some patchy necrosis; lesions in the large intestine are much more severe and are probably responsible for the diarrhea that is seen in some cases of EVA.[156]

Therapy. Treatment of EVA is primarily supportive in nature. Antipyretic analgesics may be given to lower the fever and provide some general relief. Replacement-type intravenous fluids should be given if the animal cannot keep itself hydrated properly through drinking. Corticosteroids may be given in large doses (e.g., 400 to 500 mg hydrocortisone acetate q.i.d.) only if the horse appears to be going into shock. If the case is mild, corticosteroids ought not to be used.

Prophylaxis. At present, an immunization product against EVA is not commercially available.

Bovine Virus Diarrhea (BVD)

Epidemiology. Much has been written about mucosal disease since BVD was first described by Olafson et al. in 1946. Its character within the United States has changed since then from a disease of high morbidity and low mortality to one with lower clinical incidence within a given herd, but higher mortality in clinically affected animals. With increased shipping of cattle throughout North America the virus has become widespread and many animals have serologic evidence of exposure without a history of clinical disease. It is conceivable then that exposed dams can passively immunize their calves which, as their passive immunity wears off, may contract a mild form of the disease that leaves them, in time, actively immune (preimmunized).[161] Animals that do become ill, then, may represent the highly susceptible, previously unexposed few that are open to the worst ravages of the infection.

Stock auction facilities and dealer trucks are notorious for harboring BVD virus. Another important source of infection is fecally contaminated clothing and boots, including those of veterinarians. Once established within a herd, the virus can be spread by contaminated feeding and bedding equipment as well as clothing. One to three weeks after the introduction of the BVD virus into a susceptible herd, all cows may show signs of infection within a period of a few days. In experimentally produced disease, however, the incubation period generally is 7 to 10 days.[158]

Clinical Signs. Classic signs of BVD are rapid onset of depression, high fever, fluid diarrhea that may contain flecks of blood or mucus, agalactia and mucopurulent nasal discharge. Signs of pneumonia, with cough and fever, may predominate over the gastrointestinal signs, especially in beef herds and in feedlot cattle. The development, within a day or two, of erosions in the buccal mucosa, including under the tongue, and a marked leukopenia is virtually diagnostic. Pregnant cows often abort. If the rectal temperature is monitored daily and the affected animal lives long enough, one may see a drop in temperature to near normal 3 to 4 days after the onset of signs, followed by a second fever spike at 7 to 8 days into the course of the disease.

In the field, infected animals will show varying degrees of the signs just described. Some will deteriorate and die within a few days in spite of vigorous therapeutic measures. Others will look as though they are going to die imminently but linger on, rapidly losing condition and value. Still others will gradually become normal within 7 to 10 days. There seems to be no good correlation between the extent and severity of buccal lesions and clinical course; in fact some of the sickest cows may have no oral erosions whatever.

Laboratory Findings. Severe leukopenia is the most outstanding feature of this disease. While total lymphocyte and granulocyte counts are both reduced, it is the granulocytopenia that is particularly severe. This blood count pattern differs from the leukopenia seen with salmonellosis in that the total count with BVD often bottoms out at a much lower level (sometimes to <1500 WBC/cu mm) and there is no left shift on the neutrophil series.

Both virus isolation and serology may be used to document the presence of BVD.[162,163] Fecal material and nasal swabs, plus intestinal contents from freshly deceased animals, are best to collect for virus isolation. These materials should be frozen unless they can be transferred to the laboratory immediately.

Measurement of antibody titers in the serum is only helpful if acute and convalescent sera, collected 2 weeks apart, can be compared. A rise in titer is highly suggestive that the animal in question was recently exposed to mucosal disease virus. This information must be consistent with clinical signs or necropsy findings to make the diagnosis definitive, however.

Necropsy Findings. Mucosal erosions and ulcers of varying size, number, and distribution from mouth through ileum are characteristic. The upper gastrointestinal tract seems more susceptible to mucosal damage than the lower ileum. Oral lesions tend to be quite punctate; those in the esophagus and abdomen are often linear. Gross lesions in the small intestine are most prominent in and around the Peyer's patches. Histologically, in the small intestine one may see vasculitis in the submucosa, necrosis of lymph nodules in Peyer's patches, and epithelial cell damage secondary to crypt cell necrosis.[87]

Therapy. Supportive therapy to help affected cows maintain fluid and electrolyte balance is indicated. Individual animals whose worth warrants it can be given replacement-type solutions intravenously. Electrolyte solution (Table 23–8A) should be made available for free-choice drinking. Some very sick animals may not drink and require force-fed fluids through a stomach tube. A 500-kg cow that is not milking and has normal feces requires at least 16 liters of fluid per day for maintenance. This should be a baseline figure, supplemented according to observations of degree of dehydration, milk production, and excessive fluid losses.

If cows are anorectic for more than a few days, special attention should be given to their rumen contents. These may be examined by aspiration through the stomach tube. In my experience, alfalfa meal and Brewer's yeast (Table 23–9) mixed into the fluid being given by stomach tube provide at least some substrate for the ruminal flora.

Prophylaxis. Modified-live-virus (MLV) vaccines are commercially available to provide immunity against BVD. These vaccines are quite safe and very effective when given to healthy, non-stressed, non-pregnant animals. Pregnant animals should not be immunized because the vaccine can induce congenital defects and abortion.[164,165] Cattle arriving at a feedlot should only be vaccinated immediately if there is active disease on the premises. Otherwise, they should be allowed to adapt for 3 to 4 weeks and then immunized.[166] Alternatively, if it is known that beef cattle are going to be moved to a fattening area where mucosal disease is endemic, the BVD vaccine may be included in the preconditioning program.

The question always arises—what is the optimal time to vaccinate calves born from dams known to be immune to BVD? A guideline nomogram, based upon the dam's titer, is not available for BVD as it is for distemper in dogs. It is best to wait until there is little chance that even the calf that received a very high dose of antibody in the colostrum has enough passive protection to block the active response, e.g., about 3½ to 4 months of age.[161]

In the final analysis, however, if it is at all possible to avoid using an immunizing product for BVD, do so.

Bovine Malignant Catarrh (BMC)

Epidemiology. This is an uncommon disease of cattle in North America, although herd outbreaks have been recorded here.[167,168] It has been seen worldwide, with perhaps the highest incidence being in Africa in wild ruminants. It is caused by a herpes virus which, among domestic animals, is thought to be harbored as an inapparent infection in sheep and goats.[169] Thus, there is a higher occurrence of BMC in cattle that are housed in close association with sheep, although this is not an exclusive situation.

Clinical Signs. Clinically, the major features of BMC that distinguish it from BVD are the rapid onset of marked upper respiratory and ocular disease[170] (Table 23–10). Erosions of the nasal mucosa, profuse mucopurulent nasal discharge, and stertorous breathing with marked dyspnea are characteristic. Signs of ophthalmia are seen and include severe mucopurulent ocular discharge, conjunctivitis, and blepharospasm, with eventual corneal opacity, hypopyon, and blindness. As the disease progresses, necrosis and sloughing of skin, especially on the teats, at skin-horn junctions, and in axilla and perineum occur. Terminal signs of encephalitis develop in 1 to 2 weeks. The disease is ultimately fatal; attempts to treat it are useless.

Necropsy Findings. Practically all tissues within the body have some lesions. Those in the small intestine are grossly similar to those seen with BVD. Histologically, perivascular cuffing by mononuclear cells is supposed to be quite pathognomonic.[171]

Table 23–9. Practical substrate for force-feeding anorectic cows

---

—500 g alfalfa meal
—500 g Brewer's yeast
—q.s. 20 L warm water
—If rumen moving well, add 30–60 ml propylene glycol

Feed twice a day via large-bore stomach tube.

Table 23-10. Differentiating clinical features of Bovine Virus Diarrhea (BVD), malignant catarrh (BMC), and rinderpest (R)

	Location	Dysentery	Respiratory Disease	Ocular Disease	CNS Disturbance	Skin Disease	Course	Other
BVD	Worldwide	Common	Nasal discharge Pneumonia	Very rare	Very rare	Laminitis with chronic disease	4-15 days for acute disease	When morbidity is high, mortality is low and vice versa.
BMC	Worldwide, highest in Africa	Usually	Profuse nasal discharge Lungs normal	Blepharospasm Uveitis Blindness	Tremor Incoordination Dementia	Teats Axilla Horn base	7-10 days; invariably fatal	Usually very low morbidity. Slow spread Associated with sheep
R	Mainly in Africa and Asia	Sometimes	Nasal discharge Pneumonia	Lacrimation Blepharospasm	No	Perineum Axilla Groin	6-12 days; often fatal	Rapid spread No forestomach lesions

Rinderpest

Rinderpest is a myxoviral disease of cattle and swine that occurs with greatest frequency in Africa and parts of Asia. Rare, quickly controlled outbreaks have also occurred in eastern Europe, South America and Australia. Rinderpest differs epizootically from BVD and BMC in that it spreads very rapidly throughout virtually 100% of a specific population of animals and causes high rates of mortality. (Table 23-10)

Clinical signs and laboratory findings in cattle are quite similar to those of BVD and BMC.

Necropsy reveals mucosal ulcerations of various size in the esophagus, abomasum, and small and large intestines. Histologically, marked destruction of lymphoid tissue within the intestine and in discrete nodes elsewhere is seen.

Control measures, particularly in areas where the disease is not endemic, include restricting movement of animals and fresh animal products into and out of the area. Susceptible animals within the contact area must be slaughtered whether they show signs or not. The usual strict sanitation and disinfection procedures must be applied to all affected areas.

Various attenuated vaccines against rinderpest are also available, the best of which is produced from antigen grown in tissue culture.[172] In areas that are not normally endemic, the vaccine should be used only if it appears that sanitation and slaughter procedures are ineffective, since it is undesirable to seed any environment with even an attenuated rinderpest virus.

Bluetongue in Cattle and Sheep (BT)

Epidemiology. Bluetongue (BT) is a viral disease of domestic and wild ruminants that is naturally transmitted via the flying arthropod Culicoides (sand fly). Within the domestic species, the incidence of BT is greatest in sheep; it can be seen occasionally in cattle. The disease is probably African in its origin, being first formally described in South Africa in 1880.[173] First published accounts of BT within the United States appeared in the early 1950s,[174,175] and it is still seen sporadically. It is most prevalent in southwestern and western states in late summer and early fall when vector populations are highest.

There are a number of distinct antigenic forms of the virus that apparently differ in virulence,[173] thus explaining why the disease in one locality may be less debilitating to the animals than that in another locality. Infection by one form does not confer immunity against the other forms. In sheep, immunity against any given form is short-lived (about 2 months) and it is virtually nonexistent in cattle.

Clinical Signs. Bluetongue in cattle is usually rather mild, but death loss is by no means rare. The disease will, in its severest form, cause some edema and erosions of the mouth parts with accompanying salivation and inappetence, stiffness of gait with possible laminitis, and abortion. Teat lesions in lactating beef cows may cause weaning of calves because the cows refuse to allow them to nurse.

In sheep, the clinical signs of BT range from mild disease as described previously for cattle to severe mucosal-like disease with high fever, oral erosions, salivation, diarrhea, anorexia, and hyperpnea. In later stages coronitis and myositis with severe lameness, loss of fleece, and marked deterioration of body condition will occur.[173,174] Mortality is usually low within a flock, though lambs will die in greater numbers than adults. After 10 to 15 days, animals will begin to show signs of recovery but they are often in such debilitated physical condition that it is not economical to keep them.

As seen in cattle infected with mucosal disease, both pregnant ewes and cows surviving infection with BT may deliver offspring that are hydrocephalic or have other brain abnormalities.[176]

Laboratory Findings. During the well-developed stage of the disease, clinical laboratory findings include leukopenia, which is primarily a lymphopenia. There is also an increase in SGOT and CPK secondary to the myopathy. The virus may be isolated from blood taken when the animal is very febrile and the specific serotype of the organism can be identified by serum-neutralization.[173] Fluorescent antibody and micro-gel diffusion tests have been developed to detect group-specific antibodies but these apparently are not very accurate during the viremic stage of the disease.

Necropsy Findings. Pathologically, gross lesions are seen primarily in the digestive, muscular, and cutaneous systems. The buccal mucosa is edematous, hyperemic, hemorrhagic, and eroded. The tongue may be cyanotic. Patchy hemorrhage, edema and necrosis of the ruminal and abomasal epithelia may be seen. Edema and hemorrhage occur in skeletal and cardiac muscles. Hemorrhagic streaks are found in nonpigmented hooves, with erythema and swelling around the coronet. Also subcutaneous hemorrhages may be seen.

Therapy. Treatment for BT is without effect.

Prophylaxis. The best prophylaxis against BT is control of the *Culicoides.* A vaccine is available but should not be used on pregnant ewes since it can cause congenital deformities in lambs.[177] Immunization should be repeated yearly, but not near breeding time since it will cause anestrus.[173]

Nairobi Sheep Disease (NSD)

Epidemiology. This arthropod-borne infectious viral disease of sheep is seen only in central Africa. The vector is the brown tick, *Rhipicephalus appendiculatus,* which is most active and abundant during the rainy season. Unfed adult ticks may harbor and transmit virulent virus for up to 870 days. No wild host reservoir has been identified.

Clinical Signs. Adult sheep are primarily affected. Early signs are development of a high fever, anorexia, and listlessness. After a few days diarrhea begins. At first the feces are fluid and green but in advanced stages of the disease they may contain much mucus and frank blood. There may also be swelling of the genitalia and abortion. Mortality varies from 30 to 70% and occurs within 4 to 9 days after onset of signs. Indications of impending death are a rapid onset of hypothermia and dyspnea. If diarrhea does not occur, the prognosis is much more favorable.[178]

Laboratory Findings. As with many of the acute viral diseases of ruminants that affect the gastrointestinal tract, leukopenia is a characteristic finding of NSD. Acute and convalescent sera from survivors may also be submitted for measurement of antibody titer by either CF or serum neutralization.[173] This procedure would probably be most helpful in *confirming* the presence of NSD since clinical signs and autopsy findings are quite pathognomonic in their own right.

Necropsy Findings. The combination of the presence of brown ticks in the fleece, swollen genitalia, and fecally soiled perineal region are highly suggestive of NSD. Petechial and ecchymotic hemorrhages can be seen throughout the gastrointestinal tract from the abomasum through the colon, being most concentrated around the ileocecal valve. Peyer's patches are swollen. Mesenteric lymphadenopathy and splenomegaly are often present.[173]

Therapy. There is no specific treatment for Nairobi sheep disease.

Prophylaxis. Reducing infestations by the brown tick is the aim, usually through periodic dipping. An MLV vaccine is also available which should be given yearly prior to the onset of the rainy season.

Coronavirus in Pigs and Dogs

Adult pigs and dogs[179,180] are susceptible to coronavirus (TGE) infection. The outstanding clinical signs are vomiting and diarrhea. The vomiting usually appears early in the course of the disease while diarrhea can last for 4 to 5 days. As mentioned in Part I, the adults are never as severely affected as the young animals, but the morbidity is high in all ages.

There is also an account of the isolation of a coronavirus-like agent from the feces of adult cattle with diarrhea.[181] More work needs to be done to substantiate the validity of clinically apparent infection in adult cows, but there is no reason to doubt its potentiality.

Clinical laboratory findings, pathology and supportive therapy are discussed in Part I under "Coronavirus Infection."

Parvovirus Enteritis of Dogs

A highly contagious diarrheal disease of dogs, similar in some clinical characteristics to canine coronaviral gastroenteritis (see Table 23–10A) has been associated with a very small (about 20 nM) parvo-like virus.[181a,181b] The spectrum of gut crypt epithelial necrosis and lymphoid necrosis in dogs closely resembles that which occurs in parvovirus infection of cats (feline panleukopenia, q.v.). Treatment is as described for panleukopenia. Myocarditis has been reported as a cause of sudden death in young dogs infected with parvovirus, but without diarrhea.[181c]

Table 23–10A. Clinical, Epidemiologic, and Pathologic Findings in Coronavirus and Parvovirus-infected Dogs. (Data from Appel et al.[181a] and Cooper et al.[181b])

Characteristics	Coronavirus	Parvovirus
Diarrhea	Yellow-orange, fetid, ± blood	Yellow-gray to hemorrhagic
Vomiting	Yes	Severe, protracted
Fever	Not usually	Yes
Dehydration	Severe	Severe
Anorexia	Yes	Yes
Age	All ages	All ages
Morbidity	High in kennels	High in kennels
Mortality (pups)	Low	High
Mortality (adults)	Low	Low
Leukopenia	No	Severe
Intestinal loops	Dilated, fluid-filled	Pale, turgid to severely congested
Villi	Atrophy, fusion	Epithelium attenuated
Enterocyte necrosis	No	Yes, notably in crypts
Lymphoid necrosis	No	Often present
Diagnosis	EM (feces)	EM (feces), IF(FPL), histopath

Feline Panleukopenia

Diarrhea may be a component of this viral disease which, like canine distemper, is multisystemic. Here, in contrast to canine distemper, however, the diagnosis is more easily made by the finding of leukopenia and the cause of the small intestinal dysfunction is much clearer. As stated earlier, panleukopenia virus has a predilection for rapidly proliferating cells, including the crypt cells in the small intestinal mucosa.[182] The direct result of crypt cell destruction is villous atrophy when that generation of cells is due to be mature. In fact, then, the diarrhea of panleukopenia is a malabsorptive-type diarrhea that contains excessive amounts of undigested nutrients, similar to TGE in swine. The loss of fluids from the body, through an osmotic drag of water into the gut lumen, and probably by some leakage across a disrupted mucosa, can be great enough to cause severe dehydration and electrolyte imbalance.

Cats with panleukopenia can be saved by the vigorous application of fluid therapy, including whole blood transfusions.[183] Particular attention should be paid to serum sodium concentrations. Since there is a strong osmotic component to the pathogenesis of the diarrhea, there may be a preferential water loss from the plasma. This would result in hypernatremia and in such a situation a potentially hypotonic solution, such as 0.45% NaCl/2.5% dextrose, given intravenously, might be more appropriate than an isotonic preparation. Parenteral broad spectrum antibiotic is also indicated since these animals are immunosuppressed. Feeding by gavage is not usually helpful since it abets the osmotic diarrhea and may stimulate vomiting. The older the cat, the better the prognosis.

A dog presenting with varying degrees of multisystemic disease, particularly in respiratory, gastrointestinal, and nervous system, plus a persistent fever, should be suspected of having distemper. The feces can be very fluid and flecked with mucus or fresh blood. The acute gastrointestinal signs, often including vomiting, are likely to precede the nervous system manifestations by days or even weeks.

Mycotic Infections

Epidemiology. Small intestinal mycoses in domestic animals are rare. They are most often associated with prolonged antibiotic and/or corticosteroid therapy where the normal microfloral environment of the intestine and the host's natural defenses have been severely disrupted. This is particularly applicable to the omnivores and carnivores, pigs, dogs and cats, and to young ruminants. In adult ruminants, excessive antibiotic therapy more often causes ruminal rather than intestinal mycosis.[184] In either the intestinal or ruminal disease, *Candida albicans* is the most commonly found infective agent. Various phycomycetes and Aspergillus can also cause acute gastrointestinal disease.[185,186] Another important source of intestinal mycosis is a mycotic infection elsewhere in the body, such as the skin, the guttural pouches of horses, or the mammary gland of cattle.

Clinical Signs. Systemic mycoses often involve many organ systems simultaneously, including the brain, and the animal may die without showing signs of gastrointestinal disease even though lesions are present there.[187] This has been my experience with certain equine and bovine cases.

On the other hand, mycotic enteritis may be a fulminating disease that causes severe dysentery and/or vomiting.[185,188] It is not easy to make a definitive diagnosis clinically, however, since the signs can be very similar to those of invasive bacterial enteritis.

Laboratory Findings. The persistent presence of moderate to large numbers of fungal elements in the vomitus or feces of a patient with the previously described signs should draw the clinician's attention to the possibility of a fungal gastroenteritis. Yeast bodies in large numbers seen in a Wright's stained fecal smear are also highly indicative. Likewise, culture of Candida or Aspergillus in great numbers from the feces is supportive. Should a Candida infection become septic as well, the organisms may be found in a Wright's stain of the buffy coat of a centrifuged blood sample.[189]

Necropsy Findings. Pathologically, fungi produce ulcerative lesions in the mucosa of the intestinal tract. Histologic sections of these lesions, stained with hematoxylin-eosin or special fungal stains, reveal hyphae or yeast bodies deep within the lesions. A culture of tissue deep (i.e., not exposed to intestinal contents) in such lesions should also be done. For fungal culture of either tissue or feces, a glucose-peptone broth enriched with liver or yeast extract and made selective by addition of antibiotics is recommended over Sabouraud's which lacks growth factors essential to true intestinal yeasts.[190]

Therapy. The best treatment for an animal with fungal gastroenteritis is discontinuation of antibiotic therapy or direct antifungal therapy of a recognized source of infection (e.g., guttural pouch).

In human medicine[191] nystatin has been given orally to suppress intestinal candidiasis if the causative antibiotic therapy must be continued. If the mycotic infection becomes systemic, intravenous amphotericin B is indicated; a dosage schedule recommended for dogs is outlined on page 507.

Parasitic Infections (Infestations)

Of all the diseases that afflict domestic animals, enteric parasitic infestation ought to be the *least*, rather than one of the most, troublesome. Poor sanitation, improper nutrition, and overcrowding are the basic ingredients for promoting intestinal parasitism and are some of the most controllable factors in animal management. In addition, nematodes within the intestine are readily killed by a whole variety of drugs that are, for the most part, not very toxic. Most parasitism flourishes, therefore, because it is human nature to cut corners or regard menaces casually when they are not readily apparent; occasionally it is because of complete ignorance.

Any veterinary practitioner who has dealt with intestinal parasitism for any length of time has the impression that some animals are more susceptible than others. There have been a number of studies of immune mechanisms against intestinal parasites.[192-195] In general, continued low-grade exposure in well-fed, normally stressed animals keeps the resistance high. Anything that upsets the established balance, such as reduced quality of ration, anthelmintic therapy, or poor health, will promote reduction in immunity, especially in young animals. What remains to be discovered in all gastrointestinal nematodes is the antigenic material responsible for inducing the immune response. If this can be accomplished, the next step would be to develop an effective immunizing product.

In order to break the cycle of continued helminthiasis on a property, the life cycle of the parasite in question must be well known. Basically, as has already been suggested, the cycle is broken by a combination of strategies, including anthelmintic therapy applied at a critical point in the life cycle, and improved management practices. The former reduces the number of egg-laying adults and the latter combats and removes ova or infective larvae that are already on the premises. Neither of these will be ultimately successful, however, if nutrition remains poor.

Nematodes

Strongyloidosis. Epidemiology. This is primarily a disease of young animals. Various species are host-specific for certain animals. Adult worms buried in the small intestinal mucosa cause the clinical signs. Eggs laid by the female quickly develop into first stage larvae which when defecated may become sexually mature "free living" adults or infective third stage larvae depending upon environmental conditions. The particularly insidious aspects of this parasite is that certain larvae can migrate somatically and remain dormant in a female animal until she gives birth, whereby the larvae appear in the colostrum.[132] It is postulated that this form of transmission and infection may be much more prevalent in young animals than environmental infection via either ingestion or skin penetration of infective larvae.[196,197]

Pathophysiology. Parasite penetration into the small intestinal mucosa causes epithelial cell damage. Eggs are deposited within the epithelium and are expelled into the intestinal lumen along with tissue debris, whole blood, or plasma protein. When the infestation is severe and great numbers of absorptive cells are destroyed, not only is the mucosal barrier disrupted to allow blood and plasma leakage, but maldigestion and malabsorption of nutrients also occur. The increased speed with which replacement absorptive cells are produced is governed by the degree of damage and this has implications regarding the type of maldigestion that may be seen. Very immature cell replacement in response to severe damage will not only have poor brush border formation, but also cannot produce disaccharidases and dipeptidases which are assembled within the cell and extruded into the glycocalyx where peptide hydrolysis takes place.[198]

Clinical Signs. Signs in all animal species are basically the same—diarrhea that contains varying amounts of frank blood and tissue debris, fever, weakness, depression, pale mucous membranes, vomiting (pigs, dogs, cats), and loss of body condition. At the outset, these signs might be difficult to distinguish from enteritis produced by invasive bacteria.

Laboratory Findings. The presence of ova in the feces, each containing a developed first stage larva, is diagnostic for strongyloidosis, when seen in conjunction with the signs described previously. Fresh feces only should be examined; otherwise the larvae may have hatched and are more difficult to distinguish from the usual fecal debris. As one would expect, anemia and/or hypoproteinemia are consistent features, and their degree should be assessed as a guide to therapy.

Therapy. Thiabendazole given orally at the usual dose rate of 50 mg/kg is very effective.[198,199] If gastrointestinal function is so disrupted that orally administered therapy will be vomited readily, an injectable levamisole preparation should be used.[199] Blood or plasma transfusions may be indicated either to save the life of the animal or to speed recovery in cases where the value of the patient is justified by the prospect of future gain by the client.

Strongylus vulgaris in Young Horses. *Clinical Signs.* Some young, previously unexposed horses which happen to ingest a large number of infective *S. vulgaris* larvae, either from a highly contaminated pasture or by experimental means, may develop clinical signs of diarrhea, colic, fever, depression, and anorexia within a few days.[200–202] Many of these animals will die soon after the preceding signs

appear in spite of anthelmintic and supportive therapy.

Laboratory Findings. Microscopic examination of the feces for ova will not be helpful in these cases since egg-laying adults are not involved. The presence of increased numbers (>5%) of eosinophils in the peritoneal fluid is supportive but not diagnostic while normocytic anemia and peripheral eosinophilia are also supportive.[202]

Necropsy Findings. Severe enteritis in small and large intestine and the presence of large numbers of larvae in the lumen are highly suggestive of this disease.[200] Some mesenteric arteritis may also be seen, but this is not consistent. Histologic examination reveals migrating larvae within the lamina propria and small vessels of the intestinal wall with infiltration of eosinophils and polymorphonuclear leukocytes.[201]

Therapy. Once a diagnosis has been established, usually at necropsy, all the remaining young horses having similar environmental exposure should be treated with so-called "larvicidal" doses of thiabendazole—500 mg/kg per os 2 days in a row.

Prophylaxis. General principles for control of parasite infestation are discussed in Chapter 17. In my opinion, one of the most pertinent studies on control of strongylosis in young horses in particular showed that routine worming of the mare, even as often as every 2 weeks during the early months of lactation, was the most important thing to do.[203]

Nematodirus Infections in 4—10 Week Old Lambs. Young lambs infected with large numbers of larvae of *N. battis* and *N. fillicolis* can develop a rapidly progressive severe diarrhea with dehydration. Animals may die within 2 days of the abrupt onset of signs. The diagnosis is confirmed by finding Nematodirus ova in the feces and by necropsy. It should be remembered that Nematodirus are notoriously poor egg-layers so that necropsy results are more reliable than fecal examination.[86] Principles of parasite control outlined in Chronic Enteritides or Neoplasia should be applied to such problems.

Protozoa

Coccidiosis. *Epidemiology.* Coccidiosis is a worldwide problem, primarily in young animals, although the development of increasingly intensive rearing and feeding programs has increased its incidence in older food-producing animals. All types of domestic animals can be affected with their own particular variety of *Eimeria* or *Isospora* species. The disease is most commonly encountered as a clinical problem in cattle, sheep, and dogs.[129,204-207] Its occurrence is encouraged by persistence of unsanitary environment, though occasionally, even under the best of conditions, it can be a spontaneously recurrent condition, the initiation of which is inexplicable.

With the exception of oocyst sporulations the entire life cycle of a coccidian takes place within the intestinal mucosal cells or adjacent lamina propria.[204] Low grade infections can be tolerated with no clinical signs but severe infections can be devastating, resulting in destruction of large portions of the mucosa.

According to present knowledge, infection with a coccidial agent is solely by ingestion of sporulated oocysts;[129] for all species this means via fecally contaminated feedstuffs and bedding. In addition, carnivora and omnivora may be infected by eating animal tissues that contain the oocysts. Basically, however, it is a product of poor sanitation procedures. How much the stresses of overcrowding, early weaning, or changing to artificial diets contribute to the incidence is still a matter of debate.

Clinical Signs. The outstanding sign of coccidiosis is severe hematochezia, reflecting the mucosal cell destruction. Tenesmus during defecation is a common feature. If this continues for a day or two, the animal may become very anemic and dehydrated, indicated clinically by pale mucous membranes, loss of skin turgor, hypothermia, weakness, and depression.

At this advanced stage, some feedlot cattle will convulse[205] for reasons not understood. Afflicted cattle and sheep are easily recognized by the matting of hair in the perineal region and along the caudal surface of the thighs by bloody, mucoid fecal material. Mortality can reach 50% in a group of untreated feeder animals.

Laboratory Findings. In the typical case, the most outstanding and diagnostic laboratory finding is the overwhelming number of oocysts in the feces. Unfortunately, oocysts are not always present in significant numbers (>5000/g) during the early stages of the disease when the diarrhea is at its worst.[172] Anemia and hypoproteinemia are seen in varying degrees. It is safe to say that both coccidiosis and strongyloidosis cause a much more severe anemia than any of the bacterial or viral enteritides.

Necropsy Findings. The lumen of the intestines may be filled with clotted blood. The mucosa looks alternately inflamed and eroded. Particularly indicative of coccidiosis in cattle is the presence of numerous white spots in the mucosa of the distal ileum formed by the large schizont stage of the life

cycle.[205] Numerous oocysts may be seen upon microscopic examination of mucosal scrapings even though few or none were found in the feces.

Therapy. For years coccidiosis in animals has been treated very successfully with oral sulfa drugs, sulfamethazine being one of the more commonly used in recent times. The mechanism of action against the organism is not understood but the effects are remarkably rapid if treatment is initiated before the animal is terminal. Lately the food animal industry, at the urging of the U.S. F.D.A., has looked for alternative chemotherapeutic agents that are not in the antibacterial class of drugs. An effective alternative passed for use in food-producing animals is the specific coccidiostat, amprolium, given either as a drench or in the drinking water. The recommended dosage schedules for cattle are 10 mg/kg/day for 5 days therapeutically or 5 mg/kg/day for 21 days prophylactically.[207]

Prophylaxis. Immunoprophylaxis against coccidiosis is currently being investigated.[208] The prospects look promising although commercial products for use in mammals are not yet available.

Globidiosis. Globidium is a genus of protozoa that is similar to the coccidians in morphology. The organism has also been classified as *Eimeria. Gl. gilruthi* and *Gl. fusiformis* have been reported to cause dysentery in sheep and goats in Africa and cattle in India respectively.[129] Virtually nothing is known about the endogenous development cycle of these two organisms.

Environmental Toxins

Heavy Metals

Arsenic (As), mercury (Hg), copper (Cu), and thallium (Tl) if ingested in large quantities, produce an enteritis. Highly oxidative tissues such as intestinal mucosa are particularly susceptible to damage by heavy metals, which interfere with intracellular enzyme systems. Thallium also exchanges with potassium and thus interferes with cellular metabolism. As with other agents that compromise the integrity of the mucosal barrier, invasion and toxin production by resident intestinal bacteria may cause further damage.

Potential sources of these poisons are listed in Table 23–11 along with some other details that may aid in making a definitive diagnosis. Anytime that poisoning is suspect, a detailed history and careful inspection of the premises may be much more helpful in making a diagnosis than the clinical signs. When animals are poisoned at pasture, taking note of activities that have occurred immediately adja-

Table 23–11. Potential sources of heavy metal poisons that affect the small intestine

1. Arsenic	Certain pesticides (ant and snail baits) and herbicides, insulation material such as vermiculite and Celotex, wood building materials treated with arsenical preservatives, Fowler's solution
2. Mercury	Fungicides (paints, seeds), anti-fouling paints, paper and pulp products, electrical apparatus
3. Copper	Anthelmintics, pesticides, $CuSO_4$ foot-baths, copper objects, certain plants (chronic poisoning), imbalanced mixed mineral supplements
4. Thallium	Rodenticides, certain cosmetics (?)

cent to the property in question, such as herbicidal spraying or pond treatment to reduce algae bloom is extremely important. A classic case of arsenic poisoning of cattle was caused by windblown herbicide.[209] Equally important is knowing the route of streams that may traverse the pasture, or whether there is a long unused and forgotten trash dump down in a back corner, to which the animals have access.

Clinical Signs. It must be remembered that the effect of heavy metals is not exclusively on the gastrointestinal tract. In fact, their particular effects on other systems may produce the clinical signs that provide the definitive diagnosis. For instance, profuse diarrhea or dysentery and colic are common features of arsenic, mercury, copper, or thallium poisoning, but if jaundice and hemoglobinuria are also seen, one might consider copper above the others mentioned. In general, the acute fulminating signs described in this section are due to ingestion of large amounts of heavy metal. Intake of smaller doses over a long period of time can cause a "chronic" poisoning, the signs of which are more often related to individual metal affinity for particular tissues rather than to gastroenteritis; e.g., renal disease with mercury, hepatic disease with copper, and skin disease with thallium. It should be reemphasized that there can be marked species differences in susceptibility and response to a given dose of any toxin.[210]

Necropsy Findings. Results of severe intoxication may also reflect the individual tissue affinity as well as hemorrhagic gastroenteritis, both of which will aid in making a definitive diagnosis. The gastrointestinal contents should be closely examined, particularly rumen contents, for clues regarding type and source of toxins.

Therapy. Treatment of animals with acute heavy metal poisoning is reserved primarily for those individuals whose monetary or personal value warrants it. In herd situations, it is more practical to remove the animals from the intoxicating premises until it can be detoxified. Supportive fluid, electrolyte, and nutritional therapy should always be considered, the intensiveness of which depends upon the severity of illness. Laxatives or purgatives may be used to move the toxic agent from the intestinal tract. In ruminants, rumenotomy and evacuation of rumen contents may be necessary as well to reduce the severity of intoxication. Specific antitoxic agents are available but these may produce as much discomfort in the animal as the poisoning.

Antidotes against the following heavy metals are:[211–215]

1. Arsenic: Dimercaprol (British Anti-Lewisite) given intramuscularly. This oil base may cause muscle necrosis and sloughing at the injection site.
2. Mercury: Very intensive intravenous sodium thiosulfate or intramuscular dimercaprol therapy is given. The effort is hardly warranted except for very valuable or highly prized animals.
3. Copper: No specific antidote for acute poisoning is available. Check dietary molybdenum availability. Low dietary intake of molybdenum makes an animal more prone to copper toxicity.
4. Thallium: Diphenylthiocarbazone powder is given orally, usually in gelatin capsules. The animal's potassium balance must also be closely monitored. Dimercaprol is also recommended by some.

Phosphorus

Certain rodenticides are the major source for phosphorus poisoning in domestic animals. Toxic amounts of phosphorus cause contact necrosis of the gastrointestinal mucosa resulting in violent episodes of vomiting and diarrhea. The clinical course is usually rapid with afflicted animals quickly going into shock and dying. Survivors of the acute intestinal manifestations often develop fatal renal or hepatic failure within 7 to 10 days.[172]

Necropsy Findings. Findings include hemorrhagic gastroenteritis and hepatomegaly. Liver, kidney, muscle, and gut contents collected for analysis should not be put into any sort of preservative. Fortunately, phosphorus-containing rodent baits are not used much anymore so that this type of poisoning is rare.

Plant Poisonings in Ruminants[172,216]

As a general rule, ruminants do not become poisoned by plants if left to their own devices. Some sort of human interaction usually initiates the problem. For instance, the animals may be: (1) confined in a particular area where there is little else to eat; (2) induced because of their innate behavior, to eat large amounts of a particular toxic plant, as when shrub trimmings are indiscriminately dumped into a pasture; (3) allowed to graze a pasture that is normally safe but presently toxic because of a recent fertilization; (4) exposed to lush growth of a toxic plant because of the effects of weather conditions, or a combination of the foregoing situations.

The toxic principles of a particular poisonous plant often affect more than one system in the body. Those plants that cause small intestinal disease are listed here, although the intestinal disturbance may not be manifested as the outstanding clinical signs of the introxication. If plant poisoning is suspected, a detailed history, thorough inspection of the property involved, and a complete necropsy, including careful inspection of the ingesta, will be most helpful in making a definitive diagnosis.

Bracken Fern (Pteridium aquilinium) in Cattle
1. *Toxic factor:* Unidentified
2. *Clinical signs:* High fever, hematochezia or melena, hematuria, petechial and ecchymotic hemorrhages of the mucous membranes, and prolonged bleeding time are found.
3. *Laboratory findings:* Thrombocytopenia, leukopenia, and bone marrow depression are seen.
4. *Necropsy findings:* Hemorrhaging in all organ systems, hematomas, sloughing of intestinal mucosa near hematoma, and multiple small infarcts in lungs and kidney are manifest.
5. *Treatment:* DL-batyl alcohol: 1 g/450 kg s.i.d. subcutaneously or intravenously for 4 to 5 days. Broad spectrum antibiotic. Intravenous fluids, including blood.

Nitrate/Nitrite
1. *Toxic factor:* Nitrite
2. *Clinical signs:* Ptyalism, colic, diarrhea, and vomiting, progressing to tachypnea and prostration are seen. Mucous membranes are very pale. Blood is very dark or chocolate color. Animals may die rapidly in convulsions.
3. *Laboratory findings:* Methemoglobinemia
4. *Necropsy findings:* Gastroenteritis. The blood clots poorly.

5. *Treatment:* Methylene blue in low doses 4 mg/kg as a 2 to 4% solution intravenously.

Oak (Querces Spp.)
1. *Toxic principle:* Unidentified.
2. *Clinical signs:* Colic with dysentery in the late stages; polyuria and ventral edema are seen.
3. *Laboratory findings:* Hypoproteinemia and increased serum creatinine and BUN are found.
4. *Necropsy findings:* Gastroenteritis and nephrosis.
5. *Treatment:* $Ca(OH)_2$ mixed into the ration to make up 15% of the dry weight.

Hemorrhagic Gastroenteritis

Swine (Also known as Proliferative Hemorrhagic Enteropathy or Hemorrhagic Syndrome)

This disease is apparently seen with greater frequency in Britain and Australia than in the United States. It can affect all ages but is most common in young feeder pigs and breeding stock. It was first described in detail in pigs being fed whey. Bacteriologic studies were unrevealing and it was speculated that the disease might be an allergic reaction to whey protein, although it had also been seen in animals on other types of feed.[217] Recent studies suggest that the etiology is a vibrionic agent (*Campylobacter sputorum* subsp. *mucosalis*) which also causes a more chronic intestinal adenomatosis in swine[218] (see under "Chronic Enteritides" in Part II-B).

Clinical signs vary from rapid development of pallor, collapse, and death with no specific signs of gastrointestinal disease, to marked hematochezia and anemia. Occasionally hematemesis is seen.[219,220]

The treatment and control of this disease are discussed in Part II-B.

Dogs

Hemorrhagic gastroenteritis (HGE) is a sporadically occurring affliction of dogs that is seen with high frequency in toy poodles and miniature schnauzers,[221] but can occur in all breeds and in mongrels. A few dogs seem to be prone to multiple attacks. The cause is unknown.

Clinical Signs. Signs range from mild to severe and include vomiting, hematemesis, diarrhea, and hematochezia. Tenesmus and abdominal pain are absent. Pulse rate is usually increased but temperature and respiration rate are normal. Many dogs with signs of severe gastrointestinal disease remain remarkably alert while others rapidly become depressed and even comatose.

Laboratory Findings. The most outstanding finding is a very high packed cell volume (PCV); values ranging from 50 to 86% have been recorded.[221,222] The higher the PCV at time of presentation, the more guarded the prognosis should be. Consumptive coagulopathy, consistent with a shock state, is also present as indicated by low platelet counts and prolonged prothrombin and partial thromboplastin times.

Necropsy Findings. To date the pathology of HGE in dogs has not been studied in great detail, since most cases recover and the autolysis of the gut mucosa in those that die is very rapid. At necropsy, the intestinal tract is filled with blood and all portions of the small and large intestine are a dark, reddish-black color. Hemorrhage and congestion may also be seen in the mesenteric lymph nodes.

Therapy. The treatment most indicated is fluid therapy, the vigor of which depends upon severity of presenting signs and laboratory data. Balanced plasma replacement-type solutions containing bicarbonate precursors such as acetate/propionate or lactate should be used. If the PCV is 60% or greater, the fluids should be given intravenously via cephalic or jugular vein catheters.[222] Plan on an initial administration of 80 to 90 cc/kg body weight, given rapidly until the PCV drops below 50%. Fluid infusion rate should then be maintained at 40 to 60 ml/kg/day (lesser volume for larger dogs) with proper attention to contemporary losses and maintenance requirements, until the PCV is stabilized and it appears that the episode is waning. PCV and total plasma solids should be measured at least twice daily. If additional support is deemed necessary, the fluids can be given subcutaneously at the same total daily volume in 3 to 4 divided doses. Dogs presenting with a PCV of 50% of less usually respond well to the subcutaneous therapy alone.[222] Animals should not be allowed to eat or drink for the first 2 to 3 days of hospitalization. When feeding is resumed, small amounts of a soft low-fat ration should be offered with a frequency that depends upon the patient's response.[221] Most dogs are usually back to maintaining themselves orally in 4 to 5 days.

The prognosis for successfully treating HGE in dogs is quite favorable, especially if the presenting PCV is less than 70%. The overall mortality rate of dogs with HGE in one study of 125 afflicted dogs was 8%.[221] Table 23–12 summarizes some clinical features for differentiation of acute diarrheal diseases in adult animals.

Table 23–12. Some important differential features of causes of acute, severe diarrhea in adult animals

	Fever	Dysentery*	Fecal Leukocytes	Buccal Lesions	Vomiting (Carnivora)	Blood Count	Serum Protein	Other Essential Diagnostic Procedures
Invasive bacteria	Yes	Common	Yes	No	Common	Left shift in WBC series	Decreased albumin	Fecal cultures
Entero-toxigenic bacteria	No	No	No	No	Occasionally	Very high hematocrit	Increased	Fecal pH (alkaline) Fecal culture and intestinal loop inoculations
Viruses	Yes	Variable	No	Common only in ruminants	Common	Leukopenia	Normal	Fecal and nasal cultures Serology
Nematode parasites	No[†]	Rare[†]	No[†]	No	Rare[†]	Anemia	Decreased	Fecal examination for parasites or ova
Fungi	Yes	Maybe	Yes	No	Maybe	Left shift in WBC series	Normal to increased globulin	Other signs of mycotic infection (Respiratory?) Duodenal aspiration
Heavy metals	No	Common	?	No	Common	Variable	Normal	Specific toxicology of tissue specimens

*Diarrhea containing frank blood, shreds of mucosa or both.
[†]Except Strongyloides where common.

DIFFERENTIAL DIAGNOSIS—DISEASES OF OTHER SYSTEMS, ACUTE (FULMINATING) ENTERITIDES

All Species
Organophosphate poisoning

Sheep
Bluetongue (colon)

Swine
Swine dysentery (colon)
Trichuriasis (cecum and colon)

Dogs
Acute pancreatitis
Entamoebiasis (colon and rectum)
Balantidiosis (colon)
Lead poisoning (minimal gastrointestinal lesions)

Cats
Infectious peritonitis
Entamoebiasis (colon and rectum)
Lead poisoning

CHRONIC ENTERITIDES OR NEOPLASIA

History and Signs Compatible

If Damage Not Extensive Enough to Cause Significant Malabsorption
1. Recurrent or Persistent
   —fever
   —fluid diarrhea
   —vomiting
   —anorexia
   —abdominal pain
2. Ventral Edema
   —intermandibular
   —substernal
   —extremities
3. Persistent Weight Loss
4. Thickened Intestinal Loops
5. Mesenteric Adenopathy

If Damage Extensive Enough to Cause Malabsorption Add
6. Steatorrhea (pigs and carnivora)
7. Dermatopathy

As the heading implies, this section deals with small intestinal diseases which are fairly slow in developing to a point where clinical signs are evident. With the exception of some of the parasitoses, these diseases are very resistant to symptomatic therapy and few specific treatments are known. Affected areas of intestine show absorptive cell damage and infiltration of the lamina propria with neutrophils, lymphocytes, plasmacytes, monocytes, histocytes or eosinophils, or some combination thereof. Excessive loss of plasma proteins into the bowel lumen is almost a universal feature of this group of diseases.

The occurrence of clinical evidence of maldigestion/malabsorption is dependent upon how much mucosa has been damaged. In many instances, the cause of the disease has not been determined and these afflictions are classified by the type of pathologic change present.

It remains to be elucidated in most cases how much the degree of establishment in and confinement to the gastrointestinal tract is related to the balance between level of pathogen dose, the degree of host immunologic response, or the interaction of endogenous "normal" enteric flora.

Bacterial Infections

Chronic Salmonellosis

Epidemiology. This form of salmonellosis, which causes a low grade, persistent enteritis, must be contrasted with a latent or active carrier state[65,223] where inflammation of the bowel is not routinely evident. So far as is known, there is no particular serotype of salmonella that is known to cause a persistent low grade, rather than fulminant, enteritis. Animals so afflicted are a constant health menace to all others with whom they are associated, including people.[57,224,225,226]

Signs wax and wane between periods of fever, abdominal pain, and marked diarrhea, to periods of relative quiescence where there may only be a mild or no fever and persistently poor body condition. The more active periods may be related to stressful events experienced by the animal.

Laboratory Findings. Significant findings may include moderate leukocytosis with neutrophilia, mild to moderate hypoalbuminemia, hypergammaglobulinemia and the presence of leukocytes in the feces. A high serum titer against a particular salmonella serotype is supportive, but only the culture of salmonella organisms from feces, intestinal contents, or bile is definitive. Serial fecal cultures (not rectal swabs!) taken every other day for a week or two may be necessary before the organism can be found. One should not be satisfied with a single negative culture and the laboratory should be well-equipped to cope with this elusive pathogen!

Therapy. Attempted treatment of a well-established chronic salmonella-induced enteritis is not very rewarding. Some feel that oral administration of an antibacterial agent that is found to be effective against the organism on sensitivity testing, such as nitrofurazolidone, lincomycin or trimethoprim-sulfamethoxazole is indicated.[227-229] On the other hand, there is some evidence to suggest that oral antibiotic therapy only induces a more persistent carrier state.[148,149] Effective hyperimmunization with repeated bacterin injections seems more logical but has not been tested adequately.

Prophylaxis. Monetary and sentimental value notwithstanding, euthanasia is recommended for the safety of other animals and humans on the same premises. Strict isolation is the only alternative.

Items and places exposed to the infected animal should be treated as has already been described in Part I.

Tuberculosis

Epidemiology. Tuberculosis in domestic animals of the developed countries of the world is now quite rare, but should never be forgotten. All three forms, *M. tuberculosis*, *M. bovis*, and *M. avium*, can infect animals, although there are incidence differences among animal species. Horses seem most susceptible to *M. bovis* or *M. avium*, both of which can cause intestinal disease.[230,231] Cattle are almost exclusively infected by *M. bovis* and an intestinal involvement is not common.[172] Classically, pigs develop retropharyngeal and/or miliary tuberculosis from eating infected milk or chicken carcasses. Tuberculosis control programs in the industrialized nations of the northern hemisphere have greatly reduced the incidence of TB in swine. Dogs may contract bovine or avian tubercular enteritis by eating contaminated substances, but more commonly are infected by tuberculous people.[232] Cats are very resistant but not totally immune. An interesting feature of tuberculosis is that the various species of mycobacteria must be maintained in their natural host (humans, cattle, or birds) in order for the organism to survive as an endemic threat to any species of animal;[230] that is, TB would not be seen in horses, swine, or dogs if these animals were never exposed to infected humans, cattle, or fowl.

Clinical Signs. The signs of small intestinal tuberculosis may vary greatly depending upon the amount of intestine involved. The human and bovine types tend to form discrete tubercles which may cause mucosal ulceration and diarrhea. Often the initial manifestation of TB in such cases is due to a breakaway of the organism from the primary infective site, such as the lungs, to become miliary in distribution. If the intestinal lesions are not very severe, signs of the pulmonary or peritoneal disease may predominate. Retropharyngeal lymphadenopathy is common if the original route of infection was via ingestion.

M. avium in mammals tends to be more proliferative and diffuse, not forming the typical caseated tubercles but a generalized thickening and malfunction of the small intestine and associated mesenteric lymph node enlargement. Malabsorption and excess plasma protein leakage become more severe as the lesion progresses. The affected animal becomes slowly cachectic in spite of a good appetite, may have diarrhea and steatorrhea, and will develop ventral edema if hypoalbuminemia becomes severe. The whole intestinal tract may be involved such that a proctitis may be detected and a rectal biopsy of mucosa and submucosa will be diagnostic showing the presence of acid-fast organisms within the tissue. Intradermal or subcutaneous administration of tuberculin should be done in cases where tuberculosis is suspected. Unfortunately, patients with severe infections may not react to the tuberculin, probably because they are anergic by the time the test is performed. Conversely, many horses that have no evidence of tuberculosis (if subsequently autopsied) will have reacted positively to intradermal tuberculin.[233]

Laboratory Findings. There is nothing in the results of routine tests done in patients with *intestinal* tuberculosis that is diagnostic. A blood count may show a mild to moderate leukocytosis with neutrophilia, and hypoalbuminemia with hypergammaglobulinemia would be characteristic of the serum protein pattern. The organism can be cultured from feces and biopsy material but this usually takes many weeks and is most helpful in identifying the species of mycobacterium involved. If ulcerations adjacent to tubercles are large and deep enough, some occult blood may be detected in the feces.

Necropsy Findings. Pathologically, the human and bovine forms cause the typical caseating granulomas in whatever tissue they infect, including the small intestine and its associated lymph nodes.[172] The diffuse granulomatous reaction caused by *M. avium* in the intestinal tract could not be distinguished from chronic inflammatory bowel disease, cause unknown, were it not for demonstration of the presence of acid-fast organisms or the culture of the bacillus.

Prophylaxis. Animals with tuberculosis should be destroyed and the location in which they have resided should be processed according to the guidance of state and national animal health officials.

Corynebacterium Equi *Enteritis in Young Horses*

Epidemiology. The ravages of *Corynebacterium equi* in the lungs of horses between 3 and 8 months of age are widely recognized. The intestinal component of this infection is not so well-known. The usual intestinal lesion is ulceration of the colonic mucosa within the Peyer's patches, and while this may cause some diarrhea, it is not the determining factor for survival or death. More insidious and uncommon is a chronic progressive inflammation of both small and large intestines and associated mesenteric lymph nodes. Such cases probably survive to the point where signs of chronic intestinal disease are evident because they have not been killed by the pulmonary form.

It is not yet clear whether the pulmonary or the intestinal lesions indicate the primary site of infection by *C. equi*. It is possible that both inhalation and intestinal invasion occur, the latter being aided by migrating larvae of *Strongylus vulgaris*.[234]

The predilection for *C. equi* infection in horses on certain premises suggests that the organism is hardy and probably ubiquitous on that premises. It is curious, therefore, that certain foals raised therein never contract the disease while some of their pasture mates are severely (and usually fatally) afflicted with pneumonitis. More interesting is why a few do not have pulmonary disease but instead confine the organism at the gut level where it causes the progressive debilitating enteritis.

Clinical Signs. The signs are essentially the development of chronic intractable diarrhea and persistent loss of condition. If a rectal examination can be done, enlarged lymph nodes, especially around the mesenteric root, and thickened bowel will be appreciated. However, afflicted animals are often too small to permit an extensive rectal exam. There is usually no clinical evidence of pulmonary disease, and pneumonia may or may not have been seen when the animal was younger. Persistent or recurrent low-grade fever occurs in some cases.

Laboratory Findings. The results of clinical laboratory studies of these kinds of cases are not very helpful, except perhaps to help distinguish this disease from granulomatous enteritis. In *C. equi* enteritis, serum protein concentrations are within normal limits while hypoalbuminemia is a distinct feature of granulomatous enteritis. In addition, if large numbers of corynebacteria can be seen on a Gram stain of a fecal smear, or can be easily cultured from the feces, the provisional diagnosis is supported strongly. Corynebacteria are only occasionally, if ever, found in normal equine feces.

Necropsy Findings. At autopsy, gross signs of the chronic enteric form of *C. equi* infection are confined to the intestines and mesenteric lymph nodes.[235] The nodes are enlarged and irregularly shaped. Their cut surface reveals numerous pockets within the nodal substance that are filled with cloudy grey fluid that contains numerous gram-positive rods. The normal nodal architecture is obliterated and replaced by amorphous friable material. Small and large intestines are diffusely thickened with the mucosal surface showing scattered small erosions that may exude some bloody fluid. Histologically, marked villous atrophy in the small intestine is seen, with the lamina propria and submucosa infiltrated by large macrophages. With appropriate staining these macrophages are shown to be periodic acid-Schiff (PAS) positive and contain clumps of gram-positive pleiomorphic rods, which ostensibly are the *C. equi*.

Therapy. In spite of all kinds of symptomatic treatment to reverse the progressive debilitation and stop the diarrhea, young horses with chronic *C. equi* enteritis continue to deteriorate and are usually killed for humane reasons if they do not die naturally.

Johne's Disease (Paratuberculosis) in Ruminants

Epidemiology. Johne's disease is seen in all domestic ruminants, most commonly in cattle. Horses have been experimentally infected but do not contract the disease naturally.[236] The incidence of documented cases of Johne's disease in cattle in the United States is increasing, but this may be due mainly to better diagnostic techniques and a greater tendency to report the disease (in some states, paratuberculosis is a reportable disease) than to any real increase in incidence.[237]

The causative organism is an acid-fast bacillus, *Mycobacterium paratuberculosis*, the direct pathologic effects of which are confined to the intestinal tract and associated lymph nodes. The organism is most infective for young animals although the signs of infection are not manifested until adulthood.[238] Thus, if Johne's disease becomes clinically apparent on a particular property, one can be reasonably sure that the organism is well-established there. Through epidemiologic analysis there is a suggestion that soil deficiency of phosphorus and excess of calcium may be associated with a higher incidence of paratuberculosis.[239]

Overt clinical signs are seen only in adults. The highest incidence in cattle is between 2½ and 5 years of age, although older animals may also be affected. Age incidence figures for sheep and goats are not available except that, again, it is a disease of adults. Factors that influence the timing by which Johne's disease manifests itself in a particular individual are not understood; colostrally derived antibody protection, dose of organism, age when infected, ability to mount an active immune response, diet, and mineral content of soil probably all play a part. Thus in a herd where the disease is endemic, animals may fall into one of the following four categories: (1) clinically ill, (2) asymptomatic shedder, (3) infected and asymptomatic but not shedding enough organisms in feces to be culturally detectable, or (4) uninfected.[240] One study of a large herd of Guernseys showed that a significantly higher number of fecal shedders of *M. paratuberculosis* (no overt clinical signs) were culled because of recurrent mastitis or infertility than noninfected cows in the same herd.[241] This suggests that either the animals were made more susceptible to mastitis and endometritis by *M. paratuberculosis* infection, or that they represented a group that was unable to mount an effective immune response to any number of pathogens. The former seems more likely since the institution of a practice of immediately removing newborn calves to an uninfected premises considerably reduced the incidence of mastitis and infertility in them when they became adults.

Clinical Signs. The onset of signs of paratuberculosis enteritis in cattle can be either slow and insidious or quite rapid. The signal to the producer that something is wrong is diarrhea. Initially the diarrhea may recur sporadically, becoming more watery and occurring for longer periods each time until it becomes persistent. During this time the animal begins to lose weight in spite of normal, or even increased, appetite. Sometimes, the diarrhea starts suddenly in a persistent watery form, but is never so severe that the animal is plunged into a state of severe dehydration and acidosis. This insidious disease slowly causes deterioration through malabsorptive and protein-losing enteropathy. As the disease progresses, the animals become increasingly more lethargic, anorectic, and thin. Skin elasticity is reduced and, terminally, intermandibular edema develops, reflecting the excess plasma protein loss. Sheep and goats show essentially similar signs except that diarrhea is less commonly seen.[238]

Both infected and non-infected animals react too indiscriminantly to intradermal injection of Johnin to make this test a reliable diagnostic aid. An intravenous Johnin test may be more specific, though still not perfect, and it must be supervised by a state or federal veterinarian.[240]

Laboratory Findings. The most consistent laboratory finding in a well-established case of Johne's disease is hypoproteinemia, especially hypoalbuminemia. A hypochromic normocytic anemia is also common, most likely a reflection of the malnutrition since iron stores in the marrow are often depleted and serum iron concentration is lower than normal. Numerous types of serologic tests have also been developed for diagnosing Johne's disease but their usefulness is debatable. The results of a study done in the Netherlands suggested that fluorescent antibody and complement fixation tests used together were of value in detecting subclinical infections.[242] Some workers in the United States do not have as much confidence in the usefulness of serology, especially since in their hands both complement fixation and hemagglutination inhibition tests have produced numerous false positive reactions.[243] The examination of rectal mucosal scrapings and feces of suspected cases for the presence of acid-fast organisms is also unreliable since: (1) the rectum may not be involved; and (2) there are often numerous nonpathogenic acid-fast organisms in the feces.

Fecal culture is very reliable for detecting any animal that is shedding more than 100 bacilli per gram of feces.[240] Definitive results of a culture are not available for 3 months, however. Thus this test is useful for herd screening but not very helpful in the diagnosis of a case in hand.

The most reliable method for making a quick diagnosis of Johne's disease, short of autopsy, is to biopsy the ileum and an associated lymph node through a right paralumbar laparotomy incision.

Necropsy Findings. The macroscopic intestinal lesions of Johne's disease are very characteristic. Affected intestine has thickened, stiff walls and the mucosa has a firm "corrugated" surface. Mesenteric lymphadenopathy may also be prominent.

Histologically, in both intestine and lymph node there is a loss of normal architecture due to infiltration of plasmacytes and macrophages. Giant cells are also seen, especially in the mesenteric lymph nodes. Acid-fast staining of these tissues generally reveals numerous bacilli, both intra- and extracellularly; occasionally the organisms may be difficult to find. Caseation necrosis and calcification, typical of *M. bovis*, are not seen.[171] Villous atrophy is present in affected small intestine suggesting that malabsorption occurs in at least the later stages of this disease.

Prophylaxis. At present, methods regarding attempts at control and/or eradication of Johne's disease are not unanimously agreed upon. A vaccine has been developed which is effective if given to very young calves prior to their age of greatest susceptibility. The vaccine made from killed whole cells appears to be more effective than that from fractionated cells.[244] There is also one report which claims that signs of disease in adult sheep regressed when they were vaccinated.[245] There has been some reluctance to use paratuberculosis vaccine in cattle, however, because of its tendency to provoke a positive reaction to tuberculin in some animals.

Strict adherence to a set of principles of culture and cull, immediate removal of calves to a clean premises before they have suckled, and ultrastrict sanitation procedures on the property may be a reasonable approach to eradicating Johne's disease from a given herd.[240] In many instances, however, it would be impossible for a producer to comply because he has neither the resources nor the desire to meet all the requirements.

Porcine Intestinal Adenomatosis (PIA)

Epidemiology. This fairly common disease of weaned pigs was first described in the United States in 1931.[246] In 1951 an outbreak was described in 58 animals in Denmark but unfortunately was labelled as "regional enteritis," suggesting that the lesion might be similar to Crohn's disease in humans.[247] Subsequent studies have stressed that this is not a granulomatous enteritis.

Clinical Signs. The most consistent sign of PIA is failure to grow normally.[248] Recurrent or chronic diarrhea may also be seen and frank blood may occasionally be present in the fecal material. Usually less than 1% of the group of pigs is afflicted with this chronic disease, although the whole group may have suffered from an acute self-limiting outbreak of diarrheal disease initially.[247] Thus, the signs are clinically indistinguishable from chronic salmonellosis, though the morbidity is lower.

Necropsy Findings. Pathologic changes are restricted primarily to the ileum.[247–249] Grossly the affected gut is thickened and the musosal surface is transformed into a diffuse scattering of raised hyperplastic nodules or ridges. Adjacent to the hyperplastic areas the mucosa may be eroded or ulcerated. Histologically, the mucosal epithelium is composed of proliferating immature cells lining greatly enlarged glands. There is also marked villous atrophy.[218,249] A vibrionic agent *Campylobacter sputorum* subsp. *mucosalis* can be cultured from affected mucosal cells.[250] These organisms have not been found in ileal tissue of normal pigs or of those with swine dysentery, but have been seen in some cases of necrotic enteritis (NE), a coagulative necrosis of the ileum and large intestine, and regional ileitis (RI) of pigs.[218]

RI is a combination of mucosal necrosis and smooth muscle hypertrophy of the terminal ileum. Thus, all of these pathologic manifestations may be initiated by invasion of campylobacter across the intestinal barrier. The series of events that promotes or allows the invasion remains to be discovered. It should also be noted that, to date, no successful transmission studies using the campylobacter have been reported.

Therapy. Treatment regimens for clinically affected pigs have not been developed. Even if effective methods were worked out, they might not be economically feasible. The organism is apparently sensitive to low levels of penicillin and relatively high levels of chlortetracycline in the feed. It is resistant to sulfamethazine.[251]

Prophylaxis. Because the probable etiology of PIA has only recently been discovered, no immunization products are yet available. In a large breeding/growing operation where the morbidity is continually high, any sort of effective control short of depopulation may be difficult. There is evidence suggesting resident pigs may become immune, at least to the acute hemorrhagic form of the disease, in that only newly introduced pigs develop clinical signs. The incidence has been reduced in such a case by exposing the new pigs to residents for 21 days while feeding them a non-medicated feed, then removing them and feeding a ration containing chlortetracycline (100 g/ton) and penicillin (50 g/ton).[251] This program might work for the more chronic proliferative response to the infection (PIA) as well, but this remains to be tried.

Viral Infections

Bovine Virus Diarrhea (BVD)

A rather unusual variant of BVD is characterized by chronic diarrhea, a fluctuating low grade fever, coronitis/laminitis and proliferative dermatitis. Oral and muzzle erosions may also be found, but not consistently.[163] Afflicted animals become progressively thinner and more susceptible to secondary infections, especially of the respiratory tract.

If diarrhea and wasting are the most prominent features in a particular animal, it may be difficult to distinguish chronic BVD from Johne's disease. The presence of lesions in the integumentary system and mouth, and the lack of severe hypoalbuminemia should make one more inclined to think of BVD. The finding of typical erosions within the gastrointestinal tract will make the diagnosis even more definitive; these typical lesions are not found in 100% of cases, however.

There is no effective treatment of this chronic form of BVD.

Intestinal Parasitosis

Parasitosis should always be included in the list of differential diagnoses when one is asked to examine an animal with a history of chronic gastrointestinal disease. This portion of the chapter will deal with clinically relevant aspects of intestinal helminth (i.e., nematode and cestode) and protozoal infestations that can cause chronic small intestinal dysfunction. Details regarding factors that influence the establishment of the parasitic state, and control programs can be found in Chapter 17.

Nematodes

Strongylus vulgaris Infection in Horses. The most common cause of intestinal disease in the horse is S. vulgaris. Since both small and large bowel are affected, the disease is discussed with other large bowel diseases in Chapter 24.

Trichostrongyle Infection in Ruminants. (species of Trichostrongyles, Cooperia, Nematodirus)

Epidemiology. Tissue damage by this group of worms is confined to the gastrointestinal tract, since there are no migrating larval stages of development. All ages may be afflicted but young animals are much more susceptible. Conditions have to be extremely harsh for adults to show overt signs of parasitism, but it must be remembered that the adults act as the main reservoir of infection even though they may be essentially healthy. The so-called "spring rise" phenomenon where a marked increase in fecal shedding of ova from the dam occurs following parturition is a case in point. This kind of parasitism is basically a management problem, provoked and supported by poor nutrition, poor sanitation, excessive crowding, improper pasture management, and irrational or inadequate worming procedures.[172,193]

Pathophysiology. The larvae of these worms burrow into the intestinal mucosa, mature, and re-emerge as potent adults, all species of which cause mucosal inflammation and damage. The ways in which the mucosa reacts to this insult are not fully understood but it is clear that intercellular connections are broken allowing leakage of plasma protein into the intestinal lumen, and mucosal cell absorp-

tive function is disrupted.[252] Intestinal motility is also disrupted.[253]

Clinical Signs. The sequential development of clinical signs is rather classic and insidious. First, the growth rate of young animals declines precipitously, followed by a loss of "bloom" as a progressive deterioration of conditions takes place. Haircoat loses its gloss, skin becomes dry and scaly, and the abdomen begins to contract. Watery, fetid, dark green-brown diarrhea begins and soon the animals have difficulty rising and moving about because of weakness. In terminal stages intermandibular edema ("bottle jaw") may develop. Mucous membranes become pale and dry.

Laboratory Findings. The definitive clinical laboratory finding in these ruminant parasitoses is, of course, the presence of ova in the feces. For *Trichostrongylus* and *Cooperia* 1000 eggs per gram of feces is considered significant; for *Nematodirus*, which are not as fecund, the presence of any ova at all is indicative of serious infection.[172] Anemia and hypoalbuminemia are also found, their degree depending upon duration and severity of infestation. Finally, if management conditions are such that small intestinal parasites are a problem, abomasal ostertagiasis is probably also present. When abomasal mucosa is also damaged by parasites, pepsinogen back-diffuses into the circulation and elevated serum pepsinogen concentrations can be readily measured.[254]

Necropsy Findings. If for some reason, a definitive antemortem diagnosis cannot be made, a necropsy should be done on one or two of the weakest animals in the group. If adult worms are present in profusion within the intestine, the diagnosis is unequivocal. If the worms are more difficult to find, a total count should be done. The following technique makes counting easier:[172] roll a loop of duodenum inside-out on a test tube or piece of glass rod and immerse this in an aqueous iodine solution (iodine 30 g, potassium iodide 4 g in 100 ml water) for a few minutes and then briefly into a 5% sodium thiosulfate solution. The mucosa is decolorized but iodine-stained worms retain the brown color and are easily seen. Total worm count of over 500 per intestine indicates significant infestation.

Numerous anthelmintics are available for treatment of intestinal parasites in ruminants. The type of drug should be varied periodically since parasite resistance to anthelmintics does occur. Probably more important than choice of drug is the timing of administration. It has been shown in sheep that routine directed worming is much more effective in controlling parasitism than is pasture rotation.[193,255]

The following times, recommended as best for worming sheep in England,[193] should be quite representative for most of the northern hemisphere:

1. Special dosing against nematodiriasis in the spring.
2. Dosing the ewes after lambing to control post-parturient rise in fecal egg count.
3. Dosing the lambs at weaning time and then moving them to a clean pasture, or dosing and moving both ewes and lambs in early June.
4. General dosing of every sheep on the premises in September.

Recently, some data have suggested that dairy cattle will produce more milk if given an anthelmintic even though they show no clinical signs of gastrointestinal parasitism.[256,257] This thesis needs further rigorous testing on a nationwide basis to be totally convincing, however.

Strongyloides in Swine. Strongyloides infestation in any species usually causes an acute dysenteric disease, as already described. A more chronic form of strongyloides has been seen in swine, and it manifests as a persistent diarrhea with progressive weight loss. Considering the effect of the parasite on the small intestinal mucosa, it would be reasonable to suspect that there is considerable malabsorption, but this has never been studied nor is it understood why this chronic form, rather than the acute, becomes established.

Trichuriasis in Dogs. Lesions of Trichuris infection in dogs are usually found in the cecum and colon. However, a chronic inflammatory ileitis-typhitis-colitis caused by Trichuris that resembles Crohn's disease in humans has been described.[258] The case in question had presented with a history of diarrhea and intermittent hematochezia. Ova of *Trichuris vulpis* were consistently found in the feces but treatments with phthalofyne had no effect on reversing the progressive nature of the disease. Antibiotics and steroids were also ineffective and the dog was eventually euthanatized.

Histologic examination of grossly affected intestine revealed a transmural granulomatous enteritis. Trichuris ova were found deep in the lesion and neutrophil-filled "tracts" were seen coursing from submucosa to serosa.

Hookworm Infection of Adult Dogs. Overt clinical signs of hookworm infection is rare in adult dogs, but should not be overlooked.[259] In contrast to the acute, rather fulminant, clinical course seen in hookworm infections of puppies (see Part I), the disease in adult dogs is often manifested by chronic wasting and diarrhea. The feces of these adult cases usually do not contain any gross evidence of blood. The diarrhea is probably due in part, if not totally, to small intestinal malabsorption, since there is good evidence that chronic hookworm disease causes diffuse mucosal damage and villous atrophy.[260,261]

The presence of hookworm ova in the feces of a chronically debilitated dog should put ancylostomiasis at the top of a list of differential diagnoses.

Some of the newer, orally applied, anthelmintics have replaced the painful intramuscular disophenol injections for treatment of hookworms in dogs. One recently published study shows that mebendazole given at a dose of 22 mg/kg/day for 3 to 5 days is very effective.[262]

Cestodes

Anoplocephalid Infection of Horses. *Anoplocephala perfoliata* and *magna* may be found in startling numbers in the intestines of horses that have had no history of gastrointestinal disease. On the other hand, they have been held responsible for initiating or contributing to digestive disturbances in some cases. *A. magna* is found primarily in the jejunum while *A. perfoliata* is located in the terminal ileum around the ileocecal valve.

It should be remembered that the oribatid mite is the intermediate host in equine tapeworms. The mite can be found most commonly in pastures that are overgrazed by horses.[129]

Chronic unthriftiness, intermittent colic and intermittent or persistent diarrhea may be seen. The diarrhea is never severe enough to cause marked dehydration. Mucous membranes may be paler than normal suggesting anemia. In general outward clinical signs of cestode infection in horses are not much different than those of strongylosis.

The definitive clinical laboratory result is the demonstration of tapeworm eggs in the feces; gravid segments may also be found. Unless a careful examination is made on repeated fecal samples, however, the diagnosis will be missed.[129] A blood count should also be done to evaluate the degree of anemia.

If a diagnosis of anoplocephalid infection has been substantiated, the treatment of choice is probably niclosamide, which has been found to be safe and effective at a dose of 88 mg/kg.[263]

Anoplocephalid Infection of Ruminants. *Avitellina*, *Helictometra*, *Moniezia*, *Stilesia* and *Thysanosoma* species will infect the small intestine of cattle and sheep. While there is general agreement that light infections are inconsequential to the health of an animal, there is some controversy about the effects of heavier infestations.[129] Some feel strongly that the presence of large numbers of these tapeworms will cause debilitation, intermittent diarrhea, anemia, and hair (wool) loss.[264] Thus, when faced with such a syndrome, the practitioner should at least consider trematodes and look for ova and segments in the feces. Oribatid mites are intermediate hosts.

At necropsy, large numbers of worms have been found to cause a nonspecific catarrhal enteritis so that it is reasonable to assume that malabsorption and plasma leakage could occur.

Cyclophyllidean and Pseudophyllidean Infection of Dogs and Cats. The most "civilized" tapeworm infection of dogs, and occasionally cats, is *Dipylidium caninum*, which is transmitted by fleas. The carnivora may also be infested by various species of *Taenia* by eating cysticerci-infected flesh of small wild mammals and domestic ungulates, or with *Diphyllobothrium latum* by eating certain freshwater fish.

Often rather significant tapeworm infections will be asymptomatic; sometimes they will cause perianal itching, manifested by scraping the perineum along the ground. Occasionally recurrent flatulence, vomiting, and diarrhea will be seen, the exact pathophysiology of which is not understood. Proglottids expelled either in the vomitus or feces is the most common signal of cestodiasis in dogs and cats. Ova may also be found by flotation from fecal material but a single negative fecal exam should not preclude the diagnosis.

Numerous drugs are available to rid the animal of tapeworms. Niclosamide is very effective, given orally at a rate of 155 mg/kg. Bunamidine is also very good; 25 to 50 mg/kg per os is recommended.[265]

Ridding the dog or cat of the tapeworm is only half the job. Flea control, general sanitation, avoiding feeding of raw meat, and control of hunting are all important to prevent reinfestation.

Protozoonoses

Eimeria (Globidium) in Horses and Donkeys. Epidemiology and Clinical Signs. Coccidiosis is not a major problem in the equidae; in fact it may not be *any* problem. Ponies have been experimentally given large numbers of *E. leuckarti* oocysts orally and infection has been documented histologically, yet the animals have shown no signs of gastrointestinal disease.[266] Likewise, the oocysts may be found sporadically in the feces, or gametocytes within small intestinal mucosa, of samples from clinically normal horses being screened or submitted to ne-

cropsy for other reasons.[267] On the other hand, the organism has been found, again within the small intestinal mucosal cells, of equidae suffering from diarrhea and weight loss where no recognized pathogenic agents were identified.[268,269]

Pathogenesis. Whether the *E. leuckarti* do play a part in the pathogenesis of chronic diarrhea in some horses remains to be seen. There is evidence to suggest that lesions confined to the small intestine of equids do not generally cause diarrhea because of the compensatory properties of the colon.[231] In all the reported cases of *E. leuckarti* infection, the organism has never been found within colonic mucosa. Yet in some cases where chronic diarrhea was seen, colonic lesions of some other etiology were present.[270]

Laboratory Findings. Feces from horses with chronic diarrhea should always be examined in the clinical laboratory for parasite ova of all kinds. The oocytes of *E. leuckarti* are best found by mixing a small sample of fecal material with 50% dextrose and applying the qualitative flotation techniques.

Therapy. A rational method of ridding the animal of the infection would be the oral administration of sulfamethazine; in my experience this has caused cessation of oocyst shedding in the feces but has not necessarily cured the diarrhea. The prognosis for success should be guarded, therefore, since it is not yet known how intimately the *E. leuckarti* are involved with the pathogenesis of the diarrhea. Amprolium, an effective coccidiostat in chickens and ruminants, has been given experimentally to horses where it was found to be quite toxic after long-term administration.[271] Its effectiveness against *E. leuckarti* has not been evaluated.

Giardiasis in Dogs and Cats. Epidemiology. Canine giardiasis is an uncommon disease but should always be considered when evaluating a dog or cat with chronic diarrhea. This may be one of those situations where the diagnosis might be made more often if special attention were paid to looking for the parasite.

Transmission is probably via contaminated water or coprophagia. Giardia cysts have been shown to remain viable in water for as long as 3 months.[272] After being ingested, each cyst divides to form two trophozoites (actively feeding stages). The latter can multiply by binary fission within the intestinal lumen. Electron micrographs have shown that the trophozoites attach snugly to small intestinal absorptive surface, no doubt causing the cells' early demise.[273]

Human infection has been classified into three main groups,[272] and it is reasonable to assume that canine infection could be similarly classified: (1) asymptomatic carriers, (2) patients with mild signs and minimal or no small intestinal biopsy abnormalities who respond to antiprotozoal therapy, and (3) patients with mild to severe signs and abnormal biopsies, whose response to therapy is variable. In the latter group in particular there is evidence to suggest that an underlying inability to produce IgA may account for the severity and/or persistence of the infection.[274] Immunoglobulin quantitation in infected dogs has not been done, to date.

Clinical Signs. Signs include flatulence, mild weight loss, tenesmus upon defecation, and passage of light-colored soft feces that may contain excess mucus, tar, or flecks of frank blood.[275,276] In humans, clinical signs of giardiasis are caused mainly by small intestinal malabsorption, as demonstrated by steatorrhea, decreased D-xylose absorption, and decreased serum carotene concentrations.[277] Fat balance studies in dogs with well-documented infections have not been done, but these animals will have abnormal D-xylose or D-glucose absorption.[276]

Laboratory Findings. The most important results from studies in the clinical laboratory would be the demonstration of trophozoites in feces or aspirated stomach and duodenal contents. For fecal examination, a fresh specimen is suspended in saline solution and examined directly through the microscope. If it is desired to stop the movement of the organism and delineate its morphology more clearly, add a drop of Lugol's iodine to the suspension. Intestinal aspirates should be centrifuged at 500 rpm for 5 minutes with the sediment smeared on a glass slide and examined immediately.[272] Cysts should also be looked for in the sediment preparations.

It should be stressed that inability to demonstrate trophozoites or cysts in feces or aspirates does not rule out a diagnosis of giardiasis. Jejunal biopsy and direct aspiration of contents may be necessary. In severe cases of human infection, villous atrophy is an outstanding histopathologic feature. This has not been seen in dogs, even when trophozoites are attached to the epithelium.[276]

Therapy. Most animals respond dramatically to treatment, which is in accordance with the fact that mucosal damage appears to be minimal. Recommended drugs for dogs are metronidazole, 25 mg/kg b.i.d. orally for 5 days, or quinacrine 50 to 100 mg b.i.d. orally for 3 days and repeated after a 3-day interval.[276] Metronidazole is particularly attractive because of its apparent low toxicity. In cats quinacrine hydrochloride given 10 mg/kg per os s.i.d. for up to 12 days has been effective in causing remission of clinical signs but not in eliminating the infection.[275]

Mycotic Infections

Canine Histoplasmosis

Epidemiology. This chronic systemic fungal infection invades the body via the respiratory tract. The intestinal tract is only one of the organ systems that can be affected by *Histoplasma capsulatum,* which has a predilection for reticuloendothelial tissue. The greatest prevalence of the disease is confined in North America to the Mississippi, Missouri, and Ohio River valleys, up through the Great Lakes Region and along the St. Lawrence River.[278] Histoplasmosis in humans has also been reported from Central America, South America, United Kingdom, Austria, Spain, Portugal, South America, Philippines, and Australia, although the disease in dogs has been diagnosed primarily in the United States.

It has been found that bats and wild birds can shed histoplasma in their feces.[185] The yeast-like bodies apparently become airborne when the fecal material dries. The organisms have also been seen within small intestinal mucosal lesions in bats.

Clinical Signs. Signs of systemic histoplasmosis in dogs are protean and include progressive weight loss, persistent diarrhea (often containing frank blood), chronic cough, ascites, hepatomegaly, splenomegaly, lymphadenopathy, pale mucous membranes, intermittent fever, and nasooropharyngeal ulceration.[279–281] Vomiting is rarely seen and appetite usually remains good until the terminal stages of the disease. It is the combination of chronic cough with chronic diarrhea that should make the clinician think of histoplasmosis.

Thoracic radiography will often reveal hilar lymphadenopathy and nodular miliary lesions within the lung parenchyma.

Laboratory Findings. The most definitive clinical laboratory findings are those concerned with culture of the organism. Specimens for culture should include any mucopurulent material collected from the respiratory tract, swabs of oral or nasal ulcers, and feces. On Francis's cystine blood agar incubated at 37°C the fungus appears as a small round, perhaps budding, yeast-like organism; on Sabouraud's agar at room temperature it grows as a white, cottony colony.[280]

Cytology of impressions or histologic exam of an enlarged lymph node, or smears of WBC from the buffy coat of a centrifuged blood sample, may also reveal the organism. The fungus will be engulfed in large macrophages.[281]

Complement fixation has been helpful in diagnosing histoplasmosis in humans but has proved less useful in dogs.[278] Histoplasmin for intradermal testing of specific delayed hypersensitivity is available, but there is always the chance that a chronically ill animal will be anergic.

Necropsy Findings. Typical gross lesions are numerous and readily seen. Caseation necrosis may be found in lungs, liver, spleen, and kidneys. Mesenteric lymph nodes are enlarged and mucosal ulcers may be present in any or all parts of the gastrointestinal tract. The ileal mucosa may be thickened and corrugated in a manner similar to that seen in Johne's disease of cattle. Accordingly, histologic sections of affected gut show severe PAS-positive macrophage infiltration with intracellular yeast-like bodies.[171] Specific silver stains may also be helpful.

Therapy. Amphotericin B is most commonly used for canine histoplasmosis. The drug is highly toxic to the animal and should be given with extreme care. The following regimen for amphotericin B has been recommended:[282]

1. Reconstitution is obtained by adding 10 ml sterile water for injection, U.S.P., to the 50-mg vial, thereby giving a "stock solution" containing 5 mg/ml of the drug. Amphotericin B will precipitate in saline and many other electrolyte solutions. The stock solution may be stored for 1 week at refrigerated temperatures without loss of potency.

2. Determine the total daily dose for the animal to be treated. An initial canine dosage of 0.25 mg/kg is given the first day. If the first dose is well tolerated, the dosage is increased to 0.50 mg/kg/day or 1.0 mg/kg given every other day. If a cat is to be treated, one fourth to one half the canine dosage is given.

3. The calculated dosage is withdrawn from the stock solution and placed in an appropriate amount of 5% dextrose-in-water of pH above 5.0. The volume of 5% dextrose-in-water will be determined by the size of the animal to be treated. Volumes used with success are:

Body Weight, lb	Volume of 5% Dextrose-in-Water, ml
5–15	150–200
15–30	250
>30	300–500

Fresh infusion solutions should be prepared every 48 hours.

4. An indwelling intravenous catheter is placed in the animal to be treated. Well-secured jugular catheters have been most successful.

5. The daily dosage of amphotericin B diluted in the appropriate amount of 5% dextrose-in-water is dripped as slowly as possible into the patient. Four or more hours is recommended for each administration.

6. Prior to each administration of the drug, the BUN or creatinine must be evaluated. If the BUN rises above 50 mg/100 ml, therapy is discontinued until it declines into the normal range. Abnormalities due to renal toxicity from amphotericin may be more thoroughly evaluated by additionally monitoring the PCV, urinalysis, serum potassium, and blood gases.

7. Amphotericin B is administered to effect. It may be necessary to discontinue therapy several times during the course of treatment because of renal toxicity. Therapeutic results are usually satisfactory, even when the course of therapy is interrupted. The degree of toxicity is subject to individual variation. Some patients have received 20 to 30 consecutive days of therapy with no signs of renal toxicity. Treatment is continued until clinical remission of the disease is complete. Most patients demonstrate improvement within 5 to 7 days after therapy begins and require only 2 to 3 weeks of therapy. A total dose of 4 to 5 g should not be exceeded.

8. Close observation for relapse is conducted for the first year after therapy. Additional treatment is given if necessary.

5-Fluorocyseine is a new antifungal agent that is effective against histoplasma. Its advantages are that it can be administered orally and it is relatively nontoxic; thus it can be given over a long time span. The recommended dose is 50 mg/kg/q.i.d.[278] Blood counts and BUN measurements should be done weekly during therapy. Development of resistance to this drug by the organism has been documented.[283]

Acquired Diseases of Questionable or Unknown Etiology

The group of disorders discussed in this portion of the chapter comprise some of the most enigmatic forms of intestinal disease encountered in animals. All are, essentially, classifiable as "chronic inflammatory bowel disease," though their pathologic manifestations are varied, probably dependent upon causative factor(s). Their pathogenesis is not well understood, but the types of lesions suggest the induction of some complex, persistent, immunologic phenomena. All have one clinical manifestation in common, namely, the leakage of excessive plasma protein into the bowel lumen; that is, they are all "protein losing enteropathies" of one degree or another.[284] Unfortunately, until more is known about their cause and pathogenesis, specific therapeutic principles cannot be formulated. Thus, these diseases are often difficult to treat effectively.

Granulomatous Enteritis (GE)

To date GE has been documented only in horses and dogs as far as domestic animals are concerned. The human corollary is known as Crohn's disease or regional enteritis. In humans and horses the lesion may be found anywhere along the gastrointestinal tract: in dogs, as yet, it has not been found in the stomach. As would be expected, the predominant site of the disease in a particular individual determines the pattern of clinical signs. For instance, in humans GE of the stomach may present as peptic ulcer disease; if only the colon is involved, diarrhea and hematochezia are outstanding. In horses, diarrhea is not seen unless the colon is involved.[231]

While intestinal infection by certain fungi and mycobacteria cause a granulomatous reaction, the etiology of GE is unknown in most cases. In humans, cell-mediated lymphocytotoxic reactions to numerous antigens, including cytomegalovirus and enteric anaerobes, have been implicated.[285] Transmission of human disease to rabbits has been reported by one group of investigators.[286,287] It may very well be that the lesion could be initiated by any number of antigens that would cause no reaction in most individuals, the critical factor being the patient's particular immunologic response to the antigen. The syndrome has a high familial incidence in humans,[288] further suggesting that there is an endogenous defect in response to certain agents, and that a defect may be inherited. There is no reason why a defect could not also be acquired.

Horses. Clinical Signs. Horses with granulomatous enteritis present a fairly consistent pattern of disease,[231] but by the time this pattern emerges, the disease is well established and virtually impossible to treat. The signs include progressive weight loss, hyperphagia (unless the patient is near-terminal), and sometimes ventral edema and alopecia. By rectal examination mesenteric lymphadenopathy

and/or thickened intestinal wall may be detected. Some animals may have a thin haircoat or patchy nonpruritic alopecia. Chronic diarrhea, where the feces are of a cow-manure-like consistency, may be seen but not consistently. Special efforts should be made to palpate the lymph nodes around the mesenteric root. Masses may be felt within the rectal wall itself, or the rectal mucosa may be diffusely thickened and excessively friable. If so, biopsies of rectal lesions should be taken, using a uterine biopsy instrument, for histopathologic evaluation. Diffuse mucosal involvement suggests enteric tuberculosis rather than nonspecific GE; biopsies should be submitted for acid-fast staining as well as for hematoxylin and eosin. Abdominal paracentesis should be done, with the sample being submitted for cytology, total protein determination, and evaluation of macrophage phagocytic activity. D-xylose or D-glucose studies are indicated to assess absorptive function, which is usually abnormal.[231,289]

Laboratory Findings. Outstanding clinical laboratory findings of GE in horses are hypoalbuminemia due to loss of plasma protein into the intestinal lumen, and reduced phagocytic activity of peritoneal macrophages. Up to now, macrophage phagocytosis has only been assessed by a Sano stain of peritoneal fluid,[231] which is qualitative at best. In other words, by this staining technique it is easy to find many mononuclear cells that contain phagocytosed material; in most horses with GE, such cells containing nonspecific debris can be found only with great difficulty, if at all. More quantitative studies need to be done regarding this finding.

Necropsy Findings. Gross granulomatous lesions are confined to the gastrointestinal tract and associated lymph nodes.[287] The small and large intestine may be regionally or diffusely involved. Small intestinal diverticulosis and perforation have been seen. In a few cases an associated severe strongyle larval migrans has been found. It is interesting to speculate whether this association is incidental or indicative of some immunologic defect whereby the migrating larvae provoked the granuloma formation. Histologically, granulomatous inflammation may be found in stomach and liver as well as intestines.[290] If there is neither gross nor histologic evidence of colonic involvement, the patient most likely will not have had diarrhea.

Therapy. At present, there is no formulated medical regime for treatment of GE in horses (see below under Dogs for Principles of Medical Therapy that have been developed for humans). Occasionally a lesion is localized enough that it may be surgically removed.[291] In my experience and in that of others,[289] several horses have initially responded favorably to prolonged large doses of steroids only to develop a fatal complication that may or may not have been steroid-related.

Dogs. Clinical Signs. The signs of diffuse GE in dogs usually include chronic diarrhea, ventral edema, and ascites. The dogs are usually lethargic and thin but polyphagic by the time they are finally seen for evaluation. Deep palpation of the abdomen will not be painful so that mesenteric lymphadenopathy or thickened intestines may be appreciated as long as the ascites is not too severe. D-xylose and fat absorption may be defective, but this will depend upon how severely the small intestine is involved.[292] Dogs in which the lesion is restricted to ileum may pass soft or formed feces containing large amounts of mucus and clotted blood.[293,294]

Laboratory Findings. The most consistent clinical laboratory finding in dogs with GE is hypoproteinemia in the face of normal liver and kidney profiles. Studies with intravenously injected ^{51}Cr-albumin have indicated that this is a protein-losing enteropathy,[292] although small intestinal malabsorption could also be contributing to the hypoalbuminemia. Blood counts are not helpful in making a definitive diagnosis but often show microcytic anemia.

Other Diagnostic Procedures. Regional lesions may be localized by contrast radiography using a barium swallow. Further, if the disease is affecting the intestinal tract diffusely, barium swallow may show a scalloping of the mucosal surface or thickening of the intestinal wall.[288,293] Many other disease processes can cause similar patterns, however; thus the radiographic findings must be interpreted in the context of all the results of the clinical workup and may not be worth the expense and effort.

In the final analysis, the only way canine granulomatous enteritis can be definitively distinguished from lymphangiectasia, lymphocytic/plasmacytic enteritis, lymphosarcoma, and even some cases of eosinophilic enteritis, is by intestinal biopsy. Since it is necessary to obtain full-thickness sections of the intestine, a laparotomy must be done.

Therapy. Veterinary experience with treatment of GE in dogs is extremely limited. Medical therapy for mild cases in humans has involved the use of salicylazosulfapyridine (SASP) and a corticosteroid, in combination or separately. The cleavage of the SASP at the azo- linkage by intestinal bacteria makes an antibacterial agent (sulfapyridine) and an anti-inflammatory/anti-prostaglandin synthetase agent (5 aminosalicylic acid) available close to the site of the lesion(s).[295] This drug works best, then, for disease of distal ileum and colon. Corticosteroids are used for their anti-inflammatory and immunosuppressive properties and are advocated by some as the only therapy for granulomatous enteritis in people,[288] and have been reported to be effective in dogs with regional disease.[294] Two other drugs, an antimetabolite azathioprine,[296] and an agent that kills anaerobic enteric flora, metronidazole,[297] have been reported as effective in some human cases, but not in others.

If the lesion is localized well enough, the most practical treatment would be surgical removal.

Lymphangiectasia

Lymphangiectasia refers to a group of small intestinal disorders, the outstanding histologic feature of which is marked lacteal dilatation. Lacteal dilatation may also be seen in the chronic infiltrative enteritides[292,298,299] (e.g., plasmacytic/lymphocytic, granulomatous) where there is, no doubt, restriction of lymph flow through the affected submucosa, so the sections should be examined carefully. Lymphangiectasia may also be caused by congestive heart failure where there is a general increase in pressure within the lymphatic system.[300] The cause of the lesion's occurrence as a primary entity is unknown, but there is an associated hypoprotcinemia because this is definitely a protein-losing enteropathy. It is not clear whether dilatation of the lacteals occurs first or whether it is a reflection of the hypoalbuminemia.

Intestinal lymphangiectasia in humans is associated with immunologic abnormalities such as hypogammaglobulinemia, lymphocytopenia, skin anergy, impaired allograft formation, and defective lymphocyte transformation.[300] There is a reduction of recirculation of long-lived lymphocytes into the gastrointestinal tract, resulting in a relative depletion of the population of lymphocytes necessary for in vitro blast formation.[301] Nonselective depletion of serum IgA, IgM, and IgG suggests that the hypogammaglobulinemia is due primarily to loss into the intestinal tract, while in fact their synthetic rates are normal.[284]

Small intestinal lymphangiectasia as the outstanding single lesion has rarely been reported in animals, probably because, until recently, it has not been sought. Documented cases in cattle and dogs have occurred.[298,302]

Cattle. The signs of chronic profuse diarrhea, progressive cachexia and pale mucous membranes described in one study of 10 cows with lymphangiectasia were indistinguishable from Johne's disease (paratuberculosis).[298] In fact, half of the cases were definitively diagnosed as paratuberculosis. Affected animals were hypoproteinemic and anemic. No immunoglobulin studies were done.

Definitive diagnosis of such animals would have to be made by intestinal biopsy or necropsy. Jejunum and ileum should be examined. In the study just mentioned, marked lacteal dilatation with some branched villi and irregularly shaped crypts were seen histologically in the primary cases. Intercellular spaces between absorptive cells were distended, with epithelial perforation by these dilated channels. In contrast to Johne's disease, submucosal and subserosal lymph vessels were normal. There was an associated gastritis (abomasitis), however, which is not seen in the human disease. The abomasal lesions looked like a reaction to parasite infestation though no nematodes were found.

Dogs. Clinical Signs. Signs of intestinal lymphangiectasia in dogs are essentially indistinguishable from those described for granulomatous enteritis (GE) except that vomiting is rare. If damage to mucosa and submucosa is minimal, which is not the case with GE, xylose or glucose absorption may or may not be abnormal and starch tolerance will be normal. Steatorrhea is common but the fat present is mainly in digested form.

Laboratory Findings. Clinical laboratory studies reveal that the serum concentration of both albumin and globulin is reduced. Serum protein electrophoresis has not been helpful in distinguishing among various forms of the canine protein-losing enteropathy, however. Lymphopenia is present in 50% or more of cases.[303] Serum cholesterol and triglycerides are low, probably reflecting excess leakage into the bowel, although this explanation has not been verified experimentally. Lymphopenia is also seen in cases of small intestinal malabsorption due to villous atrophy although these animals have normal serum cholesterol levels.

As mentioned, dogs with primary small intestinal lymphangiectasia have steatorrhea due mainly to increased concentration of fatty acids, which do not stain well with Sudan III. If a saline suspension of feces is mixed with a drop of glacial acetic acid and a drop of Sudan III on a slide and heated, the fatty acids will form into yellow-red radiating crystals while any triglycerides present will show as red droplets.[304] In contrast, feces from a pancreatic deficient patient will show primarily red droplets when so treated.

The only definite way known, at present, to diagnose this disease is intestinal biopsy. Jejunum and ileum should be sampled for the most accurate picture if the biopsy is via laparotomy. This would be one instance where per oral biopsy by capsule should be helpful especially if the capsule can be directed into the jejunum.

Therapy. Treatment of some of these cases can be very rewarding, though it is difficult to predict precisely which will respond and which will not. The aim of successful therapy is to reduce, or preferably eliminate, long chain triglycerides in the food (i.e., most of the fats present in regular canine diets), since these fats are absorbed directly into the intestinal lymphatic system. This involves teaching owners how to procure and properly prepare nutritious defatted foods for their dog. In order to make up for the absent triglyceride, and thus provide calories without overfilling the animal, medium chain triglycerides (MCT) may be added. MCT are as calorically dense as LCT but are split in the intestinal lumen to medium chain fatty acids and glycerol, which are absorbed into the portal venous system.[305] MCT are available commercially in an oil form. They are not as palatable as LCT but are acceptable if mixed into commercial low-fat diet (ID, Riviana Foods) or boiled meat and rice in amounts of 1 teaspoon to 1 tablespoon t.i.d.,[303] depending upon dog size. A commercial powdered mixture of vitamins, electrolytes, and MCT (Portagen, Mead-Johnson) is also useful, added to the canned low-fat dog food. This should be regarded strictly as supportive, not curative, therapy and may not always be effective. Occasional parenteral injections of fat-soluble vitamins are also indicated.

Intestinal Amyloidosis

Intestinal amyloidosis is generally part of a generalized disease process where the outstanding clinical abnormalities are more often related to renal rather than gastrointestinal dysfunction. All species are potentially vulnerable, though the lesion is seen most commonly in cattle,[306] dogs,[307] and cats.[308,309] Gastrointestinal amyloidosis in the carnivora is usually an incidental finding; for instance, four of six cats with generalized amyloid involvement had infiltration of the lamina propria of the small intestine, though the mucosa appeared normal and no signs of intestinal dysfunction were noted.[308] Cattle with amyloidosis, however, usually have a profuse watery diarrhea.[306]

Along with the diarrhea, clinical signs in cattle include progressive weight loss, and development of ventral edema. Rectal examination often reveals marked nonpainful enlargement of the kidney, which should help to distinguish amyloidosis from Johne's disease.

Affected cattle are hypoalbuminemic and uremic. The low serum albumin is due to nephropathy. Thus, there is a marked proteinuria, in contrast to Johne's disease and parasitism where the hypoproteinemia is due to a protein-losing enteropathy.

Pathologically, the intestinal tract of cattle with amyloidosis may appear grossly normal. Histologic examination reveals widespread deposition, however, especially around lymphatics and blood vessels, with lymphangiectasia of the small intestinal villi.[306]

Eosinophilic Gastroenteritis of Dogs

Eosinophilic gastroenteritis refers to a disease of stomach and/or small intestine characterized by infiltration of the lamina propria with eosinophils, without evidence of edema or vasculitis.[171] The presence of eosinophils implies that the lesion is reagin-induced, but studies in humans suggest that it is not a single reversible allergic reaction to specific foods but rather a self-perpetuating process which may be symptomatically aggravated by different foods[310] or other antigens.[311] Recently the lesion has been reported in young German Shepherds associated with visceral migration of *Toxocara canis* larvae.[312] In the majority of afflicted dogs the cause cannot be determined.

Clinical Signs. The signs are persistent or recurrent and related to the site of gastrointestinal tract involvement; that is, vomiting may be the outstanding feature in cases where the lesion is confined to stomach or upper duodenum while chronic diarrhea indicates lower small intestinal infiltration. Hematochezia may also be seen. Other signs can include variable appetite, low-grade fever, and persistent weight loss.[313–315] Thickened tender loops of bowel may be palpated. Radiology is sometimes helpful in pointing out the extent of gastric and/or intestinal involvement, while contrast studies further define the degree of thickening of the gut wall.[313] Similarly, fiberoptic endoscopy may reveal areas of submucosal infiltration and loss of organ distensibility. Unfortunately, however, in my experience, biopsy by either endoscope or capsule is rarely helpful since the lesion is too deep within the wall. If biopsy is required for a definitive diagnosis, a full-thickness section of gut must be obtained via laparotomy.

Laboratory Findings. A persistent absolute blood eosinophil count or more than 2000 cells/cmm, combined with the previously described signs, is highly suggestive of the diagnosis, but not seen in all cases.[313] Patients are usually hypoalbuminemic since this is a protein-losing enteropathy.[311] Intestinal function studies (xylose, glucose or vitamin A absorption, and fecal fat analysis) occasionally indicate some degree of malabsorption, dependent undoubtedly upon the extent of the lesion. The presence of large numbers of ascarid ova in the feces suggests visceral larval migrans-induced disease.[312]

Necropsy Findings. The lesion is grossly indicated by thickening of the bowel wall. This may occur in a patchy distribution or be diffuse within a rather large segment of bowel. The mucosal surface is raised and congested, giving it a cobblestone appearance. Histologically, the lamina propria is infiltrated with eosinophils and fibrous tissue while the overlying mucosa may show villous atrophy.[171] There is inflammatory cell infiltration of the submucosa. In those cases where visceral larval migrans (VLM) is the inciting agent, cross-section of larvae surrounded by eosinophilic granulomas may be found.[312] Mesenteric lymphadenopathy, characterized by hyperplastic cortical lymphoid follicles, and occasionally the presence of a larva, is another feature of the VLM form of the disease. Lungs and liver also give evidence of larval migration.

Therapy. Most dogs with eosinophilic enteritis respond satisfactorily to treatment with corticosteroids. Oral prednisone (2.2 mg/kg/day) tapered over a 2- to 3-week period is recommended.[313] Some cases may require long-term, persistent, low-dose therapy to remain stable, while for others intermittent (alternate day) steroid administration such as used to control some forms of skin atopy will suffice. Those dogs with VLM are regarded as more difficult to treat.[312] Perhaps adjunct treatment with large doses of thiabendazole (500 mg/kg) such as is used to treat strongyle larval migrans in horses might be helpful.

Lymphocytic/Plasmacytic Enteritis of Dogs (LPE)

Clinical Signs. This disease and lymphangiectasia probably comprise the two most common forms of protein-losing enteropathy in dogs. An mentioned before, their clinical signs are virtually indistinguishable in many cases. LPE may affect the large as well as the small bowel, however, thus causing a more severe diarrhea and dysentery.[292] Definitive diagnosis is by biopsy.

Necropsy Findings. The disease derives its name from the dense infiltration of the lamina propria by plasma cells. There are also varying degrees of submucosal infiltration, absorptive cell degeneration, villous atrophy, and lymphangiectasia. Edema is present throughout affected bowel.[292] It should be pointed out that biopsy via laparotomy is extremely risky in these patients since they have such a poor healing capacity.

Therapy. Three aspects of treatment of LPE should be considered: nutritional, antibiotic, and anti-inflammatory. As with primary lymphangiectasia, nutritional considerations include parenteral administration of B-complex and fat-soluble vitamins, and replacement of long-chain triglycerides by medium-chain triglycerides in the food. Corticosteroids are considered since this is thought to be an immune-complex disease. Reports of their effectiveness are anecdotal since no controlled therapeutic trials have been run. The antibiotic tylosin seems to be effective in some cases and does not cause any known undesirable side-effects.[316] The prognosis for a successful outcome is unfavorable, especially in long-standing cases that are hypoproteinemic and debilitated when presented for examination.

DIFFERENTIAL DIAGNOSIS—DISEASES OF OTHER SYSTEMS, CHRONIC ENTERITIDES OR NEOPLASIA

Swine, Dogs and Cats
    Pancreatic exocrine insufficiency
    Biliary obstruction
    Zollinger-Ellison syndrome (dogs)

CHRONIC NONINFLAMMATORY PANMALABSORPTIVE DISEASE

History and Signs Compatible
1. Increased appetite
2. Coprophagia
3. Persistent weight loss
4. Feces (except in horse where normal appearing if disease confined to small intestine)
    —watery
    —mushy
    —bulky
    —fetid
    —gassy
    —greasy (steatorrhea)
5. Thickened intestines
6. Increased borborygmi
7. Abdominal distention
8. Dermatopathy

In many instances, the diseases discussed in this section are clinically indistinguishable from each other. The title, "panmalabsorptive" disease, suggests that large portions of the small bowel mucosa are damaged so that malabsorption is nonselective. Reduced carbohydrate absorption (D-xylose,

D-glucose) combined with steatorrhea and increased or normal fecal trypsin content should be consistent clinical laboratory findings in pigs, dogs, and cats. Horses will also have reduced carbohydrate absorption but the feces will be normal in appearance.[317,318] Specific studies for assessing small intestinal absorptive function in ruminants remain to be developed.

Generally, intestinal biopsy is necessary for making a definitive diagnosis of diseases discussed in this section. Villous atrophy without accompanying inflammatory disease fits into this category. The emphasis here is on chronic disease, in contrast to the transient villous atrophy that occurs with some enteric viral infections. Rule-outs must include any of the chronic enteritides discussed in Chronic Enteritides or Neoplasia that may cause secondary abnormalities, the bacterial overgrowth ("stagnant loop") syndrome (see Partial (Chronic) Bowel Obstructions) and pancreatic exocrine insufficiency.

Alimentary Lymphosarcoma

Villous atrophy due to diffuse infiltration of the small intestinal wall by lymphosarcoma has been documented in many species.[313,318–322] If the mucosal damage is severe enough, signs of classic "malabsorption syndrome" may be seen. Dogs may have peritonitis due to intestinal perforation or hepatomegaly and splenomegaly.[323] Transabdominal or rectal palpation may reveal thickened intestines or mesenteric lymphadenopathy. Peripheral lymphadenopathy may also be found. The biopsy of an enlarged peripheral node may be helpful in making a definitive diagnosis. Occasionally, the animal will also be leukemic. Paracentesis abdominis should be attempted, with cytologic examination of the fluid directed at identification of tumor cells. Serology in cats is not reliable since the majority of cases of intestinal lymphosarcoma will be FeLV negative.[303]

In many instances, only small intestinal biopsy will be diagnostic. Grossly thickened bowel and enlarged mesenteric nodes should be excised for examination. If thickening of bowel is difficult to discern, sections of jejunum and ileum should be collected. Upon occasion, intestinal lymphosarcoma may be histopathologically and clinically difficult to distinguish from granulomatous enteritis, at least in horses. Nests of epithelioid cells and giant cells should be carefully sought. If present, they indicate GE. On a clinical level, protein-losing enteropathy is more severe with GE than with lymphosarcoma.

Therapy. Chemotherapy with various antimetabolites has been effective in treating some cases of lymphosarcoma in small animals. The course of treatment is long and expensive, however, and will not be discussed here.

"Idiopathic" Villous Atrophy (IVA)

In humans, villous atrophy without accompanying inflammation is referred to as "sprue." "Nontropical" sprue or "celiac disease" is due to an acquired hypersensitivity to the peptide gliadin, which is present in the gluten of many grains, especially wheat, rye, and barley.[320,324] "Tropical" sprue is thought to be due to an infectious agent (as yet unidentified) since the problem can be cured by oral tetracycline therapy.[325] With celiac disease, deficiency of fat-soluble vitamins and hypocalcemia are often found, while microcytic anemia and vitamin B_{12} deficiency are common features of tropical sprue.

Idiopathic villous atrophy has been documented in horses[317] and dogs;[319,326] there is no reason why it could not occur in all species. As yet, gliadin hypersensitivity (see Specific Food Intolerances), or any other specific cause, has not been identified in any species. Lack of accompanying lymphadenopathy and thickening of the intestinal walls would be more consistent with idiopathic villous atrophy than lymphosarcoma. As with lymphosarcoma, excessive plasma protein loss through the bowel is not a feature of IVA, which should help to distinguish it from malabsorption accompanying some of the chronic inflammatory bowel diseases. In the final analysis, however, definitive diagnosis is also dependent upon biopsy either via laparotomy or capsule passed per os (dog).[327]

Treatment of IVA with any success has been accomplished only in some canine cases. Oral antibiotics, particularly tetracycline or tylosin, oral prednisolone, or combinations of antibiotic and steroids have proven effective when applied on an empiric basis.[313] Supportive therapy with parenteral vitamin B_{12}, folic acid, and fat-soluble vitamins should also be considered. The prognosis for recovery should always be unfavorable, however, as some patients have proven to be refractory to all of the treatments mentioned.

The challenge remains to identify specific agents that cause IVA in animals in order for more rational therapy to be devised.

Chronic Ischemia

Mild malabsorption, as indicated by D-xylose absorption study, secondary to celiac arterial entrapment by the median arcuate ligament of the diaphragm, is a recognized syndrome in humans.[328] Clinical signs are primarily abdominal pain after eating; diarrhea and weight loss are not seen. The syndrome is surgically correctable.

It is possible that chronic ischemia, secondary to trauma or parasitic insult, might on rare occasions be responsible for malabsorptive disease in animals. For instance, vascular damage by migrating *Strongylus vulgaris* larvae has been postulated as one cause of D-xylose malabsorption in horses.[329]

DIFFERENTIAL DIAGNOSIS—DISEASES OF OTHER SYSTEMS, CHRONIC NONINFLAMMATORY PAN-MALABSORPTIVE DISEASE

Dogs and Cats
  Pancreatic exocrine insufficiency

Partial ("Chronic") Bowel Obstructions

History and Signs Compatible
  1. Persistent/recurrent abdominal pain
  2. Recurrent vomiting/gastric pooling
  3. Rumen distention
  4. Persistent weight loss
  5. Diarrhea
      ± melena
      ± steatorrhea ("stagnant-loop syndrome")
  6. Constipation
  7. Distended abdomen
  8. Palpable mass in abdomen
  9. Excess borborygmi

Any physical or functional abnormality which slows the passage of digesta to any degree along any portion of the small bowel over a prolonged period of time falls into this category of diseases. While obstruction occurring very high in the duodenum or accompanied by enteritis may cause vomiting or gastric/ruminal distention by fluid, the most typical clinical signs in partial small bowel obstruction are those related to malabsorption: weight loss in spite of maintained appetite, gassy, noisy bowel sounds, and chronic diarrhea (except in the horse). The signs of malabsorption are an indication of an overgrowth of enteric bacteria within the section of bowel where digesta flow is stagnated. Essentially, the bacterial flora within the stagnated loop resemble in number and species that which is normally found in the colon. Only recently have some of the more important consequences of such overgrowth been elucidated.

  1. Nutrients may be metabolized before they can

be absorbed, producing less-readily absorbable metabolites that draw water into the intestine.[330,331]

2. Bile salts are deconjugated, interfering with normal fat digestion.[332,333]

3. The small intestinal mucosa within the stagnant zone is physically altered by some of the bacterial metabolites produced, resulting in a protein-losing enteropathy and further malabsorption,[334,335] which may result in trapping of gas and fluid to cause recurrent abdominal pain.

Sometimes the presence of a stagnant-loop syndrome can be surmised by the history of previous small bowel surgery or trauma. Other times partial obstruction may be demonstrated by radiographic procedures including the oral instillation of radiopaque material. The palpation of an intra-abdominal mass along with signs of malabsorption should always increase the clinician's suspicion. Ultimately, surgical exploration of the abdomen may be necessary.

The usual absorptive studies are not helpful in definitively diagnosing a stagnant-loop syndrome. Therefore, it is no wonder that this diagnosis is not made more frequently in veterinary medicine. The techniques more recently developed in human medicine, utilizing the feeding of ^{14}C-tagged substrates (see Chapter 16) and quantitation of bacterial flora in a small bowel aspirate, need to be applied to animals.

Acquired Causes of Intestinal Stasis and Potential Bacterial Overgrowth

All Species

1. Anatomic displacements due to adhesions from previous trauma, ulcerations, or surgery.
2. Surgically created intestinal loops or blind pouches.
3. Partial devitalization of a small segment of bowel, interrupting its normal motor function, thus creating a "functional" obstruction.
4. Neoplastic[336–341] or non-neoplastic tumors (e.g., fat necrosis in cattle) that develop within the bowel wall or impinge upon it.
5. Large ascarid burden.
6. Foreign bodies and bezoars.

Special Species Considerations

1. Horses
   a. focal partial ischemia due to strongyle larval migrans damage, with recurrent colic, anterior mesenteric arteritis.
   b. diaphragmatic hernia—recurrent abdominal pain, fluid pooling in stomach.
   c. severe ascariasis—inadequate worming practice.
2. Cattle
   a. fat necrosis—palpable hard masses per rectum.
   b. partial cecal torsion—viscus dilatation just anterior to pelvic inlet.
   c. abomasal displacement—simultaneous auscultation and percussion in left flank produces a characteristic "ping."
3. Swine
   a. severe ascariasis—history of poor husbandry. Do a fecal egg count.
   b. foreign body ingestion—history?
4. Dogs
   a. cecal inversion—straining to defecate, flecks of frank blood in feces, radiographic demonstration by high barium enema.
   b. recurrent intussusception.
   c. string enteritis (may also be a peritonitis)—history of playing with stringed item; vomiting, melena, leukocytosis, and fever. If peritonitis is present, look for string caught under the base of the tongue.
   d. severe ascariasis.
5. Cats
   a. string enteritis.

Congenital Causes of Intestinal Stasis and Bacterial Overgrowth

Horse

Meckel's Diverticulum.[342] This pouching of the distal ileum is due to incomplete closure of the vitelline duct that runs between ileum and umbilicus prior to parturition.

In many cases of partial small intestinal obstruction, therapy involves surgical intervention and removal of the offending structure. Sometimes this may be impossible, even though indicated, as in advanced cases of fat necrosis in cattle where multiple loops of bowel are trapped within the mass.

If ascarids are responsible, treatment with piperazine may be all that is necessary.

In those situations where a stagnant loop has been created as a result of some surgical procedure that was necessary to save the animal's life, or where the cause is undetermined, the administration of oral antibacterial agents may alleviate the signs of malabsorption and colic. At least this is the case in human medicine; unfortunately, there is little documentation of these kinds of cases and treatment thereof in veterinary medicine to date.

Intermittent therapy may be all that is necessary. Agents which specifically reduce the number of anaerobes such as oral lincomycin or metronidazole may be more effective than tetracycline but this could depend upon which organism is overgrowing.[343,344] Initial supportive therapy with parenteral fat-soluble vitamins should also be considered.

COMPLETE BOWEL OBSTRUCTION (See also Chapter 24)

History and Signs Compatible.
1. Mild to severe abdominal pain.
2. Projectile vomiting (pigs, dogs, cats)—"fecal" vomitus.
3. Pooling of fluid in stomach (horses).
4. Rumen stasis/bloat.
5. Reduced defecation, ± melena, ± hematochezia, prominent mucus.
6. Abdominal distention.
7. Absence of intestinal sounds upon auscultation.
8. Distended 'loops" of small intestine—external or rectal palpation—marked abdominal "guarding."
9. Intra-abdominal mass appreciated upon external or rectal palpation.
10. Shock.

SPECIFIC FOOD INTOLERANCES

History and Signs Compatible.
1. Soon after eating a particular food or class of foods (consistent relationship):
   a. abdominal pain,
   b. diarrhea—± hematochezia.
   c. vomiting—± hematemesis.
2. Chronic dermatoses.

Many veterinarians have seen animals that contract a gastrointestinal disturbance every time they eat even a small amount of a certain food. When the food is withdrawn, the gastrointestinal disorder subsides. This sort of phenomenon is considered a food "intolerance," and while numerous food products have been implicated, good documentation of a specific food intolerance in veterinary medicine is rare.

Congenital Lactose Intolerance

Lactase activity within the intestinal mucosa diminishes in all species as they mature,[345,346] but certain animals may show an intolerance to milk early in life and remain particularly sensitive to milk products thereafter. Primary lactase deficiency is not indicated by any histologic lesions in the intestinal mucosa.[347] Its presence is suggested by a failure of plasma reducing substances to rise in concentration after feeding a lactose meal, and documented by the demonstration of reduced enzyme activity in small intestinal biopsy specimens (see Chapter 16).

Clinical signs of lactose intolerance are watery, frothy diarrhea which may be accompanied by mild colic due to small intestinal gaseous distention. The feces have an acid pH due to bacterial degradation of the unabsorbed sugar.

At present, true lactose intolerance has been documented only in dogs.[348] Cats and young horses also seem to be prime candidates although potentially it could occur in any species.

Protein Intolerance

In contrast to lactose intolerance, dietary protein intolerance is more likely to be a hypersensitivity where the reaction is manifested by some sort of gastrointestinal lesions. Some dogs contract vomiting and diarrhea when they eat certain red meats, probably in reaction to the meat protein.[349] Casein intolerance has been documented in young children, causing diarrhea and excessive gastrointestinal protein loss with edema formation within the intestinal wall.[350,351] There is no reason why this could not occur in domestic animals. The gliadin in gluten, a constituent of many grains, particularly wheat, rye, barley and oats, causes a severe hypersensitivity reaction in some people.[324] This is manifested by villous atrophy of the small intestinal mucosa ("nontropical sprue," "celiac sprue," "gluten-sensitive enteropathy"); the results are panmalabsorption with diarrhea, steatorrhea, and malnutrition.

In food hypersensitivity reactions, systems other than the gastrointestinal tract may also be involved. Associated skin problems seem to be especially prevalent.[352]

The most direct treatment of any food intolerance is to remove the offending dietary constituent. Often this may be difficult to identify. Once identified, replacement by a substance of similar nutritive value or palatability can be a problem. If a dog is found to be allergic to beef or horsemeat, for instance, lamb will often be tolerated.[349]

If a protein intolerance is severe and long-standing enough, the patient may have hypoproteinemia due to protein leakage from plasma to gut lumen across a reactive gut wall. In addition specific food hypersensitivity may be demonstrated in some but not all cases by skin testing.

ENTEROTOXIGENIC BOWEL DISEASE

History and Signs Compatible.
1. Normal temperature
2. Feces profuse
   —soupy
   —watery
   —fetid
   —basic pH
3. Mucous membranes pale
4. Poor capillary refill
5. Moderate to severe dehydration
6. Severe depression
7. Cool extremities
8. Coma

The pathophysiology of enterotoxigenic diarrhea in adults is the same as that in neonates (See Part I), namely, the induction of a hypersecretory state in the small bowel through increasing production of prostaglandin $F_2\alpha$ and subsequent activation of cyclic-AMP. The colon cannot compensate for the excessive water and electrolytes that spill into it, thus the watery, alkaline diarrhea ensues. There probably is also an abnormality of motility which contributes to the signs.[19]

Epidemiology. The concept that enterotoxigenic *E. coli* might even cause disease in adults has only recently been discussed in human medicine,[13,18,353,354] and has yet to be documented in animals. It is important, however, that veterinary practitioners recognize that this condition could occur. *Clostridium perfringens* type A and *Staphylococcus aureus* also produce enterotoxins and have occasionally been implicated as the cause of diarrhea in domestic animals. The major problem at present is that there is no easy way to document infection by any of the preceding agents. Simple fecal cultures are noncontributory and the organisms cause no histopathologic changes in the intestine. Special techniques are available for identifying enterotoxin production by *E. coli,* using infant mice and adrenal cell cultures,[23] and it is procedures such as these, combined with compatible clinical signs, upon which a definitive diagnosis must be based.

Clinical Signs. Profuse, watery, nondysenteric diarrhea, lack of fever and rapid dehydration are more indicative clinical signs of intestinal infection by toxigenic than invasive bacteria such as salmonellae. Absence of fecal leukocytes, normal WBC count, normal or high serum protein concentration, hyperkalemia, and marked metabolic acidosis are clinical laboratory findings that are a further indication of enterotoxigenic disease.

Therapy. Treatment should be directed primarily at correcting the water, electrolyte, and acid-base imbalances. Intravenous therapy will be necessary for severely depressed or comatose animals; the fluid of choice is an isotonic multi-electrolyte solution (MES) that contains bicarbonate precursors, such as acetate or gluconate. If the patient is severely dehydrated and depressed, 5% $NaHCO_3$ is recommended for initial intravenous therapy followed by MES. Approximations of bicarbonate deficit and rules of thumb for application of fluids are outlined in Table 23–4. If equipment for measuring blood gases is readily available, it should be used to guide initial therapy and monitor the patient's progress.

If the patient is willing to drink or is ambulatory, oral fluid replacement therapy in part or in toto may suffice. For the carnivora, a dextrose-electrolyte solution, presented in Table 23–5, is recommended. For adult horses and ruminants, the same electrolyte mixture in a concentration of 120 to 160 g per 15 liters of water, without the dextrose, can be tried. Fresh water and salt block should always be available.

The use of antibacterial drugs in the treatment of toxigenic intestinal disease is controversial. Some contend that fluids alone are indicated. Others feel that reduction of the numbers of offending organisms by oral antibiotic administration will shorten the course of the illness and that the risk of further disrupting the normal intraluminal microcosm by this therapy must be taken.

Prophylaxis. The most effective prophylaxis against enterotoxigenic intestinal disease is good management, that is, provision of a clean environment. Possible concentrated sources such as contaminated drinking water or unusual foods should also be looked for and eliminated.

REFERENCES

1. Smith, H. W.: The development of the flora of the alimentary tract in young animals. J. Pathol. Bacteriol. *90*:495, 1965.
2. Sears, H. J., Brownlee, I., and Uchiyama, J. K.: Persistence of individual strains of Escherichia coli in the intestinal tract of man. J. Bacteriol. *59*:293, 1950.
3. Craven, J. A., and Barnum, D. A.: Ecology of intestinal Escherichia coli in pigs. Can. J. Comp. Med. *35*:324, 1971.
4. Wray, C.: Factors influencing occurrence of colibacillosis in calves. Vet. Rec. *96*:52, 1975.
5. Moon, H. W.: Pathogenesis of enteric diseases caused by Escherichia coli. *In* Advances in Veterinary Science and Comparative Medicine. Edited by C. A. Brandley and C. E. Cornelius. New York, Academic Press, 1974.
6. Stevens, A. J.: Coliform infections in the young pig and a practical approach to the control of enteritis. I. Vet. Rec. *75*:1241, 1963.
7. Reisinger, R. C.: Pathogenesis and prevention of infectious diarrhea (scours) of newborn calves. J.A.V.M.A. *147*:1377, 1965.
8. Logan, E. F., and Penhale, W. J.: Studies on the immunity of the calf to colibacillosis. Vet. Rec. *91*:419, 1972.

9. Boyd, J. W., Baker, J. R., and Leyland, A.: Neonatal diarrhea in calves. Vet. Rec. *95*:310, 1974.

10. Fey, H.: Immunology of the newborn calf: its relationship to colisepticemia. *In* Neonatal Enteric Infections Caused by Escherichia Coli. Edited by B. C. Tennant. Ann. N. Y. Acad. Sci. *176*:49, 1971.

11. Barnum, D. A., Glantz, P. J., and Moon, H. W.: Colibacillosis. Ciba Vet. Mono. Series/Two, 1967.

12. Field, M.: Intestinal secretion. Gastroenterology *66*:1063, 1974.

13. Grady, G. F., and Keusch, G. T.: Pathogenesis of bacterial diarrhea. N. Engl. J. Med. *285*:831 and 891, 1971.

14. Field, M.: New strategies for treating watery diarrhea. N. Engl. J. Med. *297*:1121, 1977.

15. Donawick, W. J., and Christie, B. A.: Clinico-pathologic conference. J.A.V.M.A. *158*:501, 1971.

16. Lewis, L. D., and Phillips, R. W.: Water and electrolyte losses in neonatal calves with acute diarrhea. Cornell Vet. *62*:596, 1972.

17. Tennant, B., Harrold, D., and Reina-Guerra, M.: Physiologic and metabolic factors in the pathogenesis of neonatal enteric infections in calves. J.A.V.M.A. *161*:998, 1972.

18. DuPont, H. L., Formal, S. B., Hornick, R. B., Snyder, M. J., Libonati, J. P., Sheahan, D. G., LaBrec, E. H., and Kalaz, J. P.: Pathogenesis of Escherichia coli diarrhea. N. Engl. J. Med. *285*:1, 1971.

19. Burns, T. W., Mathias, J. R., Carlson, G. M., Martin, J. L., and Shields, R. P.: The effect of heat-labile and heat-stabile Escherichia coli enterotoxin on small intestinal motility. Clin. Res. *25*:308A, 1977.

20. Mathias, J. R., Bertiger, G. M., Martin, J. L., and Cohen, S.: Migrating action potential complex of cholera: a possible prostaglandin-induced response. Am. J. Physiol. *232*:E529, 1977.

21. Dalton, R., Fisher, E. W., and McIntyre, J.: Changes in blood chemistry, body weight and hematocrit of calves affected with neonatal diarrhea. Br. Vet. J. *121*:34, 1965.

22. Fisher, E. W.: Hydrogen ion and electrolyte disturbances in the neonatal calf. *In* Neonatal Enteric Infections Caused by Escherichia Coli. Edited by B. C. Tennant. Ann. N. Y. Acad. Sci. *176*:223, 1971.

23. Moon, H. W., Whipp, S. C., and Skartvedt, S. M.: Etiologic diagnosis of diarrheal disease of calves: frequency and methods for detecting enterotoxin and K99 antigen production by Escherichia coli. Am. J. Vet. Res. *37*:1025, 1976.

24. Giannella, R. A.: Suckling mouse model for detection of heat-stabile Escherichia coli enterotoxin: characteristics of the model. Infect. Immunol. *14*:95, 1976.

25. Sérény, B.: Experimental Shigella keratoconjunctivitis: a preliminary report. Acta Microbiol. Acad. Sci. Hung. *2*:293, 1955.

26. Moon, H. W., Nielsen, N. O., and Kramer, T. T.: Experimental enteric colibacillosis of the newborn pig: histopathology of the small intestine and change in plasma electrolytes. Am. J. Vet. Res. *31*:103, 1970.

27. Christie, B. R., and Waxler, G. L.: Experimental colibacillosis in gnotobiotic baby pigs II. Pathology. Can. J. Comp. Med. *37*:271, 1973.

28. Staley, T. E., Jones, E. W., and Smith-Staley, J. A.: The effect of E. coli enterotoxins on the small intestine with or without direct mucosal contact. Am. J. Dig. Dis. *18*:751, 1973.

29. Aserkoff, B., and Bennett, J. V.: Effect of antibiotic therapy in acute salmonellosis on the fecal excretion of salmonellae. N. Engl. J. Med. *281*:636, 1969.

30. Rosenthal, S.: Exacerbation of salmonella enteritis due to ampicillin. N. Engl. J. Med. *280*:147, 1969.

31. Barnum, D. A.: The control of neonatal colibacillosis of swine. *In* Neonatal Enteric Infections Caused by Escherichia Coli. Edited by B. C. Tennant. Ann. N. Y. Acad. Sci. *176*:385, 1971.

32. Bywater, R. J.: Evaluation of an oral glucose-glycine-electrolyte formulation and amoxicillin for treatment of diarrhea in calves. Am. J. Vet. Res. *38*:1983, 1977.

33. Dey, B. P., Blender, D. C., Burton, G. C., Mercer, H. E., and Tsutakawa, R. K.: Therapeutic responses of piglets to experimentally induced colibacillosis. Res. Vet. Sci. *23*:340, 1977.

34. Rhodes, C. S., Radostits, O. M., Wenkoff, M. S., Mitchell, M. E., and Spotswood, T. P.: Development of a rational basis for the clinical management of acute undifferentiated diarrhea in newborn calves. J.A.V.M.A. *163*:1189, 1973.

35. Reference deleted.

36. Lister, E. E., and Fisher, L. J.: Establishment of the toxic level of nitrofurazone for young liquid-fed calves. J. Dairy Sci. *53*:1490, 1970.

37. Socci, A., and Buzzi, L.: Nitrofuran poisoning in the calf (hemorrhagic syndrome). Folia Vet. Lat. *5*:670, 1975.

38. Lewis, L. D.: Calf diarrhea: causes, effects, prevention and treatment. Part III. Norden News, Spring, 1978.

39. Radostits, O. M.: Clinical management of diarrhea in calves. Bovine Pract. *8*:20, 1973.

40. Phillips, R. L., Lewis, L. D., and Knox, K. I.: Alterations in body water turnover and distribution in newborn calves with acute diarrhea. *In* Neonatal Enteric Infections Caused by Escherichia Coli. Edited by B. C. Tennant. Ann. N. Y. Acad. Sci. *176*:231, 1971.

41. Ericsson, C. D., Evans, D. G., DuPont, H. L., Evans, D. J., and Pickering, L. K.: Bismuth subsalicylate inhibits activity of crude toxins of Escherichia coli and Vibrio cholera. J. Infect. Dis. *136*:693, 1977.

42. DuPont, H. L., Sullivan, P., Pickering, L. K., Haynes, G., and Ackerman, P. B.: Symptomatic treatment of diarrhea with bismuth subsalicylate among students attending a Mexican University. Gastroenterology *73*:715, 1977.

43. McEwan, A. D., Fisher, E. W., Selman, I. E., and Penhale, W. J.: A turbidity test for the estimation of immune globulin levels in neonatal calf serum. Clin Chim. Acta *27*:155, 1970.

44. Naylor, J. M., and Kronfeld, D. S.: Refractometry as a measure of the immunoglobulin status of the newborn dairy calf: comparison with the zinc sulfate turbidity and single radial diffusion. Am. J. Vet. Res. *38*:1331, 1977.

45. Naylor, J. M., Kronfeld, D. S., Beck-Nielsen, S., and Bartholomew, R. C.: Plasma total protein measurement for prediction of disease and mortality in calves. J.A.V.M.A. *171*:635, 1977.

46. Myers, L. L.: Vaccination of cows with an Escherichia coli bacterin for the prevention of naturally occurring diarrheal disease in their calves. Am. J. Vet. Res. *37*:831, 1976.

47. Goodwin, R. F. W.: A wider view of neonatal diarrhea in the pig. Vet. Rec. *100*:26, 1977.

48. Gay, C. C.: In utero immunization of calves against coli-septicemia. Am. J. Vet. Res. *36*:625, 1975.

49. Kohler, E. M., Cross, R. F., and Bohl, E. H.: Protection against neonatal enteric colibacillosis in pigs suckling orally vaccinated sows. Am. J. Vet. Res. *36*:757,1975.

50. Kohler, E. M.: Protection of pigs against neonatal enteric colibacillosis with colostrum and milk from orally vaccinated sows. Am. J. Vet. Res. *35*:331, 1974.

51. Rutter, J. M.: Escherichia coli infections in piglets: pathogenesis, virulence and vaccination. Vet. Rec. *96*:171, 1975.

52. Kohler, E. M.: Oral vaccination of sows with enteropathogenic strains of E. coli—Reporting results of swine practitioners. Proc. Int. Pig. Vet. Soc., 4th Int. Congr., 1976, p. J.2.

53. Porter, P., Kenworthy, R., Holme, D. W., and Horsfield, S.: Escherichia coli antigens as dietary additives for oral immunization of pigs: trials with pig creep feeds. Vet. Rec. *92*:630, 1973.

54. Porter, P.: Oral immunization to prevent enteric colibacillosis of weaned pigs. Proc. Int. Pig Vet. Soc., 4th Int. Congr., 1976, p. J.3.

55. Grau, F. H., Brownlie, L. E., and Smith, M. G.: Effects of food intake on numbers of salmonellae and Escherichia coli in rumen and feces of sheep. J. Appl. Bacteriol. *32*:112, 1969.

56. Williams, L. P., and Newell, K. W.: Salmonella excretion in joy-riding pigs. Am. J. Publ. Health *60*:926, 1970.

57. Williams, B. M.: Environmental considerations in salmonellosis. Vet. Rec. *96*:318, 1975.

58. Smith, B. P., Reina-Guerra, M., and Hardy, A. J.: Prevalence and epizootiology of equine salmonellosis. J.A.V.M.A. *172*:353, 1973.

59. Bohnhoff, M., and Miller, C. P.: Enhanced susceptibility to salmonella infection in streptomycin-treated mice. J. Infect. Dis. *111*:117, 1962.

60. Morse, E. V., Duncan, M. A., Baker, J. S., Amstutz, H. E., Myhron, E. P., and Gossett, K. A.: Prevalence, clinical aspects, treatment and control of bovine salmonellosis. Bovine Pract. *11*:17, 1976.

61. Rothenbacher, H.: Mortality and morbidity in calves with salmonellosis. J.A.V.M.A. *147*:1211, 1965.

62. Nape, W. F.: Recovery of salmonellae from material in feed mills. Proc. 72nd Annu. Meet. U. S. Livestock Sanit. Assoc. 1968, p. 144.

63. Linton, A. H., Howe, K., Pethiyagoda, S., and Osborne, A. D.: Epidemiology of salmonella infection in calves (1): its relation to their husbandry and management. Vet. Rec. *94*:581, 1974.

64. Morse, E. V.: Salmonellosis—An environmental health problem. J.A.V.M.A. *165*:1015, 1974.

65. Richardson, A.: The transmission of Salmonella dublin to calves from adult carrier cows. Vet. Rec. *92*:112, 1973.

66. Jubb, K. V. F., and Kennedy, P. C.: Pathology of Domestic Animals, 2nd Ed., Vol. 2. New York, Academic Press, 1970, p. 84.

67. Smith, H. W., and Jones, J. E. T.: Observations on experimental

oral infection with *Salmonella dublin* in calves and *Salmonella choleraesuis* in pigs. J. Pathol. Bacteriol. *93*:141, 1967.

68. Jakeuchi, A.: Electron microscopic studies of experimental salmonella infection. I. Penetration into the intestinal epithelium by *Salmonella typhimurium*. Am. J. Pathol. *50*:109, 1967.

69. Giannella, R. A., Gots, R. E., Charney, A. N., Greenough, W. B., and Formal, S. B.: Pathogenesis of salmonella-mediated intestinal fluid secretion. Gastroenterology *69*:1238, 1975.

70. Kinsey, M. D., Dammin, G. T., Formal, S. B., and Gianella, R. A.: The role of altered intestinal permeability in the pathogenesis of salmonella diarrhea in the Rhesus monkey. Gastroenterology *71*:429, 1976.

71. Powell, D. W., Solberg, L. I., Plotkin, G. R., Catlin, D. H., Maenza, R. M., and Formal, S. B.: Experimental diarrhea. III. Bicarbonate transport in rat salmonella enterocolitis. Gastroenterology *60*:1076, 1971.

72. Rout, W. R., Formal, S. B., Dammin, G. J., and Gianella, R. A.: Pathophysiology of salmonella diarrhea in the Rhesus monkey: intestinal transport, morphological and bacteriological studies. Gastroenterology *67*:59, 1974.

73. Giannella, R. A., Rout, W. R., and Formal, S. B.: Effect of indomethacin on intestinal water transport in salmonella-infected Rhesus monkeys. Infect. Immun. *17*:136, 1977.

74. Giannella, R. A.: The importance of the intestinal inflammatory reaction in salmonella-mediated intestinal secretion. Gastroenterology *72*:A-39/1062, 1977 (Abst.).

75. Seaton, V. A.: Salmonellosis in the bovine animal. Bovine Pract. *11*:53, 1976.

76. O'Connor, P. J., Rogers, P. A. M., Colins, J. D., and McErlean, B. A.: On the association between salmonellosis and the occurrence of osteomyelitis and dry gangrene in calves. Vet. Rec. *91*: 549, 1972.

77. Hobbs, B. C.: Public health significance of salmonella carriers in livestock and birds. J. Appl. Bacteriol. *24*:340, 1961.

78. Gibson, E. A.: Reviews of the progress of dairy science: diseases of dairy cattle. Salmonella infection in cattle. J. Dairy Sci. *32*:97, 1965.

79. Smith, H. W.: Salmonella food poisoning in human beings. The part played by domestic animals. R. Soc. Health J. *89*:271, 1969.

80. Kampelmacher, E. H.: Salmonellosis in the Netherlands. An. Inst. Pasteur *104*:647, 1963.

81. Wilcock, B. P., and Olander, H. J.: The pathogenesis of porcine rectal stricture. II. Experimental salmonellosis and ischemic proctitis. Vet. Pathol. *14*:43, 1977.

82. Weaver, L. D.: Control of salmonellosis in calves: a clinical evaluation of dry cow vaccination. Proc. 9th Annual AABP Convention, 1976, p. 27.

83. Fisher, E. W., Martinez, A. A., Trainin, Z., and Meirom, R.: Studies on neonatal calf diarrhea. IV. Serum and faecal immune globulins in neonatal salmonellosis. Br. Vet. J., *132*:39, 1976.

84. Griner, L. A., and Bracken, F. K.: Clostridium perfringens (type C) in acute hemorrhagic enteritis of calves. J.A.V.M.A. *122*:99, 1953.

85. Griner, L. A., and Baldwin, E. M.: Further work on hemorrhagic enterotoxemia of infant calves and lambs. Proc. 91st Annu. Meet. Am. Vet. Med. Assoc., 1954, p. 45.

86. Reid, J. F. S.: The common diarrhea of sheep in Britain. Vet. Rec. *98*:496, 1976.

87. Berkholt, G. A.: Ulcerative enteritis—clostridial antigens. Am. J. Vet. Res. *36*:583, 1975.

88. Kent, T. H., and Moon, H. W.: The comparative pathogenesis of some enteric diseases. Vet. Pathol. *10*:414, 1973.

89. Mebus, C. A., Stair, E. L., Underdahl, N. R., and Twiehaus, M. J.: Pathology of neonatal calf diarrhea induced by a Reo-like agent. Vet. Pathol. *8*:490, 1971.

90. Mebus, C. A., Underdahl, N. R., Rhodes, M. B., and Twiehaus, M. J.: Calf diarrhea (scours) reproduced with a virus from a field outbreak. Nebraska Agric. Exp. Sta., Univ. of Nebraska, Lincoln, Nebr. Res. Bull. #233, 1969.

91. Flewett, T. H., Bryden, A. S., and Davies, H.: Virus diarrhea in foals and other animals. Vet. Rec. *96*:477, 1975.

92. Kanitz, C. L.: Identification of an equine rotavirus as a cause of neonatal foal diarrhea. Proc. 22nd Annual AAEP Convention, Dallas, 1976, p. 155.

93. Pearson, G. R., and McNulty, M. S.: Pathological changes in the small intestine of neonatal pigs infected with a pig Reovirus-like agent (Rotavirus). J. Comp. Pathol. *87*:363, 1977.

94. Snodgrass, D. R., Smith, W., Gray, E. W., and Herring, J. A.: Rotavirus in lambs with diarrhea. Res. Vet. Sci. *20*:113, 1976.

95. Woode, G. N., Bridger, J. C., Jones, J. M., Flewett, T. H., Bryden, A. S., Davis, H. A., and White, G. B. B.: Morphological and antigenic relationships between viruses (Rotaviruses) from acute gastroenteritis in children, calves, piglets, mice and foals. Infect. Immun. *14*:804, 1976.

96. Acres, S. D., Laing, C. J., Saunders, J. R., and Radostits, O. M.: Acute undifferentiated neonatal diarrhea in beef calves I. Occurrence and distribution of infectious agents. Can. J. Comp. Med. *39*:116, 1975.

97. McNulty, M. S., Allan, G. M., Curran, W. L., and McFerran, J. B.: Comparison of methods for diagnosis of Rotavirus infections of calves. Vet. Rec. *98*:463, 1976.

98. England, J. J., Frye, C. S., and Enright, E. A.: Negative contrast electron microscopic diagnosis of viruses of neonatal calf diarrhea. Cornell Vet. *66*:172, 1976.

99. Barnett, B. B., Spendlove, R. S., Peterson, M. W., Hsu, L. Y., LaSalle, V. A., and Egbert, L. N.: Immunofluorescent cell assay of neonatal calf diarrhea virus. Can. J. Comp. Med. *39*:462, 1975.

100. Mebus, C. A., White, R. G., Bass, E. P., and Twiehaus, M. J.: Immunity to neonatal calf diarrhea virus. J.A.V.M.A. *163*:880, 1973.

101. Mebus, C. A., Stair, E. L., Rhodes, M. B., and Twiehaus, M. J.: Neonatal calf diarrhea: propagation, attenuation, and characteristics of a corona virus-like agent. Am. J. Vet. Res. *34*:145, 1973.

102. Keenan, K. P., Jervis, H. R., Marchwicki, R. H., and Binn, L. N.: Intestinal infection of neonatal dogs with canine coronavirus 1–71: studies by virologic, histologic, histochemical and immunofluorescent techniques. Am. J. Vet. Res. *37*:247, 1976.

103. Bass, E. P., and Sharpee, R. L.: Coronavirus and gastroenteritis in foals. Lancet *2*:822, 1975.

104. Bohl, E. H., and Cross, R. F.: Clinical and pathological differences in enteric infections in pigs caused by *Escherichia Coli* and by transmissible gastroenteritis virus. *In* Neonatal Enteric Infections Caused by Escherichia Coli. Edited by B. C. Tennant. Ann. N. Y. Acad. Sci. *176*:150, 1971.

105. Moon, H. W.: Mechanisms in the pathogenesis of diarrhea: a review. J.A.V.M.A. *172*:443, 1978.

106. Mebus, C. A.: Viral calf enteritis. J. Dairy Sci. *59*:1175, 1976.

107. Morin, M., Morehouse, L. G., Solorzano, R. F., and Olson, L. D.: Transmissible gastroenteritis in feeder swine: clinical, immunofluorescence and histopathological observations. Can. J. Comp. Med. *37*:239, 1973.

108. Binn, L. N., Lazar, E. C., Keenan, K. P., Huxsoll, D. L., Marchwicki, R. H., and Straus, A. J.: Recovery and characterization of a corona-virus from military dogs with diarrhea. Proc. 78th Annu. Meet. U. S. Anim. Health Assoc., 1974, p. 359.

109. Butler, D. G., Gall, D. G., Kelly, M. H., and Hamilton, J. R.: Transmissible gastroenteritis: mechanisms responsible for diarrhea in an acute viral enteritis in piglets. J. Clin. Invest. *53*:1335, 1974.

110. Hooper, B. E., and Haelterman, E. O.: Lesions of the gastrointestinal tract of pigs infected with transmissible gastroenteritis. Can. J. Comp. Med. *33*:29, 1969.

111. Giles, N., Borland, E. D., Counter, D. E., and Gibson, E. A.: Transmissible gastroenteritis in pigs: some observations on laboratory aids to diagnosis. Vet. Rec. *100*:336, 1977.

112. Saif, L., Bohl, E. H., Kohler, E., and Hughes, J.: Immune electron microscopy of transmissible gastroenteritis virus and rotavirus of swine. Am. J. Res. *38*:13, 1977.

113. Mebus, C. A., Newman, L. E., and Stair, E. L.: Scanning, electron, light and immunofluorescent microscopy of intestine of gnotobiotic calf infected with calf diarrheal coronavirus. Am. J. Vet. Res. *36*:1719, 1975.

114. Haelterman, E. O.: Personal communication: Purdue University, West Lafayette, IN, 1978.

115. Thurber, E. T., Bass, E. P., and Beckenhauer, W. H.: Field trial evaluation of a reo-coronavirus calf diarrhea vaccine. Can. J. Comp. Med. *41*:131, 1977.

116. Store, S. S., Stark, S. L., and Phillips. M.: Transmissible gastroenteritis virus in neonatal pigs: intestinal transfer of colostral immunoglobulins containing specific antibodies. Am. J. Vet. Res. *35*:339, 1974.

117. Bohl, E. H.: Transmissible gastroenteritis. *In* Diseases of Swine, 4th ed. Edited by H. W. Dunne and A. D. Leman. Ames, Iowa University Press, 1975.

118. Lambert, G., McClurkin, A. W., and Fernelius, A. L.: Bovine viral diarrhea in the neonatal calf. J.A.V.M.A. *163*:1189, 1973.

119. Rosenquist, B. D., and Dobson, A. W.: Multiple viral infection in calves with acute bovine respiratory tract disease. Am. J. Vet. Res. *35*:363, 1974.

120. Mills, J. H. L., and Luginbuhl, R. E.: Distribution and persistence of mucosal disease virus in experimentally exposed calves. Am. J. Vet. Res. *29*:1367, 1968.

121. Lambert, G., Fernelius, A. L., and Cheville, N. F.: Experimental bovine viral diarrhea in neonatal calves. J.A.V.M.A. *154*:181, 1969.

122. Lambert, G.: Bovine viral diarrhea: prophylaxis and postvaccinal reactions. J.A.V.M.A. *163*:874, 1973.
123. Mattson, D. E.: Adenovirus infection in cattle. J.A.V.M.A. *163*:894, 1973.
124. Mattson, D. E.: Naturally occurring infection of calves with bovine adenovirus. Am. J. Vet. Res. *34*:623, 1973.
125. York, C. J., and Baker, J. A.: A new member of the psittacosis-lymphogranuloma group of viruses that causes infection in calves. J. Exp. Med. *93*:587, 1951.
126. Storz, J., Collier, J. R., Eugster, A. K., and Altera, K. P.: Intestinal bacterial changes in chlamydia-induced primary enteritis of newborn calves. *In* Neonatal Enteric Infections Caused by Escherichia Coli. Edited by B. C. Tennant. Ann. N. Y. Acad. Sci. *176*:162, 1971.
127. Doughri, A. M., Young, S., and Storz, J.: Pathologic changes in intestinal chlamydial infections of newborn calves. Am. J. Vet. Res. *35*:939, 1974.
128. Storz, J., and Bates, R. C.: Parvovirus infections in calves. J.A.V.M.A. *163*:884, 1973.
129. Soulsby, E. J. L.: Helminths, arthropods and protozoa of domestic animals (Mönnig), 6th ed. Baltimore, The Williams & Wilkins Co., 1968.
130. Meuten, D. J., and Von Kruiningen, H. J.: Cryptosporidiosis in a calf. J.A.V.M.A. *165*:914, 1974.
131. Pohlenz, J., Moon, H. W., Cheville, N. F., and Bemrick, W. J.: Cryptosporidiosis as a probable factor in neonatal diarrhea of calves. J.A.V.M.A. *172*:452, 1978.
132. Krakowka, S.: Transplacentally acquired intestinal and parasitic diseases of dogs. J.A.V.M.A. *171*:750, 1977.
133. Congdon, L. L., and Ames, E. R.: Thiabendazole for control of Toxacara canis in the dog. Am. J. Vet. Res. *34*:417, 1973.
134. Georgi, J. R.: Parasitology for Veterinarians, 2nd ed. Philadelphia, W. B. Saunders Co., 1974.
135. Soulsby, E. J. L.: Textbook of Veterinary Clinical Parasitology. Philadelphia, F. A. Davis Co., 1967.
136. Anderson, N. V.: Diseases of the small intestine. *In* Veterinary Internal Medicine. Edited by S. J. Ettinger, Philadelphia, W. B. Saunders Co. 1975.
137. Horlein, B. F.: The evaluation of various chemical agents in the treatment of soil infected with larvae of the dog hookworm (Ancylostoma caninum). North Am. Vet. *31*:253, 1950.
138. Rankin, J. D., and Taylor, R. J.: The estimation of doses of *Salmonella typhimurium* suitable for the experimental production of disease in calves. Vet. Rec. *78*:706, 1966.
139. Williams, L. P., Vaughn, J. B., and Blanton, V.: A ten-month study of salmonella contamination in animal protein meals. J.A.V.M.A. *155*:167, 1969.
140. Baker, J. R.: An outbreak of salmonellosis involving veterinary hospital patients. Vet. Rec. *85*:8, 1969.
141. Johnson, K. G.: Salmonellosis in calves due to lactose fermenting *Salmonella typhimurium*. Vet. Rec. *98*:276, 1976.
142. Kahrs, R., Bentinck-Smith, J., Bjorck, G. R., Brunner, D. W., King, J. M., and Lewis, N. F.: Epidemiologic investigation of an outbreak of fatal enteritis and abortion with dietary change and *Salmonella typhimurium* infection in a dairy herd. A case report. Cornell Vet. *62*:175, 1972.
143. Tutt, J. B., and Hoare, D. J. B.: Disease associated with *S. typhimurium* in cattle. Vet. Rec. *95*:334, 1974.
144. Hall, G. A., and Jones, P. W.: A study of the pathogenesis of experimental *Salmonella dublin* abortion in cattle. J. Comp. Pathol. *87*:53, 1977.
145. Morse, E. V., Duncan, M. A., Estep, D. A., Riggs, W. A., and Blackburn, B. O.: Canine salmonellosis: a review and report of dog to child transmission of salmonella enteritis. Am. J. Publ. Health *66*:82, 1976.
146. Caraway, C. T., Scott, A. E., Roberts, N. C., and Hansen, G. A.: Salmonellosis in sentry dogs. J.A.V.M.A. *135*:599, 1959.
147. Förster, D., and Holland, V.: Occurrence of salmonella in the dog. Zentralbl. Veterinaermed. *21B*:124, 1974.
148. See ref. 29. Reference deleted.
149. Antibiotics in gastroenteritis (Editorial). Lancet *2*:1169, 1970.
150. Fox, I. W., Hoag, W. G., and Strout, J.: Breed susceptibility, pathogenicity, and epidemiology of endemic coliform enteritis in the dog. Lab. Anim. Care *15*:194, 1965.
151. Vantrappen, G., Agg. H. O., Ponette, E., Geboes, K., and Bertrand, P.: Yersinia enteritis and enterocolitis: gastroenterological aspects. Gastroenterology *72*:220, 1977.
152. Kaneko, K., Hamada, S., and Kato, E.: Occurrence of Yersinia enterocolitica in dogs. Jpn. J. Vet. Sci. *39*:407, 1977.
153. Karstad, L., Landsverk, T., and Lassen, J.: Isolation of Yersinia enterocolitica from a dog with chronic enteritis. Acta Vet. Scand. *17*:261, 1976.

154. Scott, F. W., Kahrs, R. F., Campbell, S. G., and Hillman, R. B.: Etiologic studies on bovine winter dysentery. Bovine Pract. *8*:40, 1973.
155. Kahrs, R. F., Scott, F. W., and Hillman, R. B.: Epidemiologic observations on bovine winter dysentery. Bovine Pract. *8*:36, 1973.
156. Estes, P. C.: Equine viral arteritis. Vet. Pathol. *9*:83, 1972.
157. Larsen, S., Flagstad, A., and Aalbaek, B.: Experimental feline panleukopenia in the conventional cat. Vet. Pathol. *13*:216, 1976.
158. Baker, J. A., York, C. J., Gillespie, J. H., and Mitchell, G. B.: Virus diarrhea in cattle. Am. J. Vet. Res. *15*:525, 1954.
159. Carlson, J. H., Scott, F. W., and Duncan, J. R.: Feline panleukopenia I. Pathogenesis in germ-free and specific pathogen free cats. Vet. Pathol. *14*:79, 1977.
160. Bürki, F.: The virology of equine arteritis. *In* Equine Infectious Diseases, Vol. II. Edited by J. T. Bryans and H. Gerber. Basel, S. Karger, 1970.
161. Kendrick, J. W.: Bovine viral diarrhea: decay of colostrum-conferred antibody in the calf. Am. J. Vet. Res. *35*:589, 1974.
162. Pritchard, W. R.: The bovine viral diarrhea-mucosal disease complex. Adv. Vet. Sci. *8*:2, 1963.
163. Bruner, D. W., and Gillespie, J. H.: Hagan's Infectious Diseases of Domestic Animals. Ithaca, NY, Cornell University Press, 1973.
164. Kahrs, R. F.: Differential diagnosis of bovine viral diarrhea-mucosal disease. J.A.V.M.A. *153*:1652, 1968.
165. Kahrs, R. F.: The relationship of bovine viral diarrhea-mucosal disease to abortion in cattle. J.A.V.M.A. *159*:1383, 1971.
166. Herrick, J. B.: Preconditioning feeder cattle. *In* Bovine Medicine and Surgery. Edited by W. J. Gibbons, E. J. Catcott, and J. F. Smithcors. Wheaton, IL, American Veterinary Publications, 1970.
167. Gray, A. P., and Anthony, H. D.: Outbreak of malignant catarrhal fever in Kansas. Proc. 72nd Annu. Meet. U. S. Livestock Sanit. Assoc., 1968, p. 456.
168. Pierson, R. E., Thake, D., McChesney, A. E., and Storz, J.: An epizootic of malignant catarrhal fever in feedlot cattle. J.A.V.M.A. *163*:349, 1973.
169. Pierson, R. E., Storz, J., McChesney, A. E., and Thake, D.: Experimental transmission of malignant catarrhal fever. Am. J. Vet. Res. *35*:523, 1974.
170. Plowright, W.: Malignant catarrhal fever. J.A.V.M.A. *152*:795, 1968.
171. Jubb, K. V. F., and Kennedy, P. C.: Pathology of Domestic Animals. 2nd ed., Vol. 2, p. 27. New York, Academic Press, 1970.
172. Blood, D. C., Henderson, J. A., and Radostits, O. M.: Veterinary Medicine, 5th ed. Philadelphia, Lea & Febiger, 1979.
173. Jensen, R.: Diseases of Sheep. Philadelphia, Lea & Febiger, 1974.
174. Hardy, W. T., and Price, D. A.: Sore muzzle of sheep. J.A.V.M.A. *120*:23, 1952.
175. McKercher, D. G., McGowan, B., Howarth, J. A., and Saito, J. K.: A preliminary report on the isolation and identification of the bluetongue virus from sheep in California. J.A.V.M.A. *122*:300, 1953.
176. Griner, L. A., McCroy, B. R., Foster, N. M., and Meyer, H.: Bluetongue associated with abnormalities in newborn lambs. J.A.V.M.A. *145*:1013, 1964.
177. Shultz, G., and DeLay, P. D.: Losses in newborn lambs associated with bluetongue vaccination of pregnant ewes. J.A.V.M.A. *127*: 224, 1955.
178. Montgomery, R. E.: Tick-borne gastroenteritis of sheep and goats in East Africa. J. Comp. Pathol. Ther. *30*:28, 1917.
179. Cartwright, S., and Lucas, M.: Vomiting and diarrhea in dogs. Vet. Rec. *91*:571, 1972.
180. Binn, L. N., Lazar, E. C., Keenan, K. P., Huxsoll, D. L., Marchwicki, R. H., and Strano, A. J.: Recovery and characterization of a coronavirus from military dogs with diarrhea. Proceedings 78th Annu. Meet. U. S. Anim. Health Assoc. *78*:359, 1975.
181. Horner, G. W., Hunter, R., and Kirkbride, C. A.: A coronavirus-like agent in the feces of cows with diarrhea. N.Z. Vet. J. *23*:98, 1975.
181a. Appel, M. J. G., Cooper, B. J., Griesen, H., Scott, F. and Carmichael, L. E.: Canine viral enteritis. I. Status report on corona- and parvo-like viral enteritides. Cornell Vet., *68*:123, 1979.
181b. Cooper, B. J., Carmichael, L. E., Appel, M. J. G. and Griesen, H.: Canine viral enteritis. II. Morphologic lesions in naturally occurring parvovirus infection. Cornell Vet., *68*:134, 1979.
181c. Hayes, M. A., Russell, R. G., and Babiuk, L. A.: Sudden death in young dogs with myocarditis caused by parovirus. J.A.V.M.A., *174*:1197, 1979.
182. Carlson, J. H., and Scott, F. W.: Feline panleukopenia II. The relationship of intestinal mucosal cell proliferation rate to viral infection and development of lesions. Vet. Pathol. *14*:173, 1977.
183. Farrow, B. R. H., and Love, D. N.: Infectious diseases. *In* Textbook of Veterinary Internal Medicine. Edited by S. J. Ettinger. Philadelphia, W. B. Saunders Co., 1975.

184. Seelig, W. S.: Mechanisms by which antibiotics increase the incidence and severity of candidiasis and alter the immunologic defenses. Bacteriol. Rev. *30*:442, 1966.

185. Smith, J. M. B.: Mycoses of the alimentary tract of animals. N.Z. Vet. J. *16*:89, 1968.

186. Edds, G.T.: Acute aflatoxicosis: a review. J.A.V.M.A. *162*:304, 1973.

187. Stokes, R.: Intestinal mycosis in a cat. Aust. Vet. J. *49*:499, 1973.

188. Barsanti, J. A., Attleberger, M. H., and Henderson, R. A.: Phycomycosis in a dog. J.A.V.M.A. *167*:293, 1975.

189. Silverman, E. M., Norman, L. E., Goldman, R. T., and Simmona, J.: Diagnosis of systemic candidiasis in smears of venous blood stained with Wright's stain. Am. J. Clin. Pathol. *60*:473, 1973.

190. Van Uden, N.: The occurrence of candida and other yeasts in the intestinal tract of animals. Ann. N.Y. Acad. Sci. *89*:59, 1960.

191. Brandborg, L. L.: Other infections, inflammatory and miscellaneous diseases. *In* Gastrointestinal Disease. Edited by M. H. Sleisenger and J. S. Fordtran. Philadelphia, W. B. Saunders Co., 1973.

192. Kelly, J. D.: Mechanisms of immunity to intestinal helminths. Aust. Vet. J. *49*:91, 1973.

193. Gibson, T. E.: Recent advances in the epidemiology and control of parasitic gastroenteritis in sheep. Vet. Rec. *92*:469, 1973.

194. Soulsby, E. J. L.: Determinants of parasitism: factors in pathogenesis. *In* Pathophysiology of Parasitic Infection. Edited by E. J. L. Soulsby. New York, Academic Press, 1976.

195. Patton, S., Mock, R. E., Drudge, J. H., and Morgan, D.: Increase in immunoglobulin T concentration in ponies as a response to experimental infection with the nematode Strongylus vulgaris. Am. J. Vet. Res. *39*:19, 1978.

196. Mirck, M.: On the life cycle of Strongyloides westeri in Shetland Ponies in the Netherlands. Trop. Geogr. Med. *27*:442, 1975.

197. Stewart, T. B., Stone, W. M., and Marti, O. G.: Strongyloides ransomi: prenatal and transmammary infection of pigs of sequential litters from dams experimentally exposed as weanlings. Am. J. Vet. Res. *37*:541, 1976.

198. Enigk, K., Dey-Hazra, A., and Eduardo, S. L.: Activity of disaccharidases and dipeptidases of the intestinal mucosa of piglets during mild and severe infections with Strongyloides ransomi. J. Comp. Pathol. *86*:243, 1976.

199. Franz, K. H.: Clinical trials with thiabendazole against human strongyloidosis. Am. J. Trop. Med. Hyg. *12*:211, 1963.

200. Drudge, J. H., and Lyons, E. T.: The chemotherapy of migrating strongyle larvae. *In* Equine Infectious Diseases, II. Edited by J. T. Bryans and H. Gerber. Basel, S. Karger, 1970.

201. Duncan, J. L., and Pirie, H. M.: The pathogenesis of single experimental infections with Strongylus vulgaris in foals. Res. Vet. Sci. *18*:82, 1975.

202. Patton, S., and Drudge, J. H.: Clinical response of pony foals experimentally infected with Strongylus vulgaris. Am. J. Vet. Res. *38*:2059, 1977.

203. Duncan, J. L.: Field studies on the epidemiology of mixed strongyle infection in the horse. Vet. Rec. *94*:337, 1974.

204. Pellérdy, L. P.: Coccidia and Coccidiosis. Budapest, Akademiai Kiado, 1965.

205. Slater, R. L.: Bovine coccidiosis: A review of the problem and projected new solutions. Proceedings 6th Annual AABP Convention. 1973, p. 147.

206. Taylor, S. M., O'Hogan, J., McCracken, A., McFerran, J. B., and Purcell, D. A.: Diarrhea in intensively reared lambs. Vet. Rec. *93*:461, 1973.

207. Norcross, M. A., Seigmund, O. H., and Fraser, C. M.: Amprolium for coccidiosis in cattle: a review of efficacy and safety. V.M./S.A.C. *69*:462, 1974.

208. Rose, M. E.: Coccidiosis: immunity and prospects for prophylactic immunization. Vet. Rec. *98*:481, 1976.

209. Weaver, A. D.: Arsenic poisoning in cattle following pasture contamination by drift of spray. Vet. Rec. *74*: 249, 1962.

210. Clarke, E. G. C.: Species differences in toxicology. Vet. Rec. *98*: 215, 1976.

211. Buck, W. B., Osweiler, G. D., and Van Gelder, G. A.: Clinical and Diagnostic Veterinary Toxicology. Dubuque, IA, Kendall/Hunt Publishing Co., 1973.

212. Oehme, F. W.: A survey of poisonings commonly observed by the bovine practitioner. D.V.M. Newsmagazine, Vol. 6, March/April 1974.

213. Case, A. A.: Toxicity of various chemical agents to sheep. Am. J. Vet. Res. *164*:277, 1974.

214. Stevenson, D. E.: Pesticides and domestic animals. Vet. Rec. *97*:164, 1975.

215. Aronson, C. E.: Thallium intoxication. *In* Current Veterinary Therapy, Vol. VI. Edited by R. W. Kirk. Philadelphia, W. B. Saunders Co., 1977.

216. Kingsbury, J. M.: Poisonous Plants of the United States and Canada. Englewood Cliffs, N.J., Prentice-Hall, 1964.

217. Jones, J. E. T.: An intestinal hemorrhage syndrome in pigs. Br. Vet. J. *123*:286, 1967.

218. Rowland, A. C., and Lawson, G. H. K.: Porcine intestinal adenomatosis: a possible relationship with necrotic enteritis, regional ileitis and proliferative hemorrhagic enteropathy. Vet. Rec. *97*:178, 1975.

219. Rowntree, P. G. M.: A hemorrhagic bowel syndrome in the pig. Vet Rec. *91*:347, 1972.

220. Love, R. J., Love, D. N., and Edwards, M. J.: Proliferative hemorrhagic enteropathy in pigs. Vet. Rec. *100*:65, 1977.

221. Burrows, C. F.: Canine hemorrhagic gastroenteritis. J.A.A.H.A. *13*:451, 1977.

222. Bernstein, M.: Hemorrhagic gastroenteritis. *In* Current Veterinary Therapy, Vol. VI. Edited by R. W. Kirk. Philadelphia, W. B. Saunders Co., 1977.

223. Haddock, R. L.: Asymptomatic salmonellosis in a swine herd. Am. J. Publ. Health *60*:2345, 1970.

224. Rothenbacher, H.: Mortality and morbidity in calves with salmonellosis. J.A.V.M.A. *147*:1211, 1965.

225. Barnes, D. M., and Bergeland, M. E.: Salmonella typhisuis infection in Minnesota swine. J.A.V.M.A. *152*:1766, 1968.

226. Thomas, G. W., and Harbourne, J. F.: Salmonella paratyphi B infection in dairy cows. Vet. Rec. *91*:148, 1972.

227. Bryans, J. T., Moore, B. O., and Crowe, M. W.: Safety and efficacy of furoxone in the treatment of equine salmonellosis. V.M./S.A.C. *60*:626, 1965.

228. DeGeeter, M. J., Stahl, G. L., and Geng, S.: Effect of lincomycin on prevalence, duration, and quantity of Salmonella typhimurium excreted by swine. Am. J. Vet. Res. *37*:525, 1976.

229. Clementi, K. J.: Trimethoprim-sulfamethoxazole in the treatment of carriers of salmonella. J. Infect. Dis. *128*:S 738, 1973.

230. Frances, J.: Tuberculosis in Animals and Man. London, Cassell & Co., 1958.

231. Merritt, A. M., Cimprich, R. E., and Beech, J.: Granulomatous enteritis in nine horses. J.A.V.M.A. *169*:603, 1976.

232. Snider, W. R.: Tuberculosis in canine and feline populations: study of high risk populations in Pennsylvania. Am. Rev. Respir. Dis. *104*:866, 1971.

233. Konyha, L. D., and Kreier, J. P.: The significance of tuberculin tests in the horse. Am. Rev. Respir. Dis. *103*:91, 1971.

234. Knight, H. D.: Corynebacterial infections in the horse: problems of prevention. J.A.V.M.A. *155*:446, 1969.

235. Cimprich, R. E., and Rooney, J. R.: Corynebacterium equi enteritis in foals. Vet. Pathol. *14*:95, 1977.

236. Larsen, A. B., Moon, H. W., and Merkal, R. S.: Susceptibility of horses to Mycobacterium paratuberculosis. Am. J. Vet. Res. *33*:2185, 1972.

237. Kopecky, K. E.: Distributions of bovine paratuberculosis in the United States. J.A.V.M.A. *162*:787, 1973.

238. Larsen, A. B.: Johne's disease. *In* Bovine Medicine and Surgery. Edited by W. J. Gibbons, E. J. Catcott, and J. F. Smithcors. Wheaton, IL, American Veterinary Publications, 1970.

239. Fouquet, G., and Delaney, G.: Phosphorus and Johne's disease. Recueil Med. *136*:467, 1960.

240. Larsen, A. B.: Can Johne's disease (paratuberculosis) be eradicated? Proceedings, Annual Convention AABP, 1974, p. 46.

241. Merkal, R. S., Larsen, A. B., and Booth, G. D.: Analysis of the effects of inapparent bovine paratuberculosis. Am. J. Vet. Res. *36*:837, 1975.

242. Goudswaard, J., Gilmour, N. J. L., and Dÿkstra, R. G.: Diagnosis of Johne's disease in cattle: a comparison of five serotypical tests under field conditions. Vet. Rec. *98*:461, 1976.

243. Merkal, R. S., Larsen, A. B., Kopecky, K. E., and Neso, R. D.: Comparison of examination and test methods for early detection of paratuberculous cattle. Am. J. Vet. Res. *29*:1533, 1968.

244. Larsen, A. B., Moyle, A. I., and Humes, E. M.: Experimental vaccination of cattle against paratuberculosis (Johne's disease) with killed bacterial vaccines: a controlled field study. Am. J. Vet. Res. *39*:65, 1978.

245. Crowther, R. W., Polydoron, K., Nitti, S., and Phyrilla, A.: Johne's disease in sheep in Cyprus. Vet. Rec. *98*:463, 1976.

246. Biester, H. E., and Schwarte, L. H.: Intestinal adenoma in swine. Am. J. Pathol. *7*:175, 1931.

247. Emsbo, P.: Terminal or regional ileitis in swine. Nord. Vet. Med. *3*:1, 1951.

248. Jönsson, L., and Martinson, K.: Regional ileitis in pigs: morphological and pathogenetical aspects. Acta Vet. Scand. *17*:223, 1976.

249. Dodd, D. C.: Adenomatous intestinal hyperplasia (proliferative ileitis) of swine. Pathol. Vet. *5*:333, 1968.

250. Lawson, G. H. K., and Rowland, A. C.: Intestinal adenomatosis in the pig. A bacteriological study. Res. Vet. Sci. *17*:331, 1974.
251. Love, R. J., and Love, D. N.: Control of proliferative hemorrhagic enteropathy in pigs. Vet. Rec. *100*:473, 1977.
252. Nielsen, K.: Pathophysiology of parasitic infection: plasma protein metabolism. *In* Pathophysiology of Parasitic Infection. Edited by E. J. L. Soulsby. New York, Academic Press, 1976.
253. Bueno, L., Dorchies, P., and Ruckebusch, Y.: Electromyographic analysis of perturbations of ileal motility by gastrointestinal strongyles in sheep. C. R. Soc. Biol. (Paris) *169*:1627, 1975.
254. Thomas, R. J.: Significance of serum pepsinogen and abomasal pH levels in a field infection of O. circumcincta in lambs. Vet. Rec. *97*:468, 1975.
255. Levine, N. D., Clark, D. T., Bradley, R. E., and Kantor, S.: Relationship of pasture rotation to acquisition of gastrointestinal nematodes by sheep. Am. J. Vet. Res. *36*:1459, 1975.
256. Bliss, D., and Todd, A. C.: Milk production in Wisconsin dairy cattle after deworming with thiabendazole. V.M./S.A.C. *69*:638, 1974.
257. Bliss, D., and Todd, A. C.: Milk production by Vermont dairy cattle after deworming. V.M./S.A.C. *71*:1251, 1976.
258. Widmer, W. R., and Van Kruiningen, H. J.: Trichuris-induced transmural ileocolitis in a dog—an entity mimicking regional enteritis. J.A.A.H.A. *10*:581, 1974.
259. Turner, T., and Pegg, E.: A survey of patent nematode infections in dogs. Vet. Rec. *100*:284, 1977.
260. Migasena, S., Gilles, H. M., and Maegraith, B. G.: Studies on Ancylostoma caninum infection in dogs I. Absorption from the small intestine of amino-acids, carbohydrates, and fats. Ann. Trop. Med. Parasitol. *66*:107, 1972.
261. Migasena, S., Gilles, H. M., and Maegraith, B. G.: Studies in Ancyclostoma caninum infections in dogs II. Anatomical changes in the gastrointestinal tract. Ann. Trop. Med. Parasitol. *66*:203, 1972.
262. Guerrero, J.: Telmintic (Mebendazole Powder): a new broad spectrum anthelmintic for canine use. Pract. Vet. *49*:15, 1978.
263. Drudge, J. H.: Metazoal diseases. *In* Equine Medicine and Surgery. Edited by E. J. Catcott, and J. F. Smithcors. Wheaton, IL American Veterinary Publications, 1972.
264. Graber, N.: I.A.C.E.D. Symposium on Helminthiasis in Domestic Animals, Nairobi, Kenya, 1956.
265. Soifer, F. K.: Intestinal parasitism. *In* Current Veterinary Therapy, Vol. VI. Edited by R. W. Kirk. Philadelphia, W. B. Saunders Co., 1977.
266. Barker, I. K., and Remmler, O.: The endogenous development of Eimeria leuckarti in ponies. J. Parasitol. *58*:112, 1972.
267. Roberts, M. C., and Cotchin, E.: Globidium leuckarti in the small intestine of three horses. Br. Vet. J. *129*:146, 1973.
268. Dunlap, J. S.: Eimeria leuckarti infection in the horse. J.A.V.M.A. *156*:623, 1970.
269. Wheeldon, E. B.: Globidium leuckarti infections in a horse with diarrhea. Vet. Rec. *100*:102, 1977.
270. Mason, R. W., and King, S. J.: Eimeria leuckarti in the horse. Aust. Vet. J. *47*:460, 1971.
271. Cymbaluk, N. F., Fretz, P. B., and Loew, F. M.: Amprolium-induced thiamine deficiency in horses: clinical features. Am. J. Vet. Res. *39*:255, 1978.
272. Raizman, R. E.: Giardiasis: an overview for the clinician. Am. J. Dig. Dis. *21*:1070, 1976.
273. Erlandsen, S. L.: Scanning electron microscopy of intestinal giardiosis: lesions of the microvillus border of villus epithelial cells produced by trophozoites of giardia. Proceedings Workshop of Advances in Biomedical Applications of the SEM. Chicago, IIT Research Institute, 1974.
274. Ament, M. E., and Rubin, C. E.: Relation of giardiasis to abnormal intestinal structure and function in gastrointestinal immuno-deficiency syndromes. Gastroenterology *62*:216, 1972.
275. Brightman, A. H., and Slonka, G. F.: A review of five clinical cases of giardiasis in cats. J.A.A.H.A. *12*:492, 1976.
276. Johnson, G.: Giardiasis. *In* Current Veterinary Therapy, Vol. VI. Edited by R. W. Kirk. Philadelphia, W. B. Saunders Co., 1977.
277. Wright, S. G., Tomkins, A. M., and Ridley, D. S.: Giardiasis: Clinical and therapeutic aspects. Gut *18*:343, 1977.
278. Scott, D. W.: The systemic mycoses. *In* Current Veterinary Therapy, Vol. VI. Edited by R. W. Kirk. Philadelphia, W. B. Saunders Co., 1977.
279. Menges, R. W.: Canine histoplasmosis. J.A.V.M.A. *119*:411, 1951.
280. Ditchfield, J., and Fischer, J. B.: Histoplasmosis in the dog. A report of four Ontario cases. Can. Vet. J. *2*:406, 1961.
281. Stickle, J. E., and Hribernik, T. N.: Clinicopathological observations in disseminated histoplasmosis in dogs. J.A.A.H.A. *14*:105, 1978.
282. Richardson, R. C.: Personal communication, Purdue University, West Lafayette, IN, 1978.
283. Bennett, J. E.: Chemotherapy of systemic mycoses. N. Engl. J. Med. *290*:32 and 320, 1974.
284. Waldmann, T. A.: Protein-losing enteropathy. *In* Modern Trends in Gastroenterology. Edited by W. I. Card and B. Creamer. London, Butterworth and Co., 1970.
285. Meuwissen, S. G. M., Nadorp, J. H. S. M., and Tytgai, G. N. J.: Crohn's Disease. A review of immunopathological aspects. Neth. J. Med. *20*:78, 1977.
286. Cave, D. R., Kane, S. P., Mitchell, D. N., and Brooke, B. N.: Further animal evidence of the transmissible agent in Crohn's disease. Lancet *2*:1120, 1973.
287. Donelly, B. J., Delaney, P. V., and Healy, T. M.: Evidence for a transmissible factor in Crohn's disease. Gut *18*:360, 1977.
288. Donaldson, R. M.: Regional enteritis. *In* Gastrointestinal Diseases. Edited by M. H. Sleisenger and J. S. Fordtran. Philadelphia, W. B. Saunders Co., 1973.
289. Meuten, D. J., Butler, D. G., Thomson, G. W., and Lumsden, J. H.: Chronic enteritis associated with malabsorption and protein-losing enteropathy in the horse. J.A.V.M.A. *172*:326, 1978.
290. Cimprich, R. E.: Equine granulomatous enteritis. Vet. Pathol. *11*:535, 1974.
291. Wheat, J. D.: Personal communication, University of California, Davis, CA, 1974.
292. Finco, D. R., Duncan, J. R., Schall, W. D., Hooper, B. E., Chandler, F. W., and Keating, K. A.: Chronic enteric disease and hypoproteinemia in 9 dogs. J.A.V.M.A. *163*:262, 1973.
293. Strande, A., Sommers, S. C., and Petrak, M.: Regional enterocolitis in Cocker Spaniel dogs. Arch. Pathol. *57*:357, 1954.
294. Rechenberg, R.: Regional enteritis in the dog. Monatschr. Vet. Med. *29*:352, 1974.
295. Goldman, P., and Peppercorn, M. A.: Salicylazosulfapyradine in clinical practice. Gastroenterology *65*:166, 1973.
296. Brown, C. H., and Achkar, E.: Azathioprine therapy for inflammatory bowel disease. A preliminary report. Am. J. Gastroenterol. *54*:363, 1970.
297. Ursing, B., and Kamme, C.: Metronidazole for Crohn's disease. Lancet *1*:775, 1975.
298. Nielsen, K., and Andersen, S.: Intestinal lymphangiectasia in cattle. Nord. Vet. Med. *19*:31, 1967.
299. Campbell, R. S. F., Brobst, D., and Bisgard, G.: Intestinal lymphangiectasia in a dog. J.A.V.M.A. *153*:1050, 1968.
300. Waldmann, T. A.: Protein-losing enteropathy. Gastroenterology *50*:422, 1966.
301. Weiden, P L., Blaese, M., Strober, W., Block, J. B., and Waldmann, T. A.: Impaired lymphocyte transformation in intestinal lymphangiectasia: evidence for at least two functionally distinct lymphocyte populations in man. J. Clin. Invest. *51*:1819, 1972.
302. Mattheeuws, D., DeRick, A., Thoonen, H., and VanderStock, J.: Intestinal lymphangiectasia in a dog. J. Small Anim. Pract. *15*:757, 1974.
303. Burrows, C. F.: Personal communication, University of Pennsylvania, 1978.
304. French, A. B.: Intestinal absorptive function and its assessment. Notes from a course organized by the American College of Physicians, Ann Arbor, MI, February 23–27, 1970.
305. Holt, P. R., and Clark, S. B.: Dietary triglyceride compostion related to intestinal fat absorption. Am. J. Clin. Nutr. *22*:279, 1969.
306. Murray, M., Rushton, A., and Selman, I.: Bovine renal amyloidosis: a clinico-pathological study. Vet. Rec. *90*:210, 1972.
307. Slauson, D. O., Gubble, D. H., and Russel, S. W.: A clinicopathological study of renal amyloidosis in dogs. J. Comp. Pathol. *80*:335, 1970.
308. Clark, L., and Seawright, A. A.: Generalized amyloidosis in seven cats. Pathol. Vet. *6*:117, 1969.
309. Crowell, W. A., Goldston, R. T., Schall, W. D., and Finco, D. R.: Generalized amyloidosis in a cat. J.A.V.M.A. *161*:1127, 1972.
310. Leinbach, G. E., and Rubin, C. E.: Eosinophilic gastroenteritis: a simple reaction to food allergens? Gastroenterology *59*:874, 1970.
311. Klein, N. C., Hargrove, R. L., Sleisenger, M. H., and Jeffries, G. H.: Eosinophilic gastroenteritis. Medicine *49*:299, 1970.
312. Hayden, D. W., and Van Kruiningen, H. J.: Eosinophilic gastroenteritis in German Shepherd dogs and its relationship to visceral larval migrans. J.A.V.M.A. *162*:379, 1973.
313. Anderson, N. V.: The malabsorption syndromes. *In* Current Veterinary Therapy, Vol. VI. Edited by R. W. Kirk. Philadelphia, W. B. Saunders Co., 1977.
314. Hall, C. L.: Three clinical cases of eosinophilic enteritis. Southwest Vet. *21*:41, 1967.

315. VanKruiningen, H. J., and Hayden, D. W.: Interpreting problem diarrheas in dogs. Vet. Clin. North Am. 2:29, 1972.
316. Van Kruiningen, H. J.: Clinical efficacy of tylosin in canine inflammatory bowel disease. J.A.A.H.A. 12:498, 1976.
317. Bolton, J. R., Merritt, A. M., Cimprich, R. E., Ramberg, C. F., and Streett, W.: Normal and abnormal xylose absorption in the horse. Cornell Vet. 66:183, 1976.
318. Roberts, M. C., and Pinsent, P. J. N.: Malabsorption in the horse associated with alimentary lymphosarcoma. Equine Vet. J. 7:166, 1975.
319. Kaneko, J. J., Moulton, J. E., Brodey, R. S., and Perryman, V. D.: Malabsorption syndrome resulting in nontropical sprue in dogs. J.A.V.M.A. 146:463, 1965.
320. Jeffries, G. H., Wesen, E., and Sleisenger, M. H.: Malabsorption. Gastroenterology 56:777, 1969.
321. Novis, B. H., Bank, S., Marks, I. N., Selzer, G., Kahn, L., and Sealy, R.: Abdominal lymphoma presenting with malabsorption. Q. J. Med. 40:521, 1971.
322. Wilkinson, G. T.: Some preliminary clinical observations on the malabsorption syndrome in the cat. J. Small Anim. Pract. 10:87, 1969.
323. Chiapella, A.: Personal communication, University of Pennsylvania, 1978.
324. Kowlessar, O. D., and Sleisenger, M. H.: The role of gliadin in the pathogenesis of adult celiac disease. Gastroenterology 44:357, 1963.
325. Klipstein, F. A.: Tropical sprue. Gastroenterology 54:275, 1968.
326. Hill, F. W. G., and Kelly, D. F.: Naturally occurring intestinal malabsorption in the dog. Am. J. Dig. Dis. 19:649, 1974.
327. Batt, R., Jones, P. E., and Peters, T. J.: Peroral jejunal biopsy in the dog. Vet. Rec. 99:337, 1976.
328. Garvin, P. J., Sawyer, O., Cabol, E., Karminski, D., and Codd, J. E.: Malabsorption and abdominal pain secondary to celiac artery entrapment. Arch. Surg. 112:655, 1977.
329. Merritt, A. M., Bolton, J. R., and Cimprich, R. E.: Differential diagnosis of chronic diarrhea in horses over 6 months of age. J. S. Afr. Vet. Assoc. 46:73, 1975.
330. Chernov, A. J., Doe, W. F., and Gompertz, D.: Intrajejunal volatile fatty acids in the stagnant loop syndrome. Gut 13:103, 1972.
331. Prizant, R., Whithead, J. S., and Kim, Y. S.: Short chain fatty acids in rats with jejunal blind loops I. Analysis of SCFA in small intestine, cecum, feces, and plasma. Gastroenterology 69:1254, 1975.
332. Kim, Y. S., and Spritz, N.: Metabolism of hydroxy fatty acids in dogs with steatorrhea secondary to experimentally produced intestinal blind loops. J. Lipid Res. 9:487, 1968.
333. Gracey, M., Burke, V., Oshin, A., Barker, J., and Glasgow, E. F.: Bacteria, bile salts, and intestinal monosaccharide malabsorption. Gut 12:683, 1971.
334. Nygaard, K., and Rootwelt, K.: Intestinal protein loss in rats with blind segments on the small bowel. Gastroenterology 54:52, 1968.

335. Toskes, P. P., Giannella, R. A., Jervis, H. R., Rout, W. R., and Takeuchi, A.: Small intestinal mucosal injury in the experimental blind loop syndrome. Gastroenterology 68:1193, 1975.
336. Brodey, R. S., and Cohen, D.: Epizootiologic and clinicopathologic study of 95 cases of gastrointestinal neoplasms in the dog. Sci. Proc. 101st Annu. Meet. A.V.M.A. (July 19–23), 1964, p. 167.
337. Brodey, R. S.: Alimentary tract neoplasms in the cat: a clinicopathologic survey of 46 cases. Am. J. Vet. Res. 27:74, 1966.
338. Cotchin, E.: Tumors of farm animals: a survey of tumors examined at the Royal Veterinary College, London, during 1950–60. Vet. Rec. 72:816, 1960.
339. Simpson, B. A., and Jolly, R. D.: Carcinoma of the small intestine in sheep. J. Pathol. 112:83, 1974.
340. Patnaik, A. K., Liu, S-K., and Johnson, G. F.: Feline intestinal adenocarcinoma. Vet. Pathol. 13:1, 1976.
341. Patnaik, A. K., Hurvitz, A. I., and Johnson, G. F.: Canine gastrointestinal neoplasms. Vet. Pathol. 14:547, 1977.
342. Grant, B. D., and Tennant, B. C.: Volvulus associated with Meckel's diverticulum in the horse. J.A.V.M.A. 162:550, 1973.
343. Welkos, S., Toskes, P., and Baer, H.: The role of anaerobic bacteria in the B₁₂ malabsorption of the stasis syndrome. Clin. Res. 25:320A, 1977.
344. Welkos, S. L.: The pathogenesis of malabsorption in the stasis syndrome: the role of bacterial overgrowth. Ph.D. Thesis, University of Florida, 1977.
345. Doell, R. G., and Kretchmer, N.: Studies of small intestine during development I. Distribution and activity of β-galactosidase. Biochim. Biophys. Acta 62:353, 1962.
346. Roberts, M. C., Kidder, D. E., and Hill, F. W. G.: Small intestinal beta-galactosidase activity in the horse. Gut 14:535, 1973.
347. Welsh, J. D.: Isolated lactase deficiency in humans. Report on 100 patients. Medicine 49:257, 1970.
348. Hill, F. W. G.: Malabsorption syndrome in the dog: a study of thirty-eight cases. J. Small Anim. Pract. 13:575, 1972.
349. Plechner, A. J., and Stannon, M.: Food-induced hypersensitivity. Mod. Vet. Pract. 58:225, 1977.
350. Shiner, M., Ballard, J., and Smith, M.: The small intestinal mucosa in cows milk allergy. Lancet 1:136, 1975.
351. Brusseret, P. D.: Common manifestations of cows milk allergy in children. Lancet 1:304, 1978.
352. Marks, J., and Shuster, S.: Intestinal malabsorption and the skin. Gut 12:938, 1971.
353. Banwell, J. G., Gorbach, S. L., Pierce, N. F., Mitra, R., and Mondal, A.: Acute undifferentiated human diarrhea in the tropics II. Alterations in intestinal fluid and electrolyte movements. J. Clin. Invest. 50:890, 1971.
354. Hobbs, B. C., Rowe, B., Kendall, M., Turnbull, P. C. B., and Ghosh, A. C.: Escherichia coli 027 in adult diarrhea. J. Hyg. 77:393, 1976.

Chapter 24

THE COLON, RECTUM, AND ANUS

ROBERT A. ARGENZIO, ROBERT H. WHITLOCK,
and COLIN F. BURROWS

Primary colonic diseases in animals are accompanied by signs of obstruction or diarrhea, each with a fairly characteristic change in the pattern of fecal passage. In addition, the colon may participate secondarily in small bowel disease processes because it serves as the modulator of small bowel function; that is, the reserve of colonic absorptive function can partially compensate for inadequate absorptive function of the small intestine. If the reserve capacity of the colon is overwhelmed, however, diarrhea ensues in the face of a basically healthy colon. An overload of fermentable substrate in the colon is such an example. In the adult herbivore, the colon has the fundamentally important function of microbial digestion, but even the voluminous ascending colon of herbivores malfunctions if overloaded with fermentable substrate.

Some diseases can be attributed to functional derangements of the organ, even though the colon is not the site of specific pathologic changes. For example, impaction of the ileocecal valve of the horse results in death within 24 to 48 hours. This does not involve the colon per se but death most probably results from failure of the large volumes of digestive secretions to reach the absorptive surfaces of the colon. Thus, the animal dehydrates into its own small bowel. Therefore, factors interfering with colonic absorption may result in functional disease.

The large bowel diseases of large animals and small animals are discussed separately in order to reflect some inherent species differences in signs and findings, and in methods of examination, as well as to better serve the needs of the species-oriented reader.

Part I. Diseases of the Colon, Rectum, and Anus in the Horse, Cow, and Pig

ROBERT A. ARGENZIO, and ROBERT H. WHITLOCK

SIGNS OF COLONIC DISEASE

Abdominal Distention

A sudden abnormal increase in abdominal size in horses (pregnancy is a normal increase) is usually considered evidence of colonic disease or, less commonly, of ascites. The distention may be due to accumulated gas or fluid or ingesta in the large bowel. Distention of the small bowel rarely causes noticeable abdominal distention in the horse. Thus, visual examination of the horse can often differentiate between large bowel disease and small bowel disease in cases of colic. An exception to this might be distention or impaction of the cecum,

523

which is rarely massive enough to cause abdominal distention. Ascites associated with heart failure or neoplasia such as lymphosarcoma or squamous cell carcinoma of the stomach is much slower in onset.

Abdominal distention in cattle is more often associated with forestomach obstruction with fluid and ingesta accumulation in the rumen and occasionally in the abomasum. A right-sided abdominal distention in a cow may be caused by a distended cecum and colon if it is in the upper caudal quadrant. However, distention in the lower right quadrant is usually associated with abomasal distention (impaction). An asymmetric enlargement on the right side of the abdomen may be associated with abomasal volvulus or cecal volvulus.

Swine with prominent abdominal distention may have atresia ani if they are less than 6 weeks of age or, if older, an acquired stricture of the rectum. Rarely, an abdominal mass may be so large as to produce visible local protrusion of the pigs' abdominal wall.

Diarrhea

Diarrhea is considered to be a clinical sign of large bowel disease in adult horses, cattle, sheep, and pigs, whereas small bowel disease may not alter the fecal consistency in these large animals. This is not true in small animals such as the dog and the cat, because of the relatively small capacity of the colon in those species. As a clinical sign, diarrhea is best subdivided by duration—acute versus chronic. (Table 24–1 offers diagnostic plans.)

Horses with acute diarrhea should be considered to have salmonellosis until proven otherwise. Salmonella is the most common cause of acute diarrheal disease in the horse and every effort should be made to prove or rule out this possibility.

Chronic diarrhea in the horse is a very important clinical sign. Perhaps the most common cause of chronic diarrhea is an immunologically mediated colitis, possibly associated with a viral agent. These horses have often been treated extensively with various therapeutic agents with minimal success.

Acute diarrheal disease in stabled cattle is most commonly associated with salmonellosis, BVD, and winter dysentery (during the winter months in the northeastern United States) and with mycotoxicosis in the southeastern United States during winter as well as other seasons.

Chronic diarrhea is not as life-threatening as acute diarrhea, since there is less loss of fluid and electrolytes, but it usually leads to emaciation and cachexia. The list of diagnostic rule-outs that one

Table 24–1. Diagnostic Plans for Chronic Diarrhea in Horses and Cattle (Diagnoses Listed in Order of Decreasing Incidence)

Horses	Diagnostic Plan
1. Parasitism	Fecal counts
2. Strongyle larval migrans	Fecal counts
3. Chronic salmonellosis	Fecal culture
4. *Corynebacterium equi*	History
5. Chronic liver disease	Liver tests
6. Chronic renal disease	Renal tests
7. Abdominal neoplasia	Physical examination,
Lymphosarcoma	peritoneal tap, and
Squamous cell carcinoma	exploratory laparotomy
Mesothelioma	
Melanoma	
8. Chronic heart failure	Cardiac examination
9. Posterior vena caval mass	Exploratory laparotomy
10. Mesenteric abscesses	Exploratory laparotomy
11. Histoplasmosis	Culture, titer
12. Trichomonads	Not a cause of diarrhea in horses

Cattle	Diagnostic Plan
1. Parasitism	Fecal egg count
2. Johne's disease	Fecal culture
3. Salmonellosis	Fecal culture
4. Bovine virus diarrhea	Virus identification
5. Abdominal fat necrosis	Rectal exam
6. Chronic peritonitis	Peritoneal tap
7. Thrombosis of the posterior vena cava	Liver tests
8. Renal amyloidosis	Urinary protein
9. Heart failure	Cardiac examination
10. Abdominal neoplasia	Physical examination,
Lymphosarcoma	peritoneal tap, and
Squamous cell carcinoma	exploratory laparotomy
—stomach	
Adenocarcinoma	
—intestine	
Granulosa cell tumor	
—ovary	
11. Mycotoxicosis	Feed evaluation
12. Copper deficiency	Test for excess molybdenum
13. Bluetongue	Virus isolation
14. Ascites—any cause	Physical examination Peritoneal tap
15. Foreign materials—sand, cinders	Fecal examination
16. Magnesium excess	Evaluate ration

should consider as possible causes of chronic diarrheal disease in the cow is shown in Table 24–1.

Tenesmus

Tenesmus is defined as straining, but especially ineffectual and painful straining to defecate or urinate. Tenesmus in horses is an uncommon finding, perhaps because of the higher dry matter content of the feces and the conformation of the perineal and rectal area. Tenesmus may occur following an examination of the internal organs and especially where there have been repeated, traumatic rectal examinations which result in injury to the rectal mucosa.

Tenesmus is a common clinical sign seen in cattle with diarrheal diseases. Many cattle that have had diarrhea for several hours or days may have periods of tenesmus in which they will strain to defecate and then draw air into the rectum, which causes further irritation to the anorectal mucosa. Tenesmus is also an iatrogenic problem associated with deep rectal examination, especially in cattle with diarrhea. The tenesmus can be so violent that it will lead to further deterioration of the cows' condition. In fact, rectal examination of a bovine patient with severe diarrhea may be contraindicated. Occasionally a cow may experience vigorous (''malignant'') tenesmus, where the alternate filling and evacuation of air through the rectum becomes such a problem that she is unable to eat and in this weakened state may die. This seems to be a greater problem in the early postpartum period following rectal manipulation of the uterus.

Other causes of tenesmus that one should consider would be coccidiosis and rabies in cattle. In rabies, tenesmus may occasionally be an early clinical sign and should always be considered in the sporadic case of tenesmus in the cow, when other causes of tenesmus are not apparent.

Rectal tenesmus in swine often leads to rectal prolapse, and follows obstetric manipulation in sows. In weanlings and feeder pigs, it is associated with the inflammation of the rectum that precedes rectal stricture, with abrupt introduction to high-energy rations and with compression trauma to the abdomen.

Blood in the Feces

Blood in the feces (characteristically, bright blood) is an indication of bleeding in the colon. It may be due to any ulcerative process such as parasites or neoplasia. In cattle one should first consider coccidiosis, while in calves with fetid diarrhea and hematochezia one should consider salmonellosis. In the horse, melena is less common and rarely seen even with salmonellosis. Dark feces with digested blood are associated with gastric carcinomas in horses. However, anal bleeding can be caused by rectal examination. In cattle, this is usually of minimal importance as the rectal mucosa will heal over and possibly result in a small scar formation. In the horse any evidence of blood following a rectal examination is usually a serious clinical sign and may indeed indicate rupture of the rectal wall, which could be fatal.

Flatulence

Flatulence seems to be a more common clinical sign in horses than in any other species. It often occurs following bouts of indigestion and consumption of highly fermentable feeds. It is indicative of the resolution of a problem rather than a primary sign of colonic disease.

Pruritus Ani

Pruritus of the anus occasionally occurs in horses, usually in association with pinworms (Oxyuris equi) around the anus or as an early manifestation of an anal melanoma. Occasionally squamous cell carcinomas of the equine vagina may invade the rectal area and present as large infiltrative cauliflower-like lesions. Perirectal abscesses due to strangles may present as tumors in young foals. Any space-occupying lesion in this area may be associated with tenesmus and occasionally bleeding. Pruritus ani is uncommon in the cow.

Rectal fistulas as a cause of pruritus are most common in small animals and rarely occur in cattle or horses.

EXAMINATION OF THE COLON AND ANORECTUM

Visual Examination

Visual examination of the feces of any patient is an essential procedure to include in the physical examination. In large animals, a good way to evaluate whether the feces are normal is to compare them to feces of the herdmates on the same diet and under the same environmental conditions. The greatest variations in fecal consistency occur in cattle. Heifers on a roughage diet will have a very firm bowel movement compared to lactating adult cows on a high concentrate ration (unformed feces) and to beef cows on a lush pasture in the springtime, in which the feces are quite fluid. The fibrous coarseness of the feces varies with the diet, species, and age. Older horses with poor dentition will have coarse undigested roughage in the feces and this may be a clue to the cause of colic in the older horse.

The odor of the feces will give further information about the diet, and occasionally one can gather information to implicate a specific disease. For example, a typical ''septic-tank'' odor from bovine feces would indicate salmonellosis, whereas a ''fruity'' odor in adult dairy cattle may implicate ketosis or recent therapy with propylene glycol.

Occasionally it is advantageous to evaluate the

physical characteristics further by mixing the feces with water and allowing them to settle in a transparent container or a plastic sleeve. In this way, one can easily detect the presence of sand or cinders in the feces which otherwise may not be apparent. This is often of value in trying to ascertain the presence or absence of sand as a cause of colic in horses, and of excess soil as a herd problem in cattle with pica.

The color of the feces is often a reflection of the dietary constituents. Yellow pale feces may be indicative of milk in the diet. Occasionally the yellow color may be present when there is forestomach obstruction, with excessive bile present in the feces. Black feces (melena) are indicative of bleeding in the proximal digestive tract and suggest the presence of digested blood, as may occur with gastric ulcers in horses, cattle, or pigs.

Auscultation-Percussion

Auscultation of the colon and anorectum is of utmost value in a routine physical examination in horses and cattle. Auscultation over the cecum and colon will give an indication of borborygmus and may be interpreted to reflect intestinal contractions but not motility or transit rate. Animals with profuse diarrhea may have relatively little borborygmus; on the other hand, intense peristalsis and borborygmal sounds may present in colic but transit rate of ingesta is slowed. Horses will often have an accumulation of cecal gas during colic. Simultaneous auscultation and percussion enables one to determine the presence of gas, which occasionally may be extensive enough to necessitate trocarization. One should continue to auscult each portion of the large colon of the horse. Occasionally one can

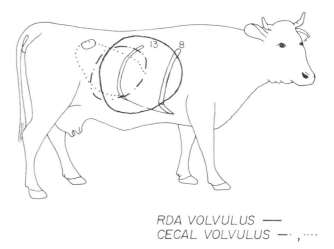

RDA VOLVULUS ——
CECAL VOLVULUS —· , ····

Figure 24–2. The circles outline the typical "ping" sites associated with an abomasal volvulus and cecal volvulus.

auscult normal borborygmal sounds on the right side and detect diminished borborygmal sounds on the left side suggestive of the impaction at the pelvic flexure. This and similar findings can also occur during thromboembolic colic, all of which help to localize the lesion.

Cattle that are anorectic for a variety of reasons will often have an accumulation of gas in the cecum and spiral colon (Fig. 24–1). Auscultation-percussion will yield a "ping" under the last rib (right side). This should not be confused with a right abomasal displacement or a cecal volvulus, both of which can occur and give rise to a "ping" in this area (Fig. 24–2). The size of the normal cecum varies from 5 to 8 cm in diameter, but up to 35 cm in diameter if severely distended. These large gas accumulations in the coiled colon and cecum give the most trouble to clinicians. Rectal examination will help differentiate these disorders. A large gas-filled viscus in the right paralumbar fossa extending downward toward the stifle or caudally toward the tuber coxa should cause one to consider cecal volvulus as a strong probability (Fig. 24–2). See Chapter 22 for details concerning right abomasal displacement.

Palpation

Palpation of the posterior abdomen is most easily carried out per rectum in the adult horse and cow because of the large size of the colon. Transabdominal palpation can be done by making a fist and gently pushing in at the abdominal wall to ascertain the presence of masses or localized pain in the colon or cecum, such as that associated with an abscess.

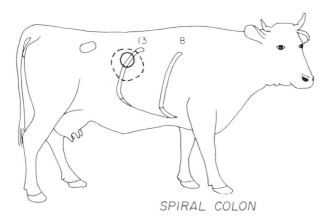

SPIRAL COLON

Figure 24–1. The small, solid circle outlines the area typically associated with a gas accumulation in the coiled colon. The dashed circle outlines the "ping" that can occur in some cattle with an atonic coiled colon.

Although relatively easy to do, it is more difficult to interpret the finding in well-muscled horses or obese cattle. Some animals are very sensitive to this procedure and may need to be sedated but sedation will diminish the response to pain. One should be able to palpate a distended colon or cecum in horses or cattle. Transabdominal palpation in pigs is limited by the heavy layer of muscle and fat in the abdominal wall.

Examination Per Rectum

Rectal examination is best carried out in large animals while the animal is adequately restrained. The rectal exam in the horse is facilitated by sedation with a tranquilizer such as acetylpromazine, promazine, or xylazine followed by 15 to 30 mg of propantheline bromide (Pro-Banthine) intravenously. One may begin the examination 5 to 10 minutes after drug administration. The feces are removed from the rectum and one can then perform a very detailed examination of the abdomen of the horse. If the cecum is distended, one may palpate the medial cecal tenia, which feels like a tight string on a banjo, from high in the right paralumbar area to the lower left flank. The inexperienced clinician may mistakenly interpret this to suggest intestinal accidents.

The pelvic flexure of the colon and the consistency of colonic contents will yield information about the possibility of an impaction colic. In cases of severe colonic impaction, the pelvic flexure will extend into the pelvic inlet.

The spleen can be palpated in most normal horses just anterior to the pelvic inlet at the left paralumbar fossa (this cannot be interpreted as gastric distention, as was once commonly thought). The stomach is rarely palpated, quite dorsal in the abdomen and anterior to the left kidney. The mesenteric artery can be palpated in most sedated horses and the detection of a fremitus may substantiate the impression of a mesenteric arteritis. However, to associate all mesenteric arteritis with clinical disease would be a mistake. The inguinal rings of the stallion and bull should be evaluated for possible intestinal incarceration as the cause of colic.

In cattle, a rectal examination is a necessary part of a complete physical and genital examination. In evaluation of the cecum, a rectal examination will confirm a diagnosis of cecal volvulus in all cases, as either the tip of the cecum or the flexed portion of a cecal volvulus will be detected as a 10- to 15-cm diameter gas- and fluid-filled viscus in the right hemi-abdomen. Such a finding is pathognomonic for a cecal volvulus or cecal dislocation. Coupled with signs of intestinal accident, such as rapid pulse and an acute decrease in milk production, the diagnosis is confirmed.

Biopsy of the rectum and colon is possible and is occasionally done in inflammatory and neoplastic diseases. In large animals the most common use for biopsy is to rule out Johne's disease. However, Johne's disease must be well-advanced before rectal biopsy is positive. Needle or wedge biopsy of masses or tumors in the area is required to make a definitive diagnosis. One must always consider melanomas in grey horses and squamous cell carcinomas in older mares or cows where the lesion has extended from the vulva to the anus.

Proctoscopic Examination

Proctoscopic examination is best carried out in large animals with the use of an aluminum or glass vaginal speculum. Epidural anesthesia and removal of all fecal contents from the rectum will facilitate the examination. This technique will allow visualization of lesions in the rectum. Proctoscopic and colonoscopic examinations are done in horses and cattle to facilitate the taking of biopsies.

DISEASES OF THE COLON, RECTUM, AND ANUS IN THE HORSE, COW, AND PIG

Specific diseases of the colon in large animals will be considered as either obstructive or diarrheal. While in many cases, the line between these two syndromes is relatively thin with respect to the cause, a characteristic pathogenesis and pathophysiology are usually elicited. These in turn lead to a diagnosis and rational treatment. Although it is not possible to discuss all of the colonic diseases in detail, the ones selected represent a wide variety of causes and manifestations of pathophysiology. Thus a critical examination of these diseases should provide a basis for the understanding of large bowel diseases in general.

Obstructive Diseases

Obstructive diseases of the large intestine can be classified into three general pathogenetic groups. These are (1) vascular obstructions, (2) mechanical obstructions, and (3) neurogenic obstructions.

Vascular obstructions arise from thrombi or emboli in the arterial supply or venous drainage from a segment of intestine. The degree of circulation which is compromised and the extent of collateral circulation and anastomotic relationships dictate the consequences of acute or chronic vascular occlusive disease. Segments of infarcted bowel become paralyzed and result in obstruction due to the inability of the ischemic musculature to contract.

Mechanical obstructions are a result of partial or complete occlusion of the lumen due to intraluminal masses or compression of the bowel wall. The former are known as obturation obstructions and include fecal impactions, enteroliths, and parasites. The latter group includes hernias, strictures, stenoses, volvulus and intussusceptions.

The neurogenic group arise from primary or reflex hypermotility (spasm) or hypomotility and stasis. The latter can be considered from the standpoint of reflex ileus due to trauma, peritonitis, or indigestion. The vague term of indigestion is considered to represent abnormal microbial fermentation characterized by tympany and stasis. Although the precise pathogenesis of this obstruction has not been defined, it will be considered in this group.

The incidence of fatal obstructive diseases for 161 cases of equine colic is shown in Table 24–2.[1] It is obvious that the colon is incriminated in a large proportion of equine colics. For example, impactions of the colon and cecum alone account for nearly 30% of all equine colics. Equally important is the high incidence of strangulation obstructions (28%), which are usually far more critical in the large bowel than are simple obstructions. Simple obstruction may develop into strangulation owing to abnormal motility of the obstructed bowel or compromise of the vasculature from distention.

The pathophysiologic consequences of obstructions will be considered before proceeding to specific diseases. For this purpose it is convenient to examine these diseases from the standpoint of simple versus strangulated obstruction.

Simple Obstruction

The circulation is not initially compromised when the gut lumen is obstructed, and the clinical manifestations are due primarily to the sequestration of fluid and gas in the gut lumen. With partial or complete obstruction, hypermotility of the segment proximal to the obstruction occurs due to neural reflexes, as discussed in Chapter 12. Thus, in the case of partial obstruction, diarrhea may be a prominent clinical sign.[2] The absence of feces indicates complete bowel occlusion.

The duration of the obstruction and progression of clinical signs depends on the site of obstruction. The amount of normally functioning proximal intestine is responsible for reabsorption of the endogenous secretions. Referring back to Chapter 12, the large intestine of the 100-kg pony must reabsorb approximately 20 liters per day. Seventy-five percent (15 liters) is reabsorbed in the cecum and ventral colon. Therefore, the higher the obstruction, the more critical will be the depletion of extracellular fluids. For example, obstruction at the ileocecal valve could result in death within 24 hours owing exclusively to dehydration and hypovolemic shock. Compensatory absorption by the small intestine may not be sufficient to sustain plasma volume if the obstruction is sudden and complete.

During high large intestinal obstructions, the proximal segments rapidly become distended with fluid and gas in the presence of a competent ileocecal valve. The distention itself creates additional problems. First, the normal propulsive action is reflexly abolished and the proximal overdistended segment becomes paralyzed.[2] Atony may

Table 24– 2.   Incidence of Classes of Equine Colic[1]

	% Total	% Class
Acute gastric dilatation	17.6	
Intestinal indigestion	5.3	
Impaction of colon and cecum	27.5	
Displacements and tumors	23.6	
volvulus of small intestine		53.5
volvulus of large colon		16.7
pedunculated lipoma—small intestine		20.0
pedunculated lipoma—small colon		6.7
herniation—small intestine		3.3
Stricture or foreign body	16.0	
Parasitism	10.0	
thrombosis of anterior mesenteric artery		33.3
thrombosis of mesenteric vessel to small intestine		9.2
chronic parasitism		58.5

[1]Modified from Coffman, 1970.

persist after the obstruction is removed and is an example of a secondary paralytic ileus. Second, the distention compromises the venous return by compression of the veins and fluid leaks into the bowel wall. If allowed to continue, gangrene and septic shock may supervene. Third, the normal absorptive mechanisms are reversed and the bowel actually secretes fluid into the lumen. In fact this secretion continues for some time after the obstruction is removed.[3] Thus, a vicious cycle is created whereby the initial cause induces a secondary ileus and not only is absorption prevented, but secretion further contributes to the already overloaded bowel. In untreated cases, perforation may occur with its catastrophic consequences. These factors emphasize the need for early treatment before secondary complications arise and also point out that supportive fluid therapy is critical even after the obstruction is removed. It becomes obvious that osmotic drugs and cathartics must be avoided unless a simple impaction can be determined with certainty.

Systemically, the prime concern in simple obstruction is the depletion of plasma volume and reduction in cardiac output.[4] Acid-base disturbances are also to be expected. Thus, the early manifestations are those of progressive hypovolemic shock as opposed to the septic shock of strangulation obstruction. If the obstruction is low, e.g., pelvic flexure or small colon, or is not complete, the systemic signs are not as severe.[5] The prime concern for support is therefore fluid replacement and acid-base therapy. Referring to the electrolyte composition of the various segments of bowel in Chapter 12, an estimate of the ions lost to the bowel can be made. In contrast to the small bowel, Cl^- is not the major deficit in colonic obstruction since most of the Cl^- is reabsorbed in the small intestine. Therefore, one may suspect that alkalosis will be a prominent feature of small bowel obstruction, while acidosis may predominate in large bowel obstructions. However, the situation is not always predictable. For example, alkalosis occurs in most obstructive bowel disease in cattle.[6] Yet, most obstructions in cattle occur proximal to the colon. In the horse, acidosis is the rule and the empiric administration of $NaHCO_3$ has been recommended.[7] Furthermore, acidosis always occurs secondary to decreased tissue perfusion and lactic acid production.

In hypovolemic shock, intense peripheral vasoconstriction is present. This reflex response maintains arterial blood pressure and perfusion of the heart and brain. Therefore, the use of such agents as promazine tranquilizers for their sedative action may be dangerous owing to their peripheral vasodilatory effects.[7] However, prolonged vasoconstriction produces anoxia of peripheral tissues and viscera. Therefore, in normotensive individuals, such vasodilatory compounds may be useful[8] if used judiciously and with extreme caution. The first and most important factor is replacement of the extracellular fluid volume. Monitoring of central venous pressure may provide a good evaluation of the effective circulatory volume and cardiac output.[7,9]

Strangulation Obstruction

In strangulation of the bowel, fluid and acid-base therapy is still of great importance but other urgent factors now become of equal concern. In general, surgical intervention is required in the majority of these cases. When the bowel becomes strangulated (volvulus or intussusception), the venous drainage becomes impaired and the bowel wall becomes edematous. Stagnation of blood flow occurs and hypoxia develops. If stagnation is severe, arterial input may also be compromised. Thus, the infarcted bowel becomes severely hypoxic and, if left untreated, gangrene develops.

The normal bowel mucosa is fairly impermeable to bacterial toxins, but the permeability of the infarcted bowel is greatly increased. Therefore endotoxin, which is produced by all gram-negative bacteria, may be absorbed leading to toxemia and septic shock.[10] The ischemic liver becomes progressively less capable of removing endotoxin from the portal blood.[11,12]

The cardiovascular manifestations of septic shock are somewhat controversial and may differ with the species. For example, some investigators have found a high cardiac output and low peripheral resistance (high output shock).[9] However, most work in the dog indicates an intense adrenergic stimulation and vasoconstriction of peripheral tissues and certain visceral organs.[11] Endotoxin becomes a potent sympathomimetic substance after interaction with the blood and furthermore elicits a massive secretion of catecholamines from the adrenal gland. The intestinal circulation is particularly vulnerable and the splanchnic viscera may become ischemic owing to intense arteriolar constriction. Extensive splanchnic pooling of blood occurs. These changes in the capillary circulation may occur within minutes in septic shock, while the same changes may take hours to develop in hypovolemic shock.[12]

Specific Obstructive Diseases

Vascular Obstructions

The diseases discussed in this section are considered to have a primary vascular pathogenesis. However, obstructive diseases that secondarily result in venous or arterial occlusion, e.g., intestinal displacements, can be expected to follow the same general pathophysiologic pattern as acute, primary vascular obstruction. The prime concern is ischemia of the bowel with subsequent necrosis, gangrene, and septic shock. In these acute episodes of infarction, segments of intestine become paralyzed and result in functional intestinal obstruction. In less severe situations, mucosal ulceration results and these are discussed in the section on diarrhea. In chronic cases, healing and scarring of these ulcerative lesions are believed to be bases for the development of strictures and stenosis.

Acute Thromboembolic Vascular Disease of Horses. This disease is primarily due to migration of strongyle larvae and specifically to their localization in the cranial mesenteric artery. Although most horses (90%) have verminous mesenteric arteritis, most do not develop severe clinical signs. Only those vermin-laden arteries that have a saccular dilatation are correctly called aneurysms. The presence of these lesions is a major factor in the predisposition to most of the large intestinal problems in the horse.[13]

Pathogenesis and Pathology. The migration of *S. vulgaris* and the associated vascular lesions are described under diarrheal diseases.

Pathophysiology. The cecum and large colon of the horse are supplied by the cranial mesenteric artery and its branches. Extensive anastomosing branches help minimize the consequences of occlusive vascular disease. The abrupt blockage of major vessels before subdivision may be responsible for ischemia of large segments of bowel. Conversely, slowly progressive vascular occlusion may permit the development of adequate collateral circulation while abrupt occlusion is more likely to cause ischemic necrosis.[14] In the horse, the ileocecocolic artery is by far the most commonly affected in the production of the acute syndrome.

Blood flow to the colon of such species as dog, cat, and man accounts for approximately 5% of the cardiac output at rest.[15] Obviously, in the horse, the percentage will be much greater. Eighty percent of the total colonic blood flow is directed to the mucosa while the remaining 20% nourishes the muscularis.[15] Therefore, in ischemic episodes, the mucosa is more vulnerable to necrosis and ulceration.

During digestion, splanchnic blood flow increases by 200% in such species as dog and cat,[16] and this increase subserves the absorptive function of the bowel. Occlusion of small arterial branches or chronic occlusion of larger branches compromises this increase in blood flow and may be responsible for many transient colics observed in horses.[17] In man, this is the basis for the syndrome of acute abdominal pain in patients with mesenteric vascular disease.[18] Thus, a large number of recurrent colics in horse and man may be of similar pathogenesis. Indeed, many believe that chronic arterial lesions are directly responsible for the underlying causes of most equine colics.[13]

Abrupt occlusion of large arterial branches results first in spasm and then in stasis of large segments of bowel.[19] The pathophysiologic consequences for the bowel are thus the same as described previously for strangulation obstruction. Tissue destruction and gangrene quickly supervene.

Three distinct morphologic types of thromboembolic disease have been described in the horse.[20] The first form is characterized by a fulminant clinical course of shock, dehydration, and early death. This peracute form occurs as a result of an acute thrombotic phenomenon in the ileocecocolic artery initiated by strongyle larvae and probably mediated by local intravascular coagulation. The second form is the more common "typical" form that most clinicians associate with verminous arteritis; i.e., a chronic relapsing, intermittent colic, and at necropsy, a segmental necrosis and thrombosis of associated vessels. The third type occurs as a result of a recent massive infestation especially in the jejunal vessels and occurs in young horses and older horses that have had minimal previous exposure to strongyle larvae. The first and third types are more common in younger horses and as a result may have negative fecal counts, which could lead all but the astute clinician astray. (The prepatent period of *S. vulgaris* is 6 months.)

Systemically, these changes are manifested by a progressive metabolic acidosis as tissue perfusion decreases. However, a decrease in arterial pH may only occur in the terminal stage since respiratory compensation lowers the arterial pCO_2. Loss of fluid into the gut and peritoneal cavity results in decreased extracellular fluid volume. Large amounts of protein also leak into the peritoneal fluid and bacterial concentration of this fluid is greatly increased.[21] The heart rate increases gradually to compensate for the decreased plasma volume and cardiac output and this reflex rate increase maintains arterial pressure until the terminal stage. Blood glucose may be elevated up to 300 mg/dl as a response to the acute stress. Death occurs within 24 to 48 hours after experimental colonic infarction.

Diagnosis. Horses with acute thromboembolic colic will usually present with signs of mild colic with dullness and depression. The vital signs may be normal or moderately increased, depending upon the degree of gut ischemia present. The clinical signs vary and may consist of pawing, stamping, kicking at the abdomen, getting up and down frequently, looking at the flank, rolling, curling the upper lip, lying on the back, carefully lying down and slowly getting up or frequently attempting to urinate. The onset of clinical signs occurs approximately 12 hours following experimental acute arterial infarction.[21] Evidence of pain is less severe in thromboembolic colic than in acute obstructive disease. The overriding manifestation may be depression and dullness compared to the obstructive colics. The abdominal size should be normal to perhaps slightly increased, associated with increased fluid in the gastrointestinal tract.

GASTROINTESTINAL SYSTEM. Auscultation of the abdomen usually shows decreased borborygmus most prominent over the area of ischemia, commonly the cecum and right dorsal colon. Simultaneous auscultation-percussion will often reveal a "ping" sound over the cecum. The gas accumulates as a result of ileus. Sustained silence (lack of borborygmi) usually suggests a grave prognosis with irreversible morphologic changes.[10] Gastric reflux is usually associated with small bowel obstruction; however approximately 50% of horses with large bowel obstruction have gastric reflux. If gastric reflux is present, medication should *not* be given by nasogastric tube.

A rectal examination in thromboembolic accidents will usually not aid in detection of definitive abnormalities. Occasionally the cranial mesenteric artery may be palpated and the presence of fibrosis, nodularity or fremitus will provide evidence of verminous arteritis. However, changes in the cranial mesenteric artery are present in many horses with colic, making interpretation difficult. Pain in the area of the mesenteric artery, determined by digital palpation, may also suggest verminous arteritis but normal horses may also resent this effort at deep palpation.[17] Most thromboembolic colics have an increased softness of the colonic contents without any obvious displacements. Many times,

the medial cecal tenia is tense and the neophyte may interpret this as a sign of strangulation. Caution must be used in the interpretation of this tense cecal tenia.

Perhaps the most rewarding aid in the diagnosis of thromboembolic colic is peritoneal centesis. Obtaining normal clear transparent yellow fluid would indicate a relatively minor lesion or no vascular lesion. The presence of the red blood cells that are not a result of contamination during the centesis procedure suggests recent strangulation or infarction of bowel. The prognosis is proportional to the severity of the erythrocyte diapedesis. As the disease progresses (veterinarians usually see the later stages), there may be less erythrocytes and the fluid becomes turbid to amber, suggesting a subacute to chronic bowel infarction with the resultant neutrophil diapedesis. The leukocyte count may be as high as 100,000 to 300,000 per mm[3]. This helps confirm the presence of peritonitis, which is most likely associated with an infarcted bowel. The protein concentration in the peritoneal fluid is easy to measure by refractometer, which gives valuable information about the severity of the situation. The greater the protein is above 3 g/dl, the more massive the lesion (infarction).

CARDIOVASCULAR SYSTEM. The loss of fluid and electrolyte into the peritoneal cavity and gut lumen initiates intense reflex cardiovascular changes. Clinically, these are recognized as cold extremities and ears, and pale mucous membranes, all of which are manifestations of intense peripheral vasoconstriction. The capillary refill time is prolonged (normal is about 2 seconds). The skin loses its turgor and the eyes become sunken. As the disease progresses and more fluid is sequestered outside the vascular system, the heart rate increases. The blood pressure decreases in terminal stages of the disease.

The hematocrit and total plasma protein are very useful parameters to evaluate, since they increase in proportion to the severity of the disease. A rising hematocrit with a lowering of total plasma proteins indicates a maldistribution of protein and is associated with massive infarcted lesions. This is a grave prognostic sign.

As tissue perfusion decreases, vasoconstriction becomes more apparent, and lactic acid production increases with an increase in plasma lactate. Plasma lactate greater than 75 mg/dl is associated with a decreased survival rate (33%). With progression of the disease, the acidosis causes an increase in rate and depth of respiration in an attempt to compensate for the metabolic acidosis. Bicarbonate concentration decreases from a normal of 25 to 10 mEq/L.

In the final stage of the disease when stagnant anoxia is present, the arterial tone is lost and circulatory collapse is imminent. At this point arterial pressure, cardiac output, and arterial pH all decrease rapidly and death results from circulatory failure.

Treatment. Treatment is primarily supportive and must be aimed at several different areas including: (1) relief of pain; (2) re-establishment of fluid volume, electrolyte, and acid-base status; and (3) improvement of visceral circulation.

Relief of pain may be accomplished by one of several analgesics such as: (1) xylazine at the rate of 300 to 500 mg/1000 lb, and (2) pentazocine at the rate of 500 to 1000 mg/1000 lb. These drugs have minimal effects on gut motility and arterial pressure compared to phenothiazine tranquilizers,[7] which are contraindicated in hypovolemic shock. Other analgesics such as phenylbutazone (2 to 4 g intravenously) or meperidine may be given (500 to 1000 mg intramuscularly or, at the most, half of the total dose intravenously). All of these drugs may be efficacious for the relief of pain, but the duration of action is relatively short, i.e., 1 to 2 hours.

A stomach tube should be passed repeatedly (or, alternatively, left in place) in an attempt to remove any refluxed bowel content, if present. Irritant and bulk cathartics are contraindicated in cases of bowel reflux into stomach.

The replacement or re-establishment of extracellular fluid and correction of the acid-base changes are the major prerequisites for an effective approach to the treatment of cardiovascular collapse due to thromboembolism. Polyionic fluids in the form of balanced electrolytes rich in bicarbonate are required. Twenty liters may easily be given over a 2- to 4-hour period in cases of severe hemoconcentration. Some clinicians advocate the use of 100 to 300 g of sodium bicarbonate as a 5% solution intravenously to correct the metabolic acidosis, followed with an isotonic polyionic fluid to replace the extracellular fluid loss. Fluid therapy should be monitored by repeated microhematocrit and total plasma protein determinations, to assess adequacy of fluid replacement and also to protect against hemodilution. The amount of fluid given is based upon the achievement of urine output, effective peripheral perfusion as determined by capillary refill, and re-establishment of normal hematocrit which may be the best single index. In our experience, it is usually unnecessary to monitor central venous pressure as most horses will tolerate 6 to 10 liters of a balanced polyionic fluid per hour. This can be achieved by gravity intravenous drip through a 16-gauge catheter.

The visceral circulation is best re-established by correction of the extracellular fluid deficit. Phenothiazine tranquilizers may be used but, if used, should be given only when extracellular fluid volume has been re-established. Blood flow may be enhanced by massive doses of corticosteroid (10 to 20 mg/kg), i.e., 9-fluoro-prednisolone.[10] The benefit of steroid in the treatment of shock in horses has yet to be confirmed by critical study. It is advantageous to add calcium to intravenous fluid, as horses become mildly hypocalcemic during intensive fluid therapy and calcium has been shown to have enhanced effect on gut motility as well as on blood flow to the intestinal tract.

Heparin or dicoumarin derivatives have also been advocated for use in the treatment of thromboembolic colic associated with disseminated intravascular coagulation. There is currently much active research in this area of veterinary medicine and the appropriate dosage and therapeutic regimes have yet to be established. We have used sodium gluconate (400 ml of a 25% solution/1000 lb and repeated at 30-minute intervals for up to 5 treatments) as a splanchnic vasodilator. Antibiotic is often used in thromboembolic colic, but probably is of more value to the clinician's peace of mind than efficacious for the horse.

Removal of the cause of the thromboembolic colic is unrewarding surgically. Large doses of thiabendazole (500 mg/kg, which is 10 times the normal dose) have been shown to be efficacious in removal of migrating larvae and adults in the intestinal tract. The importance of an adequate parasite control program should be emphasized to the owners as this will decrease the incidence of colics of all types.

The prognosis in documented cases of thromboembolic colic is unfavorable; 85% mortality is to be expected, in our practice. Surgical intervention is usually unrewarding as massive colonic lesions cannot be resected. When small bowel lesions are resected, additional areas of infarction often occur. Supportive medical care as outlined previously seems to be the most rational approach to therapy with a guarded prognosis at best. Chloramphenicol or neomycin sulfate have been recommended.[8,22]

The importance of parasite control should be emphasized, since the incidence of equine colic is markedly decreased in situations where stringent control of parasites is practiced.

Chronic Vascular Obstruction: Porcine Rectal Stricture and Ischemic Proctitis. These diseases are a result of (1) small infarctions that have produced ulcerations or (2) ulcerations of the mucosa from various causes which have subsequently healed but have injured the vascular supply. Although most areas of the colonic and rectal mucosa regenerate without complications, there are particularly susceptible areas; e.g., the rectum in some species in which clinical disease in the form of strictures and stenoses is produced. At present, the syndrome of rectal stricture is recognized only in pigs, dogs, and man. Since rectal stricture is becoming an economically important problem of increasing incidence in some midwestern swine herds the pathogenesis in pigs will be considered in some detail.

This is an acquired disease in pigs of 2 to 5 months of age. An annular fibrous constriction of the rectum results in chronic obstipation and finally complete obstruction. Herd morbidity is 1 to 5% and mortality 85 to 100%. All animals with complete stricture eventually die.[23]

Pathogenesis and Pathology. The arterial supply to the rectum is derived from the caudal mesenteric artery, which gives rise to the cranial hemorrhoidal artery. The internal pudendal artery, a branch of the internal iliac artery, contributes blood to the anus and a few millimeters of adjacent rectal mucosa. Thus, a watershed zone is created between two adjacent arterial supplies near the recto-anal junction. It is precisely in this anastomotic zone that the rectal strictures are found.

These areas of arterial anastomosis are particularly vulnerable to ischemia of a marginally adequate collateral supply. In man, similar vulnerable areas of the colon include zones that lie between the cranial and caudal mesenteric arteries and the rectosigmoid area, in which the caudal mesenteric and internal iliac arteries anastomose.[24]

While a number of primary causes may result in ischemia, such as toxic compounds in the feed, prolapsed rectum, or infectious agents, recent studies have demonstrated a convincing association between salmonellosis and rectal strictures in pigs.[24,25] This accounts for the apparently infectious nature of the disease.

The initial ulcerative proctocolitis associated with porcine salmonellosis involves most of the large intestine. The ulcerative lesions are initiated by small infarcts. Of the animals which survive acute enteric salmonellosis, many have the residual lesions of rectal stricture or maturing ulcers in the same region. Other parts of the intestine may heal without complications but the poor reparative capacity of these anastomotic zones predisposes them to a persistent cicatrizing ulcerative proctitis which progresses to rectal stricture and obstruction.[25]

Diagnosis. The clinical signs of the disease are pronounced emaciation, depression, dehydration, and tenesmus. Particularly striking is the grossly enlarged abdomen due to tremendous distention of the large intestine with fluid and gas. In animals not completely obstructed, fluid or pasty feces and flatulence may be present. In all cases, the stricture can be palpated per rectum, 3 to 5 cm from the anus.[26]

Treatment. In less severe cases, bougienage and dilatation may be effective. In more severe cases, if the animal is to be saved, surgical intervention is necessary.[27]

Mechanical Obstructions

Causes of mechanical obstructions of the large intestine are far too numerous to describe in detail. Ingestion of foreign objects, herniation of the small colon through the nephrosplenic ligament, strictures or stenoses due to inflammatory or vascular lesions, tumors, impactions from feed, bezoars or sand, and intestinal displacements account for most of the primary causes.

Except for the most simple feed impactions, the majority of these obstructions require surgical intervention. Due to the relatively high incidence of feed impactions and torsion of the large colon of the horse, these will be considered in detail.

Impactions of Large Intestine

These disorders occur primarily in horses and pigs but are most common in the horse[28] and will be discussed as such here. The type of impaction is important because it will dictate the type of treatment; i.e., medical or surgical. Feed and fecal impactions are common and these can usually be reduced with medical treatment. On the other hand, enteroliths must usually be removed surgically. The rectal examination often helps differentiate between enteroliths and fecal impactions. The latter are usually palpable. If an enterolith is not found, it is customary to treat medically and observe for a response. However, the decision to postpone the surgical procedure may reduce the patient's chances for survival. Consideration of the sequence of pathologic events indicates that a simple obstruction, if complete, may become life-threatening. This is especially true if an enterolith completely obstructs the small colon or the pelvic flexure of the colon.

Pathogenesis. The most probable sites of resistance to digesta flow in the colon of the horse are the cecocolic junction, the pelvic flexure, and the origin of the small colon. Furthermore, the resistance to flow of particles increases in the aboral direction indicating that the origin of the small colon is the most susceptible to impaction and obstruction. There is very little or no resistance to flow at the sternal or diaphragmatic flexures.

There is an exceedingly long retention time of larger particles in the dorsal colon (> 7 days). This time is sufficient for the development of large enteroliths from a nidus. Thus, most of these enterolith obstructions occur at the transverse colon or at the origin of the small colon.[29,30,31] Feed impactions are most common at the pelvic flexure, but factors other than the anatomic narrowing of this segment may be involved. Motor events occurring at this location need to be studied in detail for this may be a pacemaker zone of the colon and could account for a number of abnormal conditions associated with this location; e.g., impaction, torsion, or rupture. Impaction of the cecum is less common but is more serious as it is less responsive to medical therapy.

The cause of feed impactions is to a large degree speculative. Indigestible fibrous feedstuffs, dental diseases, motor insufficiency of the bowel, and insufficient water intake have been incriminated. Older horses are most predisposed to impactions, which may be a reflection of reduced digestive efficiency, reduced bowel motility, and dental disease.

Enteroliths require a nidus for precipitation and consist mainly of ammonium magnesium phosphate (struvite). The magnesium phosphate is probably from grain in which the salt is present in large amounts. If for some reason the salt is not ionized in the acid gastric contents, the phosphate is not absorbed in the small intestine and the magnesium and phosphate combine with ammonia formed by bacterial degradation of protein in the colon.[19]

Fibrous impactions are not uncommon. These usually consist of fibrous plant material impregnated with a phosphate salt.[19,22] Recently, the use of rubberized fencing material has resulted in an unusually high incidence of fibrous impactions in horses on those farms, resulting from the ingestion of the nylon strands of the fabric.[30] These foreign bodies may serve as a nidus for enteroliths and usually lodge in the small or transverse colon.

Diagnosis. These obstructions are usually manifested clinically by a moderate degree of abdominal pain and mildly increased heart and respiratory rates (approximately 40 to 60 per minute and 16 to 25 per minute respectively).[30] Small amounts of firm, mucus-covered feces may be passed in the case of partial obstruction. If the obstruction is complete, the presence of the impaction may be suspected based on a finding of tympany. Fortunately, the animals are usually anorectic and microbial fermentation is therefore at a minimum. Thus, the colon may be capable of supporting chronic obstruction for some time if the obstruction is low, since the cecum and ventral colon recover the majority of the endogenous fluid and electrolytes. Continued absorption of water from the proximal colon results in an impacted mass which can usually be discerned on rectal palpation. The obvious sites of importance have been described, most of which can be palpated per rectum.

Treatment. The majority of fecal impactions will respond to treatment with mineral oil (3 to 4 liters/1000 lb), which may be repeated in 12 to 16 hours if there is no evidence of gastric reflux. Another emollient cathartic is raw linseed oil at the rate of 6 to 12 ounces per os. Boiled linseed oil contains lead and should not be used therapeutically in animals. The most popular softening agent is dioctyl sodium sulfosuccinate (DSS; Permeatrate, Haver-Lockhart), which is given at the rate of 20 to 30 g (1 to 3 oz 5% solution) per os/1000 lb. Excessive doses may be toxic and cause diarrhea and death.[32]

Softening agents injected through the abdominal or rectal wall have been used[17] but are not recommended because of the inherent irritant properties of these agents if they are injected into the peritoneum or into tissue. While fibrous impactions usually have to be removed surgically,[33] the use of cellulase, which has been successful in the treatment of humans,[34] should be investigated. Parasympathomimetics are also used if the response to mineral oil is poor.

Neostigmine is a popular and relatively safe cholinergic when given at the rate of 2 to 10 mg/1000 lb subcutaneously.[35] Higher doses or intramuscular injections will cause more discomfort and are more dangerous. These should be used only when there are simple impactions and when mineral oil or some other softening agent has been previously administered.

Due to the recent interest in the pathophysiology of diarrhea, a number of cathartics and laxatives have come under careful scrutiny as to their mechanisms of action. These are worthy of mention since many of them are used extensively in veterinary medicine to treat symptomatic constipation.

The pharmacologic classification of laxatives now in use is based to a large degree on the supposed effect on motility. For example, the stimulant or irritant cathartics such as castor oil, bisacodyl, anthraquinones and phenolphthalein are presumed to stimulate motility due to their "irritant" effects on colonic mucosa. However, none of these have been shown to have a primary effect on motility. All have been shown to induce net fluid and electrolyte accumulation in the lumen. Therefore, any effects on motility are probably secondary to net fluid accumulation.[36]

Even the saline cathartics, such as magnesium salts, may have a mechanism of action other than their osmotic effects. For example, Mg^{++} is known to stimulate the release of cholecystokinin, and this hormone is capable of stimulating intestinal fluid and electrolyte secretion.[36]

The softening agent, dioctyl sodium sulfosuccinate, has been shown to induce net secretion of Na$^+$, Cl$^-$, and water into the cecum. The mechanism of action appeared to result from stimulation of cAMP.[37] Irritant cathartics such as castor oil, thought to promote catharsis by their direct irritation of the bowel, now have been shown to cause structural changes on the surface of the epithelial cells and villar tips.[38,39]

Thus, the choice of a cathartic must be carefully evaluated. If the animal is already suffering from dehydration due to the more serious intestinal obstructions, the use of such agents may further compromise the vascular compartment. On the other hand, the effectiveness of a laxative rests on its ability to increase fecal water excretion. Motor stimulants cannot result in net fluid accumulation. The premise that insufficient motility is largely responsible for impaction is questionable and most probably the primary cause is due to other factors. Furthermore, because stimulation of intense motor activity can result in rupture of the intestine over a hard fecal mass, the use of such compounds, by themselves, is theoretically unsound.

Torsion of Large Colon

The large colon of the horse is anatomically predisposed to displacement owing to its great size and free mobility. During ontogenesis, the ascending colon of herbivores becomes greatly elongated, forming the spiral colon in ruminants and pigs and the large ventral and dorsal colons of the horse. Thus, the mesentery of the ascending limb is drawn out and narrowed, becoming a ligament connecting the two limbs rather than a mesentery. Apart from the attachments on the right side, e.g., cecocolic fold and right dorsal and transverse colons, the remainder of the whole large colon is potentially mobile. Therefore, the majority of torsions involve the left colon. The mesocolon can in fact act as an axis of rotation around which dorsal and ventral colons can rotate.[40]

The smaller left dorsal colon apparently initiates the twist, moving medially or laterally and ventrally on the ventral colon. Thus, the torsion may be in either a clockwise or counterclockwise direction. Since the pelvic flexure is completely free to move, rotations of 90° are common and usually are not associated with clinical signs. Torsions of 180° may stop the flow of ingesta and at this point act as a simple obstruction. Rotations of 180° to 270° may compromise the vasculature and a torsion of 360° will occlude the vasculature and result in strangulation obstruction and ischemic necrosis.[17]

The cause of colonic torsion is entirely speculative. Factors such as the horse rolling from milder types of colic, e.g., spasmodic colic, and abnormal rates of gas production, stasis of certain segments and hypermotility of the left dorsal colon have been implicated but are difficult to prove. Sclerosis and atrophy appear to be a factor in man.[41] The dynamic participation of colonic segments would appear to be reasonable in initiating the twist. Therefore, it is quite possible that strongyle larvae-induced ischemia or dietary factors inducing tympany and abnormal motility are directly involved. A history of parasite control and feeding practices should be elicited from the owner as possible clues to the underlying cause.

The whole spectrum of pathophysiologic events discussed previously for simple and strangulated obstructions may be encountered. A diagnosis can usually be made on rectal palpation. If the apex of the gas-distended cecum can be palpated in the middle third of the abdomen, this is virtually pathognomonic for 180° torsion of the large colon.[8] Surgical reduction of the torsion is the only effective treatment.[17]

Neurogenic Obstructions

These diseases are characterized by an interference with the nervous control of motility as either a primary or secondary event. Primary neurogenic obstruction has been attributed to the absence or degeneration of autonomic ganglia such as occurs in grass sickness in horses, megacolon of pigs, and megacolon in dogs. In addition, it is speculated that verminous aneurysms of the cranial mesenteric artery in horses may produce compression on the celiac plexus resulting in stasis and obstruction of the large intestine.[42] However, a vascular pathogenesis for this disease appears more likely[19] and has been discussed previously.

The disorder in horses and cattle known as spasmodic colic has been attributed to an increase in parasympathetic tone producing intense spasms of the intestine. Loud intestinal sounds are clearly audible, and the disorder appears to be relieved by administration of parasympatholytic agents, e.g., atropine.[28] However, evidence that the autonomic nervous system is primarily involved has not been demonstrated. A fortuitous study of a pony with spasmodic colic has provided some insight into the problem.[43] This pony had electrodes implanted in several sites of the gastrointestinal tract to study motility. Acute pain and loud intestinal sounds were associated with violent electrical activity of the proximal jejunum. Inhibition of gastric and colonic motility was present. It was suggested that the pain was associated with a sudden intestinal distention coinciding with the arrival of peristaltic waves in the spastic zone. Morphine inhibited the intestinal spasm and relieved the pain. Morphine analgesia also stimulated colonic motor activity (morphine is generally contraindicated in horses).

Secondary reflex inhibition of motility is probably common but has been little studied. Paralytic ileus due to surgery in the face of peritonitis is of this origin.[44] Of more recent interest is the concern that indigestion associated with high grain feeding or dietary changes results in gastrointestinal atony. Studies of forestomach, abomasal, and cecal motility in cattle are highly convincing in this regard.[45] Whether the disorder in the large intestine is due to central or local neural reflex inhibition or to a direct effect on the muscle is not conclusive.

Colonic and Cecal Tympany

This disease primarily affects horses and cattle but also occurs in pigs. In the horse, the tympany may be primary, due to abnormal fermentation, or secondary due to obstruction. In ruminants it most commonly is associated with a relative ileus in cases where cows are anorectic for unknown reasons. In pigs, it is largely secondary to obstruction. The primary disorders of tympany can predispose to such accidents as abomasal and cecal displacements in cattle.[45,46]

Pathogenesis. Large amounts of gas are produced in the cecum and ventral colon of the horse from microbial fermentation. It has been estimated that 5 moles of organic acid per day are produced in the cecum alone in a 100-kg animal.[47] If true, it can be roughly estimated that some 100 to 150 liters of CO_2 and CH_4 will be produced by fermentation and neutralization processes under these conditions (cf. Chapter 12). While some of this gas can be ab-

sorbed, and this is an important route for removal of CO_2, it is obvious that the rate of production far exceeds the rate of absorption; therefore to prevent accumulation, the gas must be expelled to the colon and thence to the rectum.

Specific motility events of the cecum are necessary to transport gas through the relatively narrow cecocolic ostium. In fact, a special mass contraction associated only with gas transport occurs once the cranial part of the cecal base has become enormously dilated with gas.[48] Thus, it is obvious that inhibition of motility from any cause can result in rapid gas accumulation and dilation of the cecum. In addition, the shape and course of the proximal ventral colon can form a gas trap.[40]

The primary disorder is usually associated with a dietary change to a highly fermentable green feed or grain, especially corn. While these dietary changes can bring about an overproduction of gas and acid in the cecum and ventral colon, it does not appear to be the excess of gas production and distention which is responsible for decreased motility. It has now been demonstrated conclusively that the undissociated volatile fatty acids (VFA), especially butyric acid, results in a profound inhibition of forestomach, abomasal, and cecal motility in ruminants.[45,49] Reflex inhibition from distention is not necessary to elicit the response. The concentration of undissociated acid necessary to inhibit motility of the cecum can be quite easily obtained with grain feeding, even in ruminants.

Further studies with isolated rabbit duodenum indicate that motility of this preparation is also inhibited in the presence of 10 mM undissociated butyric acid.[45] These results suggest that the extrinsic reflexes, which are a feature of postoperative ileus, are not involved. The effect may be directly on the muscle or involve the intrinsic neural plexus. In vivo studies with the sheep abomasum[50] indicated that infusion of 15 mmoles of undissociated VFA was associated with a reduction or a complete absence of action potentials. However, no discernible effect on the slow wave potentials was demonstrated. Thus, it appears that the inherent, spontaneous depolarizations and repolarizations of the muscle are intact and the evidence seems to point to factors which are capable of eliciting the spike discharge.

The question arises as to why all animals subjected to these dietary changes are not similarly affected. However, as discussed previously, chronic arterial lesions have been proposed as a predisposing cause in many types of equine colic. Since the absorption of VFA (and CO_2) from the large intestine is blood-flow dependent, it is not difficult to imagine that an insufficient increase in blood flow could impair VFA absorption and lower the luminal pH. When this occurs, the relative proportion of butyric acid increases.[45]

Diagnosis. Tympany must be differentiated from other causes of colic. Abdominal distention is evident, and only the large intestine is capable of distending the abdomen to this degree in the horse.[8] A history of a change of feed is quite helpful.

Acute episodes of pain are present and intestinal sounds are reduced. A characteristic high pitched "ping" may be heard on simultaneous auscultation-percussion over the cecum. The size of the gas-filled viscus may be determined by moving the snapping finger while keeping the head of the stethoscope localized over the viscus. If cecal tympany is the cause of the pain, the "ping" area outlined will be as large as 30 to 45 cm in diameter.

If the disorder is primary, obstruction is usually not complete and large amounts of flatus may be passed. Rectal examination reveals a huge distended cecum and tense cecal tenia. The colon usually seems less distended. The severe signs of shock and changes in blood chemistry are absent if the condition has not progressed to displacement of the organs and complete obstruction. Most cases of cecal tympany in the horse are a sequel to ileus or other forms of colic.

Treatment. In severe cases trocarization is necessary. Gas in the cecum will rise to the highest point, i.e., the base. Therefore, trocarization, with a small-bore trocar, at the highest point of the bulge halfway between the tuber coxae and the last rib on the right side should be performed.[40] Anti-ferment agents represent an archaic approach as most are very irritating to the intestinal mucosa and do little to decrease fermentation. Cholinergic (neostigmine) is indicated in low doses (2 to 4 mg/1000 lb) to re-establish motility and prevent further gas accumulation.

Grass Sickness

Grass sickness is a disease of horses occurring chiefly in Europe. Three- to eight-year-old animals and animals kept outdoors are most frequently affected.[51] The disease does not appear to be contagious, although there is an association with particular premises. All breeds of horses including nondomestic equines can be affected.[52] The disease is highly fatal and, thus far, refractory to treatment.

Clinical signs include difficulty in swallowing, extensive salivation, and depressed gastrointestinal borborygmus (motility). Interestingly, abdominal pain is minimal in this disease compared to most horses with colic. Muscular tremors and fasciculations with patchy sweating over the shoulders and hindquarters are common signs. The clinicopathologic changes are consistent with dehydration except the tendency for hypochloremia and hyperglycemia in acute cases.[53]

In animals that die acutely, the stomach and small bowel are grossly dilated with fluid and gas. In many, the stomach has ruptured and is the immediate cause of death. The large colon is greatly dilated and filled with compact dry digesta. In more chronic cases, wasting occurs to such an extent that the horse resembles a Greyhound and must be destroyed. Necropsy of these chronic cases reveals a greatly shrunken gastrointestinal tract with the large intestine impacted with firm black feces. The only important histopathologic changes observed are degeneration and death of neurons in the sympathetic ganglia.[55,56,57]

Recent studies[58,59] have demonstrated that transfusion of plasma from sick animals to healthy individuals resulted in identical changes in the autonomic ganglia. Therefore, a neurotoxic factor is present. The factor has been identified as either a protein of molecular weight of 30,000 or greater, or a factor that is bound to a protein. However, in no case has the clinical disease been reproduced, suggesting that as yet unknown factors participate in the disease syndrome.

Megacolon (Hirschsprung's Disease)

Megacolon is an infrequent disease which has been described in pigs and dogs.[60,61] Absence or degeneration of the intramural plexus is the causative factor. The disease is of interest because it demonstrates the importance of the intrinsic nerves to normal colonic motility. Furthermore, many of these cases may have gone unrecognized since the syndrome is quite similar to impaction of the large intestine or acquired megacolon from other causes. In the dog, most are secondary and acquired (pseudomegacolon). In man, the primary defect occurs in one of every 5000 live births and is a familial disease.

Pathogenesis. In man, the disease is congenital and believed to arise as a consequence of failure in development of intramural ganglion cells, which proceeds from the cephalic to caudal end during embryonic development. Thus, the aganglionic segments extend proximally from the internal anal sphincter for varying distances.[62] There is an absence of intramural ganglion cells in both the submucosal (Meissner's) and the myenteric (Auerbach's) plexuses. In addition, the cholinergic, adrenergic, and purinergic innervation of the segment is abnormal.[63]

The lesion consists of a contracted aganglionic segment, with dilatation of the proximal intestine. The abnormal segment does not relax after injection of methacholine, while normally innervated segments do.[63] Therefore, it appears that the intrinsic nerves are primarily inhibitory to muscle contractions.[64] In dogs and cats an aganglionic segment is usually not present. Rather, there is generalized dilatation of the colon.

Diagnosis. In pigs, signs of the disease did not appear until after about 11 weeks of age. Therefore, the disease may be acquired in pigs. Distention and enlargement of the abdomen are the chief clinical signs. Similar signs are apparent in impaction and rectal strictures. Rectal biopsy demonstration of an absence of ganglion cells is diagnostic.[60]

Treatment. The disease in pigs is consistent with the familial, hereditary aspects of the disease and slaughter of the breeding stock whose progeny have megacolon disease is recommended.[60] Medical or surgical resection of the aganglionic segment is not only prohibitive economically but is contraindicated for breeding stock on ethical grounds.

Cecal Dislocation, Displacement, and Volvulus in Cattle

Cecal disorders in dairy cattle are increasing in incidence.[65-71] Their pathogenesis was discussed under colon and cecal tympany.

History. The owner reports a capricious appetite and diminished milk production. For example, 25 of 27 cows had an acute decrease in milk production in one affected herd.[72] These cows were on a high grain diet. Corn silage or high-moisture corn are commonly associated with cecal disorders.

Abdominal pain is often present. It varies from treading to colic manifested as restlessness, to the cow getting up and down repeatedly and to kicking at her abdomen. Severe abdominal pain was present in 22 of 38 cases in our practice, where any notation of pain was recorded.[72] Seven of the cows showed no evidence of pain.

Cecal disorders are frequently characterized by an abrupt change in the pattern of fecal passage. In our review of unpublished cases, defecation ceased in 29 of 47 cows in the several hours prior to examination, while 4 cows had diarrhea. Only 3 of the 47 cows had normal feces.

Physical Findings. Temperature and respiratory rate remain in the normal range in simple cecal dislocation. A normal pulse (60 to 80 per minute) was recorded in 20 of 45 cows, while 13 of 45 had a pulse greater than 100 per minute.[72] As the "twist" became more severe, the pulse rose proportionately. Ruminal motility is diminished in strength and rate of contraction when the cecum is diseased.

Ketone bodies are often present at moderate concentrations in the urine and milk.

A "ping" sound may be elicited by snapping the fingers against the right caudal area of the rib cage. The area involved is more caudal than that of a right abomosal displacement (Fig. 24–1).

Rectal examination will confirm the diagnosis. A gas-distended viscus (resembles a flexed human knee or a loaf of Vienna bread) is found in the pelvic inlet or just anterior to the brim of the pelvis. The finding is characteristic and diagnostic in nearly 98% of the cases. In 17 of 52 cases, the blind tip of the cecum could be palpated whereas in 35 out of 52 cases the dilated or twisted colon could be palpated.[72]

The cecum may rotate clockwise or counterclockwise when viewing the cow from the right. The severity and extent of the rotation determine the degree of vascular embarrassment and the severity of the clinical signs. The tip of the cecum may be exterior to the omental sling but usually is contained within. Most animals with a cecal volvulus have a compensated hypochloremic, hypokalemic metabolic alkalosis. (<90 mEq Cl⁻/L, <4 mEq K⁺/L, >30 mEq HCO₃⁻/L).

Treatment. Calcium gluconate (250 to 500 ml 20% solution) subcutaneously promotes intestinal motility by correcting the hypocalcemia that is often present. Cathartics may be of value in promoting defecation.

Surgical intervention to decompress the cecum and remove ingesta from the adjacent colon is necessary in all cases of cecal volvulus.

In most cases surgical intervention via a right flank laparotomy and typhlotomy is done. In all cases where surgical intervention is done, the tip of the cecum is incised and drained of fluid and gas. If gangrene is not present, the incision is simply oversewn and replaced in the abdominal cavity.

Thirteen of the previously described 47 cases had a clockwise rotation of the cecum when viewing the cow from the right, whereas 9 rotated counterclockwise.[72] The degree of rotation varied from 90 to 360° (10 cases). Typhlectomy was carried out on eight cases, with seven survivors. The overall recovery rate with surgical intervention was approximately 85%. Five of 46 cases recurred (11%).[72] The postsurgical complications were minimal.

Diarrheal Diseases

Diarrhea may ultimately result when the colon is overwhelmed by a small intestinal diarrhea, or from primary colonic disease. The latter will be examined from the standpoint of (1) mechanisms of absorptive failure and (2) active or passive secretion.

Normal Absorptive Function

Normally the colon absorbs Na⁺, VFA, and water and secretes HCO_3^-; 95% of the fluid presented to the normal colon is reabsorbed. However, perfusion studies suggest that the normal colon may be capable of absorbing 3 to 4 times this amount. For example, the colon of the 50-kg pig can absorb 8.6 liters of water, 1.9 moles of Na⁺, and 2.9 moles of VFA, and secrete 1 mole of HCO_3^- each day.[73] Similar values are obtained in goats.[74] The dog colon does not have this reserve absorptive capacity. These figures imply that in adult herbivores or omnivores, (1) massive small bowel secretion must be present to overwhelm a normal colon or (2) colonic disease must be suspected in diarrheic states. Yet small bowel disease can secondarily result in colonic malfunction, as discussed below.

Functional Changes

Alterations of Normal Microbial Flora. Alteration of the colonic flora can result in diarrhea in two ways. First, the normal bacteria suppress establishment of pathogens, as resident strains of bacteria have the advantage in competition for substrate. In addition, the end-products or end-effects of these bacteria, i.e., pH, Eh, and VFA, discriminate against the invaders. Undissociated VFA are bactericidal.[75,76] Second, alteration or suppression of the normal flora will have an effect on colonic absorptive mechanisms. The presence of an optimal pH and VFA concentration is required for maximal absorptive function in species which have been studied (cf. Chapter 12).

Thus, chronic idiopathic diarrhea in horses has responded to fecal fluid transplants from normal horses. Apparently the syndrome of chronic diarrhea was initiated by a change in the luminal environment brought about by "stress" coupled with the administration of antibiotics.[77]

Fermentative Diarrhea. In small animals and man the most important causes of osmotic diarrhea are secondary to small bowel malabsorption. However, even in the absence of small bowel malabsorption, large quantities of volatile fatty acids can be rapidly produced in the colon, especially in the horse.

Figure 24–3 shows the total volume and VFA

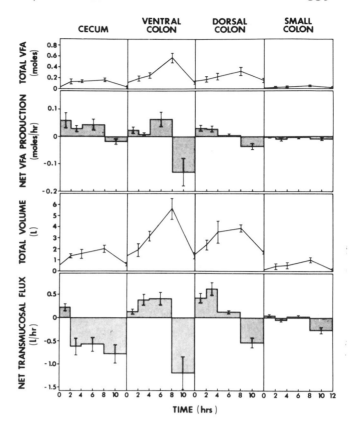

Figure 24–3. VFA content, net VFA production, volume of water and net transmucosal flux of water determined for individual segments of large intestine as a function of time. Negative values designate net absorption of VFA or H_2O.[78] (By permission of the editor, Cornell Veterinarian, and R. A. Argenzio.)

content in four segments of the equine large intestine throughout a 12-hour cycle when the animals are fed at 12-hour intervals.[78] The net increase in VFA is paralleled by a net increase in Na⁺ and water. An increase in the effective osmotic pressure cannot occur in the presence of sufficient $NaHCO_3$ buffer (see Chapter 14). However, the Na⁺ and HCO_3^- must come from somewhere, and the ileal inflow does not appear to suffice for the neutralization of VFA in the colon. Therefore, the colonic mucosa appears to add Na⁺, HCO_3^-, and water from the plasma, by an as yet unknown mechanism, and in amounts sufficient to neutralize these net increases in VFA. The pH and osmotic pressure were relatively unaffected by the large net increases in VFA.

Thus, in the 160-kg ponies cited in Figure 24–3, a net gain of 1.6 moles of acid/24 hours was present which required its equivalent of Na⁺, HCO_3^-, and water to be added from the blood. While an osmotic inflow as such was absent, the fermentation process elicits electrolyte and water movement from the plasma. These four- to five-fold volume changes which occur under normal feeding conditions imply that an overactive microbial fermentation could result in massive fluid movement from blood to lumen. When the HCO_3^- buffer capacity is exceeded, luminal acidification, hyperosmolality, and osmotic diarrhea can be expected.

Abnormal Motility. The volume increases in the preceding example did not precipitate diarrhea, primarily because a high resistance to aboral flow exists at the termination of these segments. This allows sufficient time for the reabsorption of electrolytes and water. This resistance is probably due either to sphincter-like control at the junctions (pelvic flexure and small colon) or to anti-peristaltic motility. In either case, hypomotility would likely result in diarrhea because of loss of resistance to aboral flow. Thus, in spite of previously held intuition, hypomotility and a flaccid colon appear to be associated with diarrhea in horses and probably in cattle as well.

Clinically this can be very confusing as one may often auscult increased borborygmal sounds in patients with diarrhea. However, borborygmus should not be equated with motility or effective persistalsis, in our opinion. In fact, studies have now shown that in canine colitis, the spontaneous slow wave is depressed,[79] which implies that deranged motility may be one primary cause of diarrhea in certain inflammatory conditions. On the other hand, if the luminal volumes become great enough, secondary to increased secretion or decreased absorption (as occurs in most diarrheal diseases), this may evoke mass movements of ingesta. Therefore, the primary cause of diarrhea must be carefully evaluated prior to treatment aimed at modifying intestinal motility.

Structural Changes

Edema. Referring back to Figure 14–1, it is evident that interstitial edema can occur if the filtration at the arterial end of the capillary exceeds the reabsorptive capacity at the venous or lymphatic end. One factor resulting in derangement of the capillary dynamics is a decrease in the plasma colloid osmotic pressure. This occurs due to hypoproteinemia (the total plasma protein must be less than 4.5 g/dl) caused by nephritis or nephrosis, reduced hepatic synthesis of albumin, nutritional deficiency, or parasitic invasion or by intestinal loss.[80] Second, general venous stasis (congestive heart failure), local venous stasis, lymphatic obstruction, or interference with venous return to the heart may result in intestinal edema.

The resulting increase in tissue fluid pressure increases the permeability of the intestinal mucosa and provides the driving force for passive filtration secretion. Effective net absorption is prevented and diarrhea results.

Inflammation. Inflammatory diseases of the bowel are principally due to pathogenic microorganisms. However, other disorders, e.g., ischemia and toxins ingested with food, also contribute to inflammation. The cause of a number of inflammatory diseases such as colitis X and ulcerative colitis is unknown.

While it is apparent that inflammatory edema can result in decreased absorption or increased secretion as outlined previously, a number of invasive pathogens are now known to induce active secretion in the colon even though the elaboration of an enterotoxin has not been established. For example, studies in experimental animals infected with Salmonellae have now shown that activation of adenyl cyclase and cAMP is responsible for the active electrolyte secretion.[81] Despite the extensive mucosal damage, and even though invasion by the organism is essential to its pathogenicity, the permeability of the intestinal mucosa is essentially normal. However, the inflammatory process itself seems to be necessary for the secretion to develop.[82]

Therefore, some acute inflammatory diarrheal diseases involving the colon may be a result of active secretion although the pathogenesis has not yet been defined. Two possible candidates for the activation of cAMP in the absence of enterotoxin may be the prostaglandins or vasoactive intestinal peptide (VIP) released from the inflamed intestinal mucosa. Both of these agents are present in high concentrations in colonic mucosa and both have been shown to activate the cAMP system.

Active Secretion from Other Causes

Two agents have recently been identified as inducing active secretion in the colon of man and animals. These are bile acids and fatty acids.[83,84] Although permeability changes have also been associated with these acids and other substances,[85,86] a suitable driving force for passive net secretion is not obvious. However, bile acids and fatty acids have been associated with stimulation of the cAMP secretory system of the colon. Therefore, in the presence of ileal disease or fat malabsorption, colonic involvement in the production of diarrhea should be anticipated. In fact, it has been proposed that certain antibiotics, especially those secreted into the bile, e.g., the tetracyclines and clindamycin, may inhibit the growth of normal anaerobic bacteria which dehydroxylate the bile acids and thus minimize net secretion. Hydroxylated bile acids apparently are responsible for the diarrhea associated with bile acid malabsorption.[87,88]

Specific Diarrheal Diseases

Colitis X

Colitis X is a peracute highly fatal diarrheal disease of the horse. The disease occurs sporadically at any time of the year and under all types of management. Horses of all ages and breeds can be affected. The cause is unknown. Colitis X is noncontagious and noninfectious. The mortality rate is high (at least 90% in untreated animals). Affected animals may die of shock within 3 to 24 hours.[89]

Pathogenesis. A massive shift of fluids from the extracellular space to the gut lumen occurs. Most horses have an acute, profuse, watery, nonbloody diarrhea but in some animals, fluids are sequestered in the bowel lumen without diarrhea. The mechanism of fluid loss is unknown. Several theories have been proposed to explain the "shock-colon syndrome"; however, none of these have been proven experimentally and none have considered the intestinal fluid loss to be the primary cause of shock. Among these proposed mechanisms are (1) endotoxic shock, (2) anaphylactic shock, and (3) exhaustion shock.

The intravenous injection of microgram amounts of endotoxin into experimental animals results in a highly lethal shock syndrome. Endotoxin is produced by all gram-negative bacteria including the normal colonic flora. Thus it is always present in the lumen because of bacterial death and senescence.[90] However, very little endotoxin is absorbed by the normal colonic mucosa, and what is absorbed is rapidly detoxified by the reticuloendothelial system of the liver. The intravenous injection of *E. coli* into ponies resulted in an endotoxemia and a clinical syndrome similar to that of colitis X.[91] Yet, no diarrhea occurred, even in animals maintained for as long as 25 hours. A bacteremia in cases of colitis X has not yet been demonstrated.[92]

Horses immunized with bovine serum albumin, and subsequently challenged, develop a clinical syndrome identical to colitis X.[93] The pathologic changes were also similar to colitis X and involved primarily the large intestine and the lung. These findings are supportive of the hypothesis that the equine lung and equine large intestine are the primary shock organs, but they provide no additional insight into the pathogenesis of colitis X.

Since a number of animals with colitis X have been subjected to a previous stress, e.g., transport or infection, it has been proposed that a secondary stress, for example, antibiotic treatment, could precipitate the disorder since the animals' resistance may be taxed to the limit.[94] Yet in many instances, no history of previous stress is evident and an apparently healthy animal may be affected.[92] Increased numbers of *Clostridium perfringens* have been found in the colon of some horses with clinical and necropsy findings compatible with colitis X. High dietary intake of protein, with low intake of cellulose, in combination with stress and antimicrobial therapy may have been important factors in these horses, which were collectively referred to as examples of equine intestinal clostridiosis.[94a] The association of antimicrobial therapy with colitis in these horses has a possible parallel in the circumstances preceding antibiotic-associated pseudomembranous colitis of humans,[94b] in which certain antimicrobial drugs (notably clindamycin) alter colonic microbial flora, allowing toxin-producing clostridia to proliferate.

Pathology. The pathologic changes involve the cecum and colon. The ileum is infrequently involved and no lesions are present in the stomach, duodenum, or jejunum. Grossly, the large intestine has a dull, reddish-blue to cyanotic color. A large quantity of foamy, malodorous fluid ingesta is present in the lumen. The mucosa appears intensely hyperemic with edema and hemorrhage in the submucosa. However, free blood is rarely found in the lumen.[89]

The liver is engorged with dark, non-clotting blood which oozes from the cut surface. The lung changes are compatible with alveolar emphysema, hyperemia, and varying degrees of edema. The adrenals are intensely hemorrhagic.

Upon histologic examination of the cecum and colon, the capillaries are engorged with blood with a marked dilatation of the venules and veins. Distinct evidence of sludging is present in the venous system. The small arteries of the submucosa show varying degrees of vasoconstriction and fresh dissection reveals an absence of blood in the arteries. The epithelium may have varying degrees of necrosis or may be completely normal. No significant new accumulation of inflammatory cells can be demonstrated.

These are clearly the lesions of passive congestion and stagnation of blood flow. Similar lesions are present in the large intestine when the venous drainage is blocked due to volvulus, strangulation, or incarceration.[89]

Pathophysiology. When the circulating blood volume is decreased for any reason, and this includes secretion into the lumen of the intestine or sequestration of fluid due to decreased absorption, the tonic stimulation of the baroreceptors in the carotid bodies and aortic arch is decreased. The result is a decrease in the parasympathetic tone and an increase in the sympathetic tone which results in release of norepinephrine at nerve terminals including those of the adrenal. The adrenal medulla in turn secretes more vasoactive substances, e.g., epinephrine.

The viscera and lungs (which are considered to be the primary targets in shock) are rich in α-adrenergic receptors and therefore intense arterial constriction occurs in the splanchnic region. Thus, the vascular space is reduced and total peripheral resistance is increased, ensuring blood flow to the heart and brain, which are insensitive to vasoactive substances.[11]

However, due to the increase in total peripheral resistance, the viscera become ischemic and if the ischemic anoxia is prolonged, or intense for even short periods, stagnant anoxia develops. Thus, arteriolar tone is lost and the capillaries and venules become congested owing to the increased viscosity of the blood. This effect results in immobilization of large amounts of blood in the stagnant circulation further compromising the effective blood volume. The retention of blood in the capillaries raises the hydrostatic pressure and fluid leaks into the tissue fluid compartment.[11]

While an increase in tissue hydrostatic pressure of only 4 to 5 cm H_2O is sufficient to increase the permeability of the intestinal mucosa and result in net fluid secretion,[95] it should be emphasized that the mechanism of fluid loss in this disease is unknown. A primary diarrheal disease could result in the same spectrum of events, including the pathologic changes in the last stages of shock. Unfortunately, by the time the animal comes to necropsy, visceral hypoxia has probably already developed and the lesions are not sufficient to establish whether the fluid loss is a primary or secondary event. This obviously complicates therapeutic measures, especially those involving antibiotic and vasoactive drugs.

Diagnosis. An accurate clinical diagnosis of this disease cannot usually be established with certainty. However, in any stressed horse with clinical evidence of shock and acute diarrhea, a high index of suspicion must be had for colitis X.

Clinical Signs. Explosive, watery diarrhea of abrupt onset is the chief clinical sign. Rarely, diarrhea is not present, but auscultation and percussion of the abdomen will reveal the presence of massive amounts of sequestered fluid. Paracentesis will rule out ascites which in any case is rare in the horse. Borborygmus is minimal but, when present, sound like water in a drum. The temperature may initially be slightly elevated but returns to normal or subnormal as shock progresses.[92] Often mild abdominal pain (colic) may be noted, but the overriding clinical impression is one of dullness and depression due to cardiovascular collapse.

Further examination reveals a loss of skin elasticity, congested mucous membranes, and a delayed capillary refill time up to 6 or 7 seconds; normal is 1 to 2 seconds. As deep shock approaches, there is a tachycardia (80 to 100 per minute) and a thready rapid pulse. The extremities are cool and areas of patchy sweating are present. In terminal stages, signs of central nervous system depression appear followed by prostration, cyanosis, and death.[92]

Laboratory Findings. A progressive increase in the PCV, up to 60 to 70%, is common as extracellular contraction proceeds. There is a leukopenia (<3 to $4000/mm^3$) and an inverted differential (neutropenia with a relative increase in lymphocytes). The metabolic acidosis is severe with blood pH values as low as 7.0 and bicarbonate down to 5 to 8 mEq/L. There appears to be a moderate decrease in serum Na^+ ($140 \rightarrow 125$) and Cl^- ($100 \rightarrow 85$ mEq/L) and the concentration of K^+ may be as low as 1.5 mEq/L. The serum protein is increased (8 to 10 g/dl) and the BUN is over 25 mg/dl due to prerenal azotemia. The blood glucose may be elevated to 185 mg/dl or more.[92]

Differential Considerations. The clinical signs are similar to those of endotoxic and anaphylactic shock and it is not yet established whether these are involved in colitis X. The disease must be differentiated from other acute diarrheal diseases, especially salmonellosis and to lesser degree verminous arteritis and acute peritonitis.

Colitis X is very difficult to distinguish from peracute salmonellosis clinically. Most clinicians consider colitis X first in any horse with peracute profuse diarrhea. If salmonella is isolated subsequently or the horse has a more protracted course, then other diagnoses, e.g., salmonellosis, are considered most likely. In peracute salmonellosis, high fever may be present but the acidosis of Salmonella-infected animals may not be as severe as with colitis X.[96] Both salmonellosis and colitis X have an initial leukopenia (<4000 WBC/mm^3) and if the horse survives, as in salmonellosis, a leukocytosis may occur. On occasion, other animals in the stable may have diarrhea, which would suggest salmonella, but horizontal transmission is most common in veterinary hospitals where stress is most common and the agent seems to persist.

The acute, profuse diarrhea associated with strongyle larval migration presents a similar but rarely peracute clinical picture. The acute form of strongyle migration appears much less often than the more chronic forms of strongylosis.[97] Abdominocentesis may yield an increased percentage of eosinophils, with a peripheral eosinophilia as well.[96]

Acute peritonitis should be suspected if there is a recent history of abdominal surgery or difficult rectal examination. Peritonitis can also occur secondary to rupture of the intestine from obstruction of strongyle larvae-induced ischemia. Abdominocentesis will reveal a WBC count of greater than 10,000/mm^3 with predominantly neutrophils.[96] The centesis examination is the key to ruling out this diagnostic consideration.

Treatment. Treatment of colitis X is directed at (1) replacement of electrolyte and water loss, (2) correction of the acidosis, and (3) improvement of tissue perfusion and cardiac output. The single most important factor is expansion of the extracellular fluid compartment with intravenous balanced electrolyte solutions. The amount of fluid loss can be estimated in severe dehydration to be 12% of the body weight.[92] Thus a 1000-pound horse may require 60 liters of fluid to be given at the rate of 3 to 12 liters per hour depending on the observed response (decrease in hematocrit and plasma proteins).

Although lactated Ringer's solution or glucose-NaCl solutions have been recommended, these are questionable for two reasons. First, the conversion of lactate to bicarbonate is dependent on oxidative cellular metabolism and in severe acidosis, anaerobic metabolism and lactic acid production are accelerated. Second, the administration of glucose to a hyperglycemic animal is questionable. In severe shock, the intense sympathetic activity has probably caused an outpouring of glucose from the liver. Thus, further glucose administration may cause an osmotic diuresis.

An alternative method for correction of the acidosis is direct administration of sufficient HCO_3^-. In severe acidosis with blood pH values of 7.0, the plasma bicarbonate may be about 10 mEq/L. Therefore, a deficit of 15 mEq/L is present, with a total deficit of about 2000 mEq HCO_3^- in a 450-kg (1000-lb) horse. It would require about 150 g of $NaHCO_3$ to correct this deficit. Some advocate the use of several liters of hypertonic 5% $NaHCO_3$ (600 mEq HCO_3^-/L) as initial fluid therapy to correct the severe acidosis, to be followed with an isotonic polyionic fluid.

The concentration of K^+ in the fluid requires additional comment. First, it appears that hypokalemia is present which is a peculiar manifestation in shock and acidosis in horses. The cause is unknown and could be a hypersecretion of aldosterone. Therefore, potassium-free or potassium-poor solutions will exacerbate the hypokalemia. Second, correction of the acidosis with HCO_3^- should shift K^+ into the intracellular compartment in exchange for H^+.[98] Thus, K^+ should be administered when massive amounts of HCO_3^- are given together with constant monitoring of the heart.[92] High $[K^+]$ solutions must not be given to the horse at a rate greater than 3 liters per hour.[98] Most adult horses will tolerate 40 mEq/L or up to 200 mEq/hr without untoward effects. Oral solutions of KCl are safer (up to a maximum of 1000 mEq/dose) and since the small bowel is presumably intact, oral replacement therapy may be supplementary. Most horses given oral fluid therapy, i.e., 20 to 80 liters, will develop an even more profuse diarrhea. However, an animal in severe shock must receive intravenous fluids immediately, preferably through a large bore catheter (16 to 14 gauge).

Antibiotic and Vasoactive Drugs. If a diagnosis of colitis X can be made with certainty, antibiotic therapy is questionable. In any event, the use of oral antibiotic or one primarily excreted by the biliary system is strongly contraindicated. As mentioned, antibiotic may exacerbate the disorder even if an infectious agent is present. If antibiotic is to be used, it must be given systemically and one excreted by the kidney is to be preferred.

Vasoconstrictor drugs are usually contraindicated in cases of shock unless cardiac failure is imminent. The vascular system is already under intense α-adrenergic stimulation and administration of these agents will further compromise the visceral and peripheral hypoxia which is present. The goal to achieve is increased cardiac output and increased tissue perfusion. This depends first on establishing sufficient plasma volume and second on support from α-blockers or β-adrenergic drugs, which increase perfusion of the ischemic viscera as well as cardiac output. A massive dose (10 times pharmacologic) of corticosteroid may be useful in severe shock.[92] These drugs are thought to augment tissue perfusion and cardiac output. An infectious agent, e.g., Salmonella, should be ruled out if corticosteroid is used continuously. Otherwise, systemic bactericidal antibiotic support must be given.[99]

Strongylosis (strongyle larval migrans)

Pathogenesis. The pathogenesis of strongylosis must be considered in two stages. The first is the migration of larvae from the intestine and their localization in arteries. The second is the adult stage and their localization on the mucosa of the cecum and colon.

The route of larval migration has been subject to much controversy. However, recent studies in experimentally infected horses[100] indicate that the larvae penetrate both the small and large intestine and appear in the submucosa within a few days. About 1 week after infection, fourth stage larvae are demonstrated in the lumen of submucosal arteries and then migrate up the arterial tree toward the cranial mesenteric artery. Many larvae reach this site by 3 weeks postinfection. There they develop into mature fourth stage larvae and after 3 to 4 months, the young adults migrate down the arteries towards the intestine.

Thus, the severe clinical syndrome of intestinal infarction can occur within 3 weeks after infection. Evidence of verminous mesenteric arteritis has been recorded in 10- and 18-day-old foals.[101] The acute syndrome associated with severe colic has been discussed previously under obstructive diseases. The present section is concerned with the diarrheal syndrome and is associated with occlusion of the small vessels of the mucosa of the large intestine by the migrating larvae, which leads to mucosal ulceration.

The young adults, once released back into the intestine, require a further 6 to 8 weeks to establish patency.[100] Thus, a prepatent period of approximately 6 months exists. It is very important for the clinician to remember that foals may be dying of strongylosis and have a negative fecal egg count. The adult strongyles inhabit the large intestine, where they cause massive blood loss. Thus, anemia may be a prominent finding at this stage.[100] The anemia is normocytic and normochromic with no evidence of response, as are most anemias in the horse.

Pathology. Infective larvae penetrate the mucosa of the ileum, cecum, and colon within a few days after ingestion. Submucosal hemorrhages and edema associated with the infiltration of neutrophils, mononuclear cells, and eosinophils are seen. The lymphatics are dilated with neutrophils.[102]

Nodules varying in size from pin-point to several centimeters form around the larvae in the submucosa and subserosa. When the larvae leave to enter the bloodstream, small crater-like openings are left which eventually heal by scarring. If these nodules rupture, local or general peritonitis or massive hemorrhage may occur.[19] Rarely, a massive hemoperitoneum may occur that will require blood transfusion.

Once the larvae reach the cranial mesenteric artery, a thromboarteritis may occur by adhesion of the larvae to the intima of the artery. Small thrombi are formed around the attached larvae leading to leukocyte infiltration and edema. This leads to a fibroblastic response with mononuclear cell infiltrate. At this stage the wall becomes solid and thick with a fremitus developing.[19] The nodular thickening, local pain, or the fremitus may be detected by rectal examination. Tortuosity and aneurysm of the cranial mesenteric artery are common but not invariable.

After 3 to 4 months, mature fourth stage larvae migrate from the cranial mesenteric artery toward the intestine until they reach a point where they can travel no further because of their size. At this point a nodule forms and subsequently ruptures, delivering the larvae into the intestine.[100]

In many cases, occlusion of end arteries by the larvae results in local ischemia and ulceration of the mucosa. Areas of inflammation and widespread hemorrhages may be present depending on the rate and extent of parasite migration. Extensive eosinophilic infiltration around partially and completely thrombosed vessels is present in the submucosa of the cecum and colon. The extensive ulceration, irregular in outline, is present primarily on the mesenteric side of the bowel. Many of these ulcers are deep and have necrotic areas with peripheral hemorrhages. Multiple emboli are always present in the dorsal and ventral colic arteries and the medial cecal artery. Thus, an association between the arterial lesions and ulceration of the mucosa has been demonstrated.[97]

The adult stage is characterized by attachment of the parasites to the mucosa, where they feed by sucking blood. Bleeding ulcerations may also occur from movements of the adult strongyles on the mucosa. Secondary bacterial invasion is possible leading to a catarrhal enteritis but it is rare to have clinical signs of enteritis. Strongyles in the intestine predispose to salmonellosis.

Pathophysiology. The pathologic lesions suggest malabsorption as the cause of the diarrhea. Unfortunately, little experimental work has been done and only generalizations can be made.

Abnormal d-xylose absorption is often present in cases of chronic diarrhea associated with *S. vulgaris*.[96] This would appear to correlate with the extent of small bowel damage and implies that malabsorption is also present in the large intestine, probably to a greater degree than in the small intestine. Malabsorption alone, in the horse, is associated with diarrhea.

While malabsorption of electrolytes and non-electrolytes and a decrease in disaccharidase activity is associated with a number of parasitic diseases, these functional defects are correlated only with the pathologically affected segment of bowel.[103] The intestine is capable of such compensatory function that the overall absorption by the bowel may in fact be normal. Thus, selective and sensitive tests such as D-xylose absorption appear to offer a greater degree of validity than glucose absorption.[104]

One of the common pathologic bases for an excessive enteric loss of plasma protein is ulceration of the intestinal mucosa or, less commonly, obstructive mesenteric lymphadenopathy. An accelerated loss of albumin into the gut has been demonstrated in mildly infected horses.[100] Low serum albumin associated with dehydration and subcutaneous edema has been reported in naturally occurring cases.[105] Other cases have no evidence of protein-losing enteropathy.[96] However, these differences may depend on the functional state of the bowel at the time of examination. For example, in some helminth infections an accelerated rate of protein leakage occurs only during severe clinical episodes, e.g., profuse diarrhea. During the quiescent period or during convalescence, intestinal protein loss may be decreased.[106]

Hypoproteinemia, specifically hypoalbuminemia, may be associated with this disease. It should not be regarded as a causal factor, but rather as a result of the disease. The total protein must be 4.5 g/dl or less to cause edema and even then is rarely associated with diarrhea.

Diagnosis. Clinical Findings. The diarrhea of strongylosis may be manifested as (1) an acute, profuse, diarrhea accompanied by shock, leading to death in a few hours, (2) a profuse and continuous diarrhea in which the animal may survive for weeks or months or (3) a mild diarrhea ("cow-like" feces) alternating with episodes of profuse diarrhea. In one study, 91 cases were examined and of these 56 were characterized by profuse diarrhea and 25 by chronic diarrhea.[97] Thus, very few animals seem to be affected with the shock syndrome which bears clinical signs similar to colitis X.

The signs associated with the chronic form feature a loss of body weight and condition, progressive dehydration and weakness, and finally incoordination and recumbency. Recurrent episodes of low-grade, self-limiting colic should raise the index of suspicion for this disease. Subcutaneous edema over the joints, brisket, ventral thorax and abdomen, prepuce or vulva may be present. The temperature, pulse, and respiration are normal. Rectal examination may reveal the presence of an aneurysm of the cranial mesenteric artery.[97]

On occasion, definitive diagnosis may only be made by exploratory laparotomy. A left flank approach with the horse sedated and anesthetized locally will suffice. Grossly, the presence of palpable mesenteric arteries or the formation of numerous streaks of hemametasma ilei are indicative of strongyle larval migrans. Histologic examination of intestinal biopsies of affected bowel can show varying degrees of eosinophilic infiltration of the lamina propria, villous atrophy of the mucosa, and thrombosis of arteries within the intestinal wall.[102,104] Migrating larvae may also be found in the sections.

Laboratory Findings. Egg counts of *Strongylus* spp. in the feces are of less value because of dilution when diarrhea is present. There is a moderate to severe hemoconcentration depending on the degree of dehydration, but the white cell counts (both total and differential) may be normal or increased.[97] In some cases there is an eosinophilia but in others the eosinophil count may be normal or subnormal. However, abdominocentesis may reveal an increase in eosinophils and an increase in phagocytic activity.[96]

In cases associated with edema, total serum protein is decreased to less than 4.5 g/dl, owing primarily to hypoalbuminemia as the β-globulins are often increased, which is interpreted by many as evidence of an internal parasite load. Therefore, ^{51}Cr-albumin turnover will be increased in these cases. D-xylose absorption may be decreased.

In cases involving the adult worms, the primary clinical manifestations are related to anemia and loss of condition due to the blood loss.

Treatment. Treatment must be directed at (1) replacement of electrolytes and water, (2) correction of acidosis if present, (3) improvement of collateral blood flow to the viscera, (4) nutritional therapy, and (5) elimination of the larval and adult strongyles.

In the case of acute, profuse diarrhea, dehydration and shock, the fluid therapy should be essentially the same as discussed for colitis X. Similar electrolyte problems are present, including hypokalemia.[97] If the diarrhea is acute and profuse, acidosis can be expected to develop. If anemia is severe (PCV 12%), whole blood or a plasma volume expander should be given.

In the more chronic cases, replacement of electrolytes (Na^+, K^+, and Cl^-) is still the primary aim and must be continued until the animal has recovered. Oral solutions containing 50 to 100 g $NaHCO_3$ or a commercially available electrolyte solution can be given in the drinking water each day. The animal should have unlimited access to drinking water.[97]

In cases where it is concluded that acute thrombo-occlusive vascular disease is present (cranial mesenteric aneurysm, recurrent colic), anticoagulants have been found useful.[97] In a series of 55 such cases, a 6% dextran (mol wt 70,000) solution in 5% dextrose was given and 52 of the 55 horses recovered. Of 16 horses which were not so treated, 14 had to be destroyed. An initial dose of 1500 ml should be given as a slow intravenous injection, followed by 500 ml on the following day. Dextran is a plasma volume expander and also has potent anticoagulant effects. It seems to minimize sludging of blood and improves the microcirculation. A few animals may show an untoward reaction (tachycardia, collapse and struggling for several minutes) and the first 50 to 100 ml should be given slowly, while monitoring the heart.

If prominent subcutaneous edema is present and renal, hepatic, cardiac, and dietary causes of edema are ruled out, a protein-losing state must be suspected. A high protein ration such as alfalfa, with a high protein concentrate, is recommended. Following this treatment, the edema should be reduced within a few days.[97]

The most useful anthelmintic for elimination of strongyles is thiabendazole. In the case of adult worms, this should be given at a dose of 50 mg/kg. If the larvae are still migrating, 10 times the normal dose (500 mg/kg $\simeq$ 22 g/45 kg) should be given 2 days in a row.[107] Thiabendazole is absorbed and has systemic activity against strongyle larvae at this dose. Owners should be warned that this dose may cause the horse to stop eating grain for a few days. Also, the 10 × dose of thiabendazole has caused laminitis on rare occasions. One should not expect much success in severe cases where many fourth and fifth stage larvae are present.[108]

Prophylaxis. Control of all forms of strongylosis depends primarily upon attempts to keep egg-

burdens low in pastures and paddocks. Control strategies are discussed in Chapter 17.

Salmonellosis

Salmonellosis is a disease of all animals and man. The species of Salmonella commonly encountered are *S. typhimurium* in horses, *S. typhimurium* and *S. dublin* in cattle and sheep, and *S. typhimurium* and *S. choleraesuis* in pigs.

Pathology. The primary lesions of the enteric form of salmonellosis in horses occur in the large intestine as a catarrhal enterocolitis with hyperemia and edema of the mucosa. Hemorrhagic colitis may occur in more severe cases. A combination of catarrhal enteritis, hemorrhagic typhlitis, and colitis have been described in horses,[109] characterized by superficial necrosis of the mucosa with a greyish-red, pseudo-diphtheritic membrane.

As the inflammation progresses, fibrin deposits and leukocyte margination occur between the superficial lesion and the underlying area and, in chronic cases, thickening and scarring of the bowel occurs.

Experimental *S. typhimurium* results in the most striking lesions in the colon which may be a result of delayed transit in this region.[24] In the less severe cases, a catarrhal colitis with petechial hemorrhages deep within the mucosa is observed. The luminal contents are a watery, mucofibrinous exudate with blood occasionally present. In more advanced cases, hemorrhagic areas with overlying erosions are found. These are usually focal, but in some there is a diffuse fibrinonecrotic colitis and typhlitis. The most severe lesions are an almost full-thickness necrosis of the colon and cecal wall. A diffuse and fibrinonecrotic proctitis is also observed in such cases. Discrete deep annular ulcers are common in the rectum. Similar lesions are present in field cases infected with *S. typhimurium* and *S. choleraesuis.*[24]

Pathophysiology. The number of cases of salmonellosis in the horse associated with stress and antibiotic therapy (lincomycin, erythromycin, tylosin and especially the tetracyclines) continues to mount, in our opinion. The tetracyclines are concentrated in the liver and delivered in high concentration in bile to the intestine.[110] Thus, the probability of altering the normal intestinal flora is increased and this provides a basis for establishment of pathogens. In a number of documented cases, salmonella organisms were found to be resistant to tetracyclines as well as to a number of other broad-spectrum antibiotics.[111] Any sudden alteration in dietary intake, fasting, or change in motility, as may occur in colic, will induce great change in proportions of colonic bacterial flora.[112] Massive changes in the numbers and types of organisms can occur within a period of 2 to 4 hours. Therefore, serious consideration should be given to the view that alteration of the normal flora may be an important mechanism predisposing to diarrhea, especially if the horse is a salmonella carrier or has been exposed to a salmonella-contaminated environment recently.

Clinical Signs. The clinical signs are representative of the stage of the disease, i.e., *septicemia, acute enteritis, chronic enteritis,* or *carrier states.* The septicemic form is most common in foals up to 6 months of age. In this stage there is dullness, depression, severe dehydration, and a high fever (105 to 107° F). Death may occur within 24 to 72 hours from septicemia and hypovolemic shock due to the massive fluid losses.

The acute form of enteritis is more common in foals, aged horses, and stressed or debilitated horses. In the adult horse, frank blood is rarely passed in the feces. A fever of 103 to 106° is present. Large volumes of mucoid to water-like feces are voided. The bulbar and palpebral conjunctiva are injected and severely congested. A prominent leukopenia and neutropenia occur at onset, followed by a leukocytosis and neutrophilia with a metabolic acidosis in 24 to 48 hours. In the chronic form, the diarrhea is not as severe and the feces appear similar to cow feces.[109]

In our experience, severely infected horses may develop disseminated intravascular coagulation (DIC), manifested clinically by rapid thrombosis of veins used for venipuncture, and development of laminitis. When this occurs, the prognosis is very unfavorable. The diarrhea in these acute cases is usually not bloody or flecked with tissue debris but is projectile and extremely fluid. Such animals object vigorously to rectal examination. Some horses recover completely within a week. Others, especially those with DIC, may die rapidly or linger and slowly deteriorate over a few weeks. Still others may stabilize and begin to feel better within a few days but continue to have persistent diarrhea for months.

Animals that are known to experience a short, self-limiting course of diarrhea whenever exposed to a stressful situation should be regarded with much suspicion.[113] For instance, horses known to have diarrhea whenever they race or experience an upper respiratory infection have been admitted to our practice* for an elective surgical procedure. It is

*School of Veterinary Medicine, University of Pennsylvania, Philadelphia, PA.

not uncommon for such animals to have fever and diarrhea after surgery, with culture of salmonellae from their feces where none could be cultured presurgically.

Some clinicians monitor the white cell count daily for 7 days following surgery in horses; if a leukopenia occurs, the animal is immediately isolated and given systemic antibiotic therapy.[114]

The features which distinguish colitis X, peritonitis, and strongylosis from salmonellosis have been discussed under colitis X.

Diagnosis. The most definitive diagnosis is culture of the salmonella organisms from the feces of the clinically affected patient. However, the absence of organisms on one or even three culture attempts does not rule out salmonellosis. A minimum of six negative fecal cultures for salmonella are required before one is comfortable about ruling out salmonellosis (this is assuming optimum conditions for culture). The author observed one mare that was negative for Salmonella in 10 consecutive fecal cultures, though when she died following two weeks of diarrhea, fever, and progressive hypoproteinemia, the organism was cultured from her bile. By comparison, the lack of fecal-positive salmonella cultures in cattle was especially enlightening. In one study, 18% of rumen samples in cattle were positive for salmonella compared to 10% of the fecal samples from the same group of animals.[115]

In vitro antimicrobial sensitivity tests should always be conducted with drugs having antimicrobial activity against salmonellae. Salmonellae frequently isolated from horses have the following susceptibilities, in our experience:

1. Gentamicin	100%	6. Kanamycin	58%
2. Chloramphenicol	96%	7. Tetracycline	40%
3. Furadantin	96%	8. Streptomycin	33%
4. Ampicillin	62%	9. Erythromycin	0%
5. Neomycin	58%	10. Lincomycin	0%
		11. Penicillin	0%

In some veterinary institutions, salmonella isolates are resistant to all antibiotics including gentamicin and chloromycetin, possibly owing to the selective resistance induced by promiscuous use of antimicrobial drugs.

Antimicrobic therapy for salmonellosis in the horse presents a major problem. It has been said that treatment with broad-spectrum antibiotic is without clinical benefit or is contraindicated as it prolongs the carrier state.[116] Drug sensitivity or resistance appears to have little bearing on eliminating salmonellae from the feces or organs of infected horses.[109,111] The nitrofuran drugs have been used with some success.[116] Most salmonellae from horses are susceptible to gentamicin, chloramphenicol, or nitrofurantoin, in our experience. Oral chloramphenicol (50 mg/kg split q.i.d.) may be cheaper than gentamicin (4.4 mg/kg) and both seem to be of more benefit than nitrofurans, despite the in vitro sensitivity of many salmonella isolates to nitrofuran compounds.

Treatment. Fluid therapy is the cornerstone of treatment for salmonellosis in horses. The pathophysiology of salmonellosis in experimental animals indicates a major loss of Na^+, Cl^-, and H^+ into the intestine. Therefore, only a minor acidosis may be present and this is presumably due to anaerobic tissue metabolism in the acutely dehydrated animal. Some horses with acute diarrheal problems initially have a metabolic alkalosis.[117] As the process continues, metabolic acidosis develops. Thus, the most important fluid replacement therapy consists of a balanced electrolyte solution similar in composition to the plasma. See the therapy section under colitis X for a more complete description of fluid therapy in horses.

A suspension of 480 ml (four 4-oz cupfuls) of charcoal powder in 2 liters of water, given by stomach tube b.i.d., is recommended. Charcoal treatment may be repeated for 2 to 3 days.

The studies concerning the pathophysiology of salmonellosis suggest alternative approaches to controlling a life-threatening diarrhea when antibiotic treatment is without benefit or fluid therapy is impractical. If the diarrhea is in fact mediated by prostaglandins, agents such as loperamide or indomethacin may be useful, since both have been shown to be effective in antagonizing prostaglandin-induced diarrhea.[118,119] While these drugs have not yet been used in salmonellosis of domestic animals, present-day research on this disease is providing a basis for examination of such agents in the clinical situation.

At the present time, the best method of control is prevention,[120] which includes all the necessary factors for good management and hygiene, and minimization of stress. One commercial vaccine (Paratyfol [Salmonella dublin-typhimurium]) is available and its use is advocated by some, although others regard its efficacy as unproven.

Equine Granulomatous Enteritis

This chronic wasting disease of the horse affects both the small and large bowel.[121] Diarrhea, if present, is intermittent. In a group of 12 horses with this disease, 11 were Standardbreds and one a Thoroughbred. No sex or age distribution was apparent. In one horse, *Mycobacterium tuberculosis,* avian type, was isolated from the feces; however, no etiologic agent was found in any of the other animals.[121]

Pathologic Lesions. The gross and microscopic pathology of this disease resembles Crohn's disease in man[121] and, to a lesser extent, Johne's disease in cattle. Grossly, adhesions of small and large intestine may be present. The serosal surface of the adhered bowel is red-purple and in some areas yellow-white or red fibrous plaques and firm white nodules are present. In the large colon, the mucosal surface reveals the presence of numerous linear erosions 2 to 3 mm wide and 40 mm long. The mesenteric nodes are enlarged and edematous. On cut surface of the lymph nodes, wet, grey firm tissue or many firm white nodules may be present. These are characterized histologically by a focal or diffuse infiltrate of mononuclear cells enclosed in some places by fibrous tissue.

Histologically, the ileum appears most severely affected and the large intestine least affected. Cellular infiltrate of the lamina propria is by lymphocytes and macrophages or epithelioid cells. Plasma cells and a few multinucleated giant cells are also seen. A few walled-off granulomas in the submucosa of the small bowel are found. Superficial erosions surrounded by a zone of neutrophils are seen in both the small and large intestine. Mononuclear cells extend into the muscularis but this is more common in the small bowel. One prime feature in the small intestine is a severe villous atrophy.

Pathophysiology. The disease is primarily one of protein-losing enteropathy and malabsorption. ^{51}Cr-albumin excretion is increased over normal and hypoalbuminemia is present.[122] This feature is characteristic of any small intestinal granulomatous reaction regardless of the cause.

Some of these horses may have concomitant skin lesions which have been shown to be immunologically mediated (deposits of globulins in the prickle cell layer and along the basement membrane).[123] Dermatitis herpetiformis is associated with a nontropical sprue-like disease due to a gluten hypersensitivity. These lesions are most severe in the ileum as are the lesions of granulomatous enteritis. Finding IgA deposits below the dermal basement membrane is diagnostic.[123]

Severe villous atrophy of the small intestinal mucosa is present and D-xylose and glucose malabsorption are demonstrable.[122] Malabsorption accounts for the weight loss and poor condition observed clinically. Since the ileum seems to be primarily involved, active absorption of bile acids is probably impaired, which would further exacerbate small bowel lipid malabsorption. Lipid malabsorption has been demonstrated in affected horses.[124] Both bile acids and fatty acids are capable of stimulating colonic secretion and this may account for the intermittent chronic diarrhea observed in some animals. Further investigation is needed to elucidate the pathogenesis.

Diagnosis. The most consistent abnormalities are hypoalbuminemia and reduced phagocytosis by peritoneal macrophages. Neither finding is specific for equine granulomatous enteritis.

Hypoalbuminemia may be due to protein-losing enteropathy if the urine is protein-free, the liver function is normal, the dietary intake is adequate and there is no evidence of protein accumulation in a body cavity, i.e., pleural effusion. The finding of reduced macrophage phagocytic activity is subjective at best. Rectal palpation may reveal masses in the areas of the anterior mesenteric artery. If well developed, the mass will resemble a cluster of soft large grapes. The rectal mucosa may be thickened and friable. If the rectum is involved, proctoscopy may reveal the presence of erosions which supports the diagnosis. Albumin turnover and D-xylose absorption tests are also useful. A confirmed diagnosis rests on an intestinal or mesenteric lymph node biopsy.[122] However, any horse with a severe hypoproteinemia (TP < 4.5 g/dl) and a flat oral glucose tolerance curve or decreased xylose absorption is a prime candidate for granulomatous enteritis and a defined data base should be completed.

Treatment. The use of salicylazosulfapyridine in combination with corticosteroids has been recommended.[122,124] Supportive intravenous nutritional therapy may be necessary until the small bowel mucosa regains normal function, although the complications following prolonged use of indwelling intravenous catheters are enormous. The prognosis in these patients is poor and most affected horses are euthanatized.

Equine Chronic Diarrhea of Other Causes

Chronic diarrhea in horses continues to be a clinical enigma, since many cases are not classifiable by present knowledge and techniques. In the absence of precise diagnostic criteria, the effectiveness of therapy is sometimes difficult to evaluate.

Several reports in the literature allude to an equine intestinal trichomonad that has been associated with chronic diarrhea.[125,126,127] The diagnosis of intestinal protozoal diarrhea is based on the microscopic detection of large numbers of trichomonads in the diarrheic feces. The protozoan has been referred to as *Tritrichomonas fecalis* and *Tritrichomonas equi.*[128] Perhaps the most important reason that this continues to be perpetuated in the veterinary literature is because many horses with trichomonads in their feces respond to a trichomonacidal drug.[126] This drug (iodochlorhydroxyquin) has been and continues to be an effective therapy, at least symptomatically, for many types of equine diarrhea. Many of these horses will have, and have had, diarrhea for months and occasionally years. When treated with approximately 10 g daily, there is usually a fairly prompt response in the consistency of the feces to normal ball formation. This response takes place in 3 to 5 days. However, as the drug is withdrawn, the chronic "cow-like" type of diarrhea returns, in our experience. If the dosage of the drug is gradually lowered, the diarrhea usually exacerbates.

Perhaps the most definitive evidence repudiating the causal relationship of trichomonads to chronic diarrhea was a survey of trichomonads in normal horses and horses with diarrhea.[128] Thirty-five percent of 289 normal horses had, by cultural examination, trichomonads in their feces. At necropsy another 37% of horses which had no signs of diarrhea also had evidence of trichomonads. Experimentally induced diarrhea was accompanied by a greatly increased concentration of trichomonads in the fecal effluent. Counts increased from 10,000 to 100,000 trichomonads per ml of fecal fluid. Thus, as many observers have proposed, the trichomonads associated with chronic diarrhea in the horse are a result of the decreased transit time (diarrhea) rather than a cause of chronic diarrhea.[129]

Other causes of chronic diarrhea and weight loss include histoplasmosis, in which the diarrhea can be fairly profuse but protracted in nature.[130] This diagnosis is difficult to make antemortem and is usually made only at necropsy. The gross lesions include a massive mesenteric lymphadenopathy, thickened wall of the cecum and colon and blood-stained intestinal contents.

Another parasite, *Globidium leuckarti,* has been found in the small intestine and colon in some horses and may be more disseminated throughout the equine population.[131] Its role in the pathogenesis of diarrhea remains to be investigated. However, some evidence has implicated its relationship to equine diarrhea.[132]

The alimentary form of lymphosarcoma has been reported as a cause of chronic diarrhea in two horses.[133] Both of these horses had diffuse involvement of the intestinal tract. One must be careful to differentiate alimentary lymphosarcoma from granulomatous enterocolitis, since both are similar grossly and histologically.

Numerous medical treatments have been attempted in horses with chronic diarrhea, but the most intriguing and perhaps successful is the use of oral serum therapy.[134] One liter of normal equine serum was given on 3 successive days and repeated in 3 weeks. All 12 horses so treated improved but several horses required three or four treatments. Most horses started to gain weight following the first serum ingestion. Whole blood given orally exacerbates the diarrhea, in our experience. Immunoglobulin determinations in these diarrheic horses and normal horses showed a significant increase of IgG in diarrheic horses, with IgA being about 50% less than in the control horses.[135] Evaluation of the cell-mediated immune response in these 12 horses was decreased compared to controls but improved as the diarrhea decreased. Is this a cause or an effect of the chronic diarrhea? The possibility that transient defects of cell-mediated immunity may predispose to equine chronic diarrhea is interesting and needs further study.

One unique surgical approach to the treatment of chronic diarrhea deserves notice; the use of an antiperistaltic bowel segment.[136] Segments of small colon 12 to 30 cm long were excised, reversed, and anastomosed in normal horses and horses with diarrhea.[137] The surgical procedure was successful in three of five horses. The reversed segment becomes an antiperistaltic segment and impedes digesta flow. The intestine anterior to the reversed segment becomes dilated in response to the impediment of ingesta flow.

Winter Dysentery of Cattle

Winter dysentery is a highly contagious, acute enteric disease of cattle characterized by a sudden onset of severe diarrhea and dysentery. It occurs primarily in dairy cattle in the northeastern and north central United States, and in Canada; it has also been reported in Australia, Israel, Sweden, France, and England. It occurs in the late fall after October 15, and during the winter months, through April 15. The most severely affected animals are 2- or 3-year-old pregnant or lactating heifers, while older cows usually have less severe signs. Severe dysentery and hemorrhage occurs in 5 to 10% of cattle. Mortality is uncommon but does occur and is primarily associated with a blood loss anemia.

Etiology and Pathogenesis. The etiology of winter dysentery is unknown. Early investigations indicated *Vibrio jejuni* to be the etiologic agent; but more recent studies have failed to substantiate this source. Viruses have been isolated and incriminated in some outbreaks.[138] There is no conclusive evidence to incriminate IBR, BVD, bovine parvovirus, enterovirus, or other cytopathic virus as causative agents.

The disease is transmitted easily by fomites, by contact, or by fecal suspensions and is extremely contagious. It has all the hallmarks of an infectious, contagious disease. Many bovine practitioners, cattle dealers, feed salesmen, and others have been incriminated for spreading winter dysentery from farm to farm.

Experimental transmission of the disease has been difficult as the agent does not survive freezing and therefore a constant source of infectious material is not always available. However, successful transmission has been done experimentally by oral or oronasal routes using fresh fecal suspension from cattle infected with winter dysentery.[138]

The incubation period varies between 3 and 5 days with a mean of 4.5 days. Transmission to experimental animals including suckling mice, rabbits, and guinea pigs have been unsuccessful, although some animals died.

Vaccination with *Leptospira pomona* vaccines or live virus vaccines of IBR, BVD, and PI-3 have not been shown to be effective in preventing outbreaks of winter dysentery. Similarly, there has been no evidence of seroconversion to BVD or IBR in winter dysentery. Mixed bovine bacterins are worthless in preventing the disease.

Pathology. As the disease is rarely fatal, no definitive reports have been written on the lesions associated with the disease.

Diagnosis. Because the cause is not yet known, diagnosis is made largely on the herd history and clinical findings rather than on laboratory tests.

Clinical Findings. An acute onset of profuse liquid brown diarrhea in a high proportion of cows in a herd should be presumptive evidence of winter dysentery.[139] Occasionally bloody feces are present. Many of the cows will have a nonproductive moist cough. There will be a concomitant reduction in milk production. A fever in the range of 103°F to 104°F occurs occasionally but is transient. There is no consistent relationship with fever and onset of diarrhea. Abortion is rarely associated with the disease, but one case has been reported, the cause of which was undetermined.[140] The disease is transient and feces usually return to normal in 5 to 7 days.

Laboratory Findings. Minimal laboratory work has been done in herds with winter dysentery. A moderate to severe anemia may occur rarely, and may be the cause of death in some animals.

Differential Diagnosis. The characteristic acute onset of diarrhea in stabled cattle enables easy herd and individual diagnosis to be made using the criteria outlined previously. Exposure to toxic chemicals or acute toxic indigestion must be considered in any herd outbreak of diarrhea. Oral examination may be helpful in differentiating winter dysentery from bovine virus diarrhea or rinderpest. Oral ulcers and erosions are found in the latter, but not in winter dysentery. Fecal samples and fecal cultures are needed to rule out parasitism and salmonellosis.

Treatment. The treatment in the past has been entirely empirical. Reports indicate that a variety of drug treatments have no effect on the duration or the severity of diarrhea.

Swine Dysentery (hemorrhagic dysentery, vibrionic dysentery, black scours)

Swine dysentery is a highly contagious diarrheal disease in pigs. The lesions are confined to the large intestine. Four forms of the disease can be recognized.[141] The peracute form is characterized by a sudden onset and rapid death, the cause of which is unknown. The acute form is the most common and in this stage a mucoid to watery diarrhea is present, followed by the passage of flecks of red blood. Death is due to dehydration, acidosis and hyperkalemia. The subacute and chronic forms are characterized by a less severe diarrhea, unthriftiness, and lack of growth or loss of weight. Passage of necrotic mucous membranes and dark blood in the feces is common. Swine dysentery most commonly affects 15- to 70-kg pigs, but can occur in suckling pigs or adults.

Etiology and Pathogenesis. The etiologic agent was formerly thought to be a vibrio (*V. coli*) but it has now been demonstrated conclusively that the agent is a large spirochete, *Treponema hyodysenteriae*.[142] However, when the spirochete is introduced into germ-free pigs, lesions are not produced. Therefore, either the presence of another agent is necessary for pathogenicity of *T. hyodysenteriae* or a change in the microenvironmental conditions in the colon may be involved, e.g., substrate, pH, or pCO_2 from normal microbial digestion.[143,144]

The pig is the only known reservoir for *T. hyodysenteriae* but these anaerobic bacteria have the potential to survive under a wide variety of environmental conditions.[142] Thus, transmission of the disease is prevalent unless strict measures of decontamination of infected premises are instituted.

The mode of transmission is by ingestion of fecal-contaminated feed.

Many pigs that survive the acute phase are resistant to subsequent challenge,[142] which implies that a degree of immunity is conferred by infection. However, attempts to immunize pigs orally with attenuated spirochetes have been unsuccessful. Combinations of oral dosing and parenteral inoculation are only partially successful[145] and at this time are of no practical use in prevention of the disease.

The course of the clinical disease is from 2 days to 2 weeks in the acute form, but from 3 to 4 weeks in chronic cases. The morbidity rates range from 30 to 40% to 75% depending on environmental conditions. The mortality rates range from 10% in feeder and older pigs to 60% in newly weaned pigs. However, mortality rates as high as 90% have been associated with premises in which poor sanitary conditions prevail.[141]

Pathology. The lesion is primarily a catarrhal colitis confined exclusively to the large intestine,[146] although a few instances of concurrent gastritis have been reported.[147] From the serosal surface, the colon appears hyperemic and edematous. Swollen, pale submucosal glands can be seen. The lesions are usually diffuse throughout the colon and are characterized by a mucohemorrhagic and mucofibrinous exudation. Often, a diphtheritic pseudomembrane is formed by the exudate. Blood is always found in the lumen.[146] The gross lesions were most severe at the apex of the spiral colon. Edema of the mesentery and colonic lymph nodes occurs commonly.

Microscopic examination reveals a superficial coagulative necrosis of the mucosa.[147] The epithelium may be separated from the lamina propria or completely eroded away in some areas. The eroded surface is covered with exudate containing mucus, erythrocytes, fibrin, and bacteria. Edema of the mucosa and submucosa is present with congested vessels near the lumen containing numerous neutrophils. The submucosa contains zones of hyperemia and hemorrhage with leukocytic infiltration.[147] Spirochetes morphologically compatible with *T. hyodysenteriae* were easily observed on the epithelial cell surface and in the crypts of Lieberkühn, in experimentally infected pigs 5 to 8 days postinfection.[148]

The crypts are dilated with mucus and this is associated with goblet cell hyperplasia. Numerous large spirochetes can be seen in the crypts with special stains, i.e., silver stains for spirochetes.[146]

Pathophysiology. Although spirochetes can be demonstrated within and between the epithelial cells and in the lamina propria, there is no evidence that invasion is essential for the lesions to develop.[142] Invasion beyond the lamina propria has not been demonstrated, nor has an enterotoxic substance been associated with *T. hyodysenteriae.*

The exudative and hemorrhagic process seems obviously due to increased permeability through damaged or eroded epithelium. However, studies with isolated loops of the spiral colon have shown a normal mucosal permeability, although net Na$^+$ and Cl$^-$ absorption from the colon was completely abolished. Thus, the disease appears to be one of colonic malabsorption.[149]

The clinical manifestations of acidosis and hyperkalemia are common for a number of diarrheal conditions, and probably occurs secondarily to decreased tissue perfusion.

Diagnosis. Clinical Findings. The onset of the acute phase is characterized initially by depression, contracted abdomen, and the appearance of yellow-grey soft feces, then large amounts of mucus and flecks of blood. This is followed by a watery diarrhea with blood, mucus, and shreds of mucosa. As the disease progresses, the volume of feces decreases and there is evidence of well-mixed dark blood.[142]

A febrile response may or may not be present initially but in any case disappears with the onset of diarrhea. The usual manifestations of dehydration are apparent and the pigs exhibit an increased thirst.

Laboratory Findings. A prominent left shift with high numbers of immature neutrophils (bands) is present. There is an increase in erythrocyte sedimentation rate and fibrinogen concentration. The PCV does not usually indicate significant blood loss because of concomitant dehydration. An increase in the total serum protein value is present. Serum Na$^+$, Cl$^-$, and HCO$_3^-$ concentrations are decreased. A metabolic acidosis and hyperkalemia mark the terminal stage.[146]

Differential Diagnosis. The disease must be primarily differentiated from salmonellosis.[150] Small bowel diarrheas are usually not difficult to rule out; one simply does a gross examination of the feces for endoparasites.

A positive diagnosis rests on the demonstration of large numbers of large spirochetes in the feces. While these can be detected in the feces only during the acute phase of the disease, they are always present within the mucosal lesions. The spirochetes can be viewed satisfactorily with phase or dark-field microscopy at 400 to 1000 ×. Fluorescent antibody tests are also available.[143]

Gross pathologic lesions differ primarily from salmonellosis in that (1) the swine dysentery lesions are confined to the large bowel and (2) the button ulcers of salmonellosis are absent.

Treatment. In the past, arsenical compounds were effectively used to treat the disease. However, the effectiveness of these compounds has decreased in recent years owing to the development of resistance to the compound by *T. hyodysenteriae.*[142] Therefore, in vitro sensitivity tests should be used when this is possible.

Recent studies have shown that Na arsanilate or tylosin added to the feed did not protect pigs against dysentery; in fact the pigs developed a more severe hemorrhagic diarrhea than non-treated controls. The addition of lincomycin and spectinomycin at 44 and 77 mg/kg feed prevented the disease.[151]

Medical treatment should be provided in the drinking water since sick pigs are usually anorectic. Among the effective antibiotics are streptomycin, bacitracin, neomycin, gentamicin, chlortetracycline and virginiamycin.[142] Ronidazole, a nitro-imidazole compound, has been shown to be effective at a concentration of 0.006% in the drinking water. This concentration eliminated most of the spirochetes from the colon. At higher levels, the compound may induce diarrhea.[152] Approximately one third of the treatment dose on a mg/kg/day basis would prevent the disease.

Part II. Diseases of the Colon, Rectum, and Anus in the Dog and Cat

COLIN F. BURROWS

THE COLON

The colon has two major physiologic functions in the dog and cat: (1) the absorption of water and electrolytes from the luminal contents, and (2) storage, with periodic expulsion, of the resulting fecal material.[153,154] Absorption of water and electrolytes takes place primarily in the ascending, transverse, and proximal part of the descending colon;[155,156] while storage takes place in the distal part of the organ.[153] Unlike herbivores, and possibly omnivores, there is no evidence that the colon of the dog or cat serves a significant nutritional function through the microbial digestion of luminal contents. However, the concentration of volatile fatty acids is quite high in the canine colon, regardless of the nature of the diet.[157]

Only limited data are available on normal colonic function, and little or no data on colonic function in naturally occurring colonic diseases of the dog and cat. Much of what we know, or perhaps assume, is extrapolated from studies in man and may not apply to the dog and cat. It is known that the colon serves as very efficient absorptive surface for sodium, chloride and water in all species in which it has been studied.[156,158] As in other species, the presence in the canine colon of volatile fatty acids facilitates the absorption of sodium. However, in contrast to man, the canine colon absorbs rather than secretes bicarbonate.[159] Potassium is actively secreted into the colon of all species and is exchanged for sodium under the influence of aldosterone.[160-162] This colonic sodium conservation has been shown to play a homeostatic role in some diarrheal diseases.[163] Finally, colonic mucus is very rich in potassium,[161] so that chronic mucoid diarrhea can result in potassium depletion.

The regional differences in absorption emphasize the role of colonic motility and fecal transit in the absorptive process. Since defecation is a periodic phenomenon, and input from the ileum is also probably periodic,[164] there must be some sort of coupling between colonic input and output. Subsequent provisions for orderly delays, mixing, and movement of colonic contents is necessary to facilitate the absorptive process,[154] but study of colonic motility is complicated by difficult access to the organ and by extensive anatomic and functional differences between species. These have precluded the development of an overall concept of colonic motor function.[64] Many techniques have been utilized to study colonic motility, but a clear understanding of the highly organized and complex characteristics of colonic motor function has not yet been developed. It has become clear, however, that detailed descriptions of canine and feline colonic motility based on studies in man are both unwarranted and unwise.

While distinct species differences do exist, pressure and myoelectrical recordings as well as radiographic studies have shown that the mammalian colon contracts in three basic patterns.[165-168]

Retrograde Peristalsis. This consists of ring contractions moving cephalad and is purportedly the dominant activity of the proximal colon. Although the situation is still far from clear,[166,169] retrograde peristalsis seems to occur frequently in the cat, but is reportedly absent in the dog.[170] This observation has been supported by studies of the contractile and myoelectrical activity of the normal canine colon.[171]

Segmentation. This consists of either stationary or progressive ring contractions moving over short distances in either direction, and is the dominant activity of the transverse and proximal descending colon. Segmental contractions mix the luminal contents, slow down movement of the feces in an aboral direction, and facilitate efficient electrolyte and water absorption. Intraluminal pressure studies in man have shown that there is a decrease in the degree of pressure activity in some patients with diarrhea, whereas activity is increased in constipation.[172] These findings are in agreement with the concept that the main function of colonic motor activity is to delay fecal transmit.

Mass Movements. There are strong rings of contraction moving in an aboral direction. They occur

553

at infrequent intervals in the transverse and descending colon and propel colonic contents towards the rectum. Mass movements are generated much higher in the canine colon than in the feline colon, and the entire length of the canine colon can be evacuated at will.[170] In the dog, mass movements start within 3 cm of the ileocolic junction.[171] This observation possibly explains the occasional liquid or semiliquid appearance of the terminal portion of normal canine feces.

The incidence of colonic disease in the dog is probably much higher than is generally appreciated. Experience in this practice,* where approximately 50% of the cases of chronic diarrhea in the dog are attributed to some form of colonic dysfunction, indicates that colitis is the most frequently diagnosed colonic disease. Though the practice is a referral center and thus receives a larger number of chronic diarrhea cases than the typical small animal practice, the figure of 50% does give an indication of the incidence of colonic disease, and is similar to that in man.[173]

Our experience also suggests that the general lack of awareness of the incidence of colonic disease is paralleled by a similar lack of awareness of its treatment. We see many dogs with colitis that have been treated unsuccessfully with commercially available antidiarrheal preparations such as kaolin and pectin, various antidiarrheal-antibiotic, or antidiarrheal-anticholinergic combinations. None of these drugs are particularly effective in the treatment of canine colitis. The fact that some dogs recover when treated with these agents is probably more of a tribute to the resilience of the canine colon than to the therapeutic efficacy of the commonly used antidiarrheal preparations.

Colonic disease is uncommon, and colitis extremely rare, in the cat. The reasons for this marked species difference is unclear but there are several possible explanations. Whipworm infection, a major cause of colitis in the dog, is very rare in the cat. This fact could go a long way toward explaining the difference. The cat also is more fastidious in its selection of food and thus less likely to suffer the toxic and traumatic sequelae of dietary indiscretion seen so often in the dog. The character, use, housing, and temperament of cats probably also play a role. Compared to dogs, cats lead a generally quieter, more independent, and less stressful life. Stress in its varied forms has been implicated as a major etiologic factor in colonic disease in man [153] and to a lesser extent in the dog.[174]

*University of Pennsylvania, School of Veterinary Medicine, Phila., PA 19104.

THE RECTUM AND ANUS

Fecal Continence

The rectum functions as a reservoir for feces, and plays a very important role in defecation, while the anus functions to maintain fecal continence. Fecal continence has both reservoir and sphincter components.[175] "Reservoir continence" refers to storage in the last part of the large intestine. "Sphincteric continence" refers to the seal of the anal canal. The mechanisms of fecal continence have not been well described in the dog, but it is likely that they are similar to those in man. Two experimental studies in the dog have shown that extensive removal of parts of the colon and rectum may not severely affect the fecal continence so long as a cuff of rectal muscularis and the anal sphincter musculature is preserved. The feces may become quite soft, lack cohesiveness, and be poorly formed, but continence is preserved.[176,177] The mechanisms involved in the maintenance of fecal continence are complex and include the reservoir function of the descending colon, the reservoir and sensory function of the rectum, the sphincteric mechanisms, and perhaps the sensory function of nerves in the caudal part of the medial coccygeal muscle.[178,179]

Reservoir continence is dependent upon the ability of the descending colon to adapt automatically by distention to an increasing fecal volume. There is a limit, however, for when the fecal mass reaches a certain size, peristalsis is initiated and the mass is ejected. This reservoir function is maintained even if, as in surgical ablation of the anus, all the sphincteric mechanisms have been removed.

Sphincteric continence depends on an intact nervous arc, consisting of afferent sensory nerve endings in both the rectal wall and surrounding tissue, and efferent nerves supplying the external anal sphincter. Active constriction of the striated muscle of the external anal sphincter enables it to resist the propulsive force of colonic peristalsis and to block defecation.[175]

Defecation

Normally the anus and anal canal are devoid of fecal material and in a collapsed state. Defecation commences when the rectum is distended with fecal material after colonic mass movements. This causes the internal anal sphincter to relax reflexly, allows fecal material to come into contact with receptors in the distal anal canal, and stimulates distention receptors, which are probably located in the medial coccygeal muscle or muscles of the rectal wall.[178] This response initially causes reflex contraction of the external anal sphincter and the medial coccygeal muscle and results in formation of a high pressure zone which counters the force of peristaltic movements. This reflex contraction of striated muscles prevents peristaltic expulsion of the fecal material from the anal canal. The desire or urgency to defecate is temporarily suppressed and continence is maintained.[180] The process can be repeated until the rectum is maximally distended and voluntary sphincter action can no longer hold back the fecal material.

An intact motor nerve supply to the external anal sphincter is also essential for normal defecation; spinal cord transection, peripheral nerve transection, and sphincter division may lead to a loss of continence and the ability to defecate normally.[175]

Controlled defecation can occur at any time when a moderate stimulus from the distended rectum reaches consciousness. If defecation is not convenient, active contraction of the external sphincter, in combination with rectal and colonic accommodation result in suppression of the urge to defecate. Such stimuli, if continually suppressed, as in the hospitalized dog, can lead to constipation. Alternatively, when the rectal stimulus is augmented by inflammatory diseases of the colon and rectum, urgent defecation with tenesmus takes place.[181]

Defecation involves the coordination of structures and reflexes controlled by both autonomic and somatic nervous systems. Controlled defecation necessitates controlled continence;[182] thus, intact structures are essential. During defecation, the animal assumes a squatting position, abdominal pressure is increased by closure of the glottis, the diaphragm fixates, the abdominal wall contracts and the external anal sphincter relaxes. Contraction of the medial coccygeus and other intrapelvic muscles enhances the increased abdominal pressure and contracts the rectum over the last part of the fecal bolus. The entire descending colon of the dog is usually evacuated if mass movements accompany defecation. Following defecation, the muscles of the pelvis relax and return to their normal position obliterating the rectal lumen.

The Anal Sacs

Despite a certain amount of work on the morphology and histochemistry of the anal sacs in the dog, their significance remains obscure.[179] The contents of the sacs are evacuated onto the feces either at the beginning or end of defecation or when the animal is alarmed or excited. Anatomic arrangements suggest that at defecation the overlying external sphincter squeezes the sacs against the feces in the anal canal and evacuates some of their contents. It has been suggested that the contents of the anal sacs may play a sexual or territorial marking role.[179]

SIGNS OF COLONIC AND ANORECTAL DISEASE

The many colonic and recto-anal diseases of the dog and cat have only a relatively small number of associated clinical signs (Table 24–3). Although none are pathognomonic for colonic or recto-anal disease, two predominate: diarrhea and constipation.

Diarrhea

The amount of intestinal content flowing into the colon from the ileum depends mainly on the size of the animal and nature of the diet. The colon of a 30-kg dog, for example, is reported to receive between 100 and 400 ml daily.[174] Although the total volume of fluid absorbed by the colon is calculated to be less than that absorbed by the jejunum or ileum, the absorptive efficiency of the colon is much greater,[183] so that normal feces are usually solid. In

Table 24–3. Signs of Colonic Disease and Anorectal Disease in the Dog and Cat

Diarrhea: Frequently but not invariably mucoid, less often bloody. The frequency of defecation is usually increased, and tenesmus may be present. The dog or cat may have "accidents" in the house and defecation is often associated with a sense of urgency.

Dysentery: Bloody diarrhea; blood is admixed throughout the feces or in mucus.

Hematochezia: Fresh blood on the feces is a reliable sign of colonic or rectal disease. Feces are formed to very soft.

Constipation: Caused by a number of disorders that interfere with or prevent normal colonic function and defecation. If untreated, constipation may become intractable (obstipation). Secondary changes in colonic muscle are common.

Tenesmus: Tenesmus of alimentary tract origin must be differentiated from that associated with the urogenital tract.

Vomiting: Seen in about 30% of dogs with colitis. Vomiting does not necessarily indicate gastric or small intestinal involvement in the dog with chronic vomiting and diarrhea.

Dyschezia: Painful or difficult defecation occurs with a lesion or foreign body in the rectum or anus; may lead to constipation.

Fecal Incontinence: The inability to retain feces and defecate normally. It occurs most often after surgical trauma to the rectum or anus but may also occur as a complication of neurogenic disease.

Biting the Perineal Area: Biting the skin around the anus, tail chasing, or rubbing the perineum along the ground are reliable signs of anal irritation and anal sac disease.

Weight Loss: A slowly progressive loss of weight may be seen in severe colonic diseases. It results from increased inflammatory protein loss in feces or decreased food intake.

the dog, normal feces have a moisture content of 56 to 70%.[184]

The colon is capable of absorbing much more fluid than it normally does. The human colon has been shown to have considerable absorptive reserve capacity, being able to absorb up to three times as much fluid as normal, with diarrhea resulting only when this functional reserve capacity is overwhelmed.[185-187]

Factors determining fecal consistency are poorly understood. Total water content is a major, but not the sole determinant, since in man solid feces contain between 60 and 80% water, while liquid feces contain between 70 and 90%.[188] There are no equivalent data for the dog or cat, but it is probably safe to assume that similar criteria apply. Diarrhea occurs either when there is an increase in the rate of delivery of intestinal content from the small intestine sufficient to overwhelm colonic reserve capacity, or when reserve absorptive capacity is impaired. The high efficiency of normal colonic water absorption, and the relatively small increase in fecal water required to produce diarrhea imply that only subtle changes in colonic function are needed to cause an impairment of reserve capacity.[189] Diarrhea is therefore to be expected in a wide variety of colonic diseases.

The character of colonic diarrhea and patterns of defecation vary, depending upon the underlying disease, location of the lesion and its severity. The classic description of colonic diarrhea is that it is small-volume and commonly mucoid and bloody. Defecation is frequent, often with tenesmus, and may be associated with a sense of urgency. Even a well-trained dog, if it has colitis, may defecate in the house, or suddenly beg to be let outside to defecate. While these signs are helpful in the diagnosis of diarrhea of colonic origin, it is important to realize that they are present in little more than half the cases, albeit the more severely afflicted, and their absence does not exclude colonic disease. Diarrhea does not even have to be present continuously; for example, when colonic motility is disrupted, diarrhea may alternate with periods of normal defecation.

There are four main causes of diarrhea in colonic disease (Table 24–4): (1) abnormal mucosal permeability, (2) abnormal motility, (3) abnormalities of ion transport, and (4) abnormal microbial digestion.[190] It is probable that more than one of these factors are involved concurrently in most diarrheas of colonic origin.

Abnormal colonic permeability to water and electrolytes occurs in some inflammatory diseases of

Table 24–4. A Classification of Colonic Diarrhea in the Dog and Cat

Abnormal Mucosal Permeability
- Inflammation of colonic mucosa—parasitic colitis
- Decreased colonic surface area—histoplasmosis, diffuse lymphosarcoma
- Injury to colonic mucosa—fatty acids, bile acids, laxatives

Abnormal Motility
- Psychophysiologic disorders—colonic motor dysfunction, functional diarrhea
- Infiltration of muscle—histoplasmosis
- Failure to contract normally—colitis

Abnormalities of Ion Transport
- Stimulation of colonic secretion—bile salts, fatty acids, dioctyl sodium sulfossucinate (DSS)
- Exudative diseases—colitis, severe colonic impaction, saline cathartics

Abnormal Microbial Digestion
- Bacterial overgrowth producing more osmotically active particles following small intestinal malabsorption

the colon such as parasitic colitis, in diseases which decrease surface area such as histoplasmosis or diffuse lymphosarcoma, and in situations when the colon is exposed to fatty acids and unabsorbed bile salts.[159,190]

As noted earlier, colonic motility is poorly understood and the role of abnormal transit is even more obscure. However, a significant number of dogs with chronic diarrhea show signs of colonic dysfunction, but have normal or only slightly abnormal findings on colonoscopy, and have no radiographic or biopsy abnormalities. These dogs are suspected of having some sort of colonic motor dysfunction, which has been called the irritable colon or spastic colon.[174] As in man, this syndrome may constitute part of a poorly understood group of functional diarrheas.[187] Colonic motility is probably also disrupted in inflammatory and infiltrative diseases. In experimentally induced colitis in the cat, for example, contractile activity is decreased in the acute inflammatory phase, but increased during the healing phase.[191]

Abnormalities of ion transport occur in diseases which stimulate colonic secretion. This is mediated by cyclic AMP and can be brought about by deoxycholate,[159,190] and certain dehydroxylated fatty acids.[192] Active colonic secretion has not yet been investigated to any great extent in the dog and cat. As in other species it is possible that prostaglandins could activate cyclic AMP to stimulate secretion in some types of inflammatory disease, and hydroxy-fatty acids could stimulate active secretion when excessive quantities of fat are delivered to the colon because of malabsorption in the small intestine.

Partial colonic obstructions are uncommon, but may be associated with diarrhea in which liquid feces pass the point of obstruction while more solid material is retained. It is also possible that large fecal concretions may irritate the colonic mucosa sufficiently to cause exudation. In one of the worst cases of constipation seen in a dog in this practice, the animal was, in fact, initially presented for treatment of anorexia and diarrhea.

The products of microbial digestion are essential for normal colonic absorption in several species of animals that have been studied.[190] Bacterial degradation of intraluminal contents can result, however, in an osmotic diarrhea. This condition occurs when the colonic contents become sufficiently hypertonic to retain or draw water into the colonic lumen and is associated primarily with small intestinal diseases causing malabsorption or with pancreatic exocrine insufficiency.

Constipation

Constipation means different things to different people. To many clients, for example, constipation is equated with tenesmus, a comparison that is not necessarily correct, since tenesmus may also be associated with disease in other systems. Most clinicians understand constipation to mean infrequent defecation, excessively hard or dry feces, increased straining to defecate, or too small a fecal volume.[173] Although many clients think and act otherwise, a failure to defecate is not necessarily a cause for immediate concern. The dog or cat seems to be able to retain feces in the colon for several days with no manifest adverse effects. If feces are retained for long periods, however, more water is absorbed, leaving the feces drier and harder. Defecation becomes progressively more difficult until it is virtually impossible. This intractable constipation, or obstipation, is nearly always associated with a guarded prognosis, since changes in the colon wall may be irreversible.

Constipation is often confused with megacolon, defined as a condition of extreme dilatation of the colon.[193] The two terms are *not* synonymous however, since animals with megacolon are always constipated, but constipated animals do not necessarily have megacolon. Constipation is a sign, while megacolon is a disorder of structure and function. Megacolon may be either primary or secondary. The cause of primary megacolon is still unknown in the dog and cat, but may be due to a defect in colonic smooth muscle innervation. Secondary megacolon can occur as a result of any lesion or disease that prevents normal defecation over a

Table 24–5. A Classification of the Causes of Constipation in the Dog and Cat

Dietary and Environmental
- Dietary—bones, hair, or foreign material impacted in the colon
- Lack of exercise, change of habit or environment—no litter box, hospitalization

Painful Defecation
- Anorectal disease—anal sacculitis, anal sac abscess, perianal fistula, anal stricture, anal spasm, rectal foreign body, pseudocoprostasis
- Trauma—fractured pelvis, fractured limb, or dislocated hip

Mechanical Obstruction
- Extraluminal obstruction—healed fracture of pelvis with narrowing of the pelvic canal, prostatic hypertrophy, pelvic tumor
- Intraluminal obstruction—colonic or rectal tumor, perineal hernia

Neurologic Disease
- Central nervous system dysfunction—paraplegia
- Intrinsic colonic nerve dysfunction—idiopathic megacolon

Metabolic and Endocrine Disease
- Interference with colonic smooth muscle function—hyperparathyroidism, hypothyroidism
- Debility—general muscle weakness and dehydration

prolonged period of time. Secondary megacolon is also known as pseudomegacolon, a term that should be abandoned as meaningless.

A classification of the major causes of constipation in the dog and cat is presented in Table 24–5. A large number of factors may predispose to constipation. They can be grouped into: (1) dietary and environmental, (2) those which make defecation painful, (3) obstructive, (4) neurologic, and (5) metabolic and endocrine.

The ingestion of bones, foreign material, or hair may result in large colonic fecal concretions which the animal cannot eliminate. Defecation becomes progressively more difficult as these masses slowly develop, and if unnoticed and untreated, they may eventuate in obstipation. For some animals, defecation is a routine, almost ritual act, necessitating the appropriate environment and conducive circumstances. To a dog this may mean a walk in the park, and to cats it may mean the provision of a clean litter box or other suitable location. A drastic change in environment, such as occurs when an animal is hospitalized, may lead to constipation.

Constipation also occurs in a variety of diseases associated with a painful lesion of the rectum or anus, such as anal sacculitis, anal abscesses, perianal fistulae and strictures, and rectal foreign bodies. After a few initial painful experiences the dog or cat with an anal lesion may make no further attempt to defecate. Again, if the client is not observant, severe constipation may result.

Constipation may also be brought about by several unrelated circumstances. If the adoption of the appropriate position is difficult or impossible, the animal may not be able or willing to defecate. This may be a cause of constipation in the dog or cat with a fractured pelvis, dislocated hip, or broken leg. These animals may not attempt to defecate until the pain has subsided and stabilization has occurred, by which time the feces may be very hard and treatment for the relief of constipation may be required.

Intraluminal or extraluminal obstruction of normal fecal transit inevitably results in constipation. It occurs, for example, in such disorders as perineal hernia, healed pelvic fracture with a narrowed pelvic canal, in some cases of prostatic hypertrophy, or with rectal, colonic or pelvic tumors.

Some neurologic disorders also result in constipation either through an inability of the animal to adopt the normal defecatory position or through a disturbance of colonic smooth muscle innervation and abnormal colonic motility (see Table 24–5).

Endocrine diseases may also affect intestinal smooth muscle function. Hypothyroidism is a notorious cause of constipation in man,[173] but is not a consistent finding in the hypothyroid dog. In fact, some hypothyroid dogs may present with diarrhea.[194] The hypercalcemia seen in hyperparathyroidism disrupts normal smooth muscle function and may result in constipation.[195] Finally, dehydration and debility seen in a variety of diseases may cause constipation through excessive fecal water absorption or muscle weakness.

The clinician should be aware of the many circumstances in which constipation may develop and be prepared to take either preventive or appropriate therapeutic measures in order to prevent the unfortunate sequelae of obstipation and secondary megacolon. The treatment of constipation is discussed on page 577.

Tenesmus

Tenesmus is defined as an ineffectual effort to defecate,[193] but the use of the term in veterinary medicine has been expanded to encompass severe straining due to abnormalities in or around the lower alimentary or urogenital systems, as well as straining during parturition.[196] Tenesmus is not synonymous with painful defecation, and tenesmus of alimentary origin must be differentiated by history and physical examination from diseases of other organ systems. The cat with urethral obstruction, straining to urinate, while the owner complains of the animal's constipation, is an all too familiar practice situation.

Tenesmus of alimentary tract origin is usually associated with inflammatory disease of the rectum and anus and may be seen either in diarrheal diseases or in constipation. The relationship of tenesmus to defecation may be useful in establishing a diagnosis: tenesmus before and during defecation is usually associated with constipation, whereas tenesmus after defecation is usually associated with diarrheal diseases and results from an inflamed colonic or rectal mucosa. Continuous tenesmus is rare, but when present, is most often associated with a rectal foreign body or tumor.

Vomiting

Vomiting is relatively common in severe colitis and prolonged cases of constipation. In one study, 29% of dogs with colitis had vomiting as one of the presenting signs, and it was suggested that it resulted from stimulation of the emetic center via parasympathetic afferent nerves.[197] The same parasympathetic stimulation may also cause vomiting as a consequence of constipation, since distention of the colon results in emesis.[198] Alternatively it may be due to stimulation of the chemoreceptor trigger zone by absorbed toxins.

Vomiting has no characteristic clinical presentation in colonic disease. Frequent vomiting is rare, but it can be persistent. The vomitus may be bile-stained, indicative of duodenal reflux, but is never bloody or feculent and there is no consistent temporal relationship to eating. It is unusual for the vomiting associated with colonic disease to be severe enough to cause electrolyte and acid-base imbalances.

The most important aspect of vomiting in colonic disease lies in its recognition. The dog or cat presented with a history of chronic vomiting and diarrhea does not necessarily have any gastric or small intestinal disease.

Dyschezia

Painful or difficult defecation is usually associated with lesions in or near the anus. The animal may cry out as it attempts to defecate, stop, walk around restlessly, and then repeat the process. If defecation is too painful, then fecal retention and constipation may ensue. Diseases associated with dyschezia include pseudocoprostasis, perianal fistula, anal spasm, and perineal hernia.

Hematochezia

Fresh blood in the feces is a reliable sign of colonic, rectal or anal disease. Bloody diarrhea (dysentery) is associated with severe colonic inflammatory disease, while streaks of blood in normal feces are more indicative of a bleeding lesion, such as a tumor of the distal colon, rectum, or anus.

Fecal Incontinence

This uncommon disorder is characterized by the inability to retain feces and defecate normally. Fecal incontinence occurs most frequently in the dog or cat that has undergone a surgical procedure for anorectal disease in which the structures maintaining normal fecal retention were either deliberately or accidentally damaged. It is seen, for example, as a complication of corrective surgery for perineal hernia or perianal fistulae and occasionally as a complication of perineal urethrostomy in the male cat.

Fecal incontinence can also occur as a complication of a neurologic disorder. The two most common causes in the dog and cat are spinal trauma (disc prolapse, vertebral luxation or fracture) and damage to the caudal rectal nerves.[178]

Biting the Perineal Area

Biting the skin around the anus, tail-chasing, and rubbing the perineum along the ground ("scooting") are reliable signs of anorectal irritation. Many clients associate "scooting" with "worms." This, however, is rarely the case, being most often associated with anal sacculitis or impaction. These disorders are often present in the dog with pyotraumatic dermatitis ("hot spots") over the perineal or caudal lumbar area.

Weight Loss

Insidious, progressive weight loss and debilitation are seen in the more severe colonic and anorectal diseases, such as transmural colitis, rectal adenocarcinoma, or severe colonic impaction. Weight loss may occur either directly, as a result of prolonged inappetence or anorexia, or indirectly from increased fecal protein loss in severe inflammatory processes.

DIAGNOSIS OF COLONIC AND ANORECTAL DISEASE

Colonic disease is to be considered whenever any of the signs of gastrointestinal disease are present. However, certain clusters of signs and findings bear such a high probability of being related to the colon that when they are present, it is possible to move with considerable confidence directly to the colon as the likely site of disease. Small-volume, high-frequency diarrhea with tenesmus and hematochezia would be one such example of localization of the lesion to the colon. However, absence of diarrhea and tenesmus in a dog that vomits and exhibits abdominal pain does not by any means exclude colonic disease. It simply leads one to assume that colonic disease is of lower probability for the moment, to be kept in mind as a search is made elsewhere for the diagnosis.

Armed with a sound knowledge of colonic disease in dogs and cats, one can develop improved diagnostic accuracy and efficiency by standardizing the diagnostic approach. With a few exceptions, the most certain route to a diagnosis in both distal colonic and anorectal disease is found, not in the history, but in the physical examination. This is in contrast to small bowel disease, in which even the most experienced clinician will fail to detect subtle diffuse lesions at physical examination. Granted that only the most distal segment of the colorectum is directly accessible to digital examination, it still provides an extremely valuable "window" to the colon. When combined with transabdominal palpation (one hand palpating the caudal abdomen while the other is used in rectal digital examination), much can be learned about the distal colon and rectum, the site of many lesions. Absence of findings in this region do not, of course, rule out colonic disease, but digital rectal examination may reveal such diseases as rectal stricture or foreign body, rectal adenocarcinoma, prostatic disease, and rectal dilation and sacculation. Rectal examination also allows evaluation of anal sphincter tone and the removal of a small quantity of fresh feces for examination. This fecal sample should be evaluated for abnormal color and consistency and for the presence of both foreign material and excessive mucus. A wet mount can be examined microscopically for parasites and a stained smear examined for inflammatory cells and erythrocytes.

The nature of the clinical evidence guides the workup from this point. Positive physical findings such as a mass or stenosis are studied by colonoscopy and biopsy, plain and contrast radiography, and exploratory laparotomy, usually in that order. It is often possible to excise tumors and strictures at the time of laparotomy if the preliminary workup is carefully done, providing definitive treatment while confirming the diagnosis.

A lack of specific findings at physical examination alters the diagnostic approach. Since there is greater uncertainty that a colonic lesion exists, attention shifts to more general tests that screen for abnormalities in other systems. Urinalysis, fecal examinations, and hematologic and chemistry tests take on greater meaning. It must be emphasized that repeated fecal examinations, including both direct wet mount and flotation procedures, are absolutely essential to a responsible workup of colonic (as well as small bowel) disease. Endoparasitism in dogs is so common in most parts of the world, and fecal egg concentration so variable in adults, that to neglect the homely business of fecal examination is to risk repeated professional embarrassment!

Hospitalization, feeding of the patient's usual diet, and personal observation are an essential and relatively inexpensive part of the early workup of colonic disease. Personally observing the dog defecate in the exercise run or at leash is strongly recommended. In those few minutes, the history is frequently confirmed or new observations are made that would be gained only with great difficulty, and after some delay, through the eyes of another person.

By whatever means that colonic inflammation is suspected (e.g., leukocytosis, fever, diarrhea, dysentery or hematochezia) and with endoparasitism ruled out by repeated fecal examinations, the next steps are colonoscopy and biopsy. Since even acute colonic disease is seldom life-threatening, it is usually possible to complete and assess the initial round of tests before pursuing the diagnosis with more sophisticated (and expensive) procedures. Straight-tube colonoscopy does not allow examination of the ascending colon or the ileocecocolic junction and in some patients contrast colonography may be necessary for diagnosis. Alternatively, fiberoptic colonoscopy reveals all of the colon up to and including the ileocolic junction (see Chapter 8).

Anal disease is more readily diagnosed than is colonic and rectal disease. In many cases, a history of dyschezia, tenesmus, or hematochezia indicates distal rectal or anal disease, or the client may present a dog or cat with an obvious anal lesion. The history may be misleading however, and a physical examination is just as essential for the diagnosis of anal disease as it is for colonic and rectal disease. Many German Shepherds, for example, have been treated symptomatically for weeks or months for tenesmus or dyschezia associated with chronic ''diarrhea'' or ''constipation'' when in fact they have perianal fistula, undiagnosed because nobody bothered to lift the animal's tail and examine the perineum. Visual examination of the perineum and anal area should be a routine part of the normal physical examination just as digital rectal examination should be routine in any animal with signs of colonic or anorectal disease. Visual examination may reveal the presence of tumors, perineal hernia, perianal fistula, rectal prolapse, and imperforate anus.

DISEASES WITH DIARRHEA AS THE PRINCIPAL SIGN

This category encompasses the majority of colonic disease. Two major causes are recognized: (1) inflammatory disease and (2) motility disorders.

Inflammatory Diseases

The group of diseases sharing the common factor of colonic inflammation are an important cause of chronic diarrhea in the dog. In the past there has been an unfortunate tendency to treat canine colitis as a single disease entity[197] rather than as a group of separate, albeit as yet poorly defined diseases, often needing specific individualized treatment.[199,200] Perhaps as a result of attempts to stimulate interest in some types of canine colitis as models for human disease, there has also been an overemphasis on pathologic oddities at the expense of detailed descriptions of the major types of canine colitis.

A clinical and pathologic classification based on the depth and severity of the inflammatory process into either mucosal or transmural colitis has been proposed.[201] Mucosal diseases cause inflammation of the epithelium, colonic glands, lamina propria, and superficial mucosa. In these diseases, the colon shows little change in length, pliability, or diameter, and most cases respond well to treatment. Conversely, transmural diseases cause extensive lesions that result in distortion of the colon with inflammation extending through all layers of the wall and may in some cases involve regional lymph nodes. This fortunately uncommon group responds poorly to treatment.

Inevitably some overlap exists between these two groups, depending on the individual response of the animal to the disease process and the time period from the onset of the disease to presentation. Thus, while a division into mucosal or transmural colitis may be of some prognostic significance, of more importance is the appearance of the colon at colonoscopy and biopsy, since these two factors ultimately decide the diagnosis, prognosis, and treatment.

Pathophysiology. The pathophysiology of all types of canine colitis is probably similar. Colonic inflammation brings about a disruption of salt and water transport and a change in the normal patterns of motility. In most cases of colitis these two factors probably combine to cause diarrhea.

The colonic epithelium is normally electrically polarized with the mucosal side negative to the serosa. Evidence from human and animal studies strongly suggests that this transmural potential difference is related to active sodium transport, although the exact mechanisms of its production are still unclear.[202] A marked decrease in this charge occurs in human ulcerative colitis, resulting in a loss of the characteristic ability of the colon to absorb sodium against a considerable electrochemical gradient. There is also a large increase in the plasma to lumen sodium flux rate, suggesting increased leakiness of the mucosa and a decrease in active sodium absorption.[202-204] With remission of the inflammatory process, the epithelium regains its relative impermeability to sodium and its sodium transport system reverts to normal.[202]

The motor function of the inflamed colon needs more study. There have been very few studies in the dog or cat, but it appears that colonic inflammation disrupts normal motor function in these species. In a recent study, cats with diffuse experimental colitis had a suppression of spontaneous and urecholine-stimulated contractile activity during the period of severest diarrhea, followed by an increase in activity during the period of healing and regeneration.[191] In other studies, muscle taken from the colon of cats with so-called "idiopathic summer diarrhea" showed a disruption of electrical slow wave conduction,[205] and individual colonic muscle cells in dogs with experimentally induced acute colitis had significantly deranged myoelectrical characteristics.[79] Findings of this nature may underlie the overall decrease in colonic motor activity described in ulcerative colitis in man.[206] Recent studies of colonic myoelectrical and motor responses in human ulcerative colitis, moreover, have shown an abnormal response to eating. These patients have abnormalities in smooth muscle contractility, despite relatively normal myoelectrical activity, which suggests a lack of coupling between electrical and mechanical events. It was suggested that these abnormalities in the colonic contractile apparatus may lead to postprandial diarrhea.[207]

Acute Nonspecific Colitis

This fairly common, well recognized, but poorly defined heterogenous group of diseases occurs almost exclusively in the dog. Although there are several apparent causes, they are grouped here under one heading because they have the same characteristic clinical presentation, and treatment is similar in all cases.

In most cases, the cause of the clinical signs is never known. Sometimes the history may incriminate ingestion of garbage or abrasive foreign bodies. In other cases, parasites are found upon fecal examination, or rarely, the history and laboratory studies may suggest a food-induced allergic colitis. In the case of garbage ingestion, it is likely that abrasive foreign material damages the colonic mucosa allowing secondary bacterial invasion and development of a bacterial colitis. However, with the rare exception of salmonellosis, there is no evidence that primary acute bacterial colitis occurs in the dog. Signs of colonic involvement may also accompany nonspecific acute gastroenteritis, since many of the inciting factors for acute colitis also cause gastric and small intestinal disease. The signs of colitis may coexist with those of acute nonspecific gastroenteritis or may occasionally persist after the signs of acute gastroenteritis have subsided. A small number of these cases progress to chronic colitis.

History. The syndrome is characterized by the sudden onset of severe, watery, occasionally bloody, mucoid diarrhea. Vomiting may be present in dogs with acute nonspecific gastroenteritis or with a history of scavenging or garbage ingestion. Animals are usually presented for veterinary examination within 48 hours of the onset of signs.

There is no reported age, breed, or sex predisposition, although in this practice younger dogs ($\leq$ 4 yrs) appear to be more frequently afflicted with acute nonspecific colitis than are older dogs.

Physical Findings. The physical findings depend on the severity and nature of the initial insult and on the amount of body fluid lost as vomitus and diarrhea. The dog may be depressed and, in cases of garbage ingestion, may exhibit muscle stiffness or show a change in nervous temperament.[208] A mild fever (102 to 104°F) may be present in the more severely afflicted animals. Abdominal palpation is rarely helpful in diagnosis except that pain may be elicited in some dogs with concurrent enteritis; pain can seldom be localized to the colon. Rectal examination may reveal pieces of bone, plastic, wood, or aluminum foil in those dogs whose signs have been caused by garbage ingestion.

Diagnostic Studies. The hemogram is compatible with the severity of dehydration; a leukocytosis may also be present. There will be a concomitant increase in packed cell volume and total solids in dehydrated animals, two parameters which can be used as a guide for replacement fluid therapy.[209] Abdominal radiographs are seldom specifically indicated, but may be taken to rule out other disorders. They may reveal an ileus or traces of radiopaque material in the small intestine or colon, but are not diagnostic. Colonoscopy reveals the mucosa to be hyperemic and edematous, and it may be friable and bleed readily when rubbed with the tip of the colonoscope. Small ulcers or focal areas of bleeding may be present and there is almost always a large amount of viscid tenacious mucus adhering to the mucosa and free within the lumen. The author is unaware of any published reports on the histologic appearance of the colonic mucosa in this group of diseases. The few specimens examined histologically in our practice revealed only nonspecific changes such as mucosal edema, increased vascularity, and an inflammatory cell infiltrate. Some dogs also had plasma cells or eosinophils infiltrating the mucosa and superficial submucosa.

A fecal examination is mandatory in all cases and should include both a direct smear and flotation studies for gastrointestinal parasites. When parasites are found, the possibilities that they are either the cause of the clinical signs or an incidental finding should both be considered.

Differential Diagnosis. The differential diagnosis should initially include most of the causes of acute vomiting and diarrhea in the dog. Severe whipworm and hookworm-induced colitis have a similar clinical picture. Gastrointestinal parasites and parasitic colitis are ruled out only by thorough and repetitive fecal examinations. Abdominal pain and leukocytosis are present in many cases of acute pancreatitis along with the characteristic increases in serum amylase and lipase. Hemorrhagic gastroenteritis is characterized by dysentery and is of sudden onset with a greatly increased packed cell volume. Watery or mucoid diarrhea and a smaller increase in packed cell volume are more characteristic of acute nonspecific colitis. A history of dietary sensitivity or change, an unexplained peripheral eosinophilia, and infiltration of the mucosa with eosinophils is seen in eosinophilic colitis.

Treatment. In most cases, the disease process seems to be self-limiting and treatment is supportive and symptomatic. There are many effective treatment regimens, all directed at restoring fluid and acid-base equilibrium and symptomatic treatment of the diarrhea. The extent and vigor of treatment must be tailored to the severity of the clinical signs.

If dehydration is evident, intravenous administration of a balanced electrolyte replacement solution is indicated; maintenance fluids can later be given subcutaneously.

A broad-spectrum antibiotic is indicated if the dog is febrile. Chloramphenicol, ampicillin, and tetracycline have been used effectively in our practice. Nonabsorbable oral antibiotics such as neomycin are not indicated. Oral treatment with a liquid antidiarrheal drug such as Pepto-Bismol is beneficial, as are antispasmodic drugs such as Lomotil or propantheline bromide (Probanthine). Small doses of a parenteral antiemetic such as promazine (0.25 to 0.5 mg/kg) may be given to depress the emetic center if vomiting is persistent. Since vomiting is infrequent, it is preferable to avoid the routine use of antiemetic-antidiarrheal combinations. Appropriate anthelmintic drugs should be administered if gastrointestinal parasites are present.

Dietary manipulations are quite important. The principle of resting the gastrointestinal tract in acute gastrointestinal disturbances in the dog is well established.[210] Dogs with acute enterocolitis appear to do better if starved for a minimum of 24 hours after the onset of signs, even if they show a desire to eat. Water should always be available to dogs that are not vomiting. In most cases, the dog can be offered food on the second day. Food should initially be offered in small quantities at frequent intervals and should be palatable and of high quality. It can be either home-prepared, such as cottage cheese, chicken or hamburger and rice, or a commercial canned all-meat or semimoist variety. Frequent feeding seems to be preferable to a large meal.

Prognosis. In most cases, the prognosis is good for a complete recovery. Recovery is usually rapid and the feces appear normal or near normal by the third day. However, a few dogs recover from the initial acute episode but diarrhea typical of chronic colitis persists. In these cases a more extensive set of diagnostic studies and a different therapeutic regimen is indicated. The management of this type of case is dealt with in the next section.

There will obviously be some overlap between the designations "acute" and "chronic" colitis. However, the following are discussed as chronic diseases, even if they sometimes have an acute onset, since it is their persistence that is of greatest concern to the client. This group includes chronic colitis; parasitic, eosinophilic, infectious, granulomatous, traumatic and iatrogenic colitis; and the specific but rare entity of canine histiocytic ulcerative colitis.

Chronic Colitis

This, the single most common form of canine colitis, may well be a group of as yet poorly identified separate diseases that await specific pathologic classification. There is no known cause, the clinical signs are typical of any form of chronic colitis in the dog, but unlike other forms of colitis, there is no one specific diagnostic feature.

The disease has been called idiopathic ulcerative colitis[174] and a comparison has been made in one case with human ulcerative colitis;[199] however, ulcerative colitis is probably not a good term for the disease in the dog since there is presently little evidence to justify a wide-scale comparison with the human disease. Colonic ulceration is not invariably present.

Etiology. The precise etiology and pathogenesis of chronic colitis in the dog have yet to be defined. It is possible that there is more than one cause, all resulting in a common, predictable and typical colonic response which may be self-perpetuating long after the inciting cause is removed. The disease, for example, may follow a bout of nonspecific gastroenteritis, as mentioned previously, or may be the cause of chronic diarrhea, originally attributed to whipworm or hookworm infection, but which persists long after the parasites have been eliminated. In both instances, the histologic appearance of the colonic mucosa may be similar, if not identical. If this common response is the case, perhaps rather than searching for a specific cause, one should be looking for reasons why some dogs acquire colitis, while others, in presumably identical situations, do not. As has been suggested for man,[211] it is possible that psychogenic, genetic, or immunologic factors may be involved in the development of the disease.

History. There are no data on the age, breed, sex, or seasonal incidence of the disease, but in this practice it affects dogs primarily between 6 months and 4 years of age. Many of these dogs appear to be easily excited and the onset of signs can frequently be correlated with a change in habit or environment, or with a recent attack of acute gastroenteritis. There is no evidence of any infectious component, since it is extremely rare for more than one dog in a household to be affected.

The typical history of the dog with chronic colitis is that of chronic diarrhea, often but not invariably mucoid, which in most cases has failed to respond, or responded only temporarily to conventional antidiarrheal therapy. The feces vary in consistency from semi-formed to liquid and may be bloody in the more severely affected cases. Mucus when present may be mixed with blood; in rare cases, frank dysentery is present. The frequency of defecation is increased, usually to at least twice normal and some dogs may defecate or attempt to defecate much more frequently. Defecation is often associated with a sense of urgency, unlike that of small intestinal diarrhea, which the dog seems better able to control. The individual fecal volume at each defecation is often less than normal, but the total daily fecal weight is increased significantly over that of normal dogs.[212] Tenesmus may also be present after the passage of liquid or semi-formed feces and, together with mucus in the feces, are two of the most important facts to be gained from a client when taking the history. Their presence strongly indicates some type of colitis, although their absence does not eliminate it.

Some dogs may have a history of chronic vomiting and diarrhea, and if it is not recognized that vomiting is a feature of canine colitis, the wrong diagnostic studies might be chosen at the expense of the veterinarian's time and the client's money and patience.

Weight loss and dehydration occur in the more severely affected animals and are related most often to the duration and severity of the disease. Most dogs with colitis have a normal or increased appetite. A dog with signs indicative of colitis presenting with a loss of appetite should be viewed with concern, since these animals are more severely affected and need immediate more vigorous therapy.

Physical Findings. In most cases, physical findings are not helpful in making a specific diagnosis. The dog might appear nervous, or be underweight or dehydrated. Long-haired breeds may have fecal contamination of the hair in the perineal area and a painful moist dermatitis of the skin around the perineum caused by fecal contamination. Perineal myiasis occasionally occurs in neglected long-haired dogs in warm weather. Fever is rare. Abdominal palpation does not usually yield diagnostic findings, signs of pain might occasionally be elicited on deep palpation of the caudal abdomen, and rectal examination sometimes initiates tenesmus.

In summary, the typical dog with chronic colitis appears normal at physical examination. In most cases, the only facts that the clinician has with which to initiate further studies are those obtained in a carefully taken history.

Diagnostic Studies. The disease does not appear to be a distinct histopathologic entity, since most of the microscopic features of the syndrome may be seen in other inflammatory diseases of the colon. The diagnosis therefore rests on a combination of clinical and pathologic criteria, appearance of the anatomic lesions, and exclusion of other forms of colitis.

In most cases, the hemogram is normal; however, a neutrophilia with a left-shift is present in some cases and a mild microcytic hypochromic anemia may be found if there has been persistent chronic bleeding. Serum proteins are often abnormal. The typical response is hypoalbuminemia and mild hypergammaglobulinemia, but serum protein electrophoresis has not been diagnostically useful. Microscopic examination of a fecal sample or rectal smear stained with new methylene blue or Löffler's methylene blue[213] frequently reveals erythrocytes and inflammatory cells.

Contrast radiographic studies of the colon reveal characteristic changes in the more severely affected animals or in those with long-standing disease. These changes include fine mucosal irregularities, filling defects indicative of ulcers, or changes in length and pliability (see Chapter 7). The value of this study must be weighed against the benefits likely to be gained, for it is both messy and expensive and reveals diagnostic changes in little more than half the cases studied. However, a contrast study should be considered if colonoscopic examination is negative and signs indicate large intestinal disease.

Colonoscopy is the technique of choice for diagnosis; in virtually every case, the lesions involve the descending colon and thus are readily apparent. The normal colonic mucosa appears as a smooth glistening surface, uniformly reflecting the endoscopic light from a broad area. The color of the mucous membrane is pink but the shade depends on such factors as the type of light in the endoscope and the type of preparation the patient has undergone (see Chapter 8). Soapy-water enemas induce increased mucosal blood flow and hyperemia of a sufficient degree to yield an impression of bowel irritation. Plain tepid water or saline does not alter mucosal appearance. The superficial submucosal blood vessels are usually visible through the thin translucent mucosa. Normal mucosa does not bleed when gently rubbed with the tip of the endoscope and the colon readily distends when air is insufflated.

The endoscopic features of this disease are many and varied. One of the most widespread changes is the disappearance of the submucosal blood vessels as the mucosa becomes inflamed. Mucosal thickening is irregular and results in a change in the patterns of reflected light from smooth and glistening to granular. As inflammation intensifies, the "fine" granularity appears coarser and the mucosa appears dry. Increased vascularity may be appreciated as hyperemia. Excessive amounts of viscid tenacious mucus may be seen adhering to the mucosa or free in the lumen. Unlike the normal colon, the mucosa may bleed readily when touched. Thickened plaque-like areas of lymphoid tissue may also be visible and are a normal finding unless greatly enlarged. Ulceration is variable and is not always present. Numerous small ulcers appearing as areas of pinpoint hemorrhage may be seen, or less commonly, large deep bleeding ulcers with tags of epithelial tissue around their edges are observed. Obvious granulation tissue is rare.

Although in general the extent of mucosal change seen at colonoscopy reflects the severity of the disease, the true lesion is only revealed by histologic examination of a biopsy specimen. Biopsy of focal lesions can be carried out under direct observation using uterine biopsy (alligator) forceps passed through the colonoscope.[214] These forceps cut a relatively deep segment of tissue and may damage it by crushing. Complications following biopsy are rare, but persistent arterial bleeding may develop or colonic perforation ensue if too deep a bite is taken. Bleeding is best controlled by packing the colon around the bleeding point with sponges soaked in 1:10,000 epinephrine. A safer and more efficient biopsy instrument for diagnosis of diffuse colonic disease is the Quinton suction biopsy capsule (see Chapter 8). The biopsy specimen should be placed in Bouin's solution for initial fixation for at least 8, but no more than 24 hours, and then should be placed in 70% alcohol for transfer to the pathology laboratory.

As mentioned previously, the histopathologic findings are quite varied, reflecting perhaps the stage of the disease or possibly the effect of different causes or pathophysiologic events. There seem to be no generally agreed criteria for the categorization of colonic biopsies in the dog, a situation not dissimilar from that in man.[215]

The histologic appearance is one of either an acute or chronic inflammatory reaction which is focal, invariably limited to the colonic mucosa, and rarely ulcerated. Both acute and chronic reactions may be present in a single biopsy, suggesting a progressive disease process. In the acute form the lamina propria is edematous and infiltrated with acute inflammatory cells. The colonic glands are dilated and predominantly lined by columnar epithelial cells; goblet cells are decreased in number.[216] In the chronic form the lamina propria is fibrosed and colonic glands are more separated from one another. Reactive hyperplasia characterized by an increase in length and tortuosity of the glands is frequently present.[216] As in the acute form the numbers of goblet cells are usually depleted, a finding which in man is interpreted as an important sign of active disease.[217] The cause of these changes is obscure at the present time.

Differential Diagnosis. As noted, the typical dog with chronic colitis is admitted with a history of diarrhea which is characteristically mucoid, small-volume and high-frequency. Blood may also be noted in the feces in variable amounts. The initial workup should consider all causes of chronic diarrhea; small intestinal disease can usually be eliminated by the history and by techniques noted elsewhere in this book. Colitis is differentiated from the non-inflammatory colonic diarrheal diseases by the colonoscopic and biopsy findings, and from parasitic colitis by the absence of parasite eggs in the feces and the absence of adult parasites in the colon on colonoscopy and biopsy. Colonoscopy and biopsy also differentiate chronic colitis from the other less common types of canine colitis. The presence of fecal leukocytes in a fecal smear, while helpful, is not diagnostic since these can be found in other types of canine inflammatory bowel disease.

Treatment. There is no universally effective therapeutic regimen for colitis, perhaps indicating the complexity of the disease process or its several causes. Treatment falls into three categories: antibacterial, antispasmodic, and dietary. In the severely sick animal, parenteral fluids, or perhaps even blood or plasma, may also be indicated as supportive therapy.

The drug of choice in the treatment of chronic canine colitis is sulfasalazine (Azulfidine) even though there are no controlled studies of its efficacy in the dog. This drug, a combination of sulfapyridine and 5-aminosalicylate, was initially developed for the treatment of rheumatoid arthritis in man. While of no proven efficacy against rheumatoid arthritis, sulfasalazine has been shown to be useful in the treatment and prophylaxis of ulcerative colitis in both man[218,219] and dog.[197] It appears that the drug is absorbed in the upper gastrointestinal tract, since it can be detected in the blood within 1 to 2 hours of oral intake. Little drug is excreted in the urine; most is returned to the gastrointestinal tract via the biliary system.[219] Cleavage of the azo bond, the initial step in sulfasalazine metabolism, occurs in the colon and is attributed exclusively to the action of intestinal bacteria. The drug is split into sulfapyridine, which

is absorbed and excreted in the urine, and 5-aminosalicylate, which is excreted in the feces. Rectal infusion of the separate ingredients into human patients with ulcerative colitis has shown that 5-aminosalicylate is the probable therapeutic moiety.[220] The precise mechanism of drug action is unknown but the following have been postulated:[219] (1) the drug binds to colonic connective tissue; (2) by releasing sulfapyridine and 5-aminosalicylate in the colon, the intestinal flora may allow effective concentrations of the drug(s) at their site of action; (3) the drug reduces the number of anaerobes in the feces and raises the question of the role of enteric bacteria in the pathogenesis of colitis; (4) sulfasalazine converts net sodium and water secretion into net absorption; and (5) the drug inhibits the synthesis of prostaglandins known to elicit diarrhea and affect mucosal transport.

Because of the role of intestinal bacteria in initiating the metabolism of sulfasalazine in man as well as in laboratory animals, it has been suggested that antibiotics which decrease the gut flora will disrupt the distribution of the drug or its metabolites.[219] The clinical implications of this have not been determined, but routine antibiotic therapy in colitis is probably contraindicated. However, broad-spectrum antibiotics such as chloramphenicol or tetracycline are probably indicated in those few cases in which fever is present.

Sulfasalazine is supplied in 500-mg tablets and the dose for the dog is 50 mg/kg of body weight per day, divided into four equal doses. The efficacy and dosage have not been determined in the cat; however, because of the sensitivity of this species to salicylates, it is likely that lower doses are indicated. Most dogs respond well to sulfasalazine, and need only a short (3- to 4-week) course of treatment. If the client notices an improvement, the dosage may be halved after 10 days to 2 weeks. A few dogs need long-term maintenance treatment; in these cases, the minimum dose needed to suppress signs of colitis must be found by trial and error.

Side effects of sulfasalazine in the dog are rare, but include allergic dermatitis, nausea and vomiting, and cholestatic jaundice.[197] Keratoconjunctivitis sicca has been observed in dogs treated with the maximum dose for a long period of time.[221] If drug-associated vomiting occurs, it can be reduced by use of the enteric-coated form of the drug.

Another drug that has been used in the treatment of chronic colitis in the dog is oral tylosin. This antibiotic is reportedly effective in the treatment of a wide spectrum of canine inflammatory bowel disease.[222] Dosing is imprecise, and the drug has a reported efficacy over a dose range of 11 to 200 mg/kg of body weight per day.[222] Like sulfasalazine, its mode of action is unknown. The drug has been used with some success in our practice on dogs that do not respond to sulfasalazine. Since it is reportedly more efficacious than sulfasalazine,[222] particularly for long-term usage, tylosin may eventually become the accepted drug of choice for the treatment of chronic colitis in the dog.

Metronidazole (Flagyl) is another antibacterial drug that has proven useful in the treatment of canine colitis. In addition to its antiprotozoal action, metronidazole suppresses cell-mediated immune reactions[223] and has been used in the treatment of Crohn's disease (granulomatous enterocolitis) in human patients.[224] The drug has also been shown to have a protective effect against experimental colitis.[225] Metronidazole is effective against anaerobic bacteria and has proved useful in the treatment of anaerobic infections.[220] This is relevant, since it has been postulated that the predominantly anaerobic intestinal flora may be a source of antigens participating in immunologic reactions of possible significance in inflammatory bowel disease.[224]

In our practice, the discovery of the drug's efficacy in canine colitis was serendipitous. Dogs with suspected giardiasis and concomitant inflammatory bowel disease improved dramatically when treated with metronidazole.[226] The drug is now used routinely in such cases with considerable success. Dosage is 30 mg/kg of body weight per day for 5 days.

There is no place for the routine use of anticholinergics in chronic colitis. Colonic motility is already decreased and there seems to be no point in depressing it further. In man, these drugs are of very limited efficacy in both ulcerative colitis and regional enteritis, and it is at least theoretically possible that their indiscriminate use could exacerbate or prolong diarrhea. However, their use seems warranted in those cases with excessive tenesmus or abdominal discomfort possibly associated with colonic spasm, but long-term use is to be avoided, since they provide only symptomatic relief and do not treat the underlying cause.

The use of diphenoxylate is another matter. Since this drug acts directly on colonic smooth muscle to inhibit propulsive movements and reduce diarrhea,[227] it is useful in the symptomatic treatment of colitis. It is possible that it also increases the efficacy of sulfasalazine through increased contact time in the colon. The exact dosage does not appear to have been determined in the dog, but one tablet

t.i.d. is adequate for a 35-kg dog. Long-term use of this drug is to be avoided.

The indications for corticosteroids in chronic colitis have not been clarified. In man, they result in an increased incidence of complete remission in the initial attack of ulcerative colitis or during an acute exacerbation,[211] but their beneficial effect in chronic colitis in the dog is unproven. Some dogs with colitis reportedly deteriorate when treated with steroids.[197] However, since chronic colitis is an inflammatory disease of unknown etiology, steroid use at least on a trial basis is warranted in cases unresponsive to more conventional treatment. The author has had some success with prednisolone in such cases. An initial dose of 1.0 to 2.0 mg/kg of body weight tapered over a 3- to 4-week period is the usual therapeutic regimen. Corticosteroids have proved more useful in the treatment of eosinophilic or granulomatous colitis, and their efficacy in some, but not all cases of chronic colitis calls into question the accuracy of the initial diagnosis and underlines the difficulties facing the pathologist in adequately categorizing the disease process. Dogs must be closely monitored during steroid treatment and clients warned of potential side-effects of the drug. If improvement is to take place, it is usually noted within 7 days. The drug is contraindicated in the severely debilitated animal. The need for a controlled trial of corticosteroids both as a primary and adjunctive treatment in chronic colitis in the dog is evident.

There is no specific nutritional treatment for canine colitis; the diet should, however, be nutritionally balanced and palatable. Canned all-meat dog food is preferable to dry dog food (kibble). Dry dog food, although of comparable nutritional value, causes bulkier, heavier feces in normal dogs,[228] with a correspondingly higher water content. Dry food worsens the diarrhea when colonic function is compromised in colitis. If the dog is already consuming dry dog food, any changeover must be made gradually[229] (Chapter 15).

Low-residue diets have been recommended in colitis on the premise that they decrease colonic motility.[174,210] Recent studies in the author's laboratory, however, have shown that high-residue foods decrease overall colonic motility. Normal dogs fed nutritionally balanced all-meat dog food supplemented with nonnutritive dietary fiber in the form of α-cellulose (Solka-Flok, Brown Co.) have a significant overall decrease in colonic myoelectrical and contractile activity. The feces are bulkier and fecal weight is increased on this diet, while intestinal transit time is decreased.[171] These findings support the observation that the addition of nonnutritive bulk to the diet is beneficial in some types of gastrointestinal disease.[210,226] The addition of bran to the food of some dogs with colitis brings about a reduction of diarrhea.[226] Presumably the water-absorbing properties of the bran change the nature of the feces, or perhaps the additional bulk has a beneficial effect on colonic motility. Based on the preceding evidence, and knowledge of the pathophysiology of colitis in man, we suggest that dogs with colitis receive frequent (at least t.i.d.) feedings of all-meat canned food or its home-prepared equivalent, to which has been added 1 to 3 tablespoons of coarse bran or a breakfast cereal containing bran, which some dogs find more palatable.

Prognosis. There have been no long-term studies on either the recovery rate or recurrence of canine colitis. In my experience, most dogs (about 70%) treated with the above regimen recover completely and do not have additional attacks. Some dogs, however, require long-term treatment with sulfasalazine or tylosin to control the disease, and clients should always be advised of the possibility of long-term drug treatment and its potential cost.

Parasitic Colitis

The canine colon is affected by several species of parasite. These result in colonic disease of varying severity, manifested mainly as colitis. Most important from the clinical viewpoint are whipworm and hookworm infection; much less important are entamoebiasis, giardiasis, and balantidiasis. The life cycles and pathogenesis of all gastrointestinal parasites are described in current veterinary parasitology texts;[230,231] control strategies are discussed in Chapter 17.

The high prevalence of parasitic infection in the dog mandates one or more fecal examinations in any dog admitted with a history of chronic diarrhea. The failure to rule out gastrointestinal parasitism before progressing to more complex diagnostic studies is a serious omission.

Whipworm-Induced Colitis

Whipworm-induced colitis ranks almost equally with chronic colitis in terms of incidence. However, while trichuriasis is common in the dog, not all infected dogs have overt colitis. The signs of infection, which are manifested primarily as diarrhea, seem to depend on the number of parasites and the individual response of the host.

A dog with whipworm-induced colitis may be admitted to the clinic with either acute or chronic disease. The signs and diagnosis of acute trichuriasis are similar to those of acute nonspecific colitis, except that trichuris eggs may be found in the feces. The signs of whipworm-induced colitis are similar to chronic colitis. The parasite is found primarily in the cecum and proximal and transverse colon;[230] however, in severe infections it may also be found in the distal colon and rectum where it can be seen on colonoscopy. The parasites penetrate the mucosa at least as far as the lamina propria and may cause an extensive mucosal hyperplasia and chronic inflammatory cell infiltrate, changes which readily explain the mucoid diarrhea characteristic of whipworm infection.

History. Dogs with whipworm-induced colitis have a history of diarrhea which is more often mucoid than bloody. Tenesmus is rare but in other aspects the history is similar to chronic colitis. Signs of typhlitis such as biting at the flank and irritability are occasionally reported but are unusual.

It should be emphasized that not all dogs with trichuris infection have colitis or diarrhea. Light infections can be asymptomatic or may appear as unexplained weight loss in the face of a normal or even increased appetite. Weight loss can be severe in long-standing infections.

Infection is acquired by ingestion of infective eggs and seems to recur with surprising frequency in some dogs. In these cases the history often reveals exposure to a contaminated environment such as a dirt surface or a local park frequented by a large number of dogs.

Physical Findings. As in chronic colitis, physical examination is not particularly revealing. Body weight and stage of hydration vary in proportion to the duration and severity of the infection. If diarrhea has been severe, most dogs are thin and appear slightly dehydrated. Abdominal palpation is usually not rewarding; although pain can occasionally be elicited from the mid-abdomen in the region of the cecum and ascending colon, it cannot be localized to these organs. The rectum is normal on digital examination and tenesmus is rarely elicited as the disease process seldom extends that far distally.

While the clinical signs are mostly proportional to the number of parasites in the cecum and colon, this is not necessarily so. The author has seen a few dogs with severe diarrhea, attributed to whipworm-induced colitis but which on postmortem examination had only a small number of worms in the colon. The reasons for this exaggerated response are unclear.

Diagnosis. The most important aspect of diagnosis is detection of trichuris eggs on microscopic examination of a fecal sample. Dogs with whipworm-induced colitis usually have eggs in their feces. However, shedding of eggs by the adult parasite is not continuous and at least three negative examinations must be made over a 3- to 4-day period for infection to be ruled out. This author and others[174] have seen adult whipworms in the descending colon of dogs whose fecal examinations were repeatedly negative for eggs. In some instances a smear of feces taken directly from the rectal mucosa is reportedly a better source of eggs than feces.[174,201]

Colonoscopy typically reveals the colon to be hyperemic, with excessive amounts of mucus in the lumen and adhering to the mucosa. Ulceration is rare, but areas of focal hemorrhage are occasionally present. In severe infections large numbers of creamy white adult worms about 5 to 10 mm long may be seen attached to the mucosa. Biopsy changes are nonspecific, but many cases have extensive mucosal hyperplasia. There are also eosinophil and lymphocyte accumulations in the mucosa and submucosa and an increase in mononuclear cellularity of the lamina propria. Sections of adult worms may also be present.

Hematologic and blood chemistry changes are nonspecific and nondiagnostic. A peripheral eosinophilia is not a consistent finding and, when present, other causes of eosinophilia must be considered before it is attributed to whipworm infection. Hypoalbuminemia and hypergammaglobulinemia are less common than in chronic colitis, presumably because the inflammatory response is not as severe.

Radiographic examination is seldom helpful. Plain films of the abdomen occasionally reveal an enlarged gas-filled cecum in dogs with typhlitis. Contrast radiography is a waste of time and money, except in those few dogs in which diagnosis is difficult and severe lesions may be confined to the proximal colon and cecum.

Differential Diagnosis. Whipworm-induced colitis and typhlitis are differentiated from other causes of colonic diarrhea by detecting eggs in the feces or by finding adult parasites at colonoscopy. Diagnosis can be difficult in dogs which have noninflammatory colonic diarrheal disease with a small number of parasites as an incidental finding. A primary colonic motility disorder should be considered if diarrhea continues after adequate anthelmintic and sulfasalazine therapy in these cases.

Treatment. Successful treatment is predicated upon adequate and repeated anthelmintic therapy.[232]

This is not as easy as it sounds, for whipworms are one of the most difficult parasites to eliminate, and reinfection is common if good husbandry is not practiced simultaneously.

Anthelmintics that are effective against whipworms include dichlorvos (Task, Shell Chemical), glycobiarsol (Milibis, Winthrop Labs), phthalofyne (Whipcide, Pitman Moore), mebendazole (Telmintic, Pitman Moore), and butamisole (Styquin, Cyanamid). Dichlorvos is reportedly quite effective against whipworms but at least two and frequently more doses 2 to 3 weeks apart are required. In our experience the drug is not as effective as glycobiarsol or phthalofyne, which, though having potentially more side-effects, need fewer repeat dosages for complete elimination of the parasites. There are, unfortunately, many opinions but few published facts concerning effective dosage regimens. This author prefers two doses of phthalofyne 2 weeks apart; in resistant cases glycobiarsol is also given 2 weeks later. Follow-up fecal examinations are essential to confirm that the parasites have been eliminated.

These complicated personalized dosage schedules may become obsolete if the manufacturers' claims and early anecdotal reports of the efficacy of mebendazole and butamisole prove to be well founded. These drugs promise to supersede all previous treatments and certainly merit consideration. However, more than one course of treatment is still necessary for successful elimination of the parasite.

Many clients are either unable or unwilling to take the necessary preventive sanitary measures. In susceptible dogs it is necessary, therefore, to instill in the client's mind the idea of regular fecal examinations (three times yearly—early spring, midsummer, and fall) with appropriate anthelmintic therapy as needed.

Prognosis. The prognosis for a complete recovery is usually good. However, repeat infections are common and in some apparently sensitive animals even light infections are sufficient to cause disease.

Hookworm-Induced Colitis

Hookworms are generally thought of as small intestinal parasites, but they may be found in large numbers in the colon,[233] where they cause colitis. The disease is usually chronic and characterized by mucoid, occasionally bloody diarrhea. Hookworm colitis should be suspected if a dog with chronic weight loss, diarrhea, and hookworm eggs in its feces has signs of colonic involvement (mucoid feces, increased frequency of defecation, occasional fresh blood). At colonoscopy the colonic mucosa of these dogs appears hyperemic and small ulcers are occasionally seen. Many dogs have an eosinophilia. Several drugs are effective in the treatment of hookworms; these include disophenol, dichlorvos, mebendazole, and butamisole. At least two doses 3 weeks apart are necessary to completely eliminate the parasites. If possible, management practices should be improved concurrently in order to decrease the possibility of reinfection. Treatment for hookworms is usually sufficient to control the colitis; however, as has been previously mentioned, some dogs show signs of colonic involvement long after elimination of the parasite. These patients should be treated as described for chronic colitis.

Amebic Colitis

Infection with *Entamoeba histolytica* is an occasional cause of colitis in the dog. The disease occurs sporadically in the southern part of the United States and has also been reported from India, China, Indochina, Egypt, and Panama.[234]

It has been suggested that infection may be more common in hunting and working breeds, and a coincident helminth infection may be a factor that enhances invasion of the colonic mucosa by the protozoa.[234] After ingestion, infective trophozoites pass to the colon where they invade and colonize the lamina propria and superficial submucosa, causing foci of mucosal ulceration and hemorrhage.

The disease has varying manifestations depending on the severity of infection and varying host susceptibility. These have been classified as: (1) mild: diarrhea with some blood and spontaneous recovery; (2) chronic: gelatinous mucoid feces, occasional diarrhea progressing either to subclinical infection or recurrent acute stage; (3) subacute: bloody diarrhea becoming chronic or acute; (4) acute: fulminating dysentery, terminating in death; (5) systemic: dysentery terminating in death.[81]

The most common form of presentation of the disease is the acute stage. Diagnosis is by identification of trophozoites in fresh feces suspended in physiologic saline solution, by staining with iodine or iron hematoxylin, or by colonic mucosal biopsy. Repeated fecal examinations may be necessary to detect the parasite. Colonoscopy may reveal focal ulcers of 3- to 6-mm diameter or diffuse mucosal friability and bleeding.

The disease must be differentiated from chronic colitis and other causes of dysentery, such as hemorrhagic gastroenteritis.

The optimum treatment is uncertain for the dog.

Metronidazole appears to be the drug of choice and should be combined with appropriate supportive therapy. The prognosis depends upon the severity of the infection and the stage of disease. It is thought unlikely that the dog represents an important source of infection for man.[234]

Giardiasis

Giardia canis infection in the dog is generally thought to be a small intestinal disease (Chapter 23). However, there has been one case report of giardiasis in the dog presenting as chronic ulcerative colitis.[235] The history and clinical signs of giardia-induced colitis are similar to those of chronic colitis. Diagnosis is by detection of *Giardia canis* cysts in the feces. Infection is uncommon in the cat and seems to be primarily a small intestinal disease;[236] however, rectal prolapse associated with severe diarrhea has been reported in one animal.

Treatment with quinacrine hydrochloride or metronidazole is effective. Specific therapy for colitis can be given if necessary.

Balantidiasis

Balantidium coli is a protozoal organism that normally resides in the mucus lining the colonic mucosa. The organism produces disease in man, pig, and horse, and there are sporadic case reports of infection in the dog.[237–239] In all cases, canine balantidiasis has been associated with a severe concomitant trichuris infection, with the implication that the mucosal damage caused by whipworms may allow the protozoal organism to penetrate the mucosa. Following penetration, the proteolytic secretions of *Balantidium coli* produce extensive necrosis and further ulceration of the colonic mucosa.[174] Most human and canine infections are associated with exposure to swine, and infection is acquired either by ingestion of the trophozoite or by the resistant cyst. Clinical signs include persistent, bloody diarrhea, anorexia, and dehydration. Diagnosis is by identification of the organism in a fresh fecal smear. *Balantidium coli* is 30 to 70 μ in length, and is characterized by its spiral longitudinal rows of cilia and its large oral macronucleus.

Metronidazole is effective against the organism but it appears that elimination of Trichuris alone may be sufficient to effect a cure.

Protothecal Colitis

This is an extremely uncommon cause of colitis in the dog; only three cases having been described, one in the United Kingdom[240] and two in the United States.[241,242] One additional case has been seen in our practice. The disease is caused by a pathogenic alga, *Prototheca*. The algae colonize the lamina propria and submucosa of the intestinal tract with a predilection for the colon. The inflammatory response results in constriction of the colonic lumen, focal ulceration, and segmental loss of colonic epithelium. The organism spreads via the lymphatics causing lymphadenitis which can result in lymphangiectasia. Colonoscopy reveals thickened corrugated friable mucosal folds and variable ulceration.[201] Diagnosis is made either by detection of the organism in the feces or by biopsy. There is no reported treatment.

Histoplasma Colitis

Histoplasmosis is a chronic systemic fungal infection that invades the body via the respiratory tract, although direct infection of the gastrointestinal tract is also reported to occur.[243] The general and gastrointestinal aspects of the disease are discussed in Chapter 23. The organism invades either the small or large intestine. Both may be involved simultaneously, however, for dogs with histoplasma enterocolitis are not uncommon. Histoplasma colonizes the lamina propria and submucosa of the gastrointestinal tract and elicits a prominent macrophage response. Macrophages filled with the organism distend the mucosa and submucosa to cause distortion and corrugation of the mucosa. The affected segment of intestine becomes thickened and the lumen is narrowed. The organism subsequently invades the muscle layers of the gut, the intestinal blood vessels and lymphatics, and later spreads to the regional lymph nodes and liver.[201] Progression to a disseminated disease state is generally regarded as an indication of a defective immune response by the host.[244]

History. The history of the dog with histoplasma-induced colitis is of severe chronic diarrhea and weight loss. Cough, abdominal distention and depression have also been reported in disseminated disease in which the colon was involved secondarily, and are an important diagnostic feature when present in a dog with chronic diarrhea.[245] Patients in which the disease is confined to the colon are rare. The diarrhea is typical of colonic disease, but it is frequently profuse and watery in cases with small intestine involvement and malabsorption. The presence of blood and mucus in the feces may also be reported by the client.

Physical Findings. The results of physical examination of a dog with histoplasmosis depend on the stage of the disease and the extent, if any, of systemic involvement. Most dogs are underweight and many are emaciated. Persistent fever is common. Abdominal palpation may reveal thickened intestines, hepatomegaly, or ascites. Mucous membranes are pale and a peripheral lymphadenopathy is frequently present. The dog may be dyspneic if pulmonary involvement is advanced or if there is a pleural effusion. Rectal examination may reveal a thickened mucosa with a narrow lumen. The iliac lymph nodes are frequently enlarged.

Diagnosis. Histoplasma colitis is best documented by colonoscopic examination and concomitant colonic biopsy. The mucosa appears corrugated and ulcerated and it is reported that the colon does not distend readily following insufflation of air.[201] Contrast radiography demonstrates shortening of the colon with a reduction in luminal diameter and variable serration and ulceration. A non-regenerative anemia caused either by infiltration of the bone marrow or by blood loss from gastrointestinal lesions may occur. The white cell count is usually elevated but leukopenia may be present in severe cases. Hypoalbuminemia is also frequently present. Yeast-like bodies may be present in monocytes obtained from a buffy coat smear. Organisms may also be demonstrated using Wright's stain on smears made from thoracic or abdominal effusions.[245]

A direct fecal smear rarely reveals yeast-like macrophages, and culture may be needed for confirmation.

Differential Diagnosis. The clinical picture is usually diagnostic for the disseminated form of the disease. However, in those rare cases in which the lesions are restricted to the colon, other causes of a transmural colitis should be considered and ruled out by biopsy. These include histiocytic ulcerative colitis, protothecal enterocolitis, regional colitis and enterocolitis (granulomatous colitis), and colonic lymphosarcoma.[201]

Treatment. Amphotericin B is the specific therapy and its use is discussed in Chapter 23. Other symptomatic supportive treatment is also indicated. This may include nutritional support, possibly including hyperalimentation, blood or plasma, and symptomatic antidiarrheal therapy.

Prognosis. The prognosis is unfavorable without treatment, but improved amphotericin B therapy is effective in many cases.

Granulomatous Colitis

This disease, also called regional enteritis of the colon, is reportedly analogous to regional enteritis (Crohn's disease) of man.[199,201] The disease affects both small and large intestine; aspects of small intestinal involvement including protein-losing enteropathy are discussed in Chapter 23. The disease was first described as a regional enterocolitis of Cocker Spaniel dogs in 1954.[246] It is an uncommon disease of unknown etiology characterized by patchy severe inflammation with extensive scar tissue formation in the intestinal wall. There is no apparent breed predilection; the disease has been described in the Cocker Spaniel, Weimaraner, Labrador, Dachshund, and Bassett Hound[199,247] and has been seen in Labrador Retriever, Keeshond and mixed breed dogs in our practice. A case has also been described in a Foxhound in association with an aberrant Trichuris infection.[248] Most affected dogs are under 4 years of age and there is no apparent sex predilection.

History. The dog with granulomatous colitis is usually presented with a history of chronic, bloody, occasionally mucoid diarrhea accompanied by listlessness, and weight loss. Tenesmus is also present if the distal colon and rectum are involved in the disease process. If lesions in the distal rectum and anus are sufficiently severe to cause constriction and anal fistulas, constipation, rather than diarrhea, may be the presenting complaint. An observant client might also complain of a change in shape or reduction in diameter of the feces if a rectal stricture not sufficiently severe to cause constipation is present. Vomiting may also be a complaint in some animals.

Physical Findings. The nature of the physical findings depends on the duration, location, and severity of the disease process. The physical appearance varies from normal to emaciated, although most dogs are thin with pale mucous membranes indicative of anemia. Dehydration is frequently evident and some dogs may be febrile. Abdominal palpation may reveal thickened loops of intestines if a granulomatous enteritis is present. If the rectum is involved, rectal examination may reveal a restricted lumen, thickening of the mucosa, and enlarged iliac lymph nodes.

Diagnostic Studies. The hemogram characteristically shows a mild anemia and a leukocytosis with a left shift. Some dogs have an eosinophilia, and hypoproteinemia, especially hypoalbuminemia, is often present.

Colonoscopy reveals severe granulomatous mucosal proliferation with a narrowed lumen and failure to dilate following air insufflation. The colonic mucosa appears corrugated and hyperemic, and bleeding ulcers are frequently present. The whole length of the colon need not necessarily be affected; lesions may be interspersed between relatively normal areas.

Contrast radiographs should be made if colonoscopy reveals a normal colon, since the lesions may involve only the terminal ileum, ileocolic junction, or ascending colon and may not, therefore, be visible with the commonly used short colonoscope, which permits visualization only of the descending colon. Radiographs are likely to reveal a segmental constriction of the lumen with mucosal serration and ulceration. Only biopsy is diagnostic. Published reports of the histopathology[196,246,248] describe the lesion to be characterized by ulcerations of the mucosa and submucosa. These structures are edematous with substantial infiltration of mononuclear cells, eosinophils and polymorphs. There are also lymphoid nodules and granulomatous aggregates of epithelioid cells in the submucosa. Nerve plexuses are prominent and there is inflammation and obliteration of submucosal lymphatics with transmural fissures and microabscesses leading to subserosal inflammation. Long-standing lesions may show substantial fibrosis with reduction in the surface area of the colon. This may be sufficiently severe so that colonic reserve capacity is lost and diarrhea persists in spite of treatment.

In some cases an exploratory laparotomy may be required for diagnosis; this usually reveals lymphadenopathy and characteristic thickening of the intestine.

Treatment. Surgical excision is indicated if the lesions are sparse and localized. In other cases steroids and tylosin, or steroids and sulfasalazine occasionally bring about a cure or at least retard the progression of the disease process. Symptomatic antidiarrheal and supportive fluid and electrolyte therapy are indicated in severe cases.

Prognosis. The prognosis is grave. Complete recovery is rare and there may be recurrence even after surgical excision. For these reasons many clients consider euthanasia after a course of unsuccessful or only moderately successful treatment.

Uremic Colitis

A bloody diarrhea is a fairly common finding in uremia, and while the signs of uremia rather than those of colitis are usually of most concern, blood and fluid loss from the colon can be considerable in this secondary colitis. Perhaps the most important contributing factor to this syndrome is the toxic effect of ammonia on colonic mucosal cells. The ammonia is produced by the action of bacterial urease on urea. In experimental animals the colitis can be inhibited by stimulating the production of antibodies against urease.[249] Damage to colonic mucosal cells by ammonia has also been postulated in nonuremic animals. It has been shown that urease immunization will also prevent experimentally induced colitis, and it has been suggested that eventually vaccination against urease may play a role in the treatment of other forms of colitis.[249]

This information is presently of little practical value in veterinary medicine but serves to emphasize the fact that the colonic epithelial damage and diarrhea seen in uremia cannot be reversed until the blood urea concentration is reduced.

Histiocytic Ulcerative Colitis

Canine histiocytic ulcerative colitis is a very uncommon, chronic inflammatory disease of the large intestinal mucosa. It is characterized by infiltrates of periodic-acid-Schiff (PAS)-positive macrophages and progressive, superficial ulceration.[250] Until a recent description of a case in a French Bulldog,[251] the disorder had been seen only in purebred Boxers. Histiocytic ulcerative colitis has received much more attention in the literature than its incidence deserves; it appears to be much less common now than previously and in our practice it accounts for less than 2% of all cases of colitis, with the most recent case having been seen in 1973. This decrease is probably explained at least in part by the declining popularity of the Boxer breed and by enlightened breeding programs. The recent description of histiocytic ulcerative colitis in the French Bulldog, a breed which has similar ancestry to the Boxer,[251] raises interesting questions concerning the still unknown cause and pathogenesis of the disease. The possible causes and pathogenic mechanisms have been reviewed.[174] Whatever the mechanism of epithelial injury is eventually determined to be, it is probable that a genetic predisposition underlies the disease process.[252]

History. The disease affects young Boxers of either sex, with most affected dogs showing signs before 2 years of age. The presenting complaint is often one of bloody mucoid diarrhea with maintenance of overall good body condition. The appetite is usually good, and only severe or long-standing cases are debilitated. The characteristics of the diarrhea are similar to those of other mucosal forms of colitis, with tenesmus a frequent complaint because the disease process often involves the distal colon and rectum.

Physical Findings. Physical examination is usually unrewarding with the dog appearing in very good condition. There is rarely dehydration or fever but digital rectal examination may reveal a corrugated thickened mucosa.

Diagnosis. The hemogram is usually unremarkable; however, some dogs may have a leukocytosis and mild anemia. Examination of a fecal smear stained with new methylene blue typically reveals numerous erythrocytes and neutrophils.

Colonoscopy reveals thickened mucosal folds and variable ulceration, depending upon the degree of involvement and the time from onset to examination. The findings range from mucosal hyperemia and edema to isolated or multiple strictures and deep bleeding ulcers.

Barium enema radiography demonstrates one or more of the following: shortening, loss of flexures, rigidity, eccentric reduction of lumen diameter, serration of profile edges, barium papules, and barium-filled ulcers.[201]

Biopsy is diagnostic. Microscopically there is a thickening of the lamina propria and submucosa caused by histiocytes, plasma cells, and lymphocytes, and in some cases there is ulceration and neutrophil infiltration. The majority of the histiocytes are PAS-positive and give the disease its name. The detailed histologic appearance of all stages of the disease has been described.[250,251]

Treatment. Treatment is not particularly successful, and is symptomatic. It has been reported that some cases respond favorably when treated with a combination of chloramphenicol and tylosin.[200] Relapses are common, however, and affected dogs often need lifelong treatment. Sulfasalazine has also been used with moderate success. but steroids with or without antibacterial agents seem to have little beneficial effect.

Prognosis. Mildly affected dogs may appear normal if managed correctly. The prognosis must be guarded however, since the progressive nature of the disease is not altered by present treatment methods. In view of the expense of lifelong treatment and the deteriorating condition of their pet, many clients decide on euthanasia.

Eosinophilic Colitis

Eosinophilic colitis can be either acute or chronic. In the latter case the clinical picture is similar to chronic colitis. As a specific disease entity, eosinophilic colitis is uncommon, being more frequently seen in association with eosinophilic gastroenteritis. The cause is unknown; the disease is often regarded as allergic in origin but trials of elimination diets are generally unsuccessful and other causes or manifestations of allergic reactions are rare. The characteristic findings are a circulating eosinophilia and infiltration of the colonic mucosa with eosinophils. Visceral larva migrans has been associated with a syndrome in the dog similar to eosinophilic gastroenteritis, but colonic lesions were absent.[253] Toxoplasmosis may be a cause of eosinophilic gastroenteritis in the cat. However, the role of parasites in the pathogenesis of the colonic disease remains to be elucidated and they are probably only one of several potential causes. There is no known age or breed predisposition.

History. Dogs are usually presented with a history similar to chronic colitis. Rarely, owners might associate the onset of signs with the feeding of one particular type of food. Vomiting may be a major complaint if eosinophilic gastroenteritis is also present.

Physical Findings. Dogs with eosinophilic gastroenteritis or colitis are usually normal on physical examination. Rectal examination occasionally reveals a thickened mucosa or may initiate tenesmus. Dehydration and weight loss may be evident if there is excessive fluid loss, or if the disease is particularly severe.

Diagnosis. The characteristic finding is an eosinophilia of up to 20% which cannot be attributed to any other cause. A mild anemia may also be present. Serum protein concentration varies; some cases have a hypoalbuminemia and hypergammaglobulinemia. An increase in serum IgE has been reported in human patients with eosinophilic gastroenteritis,[254] and this might prove to be an interesting avenue of investigation in similarly affected dogs.

Microscopic examination of an appropriately stained fecal smear reveals a high concentration of eosinophils.

Diagnosis is best made by colonoscopy and biopsy of the colonic mucosa. At colonoscopy the mucosa resembles that of the dog with chronic colitis; however, histologic examination of the biopsy specimen reveals numerous eosinophils in the mucosa, lamina propria, and submucosa.

Differential Diagnosis. The clinical findings resemble those of most other mucosal colitides and biopsy is essential to confirm the diagnosis. It is not unheard of for a dog with colitis to have an unrelated circulating eosinophilia, and all causes of eosinophilia, especially parasite infections, must be eliminated and a confirmatory colonic biopsy taken before the diagnosis is made. Repeated fecal examinations to rule out parasite infections are mandatory.

Treatment. If possible, any offending food must be removed from the diet. Identification of a specific dietary cause is rare and the treatment of choice is corticosteroids. High doses of prednisolone (1 to 2 mg/kg) should be given initially, gradually tapering to a maintenance dosage over a 3- to 4-week period. The lowest dose to bring about an elimination of clinical signs should be found by trial and error and this dosage should be tapered slowly after a 6- to 8-week course. Relapse is uncommon with this treatment regimen but long-term steroid therapy is required in a few cases. Oral cromoglycate has been used in the treatment of food allergy in man[225] and this alternative approach may merit a trial in those dogs which require long-term steroid therapy.

Other symptomatic and supportive treatment as described in the section on chronic colitis may be initially indicated in some dogs.

Less Common Forms of Colitis

The colon is subjected to many different types of trauma; the most common causes and their accompanying clinical syndromes have been presented in preceding sections. The reader should, however, be aware that other causes of colonic inflammation may result in an animal being admitted with signs of colitis. Most are represented only by single case reports and include mycotic colitis, traumatic colitis, antibiotic-associated pseudomembranous colitis, self-limited proctitis, lymphocytic mucosal colitis, and colitis cystica profunda.

Mycotic Colitis. Mycotic infections involving the gastrointestinal tract are rare in small animals. They usually occur either as secondary, opportunistic infections following gastrointestinal damage when the animal is debilitated, or in cases given long-term treatment with antibiotics or steroids. Mycotic infections can occur following feline infectious enteritis. One such case has been reported involving colonic infection with *Aspergillus sp.*[256] The affected animal was presented with signs compatible with infectious enteritis but later developed severe hemorrhagic diarrhea. Lesions seen radiographically in the colon were revealed at necropsy to be raised 1- to 2-cm plaques of hemorrhagic necrosis containing fungal elements identified as *Aspergillus*.

Traumatic Colitis. Colonic trauma is rare but is occasionally caused by abrasive or jagged intestinal foreign bodies. Ingested bones, sticks, wire, plastic, glass, or pieces of metal can cut or abrade the colon as they pass through. The predominant clinical sign is rectal bleeding; diarrhea is less common. The lesions are usually self-limiting following elimination of the foreign body; however an object will occasionally become lodged in the rectum, resulting in dyschezia, tenesmus, hematochezia, or constipation. Penetration of the wall may result in either a perirectal abscess or peritonitis.

Iatrogenic traumatic colitis caused by overly vigorous or inept colonoscopy is not unknown. The endoscope must always be inserted gently and not forced if resistance is met. The detailed techniques of colonoscopy are discussed in Chapter 8.

Finally, cases of rectal or colonic damage may be caused by the insertion of sticks or other objects into the rectum by perverted individuals. Anal lesions may be visible in these cases and the animal is admitted with rectal bleeding and tenesmus. In all cases treatment is symptomatic, involving antibiotics and antispasmodics. Sulfasalazine may be given if diarrhea suggestive of colitis persists.

Antibiotic-Associated Pseudomembranous Colitis. In human medicine pseudomembranous colitis has been recognized for many years as a severe gastrointestinal lesion associated with a number of conditions. In recent years the majority of cases have been ascribed to antimicrobial treatment. Clindamycin and lincomycin have been incriminated most often, but cases have been associated with a number of other antimicrobial agents. Proctoscopic examination of affected patients reveals erythematous friable mucosa covered with small sometimes confluent (1 to 5 mm) raised yellowish-white plaques. The plaques may be covered with viscid mucus, which has to be removed before the characteristic lesion can be seen. The plaque-like lesions also have a characteristic radiographic appearance.[257] One case has been seen in a dog in this practice; this animal had been treated with clindamycin for persistent osteomyelitis. Severe mucoid diarrhea typical of colonic disease started 10 days after commencement of antibiotic therapy. At colonoscopy the colon appeared identical to descriptions of the colon in human patients. Recovery occurred following withdrawal of the drug and treatment with sulfasalazine.

The lesions are thought to be caused by toxins produced by clindamycin-resistant clostridia, which proliferate when other gastrointestinal bacteria are suppressed by the drug.[94b,258]

Self-Limited Proctitis. Self-limited proctitis similar to that occurring in man has been documented in a 4-year-old Dachshund.[199] This nonspecific inflammatory process involves the rectal mucosa but not the mucosa of the more proximal colon. The clinical picture includes hematochezia, or diarrhea, tenesmus, and eosinophilia. There is hyperemia and occasional rectal ulceration. Rectal biopsy is characterized by marked congestion and hemorrhage of the lamina propria, mononuclear cell infiltration of the lamina propria, excessive mucus production, hyperplasia of crypt epithelium, frequent cystic crypts, and cystic downgrowth of crypt epithelium into submucosal lymph nodules.[199]

The disease is not severe but is difficult to eliminate. Treatment involves oral sulfasalazine and hydrocortisone retention enemas.

Lymphocytic Mucosal Colitis. This condition has been described in a 6-year-old German Shepherd dog.[199] The disease signs are similar to those of chronic colitis, and it is diagnosed by the histologic appearance of the colonic mucosa. The lesion is characterized by infiltration of the lamina propria with lymphocytes and reticulum cells and lateral splaying of displaced colon glands.[201] The condition is differentiated from lymphosarcoma by its lack of invasiveness and mitotic figures.

Colitis Cystica Profunda. This disease has been reported in an 11-month-old Boston Terrier[199] and the symptoms are similar to those of chronic colitis. The disease is characterized histologically by irregular mucosal thickness, tattered epithelium, indented mucosa, crypt epithelial cell necrosis, crypt abscesses, congestion and mononuclear cell infiltrate of the lamina propria, and abundant cystic downgrowth of hyperplastic epithelium into submucosal lymph nodules.[201]

Non-Inflammatory Colonic Diarrheal Diseases

Not all diarrheas of colonic origin are associated with inflammatory processes (see Table 24–2). In our practice about 15 to 20% of dogs with chronic diarrhea of colonic origin have no evidence of colitis on colonoscopy or biopsy and are assumed to have some sort of colonic motor dysfunction. The precise nature of this defect has not yet been defined; indeed, no definitive evidence for colonic motor dysfunction yet exists in the dog, but clinical experience strongly suggests that such a defect exists. The syndrome has been called irritable colon or spastic colon[174] and may be analogous to the irritable bowel syndrome of man. This common clinical disorder in human medicine is characterized by diarrhea or constipation in the absence of demonstrable organic bowel disease.[259] There is evidence that abnormal myoelectrical activity produces colonic dysfunction in this syndrome,[260] but there is still little objective information concerning either its cause or pathophysiology, although in man it is frequently associated with life stress and emotional tension.[261]

History. The dog with noninflammatory colonic diarrhea is admitted with a similar history to the dog with chronic colitis. The diarrhea is typically mucoid and may be intermittent but defecation is not always associated with quite the same sense of urgency as in colitis. Hematochezia, tenesmus, and vomiting are rare.

Many afflicted dogs have a long history of failure to respond to various dietary changes as well as to conventional antidiarrheal preparations, including sulfasalazine.

The disorder has a predilection for the larger breeds and appears to have an unusually high incidence in working breeds such as Seeing Eye, guard, and police dogs. Afflicted dogs tend to be temperamental, often easily excited or nervous and much more dependent on one person than are other dogs. An evaluation of the psychologic profile of owners of these dogs might be rewarding, since many seem to be either nervous individuals or excessively strict with their pet. It is helpful if an association can be made between the onset of diarrhea and changes in environment, use, or housing. It has been reported that signs may be evident only during periods of separation from the owner, or following the birth of a child into the family.[174] This author has seen diarrhea start when a new dog was brought into the household and in another case diarrhea occurred only when the owner's husband, a traveling salesman, was home on weekends.

Physical Examination. Physical examination in a dog with noninflammatory colonic diarrhea is not helpful in making the diagnosis, inasmuch as there are few detectable abnormal findings. Some dogs appear underweight in the face of reportedly good food intake. Abdominal palpation is not remarkable but digital rectal examination occasionally elicits rectal spasm.

Diagnostic Studies. Until the establishment of objective diagnostic criteria for this disease, diagnosis must be made by the exclusion of organic colonic disease and other functional diarrheas.

There are no hematologic or blood chemical changes. Microscopic examination of the feces reveals an absence of inflammatory cells and erythrocytes, and parasite eggs when present are only an incidental finding.

Colonoscopic examination and biopsy are essential for diagnosis in that they rule out all organic colonic disease. At colonoscopy the colonic mucosa may appear normal. More often, however, there is generalized hyperemia of varying severity, together with large amounts of mucus adhering to the mucosa and free in the lumen. Ulcers are absent, areas of petechial hemorrhage are rare, and the mucosa does not bleed when gently rubbed with the tip of the colonoscope. The colon may appear hypermotile even in the heavily sedated dogs, and distention of the mucosa by air insufflation or even upon insertion of the colonoscope may be difficult because of active contraction of the muscles in the colon wall.

Biopsy is usually normal. There may be mucosal hyperplasia, thickening of the lamina propria and engorgement of submucosal blood vessels with erythrocytes.

There is little recorded experience with contrast radiography in this disease. It is probable that the colon will appear normal if the dog is anesthetized for examination. Colonic spasm may be present, but distinctive lesions and filling defects as described for colitis are absent.

Treatment. Treatment consists of a combination of anticholinergics, sedatives, and dietary modification. An attempt should also be made to alleviate any contributing environmental factors. No presently available treatment is curative and the client must be advised of the probable necessity for long-term drug therapy.

Anticholinergic drugs much as propantheline bromide or clidinium (Quarzan, Roche Labs) are effective in many cases, but in some patients may need to be combined with light sedation. Chlordiazepoxide in combination with clidinium (Librax, Roche Labs) appears to be an effective drug for long-term control. A dose of one–two capsules b.i.d. or t.i.d. is usually sufficient for a 35-kg dog. Phenobarbital or chlorpromazine may also be used in excessively nervous dogs, especially before periods of anticipated stress.

Lomotil is effective for short-term control of occasional bouts of severe diarrhea associated with this syndrome. All other classes of antidiarrheal agents yield disappointing results.

The addition of fiber to the diet of dogs with this syndrome has proved beneficial. Fiber is currently of considerable public and scientific interest in that inadequate intake has been associated with a number of common diseases of man,[262] some of which are associated with abnormal colonic motor activity,[263,264] including the irritable bowel syndrome.[265,266] However, the therapeutic value of dietary fiber in the irritable bowel syndrome of man is still unresolved. In one study of patients placed on a high wheat-fiber regimen there was a significant improvement in symptoms together with an objective change in colonic motor activity;[265] however, in another study no such beneficial result was observed.[267] It has become apparent that fiber type is important since coarse bran has been shown to be much more effective than finely ground bran in changing colonic function.[268]

There are a few anecdotal reports but no published data on the effect of dietary fiber on colonic function in the dog. A low fiber diet has been recommended for the treatment of gastrointestinal disturbances;[269] increasing fecal bulk has been advocated as a treatment for both diarrhea and constipation in the dog;[210] and sterculia gum, a bulking agent with the capacity to absorb large amounts of water, reportedly has the same effect.[270] The addition of dietary fiber in the form of wheat bran to the diet of dogs with noninflammatory colonic diarrhea seems in many cases to bring about symptomatic improvement. The effect may be nonspecific, however, since bran also has a beneficial effect in some cases of colitis. Some dogs given bran can be maintained free from diarrhea for long periods without the routine use of anticholinergic drugs.[226]

The exact dose of bran in the dog is still uncertain; based on studies in man, 1–2 g of coarse bran/5 kg of body weight (3 tablespoonfuls for a 35-kg dog) appears to be appropriate and is used in this practice. Palatability is a problem if the dog is routinely fed kibble or semimoist food, but this amount can be mixed with moist canned foods without markedly decreasing palatability. An alternative approach is to use an equivalent amount of a bran-containing breakfast cereal mixed with the food for those dogs which will not accept supplementation with coarse brans.[226]

Prognosis. The prognosis is guarded inasmuch as treatment is symptomatic and dogs may need lifelong treatment. Clients should always be advised of the nature of the treatment and of its probable long-term nature. Clients are much more likely to accept the situation if the nature of the disease is adequately explained and will stop changing from one veterinarian to another in the hope of obtaining a more successful treatment and favorable prognosis. Some clients find it difficult to accept that their dogs' problems may be attributable either directly or indirectly to their relationship with the animal.

Cecal Inversion

Inversion of the cecum into the colon is an infrequent occurrence. The specific cause is unknown but seems to be associated with a weak ileocecocolic ligament. Predisposing factors include gastrointestinal parasitism and garbage ingestion.

History and Clinical Signs. The disorder is characterized by chronic, sometimes bloody, diarrhea. The nature and frequency (intermittent, variable) of the diarrhea are more characteristic of small intestinal disease (stagnant loop) rather than large intestinal disease. Tenesmus and dyschezia are not evident because the lesion does not involve the distal colon or rectum. Vomiting is infrequent unless the inverted cecum causes intestinal obstruction. Weight loss and dehydration may be profound.

Diagnosis and Treatment. Careful abdominal palpation may reveal a mass in the midcranial abdomen. This indicates the need for plain abdominal films and contrast studies (Chapter 7). Contrast radiographs reveal the inverted cecum as a filling defect at the ileocolic junction.[271] The inverted cecum can also be seen by means of the fiberoptic colonoscope. Treatment is surgical removal of the inverted cecum.

DISEASES WITH CONSTIPATION AND DYSCHEZIA AS THE PRINCIPAL SIGNS

This category includes the causes of constipation listed in Table 24–3. However, only those diseases of the colon, rectum, and anus which are associated with constipation and dyschezia will be described in this section. These include colonic impaction, idiopathic megacolon, anal stricture and spasm, perineal hernia, perianal fistula, anal sac disease, and pseudocoprostasis.

Colonic Impaction

Impaction of the colon with feces and ingested hair or foreign material such as bone or string is probably the most common cause of constipation in the dog and cat. When mixed with feces, hair, string, bone, and many other ingested materials form very hard masses which the animal finds difficult to eliminate.

Constipation is more frequent with increasing age, if the dog or cat is fed a highly purified diet or has co-existent painful rectal or anal disease. Colonic impaction is more common in the cat, presumably because this species is observed to defecate less frequently and because of its tendency to ingest hair during the grooming process. Colonic impaction can thus easily occur in these animals and be far advanced before the client notices that something is amiss. Normally, hair ingested during grooming is eliminated by vomiting a cylinder of matted hair or hair mixed with food. However, in some cats, especially the long-haired breeds or during periods of coat change, hair passes through the gastrointestinal tract and becomes incorporated in the feces.

Impaction is a recurrent problem in some apparently susceptible animals and may lead to secondary megacolon. Any disease that obstructs the normal passage of feces or causes pain on defecation can result in secondary colonic impaction. This group of diseases includes rectal stricture, colonic and rectal tumors, perineal hernia, rectal foreign bodies, perianal fistula, anal sac disease, prostatic hypertrophy, and a narrowed pelvic canal following a previous pelvic fracture.

History. The animal is presented with a history of failure to defecate for a period of time ranging from days to weeks. The client may have observed the animal making frequent attempts to defecate with little or no success. In some cases a small amount of liquid feces often containing blood or mucus may be passed with a great deal of straining. These animals might be presented with an erroneous history of diarrhea. If defecation has been unobserved, the patient might be seen only because it is dull, listless, inappetent, or anorectic and vomiting intermittently.

Diagnosis. The patient may appear depressed and is often dehydrated. Mucous membranes are frequently hyperemic and the coat may have a dull unkempt appearance. Cats may adopt a crouching hunched attitude, which is indicative of abdominal discomfort. Obvious abdominal distention is observed infrequently but abdominal palpation reveals a hard fecal mass, sometimes filling the whole length of the colon. Digital rectal examination typically reveals an empty rectum but very hard feces may be felt at the pelvic brim. Rectal examination combined with abdominal palpation is useful in localizing the fecal mass and in identifying lesions such as rectal foreign bodies, prostatic hypertrophy, or a narrowed pelvic canal which may be the underlying cause. Rectal sacculation or dilatation may also be identified by digital examination even if external signs of perineal hernia are absent.

Abdominal survey radiographs will confirm the presence of colonic dilatation and impaction and in some instances may reveal its causes, some of which are listed in Table 24–3. Following removal of the fecal mass, barium enema radiography or colonoscopy may be necessary to identify obstructive tumors, strictures or other colonic or rectal lesions.

Differential Diagnosis. In the cat, constipation should be differentiated from alimentary lymphosarcoma and idiopathic megacolon. The large tumors that sometimes occur in alimentary lymphosarcoma can be difficult to differentiate from impacted feces by abdominal palpation alone but radiographs are diagnostic. Idiopathic megacolon is identified by the extreme dilatation of the colon and the chronic history.

Treatment. Treatment of colonic impaction consists of gentle removal of the fecal concretions and, if possible, of identification and removal of any underlying cause. Most specific treatments are surgical, and range from castration in the case of prostatic hypertrophy, to resection of colonic tumors or realignment of an old pelvic fracture.

Breakdown and removal of fecal masses impacted in the colon should be accomplished as slowly and gently as possible. It is less traumatic for the patient if the feces are softened and removed over a 2- to 4-day period than if complete removal is attempted at one time. The severely constipated animal is often cachectic and dehydrated and must have corrective fluid and electrolyte therapy before any attempt is made to remove the impaction. Animals that have been inappetent or anorectic for a prolonged period of time are hypokalemic and need potassium supplementation. Potassium can be given either orally as potassium gluconate (Kaon, Warren-Teed Pharmaceuticals) or parenterally as potassium chloride. Means of defining the potassium deficit have not been precisely defined in the dog or cat, but clinical experience indicates that a daily dose of about 2 mEq/kg body weight is an adequate oral dose and 40 mEq added to each liter of maintenance fluids is an adequate and safe parenteral dose for most patients.[209]

Impaction can be treated with oral laxatives, with enemas, or by manual removal of the feces under general anesthesia following administration of enemas and laxatives. Simple impaction of relatively short duration is best dealt with by oral administration of a softening agent and lubricant such as mineral oil. This can be given alone or in combination with dioctyl sodium sulfosuccinate (DSS), which is a wetting agent and colonic irritant. DSS stimulates colonic secretion,[37] and it is therefore important that the patient be well hydrated before compounds containing this substance are administered. As a last resort in very severe cases it may be necessary to remove the fecal concretions manually with the aid of a small pair of whelping forceps or sponge forceps while the patient is anesthetized. In cats and small dogs this procedure is facilitated by "milking" the feces caudally by digital manipulation through the abdominal wall.

Once the underlying cause has been treated and the fecal concretions removed, attention should be directed to prevention of recurrence. Bones should be eliminated from the diet, regular grooming instituted, and the opportunity provided for regular defecation. Prevention may be difficult in long-standing cases which have developed secondary megacolon. In every case the therapeutic goal should be to have the patient form soft feces and defecate regularly. To this end fecal bulking and softening agents containing methycellulose, psyllium hydrophilic mucilloid (Metamucil), or DSS can be added to the diet. Dietary fiber supplements in the form of bran are also useful. Commercially available veterinary laxatives containing petrolatum as the active ingredient are especially useful in preventing hair impaction in cats.

Prognosis. The prognosis for colonic impaction depends on the cause and the duration of the disease. It is good in mild cases but when secondary megacolon has developed or it proves impossible to remove the underlying cause, the client should be warned of the necessity for continual laxative treatment and the possibility that colonic dilatation will worsen.

Idiopathic Megacolon

Primary or idiopathic megacolon is more common in the cat than the dog but is an unusual cause of constipation in either species. The cause is unknown but is possibly related to a degeneration or relative absence of myenteric ganglion cells in the colon wall. The disorder has erroneously been called Hirschsprung's disease but has *not* been shown to be analogous to this human disease. Hirschsprung's disease occurs in children and is caused by an absence of ganglion cells in a narrowed but otherwise apparently normal distal rectal segment. Fecal material is unable to pass through the aganglionic segment and gradually distends the proximal colon, eventually causing severe constipation. The internal sphincter also functions abnormally in this disease, contracting instead of relaxing when stimulated by rectal distention.[272] Neither the absence of ganglion cells in the colon wall nor abnormal anal sphincter function has been demonstrated in the dog or cat.

History. Idiopathic megacolon may present in the cat at any age from approximately 6 years onwards. The patient is usually presented with a history similar to that described for colonic impaction. Depression, loss of appetite, and occasional vomiting are the common complaints. The disease is insidious in onset and seemingly progressive in nature, for recurrent episodes of constipation of increasing severity and frequency may occur in some cats before their significance is realized. The history of the disease in the dog is similar but signs tend to occur at an earlier age. Several cats with idiopathic megacolon seen in this practice have been infected with feline leukemia virus; the significance of this finding is unknown.

Diagnosis. Most cats are depressed and have an unkempt appearance. The rectum is usually empty and dilated on rectal examination, but a mass of hard feces is felt at the pelvic inlet. Abdominal palpation confirms the presence of a large mass of feces in the colon. The whole length of descending colon and even the ascending and transverse colon may be impacted and in severe cases may be 4 to 5 cm in diameter. Abdominal radiographs are confirmatory and help to differentiate the disease from alimentary lymphosarcoma. Long-standing cases are hypokalemic and anemic.

Treatment. Treatment is as for colonic impaction but should be individualized. Preventive measures are needed for the duration of the animal's life and include dietary modifications and the regular administration of laxatives. The diet should include laxative foods such as raw liver, and bulking agents such as methylcellulose or bran.

Surgical resection of the atonic colon has been described,[273] but surgery should probably be considered only as a last resort since the complications may be worse than the disease.

Prognosis. The prognosis is guarded and depends on the stage of the disease at first examination and the ability of the client to persist with preventive and ongoing therapeutic measures.

Rectal and Anal Strictures

Strictures of the rectum and anus are rare in the dog and cat. When they do occur, it is usually as a complication of an inflammatory disease such as perianal fistula, anal sac disease, or anorectal trauma. They may also be an iatrogenic complication of anorectal surgery. Strictures are reportedly more common in German Shepherds, Beagles, and Poodles.[274] In severe cases scar tissue formation may be circumferential with varying degrees of involvement of the external anal sphincter.[178]

The animal is admitted to the clinic with a history of tenesmus, dyschezia, and hematochezia. Secondary colonic impaction may be present, and an observant client may complain of a change in shape of the feces. There may be a history of previous surgery or trauma to the anorectum.

Diagnosis is made by digital rectal examination when a firm constricting fibrous band or stenotic segment is palpated. Contrast radiographs may be indicated to define the extent of the lesion if its full extent cannot be palpated. In extreme cases the lesion may be several centimeters or more in length.[275] Biopsy allows differentiation of strictures from constricting tumors such as a scirrhous adenocarcinoma.

Mild cases may respond to dilatation but surgical correction is usually required. This involves either a myotomy of the external anal sphincter or rectal musculature, or resection of the stricture.[274] Fecal incontinence and additional scar tissue formation are complications of these surgical procedures.[178]

Rectal and Anal Foreign Bodies

Ingested sewing needles, bones, and pieces of stick or metal can traverse the gastrointestinal tract without harm, only to become lodged transversely in the distal rectum. Defecation is extremely painful or impossible in afflicted animals. The dog or cat may yelp or scream as defecation is attempted and after a few unsuccessful attempts, the animal may cease to strain. Secondary colonic impaction may occur if the disorder is untreated and long-standing cases may develop rectal strictures, fistulae, or perirectal abscesses if the rectal wall is perforated. Sometimes a thread attached to a needle may be seen protruding from the anus, thus making diagnosis relatively easy. In other cases digital rectal examination is diagnostic. General anesthesia is often required for removal of the foreign body. Other treatment is symptomatic and consists of cleansing, debridement and drainage when necessary, together with parenteral antibiotic therapy.

Anal Spasm

Anal spasm is an uncommon disease, apparently confined to German Shepherds, in which the anal sphincter contracts when the animal attempts to defecate. Distention of the external anal sphincter is extremely painful and the animal may cry out when defecation is attempted. Tenesmus, dyschezia, and constipation are common. The cause is unknown but seems to be related to an abnormal response of the muscles in the external anal sphincter to stretch. Digital rectal examination is vigorously resented by the patient and the anus feels very constricted. Secondary rectal dilatation is often present. The disorder is differentiated from anal strictures by the normal smooth texture of the anal and rectal mucosa, the absence of inflammatory tissue, and the fact that the anus can be readily distended when the dog is anesthetized. Treatment is palliative and consists of section of one or possibly both branches of the pudendal nerves that innervate the external anal sphincter.[276] Fecal incontinence is a common postoperative problem especially if both left and right nerve branches are sectioned.

Feline Fecoliths

A syndrome has been described in the older cat characterized by frequent and very painful attempts to defecate. It is caused by the incarceration of a "knob" of feces of normal size and of firm but not hard consistency in the anus between the internal and external sphincter.[277]

Abdominal palpation readily differentiates the condition from colonic impaction and megacolon, but clients frequently present the cat with a complaint of constipation. Treatment is digital expression of the fecal mass by pressure on either side of the anus as for emptying the anal sacs.

Anal Injuries

Injuries to the anus and perineum are comparatively common in the cat, less so in the dog. They are usually the result of a bite wound inflicted by an opponent when the animal turns to flee. There may be varying degrees of laceration and penetration of the anal sphincter. Treatment is symptomatic, consisting of cleansing, debridement, drainage, and if necessary reconstruction of the anal ring. Bite wounds are heavily infected, so intensive antibiotic therapy is indicated. An anal fistula is a rare complication of a bite wound but may occur if the anal wall is penetrated. The animal presents with a small draining fistula and inflammation of the skin of the perianal area. Treatment is by surgical excision of the fistulous tract.

Perineal Hernia

Perineal hernia is a well-recognized entity in the dog and is thought to result from a weakness of the pelvic diaphragm, which is composed of the muscles that form a caudal limit to the pelvic canal. Perineal hernia has been defined as herniation of a rectal diverticulum or abdominal or pelvic contents through an opening created by the separation of the muscles lateral to the anus and tailhead and dorsal to the ischium[278] or, more simply, as a failure of the supporting structures of the pelvis outlet to contain the pelvic organs.[279]

Such hernias occur almost exclusively in the older (over 7-year-old) male dog and have a significant predilection for Collies, Dachshunds, and the naturally docked breeds.[280,281]

The hernia can be either unilateral or bilateral with unilateral hernias occurring predominantly on the right side. The cause of the disease is unknown, as are the reasons for the breed predilection and predominantly right-sided occurrence.

History. Most dogs with perineal hernia are presented because of difficulty in defecation and an obvious swelling lateral to the anus. Tenesmus and constipation are common, and fecal incontinence occurs in about 10% of afflicted dogs. Occasionally the urinary bladder retroflexes into the hernia and the animal is seen with signs of acute urinary obstruction.

Diagnosis. Digital rectal examination reveals a right- or left-sided rectal dilatation or sacculation which is almost invariably filled with inspissated feces. The rectum feels slack and no longer firmly anchored and there may be varying degrees of rectal deviation. If the finger is moved laterally, it may be observed to move the skin medial to the ischial tuberosity. The flaccid dilated rectal wall tends to envelop the finger and prevent free movement, readily revealing why the dog has difficulty defecating. Some dogs may present with dyschezia and tenesmus, but have only a rectal dilatation and no obvious perineal swelling, although close examination of the perineum in short-haired dogs may reveal a slight bulge in the perineum. These animals also have perineal hernia, however, since the rectum can dilate only if the muscles of the pelvic diaphragm (mainly the levator ani) are weakened. Rectal dilatation and sacculation are not separate entities from perineal hernia, but are probably different stages of the same disease process. In rectal dilatation, there is reportedly a flaw in the rectal muscle allowing mucosal prolapse, while in sacculation the muscles are intact and the whole rectum deviates and expands to fill the space formed by the weakened pelvic diaphragm.[274,275] The rectal muscle is intact in most dogs with perineal hernia and thus rectal sacculation is more common than rectal dilatation.

Treatment. The conventional treatment is surgical repair of the hernia, but medical treatment should be tried first since about 20% of dogs can be maintained free of signs by the use of fecal softeners and occasional enemas. If dyschezia persists after medical treatment, a perineal herniorrhaphy should be carried out. The technique has been described in detail[280,282] and consists of anastomosis of the external anal sphincter to the coccygeal muscle dorsally and laterally, the sacrotuberous ligament laterally, and the internal obturator muscle ventrally. The procedure leaves much to be desired, however, for recurrence is common, even for experienced surgeons, and ranges from 37 to 46% over a follow-up period of 5 years.[280,281] Most breakdowns occur more than 12 months after the initial repair, and

clients should be advised of this before surgery, as well as of the potential complications such as fecal incontinence and rectal prolapse. It is essential that fecal softeners be continued after surgery since defecation may contine to be difficult for those animals with a dilated or deviated rectum.

The benefits of castration, both in the prophylaxis of perineal hernia as well as in the prevention of recurrence after surgical repair, remains to be proven. There are conflicting reports of statistical studies of the effects of castration. Two studies failed to demonstrate any beneficial effect,[280,281] while a study of a much larger population demonstrated a significant sparing effect of castration on recurrence of perineal hernia.[282] Even though the benefits of castration are not proven, it is a relatively innocuous procedure, and has been shown to be useful in the treatment of perianal gland neoplasms,[311] as well as in the prophylaxis of testicular tumors. Both are common diseases of the older male dog and the use of castration as part of the overall treatment of perineal hernia seems indicated.

Anal splitting is an alternative surgical treatment to perineal herniorrhaphy in dogs with excessive tenesmus, a large rectal sacculation, and little other tissue in the hernia.[284,285] In this procedure two fingers are placed through the anus into the rectum and an incision is made from the anal opening through the skin, external anal sphincter muscle, and rectal wall. This lays open the rectum, the edge of which is then sutured to the skin edge. The incision must be carefully placed to avoid the pudendal nerve and anal sac.

The prognosis must be guarded in view of the tendency for breakdown of the surgical repair, the need for persistent treatment, and the post-surgical complications. In one survey only 42% of clients were completely satisfied with the results of surgery.[280]

Imperforate Anus and Rectal Aplasia

These uncommon congenital abnormalities occur when the cloacal membrane fails to rupture or when the anorectal septum fails to complete the division of the primitive cloaca. Rectal aplasia differs from imperforate anus only in that the rectum ends blindly at a variable distance from the rectal membrane with the intervening space filled with connective tissue.

There is no known breed or sex predilection, and the clinical signs, characterized by abdominal enlargement and discomfort, tenesmus, inappetence, restlessness and occasional vomiting are noted within a few days to a few weeks of birth. Diagnosis is based on the absence of an anal opening and the usually bulging cloacal membrane. Imperforate anus may be differentiated from rectal atresia by radiography. If the patient is held upside down by its hind feet and a horizontal radiograph taken, rectal and colonic gas will migrate to the distal rectum in dogs with imperforate anus.[274]

The external anal sphincter and its nerve supply are usually intact as these two structures develop independently from the anorectal canal.[286] Surgical treatment of the imperforate anus consists of a stab or cruciate incision into the anus and excision of the cloacal membrane.[274] Rectal atresia is more difficult to correct. The greater distance between the blind-ended rectum and the anus requires a rectal pull-through in a combined abdominoperineal approach. The potential for damage to the external anal sphincter is greatly increased and thus the prognosis is correspondingly unfavorable.[178]

Rectovaginal Fistula

Rectovaginal fistula is a very rare congenital disorder which occurs less frequently than imperforate anus. The anus is usually also imperforate in this condition however, with the fecal material being expelled through the vagina.[286,287] In those dogs in which the anus remains open, the feces pass through both the anus and vulva. Fecal incontinence and subsequent contamination of the perineum lead to severe perianal and perivulvar dermatitis. A barium enema establishes the diagnosis since barium flows through the fistula into the vagina. The signs of colonic impaction observed in puppies with imperforate anus or rectal aplasia are not usually present until the animal begins to digest solid food, at which time colonic obstruction becomes more obvious.[174]

Treatment is surgical and is directed at restoring the integrity of both the vagina and anus. The fistula must be identified and removed in its entirety with separate closure of the openings into the rectum and vagina. Complications are frequent and include fecal and urinary incontinence and constipation.[287] The prognosis is guarded.

Perianal Fistula

Perianal fistula, also known as anal furunculosis, is a well-recognized entity in the dog. The disease occurs mainly in the German Shepherd, but has also been reported in Shepherd crosses, Irish Setters, Retrievers, Collies, Spaniels, and Samoyeds.[288,289] There is no sex predisposition but the disease

occurs most often in dogs older than 2 years of age. Perianal fistula is characterized by chronic ulcerating sinus tracts in the perianal tissues, which almost invariably have a malodorous purulent discharge. The specific cause is unknown but the histopathologic findings suggest that the disease results from infection and abscessation of the circumanal glands, hair follicles, and other glands in the perianal skin.[288] This infection results in necrosis, ulceration, and acute and chronic inflammation of the perianal area with development of excessive granulation tissue and fibrosis. The anal sacs are involved only secondarily in the disease process.[290] The broad tail base and low tail carriage of the German Shepherd probably account for the high incidence of the disease in this breed. These factors combine to cause poor ventilation of the anal area, the development of an overlying film of fecal material and anal sac secretions, and a moist environment which permits epidermal erosion, infection and eventually results in necrosis and fistula formation.[288,289] The disease is markedly different from the disease of the same name in man.[288]

History. The dog with perianal fistula is usually seen with one or more of the following complaints: excessive licking of the anal area, dyschezia, constipation, "scooting," hematochezia, a foul-smelling mucopurulent discharge, and tenesmus. Other signs that might occur as the disease progresses are mild fecal incontinence, intermittent diarrhea, anorexia, and weight loss. In most cases the disease is well advanced before veterinary advice is sought.

Physical Findings. Examination of the perianal area is diagnostic. The lesion is very painful and even lifting the tail may be vigorously resented. The area is usually covered with a thin film of mucopurulent exudate which, after removal by gentle cleansing, reveals ulcers, granulation tissue, and suppurating tracts. The extent of the lesions vary according to the duration of the disease process. In long-standing cases the lesions may involve the entire perianal area and tail base, and are frequently most severe in the area surrounding the opening of the ducts of the anal sacs.

Gentle probing reveals that the lesions interconnect and under-run the skin.[289] In some cases true fistulae are present between the skin and the columnar zone of the anal sphincter, while in others sinus tracts extend deeply into the perirectal tissues. The extent of the diseased tissue is therefore much greater than the superficial lesions suggest. Digital rectal examination may be vigorously resented, and in some cases anal stricture may be present as a result of excessive fibrosis. Prolonged dyschezia may result in colonic impaction.

Differential Diagnosis. The appearance of the lesion is usually diagnostic, especially if it occurs in a German Shepherd. However milder cases may be confused with chronic anal sac abscesses and perianal adenocarcinomas. In anal sac abscesses, fistulae originate in the anal sacs and are usually less extensive than in perianal fistula. Adenocarcinomas generally have a proliferation of tissue which has distinct histologic characteristics.

Treatment. Medical treatment consists of clipping the hair around the tail base and gentle cleansing. Topical antibiotic and steroid preparations have proved useful only in palliation and are not curative.

Surgical treatment provides the best chance of effecting a permanent cure. Many surgical techniques have been described.[178,274,288,289,291,292,293]

In all cases the objective is to preserve healthy tissue, and either remove diseased tissue or stimulate it to heal by granulation.

Surgical excision of all diseased tissue has been advocated as the treatment of choice.[274,288,291] However, because of the often extensive and invasive nature of the lesion, resection can lead to serious and frequently unacceptable complications. Reported complications of radical excision include flatulence, fecal incontinence, diarrhea, tenesmus, constipation, stenosis, and recurrence of the lesion. In one survey 45% of the cases developed recurrent lesions, and in 21% the results were considered unacceptable by the owner because of the complications.[288] This high recurrence rate and the severity of the complications have stimulated a search for more acceptable surgical techniques.

A method of complete debridement and anal sacculectomy followed by chemical cautery of the base of the diseased tissue has been described.[289] This technique markedly reduced the incidence of complications, but the recurrence rate was still 16.5%, and dogs with extensive anal sphincter involvement had difficulty terminating a bowel movement.

Cryosurgery combined with anal sacculectomy seems to offer some advantages over this technique inasmuch as the incidence of recurrence is less.[293] Many dogs require more than one treatment, however, and immediate complications include swelling, edema, hemorrhage, and the smell of sloughing necrotic tissue. Long-term complications include recurrence and scarring in response to severe tissue destruction caused during freezing of the deeper lesions. Scarring may be severe enough to cause

anal stenosis.[178,292] The cryosurgical technique is important; liquid nitrogen spray gives less favorable results than the carefully controlled use of a cryoprobe. In one series of 200 dogs cryosurgery achieved an 86% success rate with few complications.[294]

Another technique is a combination of anal sacculectomy and thorough debridement as previously described, followed by fulguration of the base of the diseased tissue by electrocautery.[178] This method reportedly results in less tissue damage than surgical excision or cryosurgery, fewer complications, and relatively rapid postoperative recovery. Recurrence still occurs with this technique, but fecal incontinence, flatulence, and anal stenosis are avoided as there is minimal damage to vital structures.[178]

The nature of the disease process and the site of the lesion probably mean that no surgical treatment will ever be totally effective. However, regardless of the type of treatment, one of the most important factors affecting the outcome and prognosis is the thoroughness of postoperative care. Animals whose owners are prepared to wash the perianal area regularly and cleanse it with an antibacterial soap such as Betadine or Phisohex do much better than those that are totally ignored. The area should be washed three or four times daily while healing and thereafter thoroughly cleaned on a daily basis. Dyschezia can be minimized by the use of a fecal softening and bulking agent such as Metamucil, and the chronic nonspecific diarrhea so common in German Shepherds should be controlled either by dietary modification such as the addition of coarse bran to the diet or by the use of specific antidiarrheal drugs. Recurrence is much reduced when postoperative care is adequate.

Anal Sac Disease in the Dog

Anal sac disease is by far the most common anal disorder of the dog. The reported incidence ranges from 2.0%[290] to 12.5%[295] in dogs presented for veterinary examination. The disease has no age or sex predisposition[295] but the question of breed predisposition is unresolved. One study showed no breed predisposition,[295] while another revealed a high incidence in Miniature Poodles, Toy Poodles, and Chihuahuas, and a lower than expected incidence in German Shepherds.[290]

Anal sac disease may be divided into three types: impaction, sacculitis, and abscesses. These have slightly different clinical manifestations but most likely represent different points on the spectrum of the same basic disease process rather than being separate diseases.

The specific cause of anal sac disease is unknown, but possible predisposing factors include a change in character of the glandular secretion, chronically soft feces or a recent bout of diarrhea, glandular hypersecretion associated with generalized seborrhea, and poor muscle tone in small or obese dogs.[178] Prolonged retention of normal anal sac secretion may result in fermentation, secondary bacterial infection, and abscessation.[290] An immunologic reaction following bacterial infection and toxin release has also been suggested to play a role in the pathogenesis of the disease.[296] Anal sac disease has been produced experimentally by introducing pathogenic bacteria directly into the sac or by ligating the duct from the sac.[297]

History. Certain characteristic complaints should alert the clinician to the possibility of anal sac disease. Halnan[298] listed those clients' descriptions which have specific diagnostic significance, and divided them into three specific groups.

Group 1. The signs are directly related to the discomfort associated with anal sac infection or impaction. These include tenesmus, discomfort when sitting down, licking or biting at the anal areas, "scooting," tail chasing, a perianal discharge following abscess rupture, rubbing the back against a chair or table, obsessive licking of an unrelated area of the body, and a marked change in temperament.

Group 2. The signs are not necessarily related directly to anal sac disease but are frequently present in chronic cases. They include a "rash" on the abdomen, axilla or groin, self-inflicted trauma to the skin of the lumbosacral area, and interdigital dermatitis.

Group 3. Specific behavioral changes associated with perianal irritation include jumping up suddenly while at rest as if pricked by a pin, and periodically staring at the anal area.

The history may also reveal contributing factors such as estrus or a recent bout of diarrhea.

Diagnosis. The diagnosis already indicated from the history is confirmed by examination of the perineum and perianal area. There may be obvious areas of pyotraumatic dermatitis of these areas or of the tail base or lumbosacral region, and the anal sacs are usually swollen and tender. Assessment of enlargement is somewhat subjective, but the sacs are generally considered to be enlarged when they can be easily palpated through the skin of the anal region.[298] The enlargement may be either unilateral or bilateral, with most cases being bilateral; unilateral enlargement is most often associated with an anal sac abscess rather than with impaction or sacculitis.

After assessing the size of the sacs, the veterinarian should evacuate their contents. In a 17-kg dog the normal volume is about 0.25 to 0.5 ml, and the contents should be almost clear and pale yellow-brown. Findings of turbidity, granular material, unusual coloration and pus are abnormal.[298] Abnormal fluid is always turbid because of the increased cell content.

Impaction is usually characterized by a thick pasty brown or greyish brown secretion. If this material becomes inspissated, it can be evacuated only with a great deal of difficulty as a thin ribbon. The duct may occasionally be blocked by a plug of extremely dry material which must be dislodged before the sacs can be expressed.

Anal sacculitis is characterized by a thin greenish-yellow or creamy-yellow secretion which may be flecked with blood.

Anal sac abscesses are characterized by fever and an inflamed and often hairless area over the sac. Many dogs are presented with a discharging sinus after the abscess has spontaneously ruptured.

Treatment. Manual evacuation of the contents of the sacs is an essential step in treatment of impaction or infection, and the establishment of free drainage may be all that is needed to obtain a cure. The anal sacs can be evacuated either internally, by digital pressure exerted through the rectum, or externally by pressure exerted through the perianal skin. The internal method is usually necessary in obese or tailless dogs and should be routine in those dogs in which the signs are not obviously caused by anal sac disease, since evacuation can be coupled with digital rectal examination. Rectal examination also has the advantage of permitting definition of the size, configuration, and consistency of the sacs. To empty the sac, it is simply squeezed between the finger in the rectum and the thumb externally. To evacuate the sacs from the outside, the tail is lifted with one hand and the finger and thumb of the other hand are placed on the skin of the perineum just lateral to the sacs. Inward pressure allows the finger and the thumb to move slightly behind and under the sacs, which are then evacuated with a firm squeezing movement and an upward and outward rotation of the wrist. The internal method is less painful to the dog, and the sac can be more completely evacuated.

Resolution of anal sacculitis is facilitated by instillation of an antibiotic solution into the sacs. In large dogs this can be accomplished by placing the nozzle of a tube of intramammary or otic antibiotic preparation into the duct of the gland. In smaller dogs it is easier to instill the antibiotic solution through a lacrimal needle. Many preparations are effective, but compounds containing ampicillin, chloramphenicol, or streptomycin are most effective. Panolog is also an effective preparation. In cases of recurrent infection, the secretion should be cultured and an antibiotic sensitivity test carried out. Many different bacteria with widely disparate patterns of antibiotic sensitivity have been cultured from infected glands, but *Escherichia coli, Streptococcus fecalis, Clostridium welchii* and *Proteus sp.* predominate.[298] Systemic antibiotic therapy is rarely needed for simple impaction or infection. If reinfection is a frequent occurrence, the sacs should be cauterized or removed.

Anal sac abscesses are treated slightly differently. When the infected sac is swollen and painful, the frequent application of hot packs is useful in bringing the abscess to a point at which it can be lanced. Systemic antibiotic should be given if the patient is febrile or if inflammation is extensive. After lancing, the contents of the sac should be evacuated, the sac irrigated with a solution of povidone-iodine (Betadine) or dilute hydrogen peroxide, and then filled with an antibiotic solution. The client should be instructed to clean the area at least once daily and to instill an antibiotic solution or ointment through the wound for 2 to 3 days. This keeps the wound open to allow drainage.

Recurrent anal sac abscesses are an indication for anal sac excision. Various surgical techniques have been described,[274,299] but similar basic principles apply in all cases. First the sacs must be checked to ensure that the walls are intact and then the extent of each sac is delineated with a probe or with an impregnating material such as paraffin wax. A delicate dissection follows using fine scissors or a small scalpel. The wound may be closed in one or more layers or may be left open.

An alternative to open surgery in cases where abscessation has not occurred is the ablation of the sacs by chemical cautery.[300] The technique is easier than surgical excision and has fewer postoperative complications. The detailed technique has been described.[299] It consists of lavaging the sacs sequentially with solutions of 1% cetrimide, 40% formaldehyde, or three parts methyl alcohol to one part glacial acetic acid, 1% cetrimide again, and finally local anesthetic. The sacs show an intense

reaction for about 12 hours and subsequently sclerose to form a linear scar within the muscle.

Anal Sac Disease in the Cat

The anal sacs of the cat are situated in a similar location to those of the dog but the ducts open in the circumanal tissue and are directed posteriorly; the opening of the duct is marked by a small papilla.

The incidence of feline anal sac disease is much lower than in the dog. Impaction is the most common complaint; infection and abscesses are extremely rare.

The signs of impaction are similar to those in the dog and evacuation affords relief. The secretion is frequently inspissated and must be evacuated slowly and gently.

Pseudocoprostasis

Pseudocoprostasis occurs in both the dog and cat when the hair surrounding the anus becomes matted with feces. This can completely obstruct the anal opening, impair the passage of feces, and may lead to colonic impaction. The mass of feces and hair excoriates the perianal skin and causes an acute dermatitis. During warm weather the mass serves as a nidus for deposition of fly eggs, which, when hatching into maggots, may cause extensive debridement of the anal area. Pseudocoprostasis is especially prevalent in Poodles, Schnauzers, Pekingese, and long-haired cats and dogs of all breeds. It is exacerbated if the animal has diarrhea.

The signs are mainly those of anal irritation. The animal makes frequent attempts to lick or bite the anal area and may make sudden running movements, holding the tail to one side or clamped tightly down. There is an unmistakable fecal odor to the patient; inspection of the anal area is sufficient for diagnosis.

The treatment is to clip away all matted hair and feces, clean the skin of the region, and apply a soothing dressing. Maggots can be manually removed or killed by a light dusting of flea powder and washed away. Client education is an important part of prevention.

Rectal Prolapse

Rectal prolapse is a disorder characterized by the protrusion of one or more layers of the rectum through the anus. It may be either partial or complete depending on the structures involved. Only the rectal mucosa protrudes in partial prolapse whereas all the layers of the rectum are involved if the prolapse is complete.[274] The disorder can occur whenever there is persistent straining from intestinal, anorectal, or urogenital disease. Rectal prolapse occurs in dogs and cats of any age, breed, or sex but is seen most frequently in young animals with severe diarrhea. Rectal foreign bodies can also cause severe straining and prolapse. Other predisposing factors include tumors of the distal colon or anorectum, dystocia, cystitis, urethral obstruction, prostatitis, prostatic hypertrophy, colitis, and proctitis. Defects in the pelvic musculature such as are found in perineal hernia also predispose to prolapse as does mechanical interference with the external anal sphincter.[286]

At physical examination the prolapse is obvious as a dark red edematous mass protruding from the anus. However, rectal prolapse must be differentiated from prolapse of the ileum in an ileocolic intussusception. This is achieved by an attempt to insert the finger or a blunt instrument such as a thermometer between the prolapsed mass and the anal margin. Inability to insert the instrument indicates a rectal prolapse.

Treatment is based on the identification and correction of the underlying cause and reduction of the prolapse. The various techniques for treatment of rectal prolapse have been described in detail[274] and range from simple reduction to resection. Partial prolapse usually responds well to medical treatment. The mucosa is gently replaced and antibiotic-steroid ointments are applied topically for at least 1 week. If needed, a purse-string suture can be placed around the anus. Concomitant treatment of the underlying cause is mandatory. The prolapse should be resected only if nonsurgical methods fail or if the tissue becomes necrotic. The prognosis is usually good provided that the underlying cause can be corrected.

Dog Pox

A disorder characterized by papular eruptions 1 to 1.5 mm in diameter on the mucous membranes of the dog has been described in the United Kingdom.[301] The disease occurs in dogs of all ages and is thought to be caused by a herpes virus; the name "dog pox" is therefore a misnomer. Papules occur on the penis, conjunctiva, and vulva and in the colon, rectum, and anus. It is the lesions of the lower gastrointestinal tract that reportedly cause the most severe clinical signs.[275,301] The most prominent signs are severe anorectal irritation such as occurs in anal sac disease, intractable diarrhea, and tenesmus.

Careful digital rectal palpation reveals small raised areas on the rectal mucosa. The lesions are extremely sensitive since palpation causes signs of intensive irritation, often to the extent of frenzy. Colonoscopy is reported as unrewarding, since the rectal lesions are difficult to see, but they may be readily seen on the base of the penis where they apparently cause the animal little concern.[275]

Treatment is symptomatic and not particularly successful, but spontaneous remissions do occur. A chlortetracycline-hydrocortisone preparation introduced into the rectum reportedly affords symptomatic relief.

Tumors of the Colon, Rectum, and Anus

Colonic and Rectal Tumors

Large intestinal tumors are relatively uncommon in the dog and cat, but most are malignant and have usually metastasized by the time they are diagnosed. Adenocarcinomas occur most frequently, but carcinomas, leiomyosarcomas, lymphosarcomas, carcinoid tumors, and anaplastic sarcomas have also been reported.[302-304] Benign tumors are mostly adenomatous polyps or leiomyomas.[302,302a] The location varies in different species. In the cat most tumors occur in the ileocecal area,[304] while in the dog the majority are found in the rectum.[303,305]

Adenocarcinomas have been classified into three main types based on their gross characteristics:[306] infiltrative, ulcerative and proliferative. The infiltrating tumor spreads within the rectal or colonic wall causing fibrosis which results in stricture formation of variable length. The ulcerative type produces a typical malignant ulcer with a hard base and raised edge, while the proliferative type has a wart-like appearance. All three types are slow growing and may be present for months or even years before diagnosis. The tumor eventually spreads through the rectal wall, penetrates the lymphatics, and metastasizes to the local lymph nodes, lungs, and liver. Adenocarcinomas occur predominantly in dogs older than 9 years of age,[307] more frequently in males than females, and have a particularly high incidence in Collies and German Shepherds.[303]

Colonic and rectal lymphosarcomas are uncommon and can occur either as a discrete mass or as diffuse infiltrations through the wall. This tumor occurs most frequently in dogs less than 4 years of age.

Carcinoid tumors, though rare, occur in both the small and large intestine.[303,308] The tumor is associated with diarrhea and gastrointestinal hemorrhage, and as a result of its secretion of serotonin, with systemic vasomotor effects.

Adenomatous polyps are the most common benign neoplasms of the colon and rectum with most being found in the rectum.[302,302a] There appears to be a breed predilection in collies.[302a] Carcinomas may arise within adenomatous polyps in the canine rectum;[302a,309] and several cases have been seen in our practice.

History and Physical Findings. Dogs and cats with large intestinal tumors usually have a history of dyschezia, hematochezia, tenesmus, and diarrhea. As with most malignant tumors, afflicted animals appear chronically ill and debilitated. The specific signs depend upon the tumor location and type. All three types of adenocarcinoma cause tenesmus with the frequent passage of small amounts of feces. Tenesmus worsens as the lesion develops, especially in the proliferative or obstructive type; eventually the passage of feces may be completely obstructed causing secondary colonic impaction. If the tumor does not cause an obstruction, its presence may change the character of the feces. A thin ribbon of feces is not at all uncommon with infiltrating adenocarcinomas, and hematochezia is a frequent complaint in the ulcerating type. Rectal irritation causes a mucoid diarrhea or mucus-covered feces. Digital rectal examination typically reveals a painful ringlike mass or stenotic area, the so-called "napkin-ring lesion," anterior to which hard feces frequently are palpated.

If diffusely infiltrated through the colon wall, lymphosarcomas of the large intestine cause a chronic unresponsive diarrhea similar to that seen in chronic histoplasmosis. Occasionally a single focus of lymphosarcoma may be found, and in these cases the signs resemble those of an adenocarcinoma.

Dogs with colonic or rectal polyps are not as debilitated as dogs with malignant tumors. In these animals the predominant signs are tenesmus following defecation and a chronic, unresponsive bloody or mucoid diarrhea. If tenesmus is particularly severe, animals are sometimes presented with the tumor prolapsed from the rectum.

Diagnosis. Digital rectal examination is sufficient to confirm the presence of a rectal mass and biopsy is diagnostic. Colonic tumors are diagnosed by colonoscopy or contrast radiography. Since lymphosarcoma seldom involves the mucosa, superficial mucosal biopsy may be negative, even though a mass is palpated, or the mucosa appears abnormal on contrast radiographs. Polyps appear as lobulated grapelike masses with a pedunculated sessile base.

These tumors are quite friable, and palpation or slight trauma from the colonoscope is sufficient to cause bleeding. Colonoscopy may be difficult or impossible when the tumor causes rectal stenosis.

Treatment. Surgical resection of carcinomas and adenocarcinomas can be attempted, although it is usually unrewarding because of the tendency for metastasis.

About 75% of polyps are accessible through the anus and can be easily exposed if the rectal mucosa is everted by gentle traction. The polyps can be removed either by ligation of the stalk and excision or by electrocautery. Polyps located more proximally can be excised with an electrocautery snare passed through the colonoscope or, as a last resort, via a colectomy. The prognosis is good if biopsy reveals the tumor to be a benign polyp.

Anal Tumors

The most common and clinically important tumor of the anal region is the perianal gland adenoma. Other benign neoplasms are occasionally found in the anal and perianal area of the dog. These include lipomas, melanomas, and leiomyomas. Malignant tumors of the anus are rare. They include squamous cell carcinoma, malignant melanoma, perianal adenocarcinoma, and anal gland adenocarcinoma.

Perianal Gland Adenomas. Perianal gland adenomas arise from the perianal and circumanal glands of the dog and occur most often in intact males older than 6 years. They occur infrequently in females and younger males.[274] The tumors are benign, but cause client concern because of their tendency for ulceration and hemorrhage, their unsightliness, their interference with defecation, and the animals excessive licking of the perineum.

Perianal gland adenomas occur most often in the skin surrounding the anus but can be found almost anywhere on the perineum or external genitalia.[306] The tumors begin as small, firm, well-circumscribed nodules, but can grow quite large and may eventually ulcerate, bleed, and necrose. Diagnosis is confirmed by biopsy. The tumors have been reported as an ectopic source of a parathyroid hormone-like substance which causes polydipsia, polyuria, and other signs of pseudohyperparathyroidism.[310]

The tumors are hormone-sensitive and their development can be impaired with estrogen therapy. Long-term estrogen treatment is to be avoided, however, because of the hormones' adverse effect on the bone marrow. Definitive treatment consists of surgical excision and castration.[311] Removal of the source of male hormones by castration causes regression of the tumors and lessens the chance of new tumors developing.[178] Radiation therapy is also highly effective[312] as is cryosurgery, which, if available, is perhaps the treatment of choice.[313] The prognosis is favorable with all forms of treatment.

Malignant Anal Tumors. Squamous cell carcinoma of a distinct cloacogenic type has been reported as occurring in the anal canal of the dog.[306] The tumor resembles a transitional cell carcinoma of the bladder and is highly malignant. Squamous cell carcinoma of the cutaneous portion of the anus may also be encountered infrequently. The tumor initially appears as a small indurated ulcer which progresses to a cauliflower-like ulcerated mass with irregular edges.[26] The tumor metastasizes readily, and early radical excision is essential if a cure is to be effected.[178]

Perianal adenocarcinomata resemble an ulcerated perianal gland adenoma but may occasionally involve the entire anal area with extensive ulceration and fistula formation. These latter lesions resemble perianal fistula but differ on digital rectal examination in that the anal ring is greatly thickened. The prognosis is fair if the tumor is excised early but most are already well advanced at the time of presentation.

A malignant melanoma occasionally occurs as a flat to round nodule on the anus, especially in breeds with heavily pigmented skin. Most, but not all are pigmented; unpigmented tumors resemble perianal gland adenomas.

The major problem associated with malignant anal tumors is their propensity for extensive local invasion and early metastasis. The primary lesion must always be evaluated carefully in order to ascertain the degree of local involvement. The iliac lymph nodes, liver, and lungs should all be evaluated for metastasis. The prognosis is almost always poor since even radical excision is frequently ineffective and is associated with complications such as fecal incontinence.

REFERENCES

1. Coffman, J. R.: Diagnosis and management of acute abdominal diseases in the horse. V.M./S.A.C. 65:669, 1970.
2. Rosato, E. F. Intestinal obstruction. *In* Gastrointestinal Pathophysiology. Edited by F. P. Brooks. New York, Oxford University Press, 1974, p. 286.
3. Bury, K. D., McClure, R. L., and Wright, H. K.: Reversal of colonic net absorption to net secretion with increased intraluminal pressure. Arch. Surg. 108:854, 1974.
4. Billig, D., and Jordan, P.: Hemodynamic abnormalities secondary to extracellular fluid depletion in intestinal obstruction. Surg. Gynecol. Obstet. 128:1274, 1969.
5. Datt, S. C., and Usenik, E. A.: Intestinal obstruction in the horse. Physical signs and blood chemistry. Cornell Vet. 65:152, 1975.
6. Whitlock, R. H., Tasker, J. B., and Tennant, B. C.: Hypochloremic, metabolic alkalosis and hypokalemia in cattle with upper-gastrointestinal obstruction. Am. J. Dig. Dis. 20:595, 1975.
7. Donawick, W. J.: Metabolic management of the horse with acute abdominal crisis. J. S. Afr. Vet. Assoc. 46:107, 1975.
8. Coffman, J. R.: Monitoring and evaluating the physiological changes in the horse with acute abdominal disease. J. S. Afr. Vet. Assoc. 46:111, 1975.
9. Baue, H. E.: Recent developments in the study and treatment of shock. Surg. Gynecol. Obstet. 127:849, 1968.
10. Coffman, J. R., and Garner, H. E.: Acute abdominal diseases of the horse. J.A.V.M.A. 161:1195, 1972.
11. Fine, J.: The intestinal circulation in shock. Gastroenterology 52:454, 1967.
12. Lillehei, R. C., Dietzman, R. H., and Movsas, S.: The visceral circulation in shock. Gastroenterology 52:468, 1967.
13. Bennett, D. G.: Predisposition to abdominal crisis in the horse. J.A.V.M.A. 161:1189, 1972.
14. Ockner, R. K.: Blood supply of the gut and pathophysiology of ischemia. *In* Gastrointestinal Disease. Edited by M. H. Sleisenger and J. S. Fordtran. Philadelphia, W. B. Saunders Co., 1973. p. 378.
15. Hulten, L., Jodal, M., Lindhagen, J., and Lundgren, O.: Colonic blood flow in cat and man as analyzed by an inert gas washout technique. Gastroenterology 70:36, 1976.
16. Svanvik, J., and Lundgren, O.: Gastrointestinal circulation. *In* Gastrointestinal Physiology, Vol. II. International Review of Physiology. Edited by R. K. Crane. Baltimore, University Park Press, 1977, p. 1.
17. Wheat, J. D.: Causes of colic and types requiring surgical intervention. J. S. Afr. Vet. Assoc. 46:95, 1975.
18. Ockner, R. K.: Vascular diseases of the bowel. *In* Gastrointestinal Disease. Edited by M. H. Sleisenger and J. S. Fordtran. Philadelphia, W. B. Saunders Co., 1973, p. 1560.
19. Jubb, K. V. F., and Kennedy, P. C.: Pathology of Domestic Animals, 2nd ed., Vol. 2. New York, Academic Press, 1970, p. 84.
20. Rooney, J. R.: Autopsy of the Horse. Technique and Interpretation. Baltimore, The Williams & Wilkins Co., 1970.
21. Nelson, A. W., Collier, J. R., and Griner, L. A.: Acute surgical colonic infarction in the horse. Am. J. Vet. Res. 29:315, 1968.
22. Boles, C.: Post-operative management of equine abdominal patients. J. S. Afr. Vet. Assoc. 46:123, 1975.
23. Lillie, L. E., Olander, H. J., and Gallina, A. M.: Rectal stricture of swine. J.A.V.M.A. 163:358, 1973.
24. Wilcock, B. P., and Olander, H. J.: The pathogenesis of porcine rectal stricture. I. The naturally occurring disease and its association with salmonellosis. Vet. Pathol. 14:36, 1977.
25. Wilcock, B. P., and Olander, H. J.: The pathogenesis of porcine rectal stricture. II. Experimental salmonellosis and ischemic proctitis. Vet. Pathol. 14:43, 1977.
26. Saunders, C. N.: Rectal stricture syndrome in pigs: a case history. Vet. Rec. 94:61, 1974.
27. Greiner, T. P.: Surgery of the rectum and anus. Vet. Clin. North Am. 2:167, 1972.
28. Blood, D. C., Henderson, J. A., and Radostits, O. M.: Veterinary Medicine, 5th ed. Philadelphia, Lea & Febiger, 1978.
29. Vaughan, J. T.: Surgical management of abdominal crisis in the horse. J.A.V.M.A. 161:1199, 1972.
30. Boles, C. L., and Kohn, C. W.: Fibrous foreign body impaction colic in young horses. J.A.V.M.A. 171:193, 1977.
31. Greatorex, J. C.: Observations on the diagnosis of gastrointestinal disorders in the horse. Ir. Vet. J. 25:229, 1972.
32. Moffatt, R. E., Kramer, L. L., Lerner, D., and Jones, R.: Studies on dioctyl sodium sulfosuccinate toxicity: clinical, gross and microscopic pathology in the horse and guinea pig. Can. J. Comp. Med., 39:434, 1975.
33. Hines, J. R., Guerkink, R. E., Gordon, R. T., and Weinermann, P.: Phytobezoar: a recurring abdominal problem. Am. J. Surg. 133:672, 1977.
34. Lee, S. P., Holloway, W. D., and Nicholson, G. I.: The medical dissolution of phytobezoars using cellulase. Br. J. Surg. 64:403, 1977.
35. Davis, L. E., and Knight, A. P.: Review of the clinical pharmacology of the equine digestive system. J. Equine Med. Surg. 1:27, 1977.
36. Binder, H. J., and Donowitz, M.: A new look at laxative action. Gastroenterology 69:1001, 1975.
37. Donowitz, M., and Binder, H. J.: Effect of dioctyl sodium sulfosuccinate on colonic fluid and electrolyte movement. Gastroenterology 69:941, 1975.
38. Gaginella, T. S., Lewis, J. C., and Phillips, S.: Ricinoleic acid effects on rabbit intestine: an ultrastructural study. Mayo Clin. Proc. 51:569, 1976.

39. Gaginella, T. S., Chadwick, V. S., Debongnie, J. C., Lewis, J. C., and Phillips, S. F.: Perfusion of rabbit colon with ricinoleic acid: dose-related mucosal injury, fluid accumulation and increased permeability. Gastroenterology 73:95, 1977.

40. deBoom, H. P. A.: Functional anatomy and nervous control of the equine alimentary tract. J. S. Afr. Vet. Assoc. 46:5, 1975.

41. Budd, D. C., Nirdlinger, E. L., Sturtz, D. L., and Fouty, W. J.: Transverse colon volvulus associated with scleroderma. Am. J. Surg. 133:370, 1977.

42. Rous, R. C.: Mesenteric thrombosis. J. S. Afr. Vet. Assoc.: 46:79, 1975.

43. Phaneux, L. P., Grivel, M. L., and Ruckebusch, Y.: Electromyoenterography during normal gastro-intestinal activity, painful and non-painful colic and morphine analgesia, in the horse. Can. J. Comp. Med. 36:138, 1972.

44. Smith, J., Kelly, K. A., and Weinshilboum, R. M.: Pathophysiology of postoperative ileus. Arch. Surg. 112:203, 1977.

45. Svendsen, P.: Experimental studies of gastro-intestinal atony in ruminants. In Digestion and Metabolism in the Ruminant. Edited by I. W. McDonald and A. C. I. Warner. Armidale, University of New England Publishing Unit, 1975, p. 563.

46. Duelke, B. E., and Whitlock, R. H.: Persistent cecal dilatation in a lactating dairy cow. Cornell Vet. 66:301, 1976.

47. Glinsky, M. J., Smith, R. M., Spires, H. R., and Davis, C. L.: Measurement of volatile fatty acid production rates in the cecum of the pony. J. Anim. Sci. 42:1465, 1976.

48. Dyce, K. M., and Hartman, W.: A cinefluoroscopic study of the caecal base of the horse. Res. Vet. Sci. 20:40, 1976.

49. Svendsen, P.: Inhibition of cecal motility in sheep by volatile fatty acids. Nord. Vet. Med. 24:393, 1972.

50. Bolton, J. R., Merritt, A. M., Carlson, G. M., and Donawick, W. J.: Normal abomasal electromyography and emptying in sheep and the effects of intraabomasal volatile fatty acid infusion. Am. J. Vet. Res. 37:1387, 1976.

51. Gilmour, J. S., and Jolly, G. M.: Some aspects of the epidemiology of equine grass sickness. Vet. Rec. 95:77, 1974.

52. Ashton, D. G., Jones, D. M., and Gilmour, J. S.: Grass sickness in two non-domestic equines. Vet. Rec. 100:406, 1977.

53. Stewart, J., Gordon, W. S., and McCallum, J. W.: Grass sickness in horses, biochemical investigation. Vet. Rec. 52:237, 1940.

54. Reference deleted.

55. Mahaffey, L. W.: Ganglionic lesions in grass sickness of horses. Vet. Rec. 71:170, 1959.

56. McHowell, J., Baker, J. R., and Ritchie, H. E.: Observations on the caelico-mesenteric ganglia of horses with and without grass sickness. Br. Vet. J. 130:265, 1974.

57. Obel, A-L.: Studies on grass disease. The morphological picture with special reference to the vegetative nervous system. J. Comp. Pathol. 65:334, 1955.

58. Gilmour, J. S.: Experimental reproduction of the neurological lesions associated with grass sickness. Vet. Rec. 92:565, 1973.

59. Gilmour, J. S., and Mould, D. L.: Experimental studies of neurotoxic activity in blood fractions from acute cases of grass sickness. Res. Vet. Sci. 22:1, 1977.

60. Osborne, J. C., Davis, J. W., and Farley, H.: Hirschsprung's disease: a review and report of the entity in a Virginia swine herd. V.M./S.A.C. 63:451, 1968.

61. Hoskins, H. P., Lacroix, J. V., and Meyer, K. (Eds.): Canine Medicine, 2nd ed. Wheaton, IL, American Veterinary Publications, 1959, p. 116.

62. Davidson, M., and Sleisenger, M. H.: Megacolon. In Gastrointestinal Disease. Edited by M. H. Sleisenger and J. S. Fordtran. Philadelphia, W. B. Saunders Co., 1973, p. 1463.

63. Brooks, F. P.: Hirschsprung's disease. In Gastrointestinal Pathophysiology. Edited by F. P. Brooks. New York, Oxford University Press, 1974, p. 274.

64. Weisbrodt, N. W.: Gastrointestinal motility. In Gastrointestinal Physiology. MTP International Review of Science, Vol. 4. Edited by E. D. Jacobson and L. L. Shanbour. Baltimore, University Park Press, 1974, p. 139.

65. Dirksen, G.: Dilatation and torsion of the cecum in the ox. D. T. W. 69:409, 1962.

66. Espersen, G.: Cecal dilatation and dislocation. Mod. Vet. Pract. 42:25, 1961.

67. Jones, E. W., Johnson, L., and Morre, C. C.: Torsion of the bovine cecum. J.A.V.M.A. 130:167, 1957.

68. Oehme, F. W.: Torsion of the cecum in a cow. J.A.V.M.A. 150:171, 1967.

69. Pearson, H.: Dilatation and torsion of the bovine cecum and colon. Vet. Rec. 75:961, 1963.

70. Rines, M. P.: Studies relative to torsion of the bovine cecum. M. S. Thesis, Michigan State University, 1958.

71. Svendson, P., and Kristensen, B.: Cecal dilatation in cattle. Nord. Vet. Med. 22:572, 1970.

72. Whitlock, R. H.: Cecal Volvulus in Dairy Cattle. Proceedings 9th International Congress on Cattle Diseases, Paris, France. 1976, p. 69.

73. Argenzio, R. A., and Whipp, S. C.: Interrelationship of sodium, chloride, bicarbonate and acetate transport by the colon of the pig. J. Physiol. 295:365, 1979.

74. Argenzio, R. A., Miller, N., and von Engelhardt, W.: Effect of volatile fatty acids on water and ion absorption from the goat colon. Am. J. Physiol. 229:997, 1975.

75. Grady, G. F., and Keusch, G. T.: Pathogenesis of bacterial diarrheas. N. Engl. J. Med. 285:831, 1971.

76. Meynell, G. G.: Antibacterial mechanisms of the mouse gut. II. The role of Eh and volatile fatty acids in the normal gut. Br. J. Exp. Pathol. 44:209, 1963.

77. Manahan, F. F.: Diarrhoea in horses with particular reference to a chronic diarrhoea syndrome. Aust. Vet. J. 46:231, 1970.

78. Argenzio, R. A.: Functions of the equine large intestine and their interrelationship in disease. Cornell Vet. 65:303, 1975.

79. Duff, W. M.: Intracellular recordings of slow waves from inflamed smooth muscle of the colon. Gastroenterology 72:A-29/1052, 1977 (Abst.).

80. Smith, H. A., Jones, T. C., and Hunt, R. D.: Veterinary Pathology, 4th ed. Philadelphia, Lea & Febiger, 1972, p. 104.

81. Giannella, R. A., Gots, R. E., Charney, A. N., Greenough, W. B., and Formal, S. B.: Pathogenesis of salmonella-mediated intestinal fluid secretion. Gastroenterology 69:1238, 1975.

82. Giannella, R. A.: The importance of the intestinal inflammatory reaction in salmonella-mediated intestinal secretion. Gastroenterology 72:A-39/1062, 1977 (Abst.).

83. Bright-Asare, P., and Binder, H. J.: Stimulation of colonic secretion of water and electrolytes by hydroxy fatty acids. Gastroenterology 64:81, 1973.

84. Binder, H. J., Filburn, C., and Volpe, B. T.: Bile salt alteration of colonic electrolyte transport: role of cyclic adenosine monophosphate. Gastroenterology 68:503, 1975.

85. Nell, G., Forth, W., Rummel, W., and Wanitschke, R.: Pathway of sodium moving from blood to intestinal lumen under the influence of oxyphenisatin and deoxycholate. Arch. Pharmacol. 293:31, 1976.

86. Cline, W. S., Lorenzsonn, V., Benz, L., Buss, P., and Olsen, W. A.: The effects of sodium ricinoleate on small intestinal function and structure. J. Clin. Invest. 68:380, 1976.

87. Hofmann, A. F.: Bile acids, diarrhea, and antibiotics: data, speculation, and a unifying hypothesis. J. Infect. Dis. 135:126, 1977.

88. Gorbach, S. L., and Bartlett, J. G.: Colitis associated with clindamycin therapy. Pseudomembranous enterocolitis: a review of its diverse forms. J. Infect. Dis. 135:89, 1977.

89. Rooney, J. R., Bryans, J. T., and Doll, E. R.: Colitis "X" of horses. J.A.V.M.A. 142:510, 1963.

90. Brandborg, L. L.: Other infectious, inflammatory, and miscellaneous diseases. In Gastrointestinal Diseases. Edited by M. H. Sleisenger and J. S. Fordtran. Philadelphia, W. B. Saunders Co., 1973. p. 909.

91. Burrows, G. E., and Cannon, J.: Endotoxemia induced by rapid intravenous injection of Escherichia coli in anesthetized ponies. Am. J. Vet. Res. 31:1967, 1970.

92. Vaughan, J. T.: The acute colitis syndrome: colitis "X". Vet. Clin. North Am. 3:301, 1973.

93. Mansmann, R. A.: Equine anaphylaxis. Fed. Proc. 31:661, 1972. Abstract.

94. Rooney, J. R., Bryans, J. T., Prickett, M. E., and Zent, W. W.: Exhaustion shock in the horse. Cornell Vet. 56:220, 1966.

94a. Wierup, M.: Equine intestinal clostridiosis. Acta Vet. Scand., Suppl. 62, 1, 1977.

94b. Bartlett, J. A., Chang, T. W., Gurwith, M., Gorbach, S. L., and Onderdonk, A. B.: Antibiotic-associated pseudomembranous colitis due to toxin producing clostridia. N.Engl. J. Med. 298:531, 1978.

95. Yablonski, M. E., and Lifson, N.: Mechanism of production of intestinal secretion by elevated venous pressure. J. Clin. Invest. 57:904, 1976.

96. Merritt, A. M., Bolton, J. R., and Cimprich, R.: Differential diagnosis of diarrhea in horses over six months of age. J. S. Afr. Vet. Assoc. 46:73, 1975.

97. Greatorex, J. C.: Diarrhea in horses associated with ulceration of the colon and caecum resulting from S. vulgaris larval migration. Vet. Rec. 97:221, 1975.

98. Tasker, J. B.: Acid-base and electrolyte disturbances in acute diarrheal disease in the horse. A.A.E.P. Newsletter 2:56, 1976.

99. Clinical Pathological Conference. Cornell Vet. 59:648, 1969.

100. Duncan, J. L., and Dargie, J. D.: The pathogenesis and control of strongyle infection in the horse. J. S. Afr. Vet. Assoc. 46:81, 1975.

101. Cohrs, P.: Textbook of the Special Pathological Anatomy of Domestic Animals. New York, Pergamon Press, 1967, p. 61.

102. Duncan, J. L., and Pirie, H. M.: The pathogenesis of single experimental infections with Strongylus vulgaris in foals. Res. Vet. Sci. 18:82, 1975.

103. Symons, L. E. A.: Malabsorption. In Pathophysiology of Parasitic Infection. Edited by E. J. L. Soulsby. New York, Academic Press, 1976, p. 11.

104. Bolton, J. R., Merritt, A., M., Cimprich, R. E., Ramberg, C. F., and Street, W.: Normal and abnormal xylose absorption in the horse. Cornell Vet. 66:183, 1976.

105. Blackwell, N. J.: Colitis in equines associated with strongyle larvae. Vet. Rec. 93:401, 1973.

106. Nielsen, K.: Pathophysiology of parasitic infection. Plasma protein metabolism. In Pathophysiology of Parasitic Infection. Edited by E. J. L. Soulsby. New York, Academic Press, 1976, p. 23.

107. Drudge, J. H., and Lyons, E. T.: The chemotherapy of migrating strongyle larvae. In Equine Infectious Diseases, Vol. II. Edited by J. T. Bryans and H. Gerber. Basel, S. Karger, 1970.

108. Drudge, J. H.: Personal communication. University of Kentucky, Lexington, 1978.

109. Bryans, J. T., Fallon, D. H., and Shephard, B. P.: Equine salmonellosis. Cornell Vet. 51:467, 1961.

110. Owen, R. ap R.: Post stress diarrhoea in the horse. Vet. Rec. 96:267, 1975.

111. Morse, E. V., Duncan, M. A., Page, E. H., and Fessler, J. F.: Salmonellosis in equidae: a study of 23 cases. Cornell Vet. 66:198, 1976.

112. Linerode, P. A., and Goode, R. L.: Effects of Colic on Microbial Activity of the Equine Large Intestine. A.A.E.P. Proc. 16:321, 1971.

113. Whitlock, R. H.: Acute Diarrheal Disease in the Horse. Proc. A.A.E.P. 21:390, 1975.

114. Dorn, C. R., Coffman, J. R., Schmidt, D. A., Garner, H. E., Addison, J. B., and McCune, E. L.: Neutropenia and salmonellosis in hospitalized horses. J.A.V.M.A. 166:65, 1975.

115. Daleel, E.E., and Frost, A. J.: The isolation of salmonella from cattle at Brisbane abattoirs. Aust. Vet. J. 43:203, 1967.

116. Tennant, B.: Acute enterocolitis in the horse. A.A.E.P. Newsletter 2:34, 1976.

117. Carlson, G. P.: Colitis X syndrome in horses. A.A.E.P. Newsletter 2:38, 1976.

118. Karim, S. M. M., and Adaikan, P. G.: The effect of loperamide on prostaglandin induced diarrhoea in rat and man. Prostaglandins 13:321, 1977.

119. Giannella, R. A., Rout, W. R., and Formal, S. B.: Effect of indomethacin on intestinal water transport in salmonella-infected Rhesus monkeys. Infect. Immun. 17:136, 1977.

120. Smith, B. P., Reina-Guerra, M., and Hardy, A. J.: Prevalence and epizootiology of equine salmonellosis. J.A.V.M.A. 172:353, 1978.

121. Cimprich, R. E.: Equine granulomatous enteritis. Vet. Pathol. 11:535, 1974.

122. Merritt, A. M., Cimprich, R. E., and Beach, J.: Granulomatous enteritis in nine horses. J.A.V.M.A. 169:603, 1976.

123. Whitlock, R. H.: Personal communication, 1979.

124. Meuton, D. J., Butler, D. G., Thompson, G. W., and Lumsden, J. H.: Chronic enteritis associated with malabsorption and protein-losing enteropathy in the horse. J.A.V.M.A. 172:326, 1978.

125. Bennett, S. P., and Franco, D. A.: Equine protozoal diarrhea (equine intestinal trichomoniasis) at Trinidad racetracks. J.A.V.M.A. 154:58, 1969.

126. Stoner, J. C.: Treatment of protozoal equine diarrhea. V.M./S.A.C. 63:660, 1968.

127. Laufenstein, H., and Nasti, E.: Equine intestinal trichomoniasis. Proc. 9th Annu. Conv. Am. A. Equine Pract, 1963, p. 19.

128. Damron, G. W.: Gastrointestinal trichomonads in horses: occurrence and identification. Am. J. Vet. Res. 37:25, 1976.

129. Rooney, J. R.: Trichomoniasis as a cause of equine diarrhea—a hypothesis. J.A.V.M.A. 157:1138, 1970.

130. Dade, A. W., Lickfeldt, W. E., and McAllister, H. A.: Granulomatous colitis in a horse with histoplasmosis. V.M./S.A.C. 68:279, 1973.

131. Roberts, M. C., and Cotchin, E.: Globidium leuckarti in the small intestine of three horses. Br. Vet. J. 129:146, 1973.

132. Wheeldon, E. B., and Greig, W. A.: Globidium leuckarti infection in a horse with diarrhea. Vet. Rec. 100:102, 1977.

133. Wiseman, A., Petrie, L., and Murray, M.: Diarrhea in the horse as a result of alimentary lymphosarcoma. Vet. Rec. 95:554, 1974.

134. Targowski, S. P.: Treatment of horses with chronic diarrhea: immunologic status. Am. J. Vet. Res. 37:29, 1976.

135. Targowski, S. P.: Serum immunoglobulin, dermal response, and lymphocyte transformation studies in horses with chronic diarrhea. Infect. Immun. 12:48, 1975.

136. Madding, G. F., Kennedy, P. A., and McLaughlin, R. T.: Clinical use of antiperistaltic bowel segments. Ann. Surg. 161:601, 1965.

137. Mansmann, R. A., and Gourley, I. M.: Antiperistaltic small colon segments in the horse. J.A.V.M.A. 157:1313, 1970.

138. Scott, F. W., Kahrs, R. F., Campbell, S. G., and Hillman, R. B.: Etiologic studies on bovine winter dysentery. Bovine Pract. 6:40, 1973.

139. Roberts, S. J.: Winter dysentery in dairy cattle. Cornell Vet. 47:372, 1957.

140. Kahrs, R. F., Scott, F. W., and Hillman, R. B.: Epidemiologic observations on bovine winter dysentery. Bovine Pract. 6:36, 1973.

141. Songer, J. G.: Epidemiology of swine dysentery: development and evaluation of cultural and serological methods for the detection of Treponema hyodysenteriae infection. Thesis. Iowa State University, Ames, 1976.

142. Harris, D. L., and Glock, R. D.: Swine dysentery. In Diseases of Swine, 4th ed. Ames, Iowa State University Press, 1975, p. 541.

143. Harris, D. L.: Current status of research on swine dysentery. J.A.V.M.A. 164:809, 1974.

144. Meyer, R. C., Simon, J., and Byerly, C. S.: The etiology of swine dysentery. I. Oral inoculation of germ-free swine with Treponema hyodysenteriae and Vibrio coli. Vet. Pathol. 11:515, 1974.

145. Hudson, M. J., Alexander, T. J. L., Lysons, R. J., and Prescott, J. F.: Swine dysentery: protection of pigs by oral and parenteral immunization with attenuated Treponema hyodysenteriae. Res. Vet. Sci. 21:366, 1976.

146. Glock, R. D., and Harris, D. L.: Swine dysentery. II. Characterization of lesions in pigs inoculated with Treponema hyodysenteriae in pure and mixed culture. V.M./S.A.C. 67:65, 1972.

147. Hughes, R., Olander, H. J., and Williams, C. B.: Swine dysentery: pathogenicity of Treponema hyodysenteriae. Am. J. Vet. Res. 36:971, 1975.

148. Kennedy, G. A., and Strafuss, A. C.: Scanning electron microscopy of the lesions of swine dysentery. Am. J. Vet. Res. 37:395, 1976.

149. Whipp, S. C., and Argenzio, R. A.: Pathophysiology of swine dysentery. I. Alterations in colonic permeability. Unpublished data.

150. Alexander, T. J. L., and Taylor, D. J.: The clinical signs, diagnosis and control of swine dysentery. Vet. Rec. 85:59, 1969.

151. Olsen, L. D., and Rodabaugh, D. E.: Prevention of swine dysentery with a combination of lincomycin and spectinomycin and resistance of swine dysentery to tylosin and sodium arsanilate. Am. J. Vet. Res. 37:769, 1976.

152. Taylor, D. J.: Ronidazole in the treatment of experimental swine dysentery. Vet. Rec. 95:215, 1974.

153. Smith, F. W., and Sleisenger, M. H.: Physiology of the colon. In Gastrointestinal Disease, 2nd ed. Edited by M. H. Sleisenger and J. S. Fordtran. Philadelphia, W. B. Saunders Co., 1978, p. 1523.

154. Daniel, E. E.: Electrophysiology of the colon. Gut 16:298, 1975.

155. Levitan, R., Fordtran, J. S., Burrows, B. A., and Ingelfinger, F. J.: Water and salt absorption in the human colon. J. Clin. Invest. 41:1754, 1962.

156. Phillips, S. F.: Absorption and secretion by the colon. Gastroenterology 56:966, 1969.

157. Banta, C. A., Clemens, E. T., Kronsky, M. M., and Sheffy, B. E.: Sites of organic acid production and patterns of digesta movement in the gastrointestinal tract of dogs. J. Nutrition 109:1592, 1979.

158. Levitan, R.: Colonic absorption of water and electrolytes. Am. J. Clin. Nutr. 22:315, 1969.

159. Mekhjian, H. S., and S. F. Phillips: Perfusion of the canine colon with unconjugated bile acids. Gastroenterology 59:120, 1970.

160. Phillips, S. F., and Code, C. F.: Sorption of potassium in the small and large intestine. Am. J. Physiol. 211:607, 1966.

161. Giller, J., and Phillips, S. F.: Electrolyte absorption and secretion in the human colon. Am. J. Dig. Dis. 17:1003, 1972.

162. Silva, P., Charney, A. N., and Epstein, F. H.: Potassium adaptation and Na-K-ATPase activity in mucosa of colon. Am. J. Physiol. 229:1576, 1975.

163. Rubens, R. D., and Lambert, H. P.: The homeostatic function of the colon in acute gastroenteritis. Gut 13:915, 1972.

164. Weinbeck, M., and Janssen, H.: Electrical control mechanisms at the ileo-colic junction. Proc. IVth Int. Conference on Gastrointestinal Motility. Vancouver, B.C., Mitchell Press, 1974, p. 97.

165. Chaudhary, N. A., and Truelove, S. C.: Colonic motility: a critical review of methods and results. Am. J. Med. *31*:86, 1961.
166. Christenson, J.: Myoelectric control of the colon. Gastroenterology *68*:607, 1975.
167. Misiewicz, J. J.: Colonic motility. Gut *16*:311, 1975.
168. Truelove, S. C.: Movements of the large intestine. Physiol. Rev. *46*:457, 1966.
169. Weinbeck, M.: The electrical activity of the cat colon in vivo. I. The normal electrical activity and its relationship to contractile activity. Res. Exp. Med. *158*:268, 1972.
170. Elliot, T. R., and Barclay-Smith, E.: Antiperistalsis and other muscular activities of the colon. J. Physiol. *31*:212, 1904.
171. Burrows, C. F.: Unpublished observations, University of Pennsylvania, 1978.
172. Connell, A. M.: Motility of the pelvic colon. Part II. Paradoxical motility in diarrhoea and constipation. Gut. *3*:342, 1962.
173. Polish, E. O.: The pathophysiology of common gastrointestinal symptoms. *In* Gastrointestinal Pathophysiology. Edited by F. P. Brooks. New York, Oxford University Press, 1974, p. 7.
174. Lorenz, M. D.: Disorders of the large bowel. *In* Textbook of Veterinary Internal Medicine. Edited by S. J. Ettinger. Philadelphia, W. B. Saunders Co., 1975, p. 1212.
175. Gaston, E. A.: Physiological basis for preservation of fecal continence after resection of rectum. J.A.M.A. *146*:1486, 1951.
176. Karlan, M., McPherson, R. C., and Watman, R. N.: An experimental evaluation of fecal continence—sphincter and reservoir function in the dog. Surg. Gynecol. Obstet. *119*:1312, 1964.
177. Peck, D. A., and Hallenbeck, G. A.: Fecal continence in the dog after replacement of rectal mucosa with ileal mucosa. Surg. Gynecol. Obstet. *119*:1312, 1964.
178. Walshaw, R. W., and Harvey, C. E.: The pathophysiology of rectal and anal diseases. *In* Pathophysiology in Small Animal Surgery. Edited by M. J. Bojrab. Philadelphia, Lea & Febiger. In press.
179. Ashdown, R. R.: Symposium on canine recto-anal disorders. I. Clinical anatomy. J. Small Anim. Pract. *9*:315, 1968.
180. Scharli, A. F., and Kiesewetter, W. B.: Defecation and continence: some new concepts. Dis. Colon Rectum *13*:81, 1970.
181. Duthie, H. L.: Dynamics of the rectum and anus. Clin. Gastroenterol. *4*:467, 1975.
182. Schuster, M. M.: The riddle of the sphincters. Gastroenterology *69*:249, 1975.
183. Phillips, S. F.: Diarrhea: a broad perspective. Viewpoints on Dig. Dis., 7:(No. 5), November, 1975. American Gastroenterological Assn. C. B. Slack, Inc., Thorofare, NJ.
184. Banta, C.: Personal communication. Allen Products Company, Allentown, PA, 1978.
185. Schedl, H. P.: Water and electrolyte transport: clinical aspects. Med. Clin. North Am. *58*:1429, 1974.
186. Debongnie, J. C., and Philips, S. F.: Functional reserve capacity of the human large bowel (Abst.). Gastroenterology *70*:A18/876, 1976.
187. Matseshe, J. W., and Phillips, S. F.: Chronic diarrhea—a practical approach. Med. Clin. North Am. *62*:141, 1978.
188. Phillips, S. F.: Diarrhea: pathogenesis and diagnostic techniques. Postgrad. Med. *57*:65, 1975.
189. Phillips, S. F.: Diarrhea: a current view of the pathophysiology. Gastroenterology *63*:495, 1972.
190. Argenzio, R. A.: Physiology of diarrhea—large intestine. J.A.V.M.A. *173*:667, 1978.
191. MacPherson, B. R., Shearin, N. L., and Pfeiffer, C. J.: Experimental diffuse colitis in cats: observations on motor changes. J. Surg. Res. *25*:42, 1978.
192. Binder, H. J.: Fecal fatty acids—mediators of diarrhea? Gastroenterology *65*:847, 1973.
193. Stedmans Medical Dictionary, 23rd ed. Baltimore, The Williams & Wilkins Co., 1976.
194. Belshaw, B. E., and Rijnberk, A.: Hypothyroidism. *In* Current Veterinary Therapy, Vol. VI. Edited by R. W. Kirk. Philadelphia, W. B. Saunders Co., 1977, p. 1017.
195. Capen, C. C., and Martin, S. L.: Parathyroid glands and calcium metabolism. *In* Current Veterinary Therapy, Vol. VI. Edited by R. W. Kirk. Philadelphia, W. B. Saunders Co., 1977, p. 1038.
196. Weaver, A. D.: Differential diagnosis of tenesmus in the dog. J. Small Anim. Pract. *15*:609, 1974.
197. Ewing, G. O., and Gomez, J. A.: Canine ulcerative colitis. J.A.A.H.A. *9*:395, 1973.
198. Feldman, M., and Fordtran, J. S.: Vomiting. *In* Gastrointestinal Disease, 2nd ed. Edited by M. H. Sleisenger and J. S. Fordtran. Philadelphia, W. B. Saunders Co., 1978, p. 200.
199. Van Kruiningen, H. J.: Canine colitis comparable to regional enteritis and mucosal colitis of man. Gastroenterology *62*:1128, 1972.
200. Van Kruiningen, H. J.: Letter to the editor. J.A.A.H.A. *10*:210, 1974.
201. Van Kruiningen, H. J., and Hayden, D. W.: Interpreting problem diarrheas in dogs. Vet. Clin. North Am. 2:29, 1972.
202. Edmunds, C. J., and Pilcher, D.: Electrical potential difference and sodium and potassium fluxes across rectal mucosa in ulcerative colitis. Gut *14*:784, 1973.
203. Rask-Madsen, J., and Jensen, B.: Electrolyte transport capacity and electrical potentials of the normal and the inflamed human rectum in vivo. Scand. J. Gastroenterol. *8*:169, 1973.
204. Rask-Madsen, J.: Simultaneous measurement of electrical polarization and electrolyte transport by the entire normal and inflamed human colon during in vivo perfusion. Scand. J. Gastroenterol. *8*:327, 1973.
205. Christensen, J., Weisbrodt, N. W., and Hauser, R. L.: Electrical slow wave of the proximal colon of the cat in diarrhea. Gastroenterology *62*:1167, 1972.
206. Spriggs, E. A., Code, C. F., Bargen, J. A., Curtiss, R. K., and Hightower, N. C.: Motility of the pelvic colon and rectum of normal persons and patients with ulcerative colitis. Gastroenterology *19*::480, 1951.
207. Snape, W. J., Matarazzo, S. A., and Cohen, S.: Abnormal colonic myoelectrical and motor responses to eating in ulcerative colitis (Abst.). Gastroenterology *74*:1097, 1978.
208. Suddeth, W. H.: Enterotoxemia. *In* Current Veterinary Therapy, Vol. IV. Edited by R. W. Kirk. Philadelphia, W. B. Saunders Co., 1971, p. 80.
209. Burrows, C. F., Kolata, R. J., and Soma, L. R.: Shock: pathophysiology and management. *In* Current Veterinary Therapy, Vol. VI. Edited by R. W. Kirk. Philadelphia, W. B. Saunders Co., 1977, p. 26.
210. Strombeck, D. R.: Dietary management of gastrointestinal problems. *In* Diet and Disease in Dogs. Edited by D. S. Kronfeld and D. G. Low. Irvine, CA, University of California, 1975.
211. Cello, J. P., and Meyer, J. H.: Ulcerative colitis. *In* Gastrointestinal Disease, 2nd ed. Edited by M. H. Sleisenger and J. S. Fordtran. Philadelphia, W. B. Saunders Co., 1978, p. 1597.
212. Burrows, C. F., Merritt, A. M., and Chiapella, A.: Determination of fecal fat and trypsin output in the evaluation of chronic canine diarrhea. J.A.V.M.A. *174*:62, 1979.
213. Harris, J. C., Dupont, H. L., and Hornick, R. B.: Fecal leukocytes in diarrheal illness. Ann. Intern. Med. *76*:697, 1972.
214. Anderson, N. V.: Biopsy of the gastrointestinal system. Vet. Clin. North Am. *4*:317, 1974.
215. Morson, B. C.: Rectal biopsy in inflammatory bowel disease. N. Engl. J. Med. *287*:1337, 1972.
216. Kelly, A.: Personal communication, University of Pennsylvania, 1978.
217. Morson, B. C.: Pathology of ulcerative colitis. Proc. R. Soc. Med. *64*:976, 1971.
218. Das, K. M., and Sternlieb, I.: Salicylazosulfapyridine in inflammatory bowel disease. Am. J. Dig. Dis. *20*:971, 1975.
219. Goldman, P., and Peppercorn, M. A.: Sulfasalazine. N. Engl. J. Med. *293*:20, 1975.
220. Khan, A. K. A., Piris, J., and Truelove, S. C.: An experiment to determine the active therapeutic moiety of sulfphasalazine. Lancet *2*:892, 1977.
221. Aguirre, G.: Letter to the editor. J.A.V.M.A. *162*:8, 1973.
222. Van Kruiningen, H. J.: Clinical efficacy of tylosin in canine inflammatory bowel disease. J.A.A.H.A. *12*:498, 1976.
223. Grove, D. I., Mahmoud, A. A. F., and Warren, K. S.: Suppression of cell-mediated immunity by metronidazole. Int. Arch. Allergy Appl. Immunol. *54*:422, 1977.
224. Ursing, B., and Kamme, C.: Metronidazole for Crohn's disease. Lancet *1*:775, 1975.
225. Onderdonk, A. B., Hermos, J. A., Dziuk, J. L., and Bartlett, J. A.: Protective effect of metronidazole in experimental ulcerative colitis. Gastroenterology *74*:521, 1978.
226. Chiapella, A. M.: Personal communication, University of Pennsylvania, 1978.
227. Sleisenger, M. H.: Clinical pharmacology. *In* Gastrointestinal Disease. Edited by M. H. Sleisenger and J. S. Fordtran, Philadelphia, W. B. Saunders Co., 1973, p. 418.
228. Merritt, A. M., Cowgill, L. D., Burrows, C. F., and Streett, W.: Quantitation of canine fecal fat and trypsin output from normal dogs on a meat-base or cereal-base diet. J.A.V.M.A. *174*:59, 1979.
229. Kronfeld, D. S.: Nature and use of commercial dog foods. *In* Diet and Disease in Dogs. Edited by D. S. Kronfeld and D. G. Low. Irvine, University of California, 1975.
230. Soulsby, E. J. L.: Helminths, Arthropods and Protozoa of Domesti-

cated Animals (Mönnig), 6th ed. Baltimore, The Williams & Wilkins Co., 1968.
231. Georgi, J. R.: Parasitology for Veterinarians, 2nd ed. Philadelphia, W. B. Saunders Co., 1974.
232. Soifer, F. K.: Intestinal parasitism. In Current Veterinary Therapy, Vol. VI. Edited by R. W. Kirk. Philadelphia, W. B. Saunders Co., 1977, p. 458.
233. Migasena, S., Gilles, H. M., and Maegraith, B. G.: Studies in Ancylostoma caninum infection in dogs. II. Anatomical changes in the gastrointestinal tract. Ann. Trop. Med. Parasitol. 66:203, 1972.
234. Jordan, H. E.: Amebiasis (Entamoeba histolytica) in the dog. V.M./S.A.C. 67:61, 1967.
235. Ewing, G. O., and Aldrete, A. V.: Canine giardiasis presenting as chronic ulcerative colitis: a case report. J.A.A.H.A. 9:52, 1973.
236. Brightman, A. H., and Slonka, G. F.: A review of five clinical cases of giardiasis in cats. J.A.A.H.A. 12:492, 1976.
237. Hayes, F. A., and Jordan, H. E.: Canine helminthiasis complicated with Balantidium species. J.A.V.M.A. 129:161, 1956.
238. Bailey, W. S., and Williams, A. G.: Balantidium infection in the dog. J.A.V.M.A. 114:238, 1949.
239. Ewing, S. A., and Bull, R. W.: Severe chronic canine diarrhea associated with Balantidium-Trichuris infection. J.A.V.M.A. 149:519, 1966.
240. Povey, R. C., Austwick, P. K. C., Pearson, H., and Smith, K. C.: A case of prototothecosis in a dog. Pathol. Vet. 6:396, 1969.
241. Van Kruiningen, H. J., Garner, F. M., and Schiefer, B.: Prototothecosis in a dog. Pathol. Vet. 6:348, 1969.
242. Van Kruiningen, H. J.: Prototothecal enterocolitis in a dog. J.A.V.M.A. 157:56, 1970.
243. Ditchfield, W. J. B.: Mycotic diseases. In Canine Medicine. Edited by E. J. Catcott. Santa Barbara, CA, American Veterinary Publications, 1968, p. 172.
244. Berry, C. L.: The development of the granuloma of histoplasmosis. J. Pathol. 97:1, 1969.
245. Stickle, J. E., and Hribernik, T. N.: Clinicopathological observations in disseminated histoplasmosis in dogs. J.A.A.H.A. 14:105, 1978.
246. Strande, A., Sommers, S. C., and Petrak, M.: Regional enterocolitis in Cocker Spaniel dogs. Arch. Pathol. 57:357, 1954.
247. Rechenberg, V. R.: Enteritis Regionalis bein Hund. Monatschr. Vet. Med. 29:352, 1974.
248. Widmer, W. R., and Van Kruiningen, H. J.: Trichuris-induced transmural ileocolitis in a dog—an entity mimicking regional enteritis. J.A.A.H.A. 10:581, 1974.
249. LeVeen, E., Falk, G., Ip, M., Mazzapica, N., and LeVeen, H.: Urease as a contributing factor in ulcerative lesions of the colon. Am. J. Surg. 135:53, 1978.
250. Gomez, J. A., Russell, S. W., Trowbridge, J. O., and Lee, J.: Canine histiocytic ulcerative colitis. Am. J. Dig. Dis. 22:485, 1977.
251. Van der Gaag, I, Van Trorenburg, J., Voorhart, G., Happe, R. R., and Aalfs, R. H. G.: Histiocytic ulcerative colitis in a French Bulldog. J. Small Anim. Pract. 19:283, 1978.
252. Russell, S. W., Gomez, J. A., and Trowbridge, J. O.: Canine histiocytic ulcerative colitis. Lab. Invest. 25:509, 1971.
253. Hayden, D. W., and Van Kruiningen, H. J.: Eosinophilic gastroenteritis in German Shepherd dogs and its relationship to visceral larval migrans. J.A.V.M.A. 162:379, 1973.
254. Caldwell, J. H., Tennenbaum, J. H., and Bronstein, H. A.: Serum IgE in eosinophilic gastroenteritis. Response to intestinal challenge in two cases. N. Engl. J. Med. 292:1388, 1975.
255. Vaz, G. A., Tan, L. K. T., and Gerrard, J. W.: Oral cromoglycate in treatment of adverse reaction to foods. Lancet 1:1066, 1978.
256. Bolton, G. R., and Brown, T. T.: Mycotic colitis in a cat. V.M./S.A.C. 67:978, 1972.
257. Tedesco, F. J., Stanley, R. J., and Alpers, D. H.: Diagnostic features of clindamycin-associated pseudomembranous colitis. N. Engl. J. Med. 290:841, 1974.
258. Reference deleted.
259. Snape, W. J., Carlson, G. M., and Cohen, S.: Colonic myoelectric activity in the irritable bowel syndrome. Gastroenterology 70:326, 1976.
260. Snape, W. J., Carlson, G. M., Martarrazo, S. A., and Cohen, S.: Evidence that abnormal myolectrical activity produces colonic motor dysfunction in the irritable bowel syndrome. Gastroenterology 72:383, 1977.
261. Almy, T. P. : Wrestling with the irritable colon. Med. Clin. North Am. 62:203, 1978.
262. Burkitt, D. P., Walker, A. R. P., and Painter, N. S.: Effect of dietary fibre on stools and transit times and its role in the causation of disease. Lancet 2:1408, 1972.

263. Reilly, R. W., and Kirsner, J. B.: Fiber Deficiency and Colonic Disorders. New York, Plenum Press, 1975.
264. Dwyer, J. T., Goldin, B., Gorbach, S., and Patterson, J.: Drug therapy reviews: dietary fiber and fiber supplements in the therapy of gastrointestinal disorders. Am. J. Hosp. Pharm. 35:278, 1978.
265. Manning, A. P., Heaton, K. W., Harvey, R. F., and Uglow, P.: Wheat fiber and the irritable bowel syndrome. Lancet 2:417, 1977.
266. Grimes, D. S.: Refined carbohydrate, smooth-muscle spasm and disease of the colon. Lancet 1:395, 1976.
267. Soltoft, J., Gudmand-Hoyer, E., Krag, B., Kristensen, E., and Wulff, H.: A double blind study of the effect of wheat bran on symptoms of irritable bowel syndrome. Lancet 1:270, 1976.
268. Kirwan, W. O., Smith, A. N., McConnell, A. A., Mitchell, W. D., and Eastwood, M. A.: Action of different bran preparations on colonic function. Br. Med. J. 4:187, 1974.
269. Amand, W. B.: Diet and gastrointestinal problems. In Canine Nutrition. Edited by D. S. Kronfeld. Philadelphia, University of Pennsylvania, 1972.
270. Fennell, C.: The use of sterculia gum for controlling intestinal tone in the dog and cat. J. Small Anim. Pract. 17:543, 1976.
271. Guffy, M. M., Wallace, L., and Anderson, N. V.: Inversion of the cecum into the colon of a dog. J.A.V.M.A. 156:183, 1970.
272. Toben, F., Reid, N. C. R. W., Talbert, J. L., and Schuster, M. M.: Nonsurgical test for the diagnosis of Hirschsprung's disease. N. Engl. J. Med. 278:188, 1968.
273. Yoder, J. T., Dragstedt, L. R., and Starch, C. J.: Partial colectomy for correction of megacolon in a cat. V.M./S.A.C. 63:1049, 1968.
274. Greiner, T. P., and Betts, C. W.: Disease of the rectum and anus. In Textbook of Veterinary Internal Medicine. Edited by S. W. Ettinger. Philadelphia, W. B. Saunders Co., 1975, p. 1307.
275. Lewis, D. G.: Symposium in canine recto-anal disorders—III: clinical management. J. Small Anim. Pract. 9:329, 1968.
276. Harvey, C. E.: Personal communication, University of Pennsylvania, Philadelphia, PA, 1978.
277. Joshua, J. O.: Chapter 8. The alimentary tract. In Clinical Aspects of Some Diseases of Cats. Edited by Joan O. Joshua. London, Heineman, 1965.
278. Ellet, E. W., and Archibald, J.: Hernia. In Canine Surgery, 1st Archibald ed. Wheaton, IL, American Veterinary Publications, 1965, p. 487.
279. Blakely, C. L.: Perineal hernia. In Canine Surgery, 4th ed. Wheaton, IL, American Veterinary Publications, 1957, p. 458.
280. Burrows, C. F., and Harvey, C. E.: Perineal hernia in the dog. J. Small Anim. Pract. 14:315, 1973.
281. Harvey, C. E.: Treatment of perineal hernia in the dog—a reassessment. J. Small Anim. Pract. 18:505, 1977.
282. Hayes, H. M., Wilson, G. P., and Tarone, R. E.: The epidemiologic features of perineal hernia. J.A.A.H.A. 14:703, 1978.
283. Dietrich, H. F.: Perineal hernia repair in the canine. Vet. Clin. North Am. 5:383, 1975.
284. Whittlestone, J. F.: Letter to the editor. J. Small Anim. Pract. 14:828, 1973.
285. Harvey, C. E.: Anal splitting in dogs with perineal hernia: technique and results. J.A.A.H.A. 14:243, 1978.
286. Amand, W. B.: Non-neurogenic disorders of the anus and rectum. Vet. Clin. North Am. 4:535, 1974.
287. Rawlings, C. A., and Capps, W. F.: Rectovaginal fistula and imperforate anus in a dog. J.A.V.M.A. 159:320, 1971.
288. Harvey, C. E.: Perianal fistula in the dog. Vet. Rec. 91:25, 1972.
289. Robins, G. M., and Lane, J. G.: The management of anal furunculosis. J. Small Anim. Pract. 14:333, 1973.
290. Harvey, C. E.: Incidence and distribution of anal sac disease in the dog. J.A.A.H.A. 10:573, 1974.
291. Christie, T. F.: Perianal fistula in the dog. Vet. Clin. North Am. 5:353, 1975.
292. Liska, W. D., Greiner, T. P., and Withrow, S. J.: Cryosurgery in the treatment of perianal fistulae. Vet. Clin. North Am. 5:449, 1975.
293. Lane, J. G., and Burch, D. G. S.: The cryosurgical treatment of canine anal furunculosis. J. Small Anim. Pract. 16:387, 1975.
294. Lane, J. G.: Personal communication, University of Bristol, 1978.
295. Halnan, C. R. E.: The frequency of occurrence of anal sacculitis in the dog. J. Small Anim. Pract. 17:537, 1976.
296. Halnan, C. R. E.: The anal sacs of the dog. FRCVS Thesis. Royal College of Veterinary Surgeons. London, England, 1973.
297. Halnan, C. R. E.: The experimental reproduction of anal sacculitis. J. Small Anim. Pract. 17:693, 1976.
298. Halnan, C. R. E.: The diagnosis of anal sacculitis in the dog. J. Small Anim. Pract. 17:527, 1976.
299. Halnan, C. R. E.: Therapy of anal sacculitis in the dog. J. Small Anim. Pract. 17:685, 1976.

300. Halnan, C. R. E.: Canine anal sac disease. Veterinary Annual No. 18. Edited by C. S. Grunsell and F. W. G. Hill. Bristol, England, Scientechnica, 1978, p. 225.
301. Joshua, J. O.: "Dog pox": some clinical aspects of an eruptive condition of certain mucous surfaces in dogs. Vet. Rec. 96:300, 1975.
302. Hayden, D. W., and Nielsen, S. W.: Canine alimentary neoplasia. Zentralbl. Veterinaermed. A20:1, 1973.
302a. Seiler, R.J.: Colorectal polyps of the dog: A clinicopathologic study of 17 cases. J.A.V.M.A. 174:12, 1979.
303. Patnaik, A. U., Hurvitz, A. I., and Johnson, G. F.: Canine gastrointestinal neoplasms. Vet. Pathol. 14:547, 1977.
304. Brodey, R. S.: Alimentary tract neoplasms in the cat: a clinicopathologic survey of 46 cases. Am. J. Vet. Res. 27:74, 1966.
305. Brodey, R. S., and Cohen, D.: An Epizootiologic and Clinicopathologic Study of 95 Cases of Gastrointestinal Neoplasms in the Dog. Proc. 101st Annu. Meet. Am. Vet. Med. Assoc. 1964, p. 167.
306. Levene, A.: Symposium on canine recto-anal disorders—II: The surgical pathology of ano-rectal disease in the dog. J. Small Anim. Pract. 9:323, 1968.
307. Schäffer, E., and Schieffer, B.: Incidence and types of canine rectal carcinomas. J. Small Anim. Pract. 9:491, 1968.
308. Giles, R. C., Hildebrandt, P. K., and Montgomery, C. A.: Carcinoid tumor in the small intestine of a dog. Vet. Pathol. 11:340, 1974.
309. Silverberg, S. G.: Carcinoma arising in adenomatous polyps of the rectum in a dog. Dis. Colon Rectum 14:191, 1971.
310. Rijnberk, A.: Pseudohyperparathyroidism in the dog. Tijdschr. Diergeneeskd. 95:515, 1970.
311. Wilson, A.P., and Hayes, H.M.: Castration for treatment of perianal gland neoplasms in the dog. J.A.V.M.A. 174:1301, 1979.
312. Gillette, E. L.: Veterinary radiotherapy. J.A.V.M.A. 157:1707, 1970.
313. Liska, W. D., and Withrow, S. J.: Cryosurgical treatment of perianal gland adenomas in the dog. J.A.A.H.A. 14:457, 1978.

Chapter 25

DISEASES OF THE LIVER

BUD C. TENNANT and WILLIAM E. HORNBUCKLE

The liver plays a central role in numerous metabolic processes, and the broad spectrum of clinical signs in patients with liver disease are the result of disturbances in these multiple synthetic, excretory, and digestive functions. The liver has great reserve capacity, and significant liver disease can be present but remain clinically "silent" as long as this functional reserve is maintained. Hepatic insufficiency or hepatic failure occurs only after most of the hepatic parenchyma has been lost. An understanding of the pathophysiologic disturbances which occur in liver disease is critical in the elucidation of the mechanisms responsible for clinical signs, in diagnosis, and in the initiation of rational therapy.

CLINICAL SIGNS OF HEPATIC INSUFFICIENCY

Liver disease is usually quite advanced before these clinical signs appear. Recognition of one or more of these signs not only directs attention to the liver as the probable site of disease, but also helps the clinician focus the laboratory studies more effectively.

Icterus

The clinical sign of *icterus* or *jaundice* develops when the yellow pigment bilirubin accumulates in plasma and other tissues. Bilirubin is derived primarily from hemoglobin during the normal removal of aged erythrocytes by reticuloendothelial cells. In the plasma, bilirubin is in unconjugated form, bound to albumin. Hepatocytes remove the unconjugated pigment and form bilirubin diglucuronide and other water-soluble conjugates which are excreted in the bile. The plasma bilirubin concentration increases (hyperbilirubinemia) if production of bilirubin exceeds the excretory capacity of the liver. Overproduction of bilirubin is responsible for the icterus observed in acute hemolytic anemia. Defective excretion of bilirubin occurs either in hepatocellular dysfunction or in obstruction of the biliary tract.

Yellow discoloration of tissues can first be noted by careful observation when the plasma bilirubin value exceeds 2 to 3 mg/dl and can be appreciated even by an untrained observer when the concentration reaches 7 to 8 mg/dl. The correlation between the plasma bilirubin value and the degree of clinical icterus is by no means perfect. Elevated plasma bilirubin values are usually present for one or more days before clinical icterus is apparent, and there may be a similar delay between the time plasma bilirubin returns to normal and the clearance of the yellow discoloration of tissues. It is said that conjugated bilirubin has a greater affinity for connective tissue than the unconjugated pigment, so the degree of icterus is greater in cholestatic liver disease for any given serum bilirubin concentration because of the predominantly conjugated hyperbilirubinemia.[1] Apparent tissue affinity may be related to albumin binding and the relative ability of conjugated and unconjugated pigments to diffuse from plasma; i.e., unconjugated bilirubin is much more tightly bound to albumin than conjugated bilirubin, which would be a greater impedance to passage into the interstitial space.

Visible yellow discoloration of tissues is most readily recognized in animals in the unpigmented sclera. The normal red color of the visible mucous membranes makes detection of a slight yellow cast more difficult. It is possible to apply pressure to the mucous membranes of the lip and temporarily reduce blood flow to the area, so that the underlying color of the tissue can be better visualized.

The color of plasma (icteric index) may be useful clinically in the evaluation of icterus. Normal canine, feline, and ovine plasma is free of yellow color. The finding of yellow plasma in these species is highly suggestive of hyperbilirubinemia. Cattle absorb and transport significant quantities of carotene in plasma and, because the icteric index varies with the dietary intake of carotene, the index is of little use in this species. Normal horse plasma has a high icteric index, which in part is due to a plasma bilirubin concentration that is usually higher than in other species.

Notable species differences occur in the frequency with which icterus is observed in association with liver disease. In sheep and cattle dying of terminal hepatic insufficiency, there usually is a significant clinical elevation in plasma bilirubin but the value may not be high enough to produce clinical icterus.[2,3] This is owing either to the apparent reserve capacity of the liver to excrete bilirubin or to the adaptation of extrahepatic mechanisms for bilirubin excretion and/or degradation. Clinical icterus, when present in ruminants, is most frequently associated with hemolytic anemia where acute overproduction of bilirubin exceeds excretory capacity, e.g., anaplasmosis (cattle) and copper poisoning (sheep).

The clinical significance of icterus in the horse is somewhat more difficult to evaluate than in other species. The sclera and visible mucous membranes of most normal horses do not appear icteric. In 10 to 15% of normal horses, however, a slight but definite (1/4) yellow discoloration of the sclera and/or oral mucous membranes can be detected.[4] Scleral icterus of a moderate degree (2/4) may also be observed in horses with a variety of illnesses which do not appear to involve the liver directly, e.g., pneumonia, impaction of the large intestine, and enteritis. Reduction in food intake is a common factor in such disorders and fasting is known to produce a rapid increase in plasma bilirubin concentration.[4,5] In both hemolytic anemia and hepatic failure in the horse, the degree of icterus is usually remarkably greater than that seen under physiologic conditions or associated with reduced food intake. In the horse, severe icterus is almost invariably present in acute hepatic necrosis.[4,6] However, in chronic hepatic disease, icterus may be a more variable sign. In a series of 34 cases of cirrhosis in the horse, significant icterus was a presenting sign of 70%.[4] Icterus was even less frequent (40%) in another series of cirrhotic horses.[7]

The dog and cat appear to be intermediate between ruminants and the horse in the development of clinical icterus. Hemolytic disease, hepatocellular dysfunction, and extrahepatic bile duct obstruction are characteristically associated with icterus in these species. In experimental extrahepatic bile duct obstruction in the dog, the plasma bilirubin increases at once following surgical procedure and clinical icterus is observed within 1 to 3 days. After 2 to 3 weeks, however, the plasma bilirubin of some dogs begins to decline and clinical icterus may disappear. As in sheep and cattle, this may be related to the adaptation of extrahepatic mechanisms of bilirubin excretion, particularly in the kidney. The kidney of the dog is capable of adapting so that the rate of renal excretion of bilirubin equals the rate of formation. In cats with complete extrahepatic bile duct obstruction, however, no such decrease is observed but persistent hyperbilirubinemia and deep icterus are characteristic.[8]

Encephalopathy

The disturbances of cerebral function that accompany hepatic insufficiency are collectively referred to as hepatic encephalopathy. The severity of neurologic signs may vary from subtle and intermittent behavioral changes to lethargy or stupor to bizarre behavior with maniacal signs, seizures and coma (hepatic coma).

Occurrence and Clinical Signs

Hepatic encephalopathy is a prominent clinical feature of hepatic failure in the horse. In one series of cases, 82% of the horses with acute hepatitis and 32% of those with cirrhosis presented with prominent neurologic signs.[9] Varying degrees of central nervous derangement may be observed. Some horses stand quietly with the feet spread apart and the head lowered, occasionally nodding the head or jerking the head and neck up into a normal position. Briefly, the horse may appear more alert as if startled, but within moments, the head may be lowered to its previous position and the somnolent appearance returns. Generalized or local muscle tremors are seen in some cases and there may be twitching of the muzzle and lips. The pupillary response to light is normal or moderately sluggish, but in some cases vision appears defective.

Incoordination and dysmetria are observed commonly. Compulsive walking, either in a circle or in a single direction, is seen frequently. In the latter case, the horse appears completely oblivious to its surroundings, walking over or through objects in its path ("walking disease").

Acute fulminant cases may become delirious. The head may be pressed forcibly against a wall for long periods of time. The horse may fall suddenly to the ground and assume a variety of unusual positions. There may be numerous unproductive attempts to rise and periods of violent thrashing. When the horse successfully rises, it may be completely uncontrollable; forward lunging movements may be so violent that the horse becomes a menace to personnel and equipment. In some cases, the violent rolling and assumption of unnatural positions may resemble the signs seen in acute intestinal obstruction. It is possible that part of the clinical picture in such cases is the result of abdominal pain originating from the liver.

In cattle, the syndrome of hepatic encephalopathy typically has an abrupt onset but is actually a terminal manifestation of chronic cirrhosis.[10,11] In a herd outbreak of megalocytic hepatopathy involving 13 fatal cases,[3] the clinical signs in all calves were similar. Calves first were noted to be dull, to stand apart from other calves, and to be anorectic. Other behavioral abnormalities included charging riders on horseback and unusual, unrestrained bawling. Head pressing and circling were not observed. Progressive dysmetria and ataxia developed and the calves became laterally recumbent, unable to rise or to assume a sternal position. While down, they continued to bawl. The tongue protruded and excessive salivation was noted. Tremors of the muscles of the shoulders and thighs were noted. Involuntary jerking of the limbs also occurred, followed intermittently by uncontrolled running movements. Tenesmus was a prominent clinical feature and frequently resulted in prolapse of several centimeters of rectal mucosa. Small quantities of urine dribbled from the vulva each time the calf strained. There was no apparent anesthesia of the perineum or paralysis of the tail. Death occurred within 48 hours of the onset of the central nervous system disturbance.

Hepatic encephalopathy is observed frequently in the dog with congenital or acquired portosystemic vascular shunts and may be one of the most prominent presenting clinical features of this form of liver disease.[12–15] Neurologic signs often are episodic in nature and may be present for many months before recognition of the underlying hepatic disturbance. Depression and stupor with amaurotic blindness have been observed in more than half the reported cases of congenital portacaval shunts in dogs, with circling, head pressing, and intermittent seizures being observed somewhat less frequently. Hepatic encephalopathy also has been associated with other primary diseases of the canine liver,[16,17] including in two cases an apparent deficiency of arginosuccinate synthetase, an enzyme of the Krebs urea cycle.[18]

The clinical differentiation between hepatic encephalopathy and primary inflammatory, degenerative, or neoplastic diseases of the brain is based on the demonstration of severe underlying hepatic disease. In the horse with acute hepatitis, clinical icterus almost always is present at the time neurologic signs are observed. In the dog and in cattle, frank clinical jaundice is observed infrequently in animals with hepatic encephalopathy so that liver function tests and/or liver biopsy are required for confirmation. However, in cases of primary hyperammonemia due to deficiency of urea cycle enzymes, standard liver function tests may be normal.[18]

Pathogenesis

The factors responsible for development of the encephalopathy observed in hepatic failure are only partially understood. One of the important functions of the liver is the synthesis of urea from ammonia. Ammonia is present in peripheral blood in a concentration of 2 to 5 mM/L and in portal venous blood the concentration may be five times as high. Most of the portal ammonia is removed by the normal liver to form urea, with only a small fraction passing into the systemic circulation.

Hepatic synthesis of urea is reduced in hepatic failure, and in the horse[4,19,20] and dog[15,17] significant elevations of blood ammonia have been demonstrated. Ammonia has potent neurotoxic effects, and many of the neurologic signs of hepatic encephalopathy can be observed when toxic doses of ammonium salts are administered intravenously.[21]

The reactions of blood ammonia are determined by the physicochemical laws which apply to gases in solution and to the dissociation of weak bases. The ammonia:ammonium ion buffer system of blood can be described by the Henderson-Hasselbalch equation:

$$pH = pKa - \log \frac{NH_3}{NH_4^+}$$

The pKa for this system has been determined to be approximately 9.1 in the dog.[22] This means that at the physiologic pH of 7.4, almost all of the ammonia of blood is in ionized form (NH_4^+). As the blood pH increases, the relative amount of free ammonia (NH_3) increases, and as the pH decreases, the amount of NH_3 decreases ($NH_3 + H^+ \rightleftarrows NH_4^+$). The cells of the body are almost impermeable to NH_4^+ but are permeable to NH_3, which can pass through membranes by non-ionic diffusion.[23,24,25] These principles are important in determining the amount of ammonia absorbed from the gastrointestinal tract or the amount which can pass from blood into brain tissue.

The potassium status, because of its influence on acid-base parameters, may be an important determinant in NH_3 toxicity. Potassium deficiency ultimately results in the development of metabolic alkalosis causing a shift in the $NH_3 \rightleftarrows NH_4^+$ equilibrium in the direction of the more toxic, free ammonia.

Blood ammonia ultimately is derived from dietary nitrogen. The gastrointestinal tract is believed to be the major source of blood NH_3 but it also is produced by other tissues, e.g., muscle and kidney. Renal ammonia is produced from glutamine and to a lesser extent from other amino acids. Ammonium production by the kidney is one of the normal physiologic mechanisms for H^+ excretion, and the excretion of NH_4^+ is directly related to the pH gradient between blood and urine. In acid urine, the total urinary excretion of NH_4^+ is high and with alkaline urine, NH_4^+ excretion in the urine is low.

The conclusion that the gastrointestinal tract is the major source of blood NH_3 is based on the high concentration of NH_3 found in portal blood. Part of the portal ammonia is derived from the action of bacterial enzymes on dietary amino and amide nitrogen and part is derived from urea, which is present in the normal secretions of the alimentary canal and is hydrolyzed by the enzyme urease within the lumen of the bowel, primarily in the large intestine. The question of whether intestinal urease is produced in part by mammalian cells or whether it is entirely of bacterial origin has been the subject of controversy for many years. The classic study using germ-free rats demonstrated that intestinal urease was exclusively bacterial in origin,[26] an observation confirmed recently in germ-free dogs.[27]

The relative importance of NH_3 produced by intestinal bacteria and that produced from nonbacterial sources is still not fully known. Nance et al.[28] and Nance and Kline[29] have demonstrated that germ-free dogs with Eck fistulae develop hyperammonemia and evidence of "encephalopathy" suggesting that endogenous NH_3 production also may contribute significantly. It has been shown that the intestine can metabolize significant quantities of glutamine independent of intestinal bacteria and that approximately 30% of the glutamine nitrogen appears as NH_3 in the portal blood.[30]

Hepatic encephalopathy has on occasion been associated with profound hypoglycemia. The liver plays a central role in maintenance of the blood glucose concentration. In fulminant hepatic failure in the horse, the blood glucose has been reported in some cases to decrease to 20 mg/dl or less.[3,4,31] Hypoglycemia also has been observed in a small number of cases of dogs with chronic hepatic insufficiency.[12,13]

Other potentially neurotoxic substances have been suggested as having a role in the syndrome of hepatic encephalopathy. Indole and indolyl derivatives which are formed by intestinal bacteria from tryptophan have been suggested as encephalotoxic compounds capable of inducing "hepatic coma."[32] Other studies have incriminated short chain fatty acids. In experimental hepatic failure, total volatile fatty acid (VFA) increases significantly prior to death.[33] Increased plasma VFA concentrations have also been observed in spontaneous hepatic encephalopathy. When infused intravenously into experimental animals, VFA produces cerebral depression followed by coma.[34]

Histopathology of the Brain

There is now generally good agreement that histologic lesions can be demonstrated in the brain of animals with hepatic encephalopathy (Fig. 25–1a-c). "Spongy degeneration" or polymicrocavitation of the brain has been described in sheep and cattle with pyrrolizidine alkaloid toxicosis.[3,21] Although it had been suggested that these lesions were the direct result of the alkaloid,[35] their development closely paralleled the development of the hepatic lesions[3] and the lesion has been reproduced by intravenous administration of ammonium acetate.[21] Polymicrocavitation has also been observed in the dog with hepatic encephalopathy.[15] Dogs, in contrast to cattle, develop astrocytosis but the Alzheimer type II astrocytes which are characteristic of hepatic encephalopathy in man are only occasionally observed in the dog. In horses, Alzheimer type II astrocytes have been seen in cases of hepatic encephalopathy but polymicrocavitation is very unusual. The lesions of the brain in hepatic encephalopathy of domestic species have been described and reviewed recently.[36–39]

Photosensitization

The term photosensitivity is used to describe the state of hyperreactivity to sunlight.[40] The clinical signs of *photosensitization* develop when photosensitive animals are exposed to light and are characterized by inflammation and necrosis of the unpigmented skin (photodermatitis). A distinction should be made between sunburn and photosensitization. Animals with unpigmented skin, when maintained for long periods of time indoors, develop sunburn when there is unaccustomed exposure to sunlight. Sunburn is a reaction of the unpigmented and unprotected skin of otherwise normal animals to ultraviolet radiation (320 mμ). Photosensitization is usually a much more severe reaction of skin which requires the presence of a photodynamic substance. The effective wavelength of light in photosensitization is determined by the absorption spectrum of the sensitizing compound, which, unlike sunburn, usu-

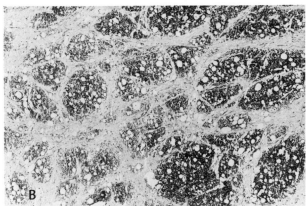

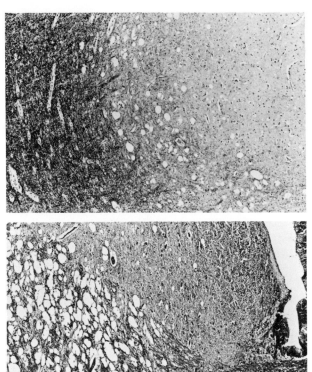

Figure 25–1. Polymicrocavitation in the deep cortex and juxtacortical white matter (**A**), in the internal capsule (**B**) and in tracts adjacent to the third ventricle of a Holstein-Friesian heifer with cirrhosis of the liver caused by ingestion of pyrrolizidine alkaloids and showing signs of hepatic encephalopathy. Brain tissue was perfused in situ with 10% buffered formal saline solution through the carotid arteries immediately following euthanasia to eliminate postmortem artifacts. **A** and **B**—Luxol fast blue/periodic acid Schiff stain × 22.5. **C**—Hematoxylin and eosin. (From Finn and Tennant.[3])

ally extends into the region of visible light. Another fundamental difference between sunburn and photosensitization is that sunburn can apparently occur in the absence of molecular oxygen[41] whereas photosensitization effects can be demonstrated only in the presence of molecular oxygen.[42,43] In sunburn, there also is a characteristic delay between exposure to light and the development of erythema of the skin and evidence of soreness or pruritus. In photosensitization, the first signs may be noted within minutes following exposure to light.[44]

There are three principal types of photosensitization recognized in domestic animals.[40] Primary photosensitivity is caused by ingestion of significant amounts of photodynamic substances which are not normally present in the diet. Within this group are the diseases caused by ingestion of the poisonous plants *Hypericum perforatum* (St. John's wort, Klamath weed) and *Fagopyrum esculentum* (buckwheat). Photosensitization caused by the administration of the parasiticide phenothiazine also is considered to be a form of primary photosensitization. The photosensitizing compound is phenothiazine sulfoxide, which has the unusual characteristic of penetrating the aqueous humor as well as the skin, thereby producing severe keratitis.

The second type of photosensitization is due to aberrant pigment production from endogenous sources. Congenital porphyria (pink tooth) of cattle is the best known of this group of diseases although porphyria associated with photosensitization has also been observed in cats and swine. In cattle, there is a marked increase in production of the uroporphyrin I isomer, which is deposited in the teeth and bones and excreted in large quantities in the urine. There is also an increase in the protoporphyrin content of erythrocytes. The photodermatitis and hemolytic anemia which are present in the disease appear to be directly related to the photodynamic effects of these porphyrins.[45]

The third group of diseases characterized by photosensitivity are those which develop secondarily to liver disease (hepatic photosensitization) (Fig. 25–2). Photodermatitis associated with liver disease is recognized clinically only in herbivorous animals. Hepatic photosensitivity may be observed in both acute and chronic liver diseases in which there are morphologic and functional changes or, in Southdown sheep with congenital photosensitivity, in which there are no morphologic abnormalities, but significant biochemical defects in excretory function.[46]

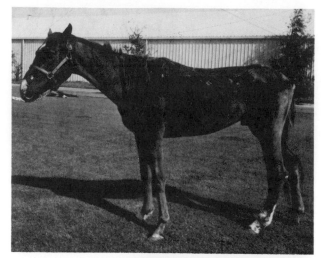

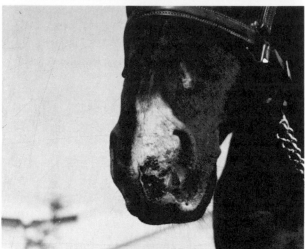

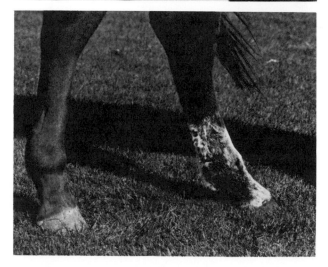

Figure 25–2. Two-year-old gelding with cirrhosis caused by pyrrolizidine alkaloid ingestion showing weight loss (top) and photodermatitis of the unpigmented muzzle (middle) and left rear fetlock (bottom). (From Tennant, et al.[9])

Pathogenesis

The photosensitizing agent in hepatic photosensitivity is phylloerythrin, a porphyrin derivative of chlorophyll.[44,47,48] Phylloerythrin is produced by intestinal microorganisms which remove the magnesium atom from the chlorophyll molecule and hydrolyze the phytyl and carboxymethoxy side chains[49] leaving the porphyrin nucleus intact. Most of the phylloerythrin produced each day is excreted in the feces but a part is absorbed into the portal circulation. In normal animals, plasma phylloerythrin is effectively removed by the liver and excreted in the bile. Phylloerythrin is found not only in the bile and feces of herbivores but also in other species if the diet contains chlorophyll. The comparatively large amounts excreted by ruminants is attributed to a high chlorophyll intake and to the apparently more favorable conditions for microbial action in the forestomachs.[40]

In hepatic insufficiency, phylloerythrin is diverted to the general circulation and ultimately accumulates in the skin. In the superficial layers of the skin, phylloerythrin absorbs radiant energy from the sun resulting in free radical formation. It is believed that by causing peroxidation of cellular lipids and other cellular components, free radicals damage cell organelles including lysosomes. Inflammation and necrosis of the skin are thought to be due to these direct cellular effects and to the secondary action of lysosomal enzymes.[50] The critical range of wavelengths (action spectrum) that produce photodermatitis in hepatic photosensitivity was shown in geeldikkop to be 380 nm to 650 nm[51] and in facial eczema 400 nm to 620 nm.[48] These ranges are consistent with the known absorption spectrum of phylloerythrin (Fig. 25–3).

Clinical Signs and Distribution of Lesions

Although the types of hepatic disease associated with photosensitivity vary considerably, the effects directly attributable to the photodynamic action of phylloerythrin are qualitatively similar. The nature and severity of the cutaneous lesions are dependent upon the amount of phylloerythrin in the skin, intensity of light, and duration of exposure. In the horse (see Fig. 25–2), the most common site of photodermatitis is the muzzle, which has a sparse protective covering of hair and often is unpigmented. Unpigmented areas of the distal extremities also are frequently affected.[9,51] In cattle, unpigmented areas of the muzzle, back, escutcheon, and teats appear to be especially susceptible.

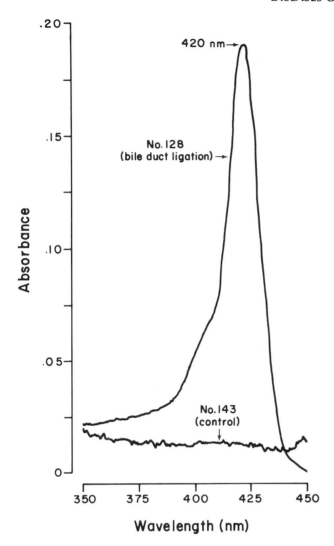

Figure 25–3. Spectrophotometric scan of extract from plasma of mature sheep with experimental bile duct obstruction (8 days' duration) compared to normal sheep. A substance is demonstrated in the plasma of the sheep with bile duct obstruction which has an absorption maximum of 420 nm, a characteristic of phylloerythrin. (Courtesy of B. H. Baldwin and D. Levy.)

As in cattle and horses, the areas of skin affected in sheep are those which receive the greatest exposure to light and which lack protection of pigment or wool. These include the ears, eyelids, face, lips, and coronets.[52]

The first clinical signs of photodermatitis may be apparent restlessness with shaking of the head or rubbing of affected parts. Individual animals may seek relief in the shade. Erythema and edema are the first cutaneous manifestations of photosensitization. In sheep, the swelling of the lips, ears, and face have led to the descriptive terms "big head" and "facial eczema." Following edema, serum may ooze from affected skin. Ultimately, second or third degree burns may develop, and, in severe cases, the morbidity and mortality attributable to the lesions of the skin may result in greater loss than that due to the primary liver disease.

Ascites

When associated with liver disease, ascites is indicative of a chronic process and one which almost always is characterized by cirrhosis. There are important species differences in the frequency of occurrence of ascites. In dogs and cats with advanced cirrhosis, ascites is a relatively common sign but is almost never observed in horses.[4] Conspicuous ascites also is unusual in cattle with cirrhosis[3,53] but has been observed at necropsy.[11] Ascites has been reported in association with liver abscess in cattle where thrombosis of the hepatic vein adjacent to the abscess causes marked hepatomegaly.[54,55] In sheep, ascites has been observed in cirrhosis, but is unusual with the sclerosing cholangitis which accompanies fascioliasis.[2]

Physical Findings

Excessive abdominal fluid is not difficult to detect when the volume is large. In such cases, abdominal paracentesis is usually diagnostic. Palpatory percussion also may be useful. Using the fingers of one hand, the flank is struck abruptly to induce a fluid wave which, following a momentary pause, is palpated or "caught" in the opposite flank with the palm of the other hand. Such a fluid wave can often be induced in the most ventral portions of the flanks in clinically normal animals but, when induced in the midflank region or above, is indicative of free abdominal fluid.

The so-called "puddle sign" has been described in the dog for identification of minimal ascites.[56] Auscultatory percussion is used with the percussion note being induced in the lower flank of the dog while in a standing position. The head of the stethoscope is placed over the other flank opposite the point of percussion. As percussion is continued at the same point, the stethoscope is moved dorsally and an abrupt change in resonance is used to identify the fluid line. Excessive fluid within the lumen of the intestine does not produce this characteristic line of demarcation.

Examination of Ascitic Fluid

It is important to differentiate between ascites caused by liver disease and ascites from other primary diseases. The distinction is usually made based on the examination of ascitic fluid and the results of biochemical, radiologic, and surgical tests for evaluation of the hepatobiliary system.

Biochemical and cytologic examinations of ascitic fluid may be useful but seldom are diagnostic. Low protein concentration (<1.5 to 2.0 g/dl of fluid) are unusual in ascites caused by inflammation or neoplasia. The protein concentration of ascitic fluid in cirrhosis is variable depending on the protein concentration in peripheral blood but typically exceeds 2 to 2.5 g/dl because it is largely a reflection of high-protein lymph exuded from liver. Total nucleated cell counts in ascitic fluid from dogs with cirrhosis are seldom greater than 1000 to 2000/μl. Bloody or turbid fluid typically results from inflammatory or neoplastic processes, e.g., feline infectious peritonitis or lymphosarcoma. Fluid deeply stained with bile pigment indicates a direct communication between the biliary system and the peritoneal cavity. In domestic animals, so-called "bile ascites" or bile peritonitis is primarily a problem of the dog and cat and is the result of trauma.

Pathogenesis of Ascites in Cirrhosis

Under physiologic conditions there is significant bidirectional movement of fluid, electrolytes, and, to a lesser degree, protein across the portal capillary bed, through the interstitial space, and across the peritoneal membrane into the peritoneal cavity. These movements are determined by osmotic and hydrostatic forces that, under normal conditions, are described by Starling's equation. In the equation, plasma colloidal osmotic pressure minus ascitic fluid colloidal osmotic pressure equals portal capillary pressure minus the intra-abdominal hydrostatic pressure. Normal portal capillary pressure on the arterial side of the capillary bed favors filtration of a nearly protein-free tissue fluid. Reabsorption of interstitial fluid occurs on the venous side of the capillary bed because hydrostatic pressure drops below that of the colloidal osmotic pressure of plasma proteins.

During investigations of the role of mechanical factors in the formation of lymph, Starling[57] observed that obstruction of hepatic venous flow (by constriction of the thoracic vena cava cranial to the hepatic vein) produced a great increase in lymph flow through the thoracic duct and production of lymph high in protein. Portal vein obstruction produced increased thoracic duct lymph but with a distinctively low protein content. He concluded that the increased flow of thoracic duct lymph following ligation of the thoracic vena cava arose from hepatic

lymph, and, after portal vein ligation, thoracic duct lymph originated from the mesenteric capillary bed.

Hepatic lymph is produced primarily in the sinusoids (90%) and normally accounts for 25 to 50% of thoracic duct lymph flow.[58] In the dog, hepatic lymph from a much higher protein content than lymph from other tissues because of the unique permeability of the sinusoid to plasma proteins.[59] In experimental cirrhosis in the dog and other species, the flow rate of thoracic duct lymph is increased 2 to 5 times, and the protein content also is increased significantly.[60,61]

For many years, it was assumed that ascites associated with cirrhosis was caused by increased portal vein pressure secondary to vascular obstruction within the liver. Ligation of the portal vein before its entry into the liver, however, produces only minimal and transient ascites or no ascites.[62,63,64] Ligation of either the hepatic vein[65-69] or the caudal vena cava at a site cranial to the hepatic vein[62,64,70-72] produces prompt and intractable as-

NORMAL

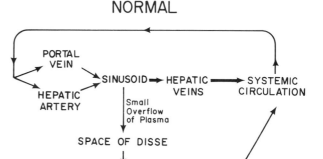

CIRRHOSIS

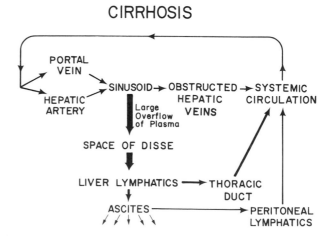

Figure 25–4. Diagram summarizing the hemodynamic factors involved in the normal and cirrhotic liver. (Redrawn after Orloff et al.[69])

cites in the dog. Lymph fluid has actually been visualized to form droplets which "weep" from the surface of the liver following obstruction of hepatic vein outflow.[73] The protein content of such ascitic fluid is 3.0 to 3.5 g/dl or higher because of its origin as hepatic lymph. This observation is consistent with the clinical finding that the protein content of ascitic fluid in cirrhosis is characteristically higher than that of other transudates (modified transudate), and it is now believed that much of the ascitic fluid in cirrhosis is derived directly from the liver (Fig. 25–4).

Although experimental portal obstruction per se does not result in ascites, only transient portal hypertension is actually produced. When persistent portal obstruction is produced experimentally by aortic-portal anastomosis, hypertension develops.[71,72] The ascitic fluid has a characteristically low protein content because of its origin in the mesenteric capillary bed. It is probable that in most cases of cirrhosis, both hepatic lymph (high protein) and mesenteric lymph (low protein) are produced at an increased rate and that ascites develops when the return of lymph to the systemic venous circulation fails to keep pace.[74]

The protein content of ascitic fluid in hepatic disease will be influenced by the relative proportions of ascitic and hepatic lymph which contribute to ascites. The protein content of hepatic lymph is determined by the circulating plasma protein concentration. In advanced cirrhosis, when hypoproteinemia has developed, the protein content of ascitic fluid can be expected to be proportionately lower.

Serum albumin is the major component of plasma and tissue fluid oncotic pressure and is produced exclusively in the liver. The hypoalbuminemia associated with chronic liver disease has been considered to be a contributing factor to development of ascites but current evidence suggests its role is minimal. The intravascular and total body albumin pools may actually not be greatly altered in cirrhosis although plasma albumin may be low.[75] Because of the unique permeability of the liver sinusoid to plasma proteins, oncotic pressure has essentially no effect on hepatic lymph flow and would not be expected to influence the hepatic component of ascites. It has further been demonstrated that the oncotic pressure of mesenteric tissues actually favors the movement of tissue fluid into the vascular system.[76]

In order for ascites to develop, there must be a proportional expansion in total body sodium and water. It is known that excessive salt intake greatly exaggerates ascites formation[64] and it is believed the development of ascites is preceded by increased sodium retention by the kidney. Aldosterone levels are significantly increased in dogs with ascites due to hepatic vein obstruction[77] but the underlying mechanisms of this steroid response are still unsolved.[78,79] The liver is the primary site of renin degradation, and it has been suggested that decreased degradation of renin by the diseased liver results in increased production of bradykinin, which in turn stimulates aldosterone release from the adrenal cortex.

LABORATORY ASSESSMENT OF HEPATIC FUNCTION

Numerous laboratory tests are available for the evaluation of hepatic function. In general, such tests are used to (1) detect subclinical hepatic disease, (2) aid in the differential diagnosis of icterus, (3) assess total hepatocellular mass, and (4) evaluate hepatic function during the course of hepatic disease. The tests are based on (1) the measurement of substances in the plasma which are normally synthesized or excreted by the liver, (2) demonstration of enzymes the activities of which are related to abnormal liver function, and (3) the study of the rate of plasma removal of certain test-dyes which are excreted by the liver. In most cases, no individual laboratory test is diagnostic but, taken together, the results of a group of liver function tests may be of significant help in the differential diagnosis and clinical management of liver disease.

Tests of Bile Pigment Excretion

Bile Pigment Metabolism

Origin of Bilirubin. Bilirubin is a yellow pigment which is a product of the enzymatic degradation of heme. In normal animals, approximately 80% of the bilirubin is produced from hemoglobin heme following removal of aged erythrocytes from the circulation by reticuloendothelial cells.[80,81] Heme from other sources (e.g., myoglobin, the cytochromes, peroxidase, and catalase) accounts for the remaining bilirubin production. The liver contains large amounts of the microsomal cytochromes P-450 and b_5 and appears to be the most important source of the bilirubin derived from non-erythroid sources.

The initial step in bilirubin formation is the opening of the heme (ferroprotoporphyrin) ring at the α-methene bridge (Fig. 25–5). This reaction is catalyzed by microsomal heme oxygenase,[82] which has the characteristics of the mixed function

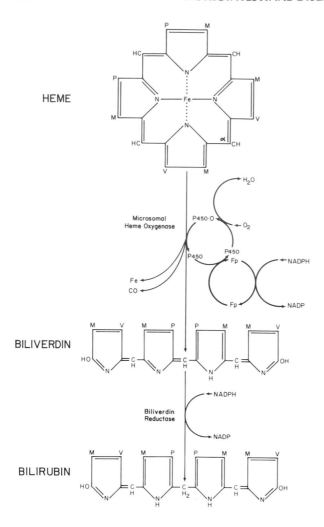

HEME

Microsomal
Heme Oxygenase

BILIVERDIN

Biliverdin
Reductase

BILIRUBIN

Figure 25–5. Enzymatic steps in the formation of bilirubin from heme (ferroprotoporphyrin).

oxidases. Cytochrome P-450 serves as the terminal oxidase and there is an obligatory requirement for molecular oxygen and reduced nicotinamide adenine dinucleotide phosphate (NADPH). The products of the heme oxygenase reaction are equimolar amounts of iron, biliverdin, and carbon monoxide. As far as is known, this is the only reaction in mammalian tissues in which carbon monoxide is produced and quantitation of the rate of carbon monoxide excretion has been used as an index of the rate of heme catabolism and of bilirubin production.

The second step in formation of bilirubin is the reduction of biliverdin by the cytosolic enzyme biliverdin reductase which, like heme oxygenase, requires NADPH.[83] In most mammals, biliverdin reductase is present in excess and, therefore, is not normally rate limiting as far as bilirubin synthesis is

concerned. Biliverdin reductase activity, however, is almost completely lacking in birds and in avian species biliverdin is the major pigment of bile. Biliverdin also is found in significant quantities in the bile of certain mammalian species such as the rabbit, presumably because of biliverdin reductase "deficiency."

Heme oxygenase is most active in the tissues which are normal sites of erythrocyte removal and heme degradation. The spleen appears to be most important in this regard, followed by the liver and bone marrow.[84] The kidney normally plays a minor role in this process but in hemolytic disorders, when there is intravascular hemolysis and hemoglobinuria, the kidney assumes a quantitatively more important role.

When there is intravascular hemolysis, glomerular filtration of hemoglobin is initially prevented because of the binding of hemoglobin to the plasma protein haptoglobin. When the haptoglobin binding capacity is exceeded, glomerular filtration occurs and, depending on the amount of hemoglobin filtered, part or all is reabsorbed by the tubular epithelium. There is then rapid induction of heme oxygenase activity in the tubule and significant bilirubin formation by the kidney.[85-87] Renal degradation of hemoglobin has been suggested as having a homeostatic function intended to conserve iron and to minimize renal injury in hemoglobinuric nephropathy.[88]

Hepatic Excretion of Bilirubin. Unconjugated bilirubin is a nonpolar compound which is almost completely insoluble at physiologic pH. In plasma, unconjugated bilirubin is bound to albumin, which allows transport in stable aqueous solution to the liver.

The mechanisms involved in the hepatic excretion of bilirubin are similar to those utilized by most other organic anions. The initial step is uptake of bilirubin by the hepatocyte. The exact mechanism of transfer across the plasma membrane is poorly understood, but bilirubin appears to dissociate from albumin and then to cross the plasma membrane by non-ionic diffusion.[89] The rate of hepatic uptake of bilirubin is regulated in part by ligandin (Y-protein), a low molecular weight cytosolic protein (44,000 to 46,000) which makes up approximately 5% of the protein of liver cytoplasm. In neonatal liver the concentration of ligandin is low and there is an associated decreased capacity to excrete bilirubin. Ligandin synthesis can be induced by drugs such as phenobarbital, which stimulates bilirubin excretion. Ligandin also binds other organic anions (e.g., porphyrins, sulfobromophthalein (BSP), indocyanine green, and certain steroid hormones such as cortisol), and intracellular binding is believed to be important in their hepatic uptake. Purified ligandin has significant S-aryl transferase activity and recently was shown to be identical to glutathione transferase B, which is responsible for the enzymatic conjugation of BSP with glutathione.[90,91]

The second step in hepatic excretion of bilirubin is the formation of polar conjugates such as bilirubin diglucuronide. Conjugation with glucuronic acid is catalyzed by glucuronyl transferase, a microsomal enzyme which requires uridine diphosphoglucuronic acid (UDPG). Glucuronic acid esters of bilirubin have been identified in the bile of a variety of species including the dog,[92] rat,[93] guinea pig,[94] and also in the bile of the horse, pig, cat, sheep, and cattle.[95]

Gordon et al.[96] recently have confirmed that bilirubin diglucuronide is the major conjugate excreted in canine bile. There is evidence, however, that the bile of dogs[97-99] and other species[100] contains significant amounts of bilirubin conjugates of several carbohydrates including glucose and xylose.

The final and rate-limiting step in hepatic excretion of bilirubin is the transport of conjugated bilirubin across the bile canaliculus into the biliary tree. The mechanism for the final transport of conjugated bilirubin into bile appears to be separate from that of the bile salts.[101] Bile salts, however, enhance the flow of bile and in so doing, increase the maximum transport capacity for bilirubin.[102]

Following excretion by the liver, conjugated bilirubin enters the intestine. Unlike the unconjugated pigment, conjugated bilirubin is poorly absorbed in the small intestine and passes to the large intestine where it is reduced to a series of colorless derivatives collectively called urobilinogens (stercobilinogens). Reduction is catalyzed by the dehydrogenases of anaerobic colonic bacteria. In germ-free animals lacking intestinal microorganisms, bilirubin is passed unaltered in the feces and no urobilinogen is produced.[103]

Most of the urobilinogen formed in the colon is passed in the feces. The remainder enters the portal circulation, passes to the liver and is excreted again in the bile. A small fraction of the absorbed urobilinogen (1 to 5%) passes into the general circulation and is excreted by the kidney. In the dog, renal excretion of urobilinogen occurs by glomerular filtration and tubular secretion, the latter being enhanced significantly by acidification of the urine.[104]

Extrahepatic Conjugation and Excretion of Bilirubin. Although the liver is the principal site of

bilirubin conjugation and excretion, alternate pathways have been demonstrated. In normal animals, these alternate mechanisms are of minor significance but may become quantitatively more important in liver disease. For example, after total hepatectomy, dogs have been shown to develop moderate hyperbilirubinemia and bilirubinuria.[105] In addition to unconjugated bilirubin, the plasma of hepatectomized dogs contains the monoglucuronide[106] and, in some studies, the diglucuronide of bilirubin.[107] The kidney and intestine have been shown to be sites of conjugation of infused bilirubin.[108]

Determination of Serum Bilirubin

Bilirubin is determined by the *van den Bergh* or *"diazo"* reaction in which bilirubin is coupled with diazotized sulfanilic acid. The products of the reaction are dipyrroles called *azo pigments.* The azo pigments are stable compounds, a characteristic which has been useful in recent studies of the structure of bilirubin conjugates.

Conjugated bilirubin reacts with diazotized sulfanilic acid in aqueous solution (van den Bergh "direct reaction") whereas unconjugated bilirubin reacts very slowly. Only after addition to the aqueous solution of an accelerator such as methyl or ethyl alcohol is the diazotization of unconjugated bilirubin complete ("indirect reaction"). It is said that approximately 10% of the unconjugated bilirubin in plasma will give a false "direct" reaction.[89]

It has been assumed that the requirement of an organic solvent for the reaction of unconjugated bilirubin was related to the water insolubility of the pigment. Evidence reviewed recently,[109] however, suggests that intramolecular hydrogen bonding may be a factor more important than actual solubility in preventing the reaction of unconjugated bilirubin with the diazo reagent.[110,111] The intramolecular hydrogen bonds of unconjugated bilirubin appear to inhibit the diazo reaction. In conjugated bilirubin, the two propionic acid side chains are esterified with glucuronic acid or other carbohydrates disrupting the intramolecular hydrogen bonding[110] and allowing the direct diazo reaction. Accelerators may have a similar effect on the intramolecular hydrogen bonds of the unconjugated pigment.

Pathophysiologic Mechanisms in Hyperbilirubinemia and Interpretation of the van den Bergh Test

Table 25–1 summarizes the pathophysiologic mechanisms which are responsible for the development of hyperbilirubinemia. Unconjugated

Table 25–1. Pathophysiologic Mechanisms in Hyperbilirubinemia

	Plasma Bilirubin		Urine Bilirubin	Urine Urobilinogen
	unconjugated	conjugated		
Increased bilirubin production hemolytic anemia hematoma resorption	↑	N	0	↑
Impaired hepatic uptake of unconjugated bilirubin neonatal hyperbilirubinemia fasting hyperbilirubinemia benign unconjugated hyperbilirubinemia of horses congenital photosensitivity (Southdown sheep)	↑	N	0	N
Impaired conjugation of bilirubin glucuronyl transferase deficiency (Gunn rat) neonatal hyperbilirubinemia	↑	N	0	N
Impaired biliary excretion of bilirubin intrahepatic cholestasis black liver disease (Corriedale sheep) congenital photosensitivity (Southdown sheep) biliary cirrhosis bile duct obstruction	↑	↑	↑	↓ or 0

N, normal; 0, absent; ↑, increased; ↓, decreased

hyperbilirubinemia is observed when there is increased production of bilirubin, e.g., hemolytic disease (prehepatic icterus), or when hepatic uptake or conjugation of bilirubin is decreased. Although the unconjugated bilirubin of plasma may be significantly increased in such disorders, the pigment is tightly bound to albumin and essentially none is filtered by the glomerulus. Consequently, bilirubin does not appear in the urine of patients with unconjugated hyperbilirubinemia. In hemolytic disease, the amount of bilirubin excreted by the liver and therefore the amount which reaches the intestine may be remarkably increased. This results in increased urobilinogen formation and increased urinary excretion.

Conjugated hyperbilirubinemia is a characteristic of either intrahepatic cholestasis or of extrahepatic bile duct obstruction (posthepatic icterus). When the primary defect is impaired excretion of bilirubin, uptake and conjugation may proceed at relatively normal rates but the conjugated pigment is refluxed into the plasma. The plasma concentration of bilirubin increases and the conjugated pigment, which is water soluble and less firmly bound to albumin, is filtered by the glomerulus resulting in bilirubinuria.[112,113] Because bilirubin excretion into the intestine is either significantly reduced or absent, the formation of urobilinogen by intestinal bacteria is remarkably reduced and the urinary urobilinogen test is characteristically negative in complete extrahepatic obstruction. Broad-spectrum antibiotic therapy decreases the metabolic activity

of intestinal bacteria and may cause a spuriously negative urobilinogen test.

The biochemical differentiation between unconjugated and conjugated hyperbilirubinemia using the van den Bergh reaction can be useful in differentiating between prehepatic and posthepatic causes of icterus. In primary hepatocellular disease (hepatitis, cirrhosis) all excretory steps (uptake, conjugation, and excretion) may be deranged resulting in elevations of both conjugated and unconjugated pigment.

Important species characteristics must be taken into account when interpreting results of the van den Bergh reaction. In general, the interpretation in dogs and cats is similar to that in human subjects. Typically, in cholestatic disease, the conjugated fraction is elevated, representing 50 to 75% of the total serum bilirubin. The horse has a higher normal serum bilirubin than any of the other domestic species, and values as high as 4.0 mg/dl or higher have been observed in otherwise healthy individuals. In addition to hepatic and hemolytic diseases, hyperbilirubinemia is observed in horses with intestinal obstruction and a variety of other serious systemic diseases. Starvation alone causes an abrupt increase in the unconjugated serum bilirubin value in the horse,[4,5] and reduced food intake is the probable cause of the "nonspecific" hyperbilirubinemia observed in horses with other than hepatic or hemolytic diseases (Fig. 25–6).

In cattle and sheep, hyperbilirubinemia of sufficient severity to produce clinical icterus (≥ 3

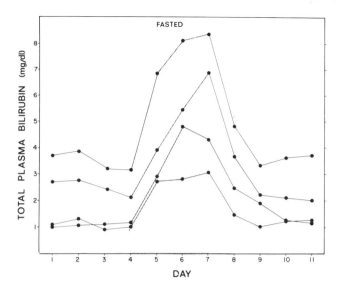

Figure 25–6. Influence of starvation on the plasma bilirubin of horses. (From Tennant et al.[4])

mg/dl) is caused most frequently by hemolytic disease. Moderate biochemical hyperbilirubinemia (< 3 mg/dl) without clinical icterus is observed in both species with the fatty liver associated with ketosis or acetonemia. In this case the unconjugated pigment predominates. Mild conjugated hyperbilirubinemia has been observed in sheep with sclerosing cholangitis caused by *Fasciola hepatica* infestation,[2] and in cattle with cirrhosis.[3]

Serum Enzyme Determinations

Measurements of enzyme activity in serum have been utilized in the diagnosis of liver disease for many years. Alkaline phosphatase was shown to be useful in the diagnosis of biliary tract disease more than 35 years ago, and aminotransferases (transaminases) were introduced in the mid-1950s for the diagnosis of hepatocellular disease. Since then, numerous advances have been made to increase specificity and usefulness by determining the origin of enzymes within cells or organs and by identifying kinetic and other specific characteristics of serum enzymes of hepatic origin.

Serum Aminotransferase (Transaminase)

The serum aspartic aminotransferase (glutamic-oxalacetic transaminase, GOT) and alanine aminotransferase (glutamic-pyruvic transaminase, GPT) are the enzymes in most general use as indicators of hepatocellular damage. The GOT is present in numerous tissues other than the liver, and elevations in serum activity are therefore not specific for

liver disease. Taken together with other abnormal liver function tests, however, the elevated serum GOT can be of significant value.

The GOT is present both in mitochondria and in the cytosol, and the isozymes can be separated electrophoretically.[114] In reversible metabolic or inflammatory disorders associated with increased hepatocyte permeability, only the cytosolic isozyme increases in the serum. In massive necrosis both mitochondrial and cytosolic fractions are elevated.[115]

The GPT is a cytosolic enzyme present in highest concentration in the liver, and an elevation in the serum GPT can be taken as specific evidence of hepatocellular damage. Unfortunately, of the domestic species, only the dog[116] and cat[117] have sufficient hepatic activity of GPT to demonstrate significant elevations in hepatic disease. In these species the serum GPT has proven useful,[118,119] moderate hepatic necrosis being suggested by values of 50 to 400 IU/dl and severe necrosis by values above 400 IU/dl.

Serum Alkaline Phosphatase (SAP)

The alkaline phosphatases are a group of zinc metalloenzymes which are present in most tissues. High concentrations are found in the intestine, kidney, bone, and liver. Light and electron microscopic studies have demonstrated that alkaline phosphatase activity is highest on the absorptive or secretory surfaces of cells.[120] Within liver cells, alkaline phosphatase is bound to membranes and, when liver homogenates are subjected to high-speed centrifugation, alkaline phosphatase activity sediments primarily with the microsomal and plasma membrane fractions.[121]

The actual physiologic function(s) of alkaline phosphatase remains uncertain. The localization of the enzyme to cell surfaces known to be responsible for active secretion or absorption suggests a role in membrane transport. There is circumstantial evidence that the alkaline phosphatase of osteoblasts may be involved in bone calcification. It has been suggested that intestinal calcium-stimulated adenosine triphosphatase, which may have a role in active calcium transport, and alkaline phosphatase are different activities of the same enzyme.[122] A similar relationship appears to exist between alkaline phosphatase and other enzymes involved in active transport; e.g., sodium, potassium-stimulated adenosine triphosphatase of several tissues including liver have significant hydrolytic activity against alkaline phosphatase substrates such as p-nitrophenyl phosphate.[123]

The SAP in normal animals originates primarily from liver and bone.[124–126] Elevations in SAP are observed in normal growing animals or in adult animals with increased osteoblastic activity. The SAP may be elevated in both acute and chronic liver diseases but great elevations are indicative of cholestasis, with the highest plasma concentrations observed in animals with cholangitis, biliary cirrhosis, or extrahepatic bile duct obstruction.

The alkaline phosphatase isozymes of various tissues may be differentiated on the basis of relative differences in heat stability, inhibition of L-phenylalanine, or electrophoretic mobility.[125,127,128] Alternatively, other serum enzymes which are more specific for biliary tract disease may be utilized in the diagnostic workup. These include leucine aminopeptidase,[129] gamma glutamyltransferase, and 5'nucleotidase.[130] When the serum alkaline phosphatase is significantly elevated, other clinical signs will usually allow separation of diseases of the liver from those of other tissues, such as bone.

Unlike serum GOT and GPT, elevations in SAP are not due simply to leakage of enzyme through damaged cells. Although there has been evidence to the contrary available for many years, it generally has been accepted that the liver excreted alkaline phosphatase produced in other tissues and that the high SAP levels observed in cholestatic liver disease were the result of a decrease in hepatic excretion.[131] It now is known that experimental obstruction of bile flow stimulates de novo synthesis of hepatic alkaline phosphatase,[132,133] and the newly synthesized enzyme is refluxed into the circulation. Partial hepatectomy also stimulates increased synthesis of alkaline phosphatase in the remaining hepatic tissue.[134] Similar mechanisms undoubtedly are involved in clinical extrahepatic bile duct obstruction, in intrahepatic cholestasis or in infiltrative diseases of the liver (e.g., lymphoma) in which the terminal branches of the biliary tree are obstructed, and in regenerative processes following hepatic injury.

Until recently, most sources reported that cats differed from other species by not developing an increased SAP in extrahepatic bile duct obstruction or in other cholestatic liver diseases. Although excellent experimental data to the contrary have been available since 1948,[135] the results most frequently cited state that extrahepatic obstruction in cats produces "inconsistent" elevations of SAP[136] or "negligible" elevations, reportedly due to urinary excretion of alkaline phosphatase.[137] However, other studies have established that cholestatic liver disease in cats can be expected to cause significant elevations in SAP.[129,135] The induction of alkaline phosphatase synthesis by bile duct obstruction also appears to occur in the cat as in other species.[138]

Dye Excretion Tests

The liver can excrete many organic anions including the following dyes: rose bengal, indocyanine green, and sulfobromophthalein (Bromsulphalein, BSP). Of these, sulfobromophthalein is most frequently used in liver function studies. Following intravenous administration, the dye is removed rapidly from the plasma primarily by the liver, and subsequently is excreted in the bile. Delayed plasma clearance is used as an indicator of hepatocellular or biliary tract disease.

The overall process of hepatic excretion of BSP is similar but not identical to that of bilirubin. BSP and bilirubin appear to be transported across the plasma membrane by different routes in that membrane binding sites are not shared.[139] Within the cell, however, bilirubin and BSP compete for binding on the cytosolic protein, *ligandin*. Ligandin, by serving as an ion "sink," is thought to be an important driving force in the overall process of hepatic uptake.[140] The conjugation mechanisms for bilirubin and BSP are completely separate. BSP is conjugated with glutathione by action of the cytosolic enzyme S-aryl transferase-B. Although conjugation facilitates excretion of BSP, it is not an obligatory step since approximately 50% of the BSP in bile is unconjugated. Conjugation of bilirubin with glucuronic acid or other sugars requires one of the glycosyl transferases which are microsomal enzymes. Conjugation appears to be critical in the hepatic excretion of bilirubin. The canalicular transport of BSP is similar to that of conjugated bilirubin, but whether there is competition between the two for a carrier mechanism is unknown.

In the icteric patient, the question arises whether competition between BSP and bilirubin will alter the results of the BSP excretion test. In general, the BSP test is seldom justified in such patients since hepatic disease is evident and no important additional information is likely to be provided. In general, the BSP test is most useful for situations in which a suggestion of occult liver disease exists but in which the results of other liver function tests are equivocal. The net competitive effect of bilirubin on BSP excretion is not great. For example, horses starved for 72 hours developed a three-fold elevation in total bilirubin but BSP excretion was prolonged less than 25%.[141]

In the dog and cat, a standard dose of 5 mg/kg of

BSP is administered as an intravenous bolus. A sample of blood is removed at 30 minutes and the BSP concentration is determined spectrophotometrically. It is assumed that the original dose of BSP (5 mg/kg) is distributed in a plasma volume of 5 ml/kg so that the concentration of BSP in plasma at time zero is (by definition) 1 mg/ml. The percent retention at 30 minutes is calculated from the ratio of the concentration at time zero and at 30 minutes. Retention of 5% or less is considered to be within normal limits.[142]

In the large domestic species, it often is difficult or inconvenient to obtain body weight measurements. Because the initial slope of the disappearance curve is independent of BSP dose, a standard 1-g dosage is administered to normal-sized horses (450 kg) and 0.5 g to smaller-sized horses. Blood samples are obtained at 6, 9, and 12 minutes following injection, the BSP concentration is determined in each, and the fractional clearance rate or plasma half time ($T_{1/2}$) is calculated. In the horse, normal plasma $T_{1/2}$ values vary between 2.5 and 3.5 minutes. In cattle, BSP excretion rate is similar to the horse. Sheep have a more rapid excretion rate requiring samples to be taken at 3, 5, and 7 minutes following injection. Normal $T_{1/2}$ values range from 1.6 to 2.7 minutes.[142]

The BSP test is safe although the dye is very irritating if infiltrated perivascularly. The test should be used only when cardiovascular function is normal. If hypovolemia or hypotension is present, hepatic perfusion will be reduced and erroneously prolonged clearance rates may be observed.

HEPATIC DISEASES

Acute Equine Hepatitis

Acute hepatitis is frequently observed as a clinical syndrome in the horse. In this species, the disease (Theiler's disease, serum hepatitis, infectious hepatitis) may occur sporadically in individuals or in epizootic form, with several cases on an individual farm or in the same veterinary practice setting.

The cause of the disease is unknown. Its occurrence in patients following the prophylactic or therapeutic use of serum from other horses has led to the suspicion that the disease is infectious and possibly due to a viral agent similar to that causing human hepatitis B.[143,144] While it is possible that such an infectious disease does occur in horses, there is no direct scientific evidence which adequately proves such a hypothesis. Attempts to transmit hepatitis to experimental horses using the

blood or other tissues of clinical cases have been uniformly unsuccessful. A total of 28 individual transmission experiments have been reported by five separate research groups.[6,145-149] In only one of these experimental horses was acute hepatitis observed following inoculation.[145] Because no experimental control animals were utilized, the investigator (Sir Arnold Theiler) concluded that the horse could ". . . have contracted the disease spontaneously. . . ."

In past years, several outbreaks of acute hepatitis have been reported which involved large numbers of horses. In some cases, investigators associated hepatitis with the prophylactic administration of antiserum of equine origin,[146-154] but similar outbreaks have been observed in which antiserum administration was not a factor.[31,155,156] Sporadic cases of acute hepatitis also have been observed following administration of tetanus antitoxin.[156-159] In most of these reports, it is impossible to establish a cause-effect relationship. Most cases of acute equine hepatitis seen today do not present with histories of injection of equine serum prior to onset of illness.[9,160] It is possible that an infectious agent causing hepatitis could be transmitted from horse to horse directly, or by indirect methods other than by injections of serum. It also seems likely that currently unrecognized factors, e.g., environmental or dietary toxins, may play significant roles in the pathogenesis of acute hepatitis in horses.[161]

In most cases of acute hepatitis, the onset of clinical signs is abrupt, with anorexia and lethargy being followed by signs of central nervous system disturbance. Affected horses may walk in circles or press the head against the wall or other objects. Others may walk compulsively through or over objects in their path as if completely oblivious to the surroundings. Violent seizure activity may be observed terminally in some cases. Death ordinarily is preceded by deep coma. Signs of encephalopathy may be the first clinical abnormalities noted by the owner. The fatality rate has been reported to vary from 25%[154] to 89%.[151]

Jaundice is almost invariably present in cases of acute hepatitis.[4,162,163] Voided urine typically is dark brown, or when intravascular hemolysis occurs, may be dark red.[164-166] In horses with unpigmented skin, the initial signs of photodermatitis may be referrable to pruritus of affected areas, e.g., frequent rubbing of the unpigmented muzzle on the ground or other objects. Within 24 to 48 hours, the superficial layers of affected skin become dry, leathery, and eventually slough.[9]

The diagnosis of acute hepatitis should be suspected on the basis of history and clinical signs. Active hepatic necrosis always is associated with elevations in the serum GOT, and in the more "liver specific" enzymes, sorbitol dehydrogenase and ornithine-carbamyl transferase. The serum bilirubin concentration also is consistently elevated in acute hepatitis. Although useful, these tests, like clinical signs, indicate only the presence of liver disease and must be used cautiously even to distinguish acute from chronic hepatic insufficiency. They never can be used to establish the cause of hepatic insufficiency.

The percutaneous liver biopsy is perhaps the most useful of all the diagnostic methods available in a differential diagnosis of equine hepatic disease. In clinical cases of acute hepatitis, there is either severe central lobular necrosis or massive necrosis. The inflammatory reaction which accompanies the death of hepatocytes, particularly in fatal cases, may be surprisingly minimal. In the portal areas, a mild round cell infiltration is often observed with mild bile duct proliferation. Such lesions are not specific for any given cause of hepatitis but would be expected with toxicoses as well as infectious causes.

The clinical management of horses with acute hepatitis is directed toward temporary nutritional support of the patient and control of signs of encephalopathy. Sedation often is necessary and for this purpose, the phenothiazine tranquilizers are useful. Efforts to control encephalopathy also are directed toward reduction in the production of ammonia and other suspected neurotoxic substances by colonic bacteria. Cathartics such as mineral oil or dilute dioctyl sodium sulfosuccinate-glycerin solution can be administered to prevent intestinal stasis. Bacterial activity can be reduced by the oral administration of a nonabsorbable broad-spectrum antibiotic. Neomycin in an oral dose of 10 to 15 g four times per day can be useful. In anorectic horses, special attention must be given to provision of exogenous carbohydrate for maintenance of blood glucose. In patients which have developed hypoglycemia or in which hypoglycemia is considered a risk, it is advisable to provide a continuous intravenous drip of 5% dextrose.[9]

Infectious Canine Hepatitis

Infectious canine hepatitis (ICH) or Rubarth's disease was described originally in 1947.[167] The causative agent, which has been classified as Canine Adenovirus Type I, grows readily in tissue culture, and strains with modified virulence have been used to produce effective vaccines.[168,169]

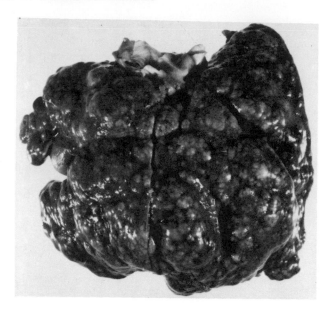

Figure 25–7. Gross appearance of liver of a dog admitted to the clinic with signs of terminal hepatic failure. Histologic examination demonstrated morphologic features of chronic active hepatitis.

In areas where vaccination programs are well established, the clinical diagnosis of ICH is very unusual. The decreasing frequency of ICH is reflected in the numbers of postmortem diagnoses made between 1953 and 1974 in our practice. Of 75 dogs diagnosed as having ICH during this 21-year period, 57% were observed during the first 7 years of the study; only 7 (9%) were seen between 1970 and 1974.

The clinical manifestations of ICH vary widely. An acute, fulminant form is recognized in which the mortality rate is very high. The clinical signs in spontaneous clinical cases are similar to those seen experimentally. Characteristically, there is fever, malaise, tonsillitis, multifocal vasculitis with associated hemorrhages, leukopenia, proteinuria, and clinical and biochemical evidence of severe hepatocellular necrosis and insufficiency. Typically, clinical icterus is not observed. Although the acute form of ICH which is recognized clinically has a high fatality rate, most infections are actually clinically mild or inapparent and, unless tests for seroconversion are performed, cannot be recognized as ICH.

Approximately 20% of dogs recovering from ICH infection develop acute uveitis and leucoma during early convalescence (9 to 14 days following inoculation). The so-called "blue eye" of hepatitis has been shown to be the result of an immune-mediated inflammatory response of the Arthus type.[170–172]

Immune-mediated uveitis also is seen in dogs following vaccination against ICH with modified live virus vaccines, in approximately the same frequency and at the same time following administration of virus. Recent studies suggest that Canine Adenovirus Type II can be used to vaccinate against the pathogenic Type I without the ocular complications.[173]

In most cases, the inflammatory reaction of the uveal tract is self-limiting, responding to topical mydriatic treatment and to corticosteroids with complete resolution in less than 1 month. Rarely, exudate occluding the anterior drainage angle requires special treatment for glaucoma.

Following experimental infection, ICH virus can be isolated from blood, spleen, kidney, and liver. Acidophilic intranuclear inclusion bodies, typical of the ICH virus, can be identified in tissues.[174] Using fluorescent antibody techniques, ICH antigen could be demonstrated in liver for only 7 to 10 days after virus inoculation,[175] but the virus is shed in the urine for many weeks following infection.

It was believed that the abnormal coagulation of blood observed in acute hepatic failure was due primarily to lack of hepatic synthesis of the protein factors responsible for coagulation. Recent experimental studies suggest that the coagulopathy in ICH is comparable in important ways to disseminated intravascular coagulation (DIC).[176] Thrombocytopenia, abnormal platelet function, prolonged prothrombin time, and increased fibrin degradation products were observed terminally in experimental ICH. The presence of DIC in clinical subjects also has been demonstrated in acute hepatitis[177] and in aflatoxin-induced hepatopathy.[178]

It has been assumed that, following acute ICH infection, recovery is uncomplicated except for transient uveitis and that permanent immunity is conferred. Some experimental studies, however, suggest that, under certain conditions, convalescence may be far more complicated.[175] In these studies, 49 experimental dogs with varying ICH antibody titers were infected with virulent virus. In 19 with antibodies of 1:500 or higher, complete protection from the infection was observed, and the dogs remained clinically normal. In another group of 19 dogs, ICH antibody titers were 1:4 or less, and dogs died between 4 and 9 days following inoculation of typical acute hepatitis.

A third group of 11 dogs was studied which had intermediate ICH antibody titer (1:16 to 1:500). Each of these dogs developed clinical illness, but the incubation period was significantly longer than in the group with lowest antibody titers. Four of the 11 dogs died between 8 and 21 days with extensive lesions of hepatitis. The remaining 7 dogs developed chronic progressive hepatitis characterized by infiltration of the portal areas with lymphocytes and plasma cells and by fibrosis.[175,179,180] More recently, highly susceptible dogs were given hyperimmune serum sufficient to produce intermediate ICH antibody titers and challenged with ICH virus. Again, a chronic active form of hepatitis resulted.[181]

Although the evidence for ICH-induced chronic hepatitis is entirely experimental at this time, there are clinical circumstances during which dogs are known to have moderately low antibody titers and could be exposed to field strains of ICH virus. These include the young dog which has a decreasing maternal antibody titer prior to receiving active immunization, and the dog which receives hyperimmune serum prophylactically in anticipation of future active immunization.

A spontaneous, chronic disease similar to that observed in the experimental work previously described is not common in dogs. Cases of unexplained chronic hepatitis are observed, however, and it is possible that in some the ICH virus plays a role in pathogenesis.[182] Proof of such a relationship will be extremely difficult. In the experimental dogs which developed chronic hepatitis, ICH viral antigen disappeared from the liver early in the course of the disease. Therefore, one might not expect to demonstrate ICH antigen in the end-stage chronic hepatitis even though ICH virus may play an early pathogenic role.

Chronic Active Liver Disease

Chronic active liver disease, often of unknown cause, is recognized clinically in all species of domestic animals but is most seen in the dog and cat. It is generally regarded as a chronic inflammatory process accompanied by varying degrees of hepatocyte necrosis and often associated with progressive fibrosis. Cholestasis may or may not be a dominant clinical feature. In many patients, liver disease may be clinically silent for long periods of time.

The cause of chronic active liver disease is speculative. In the case of the dog and based on experimental studies described previously,[175,179–181] it is possible that some cases have resulted from infection with ICH virus.[182] The presumption that the cumulative effects of environmental toxin(s) are important in some cases of chronic liver disease in the dog and cat is based on the similarity of the lesions of clinical cases and certain types of experimental toxicoses.[178] In cats, chronic active liver disease may vary from lesions limited to pericholangeal mononuclear cellular infiltrations to cholangitis and to sclerosing cholangitis and biliary cirrhosis. Interstitial fibrosing pancreatitis is a concomitant finding in some of these same feline patients.

An animal with chronic active liver disease may or may not have signs of liver insufficiency, but chronic active liver disease should be suspected in animals with recurrent histories of illness associated with abnormal liver function tests. Increased SGPT and SAP values associated with hyperbilirubinemia and with frank bilirubinuria often are present. Change in liver size and contour based on physical and/or radiographic examination also should raise the question of active, progressive liver disease. A liver biopsy is necessary to establish the diagnosis and to eliminate other specific types of liver disease.

In selected cases, periodic liver biopsies will assist in establishing the pattern of change and response to therapy.

Chronic Progressive Hepatitis of Bedlington Terriers

A chronic, progressive form of hepatitis has been described in Bedlington Terriers.[183] The disease apparently is confined to the Bedlington breed and is believed to be inherited. The incidence of clinical and biochemical signs of hepatic disease in Bedlingtons suggests a high gene frequency.

The disease is observed characteristically in adult dogs of both sexes. Initially, clinical signs of chronic illness may be minimal. Typically, clinical signs of hepatic failure develop abruptly and then the clinical course is short. The biochemical abnormalities are those of chronic cholestasis and abnormalities including moderate to marked elevations in SGPT, SAP, and serum bilirubin, particularly the "direct reacting" fraction. The serum albumin is decreased, and the gamma globulin fraction is elevated.[183]

The chronic, progressive hepatitis and cirrhosis which develop in Bedlingtons is clinically similar to the end-stage cirrhosis seen from time to time in other breeds of dogs. The nodular gross appearance (post-necrotic scarring) is also similar. The pathogenesis of the Bedlington disease, however, appears to be unique and related directly to the accumulation of copper in hepatocytes. Recent studies indicate that copper accumulation begins in affected dogs at an early age and progresses throughout life. Copper-containing pigment can be identified within the cytoplasm of hepatocytes in biopsy specimens using a rubeanic acid stain. It is believed that affected Bedlingtons have a primary defect in copper excretion similar to that occurring in Wilson's disease (hepatolenticular disease) of humans. Copper accumulation is believed to lead to the inflammatory changes and ultimately to cirrhosis. Because the disease has been recognized only recently, no effective method of treatment or control has been reported. It has been suggested that drugs such as D-penicillamine, a potent chelator of copper, could be used to mobilize hepatic copper and promote renal excretion.[183]

Suppurative Cholangitis

In normal animals, a relatively sterile biliary duct system is maintained by the regular flow of bile from the gallbladder and biliary tree, through the sphincter of Oddi into the intestine. Biliary infection occurs primarily when there is some degree of obstructed bile flow. Enteric bacteria are the most frequently encountered microorganisms, suggesting that infection frequently is ascending.

In the horse, approximately half of the cases of chronic cholangitis are associated with bile duct obstructions. Such patients characteristically are admitted with protracted histories of intermittent fever, jaundice, and vague, recurrent abdominal pain. At necropsy, the remaining patients have no gross lesions which can account for the finding that bile is under significant pressure. Some type of functional obstruction of the sphincter of Oddi, however, is the most reasonable explanation. Sclerosing cholangitis eventually develops in which all major bile ducts are thickened with dense fibrous connective tissue. Biliary cirrhosis also may be a sequela to chronic cholangitis. In this type of cirrhosis, the connective tissue uniformly encircles each lobule, and there is prominent proliferation of bile ductules.

The clinical diagnosis of suppurative cholangitis is suggested by the findings of fever, leukocytosis, and jaundice. Cholestasis is indicated by significant elevations in SAP and in the direct reacting (conjugated) fraction of the van den Bergh bilirubin test. Percutaneous liver biopsy may demonstrate a suppurative reaction in the portal areas or, in advanced cases, biliary cirrhosis.

Liver Fluke Infections

By far the most frequent type of severe cholangitis encountered in animals is that caused by liver flukes. *Fasciola hepatica* is the most common species, although *Fasciola gigantica* and species of *Fascioloides*, *Dicrocoelium*, and *Paramphistoma* also infect domestic species.

Hepatic fascioliasis occurs throughout the world

where climatic conditions are suitable for snails, which are the intermediate host of *F. hepatica.* Important host snails are *Lymnea truncatula* (Great Britain) and *Galba bulimoides* or *G. techella* (United States). Low swampy areas provide an ideal environment for perpetuation of the parasite. Pastures irrigated by frequent flooding also provide suitable conditions for outbreaks.

Clinical manifestations of fascioliasis are observed primarily in sheep. Clinical signs of fascioliasis are unusual in cattle, and this species is preferred for pasturing areas known to produce severe losses in sheep.[184]

Signs of acute hemorrhagic necrosis of the liver occur when immature flukes penetrate the liver capsule and begin migration. Hepatic migration of flukes is believed to be important in activation of *Clostridium novyi* spores and in the production of black disease, a uniformly fatal toxemia. Such spores lie dormant in the parenchyma until necrosis of the liver results in conditions favorable for vegetative growth. Fluke-induced liver damage also is considered critical in the pathogenesis of bacillary hemoglobinuria. In this disease, the growth of *Cl. hemolyticum* in the liver is favored because of fluke-induced necrosis.

The signs of chronic fascioliasis are caused by the activity of mature flukes in the bile ducts, and the severity of signs is dependent on the parasite burden. Severe weight loss is characteristic in advanced cases. There is profound anemia due to fluke-induced blood loss directly through the biliary tract.[185] Hypoproteinemia results in facial and intermandibular edema, with abdominal distention due to ascites being observed less frequently.

The course of the natural disease may be 1 to 3 months. Some sheep may survive severe fascioliasis but remain cachectic for long periods of time. In addition to overt clinical illness and mortality, chronic fascioliasis produces important production losses in apparently healthy cattle[186] and sheep.[187]

The clinical diagnosis of chronic fascioliasis often is suggested by the clinical signs and the history of disease on affected pastures. Fluke eggs can be identified in the feces in chronic infections, but sheep from affected farms often have a frequency of infection approaching 100%. A similar problem occurs in evaluating lesions found at necropsy. The quantitative severity of lesions must be evaluated to determine whether fascioliasis is the primary clinical problem. There may be concurrent intestinal parasitism, e.g., *Ostertagia, Haemonchus,* which can complicate the diagnostic process.

The control of fascioliasis is directed toward elimination of egg-laying adult flukes from the ruminant host and eradication of the snail. The adult fluke can be effectively removed by administration of carbon tetrachloride or hexachlorethane. In chronic fascioliasis, however, most of the damage to the major bile ducts is irreversible. Snail eradication has become progressively more difficult because of environmental restrictions on the use of molluscacides such as copper sulfate. For this reason and because of cost and difficulties in application, low wet areas that would be ideal for snail growth can be fenced to prevent pasturing. It also is useful to prevent cattle and sheep from being pastured together. Clinically normal cattle can serve as an important source of contaminating fluke eggs for sheep.[187]

Hepatobiliary disease produced by liver flukes also is observed in other domestic species. Although not considered to be a major problem in the United States, in certain areas of the world liver flukes may produce significant disease in pet animals; e.g., the liver fluke, *Platynosomum fastosum,* is considered to be the most important disease of cats in the Bahamas.[188] Clinical signs caused by progressive liver disease include dullness, anorexia, weight loss, variable degrees of jaundice, and, in some cases, abdominal distention due to ascites. Hepatomegaly is associated with sclerosing cholangitis.[189] *Amphimerus pseudofelineus,*[190] *Opisthorchis tenuicollis,*[188] and *Parametorchis* spp.[191] have been reported in the United States. In addition to snails, the life cycle of these flukes frequently involves species of fish as a second intermediate host, and it is possible to control infection by limiting ingestion of fresh fish.

Liver Abscess—Suppurative Hepatitis

Abscesses of the liver occur in all species but produce clinical disease most frequently in cattle. In this species they may occur in multiple sites within the parenchyma or as a single large abscess located near the hilus of the liver.

Multiple abscesses are observed with significant frequency in slaughtered cattle which have been fattened in feedlots and fed high concentrate rations. In one series of 1807 fat cattle, 322 (17.8%) had liver abscesses.[192] The organism most frequently isolated from such abscesses is *Spherophorus necrophorous,*[193,194] and the condition sometimes is called *necrobacillosis.* The distribution of lesions has suggested a metastatic origin of the initial hepatic lesion, and evidence has been provided to support the view that the causative organism enters the portal circulation through focal lesions of rumenitis.[195]

Ruminal ulcers are observed with increased frequency in cattle fed high concentrate rations. Such abscesses are usually found incidentally at slaughter. It is unusual for this type of liver abscess to produce obvious clinical disease. The economic loss incurred by condemnation of affected livers, however, is very important.

Clinical manifestations are more frequently observed in cattle with one or two large abscesses near the hilus of the liver. In such abscesses, *Corynebacterium pyogenes* or *Escherichia coli* are more frequently isolated. Several distinctly different clinical syndromes can result. There may be local inflammation and peritonitis adjacent to the abscess, resulting in anterior abdominal pain and in an illness which clinically is difficult to distinguish from traumatic reticuloperitonitis. In other cases, the abscess may dissect into either the hepatic vein or the caudal vena cava with associated thrombus formation.[55] The introduction of pus directly into the bloodstream causes an acute, frequently fatal, anaphylactoid reaction characterized by urticaria and respiratory distress, a manifestation of severe pulmonary edema. In some cases, there is metastasis from liver abscesses and an associated thrombus of the vena cava to the lung where the septic emboli cause aneurysmic changes in the affected branches of the pulmonary artery. Occasionally, such infected aneurysms rupture into adjacent bronchi producing epistaxis. Epistaxis may be recurrent resulting in anemia, or there may be a single massive, fatal hemorrhage. Rarely, hepatic abscesses cause obstruction of hepatic vein outflow resulting in marked congestion of the liver, hepatomegaly, and, in some cases, ascites.[54,55]

Congenital Anomalies of the Portal Vein (Portacaval Shunts)

In 1974, a series of dogs with hepatic insufficiency were reported in which disturbed liver function was attributed to congenital abnormalities of the portal vein.[12] In these dogs, radiographic demonstrations showed functional vascular shunts which allowed portal blood to bypass the liver and to flow directly into the systemic circulation. Patency of the ductus venosum accounted for half of these portacaval shunts. Other vascular abnormalities included portal vein atresia with functional collateral portasystemic shunts, and anomalous anastomotic shunts from the portal vein to the caudal vena cava (Fig. 25–8) or the azygous vein.

A total of 36 similar canine cases of portasystemic anastomoses now have been reported.[12,13,15,196,197] Portasystemic shunting was reported recently in a dog with situs inversus.[198] Portacaval anastomosis also has been described in the horse.[199]

Of 36 cases of portacaval anastomoses, 31 were purebred dogs representing 22 breeds. Six of the 36 were German Shepherds (17%) and 4 were Miniature Schnauzers (11%). Clinical recognition of the disorder occurred in dogs from 6 weeks to 4½ years of age. Both sexes appeared to be equally affected.

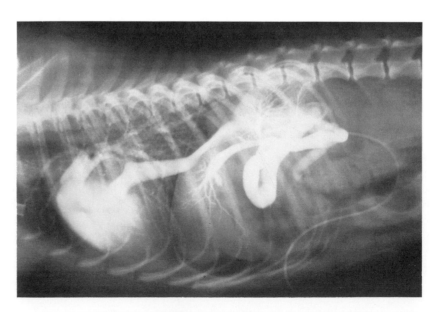

Figure 25–8. Portal venogram of a 4-year-old Miniature Schnauzer with large, tortuous portacaval shunt. Intrahepatic vessels and caudal vena cava were visualized simultaneously following infusion of contrast material into small jejunal vein. (From Barrett et al.[15])

Young affected dogs often are small for their age, and their growth is said to be "stunted." Older dogs are admitted to the clinic with histories of weight loss and gastrointestinal complaints including inappetence, vomiting and/or diarrhea, and gaseous abdominal distention following eating. Polydipsia and polyuria also are frequent historic complaints. More than half the patients with shunts are admitted with obvious signs of central nervous system disturbance which may include the following: ataxia, circling movements, head pressing, stupor, seizures, and amaurotic blindness.

Presenting physical findings other than those suggested by the history often are unremarkable. Clinical jaundice is almost always absent. Radiologic examination of the abdomen may demonstrate a remarkably small liver shadow, but this is difficult to appreciate by abdominal palpation. Clinical ascites has been reported in three of six dogs in one series[13] but has not been observed by others.

Typically, the SGPT and SAP levels are moderately but significantly elevated. In almost all cases, BSP retention is increased from a normal of 5% or less at 30 minutes to 15 to 40% retention. Fasting blood ammonia values often are elevated, but this is not an invariable finding. We have compared the ammonia levels before eating to those 1 and 2 hours following a protein-containing meal. In normal dogs, there is less than a two-fold increase in postprandial blood ammonia, and often no increase is observed. In dogs with portacaval shunts, the postprandial blood ammonia value usually exceeds the fasting value by more than a factor of 2. However, we also have seen dogs with shunts that have had normal blood ammonia values following feeding.

The definitive diagnosis of functional portacaval anastomoses is based on radiologic examination using portovenography. Splenoportograms are used in some clinics with contrast medium injected directly into the splenic pulp or into a catheterized splenic vein. Catheterization of a small jejunal vein also is satisfactory (Fig. 25–9). In both cases, contrast medium pacifies the normal liver within 2 to 4 seconds following bolus injection. Radiographs taken at 4 and 8 seconds following injection can be used to identify the functional shunts.

Treatment has been primarily palliative using supportive therapy and dietary manipulations to control signs of hepatic encephalopathy. Recently, a partial surgical closure of a shunt was said to have had a satisfactory clinical outcome. An earlier case died following complete surgical closure of the shunt.[200]

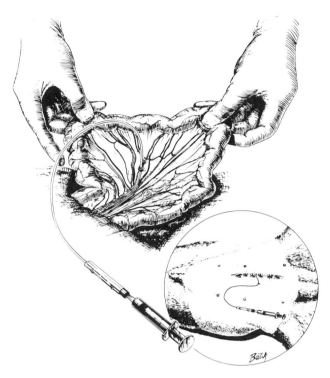

Figure 25–9. Schematic drawing of the isolation and catheterization of the jejunal vein in preparation for portal venography. (From Barrett et al.[15])

Intrahepatic Arteriovenous Fistula

Intrahepatic arteriovenous fistulae have been reported in the dog[201–203] and in the cat.[204] The canine patients so far reported all began to show clinical signs of hepatic disease during the first months of life and were assumed to have congenital arteriovenous fistulae (vascular hamartoma).

The fistulae produce portal hypertension with ascites of low protein content a prominent clinical feature (see earlier section, Clinical Signs of Hepatic Insufficiency). With very large fistulae, blood flow in the portal vein is completely reversed and prominent collateral vessels develop. Because they are seen in young dogs with moderate increases in alanine aminotransferase and in BSP retention and with suspicion of liver disease, arteriovenous fistulae must be differentiated from primary portacaval shunts. In some cases, palpation of the abnormal vascular structure is possible, and this may induce abdominal pain.

Diagnosis is most often established at exploratory laparotomy. The only treatment is complete surgical removal of the fistulae, which, because of size and complicated vascular connections, may be extremely difficult.

Drug-Induced Hepatic Toxicity

Two basic types of liver injury are produced by drugs and other hepatotoxins. Acute necrosis of hepatocytes is the characteristic effect of some, while others produce a cholestatic-cholangiolytic syndrome sometimes associated with inflammation of portal tracts and cirrhosis.

Carbon tetrachloride is one of the most extensively investigated hepatotoxic substances. A single toxic dose produces centrilobular necrosis and diffuse fatty infiltration. Biochemical and ultrastructural studies have demonstrated functional and morphologic changes of cell organelles as early as 1 to 5 hours following administration, with maximum damage occurring within 24 to 48 hours.[205] It is believed that actual damage is caused by a toxic metabolite of carbon tetrachloride, a free radical produced in the endoplasmic reticulum.[207] Drugs which stimulate proliferation of the smooth endoplasmic reticulum and increase the activity of many drug metabolizing enzymes, e.g., phenobarbital and DDT, significantly enhance the toxicity of carbon tetrachloride.[205,207] Starvation and other dietary changes also significantly alter the severity of damage produced by a given dosage of carbon tetrachloride.[207-209]

Several groups of therapeutic agents have been found to interfere with formation and/or excretion of bile. Therapeutic doses of primidone[210] and other anticonvulsants[211] have been reported to produce severe liver disease occasionally. Evidence of cholestasis also has been demonstrated in normal dogs receiving phenobarbital, primidone, or diphenylhydantoin.[212] The toxic effects of many drugs are variable, depending on the species studied. The dog, at least under special circumstances, develops cholestasis on dosages of drugs which do not affect other species.[213]

Treatment of dogs with glucocorticoids has been reported recently to induce hepatic disease.[214] Hepatomegaly was recognized clinically. Such dogs had moderate elevations in SGPT and SAP and often had prolonged retention of BSP. Histologically, there was centrilobular vacuolization and focal necrosis. Complete reversal of biochemical and morphologic abnormalities occurred following withdrawal of corticosteroid therapy. The importance of this form of toxic hepatopathy is that it be recognized during prolonged steroid therapy so that it is not confused with other primary forms of hepatopathy.

CLINICAL MANAGEMENT OF HEPATIC INSUFFICIENCY AND HEPATIC FAILURE

The medical treatment of liver disease generally is directed toward support of the patient and is dictated by existing or anticipated signs of hepatic insufficiency including encephalopathy, ascites, photosensitization, or coagulation disorders and a variety of less conspicuous signs. Nutritional management usually involves providing rations that are relatively low in protein but high in biologic protein quality, high in carbohydrate, but moderate in amounts of fat. Adjustments in diet are required when there is intolerance to protein, salt, and occasionally fat. Dietary protein, particularly meat, should be eliminated in the acute or active stages of canine hepatic encephalopathy and added in adjusted amounts during periods of remission. Roughages or concentrates high in protein should be reduced in horses with similar signs. Complete intolerance to dietary protein should be considered an unfavorable prognostic sign. Sodium restriction is important in cases of hepatic insufficiency with ascites and/or edema. Intolerance to fat usually is characterized by diarrhea and/or steatorrhea, and these signs can be partially controlled by fat restriction.

Specific types of liver disease may require special diet therapy. For example, in Bedlington terriers in which copper retention is believed to play a critical role in the pathogenesis of chronic hepatitis and cirrhosis, restriction of dietary copper clearly is indicated. The administration of D-penicillamine also has been recommended in this disease at a dose of 250 mg per day in one or in two divided doses.[215] This drug is a potent chelator of copper in that it mobilizes stored copper and facilitates urinary excretion.

The maniacal signs frequently encountered in horses with hepatic encephalopathy must be controlled with sedatives, and for this purpose, the phenothiazine tranquilizers are valuable. Other therapy in hepatic encephalopathy is aimed at reducing the production of ammonia and other suspected neurotoxins produced by intestinal bacteria. Cathartics or enemas with dilute dioctyl sodium sulfosuccinate (DSS) can be administered to prevent intestinal stasis, reducing contact time of colonic contents and decreasing ammonia absorption.[9] In addition to dietary restriction of protein, ammonia production by intestinal bacteria can be reduced by the administration of nonabsorbable broad-spectrum antibiotics such as neomycin. A dose of 50 to 100 mg/kg of neomycin sulfate can be used in horses and dogs and is sufficient to depress bacterial growth and metabolism. Nonabsorbable, soluble carbohydrates such as lactulose (1, 4-galactosidofructose) also have been recommended for use in dogs.[216] Such carbohydrates pass unaltered to the colon and are fermented by colonic bacteria to organic acids, e.g., volatile fatty acids and lactic acid. This results in acidification of the colonic contents which favors the conversion of free ammonia to ammonium ion, which is poorly absorbed, consequently reducing the amount of ammonia reaching the liver via the portal vein.[217] Lactulose also acts as an osmotic cathartic. In controlled studies with human subjects, neomycin and lactulose appear to be equally effective in controlling signs of hepatic encephalopathy.[218]

The liver plays a central role in maintenance of the blood glucose concentration. In advanced hepatic failure, hypoglycemia may develop and contribute to the pathogenesis of hepatic encephalopathy. In such cases, glucose may be administered orally or in a continuous intravenous infusion of 5 or 10% dextrose.

If massive ascites is present, symptomatic relief of respiratory distress or the sheer weight of the fluid may be obtained by abdominal paracentesis. Only a fraction of the fluid should be removed initially. Rapid and complete removal may precipitate changes in the distribution of the circulating blood volume leading to hypotension and possible peripheral vascular collapse. After initial removal of fluid, there is little indication for continued paracentesis because of the loss of plasma protein and the risk of peritonitis.

The medical management of ascites of hepatic origin is similar to that recommended for congestive heart failure. Dietary sodium should be reduced. Diuretic therapy should be administered to produce reasonably slow diuresis in which the excess body sodium is eliminated but metabolic complications (e.g., hypokalemia) are avoided. The ability to excrete ascitic fluid is limited, and a loss of more than 5% of body weight per week can result in the reduction in volume of body fluid compartments other than the extracellular fluid. The potent natriuretic diuretics such as furosemide have been recommended using the smallest and least frequent dose found to be effective in mobilizing ascitic fluid. Diuretic-induced hypovolemia accompanied by azotemia and hypokalemia can aggravate potential

or existing encephalopathy. Diuretics that inhibit carbonic anhydrase increase renal production of ammonia. If alkalemia results, problems of management of encephalopathy are compounded.[217]

Portacaval anastomosis has been used in the control of ascites associated with liver disease.[219] Such a surgical approach should be recommended with care because of the possibility of inducing hepatic encephalopathy (vide supra).

Supplementation with fat and water-soluble vitamins is considered to be empirical but is accepted clinical practice. Vitamin K is particularly indicated in cases with severe, diffuse hepatocellular disease or with long-standing cholestasis. The synthesis of coagulation factors II, VI, IX, and X is dependent on vitamin K. In the presence of sufficient functional hepatic mass, the administration of vitamin K can rapidly and dramatically decrease the prothrombin time in dogs with liver disease.

An animal on a balanced ration has little need for lipotrophic medication, but lipotrophic substances have been used empirically in the management of hepatic disease for many years. Most proprietary preparations include choline, methionine, and inositol. The amino acid methionine can replace dietary choline as precursor of phosphorylcholine, which is important in lipoprotein formation and fat transport mechanisms. Methionine should be used cautiously where encephalopathy is existent or is anticipated, because it is metabolized within the intestine to mercaptans which may act synergistically with ammonia to aggravate encephalopathy.[32]

The medical management of chronic active hepatitis requires prudent clinical decision and is guided by laboratory examinations and/or clinical signs expressed by the affected animal. Treatment is generally supportive with an emphasis on good nutrition. Dietary adjustments are sometimes necessary to accommodate hypoproteinemia, encephalopathy, ascites, and hypoglycemia. Glucocorticoids are indicated in selected cases because of their anti-inflammatory, immunosuppressive, or euphoric effects. Prednisolone is the preferred form.[182] Continuous administration of glucocorticoid is justified only after histopathologic examination of liver tissue obtained at biopsy and/or observation of symptomatic benefit to the affected animal. Periodic hematologic examinations will aid in the prediction of excessive glucocorticoid effects. Overdosage is possible because the catabolism of both endogenous and exogenous steroids by the diseased liver may be slower than normal.[182] The potential toxicity of glucocorticoids (i.e., steroid-induced hepatopathy) has been alluded to earlier. Additional emphasis on the importance of performing a liver biopsy prior to administration of glucocorticoid is made because the historic and laboratory features of chronic active hepatitis often resemble those of other forms of liver disease (e.g., lipidosis and neoplasia).

The high mortality observed in most forms of hepatic insufficiency is evidence of the inadequacy of current therapeutic methods. Clearly, effort may be more fruitful if applied to the prevention of hepatic disease. In the case of the pyrrolizidine alkaloid- and aflatoxin-induced hepatopathy, proper control of pastures and prevention of the consumption of contaminated hay, grain, or other food seem to be practicable procedures. The incidence of acute hepatitis in dogs, as pointed out previously, has been remarkably reduced by ICH vaccination. Much remains to be learned about the pathogenesis of chronic hepatitis in dogs, however, and about acute hepatitis in horses. Such knowledge should provide improved methods for control and prevention in the future.

REFERENCES

1. With, T. K.: Bile Pigments, Chemical, Biological and Clinical Aspects. New York, Academic Press, 1968.
2. Hjerpe, C. A., Tennant, B. C., Crenshaw, G. L., and Baker, N. F.: Ovine fascioliasis in California. J.A.V.M.A. *159*:1266, 1971.
3. Finn, J. P., and Tennant, B.: Hepatic encephalopathy in cattle. Cornell Vet. *64*:136, 1974.
4. Tennant, B., Baldwin, B., Evans, C. D., and Kaneko, J. J.: Diseases of the equine liver. Proc. Am. Assoc. Equine Pract., 21st Annu. Meet., Boston, 1975, p. 410.
5. Gronwall, R., and Mia, A. S.: Fasting hyperbilirubinemia in horses. Am. J. Dig. Dis. *17*:473, 1972.
6. Thomsett, L. R.: Acute hepatic failure in the horse. Equine Vet. J. *3*:15, 1971.
7. Gibbons, W. J., Hokanson, J. F., Wiggins, A. M., and Schmitz, M. B.: Cirrhosis of the liver in horses. North Am. Vet. *31*:229, 1950.
8. Center, S. A., Baldwin, B. H., and Tennant, B.: Unpublished data.
9. Tennant, B., Evans, C. D., Schwartz, L. W., Gribble, D. H., and Kaneko, J. J.: Equine hepatic insufficiency. Vet. Clin. North Am. *3*:279, 1973.
10. Fowler, M. E.: Pyrrolizidine alkaloid poisoning in calves. J.A.V.M.A. *152*:1131, 1968.
11. Pearson, E. G.: Clinical manifestations of tansy ragwort poisoning. Mod. Vet. Pract. *58*:421, 1977.
12. Ewing, G. O., Suter, P. F., and Bailey, C. S.: Hepatic insufficiency associated with congenital anomalies of the portal vein in dogs. J.A.A.H.A. *10*:463, 1974.
13. Cornelius, L. M., Thrall, D. E., Halliwell, W. H., Frank, G. M., Kern, A. J., and Woods, C. B.: Anomalous portosystemic anastomoses associated with chronic hepatic insufficiency in six young dogs. J.A.V.M.A. *167*:220, 1975.
14. Audell, A., Jönsson, L., and Lannek, B.: Congenital porta-caval shunts in the dog. A description of three cases. Zentralbl. Veterinaermed. [A] *21*:797, 1974.
15. Barrett, R. E., deLahunta, A., Roenigk, W. J., Hoffer, R. E., and Coons, F. H.: Four cases of congenital portacaval shunt in the dog. J. Small Anim. Pract. *17*:71, 1976.
16. Oliver, J. E.: Hepatic neuropathies—a review with two case histories. V.M./S.A.C. *60*:498, 1965.
17. Strombeck, D. R., Weiser, M. G., and Kaneko, J. J.: Hyperammonemia and hepatic encephalopathy in the dog. J.A.V.M.A. *166*:1105, 1975.
18. Strombeck, D. R., Meyer, D. J., and Freedland, R. A.: Hyperammonemia due to a urea cycle enzyme deficiency in two dogs. J.A.V.M.A. *166*:1109, 1975.
19. Rose, A. L., Gardner, C. A., McConnell, J. D., and Bull, L. B.: Field and experimental investigation of "walk-about" disease of horses (Kimberly horse disease) in Northern Australia: crotalaria poisoning in horses. Part II. Aust. Vet. J. *33*:49, 1957.
20. Cornelius, C. E., Gazmuri, G., Gronwall, R., and Rhode, E. A.: Preliminary studies on experimental hyperbilirubinemia and hepatic coma in the horse. Cornell Vet. *55*:110, 1965.
21. Hooper, P. T.: Spongy degeneration in the brain in relation to hepatic disease and ammonia toxicity in domestic animals. Vet. Rec. *90*:37, 1972.
22. Bromberg, P. A., Robin, E. D., and Forkner, C. E.: The existence of ammonia in blood *in vivo* with observations on the significance of the NH_4^+-NH_3 system. J. Clin. Invest. *39*:332, 1960.
23. Stabenau, J. R., Warren, K. S., and Rall, D. P.: The role of pH gradient in the distribution of ammonia between blood and cerebrospinal fluid, brain and muscle. J. Clin. Invest. *38*:373, 1959.
24. Warren, K. S., and Nathan, D. G.: The passage of ammonia across the blood-brain barrier and its relation to blood pH. J. Clin. Invest. *37*:1724, 1958.
25. Castell, D. O., and Moore, E. W.: Ammonia absorption from the human colon. The role of nonionic diffusion. Gastroenterology *60*:33, 1971.
26. Levenson, S. M., and Tennant, B.: Some metabolic and nutritional studies with germfree animals. Fed. Proc. *22*:109, 1963.
27. Nance, F. C., Kaufman, H. J., and Kline, D. G.: Role of urea in the hyperammonemia of germ-free Eck fistula dogs. Gastroenterology *66*:108, 1974.
28. Nance, F. C., Batson, R. C., and Kline, D. G.: Ammonia production in germ-free Eck fistula dogs. Surgery *70*:169, 1971.
29. Nance, F. C., and Kline, D. G.: Eck's fistula encephalopathy in germfree dogs. Ann. Surg. *174*:856, 1971.
30. Windmueller, H. G., and Spaeth, A. E.: Uptake and metabolism of plasma glutamine by the small intestine. J. Biol. Chem. *249*:5070, 1974.
31. Hjerpe, C. A.: Serum hepatitis in the horse. J.A.V.M.A. *144*:734, 1964.
32. Zieve, L., Doizaki, W. M., and Zieve, F. J.: Synergism between mercaptans and ammonia or fatty acids in the production of coma: a possible role for mercaptans in the pathogenesis of hepatic coma. J. Lab. Clin. Med. *83*:16, 1974.
33. Zieve, L., Nicoloff, D. M., and Mahadevan, V.: Effect of hepatectomy on volatile free fatty acids of the blood. Gastroenterology *54*:1285, 1968 (Abst.).
34. Takahashi, Y., Muto, Y., Nakao, K., and Okinaka, S.: Volatile fatty acids in hepatic coma. Proc. 3rd World Congr. Gastroenterol. [Tokyo] *3*:510, 1966.
35. Jubb, K. V. F., and Kennedy, P. C.: The Pathology of Domestic Animals, Vol. 2. New York, Academic Press, 1970, p. 216.
36. Hooper, P. T., Best, S. M., and Murray, D. R.: Hyperammonaemia and spongy degeneration of the brain in sheep affected with hepatic necrosis. Res. Vet. Sci. *16*:216, 1974.
37. Hooper, P. T.: Spongy degeneration in the central nervous system of domestic animals. Part I: Morphology. Acta Neuropathol. *31*:325, 1975.
38. Hooper, P. T.: Spongy degeneration in the central nervous system of domestic animals. Part II. Chemical analysis and vascular permeability studies. Acta Neuropathol. *31*:335, 1975.
39. Hooper, P. T.: Spongy degeneration in the central nervous system of domestic animals. Part III: Occurrence and pathogenesis—hepatocerebral disease caused by hyperammonaemia. Acta Neuropathol. *31*:343, 1975.
40. Clare, N. T.: Photosensitization in Diseases of Domestic Animals. England, Commonwealth Agricultural Bureaux, 1952.
41. Blum, H. F., Watrous, W. G., and West, R. J.: On the mechanism of photosensitization in man. Am. J. Physiol. *113*:350, 1935.
42. Cook, J. S., and Blum, H. F.: Dose relationships and oxygen dependence in ultraviolet and photodynamic hemolysis. J. Cell. Comp. Physiol. *53*:41, 1959.
43. Schothorst, A. A., Van Steveninck, J., Went, L. N., and Suurmond, D.: Protoporphyrin-induced photohemolysis in protoporphyria and in normal red blood cells. Clin. Chim. Acta *28*:41, 1970.
44. Clare, N. T.: Photosensitivity diseases in New Zealand. IV. The photosensitizing agent in Southdown photosensitivity. N. Z. J. Sci. Tech. *27A*:23, 1945.
45. Kaneko, J. J., Zinkl, J. G., and Keeton, K. S.: Erythrocyte porphyrin and erythrocyte survival in bovine erythropoietic porphyria. Am. J. Vet. Res. *32*:1981, 1971.

46. Cornelius, C. E., and Gronwall, R. R.: Congenital photosensitivity and hyperbilirubinemia in Southdown sheep in the United States. Am. J. Vet. Res. *29*:291, 1968.

47. Rimington, C., and Quin, J. I.: Studies on the photosensitisation of animals in South Africa. VII. The nature of the photosensitising agent in geeldikkop. Onderstepoort J. Vet. Sci. Anim. Ind. *3*:137, 1934.

48. Clare, N. T.: Photosensitivity diseases in New Zealand. III. The photosensitizing agent in facial eczema. N. Z. J. Sci. Tech. *25A*:202, 1944.

49. Quin, J. I., Rimington, C., and Roets, G. C. S.: Studies on the photosensitisation of animals in South Africa. VIII. The biological formation of phylloerythrin in the digestive tracts of various domesticated animals. Onderstepoort J. Vet. Sci. Anim. Ind. *4*:463, 1935.

50. Slater, T. F., and Riley, P. A.: Lysosomal damage and photosensitization produced by phylloerythrin. Biochem. J. *96*:39P, 1965.

51. Riemerschmid, G., and Quin, J. I.: Studies on the photosensitisation of animals in South Africa. XI. The reaction of the sensitised merino skin to radiation in different regions of the spectrum. Onderstepoort J. Vet. Sci. Anim. Ind. *17*:89, 1941.

52. Fowler, M. E.: Clinical manifestations of primary hepatic insufficiency in the horse. J.A.V.M.A. *147*:55, 1965.

53. Whitlock, R. H., and Brown, W. R.: Chronic cholangiohepatitis in a dairy cow. Cornell Vet. *59*:515, 1969.

54. Breeze, R. G., Pirie, H. M., Selman, I. E., and Wiseman, A.: Pulmonary arterial thrombo-embolism and pulmonary arterial mycotic aneurysms in cattle with vena caval thrombosis: a condition resembling the Hughes-Stovin syndrome. J. Pathol. *119*:229, 1976.

55. Selman, I. E., Wiseman, A., Petrie, L., Pirie, H. M., and Breeze, R. G.: A respiratory syndrome in cattle resulting from thrombosis of the posterior vena cava. Vet. Rec. *94*:459, 1974.

56. Lawson, J. D., and Weissbein, A. S.: The puddle sign—an aid in the diagnosis of minimal ascites. N. Engl. J. Med., *260*:652, 1959.

57. Starling, E. H.: The influence of mechanical factors on lymph production. J. Physiol. *16*:224, 1894.

58. Brauer, R. W.: Liver circulation and function. Physiol. Rev. *43*:115, 1963.

59. Field, M. E., Leigh, O. C., Heim, J. W., and Drinker, C. K.: The protein content and osmotic pressure of blood serum and lymph from various sources in the dog. Am. J. Physiol. *110*:174, 1934.

60. Nix, J. T., Flock, E. V., and Bollman, J. L.: Influence of cirrhosis on proteins of cisternal lymph. Am. J. Physiol. *164*:117, 1951.

61. Nix, J. T., Mann, F. C., Bollman, J. L., Grindlay, J. H., and Flock, E. V.: Alterations of protein constituents of lymph by specific injury to the liver. Am. J. Physiol. *164*:119, 1951.

62. Schilling, J. A., McCoord, A. B., Clausen, S. W., Troup, S. B., and McKee, F. W.: Experimental ascites. Studies of electrolyte balance in dogs with partial and complete occlusion of the portal vein and of the vena cava above and below the liver. J. Clin. Invest. *31*:702, 1952.

63. Volwiler, W., Grindlay, J. H., and Bollman, J. L.: The relationship of portal vein pressure to the formation of ascites—an experimental study. Gastroenterology *14*:40, 1950.

64. Berman, J. K., and Hull, J. E.: Experimental ascites—its production and control. Surgery *32*:67, 1952.

65. Orloff, M. J., and Snyder, G. B.: Experimental ascites. II. The effects of portacaval shunts on ascites produced with an internal vena cava cannula. Surgery *50*:220, 1961.

66. Orloff, M. J., and Snyder, G. B.: Experimental ascites. I. Production of ascites by gradual occlusion of the hepatic veins with an internal vena cava cannula. Surgery *50*:789, 1961.

67. Orloff, M. J., Wall, M. H., Hickman, E. B., and Spitz, B. R.: Experimental ascites. III. Production of ascites by direct ligation of hepatic veins. Surgery *54*:627, 1963.

68. Orloff, M. J., Spitz, B. R., Wall, M. H., Thomas, H. S., and Halasz, N. A.: Experimental ascites. IV. Comparison of the effects of end-to-end and side-to-side portacaval shunts on intractable ascites. Surgery *56*:784, 1964.

69. Orloff, M. J., Wright, P. W., DeBenedetti, M. J., Halasz, N. A., Annetts, D. L., Musicant, M. E., and Goodhead, B.: Experimental ascites. VII. The effects of external drainage of the thoracic duct on ascites and hepatic hemodynamics. Arch. Surg. *93*:119, 1966.

70. Witte, C. L., Witte, M. H., Dumont, A. E., Frist, J., and Cole, W. R.: Lymph protein in hepatic cirrhosis and experimental hepatic and portal venous hypertension. Ann. Surg. *168*:567, 1968.

71. Witte, C. L., Chung, Y. C., Witte, M. H., Sterle, O. F., and Cole, W. R.: Observations on the origin of ascites from experimental extrahepatic portal congestion. Ann. Surg. *170*:1002, 1969.

72. Witte, M. H., Dumont, A. E., Cole, W. R., Witte, C. L., and Kintner, K.: Lymph circulation in hepatic cirrhosis: effect of portacaval shunt. Ann. Intern. Med. *70*:303, 1969.

73. Hyatt, R. E., Lawrence, G. H., and Smith, J. R.: Observations on the origin of ascites from experimental hepatic congestion. J. Lab. Clin. Med. *45*:274, 1955.

74. Witte, M. H., Witte, C. L., and Dumont, A. E.: Progress in liver disease: physiological factors involved in the causation of cirrhotic ascites. Gastroenterology *61*:742, 1971.

75. Rothschild, M. A., Oratz, M., and Schreiber, S. S.: Albumin metabolism. Gastroenterology *64*:324, 1973.

76. Witte, C. L., Witte, M. H., Kintner, K., Cole, W. R., and Dumont, A. E.: Colloid osmotic pressure in hepatic cirrhosis and experimental ascites. Surg. Gynecol. Obstet. *133*:65, 1971.

77. Orloff, M. J., Ross, T. H., Baddeley, R. M., Nutting, R. O., Spitz, B. R., Sloop, R. D., Neesby, T., and Halasz, N. A.: Experimental ascites. VI. The effects of hepatic venous outflow obstruction and ascites on aldosterone secretion. Surgery *56*:83, 1964.

78. Orloff, M. J., Lipman, C. A., Noel, S. M., Halasz, N. A., and Neesby, T.: Hepatic regulation of aldosterone secretion by a humoral mediator. Surgery *58*:225, 1965.

79. Howards, S. S., Davis, J. O., Johnston, C. I., and Wright, F. S.: Steroidogenic response in normal dogs receiving blood from dogs with caval constriction. Am. J. Physiol. *214*:990, 1968.

80. Robinson, S. H., Tsong, M., Brown, B. W., and Schmid, R.: The sources of bile pigment in the rat: studies of the "early-labeled" fraction. J. Clin. Invest. *45*:1569, 1966.

81. Landaw, S. A., and Winchell, H. S.: Endogenous production of ^{14}CO: a method for calculation of RBC life span *in vivo*. Blood *36*:642, 1970.

82. Tenhunen, R., Marver, H. S., and Schmid, R.: Microsomal heme oxygenase: characterization of the enzyme. J. Biol. Chem. *244*:6388, 1969.

83. Tenhunen, R., Ross, M. E., Marver, H. S., and Schmid, R.: Reduced nicotinamide-adenine dinucleotide phosphate dependent biliverdin reductase: partial purification and characterization. Biochemistry *9*:298, 1970.

84. Tenhunen, R., Marver, H. S., and Schmid, R.: The enzymatic catabolism of hemoglobin: stimulation of microsomal heme oxygenase by hemin. J. Lab. Clin. Med. *75*:410, 1970.

85. Pimstone, N. R., Engel, P., Tenhunen, R., Seitz, P. T., Marver, H. S., and Schmid, R.: Inducible heme oxygenase in the kidney: a model for the homeostatic control of hemoglobin catabolism. J. Clin. Invest. *50*:2042, 1971.

86. de Schepper, J., and Van Der Stock, J.: Increased urinary bilirubin excretion after elevated free plasma haemoglobin levels. I. Variations in the calculated renal clearances of bilirubin in whole dogs. Arch. Int. Physiol. Biochim. *80*:279, 1972.

87. de Schepper, J., and Van Der Stock, J.: Increased urinary bilirubin excretion after elevated free plasma haemoglobin levels. II. Variations in the calculated renal clearances of bilirubin in isolated normothermic perfused dog's kidneys. Arch. Int. Physiol. Biochim. *80*:339, 1972.

88. Pimstone, N. R.: Renal degradation of hemoglobin. *In* Physiology and Disorders of Hemoglobin Degradation. Edited by R. Schmid, E. R. Jaffé, and P. M. Miescher. New York, Grune and Stratton, 1972, p. 31.

89. Arias, I. M.: Bilirubin metabolism. II. Excretion of bilirubin. *In* The Liver and Its Diseases. Edited by F. Schaffner, S. Sherlock, and C. M. Leevy. New York, Intercontinental Medical Book Corp., 1974, p. 97.

90. Habig, W. H., Pabst, M. J., Fleischner, G., Gatmaitan, Z., Arias, I. M., and Jakoby, W. B.: The identity of glutathione S-transferase B with ligandin, a major binding protein of liver. Proc. Natl. Acad. Sci. *71*:3879, 1974.

91. Kaplowitz, N., Percy-Robb, I. W., and Javitt, N. B.: Role of hepatic anion-binding protein in bromsulphthalein conjugation. J. Exp. Med. *138*:483, 1973.

92. Talafant, E.: Properties and composition of the bile pigment giving a direct diazo reaction. Nature *178*:312, 1956.

93. Grodsky, G. M., and Carbone, J. V.: The synthesis of bilirubin glucuronide by tissue homogenates. J. Biol. Chem. *226*:449, 1957.

94. Schmid, R.: Direct-reacting bilirubin, bilirubin glucuronide, in serum, bile and urine. Science *124*:76, 1956.

95. Cornelius, C. E., Kilgore, W. W., and Wheat, J. D.: Chromatographic identification of bile pigments in several species. Cornell Vet. *50*:47, 1960.

96. Gordon, E. R., Goresky, C. A., Chang, T.-H., and Perlin, A. S.: The isolation and characterization of bilirubin diglucuronide, the major bilirubin conjugate in dog and human bile. Biochem. J. *155*:477, 1976.

97. Fevery, J., Van Hees, G. P., Leroy, P., Compernolle, F., and Heirwegh, K. P. M.: Excretion in dog bile of glucose and xylose conjugates of bilirubin. Biochem. J. *125*:803, 1971.

98. Heirwegh, K. P. M., Fevery, J., Michiels, R., Van Hees, G. P., and Compernolle, F.: Separation by thin-layer chromatography and structure elucidation of bilirubin conjugates isolated from dog bile. Biochem. J. *145*:185, 1975.

99. Noir, B. A.: Bilirubin conjugates in bile of man, rat, and dog. Biochem. J. *155*:365, 1976.

100. Cornelius, C. E., Kelly, K. C., and Himes, J. A.: Heterogeneity of bilirubin conjugates in several animal species. Cornell Vet. *65*:90, 1975.

101. Alpert, S., Mosher, M., Shanske, A., and Arias, I. M.: Multiplicity of hepatic excretory mechanisms for organic anions. J. Gen. Physiol. *53*:238, 1969.

102. Goresky, C. A., Haddad, H. H., Kluger, W. S., Nadeau, B. E., and Bach, G. G.: The enhancement of maximal bilirubin excretion with taurocholate-induced increments in bile flow. Can. J. Physiol. Pharmacol. *52*:389, 1974.

103. Gustaffson, B. E., and Lanke, L. S.: Bilirubin and urobilins in germfree, ex-germfree, and conventional rats. J. Exp. Med. *112*:975, 1960.

104. Levy, M., Lester, R., and Levinsky, N. G.: Renal excretion of urobilinogen in the dog. J. Clin. Invest. *47*:2117, 1968.

105. Bollman, J. L., and Mann, F. C.: Studies of the physiology of the liver. XXII. The van den Bergh reaction in the jaundice following complete removal of the liver. Arch. Surg. *24*:675, 1932.

106. Hoffman, H. N., Whitcomb, F. F., Butt, H. R., and Bollman, J. L.: Bile pigments of jaundice. J. Clin. Invest. *39*:132, 1960.

107. Royer, M., Noir, B., de Walz, A. T., and Lozzio, B.: Conjugaison de la bilirubine chez le chien hepatectomise. Rev. Int. Hepat. *15*:1351, 1965.

108. Royer, M., Noir, B. A., Sfarcich, D., and Nanet, H.: Extrahepatic bilirubin formation and conjugation in the dog. Digestion *10*:423, 1974.

109. Schmid, R.: Bilirubin metabolism. I. Formation of bilirubin. *In* The Liver and Its Diseases. Edited by F. Schaffner, S. Sherlock, and C. M. Leevy. New York, Intercontinental Medical Book Corp., 1974, p. 85.

110. Fog, J., and Jellum, E.: Structure of bilirubin. Nature *198*:88, 1963.

111. Nichol, A. W., and Morrell, D. B.: Tautomerism and hydrogen bonding in bilirubin and biliverdin. Biochim. Biophys. Acta *177*:599, 1969.

112. Fulop, M., Sandson, J., and Brazeau, P.: Dialyzability, protein binding, and renal excretion of plasma conjugated bilirubin. J. Clin. Invest. *44*:666, 1965.

113. Laks, M. M., Pincus, I. J., and Goldberg, D.: Renal excretion of bilirubin in the common duct ligated dog. Gastroenterology *44*:469, 1963.

114. Wada, H., and Morino, Y.: Comparative studies on glutamic-oxalacetic transaminases from the mitochondrial and soluble fractions of mammalian tissues. Vitam. Horm. *22*:411, 1964.

115. Wilkinson, J. H.: Clinical applications of isoenzymes. Clin. Chem. *16*:733, 1970.

116. Cornelius, C. E., Bishop, J., Switzer, J., and Rhode, E. A.: Serum and tissue transaminase activities in domestic animals. Cornell Vet. *49*:116, 1959.

117. Cornelius, C. E., and Kaneko, J. J.: Serum transaminase activities in cats with hepatic necrosis. J.A.V.M.A. *137*:62, 1960.

118. Hoe, C. M., and Harvey, D. G.: An investigation into liver function tests in dogs. Part I—serum transaminases. J. Small Anim. Pract. *2*:22, 1961.

119. Hoe, C. M., and Jabara, A. G.: The use of serum enzymes as diagnostic aids in the dog. J. Comp. Pathol. *77*:245, 1967.

120. Kaplan, M. M.: Alkaline phosphatase. Gastroenterology *62*:452, 1972.

121. Emmelot, P., Bos, C. J., Benedetti, E. L., and Rumke, P. H.: Studies on plasma membranes. I. Chemical composition and enzyme content of plasma membranes isolated from rat liver. Biochim. Biophys. Acta *90*:126, 1964.

122. Haussler, M. R., Nagode, L. A., and Rasmussen, H.: Induction of intestinal brush border alkaline phosphatase by vitamin D and identity with Ca-ATPase. Nature (Lond.) *228*:1199, 1970.

123. Ahmed, K., and Judah, J. D.: Preparation of lipoproteins containing cation-dependent ATPase. Biochim. Biophys. Acta *93*:603, 1964.

124. Rogers, W. A.: Source of serum alkaline phosphatase in clinically normal and diseased dogs: a clinical study. J.A.V.M.A. *168*:934, 1976.

125. Nagode, L. A., Koestner, A., and Steinmeyer, C. L.: Organ-identifying properties of alkaline phosphatases from canine tissues. Clin. Chim. Acta *26*:45, 1969.

126. Hoffmann, W. E., and Dorner, J. L.: Separation of isoenzymes of canine alkaline phosphatase by cellulose acetate electrophoresis. J.A.A.H.A. *11*:283, 1975.

127. Nagode, L. A., Koestner, A., and Steinmeyer, C. L.: The effects of purification and serum proteins on the organ-identifying properties of alkaline phosphatases from canine tissues. Clin. Chim. Acta *26*:55, 1969.

128. Ruegnitz, P. C., and Schwartz, E.: Effects of chemical inhibition of alkaline phosphatase isoenzymes in the dog. Am. J. Vet. Res. *32*:1525, 1971.

129. Everett, R. M., Duncan, J. R., and Prasse, K. W.: Alkaline phosphatase, leucine aminopeptidase, and alanine aminotransferase activities with obstructive and toxic hepatic disease in cats. Am. J. Vet. Res. *38*:963, 1977.

130. Righetti, A. B.-B., and Kaplan, M. M.: Disparate responses of serum and hepatic alkaline phosphatase and 5'nucleotidase to bile duct obstruction in the rat. Gastroenterology *62*:1034, 1972.

131. Gutman, A. B., Hogg, B. M., and Olson, K. B.: Increased serum phosphatase activity without hyperbilirubinemia after ligation of hepatic ducts in dogs. Proc. Soc. Exp. Biol. Med. *44*:613, 1940.

132. Kaplan, M. M., and Righetti, A.: Induction of liver alkaline phosphatase by bile duct ligation. Biochim. Biophys. Acta *184*:667, 1969.

133. Kaplan, M., and Righetti, A.: Induction of rat liver alkaline phosphatase: the mechanism of the serum elevation in bile duct obstruction. J. Clin. Invest. *49*:508, 1970.

134. Pekarthy, J. M., Short, J., Lansing, A. I., and Lieberman, I.: Function and control of liver alkaline phosphatase. J. Biol. Chem. *247*:1767, 1972.

135. Dalgaard, J. B.: Phosphatase in cats with obstructive jaundice. Acta Physiol. Scand. *15*:290, 1948.

136. Cantarow, A., Stewart, H. L., and McCool, S. G.: Serum phosphatase in cats with total bile stasis. Proc. Soc. Exp. Biol. Med. *35*:87, 1936.

137. Flood, C. A., Gutman, E. B., and Gutman, A. B.: Serum and urine phosphatase activity in the cat after ligation of the common bile duct. Am. J. Physiol. *120*:696, 1937.

138. Sebesta, D. G., Bradshaw, F. J., and Prockop, D. J.: Source of the elevated serum alkaline phosphatase activity in biliary obstruction: studies utilizing isolated liver perfusion. Gastroenterology *47*:166, 1964.

139. Cornelius, C. E., Ben-Ezzer, J., and Arias, I. M.: Binding of sulfobromophthalein sodium (BSP) and other organic anions by isolated hepatic cell plasma membranes *in vitro*. Proc. Soc. Exp. Biol. Med. *124*:665, 1967.

140. Levi, A. J., Gatmaitan, Z., and Arias, I. M.: Two hepatic cytoplasmic protein fractions, Y and Z, and their possible role in the hepatic uptake of bilirubin, sulfobromophthalein, and other anions. J. Clin. Invest. *48*:2156, 1969.

141. Tennant, B.: Unpublished data.

142. Cornelius, C. E.: Liver function. *In* Clinical Biochemistry of Domestic Animals, Vol. I. Edited by J. J. Kaneko and C. E. Cornelius. New York, Academic Press, 1970, p. 161.

143. Panciera, R. J.: Serum hepatitis in the horse. J.A.V.M.A. *155*:408, 1969.

144. Qualls, C. W., and Gribble, D. H.: Equine serum hepatitis: a morphologic study. Lab. Invest. *34*:330, 1976 (Abst.).

145. Theiler, A.: Acute liver atrophy and parenchymatous hepatitis in horses. 5th and 6th Rep. Dir. Vet. Res., Dept. Agr., Union South Africa, 1919, p. 7.

146. Slagsvold, L.: Ikterus hos hester behandlet med miltbrandserum. Nor. Vet. Tidsskr. *30(2)*:69, 1938.

147. Shahan, M. S., Giltner, L. T., Davis, C. L., and Huffman, W. T.: "Secondary" disease occurring subsequent to infectious equine encephalomyelitis. Vet. Med. *34*:354, 1939.

148. Schofield, F. W., and Potter, H. R.: A report on the investigation into suspected outbreaks of encephalomyelitis during the summer and fall months of 1938. Report—Ont. Vet. College for 1938, 1940, p. 16.

149. Reference deleted.

150. Madsen, D. E.: Equine encephalomyelitis. Utah Acad. Sci. Arts Letters *11*:95, 1934.

151. Marsh, H.: Losses of undetermined cause following an outbreak of equine encephalomyelitis. J.A.V.M.A. *91*:88, 1937.

152. Marsh, H.: Supplementary note to article on equine encephalomyelitis. J.A.V.M.A. *91*:330, 1937.

153. Cox, H. R., Philip, C. B., Marsh, H., and Kilpatrick, J. W.: Observations incident to an outbreak of equine encephalomyelitis in the Bitterroot Valley of Western Montana. J.A.V.M.A. *93*:225, 1938.

154. Findlay, G. M., and MacCallum, F. O.: Hepatitis and jaundice

associated with immunization against certain virus diseases. Proc. R. Soc. Med. *31*:799, 1938.

155. Stenius, P. I.: Equine liver and brain disease in Finland in 1933. Skandinavisk Veterinartidskrift *31*:193, 1941.

156. Forenbacher, S., Marzan, B., and Topolnik, E.: Liver necrosis (dystrophia hepatis) in horses with particular consideration of etiology and therapy. Vet. Arch. *29*:322, 1959.

157. Robinson, M., Gopinath, C., and Hughes, D. L.: Histopathology of acute hepatitis in the horse. J. Comp. Pathol. *85*:111, 1975.

158. Rose, J. A., Immenschuh, R. D., and Rose, E. M.: Serum hepatitis in the horse. Proc. A.A.E.P. *20*:175, 1974.

159. Howarth, L., and Shires, M.: Serum hepatitis in a horse. Iowa State Univ. Vet. *38*:28, 1976.

160. Reference deleted.

161. McGavin, M. D., and Knake, R.: Hepatic midzonal necrosis in a pig fed aflatoxin and a horse fed moldy hay. Vet. Pathol. *14*:182, 1977.

162. Reference deleted.

163. Tennant, B., Baldwin, B. H., Silverman, S. L., and Makowski, C.: Clinical significance of hyperbilirubinemia in the horse. Proc. 1st Int. Symp. Equine Hematol., May 1975, p. 246.

164. Tennant, B. C., Evans, C. D., Kaneko, J. J., and Schalm, O. W.: Intravascular hemolysis associated with hepatic failure in the horse. Calif. Vet. *27*:15, 1972.

165. Tennant, B. C., Evans, C. D., Kaneko, J. J., and Schalm, O. W.: Hepatic failure in the horse. Mod. Vet. Pract. *53*:40, 1972.

166. Fowler, M. E.: Clinical manifestations of primary hepatic insufficiency in the horse. J.A.V.M.A. *147*:55, 1965.

167. Rubarth, S.: An acute virus disease with liver lesion in dogs (hepatitis contagiosa canis): a pathologico-anatomical and etiological investigation. Acta Pathol. Microbiol. Scand. (Suppl.) *69*:1, 1947.

168. Gillespie, J. H.: Infectious canine hepatitis. J.A.V.M.A. *132*:1, 1958.

169. Cabasso, V. J.: Infectious canine hepatitis virus. Ann. N. Y. Acad. Sci. *101*:498, 1962.

170. Carmichael, L. E.: The pathogenesis of ocular lesions of infectious canine hepatitis: 1. Pathology and virological observations. Pathol. Vet. *1*:73, 1964.

171. Carmichael, L. E.: The pathogenesis of ocular lesions of infectious canine hepatitis. II. Experimental ocular hypersensitivity produced by the virus. Pathol. Vet. *2*:344, 1965.

172. Aguirre, G., Carmichael, L. E., and Bistner, S. I.: Corneal endothelium in viral induced anterior uveitis. Ultrastructural changes following canine adenovirus type 1 infection. Arch. Ophthalmol. *93*:219, 1975.

173. Appel, M., Bistner, S. I., Menegus, M., and Carmichael, L. E.: Pathogenicity of low-virulence strains of two canine adenovirus types. Am. J. Vet. Res. *34*:543, 1973.

174. Givan, K. F., and Jeqeguel, A.: Infectious canine hepatitis: A virologic and ultrastructural study. Lab. Invest. *20*:36, 1969.

175. Gocke, D. J., Preisig, R., Morris, T. Q., McKay, D. G., and Bradley, S. E.: Experimental viral hepatitis in the dog: production of persistent disease in partially immune animals. J. Clin. Invest. *46*:1506, 1967.

176. Wigton, D. H., Kociba, G. J., and Hoover, E. A.: Infectious canine hepatitis: animal model for viral-induced disseminated intravascular coagulation. Blood *47*:287, 1976.

177. Strombeck, D. R., Krum, S., and Rogers, Q.: Coagulopathy and encephalopathy in a dog with acute hepatic necrosis. J.A.V.M.A. *169*:813, 1976.

178. Greene, C. E., Barsanti, J. A., and Jones, B. D.: Disseminated intravascular coagulation complicating aflatoxicosis in dog. Cornell Vet. *67*:29, 1977.

179. Preisig, R., Gocke, D., Morris, T., and Bradley, S. E.: Chronic hepatic injury following experimental viral hepatitis in the dog. Experientia *22*:701, 1966.

180. Gocke, D. J., Morris, T. Q., and Bradley, S. E.: Chronic hepatitis in the dog: the role of immune factors. J.A.V.M.A. *156*:1700, 1970.

181. Morris, T. Q., and Gocke, D. J.: Modified acute canine viral hepatitis—A model for physiologic study. Proc. Soc. Exp. Biol. Med. *139*:32, 1972.

182. Strombeck, D. R., Rogers, W., and Gribble, D.: Chronic active hepatitis in a dog. J.A.V.M.A. *169*:802, 1976.

183. Hardy, R. M., Stevens, J. B., and Stowe, C. M.: Chronic progressive hepatitis in Bedlington terriers associated with elevated liver copper concentrations. Minn. Vet. *15*:13, 1975.

184. Ross, J. G., and Todd, J. R.: Epidemiological studies of fascioliasis: a third season of comparative studies with cattle. Vet. Rec. *82*:695, 1968.

185. Sinclair, K. B.: The effect of splenectomy on the pathogenicity of *Fasciola hepatica* in the sheep. Br. Vet. J. *126*:15, 1970.

186. Olsen, O. W.: Liver flukes in cattle: diagnosis for treatment and prevention. Proc. U.S.L.S.A. *52*:79, 1948.

187. Roseby, F. B.: The effect of fasciolosis on the wool production of Merino sheep. Aust. Vet. J. *46*:361, 1970.

188. Todd, K. S. Jr.: Internal metazoal and protozoal diseases. In Feline Medicine and Surgery, 2nd ed. Edited by E. J. Catcott. Santa Barbara, American Veterinary Publications, 1975, p. 105.

189. Robinson, V. B., and Ehrenford, F. A.: Hepatic lesions associated with liver fluke (*Platynosomum fastosum*) infection in a cat. Am. J. Vet. Res. *23*:1300, 1962.

190. Rothenbacher, H., and Lindquist, W. D.: Liver cirrhosis and pancreatitis in a cat infected with *Amphimerus pseudofelineus*. J.A.V.M.A. *143*:1099, 1963.

191. Georgi, J. R.: Personal communication.

192. Smith, H. A.: Ulcerative lesions of the bovine rumen and their possible relation to hepatic abscesses. Am. J. Vet. Res. *5*:234, 1944.

193. Newsom, I. E.: A bacteriologic study of liver abscesses in cattle. J. Infect. Dis. *63*:232, 1938.

194. Madin, S. H.: A bacteriologic study of bovine liver abscesses. Vet. Med. *44*:248, 1949.

195. Jensen, R., Deane, H. M., Cooper, L. J., Miller, V. A., and Graham, W. R.: The rumenitis-liver abscess complex in beef cattle. Am. J. Vet. Res. *15*:202, 1954.

196. Audell, L., Jonsson, L., and Lannek, B.: Congenital porta-caval shunts in the dog. Zentralbl. Veterinaermed. A. *21*:797, 1974.

197. Reference deleted.

198. Lohse, C. L., Selcer, R. R., and Suter, P. F.: Hepatoencephalopathy associated with situs inversus of abdominal organs and vascular anomalies in a dog. J.A.V.M.A. *168*:681, 1976.

199. Beech, J., Dubielzig, R., and Bester, R.: Portal vein anomaly and hepatic encephalopathy in a horse. J.A.V.M.A. *170*:164, 1977.

200. Strombeck, D. R., Breznock, E. M., and McNeel, S.: Surgical treatment for portosystemic shunts in two dogs. J.A.V.M.A. *170*:1317, 1977.

201. McGavin, M. D., and Henry, J.: Canine hepatic vascular hamartoma associated with ascites. J.A.V.M.A. *160*:864, 1972.

202. Easley, J. C., and Carpenter, J. L.: Hepatic arteriovenous fistula in two Saint Bernard pups. J.A.V.M.A. *166*:167, 1975.

203. Rogers, W. A., Suter, P. F., Breznock, E. M., Olivieri, M., and Ruebner, B. M.: Intrahepatic arteriovenous fistulae in a dog resulting in portal hypertension, portacaval shunts, and reversal of portal blood flow. J.A.A.H.A. *13*:470, 1977.

204. Legendre, A. M., Krahwinkel, D. J., Carrig, C. B., and Michel, R. L.: Ascites associated with intrahepatic arteriovenous fistula in a cat. J.A.V.M.A. *168*:589, 1976.

205. Recknagel, R. O.: Carbon tetrachloride hepatoxicity. Pharmacol. Rev. *19*:145, 1967.

206. Recknagel, R. O., and Ghoshal, A. K.: Lipoperoxidation as a vector in carbon tetrachloride hepatotoxicity. Lab. Invest. *15*:132, 1966.

207. McLean, A. E. M., and McLean, E. K.: Diet, microsomal enzymes and carbon tetrachloride toxicity. Biochem. J. *97*:31P, 1965.

208. Campbell, R. M., and Kosterlitz, H. W.: The effects of short-term changes in dietary protein on the response of the liver to carbon tetrachloride injury. Br. J. Exp. Pathol. *29*:149, 1948.

209. Krishnan, N., and Stenger, R. J.: Effects of starvation on the hepatotoxicity of carbon tetrachloride. A light and electron microscopic study. Am. J. Pathol. *49*:239, 1966.

210. Jennings, P. B., Utter, W. F., and Fariss, B. L.: Effects of long-term primidone therapy in a dog. J.A.V.M.A. *164*:1123, 1974.

211. Nash, A. S.: Phenytoin toxicity: a fatal case in a dog with hepatitis and jaundice. Vet. Rec. *100*:280, 1977.

212. Sturtevant, F., Hoffmann, W. E., and Dorner, J. L.: The effect of three anticonvulsant drugs and ACTH on canine serum alkaline phosphatase. J.A.A.H.A. *13*:754, 1977.

213. Conning, D. M., and Litchfield, M. H.: Increase of serum alkaline phosphatase activity due to enzyme "induction" in the liver of Beagle dogs. J. Pathol. *103*: P. xii, 1971.

214. Rogers, W. A., and Ruebner, B. H.: A retrospective study of probable glucocorticoid-induced hepatopathy in dog. J.A.V.M.A. *170*:603, 1977.

215. Hardy, R. M., and Stevens, J. B.: Chronic progressive hepatitis in Bedlington terriers (Bedlington liver disease). In Current Veterinary Therapy VI. R. W. Kirk, Editor. W. B. Saunders Company, pp. 995–998, 1977.

216. Rogers, W. A.: Treatment of liver disease in small animal medicine. Proceedings of the Kal-Kan Symposium for the Treatment of Dog and Cat Diseases, September 19–20, 1977, p. 2.

217. Pirotte, J., Guffens, J. M., and Devos, J.: Comparative study of basal arterial ammonemia and of orally-induced hyperammonemia in

chronic portal systemic encephalopathy, treated with neomycin, lactulose, and an association of neomycin and lactulose. Digestion *10*:435, 1974.

218. Conn, H. O., Leevy, C. M., Vlahcevic, Z. R., Rodgers, J. B. Maddrey, W. C., Seeff, L., and Levy, L. L.: Comparison of lactulose and neomycin in the treatment of chronic portal-systemic encephalopathy. Gastroenterology *72*:573, 1977.

219. Furneaux, R. W., and Mero, K. N.: End-to-side portacaval anastomosis for correction of ascites in a terrier dog. J.A.A.H.A. *9*:562, 1973.

Chapter 26

THE PANCREAS

ROBERT M. HARDY and GERALD F. JOHNSON

Part I. Inflammatory Pancreatic Disease

ROBERT M. HARDY

Exocrine pancreatic diseases represent an extremely diverse group of clinical disorders. Inflammatory disorders are most frequently encountered and present the widest variability in clinical signs. As clinicians have increased their awareness of the signs associated with pancreatitis, the frequency with which it is diagnosed appears to be increasing. The association of diabetes mellitus with pancreatitis is also commonly observed. Inflammatory pancreatitis may result in injury to islet cells so that hypoinsulinism results.

Exocrine pancreatic insufficiency, whether due to an acquired or congenital abnormality, is a relatively uncommon clinical entity. In general, it is a benign process associated with a protracted, clinical course.

Pancreatic neoplasia presents a much different type of clinical picture. Tumors of the exocrine pancreas are often widely disseminated prior to diagnosis and are rarely associated with clinical signs referable to the pancreas. Functional islet cell tumors of the endocrine pancreas most often are manifested by signs referable to the central nervous system.

Classification of Exocrine Pancreatic Disease

From the clinician's viewpoint, pancreatic diseases are most logically considered as either inflammatory or noninflammatory in nature. Inflammatory pancreatitis may, in some cases, be further characterized as either acute or chronic (relapsing). The first time a patient is diagnosed as having an attack of inflammatory pancreatic disease, the process is classified as an acute pancreatitis. Should subsequent attacks of a similar nature develop, the patient is considered to be suffering from chronic recurrent pancreatitis. Clinically and biochemically,

there may be little, if any, difference between these two syndromes. A clinical separation is important primarily from a prognostic standpoint. In cases where animals are known to have survived several attacks of recurrent acute pancreatitis, clients should be informed of the likelihood that still further bouts may occur and/or that diabetes mellitus and pancreatic insufficiency are common sequelae in such patients. Further subdivisions into edematous or hemorrhagic necrotic pancreatitis are usually speculative unless based on specific laboratory results (methemalbumin) or biopsy information.

Noninflammatory pancreatic diseases make up approximately one third of the total number of pancreatic problems encountered by veterinarians.[1] Included in this group are diabetes mellitus, juvenile pancreatic atrophy (also called pancreatic hypoplasia), end-stage pancreatitis, and pancreatic neoplasia. Juvenile atrophy and end-stage pancreatitis appear clinically as pancreatic insufficiency states, unassociated with significant upper intestinal signs.

Diabetes mellitus occurs commonly as a result of severe, recurrent destructive pancreatitis.[2] Once a diagnosis of pancreatitis has been established, every attempt should be made to prevent recurrences in order to reduce the chance of diabetes developing. Conversely, severely ill diabetics should always be suspected of having acute pancreatitis. Many diabetic animals will be first presented for evaluation because a previously mild form of diabetes has been decompensated by an attack of acute pancreatitis.

Pancreatic neoplasia may be of exocrine or endocrine origin. In either case, clinical signs are rarely those referable to primary pancreatic disease. Exocrine tumors are highly malignant and usually exhibit signs or biochemical evidence of hepatic

621

metastases. Local intestinal infiltration is also common. Functional endocrine pancreatic tumors, principally islet cell carcinomas, manifest themselves clinically with signs attributable to hypoglycemia. Metastases are also common with these tumors.

PANCREATIC INFLAMMATION

Etiopathogenesis

Naturally occurring acute pancreatitis was first described in the dog in 1908.[3] Since that time, an ever-lengthening list of causes and mechanisms of pancreatic injury has been proposed. At times it would appear that we are no closer to understanding the disease now than we were 70 years ago.

The pancreas, like many organs, is limited in its ability to respond to injury. Thus, it is likely that a number of causes are responsible for initiating the clinical syndrome. However, the nature of the initiating pancreatic insult may dictate the clinical severity.

Volumes of experimental and clinical data have been accumulated in the past 50 years in an attempt to elucidate the causes of pancreatitis and the mechanisms responsible for its progression. The dog has been utilized as a convenient animal subject in which to test multiple theories regarding the causes of this disease. It is hard to imagine how an organ could have been more manipulated, traumatized, injected, abused, or otherwise assaulted than has the dog pancreas. As a result of these many clinical observations and experimental results, a number of proposed causes have attained prominence. From a conceptual standpoint, most of these proposed causes may be classified as inducing either large duct pancreatitis (obstructive) or small duct pancreatitis (metabolic, toxic, drug-induced).[4] The causes of each type, although quite different, result in similar pathogenetic processes and degrees of clinical illness. In spite of the impressive number of possible causes for pancreatitis, in the majority of cases a definitive etiology is never identified, even at the necropsy table.[5]

Since so few cases of pancreatitis in domestic animals have a definitive cause identified, most of the etiologic discussion to follow will relate to the human syndrome. It is hoped that this will prove valuable as an aid to future diagnostic approaches used in animals with spontaneous pancreatitis.

Alcoholism and biliary tract disease, especially cholelithiasis,[6] are by far the most common causes for pancreatitis in man. Neither of these diseases occurs with significant frequency in domestic animals. Nevertheless, from a conceptual standpoint the mechanisms by which cholelithiasis and alcoholism are thought to induce human pancreatitis may apply, at least in part, to domestic animals.

Bile reflux into the pancreatic ducts has long been proposed as at least one mechanism whereby obstruction to outflow of pancreatic and biliary secretions may lead to pancreatitis. A shared opening for both the common bile duct and major pancreatic duct is present in 60 to 90% of humans.[6] Forty percent of these individuals can be shown to have bile reflux into the pancreatic duct during cholangiography. Furthermore, in 10 to 15% of humans with both cholelithiasis and pancreatitis, a stone can be found in the ampulla of Vater. Since the major pancreatic duct in most dogs enters the duodenum at some distance from the ampulla of Vater, the likelihood that a common duct stone could lead to pancreatitis is quite low.[7] The cat, although having an anatomic arrangement much like man but without a common ampulla, has a very low incidence of acute pancreatitis. In general, following ligation of the common opening of the bile and pancreatic ducts, pressures in the pancreatic duct exceed those in the biliary tract for approximately 24 hours, preventing bile reflux into the pancreatic duct. Following this time period, however, pancreatic duct pressures decline, while biliary tract pressures increase, theoretically making it possible for bile to enter the pancreatic ductular system and induce pancreatitis.[6] Factors in addition to biliary calculi which may occlude biliary drainage include ampullary spasms, local intestinal edema, neoplasia, and parasites. Although reports of pancreatitis associated with major bile duct occlusion have appeared in the veterinary literature,[8] they are rare. In general, available evidence does not support the "common channel" theory of pancreatitis as having much clinical validity in animals.

Occlusion of the major pancreatic ducts in the absence of impaired bile duct flow may be a more likely cause for pancreatitis in the dog. Simple ligation of pancreatic ducts leads to glandular atrophy with no signs of inflammation. If, however, pancreatic outflow is impaired and simultaneously the gland is stimulated to secrete, varying degrees of edematous pancreatitis result.[6,9,10] Natural stimuli to exocrine pancreatic secretion such as feeding, or experimental secretagogues, i.e., pilocarpine, secretin, and hydrochloric acid, all produce edematous pancreatitis when given to duct-ligated dogs. If the vascular supply to the pancreas is also compromised, then the edematous pancreatitis progresses to a severe, hemorrhagic type. Multiple factors may result in partial or complete obstruction to pancreatic exocrine outflow, i.e., edema or spasms of the duodenal papilla or sphincter, inflammation of the duodenal mucosa, neoplasia, metaplasia of ductular epithelium (drug-induced), and parasitic migration into the major pancreatic duct. Reports of the cat liver fluke, *Amphimerus pseudofelineus*, invading the pancreatic ducts have appeared in the veterinary literature.[11,12] Although the presence of these flukes within the pancreatic ducts produced ductular hyperplasia and fibrosis, few if any signs referable to the pancreas were noted.

Reflux of duodenal contents into the pancreatic ducts has been proposed as another method whereby pancreatitis may be initiated.[13,14,15,16] This concept was based on an experimental closed duodenal loop preparation in dogs first described by Pfeffer in 1957. Hemorrhagic pancreatitis routinely developed in these surgically prepared dogs. Duodenal chyme in these animals contains activated pancreatic enzymes, bile acids, bacteria, lysolecithin, and emulsified fat, all products known to induce experimental pancreatitis when injected into the pancreatic ducts. It is hypothesized that in naturally occurring pancreatitis a structural or functional change occurs in the sphincters of the pancreatic ducts making them continuously patent with the duodenum. An open duct combined with increased pressures within the duodenum is thought to result in reflux of duodenal contents into the pancreas, initiating an inflammatory process.[13] At present, no conclusive evidence exists that this process actually occurs in spontaneous canine or feline pancreatitis.[17]

Nutrition also plays a role in the etiology of pancreatitis. Obesity is a frequent finding in animals with pancreatitis. Experimental animals maintained on high fat diets for extended periods are prone to a more severe form of pancreatitis than those maintained on normal diets. High protein or high carbohydrate diets did not produce this effect.[18,19,20] The intrapancreatic concentrations of proelastase and trypsinogen, both important in the pathogenesis of pancreatitis, were found to be decreased in malnourished dogs when compared to dogs on high planes of nutrition.[21] The mechanism of injury associated with feeding of a high fat diet may be related to an increased permeability of the pancreatic acinar cell membrane. This leads to greater susceptibility to both external and internal autodigestive processes. Further support for the importance of dietary factors in the etiology of pancreatitis is the common clinical association of overindulgence in

food (animals) and drink (man) just prior to the attack.

Bacteria as a cause of pancreatitis in domestic animals is of uncertain importance. Bacteria isolated from the pancreas come from four main sources: blood; lymphatics, particularly those draining the gallbladder and bile ducts; duodenum, ascending via pancreatic ducts; and proliferation of normal pancreatic flora.[10,22] Clostridial organisms are normal inhabitants of the pancreas and assume primary importance only after pancreatitis has been initiated. Once vascular compromise has taken place, these anaerobic organisms may proliferate, aggravating the disease.

Intestinal bacteria or their toxins which gain entry into the pancreatic ducts are capable of initiating pancreatitis. Much of the injury associated with the closed duodenal loop preparation mentioned previously can be eliminated by sterilizing the duodenal contents. The simultaneous occurrence of cholangitis and pancreatitis has been reported in the cat.[1] Lymphogenous spread of bacteria from the bile ducts to the pancreas or vice versa may have taken place in these animals.[22]

Interconnections between lymphatic channels of the extrahepatic biliary tract and pancreas may be important in the etiology of canine pancreatitis.[22] The main lymph drainage of the pancreas is through the paraduodenal nodes and then through the cysterna chyla or thoracic duct. Retrograde lymph flow may occur, however, from the extrahepatic biliary system into pancreatic lymphatics. The lymphatic system may thus transport inflammatory products from one part of the biliary-pancreatic complex to the other. Pancreatic lymphatics play a minor role in efferent drainage of the normal gland, venous outflow being of major importance. During pancreatitis this situation changes. The lymphatics serve to help eliminate toxic interstitial wastes that a compromised venous system cannot effectively remove. Once lymphatics become clogged with inflammatory debris, this avenue of pancreatic drainage is lost, aggravating the disease process.

Viruses have occasionally been associated with pancreatitis in humans.[4,23,24] Fulminant viral hepatitis is associated with a mild pancreatitis in some cases. Other human viruses incriminated as etiologic agents of pancreatitis include those causing mumps, mononucleosis, and the coxsackie-B_3 and B_4 viruses. The significance of viruses as causative agents of pancreatitis in domestic animals is unknown.

Autoimmune or allergic mechanisms may have a role in the initiation of pancreatitis but it remains speculative. An Arthus-type sensitization technique used on rabbits leads to a severe hemorrhagic pancreatitis.[25] Isoantibodies against pancreatic tissue have also been isolated from dogs following the production of experimental pancreatitis.[26] Current philosophies hold that such isoantibodies develop as a result of the disease and are not involved in initiation of the disease process.

Trauma as a cause of pancreatitis is uncommon. Although postoperative pancreatitis is frequent in man, dogs and cats appear to be relatively resistant. Surgical manipulations of the gland are usually well tolerated and minor surgical procedures on the pancreas are associated with mild, transient increases in serum enzymes.

Drug-induced pancreatitis may be much more prevalent in veterinary medicine than is currently appreciated. A large number of therapeutic agents have been incriminated as a cause of human pancreatitis. Such associations remain speculative in our field at the present time. In any discussion of a drug-induced disease, one must be cautious in assuming that because a drug was given and subsequently a disease developed, a cause and effect relationship exists. On the other hand, to continue to ignore the possibility as speculation while more and more cases are recorded (particularly with glucocorticoids) would seem unreasonable. The human literature contains at least 112 instances of drug-induced pancreatitis.[27] Nearly 50% were associated with glucocorticoid or ACTH administration. Other agents incriminated in man include diuretics, chemotherapeutics, estrogens, azathioprine, calcium, clonidine and phenformin, warfarin, salicylates, l-asparaginase, and d-propoxyphene.[27,28]

Glucocorticoids and ACTH are the most important and best documented drugs causing pancreatitis in man. No correlation between dose and duration of therapy has been detected.[27] I have observed multiple cases of pancreatitis in dogs in which the disease developed within a short time following the administration of glucocorticoids. In several dogs, each time steroids were readministered, a similar syndrome occurred. It would seem prudent for all veterinarians to be alert to the possibility that patients that have been given glucocorticoids and subsequently develop gastrointestinal signs may have steroid pancreatitis.

Glucocorticoids have two known effects on the pancreas that are thought to predispose to pancreatitis.[13,29] One involves an increase in viscosity and inspissation of pancreatic secretions. The second effect that steroids induce involves a proliferation of the ductular epithelium, thus reducing the luminal diameter of the ducts. Both effects would impair normal drainage of the acinar tissue and theoretically predispose to a large-duct type of pancreatitis.

Estrogen is associated with pancreatitis, in pregnant women and women receiving estrogens, at a higher incidence than in the general population. An increase in gallstone formation during late pregnancy is considered responsible for some of these cases, leading to an obstructive pancreatitis.[13] A second mechanism involves a subclinical familial type of hyperlipidemia[30] (Frederickson Type IV), which is converted to a Type V hyperlipidemia state following exposure to endogenous or exogenous estrogens.[4,27] The proposed mechanisms by which hyperlipemia causes pancreatitis will be discussed in the section on metabolic diseases.

Antimicrobial drugs that have been associated with occasional bouts of pancreatitis in man include tetracyclines, salicylazosulfapyridine, and rifampicin.[13,24,27] No evidence is available in the veterinary literature supporting similar associations.

Diuretics, particularly the chlorthiazides, furosemide and ethacrynic acid, have been reported to cause occasional cases of human pancreatitis.[27] The mechanism is unknown.

Metabolic disorders of man, notably hyperlipidemic states, uremia and hypercalcemia, are associated with an increased incidence of pancreatitis. Hyperlipidemia implies that increased concentration of circulating lipids is present, while hyperlipemia refers to a type of hyperlipidemia in which a visible lactescence of the serum is present. Hyperlipemia is visible when serum triglycerides exceed 300 to 400 mg/dl;[31] however, concentrations often exceed 1000 mg/dl[4] in man. Hyperlipemia is observed fairly often in canine acute pancreatitis.[7] In man, hyperlipemia seen with pancreatitis is considered to have one of three associations.[4,32,33] The hyperlipemia may be a primary metabolic disorder, precede the bout of pancreatitis, and be responsible for its initiation; the hyperlipemia may be secondary to the pancreatitis and causally unrelated; or it may be an incidental finding, unrelated to either cause or effect of the disease. Type I and Type V familial hyperlipidemias of man are known to predispose to pancreatitis.[4,13] Both disorders have marked increases in chylomicrons and produce a visible hyperlipemia. Pancreatitis is hypothesized to result from a combination of embolization of the pancreatic microcirculation by lipid particles and fatty acid-induced injury to capillaries.[13,27,32] In familial hyperlipidemia, the lipemia persists long after evidence for pancreatitis has disappeared. Control of serum triglycerides by using low fat diets has significantly reduced the rate of recurrence of this type of pancreatitis in human patients.[31,34] Limited lipid studies of both experimental and spontaneous canine pancreatitis have documented increases in serum glycerides but none of the evaluated animals had visible lipemia.[35,36] A family of Schnauzers with an idiopathic hyperlipidemia and marginally elevated serum amylase values has been described.[37] The significance of the hyperamylasemia was questioned.

Pancreatic lesions are stated to occur fairly often in uremic humans,[13,38] although the true morbidity of pancreatic disease in human renal failure is unknown.[39] It is most often assumed that increases in amylase and lipase that occur in dogs with primary renal failure are secondary to impaired renal elimination and not primary pancreatic disease. Until detailed histopathologic studies of the pancreas from dogs with renal failure are performed, the significance of hyperamylasemia in canine renal failure will remain speculative.

The last metabolic disease with a known increased incidence of pancreatitis is primary hyperparathyroidism. Seven percent of humans with this disease develop an associated pancreatitis.[13] Hypothesized mechanisms by which hypercalcemia causes pancreatitis include intraductal calculi formation, activation of trypsin within the pancreas, and hypercalcemia-induced vasculitis.[13] In addition to endogenous hypercalcemia, exogenously administered calcium solutions have been reported to induce pancreatitis in both animals[40] and man.[27]

Hereditary pancreatitis has recently been reported in man.[41,42] An autosomal dominant mode of inheritance is suspected. Familial pancreatitis has not been described in animals as yet, although heavily inbred lines of dogs and cats would seem likely to express such a disorder.

Pathogenesis

The pathogenesis of pancreatitis involves an extremely complex sequence of events, about which much still remains to be learned. The pancreas is a large storehouse of potent digestive enzymes. This gland has 13 times the combined protein-synthesizing capacity of the liver and reticuloendothelial system.[43] Interactions between this multitude of pancreatic enzymes combined with alterations in pancreatic microcirculation result in the wide spectrum of clinical and pathologic signs characteristic of pancreatitis. Pancreatitis ranges in severity from the mildest edematous or interstitial type to the fulminant, often fatal, hemorrhagic

necrotic pancreatitis. The proportion of the gland affected varies from isolated focal lesions to massive destruction of the entire gland. Repeated acute attacks may occur, as in chronic relapsing pancreatitis, with the eventual destruction of all functional acinar and possibly islet tissue. This process eventually results in pancreatic exocrine insufficiency and/or diabetes mellitus.[44]

The development of pancreatitis occurs in two stages.[16] The first involves the initiation of the disease process during which glandular defense mechanisms are overcome and the acini are damaged. The second stage involves the induction of autodigestion and eventual glandular necrosis once the initial insult has occurred. The initial injurious mechanisms were discussed in the previous section.

Activation of intrapancreatic enzymes is a key step in pancreatic autodigestion. Normally, pancreatic enzymes are present as inactive precursors within the pancreatic acinar cell. The concentration of activated enzymes within the pancreatic interstitium and their rate of delivery to damaged areas dictate the severity of the disease process.[6]

Trypsin is almost universally incriminated as playing a significant role in the pathogenesis of pancreatitis. Trypsin is normally present as inactive trypsinogen while within the pancreas. It is converted to trypsin within the duodenum by a duodenal mucosal hormone, enterokinase. In vitro studies have indicated that trypsinogen can be converted to trypsin by bile salts, tissue juice, calcium ions, alkaline pH and autocatalysis.[10,45] From a physiologic standpoint, in vivo autoactivation probably does not occur, being prevented by electrostatic mechanisms.[46] The effects of intrapancreatic trypsin activation are normally prevented by naturally occurring circulating trypsin inhibitors. The trypsin inhibitor (alpha-l-antitrypsin) plays a protective role, normally preventing spontaneous trypsin activation from causing significant pancreatic injury. Although large quantities of active trypsin have not been detected within the inflamed pancreas, indirect evidence supports the theory that significant amounts of trypsin have been inactivated during the disease process.[47] It is believed that trypsin in very small quantities serves as an initiator or activator of even more potent and destructive enzymes, rather than being directly involved in the autodigestion.[13,48,49]

Trypsin is capable of activating all the known pancreatic zymogens which take part in pancreatitis. The most important are chymotrypsinogen, prophospholipase-A, and proelastase.[13,46] Experimental support for the importance of chymotrypsin is gained from pathologic studies on the canine pancreas following intraductal injection of chymotrypsin. Lesions identical to those produced by trypsin were present, and significant intrapancreatic chymotrypsin concentrations were measured in trypsin-induced canine pancreatitis.

Phospholipase-A is an extremely potent cytotoxic enzyme. In the dog it is capable of inducing severe central nervous system damage, decreased pulmonary function, and hemolysis.[6] Phospholipase-A directly attacks the phospholipid component of cell membranes converting them into lysophospholipids, themselves highly cytotoxic.[12] Lysolecithin, a by-product of phospholipase-A degradation of bile lecithin, has a profound toxic effect on most cells throughout the body. Phospholipase-A is considered ultimately responsible for the necrosis of pancreatic acinar cells and adipose tissue.[49]

Trypsin conversion of proelastase to elastase has a profound effect upon pancreatic vasculature. In addition to a nonspecific proteolytic effect, elastase dissolves elastic fibers of pancreatic blood vessels producing hemorrhage and thrombosis.[50,51] This combination of phospholipase-A and elastase is considered responsible for the hemorrhage and necrosis observed in the more severe forms of pancreatitis.[49]

Trypsin also liberates two important vasoactive polypeptides, kallekrein and bradykinin, during acute pancreatitis. Both compounds are present in high concentration within the pancreas. An increase in circulating bradykinin levels is detectable within 3 hours following induction of experimental canine pancreatitis.[52] Both compounds are known to produce vasodilatation, increased capillary permeability, hypotension, leukocyte infiltration, and pain.[16,52]

Recent investigations have determined that prostaglandin-E-like material is present in high concentrations in pancreatic venous effluent and ascitic exudate formed during pancreatitis.[16,53] This substance may also play a role in the hypotension and pain of pancreatitis.

The importance of pancreatic lipase in the pathogenesis of pancreatitis has been long debated. Recent evidence supports the hypothesis that lipase is at least partially responsible for the fat necrosis seen in pancreatitis.[13] The detergent activity of bile acids is required to permit access of pancreatic lipase to triglycerides stored within fat cells. Large amounts of free fatty acids are locally liberated and may exert a further detergent effect on cell membranes perpetuating the process which results in fat necrosis.[6,13]

The importance of maintaining an intact, viable venous and lymphatic system within the pancreas cannot be overstressed. Although pancreatic vascular and acinar necrosis requires the presence of activated enzymes, the ability to maintain an intact blood supply is the single most important factor determining whether the edematous form progresses to hemorrhagic necrotic pancreatitis.[16,51,54] The development of pancreatic autodigestion requires that a degree of vascular compromise and ischemia exist. In the absence of impaired pancreatic circulation, edematous pancreatitis is a self-limiting and relatively benign process.[6] Impairment of pancreatic microcirculation leads to prolonged retention of activated enzymes and autodigestive by-products, increasing the likelihood of further injury and perpetuation of the disease. The high metabolic rate of pancreatic acini makes them especially susceptible to ischemia. Once ischemia develops, necrosis of groups of cells occurs.[1] Maintaining an adequate pancreatic circulation allows for absorption of toxic ferments, protecting the gland from further injury.[55] Since the severity of pancreatitis is proportional to the number of vessels embolized,[56] preventing vascular stasis and thrombosis within the microcirculation is critical to halting progression of the disease.

Pancreatic embolization and venous stasis result from many factors. Some of the most important include vascular necrosis, capillary occlusion by interstitial edema, fat embolization associated with hyperlipemia, hemoconcentration with sludging of red blood cells, and the development of disseminated intravascular coagulation.[10,51,54,57] Once a significant degree of ischemia and thrombosis has occurred, a potentially self-limiting disease becomes self-perpetuating.

Necrosis or rupture of the pancreatic capsule eventually occurs, releasing digestive enzymes and the by-products of pancreatic autodigestion into the peritoneal cavity. A localized chemical peritonitis develops initially but it may become widespread as the disease progresses. Regional intestinal injury allows luminal bacteria to gain access into the peritoneal cavity, converting a sterile process into a septic peritonitis.

Hypocalcemia in human pancreatitis is considered a grave prognostic sign. The presence of a similar laboratory abnormality has also been observed fairly often in dogs with acute pancreatitis, but without the grave prognostic implications of the human disease. Although numerous theories to explain the hypocalcemia have appeared,[58,59,60] the cause of hypocalcemia in pancreatitis remains largely unresolved. Possible explanations for pancreatitis-associated hypocalcemia include complexes of fatty acids and calcium in areas of fat necrosis, hyperglucagonemia, impaired parathormone secretion, hypercalcitonism, and hypomagnesemia. Recent evaluations of human patients with hypocalcemia have determined that most cases had a relative rather than absolute decrease in serum calcium.[58] The majority of the patients had a significant decrease in serum albumin concentrations which caused the relative hypocalcemia. When serum calcium concentrations were corrected for the effect of hypoalbuminemia, only 10.9% of the patients were found to have true hypocalcemia. Recent work by Robertson[60] on patients in which ionized calcium concentrations were subnormal suggests that a relative parathormone deficiency may be responsible for the hypocalcemia.

Disseminated intravascular coagulation may play a significant role in the terminal phases of acute hemorrhagic pancreatitis. Activated pancreatic enzymes gain access into the circulation either from diffusion across the peritoneal surface or through damaged pancreatic blood vessels and lymphatics. Pancreatic enzymes, in addition to being of diagnostic significance, can result in activation of the blood coagulation system and induce a hypercoagulable state.[55,61] An increased tendency toward thrombus formation is commonly recognized in patients with pancreatitis.[61] Thrombotic tendencies may be accompanied by a hemorrhagic diathesis when the rate of consumption of clotting elements exceeds the body's ability to replace them. Intravascular trypsin may account for this phenomenon. Intravenous trypsin accelerates the conversion of prothrombin to thrombin, increasing blood coagulability.[62] Other trypsin effects on blood coagulability include platelet depression, reduction of factors V and VIII, activation of fibrinolysin, and, in high doses, increased coagulation time.[63] In summary, initial stages of the coagulation abnormalities in pancreatitis are characterized by accelerated thrombosis. If the process continues, accelerated fibrinolysis occurs and eventually defibrination, platelet consumption, and hemorrhage develop.

Hypovolemic shock makes a significant contribution to the lethal nature of pancreatitis. Severe pancreatitis is characterized by the accumulation of large amounts of fluid within the interstitium of the pancreas and the peritoneal cavity. Quantities in excess of 25% of the circulating blood volume may be lost in this manner.[43,64,65] The magnitude of fluid sequestration is related in part to a loss of vascular and lymphatic integrity. The peritoneal exudate from dogs with experimental pancreatitis has substances that greatly increase vascular permeability.[66] This substance greatly increases albumin loss from blood vessels. Smaller pancreatic blood vessels are blocked by inflammatory debris producing local venous hypertension. Portal sequestration is common, and the circulating blood volume may be further reduced by 30 to 40%.[6]

The hypotensive agents kallikrein and bradykinin, in addition to a myocardial depressant factor, all augment the severity of hypovolemic shock in pancreatitis. Hypoxia and anoxia within the pancreas are associated with the release of these substances into the general circulation.

ACUTE PANCREATITIS

A majority of the clinical problems relating to the pancreas are caused by acute and chronic pancreatitis.[1] Of our domestic animals, the dog is the most frequently affected. Occasional cases are also reported in the cat,[67,67a] cow, and horse. The clinical significance of feline pancreatitis is apparently low since cats are prone to a more chronic, low-grade interstitial type of pancreatitis that usually remains subclinical.[2]

Acute pancreatitis is a disease of extreme variability. The intensity and duration of illness range from very mild, in which anorexia may be the only sign, to the severe hemorrhagic necrotic form with signs of severe anterior abdominal distress. The overwhelming majority of patients with pancreatitis survive the illness, with or without treatment. Those with the more destructive types carry a grave prognosis, however. Data from a large series of necropsies indicated that pancreatitis was the cause of death in 3% of the cases.[68]

It is not often possible to differentiate mild from severe pancreatitis clinically, especially in the early stages. Certain laboratory evaluations, however, may support a differentiation between edematous and hemorrhagic pancreatitis. Not uncommonly, animals that appear clinically to have recovered will still have progressive low-grade inflammatory disease occurring almost continuously or be prone to recurrent bouts of the acute clinical disease over many months. The clinical diagnosis in such animals is chronic pancreatitis or chronic relapsing pancreatitis. On rare occasions, an older animal will be admitted with signs referable to end-stage pancreatitis, i.e., pancreatic insufficiency, with vague or nonexistent evidence for antecedent inflammatory pancreatic disease.

Pancreatitis may be considered a disease of domestication. It occurs most often in middle-aged, obese, sedentary female dogs. Attacks are frequently noted following a large, high fat content meal.[17] Healthy, well-exercised dogs in good physical condition rarely develop pancreatitis. High fat diets are known to predispose dogs to pancreatitis and increase the severity of the disease process once initiated. Once an attack of pancreatitis has developed, it can be expected to last approximately 3 days. Occasional cases will exhibit signs of illness for 7 days and, very rarely, signs may persist for up to 6 weeks.[69,70] The mean age for such patients is approximately 5 years,[70,71] but reported cases are from 2 months to 11 years of age. Female dogs predominate in the reported cases, but the significance of this observation is unknown.

During the past 10 years (1966 to 1976), 144 cases of pancreatitis have been diagnosed in dogs and 12 cases in cats in my practice.* Eighty percent of the canine cases were over 4 years of age and 87 were female dogs (60%).

All too often, a diagnosis of pancreatitis is made as one of those miraculous "tabletop" prognostications. The accuracy of these prognostications is challenged only if the patient dies and a necropsy is performed. This no longer need be the case. By combining a thorough history and physical examination with appropriate laboratory tests, a specific diagnosis of pancreatitis may be made with a high degree of certainty.

History

The history usually, but not invariably, reflects that abdominal disease is present. Vomiting is the primary problem with localizing value and is one of the classic signs of pancreatitis. With hemorrhagic pancreatitis, animals may vomit multiple times per hour for extended periods. In milder forms of the disease, frequency of vomiting is quite unpredictable. The absence of vomiting in a sick dog does not exclude pancreatitis from consideration. Occasional patients exhibiting clinical signs of depression, anorexia, and nausea have been found to have biochemical evidence of pancreatitis.

Nausea is a fairly specific sign for pancreatitis. Nausea in animals is expressed clinically as restlessness, a reluctance to lie down for extended periods, constant pacing, and especially by ptyalism and repeated swallowing. Salivation in some cases is so copious that the lips and forefeet are wet.

Diarrhea, although not characteristic of pancreatitis, is occasionally seen in affected dogs.

Diarrhea results from injury and involvement of peripancreatic tissues (duodenum, colon) in the inflammatory process. Other organs that may become secondarily involved in pancreatitis are the liver, stomach, spleen, and kidney.

Abdominal pain is another "classic" sign of pancreatitis. Unfortunately, the subjective nature of this sign, coupled with the marked variability of animals to react to pain, make this sign unreliable. This last point is particularly important. Many veterinarians exclude pancreatitis from diagnostic consideration in vomiting dogs because they cannot demonstrate (by history or by palpation) that abdominal pain is present. My experience indicates that abdominal pain is clinically evident in relatively few dogs with a confirmed diagnosis of pancreatitis. In those few animals in which overt pain is evident, the following signs are noted: the dog snaps at the owner when handled, walks with an arched back and exhibits a stiff, sawhorse gait, and tends to seek cool surfaces to lie upon. The pain of pancreatitis is a result of pancreatic swelling and stretching of the capsule, vasospasm and pancreatic ductular injury, increased tension on the mesenteric root, or chemical peritonitis.

Anorexia and depression are commonly noted by owners. As the severity of the disease increases, depressions may worsen.

Physical Examination

The physical examination of dogs with pancreatitis varies from unrewarding to nearly pathognomonic. Finding abdominal pain in a vomiting dog is supportive of the diagnosis, particularly if such pain is localized to the anterior right quadrant. Its absence, however, by no means rules it out. Occasionally, dogs are in such pain that even the gentlest attempts at palpation are vigorously resisted. Bloating may be observed and is a result of aerophagia, pancreatic edema, and/or exudation of inflammatory by-products into the peritoneal cavity.[1] A moderate fever in the range of 103 to 105° F is to be expected. The temperature may drop to normal or even subnormal as shock develops in severe cases.

Whenever vomiting and/or diarrhea associated with pancreatitis have been severe, varying degrees of dehydration are noted. In many, the severity of the fluid deficit does not correlate well with clinical signs of dehydration.

Rule-outs

The list of possible rule-outs considered in a case of pancreatitis may be extensive, as a number of diseases present with similar signs. The greatest

---

*Small Animal Clinic, College of Veterinary Medicine, University of Minnesota, St. Paul, Minnesota 55108.

difficulty facing the clinician in the seriously ill animal with signs suggestive of pancreatitis is deciding whether to perform an immediate laparotomy or provide supportive and symptomatic care while awaiting the results of appropriate laboratory tests. Other abnormalities associated with an acute abdomen that may be confused with pancreatitis include acute renal disease (pyelonephritis, acute nephrosis), ruptured urinary bladder, urethral obstruction, gastrointestinal perforation, gastric distention, metritis, acute prostatitis and peritonitis.[72] In milder forms of pancreatitis, the only signs of illness are occasional vomiting, depression, and anorexia. Other metabolic diseases that should be considered include chronic renal failure, hepatic failure, diabetic ketoacidosis, hypoadrenocorticism, and toxicities. Fortunately, a thorough history and physical examination often help to reduce this formidable list of possible etiologies to relatively few probable ones. The clinician may then select the most logical laboratory tests, radiographic procedures, or surgical approaches to arrive at the correct diagnosis.

Diagnostic Plans

A definitive diagnosis of pancreatitis can be established only in one of two ways, laboratory confirmation or exploratory laparotomy. All other parameters are only supportive of the diagnosis. In addition to providing diagnostic specificity, laboratory evaluations confirm the presence of disease in other adjacent organs. Pancreatitis often induces significant functional changes in the liver, intestine, kidney, and especially the endocrine pancreas.[7] Alternatively, primary disease in these other organs may be confused with pancreatitis. Each case of pancreatitis should be considered unique and capable of presenting with its own set of complicating factors.

From the laboratory point of view, exocrine pancreatic disease takes two forms: acinar cell damage and pancreatic insufficiency. Acinar cell damage occurs in edematous (interstitial), necrotic hemorrhagic pancreatitis and exacerbations of chronic pancreatitis. Pancreatic insufficiency is common to end-stage pancreatitis and pancreatic atrophy. Neoplasia of the exocrine pancreas could fall into either category, but most often it presents with signs of liver failure.[73] Detectable pancreatic functional abnormalities occur only late in the disease course.

Of the commonly available laboratory tests to assess acinar cell injury, only amylase and lipase determinations are specific enough to be of diagnostic value. Increases in serum concentrations of these two enzymes are generally indicative of pancreatic acinar cell injury. These pancreatic enzymes reach the blood via several routes and are superimposed on normal blood concentrations.

Amylase

The normal serum amylase activity in dogs and cats is of uncertain origin and has no known physiologic function. In humans, three pancreatic and three salivary isoenzymes have been identified. The dog has no salivary amylase activity. Removal of serum amylase from the blood occurs, at least in part, by the kidney. Recent evidence suggests that a major route of elimination for circulating amylase in the dog involves the liver.[74] Renal excretion of pancreatic amylase was minimal in this study.

Amylase is a small molecule (mol. wt. 50,000) which is stable at refrigerator temperatures. Amylase determinations should be run on serum as amylase activity requires the presence of calcium, which would be chelated in plasma samples. Amyloclastic methods for determining amylase activity are preferred, although newer dye-starch complex saccharogenic methods appear to be reliable in the dog. Attempts to utilize amylase/creatinine clearance ratios as a diagnostic tool in canine pancreatitis have proven unreliable.[75]

The interpretation of an elevated serum amylase concentration has been the subject of much controversy in both human and veterinary medicine. As with all laboratory tests, normal values should be established for each individual laboratory and species involved. So many different methodologies and "normal" values exist for amylase activity that one must establish normal values for the test currently in use in the practice. Although "normal" amylase values for the cat have not been firmly established, it would appear that feline amylase values are similar to values determined for normal dogs.

Amylase values are known to increase mildly in stressful conditions and following the use of certain drugs, i.e., ACTH, morphine, and cortisone.[76] Since it is now known that these drugs may themselves induce pancreatitis, rejecting the use of the amylase test in the face of stress or usage of the above drugs should no longer be considered valid. Amylase, at one time, was thought to disappear from the circulation too rapidly to be of diagnostic help in many cases. Clinical data in humans[29,77] and experimental data on dogs[78] indicate that amylase activity persists in the circulation for several days following the initiation of pancreatitis and parallels lipase activity.

Recent mention has been made in the veterinary literature that amylase may be unreliable as a diagnostic test for pancreatitis associated with diabetes. This information may have been erroneously extrapolated from humans where the hyperlipemia commonly seen in diabetes and pancreatitis is known to interfere with human amylase methodology,[34,79] yielding test results that indicate normal amylase activity. Such has not been found to be the case where amyloclastic methods are used in the dog. Should the situation arise where hyperlipemia is thought to interfere with laboratory evaluations for pancreatitis, the serum may either be cleared with diethyl ether[79] or serially diluted with normal saline solution to eliminate interference caused by elevated triglycerides.

Hyperamylasemia has been reported to occur in two non-pancreatic disorders of man, tumor hyperamylasemia[80] and macroamylasemia.[81] Tumor hyperamylasemia is reported to occur primarily with metastatic pulmonary carcinomas. Tumor amylase upon electrophoretic separation is found to correspond in migration rate to one of the human salivary isoenzymes. Macroamylasemia is a biochemical abnormality associated with elevations in serum of a macromolecular species of α-amylase. Macroamylasemia in man is not associated with any particular disease or diseases at present. The relevance of the previous two human disorders to animals is unknown at this time. Should persistent hyperamylasemia be detected in the absence of signs of pancreatic disease, such abnormalities would warrant consideration.

The effect that renal failure has on canine amylase concentrations continues to pose a diagnostic problem. Uremic dogs may have serum amylase values up to 2½ times normal in the absence of observed pancreatic lesions.[82] However, no correlation between the degree of azotemia and the degree of hyperamylasemia was found.

The interpretation of hyperamylasemia in dogs with a normal blood urea nitrogen or serum creatinine concentration is uncomplicated. However, severe pancreatitis may be associated with varying degrees of prerenal azotemia, and if hypotension is prolonged, primary ischemic renal failure may occur. The clinical separation of vomiting patients with pancreatitis and prerenal uremia, from those with primary renal failure and retention hyperamylasemia is made uncomplicated by evaluating a urine specific gravity. An elevated BUN and hyperamylasemia accompanied by a high urine specific gravity (> 1.020) is indicative of prerenal uremia. Such results are compatible with, but not pathognomonic for, acute pancreatitis complicated by shock. If the urine specific gravity is low, particularly in the isosthenuric range (1.008 to 1.012), then primary renal failure with retention hyperamylasemia is suggested. Fortunately, many patients with acute pancreatitis, even when severely dehydrated, have normal BUN concentrations. In addition, those occasional dogs with prerenal uremia and pancreatitis usually have only moderately elevated BUN levels, i.e., 40 to 90 mg/dl and quite elevated amylase concentrations.

Lipase

Serum lipase is the second enzyme with diagnostic specificity for pancreatitis. Most lipase methodologies are more time consuming and technically more involved than amylase estimation. Although at one time lipase was the preferred test for pancreatitis, this is no longer the case. Both amylase and lipase rise and persist in a parallel manner following experimental pancreatitis in dogs. In general, values of less than 1.0 sigma unit are considered normal. Recent clinical data accumulated on naturally occurring pancreatitis in dogs suggest that greater diagnostic accuracy will result if both amylase and lipase are evaluated simultaneously. False negative values have been observed in some cases. This is particularly true during the recovery phase when disparities may occur between amylase or lipase values. Results from studies of human pancreatitis also indicate that a higher degree of diagnostic accuracy is obtained using both amylase and lipase simultaneously.[77]

Whether lipase is subject to the same alterations in renal failure as amylase remains unsettled. From evaluation of a limited number of patients, lipase would not appear to be falsely elevated by renal failure as often as amylase.

Blood And Urine Glucose

Diabetes mellitus and pancreatitis commonly occur together. Often a well-compensated diabetic will be decompensated by an attack of acute pancreatitis. In still other patients, a transient diabetic state will appear during the active inflammatory disease and revert to a subclinical, "prediabetic" state once the pancreatitis is controlled. In the former situation, blood glucose concentrations will remain above 200 mg/dl on repeated evaluations. Such patients nearly always need to be treated for both diabetes mellitus and pancreatitis. Patients with latent or "prediabetes" have fasting blood glucose concentrations of 130 to 200 mg/dl. While such animals are not in need of immediate insulin therapy, they are at risk of developing overt diabetes if the pancreatitis is not controlled or if recurrent attacks occur. A complete urinalysis should be obtained on all patients with pancreatitis and if glucosuria is present, a blood glucose determination should be evaluated. Dogs with mild hyperglycemia and no urine ketones whose primary problem is pancreatitis may not need insulin therapy as islet cell injury during the inflammatory process may be at least partially reversible.

Hematology

Acute pancreatitis frequently leads to changes in the hemogram. Rarely, very mild forms show no change in the peripheral blood picture. In general, pancreatitis is associated with a leukocytosis. The magnitude of the white blood cell increase is somewhat proportional to both severity and degree of tissue damage. The leukocytosis is usually characterized as a mature neutrophilia with an eosinopenia and lymphopenia. More severe states begin to exhibit a left shift and monocytosis. A marked monocytosis tends to reflect involvement of the peritoneal cavity in the disease process. In severely ill animals a degenerative left shift will be evident and agonal thrombocytopenia may be noted.

The packed cell volume (PCV) is most often elevated in pancreatitis secondary to hemoconcentration accompanying vomiting, reduced fluid intake, diarrhea, and a shift of plasma and interstitial fluid into the peritoneal cavity. A preexisting or recent anemia may mask these PCV alterations.

Methemalbumin

Recent reports indicate that serum methemalbumin values become greatly elevated in experimental hemorrhagic pancreatitis in dogs. This rise does not occur in edematous pancreatitis. Methemalbumin forms in acute pancreatitis from the digestion of extravasated blood by pancreatic enzymes. The digested hemoglobin is oxidized to a product known as metheme. Metheme is subsequently absorbed into the circulation where it then combines with albumin to form methemalbumin.[83] Once the diagnosis of pancreatitis is established, an assessment of methemalbumin concentrations will serve as a prognostic indicator. In man, methemalbumin concentrations are known to increase not only in pancreatitis, but also in mesenteric vein thrombosis, bowel strangulation, and soft tissue trauma. Recent experimental data on the dog indicate that neither superior mesenteric vein or artery ligation, nor bowel strangulation induced significant increases in serum methemalbumin levels.[83] Normal methemalbumin levels are 0 to 8 mg/dl. In experimental canine hemorrhagic pancreatitis, serum concentrations range from 25 to 125 mg/dl. Serum methemalbumin concentrations rise within 6 hours of pancreatic injury and remain elevated for up to 6 days. Elevations persisted after amylase values had returned to normal in some cases. Diseases in addition to hemorrhagic pancreatitis that have been associated with hypermethemalbuminemia in my practice include hemolytic anemias and splenic torsion.

Serum Calcium

Severe hypocalcemia may be observed in naturally occurring canine pancreatitis.[5] At the present time, no reported incidences of clinical signs associated with this biochemical abnormality have appeared. If the human experience is to be believed, most cases of hypocalcemia occurring during pancreatitis are relative rather than absolute. A prospective study measuring serum ionized calcium, total serum calcium, and serum albumin concentrations during spontaneous pancreatitis would resolve the clinical importance of this finding. Certainly, the presence of hypocalcemia in canine pancreatitis would not seem to warrant the grave prognosis it elicits in man.

Paracentesis

Paracentesis is often indicated in abdominal emergencies. The presence of serosanguinous fluid suggests that acute pancreatitis may exist. Amylase determinations on such fluid may give extremely high readings lending further support to the diagnosis. However, fluid is often not obtained at paracentesis. Intestinal obstruction as well as infarcted small intestines can also give rise to elevated peritoneal fluid amylase. However, amylase activity is less elevated in the latter two disorders.

The cytology of such fluid is characterized by large numbers of neutrophils, red blood cells, and macrophages. If bacteria are observed, sepsis is indicated. Cytology is not helpful in differentiating peritonitis secondary to pancreatitis from other causes of peritonitis.

Liver Function

Hepatic enzymes are commonly abnormal in association with pancreatitis in dogs. Whether preexisting hepatic disease initiated the pancreatitis or vice versa is oftentimes not resolved. In experimental canine pancreatitis the following pathologic changes in the liver were noted: centrolobular necrosis; disseminated, small interstitial hemorrhages, edema in the space of Disse, and sinusoidal distention.[84] Biochemical abnormalities noted most often in clinical canine pancreatitis include elevations in serum glutamic pyruvic transaminase (SGPT) and serum alkaline phosphatase (SAP) activities as well as hyperbilirubinemia. The hyperbilirubinemia is most often transient, resulting from inflammatory hepatocellular injury and compression of the common bile duct along its intrapancreatic passage. Occasionally, pancreatic fibrosis causes permanent obstructive jaundice. In general, if the hepatic disease is secondary to pancreatitis, hepatic biochemical abnormalities should return to normal once the pancreatitis has subsided.[85] Conversely, if evidence for hepatic disease persists after the pancreatitis has resolved, primary liver disease is most likely present and may have been the cause for the pancreatitis.

Renal Function

Since animals with pancreatitis and primary renal failure may appear quite similar on a clinical basis, all patients suspected of having pancreatitis should have a BUN and urinalysis taken at the same time samples are obtained for an amylase and lipase. In addition, prerenal uremia may occur secondary to acute pancreatitis and warrants vigorous therapy to prevent ischemic renal changes from occurring.

Blood Gas Determinations

A distinct form of pulmonary membrane injury is thought to occur in human pancreatitis.[86] A diffuse loss of integrity of the alveolar-capillary membrane takes place, leading to life-threatening pulmonary edema. The exact cause for the pulmonary changes is unknown but it has been hypothesized that increases in circulating free fatty acids, phospholipase-A, or vasoactive substances liberated during acute pancreatitis are responsible for the pulmonary injury. This complication carries a poor prognosis as many patients that develop "pancreatitis lung" die. A recent report in the veterinary literature suggests that this syndrome may occur occasionally in canine pancreatitis.[87] Arterial blood gas determinations are necessary to confirm the diagnosis by indicating that severe hypoxia is present.

Radiography

Abdominal radiographs serve as an ancillary aid in the diagnosis of acute pancreatitis. In the initial diagnostic plan for any acutely vomiting patient, abdominal radiographs may be deemed necessary since they are of great localizing value. The radiographic abnormalities associated with pancreatitis are often subtle and require excellent radiographic technique to be appreciated. Radiographic signs are most likely to be diagnostic in acute rather than subacute or chronic pancreatitis.[88] In general, the radiographic appearance of pancreatitis is associated with abnormalities in size, shape, and position of structures adjacent to the pancreas; i.e., the greater curvature of the stomach, the pylorus, duodenum, and transverse colon.[88] Signs of peritonitis localized to the right upper quadrant of the abdomen are also consistent with a radiologic diagnosis of pancreatitis. A granular mottling and general loss of detail in this region are characteristic. More often than not, radiographs will not confirm a diagnosis of pancreatitis but will help in ruling out other causes of an acute abdomen.

Lipid Profiles

Hyperlipemia occurs fairly often in association with canine pancreatitis. At the present time, no studies are available which indicate the type of lipid abnormality present in these lipemic dogs. Since there is a known predisposition to pancreatitis in humans with familial hyperlipidemias (Types I and V), it would be valuable to screen hyperlipemic dogs with pancreatitis to assess whether they are predisposed to a familial lipid abnormality and, thus, prone also to pancreatitis.

Pancreatic Biopsy

Recent reports in both human[89,90] and veterinary[91] literature have alluded to the value of pancreatic biopsy. In man these are performed most often at laparotomy using fine needle aspiration or large bore needle biopsy techniques for mass lesions within the pancreas. A laparoscopic approach for biopsy of the canine pancreas has been described.[91] In the dog, pancreatic biopsy has been most useful for confirming a diagnosis of pancreatic insufficiency.

Summary of Diagnostic Plans

An initial diagnostic plan designed to rule out the presence of pancreatitis should include at least the following: complete blood count, amylase, lipase, BUN, and urinalysis. Once the results of these data are known, indications for additional laboratory or radiographic procedures will be obvious.

Therapeutic Plans

The morbidity and mortality associated with canine pancreatitis are extremely varied and often unpredictable. In addition, the total lack of any controlled therapeutic trials in veterinary medicine make any discussion of the management of canine pancreatitis subject to question. Nonetheless, certain therapeutic principles may be gained from the large volume of experimental work done on the dog and from accumulations of clinical impressions over the years. In general, therapeutic efforts are designed to provide symptomatic relief and avert the complications of the disease since the cause remains obscure in most cases. From a clinical standpoint, the most important thing is to establish an early diagnosis. Specificity of diagnosis allows appropriate therapy to be instituted and may prevent any of the serious complications or chronic sequelae of pancreatitis from developing.

Acute pancreatitis results in disruption of multiple body systems; i.e., gastrointestinal, hemolymphatic, cardiovascular, and urinary. Therapy is directed at controlling or reversing the pathologic processes occurring in each of these systems and reestablishing a state of normalcy as soon as possible. Medical therapy alone will correct over 90% of the patients with acute pancreatitis in man.[92] Similar success with medical approaches can be expected in the dog. A combined medical-surgical approach may be helpful in occasional animals. The general aims of therapy include (1) recognition and correction of shock and fluid electrolyte and acid-base abnormalities, (2) suppression of pancreatic secretion, (3) control of infection, (4) relief of pain, (5) correction of coagulation abnormalities, and (6) proper management of the recovery phase.[1,4,16,93]

Volume Replacement Therapy

Death from pancreatitis most often results from hypovolemic and/or endotoxic shock. As such, volume replacement therapy is probably the single most important form of therapy in severe pancreatitis. Attempts to correct fluid deficits should be immediate and vigorous if success is to be expected. Large amounts of fluid may be functionally lost into the pancreatic interstitium, peritoneal cavity, intestinal lymphatics, and omentum. Plasma losses in experimental canine pancreatitis approach 30 to 40%.[94] The pancreatitis patient's needs for fluid support may be likened to those of a burn patient; in fact, the term "pancreatic burn" has been applied in such cases. Owing to the relatively large quantities of plasma protein extravasated into the peritoneal cavity, correlation of clinical estimates of dehydration with hematocrit and total protein determinations often yield conflicting results.[93] The progressive fluid loss into the peritoneal cavity

coupled with the release of potent vasoactive amines (bradykinin, kallikrein, and myocardial depressant factor) along with endotoxins from a devitalized intestine all combine to produce a profound state of shock.

Several therapeutic agents may be used to combat the shock of pancreatitis. Lactated Ringer's solution is an acceptable rehydrating, balanced electrolyte solution in such cases. Large volumes should be used. In animals with normal renal function, volumes as high as 90 ml/kg/hr as an initial rapid intravenous administration are indicated. The tendency is to under-replace rather than overhydrate such animals. Usual clinical estimates of the patient's fluid needs are generally too low. Low molecular weight dextran (mol. wt. 37,000 to 43,000) has been used in man and experimental dogs with good success. This agent improves pancreatic microcirculation in addition to supporting overall blood volume and flow.[51,52] Volumes on the order of 100 ml/hr of 10% dextran were given to 20-kg dogs with experimental pancreatitis. The use of low molecular weight dextran as a plasma expander in man has been associated with occasional bleeding complications.[4] An alternative plasma expander that has had good success in man is serum. This is the ideal replacement fluid, as plasma colloids along with crystalloids are lost in this disease.[94] The relative unavailability of canine serum makes this mode of therapy infeasible in the dog.

In any patient in which large volumes of fluid are going to be administered, it is imperative that adequate renal function exists. An indwelling urethral catheter is helpful to monitor urine output, and a BUN or serum creatinine should be evaluated prior to administering fluids. In patients with prerenal uremia, rapid fluid administration should be accompanied by a vigorous diuresis. If oliguria is observed, fluid volumes should be reduced and augmented diuresis begun.

In addition to low molecular weight dextran, heparin, fibrinolysin, and vasopressin have been used to improve local pancreatic blood flow and prevent the progression of edematous to hemorrhagic pancreatitis. Adequate perfusion of the pancreatic microcirculation is critical if hemorrhage and necrosis are to be prevented.[51] Heparin prevents thrombosis by inhibiting intravascular clot formation. Fibrinolysin exerts its protective effect by lysing newly formed clots. The exact mechanism by which vasopressin prevents progression of edematous to hemorrhagic pancreatitis is unknown. It has been shown that vasopressin maintains pancreatic blood flow and perfusion in dogs with pancreatitis.[95] Several experimental studies in dogs have shown that vasopressin significantly improved survival.[96,97] All three agents prevent the accumulation of high interstitial concentrations of enzymes and digestive products.[55] The recommended dosage for heparin is 100 units per kilogram given subcutaneously twice daily. Up to one half the initial dosage may be given intravenously. Such patients should be monitored closely for signs of overdosage by checking whole blood clotting times or partial thromboplastin times. Fibrinolysin (Thrombolysin) is given in dosages of 50,000 units three times daily. Vasopressin may be administered as the aqueous product, 0.09 units/kg/min intravenously over a 6-hour period. Aqueous vasopressin is in very limited supply at the present time.

The indications for treatment of hypocalcemia in canine and feline pancreatitis are uncertain. Although hypocalcemia has been observed in a number of spontaneous cases of canine pancreatitis, no clinical signs were noted and all dogs survived. Data from man would indicate that the hypocalcemia of pancreatitis is most often relative, not absolute, being reduced as a result of hypoalbuminemia. Calcium therapy should be used with caution.

Reduction of Pancreatic Secretions

Reducing pancreatic secretions is one of the most important aspects of therapy for pancreatitis. This is accomplished by suppression of hormonal and nervous control of pancreatic secretion. Secretion of the pancreas is stimulated by both reflex and hormonal means. Reflex stimulation is via the vagus, which is excited by gastric distention from food, liquid, or gas. Hormone release occurs following the entry of gas and food into the pylorus and proximal duodenum.

Secretory suppression is accomplished by a number of means. The simplest and often very effective way is to restrict all oral intake (food, water, medication) with the possible exception of liquid protectant, antacid preparations. This should continue as long as signs of vomiting exist and usually is best prolonged for 24 to 72 hours after vomiting has ceased. Gastric suction devices, commonly used in man, are impractical for most clinical situations in veterinary medicine. The use of a pharyngostomy tube for intermittent aspiration of gastric contents may have merit in selected cases.[1]

A number of chemical agents have been used to reduce the volume and character of pancreatic secretions. Although atropine and atropine-like anticholinergics have been used most often, other drugs, including glucagon, 5-fluorouracil, carbonic anhydrase inhibitors, and antienzyme preparations, have all received some measure of support from the medical profession.

Atropine and many of its analogs have been shown experimentally to reduce gastric acid secretion significantly, as well as reducing pancreatic bicarbonate and enzyme output.[98,99,100] The dose of atropine that blocks pancreatic vagal activity is between 0.04 and 0.08 mg/kg.[17,101] Although no controlled clinical trials utilizing this drug have been performed, clinical experience indicates that they are beneficial in many patients. Alternative drugs to atropine with less objectionable effects include propantheline bromide (Probanthine) at a dosage of 7.5 to 15 mg, depending on the size of the patient, two to four times daily, or Banthine at a dosage of 5 to 10 mg/kg three times daily.

Glucagon therapy has received impressive interest in recent years as a therapy for pancreatitis. Glucagon levels were found to be increased early in pancreatitis but as patients deteriorated, these levels declined. It was concluded that glucagon may be a natural defense mechanism against the ravages of pancreatitis. Experimental work has confirmed that glucagon reduces pancreatic exocrine secretion, increases splanchnic blood flow, suppresses gastric secretion, and reduces intestinal motility.[102] All of these effects are theoretically of benefit to the pancreatitis patient. A number of uncontrolled clinical trials in man have been published.[103,104,105] The most that can be concluded is that glucagon in man subjectively reduces the pain associated with pancreatitis. Controlled experiments in dogs indicate that glucagon is no more efficacious than simple volume replacement.[102] Additionally, pancreatic hemorrhages were observed in the glucagon treated group but not in untreated controls or fluid-resuscitated dogs. Because of these results, glucagon cannot be recommended for use in canine pancreatitis at this time.

A drug which has been used experimentally to control acute pancreatitis and which may be valuable on clinical patients is the anticancer drug 5-fluorouracil (5-FU). Five-fluorouracil interferes with the synthesis of DNA and RNA and thus impairs intracellular protein synthesis. In addition, 5-FU is thought to impair enzyme release from pancreatic acinar cells.[106] When this drug was administered to dogs with severe pancreatitis, 90% survived. All the control dogs treated only with fluids and antibiotics died.[106] No permanent injury to the pancreas was observed. The dosage of 5-FU used was 15 mg/kg intravenously on day 1, then 10 mg/kg the second day, 7 mg/kg the third day, and 5 mg/kg days 4 through 7. Although preliminary results are encouraging, a controlled clinical trial is badly needed.

Carbonic anhydrase inhibitors are known to reduce pancreatic volume and enzyme secretion. Acetazolamide (Diamox) has been tried on a clinical basis in man with equivocal results.[107] No valid reasons exist at this time to recommend its use in canine pancreatitis.

Antienzyme Preparations

These preparations for the therapy of human pancreatitis continue to receive either enthusiastic or lambastic comments. Experimental work in dogs using the trypsin-kallikrein inhibitor, aprotinin (Trasylol), indicates it is only of value if given prophylactically, i.e., prior to the onset of pancreatitis.[108] Such diagnostic foresight is not the norm in veterinary medicine. In addition, this drug is not commercially available in the United States.

Antibiotic Therapy

Antibiotic therapy in acute pancreatitis is currently being questioned.[4,16,109] In some institutions, antibiotics are no longer given prophylactically for pancreatitis because the risk of developing antibiotic-resistant strains is considered greater than the risk of sepsis from pancreatitis.[110] Patients are monitored closely for signs of sepsis and antibiotics are administered accordingly. Controlled clinical trials in man have indicated that ampicillin-treated patients with alcoholic or idiopathic pancreatitis had no significant differences in their disease course from those not receiving antibiotics.[111] In more severe forms of canine pancreatitis, antibiotics have been shown to improve survival rates significantly.[112,113] Broad-spectrum antibiotics are most useful, as often both gram-positive and gram-negative organisms are isolated. Procaine penicillin and dihydrostreptomycin are an effective combination. Intravenous chloramphenicol or oxytetracycline hydrochloride are also effective. Once oral intake is tolerated, oral preparations may be instituted. It has been recommended that antibiotics be continued for 1 week after clinical recovery is complete.[1] Streptomycin, oleandomycin, kanamycin, and sulfonamides are excreted in high enough concentrations to be bacteriostatic in pancreatic juice[114] and are of value where intrapancreatic infection is a problem.

Analgesia

This treatment is indicated if pancreatitis appears quite painful. The analgesic agent of choice in pancreatitis is meperidine hydrochloride (Demerol). The dose is 2.5 to 5 mg/lb intramuscularly or subcutaneously two to three times per day. Morphine is contraindicated as it causes spasm of the pancreatic duct sphincter, increases in intraductal pressures, and hyperamylasemia.[115] Meperidine has similar disadvantages, but to a much lesser degree. Generally, analgesics do not need to be administered but if they are, it is usually only for 1 to 2 days.

Glucocorticoid Therapy

Use of glucocorticoids in the treatment of pancreatitis remains controversial. Steroid use is confirmed to cause pancreatitis in rats, rabbits, mice, and man. Hyperviscosity of pancreatic secretions and pancreatic ductular metaplasia may be responsible for initiating the disease.[116,117,118] I have observed numerous cases of pancreatitis develop in steroid-treated dogs within a short time following the onset of drug administration. Conversely, survival of dogs with experimentally induced severe hemorrhagic pancreatitis was improved using glucocorticoids alone.[119,120] At our present state of understanding concerning steroids and pancreatitis, it is recommended that glucocorticoids be used only for patients in shock. Routine use of glucocorticoids in mild forms of pancreatitis has no reasonable justification.

Nonoperative Peritoneal Lavage

As an adjunct to the medical therapy of pancreatitis, peritoneal lavage may be helpful in the dog. Experimental canine studies indicated that significantly improved survival occurred in the lavaged group. Although it has been concluded that peritoneal lavage combined with medical therapy was beneficial in a clinical trial of canine pancreatitis, no data on untreated controls were included.[121] Lavage serves as a means of removing pancreatic enzymes from the peritoneal cavity and for administration of antibiotics.[122] Complications of this technique include anemia, hypokalemia, hyponatremia, and hypoproteinemia.[121]

Surgical Intervention

Operation in pancreatitis is rarely necessary. Ninety-five percent of human patients recover satisfactorily without surgical procedure.[123] Indications for surgery include patients who are deteriorating in spite of intensive medical therapy, those patients in which a definitive diagnosis is still suspect, those that would appear on laboratory data to have a pancreatic abscess, and those in whom operative peritoneal lavage is considered important. In a controlled experiment in dogs to evaluate the value of partial pancreatectomy for pancreatitis,[124] 93% of the untreated controls died, 25% died when given fluids and whole blood alone, but 59% of the pancreatectomized dogs died. In general, surgical approaches to treat pancreatitis should be reserved for last ditch heroics.

Convalescent Therapy

This mode of treatment varies from case to case. Even so, certain general guidelines may be followed that can be modified based on patient needs. Dogs with pancreatitis may often be started back on oral liquid intake within 24 hours after the last nausea and vomiting are noted. If vomiting recurs, withhold oral intake an additional 24 hours, continuing parenteral support. Keep liquid volumes small at each offering (1 to 3 oz). Gastric distention may cause renewed vomiting or stimulate excessive pancreatic secretion. Allow liquids at frequent intervals throughout the day and then free choice as soon as the patient's condition dictates. Once free-choice water is well tolerated, bland, low-fat dog food may be offered in small quantities. An alternative method of nutritional support involves the use of so called "elemental" diets (Flexical, Mead-Johnson). Such products produce minimal pancreatic stimulation while providing needed nutritional support. They are composed of amino acids, sucrose, and medium chain triglycerides, providing 1 calorie per milliliter. Antibiotic therapy should be continued for 7 to 10 days after clinical signs of illness are gone to eliminate any foci of infection from within the pancreas. Anticholinergics also appear to improve the rate of recovery when continued several days after signs are normal.

Serum enzyme values may remain elevated for several days or longer after the patient's clinical appearance is normal. Enzyme abnormalities should not prevent convalescent therapy from being started or delay a patient's release, if the animal is not vomiting and is clinically improving. A weekly CBC and amylase and lipase value should be evaluated to determine whether continuing inflammation is occurring. A few animals continue to exhibit evidence of smoldering pancreatitis for weeks or months in spite of continued therapy. In such animals, a search should be made for one of the rare etiologies of pancreatitis (hypercalcemia, neoplasia, abscess, hepatic disease, hyperlipidemia, drugs). A fasting blood glucose or high-dose intravenous glucose tolerance test often indicates that carbohydrate intolerance exists. Pancreatitis often injures

beta cells, significantly reducing the functional mass of insulin secreting tissue.

Dietary control once the patient returns home is critical. Most commercial pet foods are not high in fat and may be used. Strict avoidance of table foods is mandatory and weight reduction is usually indicated. In problem cases where recurrences develop on commercial diets, low fat prescription diets may be helpful (r/d, Riviana Foods, Inc.). Diets for patients that have recovered from pancreatitis should be high in carbohydrate, contain moderate amounts of protein, and be low in fat.[93,125]

Many complications have the potential to develop during or subsequent to an attack of pancreatitis. Fortunately, they do not occur very often. Early, severe complications include hemorrhage, shock, sepsis, renal failure, and possibly pulmonary hypoxemia. The long-standing complications of pancreatitis are obstructive jaundice (rare), diabetes mellitus (fairly common), and end-stage pancreatitis (fairly common). Pancreatic necrosis is the most common cause of diabetes in the dog.[2] Pancreatic exocrine insufficiency will be discussed later in this chapter.

Since it is extremely difficult to determine the severity of pancreatitis with either clinical or laboratory means during initial stages of the disease, the prognosis should remain guarded. Animals surviving longer than 48 hours have a good chance for clinical recovery. Owners should always be informed about the seriousness of long-term sequelae to pancreatitis, i.e., chronic pancreatitis, diabetes mellitus, and exocrine pancreatic insufficiency.

CHRONIC PANCREATITIS

Chronic pancreatitis results from repeated attacks of the acute process with relentless, progressive destruction of glandular tissue. Etiologic factors involved in chronic pancreatitis are the same as those listed for acute pancreatitis. The chronic disease is thought to be a progressive phase of the acute problem. The process is an active one, being characterized pathologically by hyperplasia of pancreatic connective tissue, loss of parenchyma, and extensive interstitial fibrosis.[1] The source of abdominal pain in chronic pancreatitis is speculated to arise from adhesions to the liver, stomach, small intestine, and omentum.

Chronic pancreatitis is the most common form of pancreatic disease in the dog. Chronic pancreatitis is rare in cats, as is end-stage pancreatitis. A number of different disease entities have been included under the term chronic pancreatitis and thus confusion about its meaning exists. Such diseases as chronic inflammatory pancreatitis, diabetes mellitus and the exocrine insufficiency states, pancreatic fibrosis (end-stage pancreatitis), and pancreatic atrophy have been included with this term. For the purposes of this discussion, the term chronic pancreatitis refers only to those animals with biochemical evidence that active acinar injury is still occurring. Amylase and lipase values in animals with end-stage pancreatitis are normal to subnormal, since nearly all functional acinar tissue has been previously destroyed. A diagnosis of chronic pancreatitis is based upon biochemical evidence that active inflammatory pancreatic disease exists and that previous attacks are known to have taken place. The diagnosis of chronic pancreatitis is similar to that for the acute disease. The severity is usually much less, however, and therapy rarely requires the heroics of the severe acute case.

Part II. Exocrine Pancreatic Insufficiency

GERALD F. JOHNSON

The exocrine pancreas, more than any other organ, synthesizes and secretes the bulk of enzymes that digest the major classes of foodstuffs in the intestine. It also secretes water and bicarbonate, thus regulating the pH of the intestine, necessary for digestion and absorption. Exocrine pancreatic insufficiency (EPI) results from a lack of these enzymes or an inability of these enzymes to digest food.

EPI can be primary or secondary. Primary EPI results from diseases such as pancreatitis, neoplastic invasion, pancreatectomy or ligation of ducts, and pancreatic hypoplasia (also called juvenile pancreatic atrophy), which affect the exocrine gland and its ducts. Primary EPI in cats is rare.[126]

Secondary EPI can occur in three ways: (1) inadequate release of the intestinal hormones, cholecystokinin and secretin; (2) decreased intraluminal pH in the small intestine; and (3) secretion of pancreatic enzymes not coordinated with arrival of the meal.

History and Signs

In primary EPI of the dog, the outstanding clinical signs are weight loss, polyphagia, increased volume of feces, and deterioration of the haircoat. The onset of signs is usually insidious and appears over a period of weeks to months. Once present, these signs will persist in the untreated patient.

EPI resulting from pancreatitis has a higher incidence in older females.[68,71] Pancreatic hypoplasia has a marked predilection for young German Shepherd dogs.[71,127]

The chief complaint of the client with an animal that has EPI may vary from coprophagy or diarrhea to a decreasing insulin requirement in the case of a diabetic animal. Seldom will all pertinent information be volunteered; this makes perceptive recording of anamnesis by the clinician a necessity. In general, however, the chief complaints are diarrhea and weight loss.

More important than the physical examination, the adequate history contributes greatly to the diagnosis and management of the disease and aids in the exclusion of other disease entities. A history of weight loss is essential: either the owners seldom seek veterinary consultation until considerable weight loss has occurred, or the disease may not have been suspected by the veterinarian when signs were less pronounced. Pancreatic insufficiency is improbable in an obese or well-nourished animal that has had little or no weight loss. In the same vein, a thin dog with an unthrifty haircoat may simply not be getting sufficient caloric intake or may have malignant disease. Particular attention is given to the duration and onset of signs, eating and bowel habits, and diet. Because maldigestion and, therefore, malabsorption are severe with EPI, changes in eating and bowel habits are usually readily noticed.

Questioning the client regarding the pet's eating habits will reveal that the dog with EPI is extraordinarily hungry, frequently scavenges or steals food, and may develop coprophagy.

Questions regarding bowel habits often reveal a history of both increased frequency (five or more times per day) and increased volume of feces. Consistency may vary from unformed to soft to sometimes formed; the feces are often light in color and have a strong pungent odor. Clients should be asked if the feces appear greasy, and if the animal's perineum is ever oily. Feces do not contain blood or mucus, and are usually not watery unless there is a concomitant disease process.

Bowel habits and characteristics of the feces also vary with the diet being fed. In normal dogs and cats, fecal volume is greater with semimoist than with canned products and, for a given energy intake, cereal yields 2½ times as much fecal material as does meat.[128] Therefore, voluminous bowel movements do not always mean malabsorption. Steatorrhea is less likely to be noticed by the client or the veterinarian if the diet contains little fat. Thus, in taking a history, the veterinarian should consider fat, protein, caloric, and residue contents since these factors significantly change the character of the feces and eating habits.

The veterinarian should question the client about any previous episodes of pancreatitis, jaundice, neoplasia, abdominal trauma, surgery, or pancreatic endocrine disease. These may be important clues that suggest the presence of EPI as well. In chronic pancreatitis, however, signs related to inflammation of the gland, if present, often go undetected by both the client and the veterinarian until signs of EPI or diabetes mellitus appear.[70]

In cases of concomitant diabetes mellitus, those signs usually precede the onset of signs of EPI. Occasionally, signs of diabetes mellitus and EPI may coexist. Signs of EPI may not be detected until after the diabetes mellitus is managed and the animal begins eating. Overlooking EPI in the diabetic dog can lead to severe weight loss, ketosis, and lower insulin requirements.

Secondary pancreatic insufficiency, i.e., pancreatic insufficiency not due to disease involving the gland itself, has not been documented in the dog but is likely to occur. Signs due to the cause of secondary pancreatic insufficiency may not be as dramatic as those of primary pancreatic insufficiency and are more difficult to document.

As mentioned earlier, secondary pancreatic insufficiency can occur in three ways.[129] First, decreased hormonal stimulation of the pancreas results in inadequate secretion of digestive enzymes. This occurs in severe mucosal disease of the small bowel when the cells that release cholecystokinin (CCK) and secretin are damaged.[130–131] Under physiologic conditions, the limiting factor of pancreatic bicarbonate secretion is the capacity of the intestine to release secretin.[131] Second, pancreatic lipase can be irreversibly destroyed at a low pH as occurs from hypersecretion of gastric acid; the result is steatorrhea. Hypersecretion of gastric acid, occurring in association with a gastrinoma, has been documented in dogs.[132,133] Although pyloroplasty is sometimes performed in dogs, signs of secondary pancreatic insufficiency due to decreased intestinal pH or rapid gastric emptying have not been a clinical problem. Third, stimulation of the pancreas must be coordinated with release of digestive enzymes, i.e., at the same time that food is being delivered to the duodenum. When a gastrojejunostomy is performed, food leaves the stomach and enters the jejunum, bypassing the enzymes released into the duodenum. This results in diminished release of CCK and secretin by the cells located in the duodenal mucosa as well as improper mixing of the meal with pancreatic enzymes, and maldigestion.

Physical Examination

Dogs exhibiting signs of EPI appear undernourished: the animal is thin, sometimes emaciated with an unthrifty appearance of the skin and hair. Younger animals with pancreatic hypoplasia may have retarded growth and signs of nutritional bone disease. Occasionally the perineum will appear oily or greasy. The animals show no signs of distress and are usually alert and active. In the examination room, the animal may be noted to be searching for something to eat. If the patient is also an unregulated diabetic, physical findings of this disease predominate.

Rule-Outs

The veterinarian must determine whether the dog is being offered enough food. Although these points are often taken for granted, some clients simply do not offer their pets an adequate diet, yet they bring them to the clinic because they are thin and have voracious appetites. By weighing the dog and knowing how much of which type of diet is eaten, some simple calculations will quickly determine whether the caloric intake is adequate. If there is any question regarding the amounts and type of food given, an adequate diet can be suggested to the client and the progress of the dog and its weight followed.

Small breeds (less than or equal to 2 kg) should receive approximately 120 kilocalories (kcal)/kg body weight; dogs weighing 10 kg should receive approximately 74 kcal/kg body weight; dogs weighing 30 kg, 57 kcal/kg body weight; and dogs weighing 70 kg, 45 kcal/kg. These are maintenance requirements, and compensation should be made for dogs engaging in special activities, such as the lactating bitch or strenuous exercise in the working breeds. Approximate figures for various dog food preparations are as follows: dry cereal, 1000 kcal/290 g, semimoist, 1000 kcal/350 g (one patty weighs 85 g), and canned, 450 kcal/453 g.[128]

Other causes of malabsorption, such as diseases of the small intestine, infiltrative lesions, benign or neoplastic disease, and parasitic disease, must also be ruled out. Malabsorption due to decreased micellarization of fat can occur with biliary tract obstruction, but jaundice and other signs predominate so that differentiating this from EPI is usually not difficult.

Hyperthyroidism in the dog may be confused with EPI because of excessive defecation, polyphagia and weight loss, among other signs.[134] We believe that this disorder is rare in cats.

An animal can also be presented with EPI already diagnosed, having been placed on medication and not responding. Two questions should come to mind: has the diagnosis of EPI been satisfactorily established, and is the management of the animal's disease being carried out properly?

Diagnostic Plans

The ideal method for evaluating the function of the exocrine pancreas is by directly measuring pancreatic enzyme activity after secretion has been induced by administration of secretin and/or CCK, or by administering test meals which rely on reflex stimulation of the pancreas.[129] The latter method is valuable in diagnosing secondary EPI. Direct testing requires duodenal intubation and is done at few veterinary institutions. A diagnosis of EPI, therefore, is based on indirect evidence provided by an evaluation of the patient's digestive and absorptive capacities. The most frequent cause of maldigestion and malabsorption in the dog encountered by the clinician, however, is EPI, and establishing the presence of steatorrhea is a major step in the

workup. A laboratory workup is indicated in animals when the presence and cause of fat malassimilation are questioned. When EPI is not a result of pancreatic hypoplasia, it is most often encountered in the dog secondary to pancreatitis, and diabetes mellitus is often present.

Often history and signs are suggestive enough to warrant treatment, particularly if pancreatic hypoplasia is suspected in a young German Shepherd dog. Even then, steatorrhea should be documented, if only with microscopic examination of the feces.

A clinical laboratory profile, including a complete blood count, blood chemistries, urinalysis, and one or more fecal analyses for parasites and ova, should be established to provide basic information regarding the overall health of the animal. This serves to eliminate disorders which may not otherwise be suspected.

Fat Digestion

Although the pancreas secretes enzymes for the digestion of each major foodstuff, fat digestion is affected most severely in EPI.[135] The pancreas is the only major source of lipase, so the detection of steatorrhea is of major diagnostic significance.

The normal absorptive capacity of dogs has been established at 93 to 98% of ingested fat.[127,100] This is termed the "coefficient of absorption," that is, ingested fat minus fecal loss, expressed as a percentage of ingested fat. A dog consuming 1000 kcal as 300 g of dry cereal ingests 25 g of fat, nearly half as much fat as a dog consuming 1000 kcal (648 g of food, 48 g of fat) as a canned meat-type food.[128] Therefore, if these dogs had coefficients of absorption of 70%, 7 g and 13 g of fat, respectively, would be detected in their fecal samples. Obviously, when performing a microscopic examination of the feces, fat would be more apparent in the dog ingesting the diet containing more fat. Detection of smaller amounts of fat can then be even more difficult because the fat can be diluted out in the large volumes of feces produced by dogs with EPI. It then becomes obvious that the clinician must have some idea of the amounts of fat ingested when evaluating steatorrhea.

Canned prescription cat foods are among the best diets to use in evaluating steatorrhea because they contain more fat than most other diets. Still, this fat content is not enough to overwhelm the healthy dog's ability to absorb fat. The average 30-kg German Shepherd dog should receive 1700 calories for this test, or at least three cans at approximately 500 kcal/can. Thus, the dog ingests adequate calories and about 100 g of fat if the diet contains 7% fat. Healthy dogs of 12- to 25-kg body weight receiving up to 800 g of fat in the diet over a period of 3 days, still absorb 93 to 98% of ingested fat.[127,136]

Quantitating fecal fat is helpful in establishing the presence of maldigestion or malabsorption, but it does not differentiate the cause. The fat content of most commercial dog and cat foods can easily be calculated from information provided on the label. By knowing both the amount of food and fat ingested and the fat lost in the feces, the coefficient of absorption of fat can be readily calculated. This figure is more meaningful than simply comparing to an arbitrary value for fecal fat loss.

From a clinical point of view, further determinations of fecal glycerides and fatty acids is not necessary, although the diagnosis of EPI can be further substantiated when most of the fat is in the form of glycerides. What is important to determine from the 72-hour fecal fat analysis is the severity of steatorrhea, which in dogs with EPI ranges from 30 to 75% loss of ingested fat into the feces.[127]

Because quantitating fecal fat can be difficult and aesthetically unpleasant, screening tests can provide valuable information. The most useful is the Sudan III or IV stain for microscopic stool fat. This correlates well with 72-hour quantitation when steatorrhea is moderate or severe as is the case with EPI. Again, intake of fat must be adequate. The value of the microscopic examination is directly related to the experience and concern of the observer. As with other tests to evaluate fat assimilation, nonabsorbable products such as mineral oil, petroleum jelly, and castor oil will interfere with interpretation; these should not be used prior to collecting specimens.

Oral glycerides and subsequent determination of plasma turbidity[137] and the vitamin A absorption test[138] can also be used as screening tests. All phases of lipid digestion and absorption must be functional. Radiolabeled fat has limited application[139,140] and is not available to most practitioners.

Nitrogen Loss

The digestion and absorption of protein can be evaluated by determining fecal nitrogen loss over a 24-hour period. This can be done from the same aliquot used for determining fecal fat, and the two test results compared. The amount of nitrogen ingested can be calculated by multiplying the protein content of the diet by 0.16, since 6.4 g of protein contains approximately 1 g of nitrogen. Fecal

analysis on normal dogs fed a commercial dry dog food revealed a nitrogen loss of no more than 6 g.[138] As with fecal fat determination, this test does not pinpoint the defect but merely supports the presence of malassimilation.

Proteolytic Enzymes

Testing for proteolytic enzymes in the feces is another method of evaluating EPI. These tests depend on the specificity of the substrate and the sensitivity of detecting enzyme activity. Measuring trypsin and chymotrypsin activity with specific substrates of arginine and tyrosine esters, respectively, proved valuable in detecting experimental EPI in dogs.[141] Though less specific, an azocasein substrate also allows quantitation of proteolytic enzyme activity.[142] Simply using a dilutional technique and gelatin or film digestion affords some quantitation of nonspecific proteolytic enzymes in the feces. The more sophisticated the test, however, the more accurate the interpretation. Proteolytic activity in the feces can vary from day to day, false-positive results can occur due to bacterial proteolytic activity, and false-negative results can occur due to bacterial degradation of enzymes. Accuracy of the test is improved if it is performed on 3 consecutive days and the results compared.

Microscopic examination of the feces using iodine stains to detect undigested muscle fibers can also provide supportive evidence of inadequate pancreatic enzyme activity. The animal's diet, however, must have contained uncooked meat.

Carbohydrate Tolerance Test

To evaluate carbohydrate assimilation, various carbohydrate tolerance tests have been employed. Starches and other complex carbohydrates are dependent on pancreatic amylase for conversion to maltose and alpha dextrins, which are then converted to glucose by glycocalyx disaccharidases of the epithelial cells. Serum glucose determinations are then used to evaluate the status of these two enzyme systems, although a defect in one or both cannot be differentiated. Because of this nonspecificity, this test contributes little to the diagnosis of EPI.

Oral tolerance testing using monosaccharides does have a place in evaluating EPI. A normal test curve provides evidence of the integrity of the small intestinal epithelium. This indirectly incriminates the pancreas as the cause of maldigestion, once steatorrhea has been proven. Monosaccharides require no enzymatic hydrolysis prior to absorption; therefore, determinations of serum glucose concentration after an ingested load reflect the absorptive capacity of the intestinal mucosa.

Glucose and D-xylose are the two monosaccharides used for oral tolerance testing. Both tests are influenced by the motility of the gastrointestinal tract. Rapid transit or, conversely, delayed gastric emptying can interfere with interpretation of results. With oral glucose tolerance testing (OGTT), the serum glucose value can be affected by those hormones that are associated with carbohydrate homeostasis, such as insulin, glucagon and epinephrine. Since some animals with EPI also have abnormalities of pancreatic endocrine function, the value of the OGTT is limited in diabetics. With pancreatic hypoplasia, prediabetic curves have been described with both intravenous and oral tolerance testing.[143,144] This may occur because of an inability to digest the carbohydrates offered in the diet, resulting in low carbohydrate absorption. In the carbohydrate-deprived dog, a diabetic-like tolerance curve occurs, which reverts to normal when carbohydrates are incorporated in the diet.[145] Repeat tolerance testing of dogs with pancreatic hypoplasia after compensation with therapy was not associated with a return to normal glucose tolerance curves in a small series.[146] There have been rare reports of animals with pancreatic hypoplasia ultimately requiring insulin. With diffuse intestinal mucosal pathology and pancreatic endocrine disease, results will be uninterpretable because absorption will be decreased owing to the intestinal disease; yet, blood glucose values may persist in being elevated owing to the endocrine abnormality.

In contrast, D-xylose is a 5-carbon sugar that for practical purposes is metabolized slowly in the body as compared to glucose. Absorption is also dependent on transit time, and degradation of D-xylose by bacteria can occur with bacterial overgrowth in the gut.[147] D-xylose is absorbed and rapidly excreted in the urine. Oral tolerance testing with D-xylose, then, is a good indication of small intestinal absorptive integrity and it is more accurate than the OGTT. D-xylose has been studied in the dog using serum values.[148]

Hepatic Evaluation

With EPI, the liver can be affected either from earlier bouts of pancreatitis which lead to varying degrees of obstructive biliary tract disease or from secondary nutritional deficiencies which can range from lipidosis to cirrhosis. Elevations in transaminases due to hepatic lipidosis are reported in pancreatic hypoplasia.[127,149] The full range of liver

abnormalities seen in diabetics can be seen with the diabetic having concomitant EPI.

Summary

Of the numerous tests available to evaluate malassimilation of nutrients, which ones are the most useful to the veterinary clinician in evaluating an animal suspected of having EPI? It is most important to document steatorrhea, which can usually be accomplished by microscopic examination of feces. However, if results are equivocal, then quantitation of 24-hour fecal fat should be performed. Monosaccharide tolerance testing with glucose (or more ideally, D-xylose) provides evidence that the intestinal epithelium is functioning adequately. These are the more valuable tests, although fecal nitrogen, proteolytic enzyme activity in the feces, plasma turbidity, and vitamin A tolerance tests can be supportive.

Due to the specificity of therapy for EPI, response to treatment provides strong evidence in support of the diagnosis. Many tests such as quantitative fecal fat and nitrogen, starch tolerance test, and plasma turbidity can be performed before and during replacement therapy to provide additional support to the diagnosis. This is rarely necessary, is time-consuming, and brings an added expense to the client.

Surgery and laparoscopy are other methods of directly examining the pancreas that should not be overlooked. This can be a favorable alternative to euthanasia. On more than one occasion performing an ovariohysterectomy has also provided a fortuitous opportunity to examine and palpate the gland, thus ruling in/out disease of the exocrine pancreas. Precautions regarding manipulation and biopsy of the pancreas should be taken. If malassimilation has been documented prior to surgery and the pancreas appears normal, full-thickness biopsy of the intestine should be performed.

Direct Challenge Testing

Direct testing of the exocrine pancreas can be accomplished by provoking secretion with exogenous secretin and/or cholecystokinin (CCK) and collecting the secretion via duodenal intubation. The volume, bicarbonate content, and enzyme content are then determined. Thus far, this is the most accurate method of evaluating the exocrine pancreas, and has been superbly documented in 65 control dogs and 27 dogs with EPI.[149] Although this method is not practical for most veterinary clinicians, it may become available to large centers and teaching hospitals (see Table 17–6).

Therapeutic Plans

Therapy for EPI is relatively simple, but the physiologic mechanisms are somewhat complex and will be discussed first.

Before signs of EPI occur in the dog, all but a small portion of the gland is destroyed.[1,150] In humans, pancreatic enzyme secretion must be less than 10% of normal before steatorrhea or creatorrhea occur.[151] Studies have evaluated the fate of orally ingested enzymes in humans, and reported less than 22% of the ingested trypsin and less than 10% of the ingested lipase were active in the duodenum. Neither of these values was more than 3% of the enzyme activity found in normal people. There are two reasons for inactivation of orally ingested enzymes: (1) acid-peptic inactivation of the enzymes in the stomach,[152] and (2) duodenal hyperacidification resulting from lack of bicarbonate output from the diseased pancreas. Rapid gastric emptying may also be a contributing factor.[153]

Lipase is irreversibly destroyed at a pH of 4 or less.[154] Gastric and duodenal pH in animals with EPI should be investigated, although very low pancreatic bicarbonate secretion has been documented in dogs with EPI.[149]

Thus, in spite of the very low enzyme activity in EPI and the marked inactivation of orally ingested enzymes, a fraction of the normal enzyme activity is all that is needed and can be had by the oral administration of pancreatic enzyme supplement. Although absorption does not return to normal, significant improvement of maldigestion has been shown by use of pancreatic enzyme supplement in dogs.[127,155,156]

No difference was noted in humans who were medicated hourly as opposed to prandially.[157] For convenience, a prandial dosage is advantageous and has been clinically effective in the dog.[127] This is also my preference.

One factor governing the success of therapy is the commercial preparation of enzymes. Several preparations have been shown to be effective in the dog.[155,156] Recent findings deal with the quality of commercial preparations. Assays of commercial preparations showed a wide range of enzyme activity, and several preparations stand out as being superior.[152,158] Among these are pancrelipase NF (Cotazym, Organon), pancreatin (Viokase, Viobin Corp.) and KU-Zyme (Kremers-Urban Co.). Though the exact enzyme activity varies, several products are suitable because the dosage can also be varied. However, it has been demonstrated that enteric coating of commercial preparations renders them less effective.[152]

Since dogs with EPI will readily accept powdered preparations mixed with the meal, digestion may be enhanced by affording more uniform mixing with the food than capsules or tablets provide.

Bile acids are lost in the presence of pancreatic insufficiency and their loss decreases markedly with the correction of the steatorrhea.[159] Bile acid concentrations were found to be adequate in people with EPI.[160] The use of bile salts in the treatment of EPI does not seem to be indicated. Antacids in the form of sodium bicarbonate have been advocated for treating the dog with EPI. In experimental EPI of dogs, gastric acid hypersecretion was shown,[161] which theoretically should contribute to the inactivation of ingested pancreatic enzyme supplement. No objective evidence is available on animals regarding the efficacy of antacids in the regimen of therapy for EPI.

A preliminary report on humans suggests that pancreatin and cimetidine (an H_2-receptor blocking agent) corrected fat malabsorption in patients with EPI and abolished steatorrhea which persisted when pancreatic enzyme supplements alone were given.[162] A recent report on humans with EPI also showed that the administration of pancreatic enzyme supplements, cimetidine, and antacids permits normalization of digestion.[163] H_2-receptor blocking drugs deserve study for the treatment of EPI in dogs.

In summary, treatment of the dog with EPI should first include adequate nutrition and caloric intake. At least until a response to therapy is obtained, a prescription canned food of moderate fat content, such as one of the feline diets or one of the intestinal diets of lower fat content, is recommended. Second, adequate pancreatic enzyme replacement therapy should be provided. Pancreatin powder at a dosage of 1 tsp/450 g canned food or 2 tsp/450 g dry food moistened and mixed well with food 20 minutes prior to feeding is recommended. Once a response to therapy has been shown by weight gain, improvement in haircoat, satiety, decreased volume and frequency of defecation with improvement of character of the feces, the diet may be changed. By this time, the owner appreciates the goals to be accomplished and can select a different diet. Observant clients quickly learn to titrate the correct dosage of pancreatic enzymes for their animal and the diet being fed.

These animals usually require more than maintenance calories since weight gain is desirable. In addition, even with adequate therapy, digestion and absorption do not return to normal. The use of antacids, though theoretically sound, has not been objectively studied in dogs. Though most seem unpalatable for dogs, their use may contribute to the goals of therapy. Vitamins, particularly fat-soluble vitamins and mineral supplements, should be provided for the growing dog with pancreatic hypoplasia. They may also be of value in the older diabetic patient.

Prognosis

The prognosis for EPI is favorable provided that concomitant disease such as diabetes mellitus can also be controlled. Clients should be educated about the disease and the goals of therapy, being told that treatment is not a cure but is meant to manage the effects of maldigestion. They should be advised that once EPI has developed, it is likely that enzyme replacement will be required for the duration of the animal's life.

Because the malabsorption of fat is a prominent feature of pancreatic insufficiency, fat-soluble vitamin deficiencies that accompany fat malabsorption can also occur, although these are rare. Fat-soluble vitamin deficiencies are not a frequent problem because bile acids are adequate and the mucosa is functional.[164] Vitamin A, D, and E deficiencies take longer to recover than does vitamin K deficiency. Vitamin E is not stored by the body and must be absorbed each day. Rarely will an animal present with a coagulopathy or an increased prothrombin time secondary to vitamin K deficiency. A puppy with EPI that is losing deciduous teeth and has permanent teeth erupting can bleed significantly because of vitamin K deficiency secondary to pancreatic hypoplasia. Pathologic fractures and nutritional bone disease due to vitamin D deficiency may also occur in young animals. Signs of pancreatic hypoplasia can occur prior to 12 weeks of age.[165] Vitamin A deficiency becomes more apparent by watching the skin and haircoat improve after initiation of replacement therapy. "Brown dog gut," though not of clinical significance, may be occasionally detected in dogs with pancreatic insufficiency as a coincidental finding at surgery or at necropsy. This finding is associated with accumulation of lipofuscin pigment in smooth muscle. Once present, the condition persists and suggests an existing or preexisting vitamin E deficiency.

Part III. Pancreatic Neoplasia

ROBERT M. HARDY

Tumors of the pancreas arise from two primary epithelial tissues. The acinar or ductular epithelium gives rise to pancreatic adenocarcinomas and the islet tissue is the site of origin for islet cell carcinomas.[166]

Pancreatic adenocarcinomas are considered uncommon tumors in domestic animals, with the dog having the highest incidence.[167,168] Adenocarcinomas of the pancreas comprise 0.6% of all canine tumors.[168] They are quite uncommon in cats and even rarer in the horse and cow. Such tumors primarily affect very old animals. The average age at which the diagnosis is made in dogs is 10 years and in cats is 12 years of age. Four of nine reported cases in cats occurred in animals over 15 years old.[168] They occur slightly more frequently in female dogs and the only apparent breed predisposition is in Airedales.

Adenocarcinomas tend to be highly malignant tumors, often metastasizing widely prior to the time diagnosis is made. These tumors frequently metastasize to the liver, and signs relating to that organ may be the reason the animal is examined.[41,71,73] The clinical signs noted most often are weight loss, anorexia, depression, vomiting, and jaundice. In one series of ten cases,[69] metastases were present in all ten and jaundice in six. Occasionally abdominal masses may be palpated or visualized radiographically.

A definitive diagnosis is rarely made except via laparotomy. Many animals die or are euthanatized, the diagnosis being made at necropsy. Occasionally, actively infiltrating carcinomas produce signs compatible with pancreatitis and elevations in amylase and lipase will be detected. Usually these enzyme values are normal. When hepatic involvement is present, laboratory evaluations may be suggestive of obstructive jaundice, i.e., hyperbilirubinemia, mild increases in SGPT, and marked increases in serum alkaline phosphatase activity. The absence of jaundice with similar enzyme patterns suggests metastatic disease is present. Radiographs of the abdomen may reveal a mass lesion in the pancreatic region[73] although this is not specific for tumor. Another relatively safe diagnostic aid involves paracentesis, with or without lavage. Carcinoma cells tend to exfoliate readily and although their site of origin is often difficult to determine, the prognosis is not altered.

The prognosis for pancreatic adenocarcinoma is invariably unfavorable because of the tendency for early and widespread metastases. The primary goal of the clinician should be to establish a definitive diagnosis as quickly as possible to reduce any prolonged suffering by the animal. No effective therapy for pancreatic carcinoma is presently available once metastases are found. If solitary tumors are identified, surgical extirpation is indicated.

Islet cell tumors of the pancreas are even less common than acinar derived neoplasms. Only 29 were reported to the Veterinary Medical Data Program between 1964 and 1972. Twenty-seven were in dogs and two in cats.[169] Islet cell carcinomas are usually relatively small but have profound physiologic effects if functional. Seventeen of the previously reported 27 cases in dogs had signs compatible with hypoglycemia. Two breeds may be predisposed to these tumors, Boxers[166] and Standard Poodles.[169] No particular age peak has been noted. Middle-aged dogs (5 years) are more commonly affected. If anything, a slightly decreased incidence occurs past middle age. Metastases are less common with "insulinomas" than with pancreatic carcinomas, approximately 50% being malignant.[169]

Clinical signs associated with functional islet cell tumors are those caused by hypoglycemia, i.e., rear limb weakness, fatigue after exercise, generalized muscle twitching, ataxia, temperament changes, and seizures.[166] Nonfunctional tumors manifest clinically much like the pancreatic adenocarcinomas, signs relating primarily to areas of metastasis.

A diagnosis of functional islet cell tumor is usually uncomplicated if a thorough history is obtained and a prolonged fast has occurred prior to obtaining a blood glucose. Although several more complex diagnostic tests are available to confirm the presence of a functional tumor, i.e., leucine tolerance, glucagon tolerance, high-dose intravenous glucose tolerance, and serum insulin activity, it would be unusual to miss the diagnosis using fasting blood glucose concentrations alone.

Treatment is aimed at surgical removal of the tumor if metastases are not seen. Occasional patients become transiently or permanently diabetic following tumor removal even though the bulk of the pancreas remains. The possibility of using cancer chemotherapy for metastatic islet cell carcinomas opens up an additional mode of therapy.[170]

Recent reports have appeared of a non-beta cell islet tumor in dogs that secreted gastrin in excessive quantities.[132,133] Gastrin-secreting tumors stimulate gastric hypersecretion and predispose to multiple gastrointestinal ulcers. This syndrome in man has been termed the Zollinger-Ellison syndrome. Clinicians should remain attuned to examine the pancreas carefully in any dog found to have unexplained gastric ulcers.

REFERENCES

1. Anderson, N. V.: Pancreatitis in dogs. Vet. Clin. North Am. 2:79, 1972.
2. Jubb, K. V. F., and Kennedy, P. C.: Pathology of Domestic Animals, 2nd ed., Vol. 2. New York, Academic Press, 1970.
3. Anderson, N. V.: Acute pancreatitis in the dog. Proc. Am. Vet. Med. Assoc. 180:82, 1964.
4. Spiro, H. M.: Clinical Gastroenterology, 2nd ed. New York, Macmillan Publishing Co., 1977.
5. Gage, E. D., and Anderson, N. V.: Acute pancreatitis in the dog. Anim. Hosp. 3:151, 1967.
6. Schiller, W. R., Suriyapa, C., and Anderson, M. C.: A review of experimental pancreatitis. J. Surg. Res. 16:69, 1974.
7. Hardy, R. M., and Stevens, J. B.: The exocrine pancreas. In Textbook of Veterinary Internal Medicine, Vol. II. Edited by S. J. Ettinger. Philadelphia, W. B. Saunders Co., 1975.
8. Fellenbaum, S.: Surgical relief of obstructive pancreatitis in the dog. V.M./S.A.C. 69:271, 1974.
9. Lium, R., and Maddock, S.: Etiology of acute pancreatitis, an experimental study. Surgery 24:593, 1948.
10. Ivy, A. C., and Gibbs, G. B.: Pancreatitis: a review. Surgery 31:614, 1952.
11. Sheldon, W. G.: Pancreatic flukes (Eurytrema procyonis) in domestic cats. J.A.V.M.A. 148:251, 1966.
12. Rothenbacher, J., and Lindquist, W. D.: Liver cirrhosis and pancreatitis in a cat infected with Amphimerus pseudofelineus. J.A.V.M.A. 143:1099, 1963.
13. Schmidt, H., and Creutzfeldt, W.: Etiology and pathogenesis of pancreatitis. In Gastroenterology. Edited by H. L. Bockus. Philadelphia, W. B. Saunders Co., 1976.
14. Byrne, J. J., and Joison, J.: Bacterial regurgitation in experimental pancreatitis. Am. J. Surg. 107:317, 1964.
15. White, T. T.: Inflammatory diseases of the pancreas. Adv. Surg. 9:247, 1975.
16. Glazer, G.: Hemorrhagic and necrotizing pancreatitis. Br. J. Surg. 62:169, 1975.

17. Anderson, N. V.: The pancreas. J.A.A.H.A. 9:89, 1973.

18. Haig, T. H.: Pancreatic digestive enzymes: influence of a diet that augments pancreatitis. J. Surg. Res. 10:601, 1970.

19. Lindsay, S., Entenmann, C., and Chaikoff, I. L.: Pancreatitis accompanying hepatic disease in dogs fed a high fat, low protein diet. Arch. Pathol. 45:635, 1948.

20. Haig, T. H.: Cellular membranes in the etiology of acute pancreatitis. Surg. Forum 20:380, 1969.

21. Goodhead, B.: Importance of nutrition in the pathogenesis of experimental pancreatitis in the dog. Arch. Surg. 103:724, 1971.

22. Weiner, S., Gramatica, L., and Voegle, L. D.: Role of the lymphatic system in the pathogenesis of inflammatory disease in the biliary tract and pancreas. Am. J. Surg. 119:55, 1970.

23. Capner, P., Lendrum, D., Jeffries, J., and Walker, G.: Viral antibody studies in pancreatic disease. Gut 16:866, 1975.

24. Salt, W. B., and Schenker, S.: Amylase—its clinical significance: a review of the literature. Medicine 55:269, 1976.

25. Thal, A.: Studies on pancreatitis: acute pancreatic necrosis produced experimentally by the Arthus sensitization reaction. Surgery 37:911, 1955.

26. Thal, A. P., Murray, M. J., and Egner, W.: Isoantibody formation in chronic pancreatic disease. Lancet 1:1128, 1959.

27. Nakashima, Y., and Howard, J. M.: Drug-induced acute pancreatitis. Surg. Gynecol. Obstet. 145:105, 1977.

28. Nelp, W. B.: Acute pancreatitis associated with steroid therapy. Arch. Intern. Med. 108:702, 1961.

29. Trapnell, J. E.: The natural history and management of acute pancreatitis. Clin. Gastroenterol. 1:147, 1972.

30. Frederickson, D. S., Levy, R. I., and Lees, R. S.: Fat transport in lipoproteins: an integrated approach to mechanisms and disorders. N. Engl. J. Med. 276:33, 1967.

31. Cameron, J. L., Capuzzi, D. M., Zuidema, G. D., and Margolis, S.: Acute pancreatitis with hyperlipemia. Ann. Surg. 177:483, 1973.

32. Cameron, J. L., Crisler, C., Margolis, S., DeMeester, T. R., and Zuidema, G. D.: Acute pancreatitis with hyperlipemia. Surgery 70:53, 1971.

33. Greenberger, N. J.: Pancreatitis and hyperlipemia. N. Engl. J. Med. 289:586, 1973.

34. Fallat, R. W., Vester, J. W., and Glueck, C. J.: Suppression of amylase activity by hypertriglyceridemia. J.A.M.A. 225:1331, 1973.

35. Bass, V. D., Hoffman, W. E., and Dorner, J. L.: Normal canine lipid profiles and effects of experimentally induced pancreatitis and hepatic necrosis on lipids. Am. J. Vet. Res. 37:1355, 1976.

36. Rogers, W. A., Donovan, E. F., and Kociba, G. J.: Lipids and lipoproteins in normal dogs and dogs with secondary lipoproteincmia. J.A.V.M.A. 166:1092, 1975.

37. Rogers, W. A., Donovan, E. F., and Kociba, G. J.: Idiopathic hyperlipoproteinemia in dogs. J.A.V.M.A. 166:1087, 1975.

38. Baggenstoss, A. J.: The pancreas in uremia: a histopathologic study. Am. J. Pathol. 24:1003, 1948.

39. Avram, M. M.: High prevalence of pancreatic disease in chronic renal failure. Nephron 18:68, 1977.

40. Neuman, N. B.: Acute pancreatic hemorrhage associated with iatrogenic hypercalcemia in a dog. J.A.V.M.A. 166:381, 1975.

41. Bergstrom, K., Hellstrom, K., Kallner, M., and Lundh, G.: Familial pancreatitis associated with hyperglycemia. Scand. J. Gastroenterol. 8:217, 1973.

42. Kattwinkel, J., Lapey, A., di Sant'Agnese, P. A., and Edwards, W. A.: Familial pancreatitis: three new kindreds and a critical review of the literature. Pediatrics 51:55, 1973.

43. Geokas, M. C., Van Lancker, J. L., Kandell, B. M., and Macheleder, H. I.: Acute pancreatitis. Ann. Intern. Med. 76:105, 1972.

44. Perman, V., and Stevens, J. B.: Clinical evaluation of the acinar pancreas of the dog. J.A.V.M.A. 155:2053, 1969.

45. Coffey, R. J.: Diseases of the pancreas: the acute pancreatic diseases. Med. Ann. District of Columbia 11:131, 1942.

46. Hadorn, B.: Pancreatic proteinases: their activation and disturbances of this mechanism in man. Med. Clin. North Am. 58:1319, 1974.

47. Ohlsson, K., and Eddeland, A.: Release of proteolytic enzymes in bile-induced pancreatitis in dogs. Gastroenterology 69:668, 1975.

48. Banks, P. A.: Acute pancreatitis. Gastroenterology 61:382, 1971.

49. Creutzfeldt, W., and Schmidt, H.: Etiology and pathogenesis of pancreatitis. (current concepts). Scand. J. Gastroenterol. 5 (Suppl. 6):47, 1970.

50. Geokas, M. C., Murphy, D. R., and McKenna, R. D.: The role of elastase in acute pancreatitis. I. Intrapancreatic elastolytic activity in bile induced acute pancreatitis in dogs. Arch. Pathol. 86:117, 1968.

51. Goodhead, B.: Acute pancreatitis and pancreatic blood flow. Surg. Gynecol. Obstet. 129:331, 1969.

52. Satake, K., Rozmanith, J. S., Appart, H., and Howard, J. M.: Hemodynamic change and bradykinin levels in plasma and lymph during experimental acute pancreatitis in dogs. Ann. Surg. 178:659, 1973.

53. Glazer, G., and Bennett, A.: Prostaglandin release in canine acute hemorrhagic pancreatitis. Gut 17:22, 1976.

54. Nemir, P., and Drabkin, D.L.: The pathogenesis of acute necrotizing hemorrhagic pancreatitis: an experimental study. Surgery 40:171, 1956.

55. Wright, P. W., and Goodhead, B.: Prevention of hemorrhagic pancreatitis with fibrinolysin or heparin. Arch. Surg. 100:42, 1970.

56. Probstein, J. G., Joshi, R. A., and Blumenthal, H. T.: Atheromatous embolization, an etiology of acute pancreatitis. A.M.A. Arch. Surg. 75:566, 1957.

57. Bockman, D. E., Schiller, W. R., Suriyapa, C., Mutchler, J. H. W., and Anderson, M. C.: Fine structure of early acute experimental pancreatitis in dogs. Lab. Invest. 28:584, 1973.

58. Imrie, C. W., Allam, B. F., and Ferguson, J. C.: Hypocalcemia of acute pancreatitis: the effect of hypoalbuminemia. Curr. Med. Res. Opin. 4:101, 1976.

59. Weir, G. C., Lesser, P. B., Drop, L. J., Fischer, J. E., and Warshaw, A. L.: The hypocalcemia of acute pancreatitis. Ann. Intern. Med. 83:185, 1975.

60. Robertson, G. M., Moore, E. W., Switz, D. M., Sizemore, G. W., and Estep, H. I.: Inadequate parathyroid response in acute pancreatitis. N. Engl. J. Med. 294:512, 1976.

61. Kwaan, H. C., Anderson, M. C., and Gramatica, L.: A study of pancreatic enzymes as a factor in the pathogenesis of disseminated intravascular coagulation during acute pancreatitis. Surgery 69:663, 1971.

62. Clarkson, A. R., MacDonald, M. K., Fuster, V., Robson, J. S., and Cash, J.D.: Glomerular lesions in acute pancreatitis. Lancet 2:726, 1970.

63. Innerfield, I., Schwartz, A., and Angrist, A.: Intravenous trypsin: its anticoagulant, fibrinolytic and thrombolytic effects. J. Clin. Invest. 31:1049, 1952.

64. Sim, D. N., Duprez, A., and Anderson, M. C.: Alterations of the lymphatic circulation during acute experimental pancreatitis. Surgery 60:1175, 1966.

65. Ofstad, E.: Formation and destruction of plasma kinins during experimental acute hemorrhagic pancreatitis in dogs. Scand. J. Gastroenterol. 5 (Suppl. 5):1, 1970.

66. Takada, Y., Appert, H. E., and Howard, J. M.: Vascular permeability induced by pancreatic exudate formed during acute pancreatitis in dogs. Surg. Gynecol. Obstet. 143:799, 1976.

67. Kelly, D. F., Baggotti, D. G., and Gaskell, C. J.: Jaundice in the cat associated with inflammation of the biliary tract and pancreas. J. Small Anim. Pract. 16:163, 1975.

67a. Owens, J. M., Drazner, F. H., and Gilbertson, S. R.: Pancreatic disease in the cat. J.A.A.H.A. 11:83, 1975.

68. Thordal-Christensen, A., and Coffin, D. L.: Pancreatic diseases in the dog. Nord. Vet. Med. 8:89, 1956.

69. Holroyd, J. B.: Canine exocrine pancreatic disease. J. Small Anim. Pract. 9:269, 1968.

70. Anderson, N. V., and Strafuss, A. C.: Pancreatic disease in dogs and cats. J.A.V.M.A. 159.885, 1971.

71. Anderson, N. V., and Low, D. G.: Diseases of the canine pancreas: a summary of 103 cases. Anim. Hosp. 1:189, 1965.

72. Finco, D.: The acute abdomen. Seminar Synopses and Scientific Presentations, 38th Annu. Meet. A.A.H.A., 1971, p. 182.

73. Anderson, N. V., and Johnson, K. H.: Pancreatic carcinoma in the dog. J.A.V.M.A. 150:286, 1967.

74. Hiatt, N., and Bonorres, G.: Removal of serum amylase in dogs and the influence of the reticuloendothelial blockade. Am. J. Physiol. 210:133, 1966.

75. Traverso, L. W., Longmire, W. P., Jr., and Tompkins, R. K.: Evaluation of experimental canine pancreatitis. J. Surg. Res. 21:247, 1976.

76. Challis, T. W., Reid, L. C., and Hinton, J. W.: Study of some factors which influence the level of serum amylase in dogs and humans. Gastroenterology 33:818, 1957.

77. Lifton, L. J., Slickers, K. A., and Pragay, D. A.: Pancreatitis and lipase: a reevaluation with a 5 minute turbidimetric lipase determination. J.A.M.A. 229:47, 1974.

78. Brobst, D., Ferguson, A. B., and Carter, J. M.: Evaluation of serum amylase and lipase activity in experimentally induced pancreatitis in the dog. J.A.V.M.A. 157:1697, 1970.

79. Farmer, R. G., Winkelman, E. I., Brown, H. B., and Lewis, L. A.: Hyperlipoproteinemia and pancreatitis. Am. J. Med. 54:161, 1973.

80. Shimamura, J., Fridhandler, L., and Berk, J. E.: Nonpancreatic type hyperamylasemia associated with pancreatic cancer. Am. J. Dig. Dis. 21:340, 1976.

81. Imrie, C. W., King, J., and Henderson, A. R.: Macroamylasemia: a report of two cases. Scott. Med. J. 18:188, 1973.

82. Finco, D. R., and Stevens, J. B.: Clinical significance of serum amylase activity in the dog. J.A.V.M.A. 155:1686, 1969.

83. Kelly, T. R., Klein, R. L., Porquez, J. M., and Honer, G. M.: Methemalbumin in acute pancreatitis: an experimental and clinical appraisal. Ann. Surg. 175:15, 1972.

84. Seefe, L. B., and Zimmerman, H. J.: Relationship between hepatic and pancreatic disease. Prog. Liver Dis. 5:590, 1976.

85. Tuzhlin, S. A., Podolsky, A. E., and Dreiling, D. A.: Hepatic lesions in pancreatitis: clinico-experimental data. Am. J. Gastroenterol. 64:108, 1975.

86. Warshaw, A. L., Lesser, P. B., Rie, M., and Cullen, D. J.: The pathogenesis of pulmonary edema in acute pancreatitis. Ann. Surg. 182:505, 1975.

87. Lees, G. E., Suter, P. F., and Johnson, G. C.: Pulmonary edema in a dog with acute pancreatitis and cardiac disease. J.A.V.M.A., 172:690, 1978.

88. Suter, P. F., and Lowe, R.: Acute pancreatitis in the dog: a clinical study with emphasis on radiographic diagnosis. Acta Radiol. Suppl. 319:195, 1972.

89. Lightwood, R., Reber, H. A., and Lawrence, W. W.: The risk and accuracy of pancreatic biopsy. Am. J. Surg. 132:189, 1976.

90. Klein, T. S., and Neal, H. S.: Needle aspiration biopsy: a safe diagnostic procedure for lesions of the pancreas. Am. J. Clin. Pathol. 63:16, 1975.

91. Dalton, J. R. F., and Hill, F. W. G.: A procedure for the examination of the liver and pancreas in dogs. J. Small Anim. Pract. 13:527, 1972.

92. White, T. T., and Heimbach, D. M.: Sequestrectomy and hyperalimentation in the treatment of hemorrhagic pancreatitis. Am. J. Surg. 132:270, 1976.

93. McHardy, G., Craighead, C. C., Balart, L., and McHardy, R.: Current medical therapy of pancreatitis. Med. Clin. North Am. 48:389, 1964.

94. Elliot, D. W.: The mechanism of benefit derived from concentrated human serum albumin in experimental acute pancreatitis. Surg. Forum 5:384, 1955.

95. Pissiotis, C. A., Condon, R. E., and Nyhus, L. M.: Effect of vasopressin on pancreatic blood flow in acute hemorrhagic pancreatitis. Am. J. Surg. 123:203, 1972.

96. Schapiro, H., McDougal, H. D., Morrison, E. J., and Wan, H. T.: Acute hemorrhagic pancreatitis in the dog. IV. Treatment with vasopressin. Am. J. Dig. Dis. 21:286, 1976.

97. Schapiro, H., Britt, L. G., Brooks, J., Campbell, D., and Blackwell, C. F.: Acute hemorrhagic pancreatitis in the dog. II. Effect of vasopressin on survival times. Am. J. Dig. Dis. 18:1075, 1973.

98. Thomas, J. E., and Pincus, I. J.: Physiology of the pancreas. In Gastroenterology, 3rd ed. Vol. III. Edited by H. L. Bockus. Philadelphia, W. B. Saunders Co., 1976.

99. Dreiling, D., and Janowitz, H.: Inhibitor effect of new anticholinergics on the basal and secretin-stimulated pancreatic secretion in patients with and without pancreatic disease. Am. J. Dig. Dis. 5:639, 1960.

100. Varrol, M., Bretholz, A., Levesque, D., Laugier, R., Tiscornia, D., and Sarles, H.: Atropine induced inhibition of the enhanced CCK release observed in alcoholic dogs. Digestion 14:174, 1976.

101. Thomas, J. E.: Mechanism of action of pancreatic stimuli studied by means of atropine like drugs. Am. J. Physiol. 206:124, 1964.

102. Condon, R. E., Woods, J. H., Poulin, T. L., Wagner, W. G., and Pissiotis, C. A.: Experimental pancreatitis treated with glucagon or lactated Ringer's solution. Arch. Surg. 109:154, 1974.

103. Condon, J. R., Knight, M., and Day, J. L.: Glucagon therapy in acute pancreatitis. Br. J. Surg. 60:509, 1973.

104. Fleischer, K., and Kasper, H.: Observations on glucagon treatment in pancreatitis. Scand. J. Gastroenterol. 9:371, 1974.

105. Svensson, J. O.: Role of intravenously infused insulin in treatment of acute pancreatitis. Scand. J. Gastroenterol. 10:487, 1975.

106. Johnson, R. M., Barone, R. M., Newson, B. L., DasGupta, T. K., and Nyhus, L. M.: Treatment of experimental acute pancreatitis with 5-fluorouracil. Am. J. Surg. 125:211–211, 1973.

107. Anderson, M. C., and Copass, M. K.: Use of carbonic anhydrase inhibitors in the treatment of pancreatitis. Am. J. Dig. Dis. 11:367, 1967.

108. Dreiling, D. A., Leichtling, J. L., and Greenstein, A. J.: Trasylol revisited: the values of proteolytic inhibitors in the therapy of pancreatitis. Mt. Sinai J. Med. N.Y. 43:409, 1976.

109. Kodesch, R., and DuPont, H. L.: Infectious complications of acute pancreatitis. Surg. Gynecol. Obstet. 136:763, 1973.

110. Anderson, M. C., and Schiller, W. R.: Acute pancreatitis. Surg. Ann. 5:335, 1973.

111. Finch, W. T., Sawyers, J. L., and Schenker, S.: A prospective study to determine the efficacy of antibiotics in acute pancreatitis. Ann. Surg. 183:667, 1976.

112. Schweinburg, F., Jacob, S., Persky, L., and Fine, J.: Further studies on the role of bacteria in death from acute pancreatitis in dogs. Surgery 33:367, 1953.

113. Reference deleted.

114. Preston, F. W., and Kukral, J. C.: Surgical physiology of the pancreas. Surg. Clin. North Am. 42:203, 1962.

115. Bogoch, A., Roth, J. L. A., and Bockus, H. L.: Effects of morphine on serum amylase and lipase. Gastroenterology 26:697, 1954.

116. Delaney, J. P., and Grim, E.: Influences of hormones and drugs on canine pancreatic blood flow. Am. J. Physiol. 211:1398, 1966.

117. Carone, F. A., and Liebow, A. A.: Acute pancreatic lesions in patients treated with ACTH and adrenal corticoids. N. Engl. J. Med. 257:690, 1957.

118. Bencosme, S. A., and Lazarus, S. S.: Pancreas of cortisone treated rabbits. A.M.A. Arch. Pathol. 62:285, 1956.

119. Cotlar, A. M., Hudson, T. L., Kaplan, M. H., and Cohn, I., Jr.: Experimental hemorrhagic pancreatitis produced by staphylococcal toxin. Surgery 47:587, 1960.

120. Anderson, M. C., Mehn, H., and Method, H. L.: Treatment of acute hemorrhagic pancreatitis with adrenocorticosteroids. Arch. Surg. 78:802, 1959.

121. Parks, J. L., Gahring, D., and Greene, R. W.: Peritoneal lavage for peritonitis and pancreatitis in 22 dogs. J.A.A.H.A. 9:442, 1973.

122. Elmslie, R. G., and Marshall, V. R.: Acute pancreatitis: management by the use of applied physiology. Geriatrics 26:122, 1971.

123. Warren, K. W., and Hoffman, V.: Changing patterns in surgery of the pancreas. Surg. Clin. North Am. 56:615, 1976.

124. Henry, L. G., and Condon, R. E.: Ablative surgery for necrotizing pancreatitis. Am. J. Surg. 131:125, 1976.

125. Berk, J. E.: Management of acute pancreatitis. J.A.M.A. 152:1, 1953.

126. Holzworth, J., and Coffin, D. L.: Pancreatic insufficiency and diabetes mellitus in a cat. Cornell Vet. 43:502, 1953.

127. Hill, F. W. G., Osborne, A. D., and Kidder, D. E.: Pancreatic degenerative atrophy in dogs. J. Comp. Pathol. 81:32, 1971.

128. Kronfeld, D. S.: Nature and use of commercial dog foods. In Diet and Disease in Dogs. Edited by D. S. Kronfeld and D. G. Low. Irvine, University of California Press, 1975.

129. DiMagno, E. P., Go, V. L.: Exocrine pancreatic insufficiency: current concepts of pathophysiology. Postgrad. Med. 52:135, 1972.

130. DiMagno, E. P., Go, V. L., and Summerskill, W. H. J.: Impaired cholecystokinin-pancreozymin secretion, intraluminal dilution and maldigestion of fat in sprue. Gastroenterology 63:25, 1972.

131. Pascal, J. P., Vaysse, N., Augier, D., and Ribet, A.: Response of the canine pancreas to duodenal acidification and secretin. Scand. J. Gastroenterol. 3:444, 1968.

132. Straus, E., Johnson, G. F., and Yalow, R. S.: Canine Zollinger-Ellison syndrome. Gastroenterology 72:380, 1977.

133. Jones, B. R., Nichols, M. R., and Badman, R.: Peptic ulceration in a dog associated with an islet cell carcinoma of the pancreas and an elevated plasma gastrin level. J. Small Anim. Pract. 17:593, 1976.

134. Rijnberk, A., and Leav, I.: Thyroid tumors. In Current Veterinary Therapy, Vol. VI. Edited by R. W. Kirk. Philadelphia, W. B. Saunders Co., 1977.

135. Hamano, K.: Digestive and absorptive functions of the gastrointestinal tract after various operations of the pancreas, especially total pancreatoduodenectomy. Arch. Jpn. Chir. 22:500, 1953.

136. Hill, F. W. G., and Kidder, D. E.: Fat assimilation in dogs estimated by a fat balance procedure. J. Small Anim. Pract. 13:23, 1972.

137. Lorenz, M. D.: Laboratory diagnosis of gastrointestinal disease and pancreatic insufficiency. Vet. Clin. North Am. 6:663, 1976.

138. Hayden, D. W., and Van Kruiningen, H. J.: Control values for evaluating gastrointestinal function in the dog. J.A.A.H.A. 12:31, 1976.

139. Kalser, M. H.: Classification of malassimilation syndromes and diagnosis of malabsorption. In Gastroenterology, Vol. 2. Edited by H. L. Bockus. Philadelphia, W. B. Saunders Co., 1976.

140. Pimparkar, B. D., Tulsky, E. G., Kalser, M. H., and Bockus, H. L.: Correlation of radioactive and chemical fecal fat determinations in various malabsorption syndromes. II. Results in idiopathic steatorrhea and diseases of the pancreas. Am. J. Med. *30*:910, 1961.

141. Grossman, M. I.: Fecal enzymes in dogs with pancreatic exclusion. Proc. Soc. Exp. Biol. Med. *110*:41, 1962.

142. Hill, F. W. G., and Kidder, D. E.: The estimation of daily fecal trypsin levels in dogs as an indication of gross pancreatic exocrine insufficiency. J. Small. Anim. Pract. *11*:191, 1970.

143. Greve, T., and Anderson, N. V.: The high-dose intravenous glucose tolerance test (H-IVGTT) in dogs. Nord. Vet. Med. *25*:436, 1973.

144. Hill, F. W. G., and Kidder, D. E.: The oral glucose tolerance test in canine pancreatic malabsorption. Br. Vet. J. *128*:207, 1972.

145. Hill, R., and Chaikoff, I. L.: Loss and repair of glucose-disposal mechanism in dogs fed fructose as sole dietary carbohydrate. Proc. Soc. Exp. Biol. Med. *91*:263, 1956.

146. Anderson, N. V.: Personal communication, 1978.

147. Hindmarsh, J. T.: Xylose absorption: its clinical significance. Clin. Biochem. *9*:141, 1976.

148. Hill, F. W. G., Kidder, D. E., and Frew, J. A.: Xylose absorption test for the dog. Vet. Rec. *87*:250, 1970.

149. Sateri, H.: Investigations on the exocrine pancreatic function in dogs suffering from chronic exocrine pancreatic insufficiency. Acta Vet. Scand. Suppl. *53*:1, 1975.

150. Dingwall, J. S., and McDonnell, W.: Partial pancreatectomy in the dog. J.A.A.H.A. *8*:86, 1972.

151. DiMagno, E. P., Go, V. L., and Summerskill, W. H.: Relations between pancreatic enzyme outputs and malabsorption in severe pancreatic insufficiency. N. Engl. J. Med. *288*:813, 1973.

152. Graham, D. Y.: Enzyme replacement therapy of exocrine pancreatic insufficiency in man. N. Engl. J. Med. *296*:1314, 1977.

153. Long, W. B., and Weiss, J. B.: Rapid gastric emptying of fatty meals in pancreatic insufficiency. Gastroenterology *67*:920, 1974.

154. Heizer, W. D., Cleveland, C. R., and Iben, F. L.: Gastric inactivation of pancreatic supplements. Bull. Johns Hopkins Hosp. *116*:261, 1965.

155. Guilian, B. B., Mitsuoka, H., Mansfield, A. O., Trapnell, J. E., Seddon, J. A., and Howard, J. M.: Treatment of pancreatic exocrine insufficiency. II. Effects on fat absorption of pancreatic lipase and 15 commercial pancreatic supplements as measured by ^{131}I-tagged triolein in the dog. Ann. Surg. *165*:571, 1967.

156. Pairent, F. W., Trapnell, J. E., and Howard, J. M.: The treatment of pancreatic exocrine insufficiency. III. The effect of pancreatic ductal ligation and oral pancreative enzyme supplements on fecal lipid excretion in the dog. Ann. Surg. *170*:737, 1969.

157. DiMagno, E. P., Malagelada, J. R., Go. V. L., and Moertel, C. G.: Fate of orally ingested enzymes in pancreatic insufficiency: comparison of two dosage schedules. N. Engl. J. Med. *296*:1318, 1977.

158. Pairent, F. W. and Howard, J. M.: Pancreatic exocrine insufficiency. IV: the enzyme content of commercial pancreatic supplements. Arch. Surg. *110*:739, 1975.

159. Weber, A. M., Roy, C. C., Chartnand, L., Lepage, G., Dufour, O. L., Morin, C. L., and Lasalle, R.: Relationship between bile acid malabsorption and pancreatic insufficiency in cystic fibrosis. Gut *17*:295, 1976.

160. Krone, C. L., Theodor, E., Sleisenger, M. H., and Jeffries, G. H.: Studies on the pathogenesis of malabsorption. Medicine *47*:89, 1968.

161. McIlrath, D. C., Kennedy, J. A., and Hallenbeck, G. A.: Relationships between atrophy of the pancreas and gastric secretion: an experimental study. Am. J. Dig. Dis. *8*:623, 1963.

162. Regan, P. T., Malagelada, J. R., Go, V. L. W., and DiMagno, E. P.: Use of cimetidine with oral pancreatic enzyme replacement in chronic pancreatitis. Clin. Res. *24*:567A, 1976.

163. Saunders, J. H. B., Drummond, S., and Wormsley, K. G.: Inhibition of gastric secretion in treatment of pancreatic insufficiency. Br. Med. J. *1*:418, 1977.

164. Taublin, H. L., and Spiro, H. M.: Nutritional aspects of chronic pancreatitis. Am. J. Clin. Nutr. *26*:367, 1973.

165. Hill, F. W. G.: Malabsorption syndrome in the dog: a study of 38 cases. J. Small Anim. Pract. *13*:575, 1972.

166. Njoku, C. O., Strafuss, A. C., and Dennis, S. M.: Canine islet cell neoplasia. J.A.A.H.A. *8*:284, 1972.

167. Kircher, C. H., and Nielsen, S. W.: Tumors of the pancreas. Bull. WHO *53*:3430, 1976.

168. Priester, W. A.: Data from 11 U. S. and Canadian colleges of veterinary medicine on pancreatic carcinoma in domestic animals. Cancer Res. *34*:1372, 1974.

169. Priester, W. A.: Pancreatic islet cell tumors: data from 11 colleges of veterinary medicine in the U. S. and Canada. J. Natl. Cancer Inst. *53*:227, 1974.

170. Meyer, D. J.: Pancreatic islet cell carcinoma in a dog treated with streptozotocin. Am. J. Vet. Res. *37*:1221, 1976.

Section Four

SYSTEMIC DISEASES
AND THE
GASTROINTESTINAL SYSTEM

Chapter 27

PERITONITIS AND ACUTE ABDOMINAL DISEASES

J. THOMAS VAUGHAN

Peritonitis is an inflammation of the mesothelial membrane that lines the peritoneal cavity and covers the intra-abdominal viscera. Peritonitis is both a primary disease entity and a secondary feature of other diseases. It is usually but not invariably attended by signs of abdominal pain. It may be of an infectious or a noninfectious nature and arises from such diverse causes as to confound logic. The mere task of classification is an exercise in ambiguity, and the etiology is so multifactorial that one questions whether any diseases do not possess the potential for causing peritonitis.

A study of peritonitis on a truly comparative basis stands to benefit much from a review of the human literature and then a thoughtful application of these principles and observations to the many variations of the disease in animals. This approach is stated in way of explanation for the liberal reference to peritonitis in man that is used herein.

The peritoneal diseases are discussed under the headings listed in Table 27–1, followed by the clinical course, diagnosis, and treatment. Acute abdominal diseases are themselves classified in Table 27–2.

CLASSIFICATION OF PERITONITIS

All causes may be grouped under four broad categories: (1) mechanical, (2) chemical, (3) infectious, and (4) other, which includes allergies, collagen vascular diseases, neoplasms, cysts, drugs (other than irritants), and even heritable tendencies.[1,2]

Infectious causes may, in turn, be subdivided into bacterial, viral, mycotic, protozoan, and parasitic. Clinical classifications are used to determine whether the infection is primary or secondary to another disease process, whether abdominal or remote. Prognostically, it is important to know whether the infection is localized, spreading or diffuse, and whether the course of the problem is acute or chronic. Thus, due to a mechanical force which perforates the gut with leakage of bowel contents into the peritoneal cavity, the patient suffers acute bacterial peritonitis.

If the host defense mechanisms fail to localize the infection, it becomes diffuse and the patient may die of a combination of endotoxemia and septicemia leading to irreversible shock. Another patient contracts a virus infection which is manifested in disease processes of the eyes, brain, spinal cord, and peritoneal cavity, all secondary to the initial viremia.

Table 27–1. Causes of Peritonitis

A. Trauma from External Forces
   Deep contusions
   External penetrating injuries
   Clinical accidents
B. Perforations and Ruptures of the Bowel and Transmural Migration of Enterobacteria
   Acute gastric injury
   Penetrating foreign bodies
   Focal necrosis
   Thromboembolic infarction
   Strangulation necrosis
   Other acute obstructions
C. Parasitisms
   Parasitic larval migrations
   Perforating lesions
   Verminous arteritis
D. Urogenital Disease
   Obstructions of urinary tract
   Penetrating injuries
   Infections
   Nephrosis
   Complications of parturition
E. Complications of Surgery
   Wound dehiscence and anastomosis failure
   Surgical sequestration
   Contamination
   Nonviable tissue
   Excessive trauma
   Excessive hemorrhage
   Ineffective drainage
   Uncorrected or supervening obstructions
   Peritoneal irritants
   Peritoneal foreign bodies
F. Miscellaneous Causes
   Intra-abdominal abscesses
   Extra-abdominal abscesses
   Biliary and pancreatic leakage
   Septicemias
   Drugs
   Neoplasms and cysts
   Other causes

Table 27–2. Acute Abdominal Diseases and Peritonitis

Classification of Acute Abdominal Diseases and Obstructive Enteropathies

A. Obturation Obstructions
   1. Dynamic ileus
   2. Adynamic ileus
   3. Bezoars
   4. Foreign bodies
   5. Meconium
   6. Parasites
   7. Gallstones
B. Displacements
   1. Intussusceptions
   2. Torsion
   3. Volvulus
   4. Restraining bands
   5. Hernias
C. Inflammatory Lesions
   1. Abscesses
   2. Adhesions
   3. Cicatricial strictures
   4. Granulomas
D. Neoplasms
   1. Intrinsic
   2. Extrinsic
E. Angiopathies
   1. Ischemias ⎫
   2. Infarctions ⎬ related to vasculitis
   3. Hematomas ⎭   aneurysm
                      thromboembolism
F. Luminal Deformities
   1. Stenoses, dilatations, and diverticulae
   2. Muscular hypertrophy
G. Congenital Anomalies
   1. Meckel's diverticulum
   2. Anomalous mesenteric bands
   3. Atresia ani et recti
H. Ruptures and Perforations
   1. Gastrorrhexis
   2. Gastric ulcers
   3. Parasitisms
   4. Diverticulae
   5. Trauma
   6. Perforating obstructions, infarctions, and strangulations
   7. Wound dehiscence or anastomosis failure
I. Extraperitoneal Causes
   1. Retroperitoneal hematoma (e.g., mesenteric, mesometrial)
   2. Retroperitoneal abscess (e.g., pelvic)
   3. Retroperitoneal neoplasm (e.g., melanoma, carcinoma, lipoma)
   4. Pneumoperitoneum and retroperitoneal emphysema (e.g., pelvic or abdominal wall injuries)
   5. Prolapse and evisceration (dystocia, surgical, obstetric)

TRAUMA FROM EXTERNAL FORCES

Wounds of the abdomen from external forces take the form of deep contusions, penetrating injuries, and clinical accidents. Nonpenetrating injuries may cause crushing, tearing of mesenteric or omental attachments, or sudden compression which bursts hollow organs, more vulnerable to rupture when filled than when empty. Fixed organs, such as spleen, liver, stomach, segments of the colon, and the kidneys are also more susceptible to such injuries. Parenchymatous organs are fractured or shattered, sometimes with rupture of the capsule and widespread injury. Leakage of contents as well as hemorrhage contribute to the resultant peritonitis.[1]

External penetrating injuries to the abdominal wall should be considered as perforating until proven otherwise. Deep bite wounds, gunshot wounds, horn wounds, and lacerations or punctures from pointed or sharp objects are examples. Extension to the peritoneal cavity may or may not be readily apparent. Sucking sounds caused by the aspiration of air into the cavity, drainage of peritoneal fluid or bowel contents, or the obvious herniation or evisceration leave no doubt and demand immediate corrective measures. It is the concealed injury to internal organs or the unobserved inoculation of the peritoneal space that may go begging for attention until peritonitis and shock are well advanced. Hence, a case is made for thoughtful assessment of the patient's vital signs and blood values as well as a careful exploration of the depths of the wound with a high degree of suspicion of internal injuries. It may be justified, if the patient's condition warrants, to perform early exploratory laparotomy with the principal objectives of arresting hemorrhage and containing contamination. Wounds may be debrided and closed during the lag phase between bacterial contamination and frank infection of injured tissues.

Clinical accidents compensate in variety for what they may lack in numbers of cases of intra-abdominal injuries. The subject here deals with the inadvertent or the unrecognized complication of an otherwise minor procedure done for diagnostic or therapeutic purposes as opposed to complications of surgical procedures. Paracentesis abdominis for confirmation of fluid levels in the peritoneal cavity has caused perforation of the diaphragm with aspiration of bile into the pleural space.[3] Needle biopsy of the liver has caused consequential hemorrhage from hepatic circulation as well as bile leakage. Paracentesis with long bevel hypodermic needles has been blamed for laceration of distended bowel with spillage of bowel contents. Laparoscopic procedures employing electrocoagulation and biopsy techniques have resulted in similar injuries to viscera. Blind installation of peritoneal drains with long curved forceps has caused perforation of the colon. Cannulation of pelvic organs for artificial insemination and intrauterine infusion has caused perforation of the uterine wall with contamination of the peritoneum. Pelvic examination by manual palpation per rectum has been the all too frequent cause of ruptures of the rectum in horses[4] and cattle. Vaginoscopy per speculum has caused laceration of the vagina, especially when performed during tenesmus. Even the simple exercise of measuring body temperature has been associated with an outbreak of peritonitis in a hospital nursery, presumably caused by thermometer-induced rectal perforation.[5]

PERFORATIONS AND RUPTURES OF THE BOWEL AND TRANSMURAL MIGRATION OF ENTEROBACTERIA

No other category accounts for more cases of peritonitis. Acute gastric injury results from many causes. Perforating ulcers are commonplace in hogs and cattle and recognized occasionally in horses as well as other species. Vagal inhibition (Hoflund's syndrome) has been associated with chronic irritation and adhesion formation in the course of traumatic reticulitis, in turn the result of penetrating foreign bodies.[6] Subphrenic abscesses between the reticulum and the diaphragm, along with neighboring pleuritis and pericarditis,[7] compare with similar pathologic processes in humans. A predisposition to gastrorrhexis may result from unintended overeating (accidental access to a grain bin) or improper overfeeding (unlimited access to dry dog feed). In the first case, a horse overloads the stomach and, due to the underdeveloped ability to eructate or vomit, the stomach may rupture from primary overdistention. Gastric volvulus, which may also result in rupture, is associated with overfeeding in large breeds of dogs, particularly if an exercise period follows too soon after a large meal. Pregnant dairy cows on high concentrate, low roughage intake are the most frequent victims of displacements of the abomasum, the most severe form of which is volvulus. If rupture does not occur first, the organ undergoes strangulation necrosis with resultant transmural migration of enterobacteria into the peritoneal cavity.

Focal necrosis of the bowel wall occurs when an obturation obstruction remains long enough in one site to cause irreversible ischemic necrosis to a part of the gut wall, usually on the greater curvature or along the antimesenteric border where the circulatory pattern is the poorest. The ischemia results from the chronic spastic contraction around the obstructing object, e.g., an enterolith, with a blanching of the blood supply to a segment of the gut wall. Other causes are discussed elsewhere (parasitisms, surgical complications, neoplasia).

Thromboembolic infarction finds its best example in the verminous arteritis of Strongylus vulgaris seen in the equidae. A larval migration of intestinal nematodes causes extensive vasculitis of the branches of the cranial mesenteric artery primarily, with resultant thromboembolism of the blood supply to the ileum, cecum, and great colon. Infarction may be widespread affecting all the named portions of the bowel; or it may be selective. In the latter case, the segments with the most precarious blood supply, such as the pelvic flexure of the left (ascending) colon, are most vulnerable to infarction. If the gut wall separates, contamination is massive and death follows quickly. If infarction is gradual, the integrity of the gut wall may be compromised so slowly that the breach comes in the form of bacterial diapedesis across nonviable gut wall.

Strangulation necrosis is usually attended by a quite dramatic course of sudden onset and intense pain. It is refractory to nonoperative therapy no matter how vigorous the effort. Peritonitis occurs if the patient survives the associated shock and intoxication. Whether or not the organ remains intact depends upon the degree of distention, the size of the viscus, and the strength of its walls. Notable examples would include volvulus of the stomach, volvulus of the small intestine, torsion of the cecum or colon, and torsion of the uterus. To extend the list, hernias and intussusceptions often are complicated by strangulation of the hernial contents or the intussusceptum. Congenital bands of tissue, e.g., Meckel's diverticulum, mesenteric rents, and fibrous adhesions from previous bouts of local peritonitis may be the causes of strangulating "gut ties."

PARASITISMS

The ravages of S. vulgaris in the horse have been alluded to. Gastrophilus larvae were found at the site of a perforated gastric ulcer with larvae in the peritoneal cavity of a horse that died with acute diffuse peritonitis. Small, ostensibly parasitic larval perforations of the colon have been associated with the cause of similar cases of peritonitis. Extensive subperitoneal migrations and encystment of Strongylus edentatus have caused a chronic, low-grade peritonitis characterized by multiple caseous nodules and generalized "shaggy" adhesions covering the involved viscera (principally cecum and colon).

A granulomatous peritonitis in man is recognized as due to Ascaris lumbricoides larval migrations. The mechanism by which an adult worm can escape without rupturing the intestinal wall is not always apparent.[8] Strongyloides stercoralis, a usually mild parasitism of man in tropical and subtropical countries, has been incriminated as the cause of fatal peritonitis in children. One case revealed a great number of filariform larvae with heavy infiltration of the gut walls, lymphatics, and mesenterics as well as lungs, pleura, and liver. The bacterial component of the peritonitis consisted of Klebsiella and Proteus spp.[9]

UROGENITAL DISEASES

Obstructing urolithiasis and wounds of the urethra may result not infrequently in ruptures of the urinary bladder and either chemical or bacterial peritonitis. Ruptures of the urinary bladder in newborn foals may cause serious uremia without sepsis due to the sterility of the urine in the neonate. Ascending urinary tract infections with deep-seated interstitial cystitis and/or pyelonephritis may be associated with localized or spreading pelvic infections.

Penetrating injuries stem from varied causes: insemination pipettes, infusion cannulae, vaginal speculae, metal urinary catheters, mismating of disproportionate individuals, malicious acts of sadism, and even coital rupture of the vaginal fornix in the hysterectomized female with a foreshortened genital tract (an argument for simultaneous ovariectomy in the bitch).[10]

Serious genital tract infections have long been associated with peritonitis originating in the pelvic cavity and spreading to the abdomen. Advancement of knowledge in the successful management of puerperal sepsis by Ignaz Phillip Semmelweis in the early part of the 19th century must be credited along with the contributions of Joseph Lister in the introduction of the principles of aseptic operating room technique in surgery and obstetrics.[11] The vulnerability of the uterus to contamination with virulent pathogens at the time of parturition and immediately afterward has been repeatedly emphasized by the consequences of septicemia and endotoxemia. Even in the less dramatic, insidious chronic infection of the tract, causing low-grade endometritis, there are instances of peritonitis as far remote as the subphrenic (suprahepatic) space that have migrated from the genital tract by undisclosed routes other than the oviducts. A classic example is to be found in women affected by the Curtis–Fitz-Hugh syndrome[12] of endometritis-salpingitis-peritonitis and gonococcal endocervicitis. There is positive correlation of phrenohepatic adhesions with recovery of cultures of *Neisseria gonorrhoeae* from the pelvic cul-de-sac (pouch of Douglas) and from the cervix in clinical cases of human gonorrhoeae.[13]

Another model of the relationship between urogenital disease and peritonitis is that found in children suffering from the nephrotic syndrome. Treatment of the preexisting nephrosis with corticosteroids is rationalized as the cause of low serum antibody levels to the offending pathogens and of the low IgG levels exhibited by children with peritonitis complicating the glomerulonephritis and focal glomerular sclerosis. Incriminated bacteria are *Hemophilus influenzae*, Pneumococcus, *Escherichia coli*, *Streptococcus fecalis* and Pseudomonas. Reminiscent of feline infectious peritonitis, the pathology is multicentric: meningitis, septic arthritis, orbital cellulitis, epiglottitis, and pneumonitis.[14,15]

Peritonitis of ovarian origin includes a chemical granulomatous peritonitis resulting from intraperitoneal rupture of benign cystic teratoma of the ovary* which spills sebaceous material into the cavity and produces a severe chemical irritation to the peritoneum. Widespread peritoneal nodules and masses cause abdominal tenderness and may precipitate an obstruction of the bowel. Ascites is frequent and the peritoneal effusion may contain an oily discharge mixed with hair. Radiography reveals a fluid line and calcification or anomalous teeth in the pelvic area. It may be confused with the metastatic spread of ovarian carcinoma, but distinction is readily made upon biopsy.[16] Inasmuch as ovarian teratomas do occur in animals, it is conceivable that similar problems could be seen.

A somewhat related condition, mucometra, is an accumulation of mucous secretions from congenitally segmented development of the uterus. In that large quantities of mucus may distend isolated segments of the tract, predisposing to intraperitoneal rupture, this might be viewed as another potential cause of chemical peritonitis.

COMPLICATIONS OF SURGERY

The inference may be problems stemming from bad technique or other human errors, but the title is meant to imply the unavoidable as well as the preventable. Early recognition *a priori* may be lifesaving to the patient. Thus it is the intention to emphasize all surgical complications in the hope that a keener awareness will minimize the bad results.

Wound dehiscence occurs and anastomoses fail when suture material breaks, knots untie, tissues reject suture, local infection perforates the closure, or tissues die owing to strangulating sutures, sequestrating ligatures, infarcting vascular lesions, or necrotizing bacterial toxins. Correct choices of suture needles and material and good techniques of pattern and knot will greatly reduce the problem. There are times, however, when viability of tissue or integrity

---

*Pseudomyxoma peritonei results from pseudomucinous cystadenoma of the ovary.[1]

of blood supply cannot be established, or when anatomic inaccessibility or extent of the lesion may obviate as complete a resection as would be desired. Production of circulating fibrinolysins by preexisting peritonitis may prevent the formation of an early seal of the anatomosis by the normal process of peritoneal healing. Gut wall rendered friable by edema and distention may fail to support the suture. Postoperative ileus and the attendant accumulation of gas and intraluminal fluid may subject suture lines to inordinate stresses and the tissues to further devitalizing influences.

Surgical sequestration means the unintentional isolation of tissue from its blood supply by ill-placed ligatures or excessive dissection. Patterns of blood supply to the abdominal viscera and particularly the bowel consist principally of progressive ramifications from a central trunk. The final divisions, before they reach the organ, are in the form of arborizing branches or arcades—in the case of the movable segments (e.g., jejunum and descending colon) or in the form of segmental branches emanating from parallel, marginal arteries—in the case of fixed segments (e.g., ileum, ascending colon, and rectum). Interruption by ligature of major branches of an arcade of vessels to a movable segment must exactly match that amount to be resected, or else it will slough. Overzealous "freeing-up" for exteriorization of fixed segments that are to be retained may produce the same effect. An example in the latter case is infarction of the rectum days after its replacement following an extensive prolapse. The breakdown of its segmental blood supply may go unnoticed if the prolapse is not resected; thus, the error is one of judgment rather than technique. The cause of death, of course, is the ensuing peritonitis.

Uncontrolled sepsis is related either to the virulence of the pathogen (conversely, the inefficacy of the treatment) or to the continued contamination of the peritoneal cavity. Resistant organisms may cause infections that are refractory to initial regimes of chemotherapy, or polymicrobial populations may potentiate the sepsis and exceed the antibiotic spectrum. Localized abscesses may be inaccessible to all but the highest blood concentration of even the effective antibiotics.[17] From the standpoint of those indications for operative surgery, perhaps the most common is that of continuing contamination due to penetrating injuries, perforating ulcers, and ruptures of the gut wall or other viscera with uncontained leakage of septic contents into the peritoneal cavity.[18-21] Largely due to the incidence of appendicitis, this category has been credited with 62% or more of the cases of human peritonitis.[1]

Closely akin is the matter of undue surgical contamination by such means as open techniques of decompression and evacuation of obstructed bowel, open resection and anastomosis, and unnecessary exposure of movable organs. Sometimes, the operation requires such apparent breaches of asepsis, indeed cannot be done without them. Even so, in the presence of gross contamination the sharp conscience of cleanliness can be dulled and our efforts to minimize soilage somewhat diminished, with the expected outcome. Neither antibiotics, nor peritoneal lavage nor drains will supplant clean operative methods.

Bacterial infection may also spread to the peritoneum from surgical or postoperative wound infections such as occur in the open castration, in which the tunic lining the vaginal process is a direct extension by evagination of the parietal peritoneum and the vaginal cavity is in direct communication with the peritoneal space. In view of this relationship one wonders why peritonitis is such an infrequent sequela to open castrations in farm animals. Other examples are to be found in the methods of ovariectomy and cryptorchidectomy that have been practiced so commonly in farm animals since long before the advent of antibiotics, and most often under field conditions where aseptic technique is at best but a forlorn effort. Host resistance must be given a lion's share of the credit.

This introduces, then, the contribution of lowered resistance, either local or general, to the pathologic process. And it is this factor which militates against the surgeon's best efforts under controlled conditions to cope with contamination by either direct soilage or transmural migration when tissues are devitalized. Incomplete removal of nonviable tissue, such as purulent pseudomembranes, callous linings of abscesses and fistulas, ischemic segments of gut wall, unduly traumatized or desiccated visceral surfaces, and infectious deposits of fibrin serve as reservoirs of contamination to perpetuate suppuration and fuel the spreading inflammatory fire in the peritoneal space. The humoral defenses of leukocytosis and immune mechanisms cannot reach the scene because of the local ischemia, or else are simply overwhelmed by the odds. This knowledge has provoked some to take the course of radical surgical debridement in the treatment of advanced generalized bacterial peritonitis in cases where the source of contamination could be eliminated.

Hemorrhage into the peritoneal cavity in the presence of contamination works disadvantageously in several ways. The loss from the circulating blood volume depletes the oxygen quotient and favors the anaerobic processes that aggravate shock and promote abscessation, such as due to the non-sporeforming facultative anaerobes (e.g., *Bacteroides fragilis*). In an experiment on mice with intraperitoneal infections of *Klebsiella pneumoniae* and *Staphylococcus aureus*, it was observed that oxygen delivery to tissues may be impaired during infection, with animals developing acidosis and hemoconcentration. Paradoxically, the animals made hypoxic on 10% oxygen concentration (versus 20% normoxic-oxygen concentration) survived longer than those exposed to infection alone. The 10% mice developed acidosis and hemoconcentration, but the reduction in red cell 2,3 diphosphoglycerate—concerned with the oxygen transport function of red cells—was not so great as in the 20% mice.[22] This suggests the interaction between the facultative coliforms, such as *E. coli*, shown to exert a dominance in early deaths due to fecal peritonitis, and the obligate anaerobes that cause indolent abscesses and later mortality.[23] Of course, this is not to ignore the parallel experiments with isolated ischemic gut loops in which the peracute deaths in 12 hours, without gross evidence of peritonitis, were regarded as models of delayed, endotoxic shock.[24] A classic example of a natural occurrence is found in horses suffering the same type of death with massive bowel strangulations. Laboratory values prior to death reflect metabolic acidosis, hypoxia, and hemoconcentration.

Experiments have been conducted to illustrate the adjuvant action of hemoglobin on bacteria in the peritoneal cavity. Hemoglobin potentiation of pathogenicity has been attributed to its ability to delay the clearance of the bacteria from the peritoneal cavity by inhibition of the normal influx of polymorphonuclear leukocytes into the site of the infection. This blockage of leukocyte chemotaxis allowed the bacteria to proliferate free of the principal mode of early host defense.[25] In a study of animal models of human peritonitis, using dogs and rodents, intraperitoneal injections of pure cultures of *Escherichia coli*, *Proteus vulgaris*, and *Bacteroides fragilis* included either mucin or hemoglobin as adjuvant.[26] Mortality rate in peritonitis of dogs has been related to the presence of adjuvants such as mucin, gum tragacanth, hemoglobin, and an albumin-like substance in dogs with experimental pancreatitis. *E. coli* and hemoglobin were described as "a lethal combination."[27]

Mention of peritoneal drainage immediately polarizes two armed camps which are equally committed to defend their convictions and refute the others. As with most diametrically opposed posi-

tions, it is likely that the truth lies somewhere in between. Notwithstanding legitimate arguments pro and con, all can agree that it is a major problem in the surgical management of peritonitis to achieve effective drainage of septic effusions and walled-off abscesses from the numerous spaces within the boundaries of the cavity and the myriad loops of intestines. Fibrin deposits, adhesions, and ileus—all natural defense mechanisms against the spread of infection—also serve as traps for exudate. Localized abscesses contiguous to accessible parts of the body wall can be drained when located. Short of radical debridement, generalized peritonitis can be drained only partially. This is discussed further under treatment.

Intestinal obstruction is the bête noire of every surgeon, particularly when laboring in the dark recesses of the equine and bovine abdomen. It may be undetected, uncorrected, or a supervening (secondary) intestinal obstruction. One enterolith is removed from the small colon, only to close the abdomen without recognition of additional enteroliths concealed in the capacious great colon, "waiting in the wings" to reobstruct during the subsequent days of recovery. An intussusception is successfully resected and a technically sound anastomosis made, only to be the site of another intussusception days later. An abdomen is explored from length to breadth for some answer to an unyielding intestinal obstruction, with disclosure of nothing more dramatic than fluid-filled loops of small intestine, or tympanitic colon, and no more satisfactory diagnosis than ileus, that vaguest of names.

Examples of *peritoneal irritants* which may be introduced at the time of surgery are talc, starch, mineral oil, barium salts,[2,12] hypertonic solutions, and alcoholic vehicles for certain antibiotics. Classified as an aseptic, granulomatous peritonitis[1] there are some similarities to other forms, such as that resulting from rupture of ovarian cysts and teratomas,[1,16] and the sclerosing mesenteritis-peritonitis induced by certain vasoactive drugs (practolol).[28-31] These must be differentiated from the sclerosing mesenteritis of *Mycobacterium tuberculosis* and *E. coli*, described as a protracted panniculitis with resultant fibrosis,[32] and from disseminated neoplasms (e.g., lymphosarcoma, mesothelioma, and carcinoma).[1] Starch peritonitis has been studied extensively, since it has been used to replace talc for surgical glove powder. Rice starch proved worse than corn starch. The granulomatous reaction in the tissues has been characterized: the starch granules are first isolated by fibrin, then incorporated into histiocytic, multinuclear, foreign body giant cells, eventually fragmented and transported to regional lymphatics. Diagnosis is easily made on tissues* stained with periodic acid-Schiff (PAS) reagent. Viewed at 250× magnification, the starch granules stain bright red; and under polarized light 250 to 400×, the granules demonstrate a typical Maltese cross configuration. Clinical signs derive from the associated adynamic ileus as well as the granulomatous masses.[33] In one recent study, two human patients with histologically diagnosed starch peritonitis demonstrated a cell-mediated immunity to corn starch using techniques of macrophage migration inhibition and lymphocyte DNA synthesis. This cell-mediated immunity was suspected as contributing to the pathogenesis of starch granuloma.[34] Interestingly, the other workers observed an elevated leukocyte count with a left shift, but no eosinophilia, and regarded intradermal skin tests for sensitivity as unreliable. Nevertheless, one of the respected treatments is corticosteroid therapy. Current investigations give promise to the use of sodium bicarbonate, especially in starch sensitive patients.[33]

Mineral oil has been used in attempts to prevent peritoneal adhesions before it was found to cause oleogranuloma.[20] Barium salts used for contrast radiography of the gastrointestinal tract have been found to be highly irritating to the peritoneum if they escape, for example, through a small perforating ulcer or as an untoward result of barium enema.[2,12] Hypertonic salt solutions are known to be irritating, and have been used even at normal strength to induce experimental sterile peritonitis in rabbits. Peritoneal exudate taken 8 hours following intraperitoneal infusion contained $23,751 \pm 3039$ granulocytes/cmm.[35] Certain antibiotic solutions of neomycin sulfate and oxytetracycline hydrochloride are irritating to the peritoneum, and intraperitoneal infusions in the conscious animal have been attended by violent colic. It can be understood that solutions intended for intraperitoneal use—whether for irrigation, for dialysis, or for chemotherapy—should be those tested and proven for that purpose.

Peritoneal foreign bodies related to surgery can scarcely be attributed to anything other than error. Surgical instruments, gauze sponges, laparotomy pads and drains or catheters that have broken off inside probably account for the majority of such items. Anticipating that such events may be inevitable in the course of human endeavor, especially in the oftentimes emotion-charged atmosphere of the operating room, many manufacturers include radiopaque threads, lines, and other indicators in

expendable supplies or software. Instruments, of course, are clearly identifiable on radiographs. The resultant problems may be sterile, granulomatous reactions or septic processes, usually abscesses. The most that can be hoped for is that the reaction is close to the body wall and accessible through a secondary incision. Regrettably, the patient suffers the consequences, but the surgeon certainly shares the grief. Sponge counts and instrument counts are de rigueur in human hospitals. Drains and catheters, attended to by nurses or technicians, may be lost internally during postoperative wound care, which underscores the need for the surgeon either to dress the wound personally or to verify that proper care has been administered. Drains, especially soft rubber Penrose drains which may become torn and break off upon manipulation or removal, should be measured in length upon installation and, when removed, should be saved for the surgeon's inspection.

Contaminated nonabsorbable sutures used in the laparotomy closure may act as foreign bodies and cause mural abscesses, which must be treated thoughtfully to guard against dehiscence on the one hand or extension of infection on the other. Cellulitis of the wound closure is no small matter to be delegated to assistants. Stitch abscesses may necessitate reoperation of the incision for removal and debridement. Weakening of the abdominal wall may predispose to evisceration or incisional hernia. The problem can be averted in most instances by the use of impervious wound protector drapes and careful decompression or evacuation per enterotomy so as to avoid soilage of the wound margins. If this should occur, vigorous toilet with copious amounts of antibiotic saline solutions may still control the contamination. Also, protective sterile absorbent bandages, changed as frequently as they become wet from drainage, and reliable wound support provided with corset binders are indicated. Possibly, the only exceptions are the lateral flank incisions in the large animal. Even here, clean premises and close observation are minimal care.

MISCELLANEOUS CAUSES

The remaining causes are a diverse lot, each of which might constitue a separate category, therefore the decision to group them under the common heading. They include the infectious and noninfectious, and those initiated by external injury as well by internal events.

Abscesses are either intra-abdominal or extra-abdominal in relation to the boundaries of the peritoneal cavity. The abdomen is divided into xiphoid, central, umbilical, inguinal, pubic, flank,

---

* Specimens taken by biopsy or paracentesis.

hypochondriac and paralumbar anatomic regions and these may be used to designate locations of abscesses. The abdomen may be divided into quadrants by imaginary frontal and sagittal planes, and into cranial and caudal abdomen by transverse plane. The peritoneal cavity is divided into compartments by the transverse colon, the great mesentery of the small bowel, and the pelvic brim. It is, in turn, subdivided into spaces by organs juxtaposed to boundaries, omenta, mesenteries, and other organs, e.g., the phrenoreticular space involved in the reticuloperitonitis of "hardware disease" of cattle. Further specification is by specific organ or structure, e.g., hepatic or mesenteric. Mural abscesses are those located in the wall of an organ or, simply, the abdominal wall. In the latter case they usually originate from extra-abdominal causes such as penetrating wounds, contaminated suture lines, and improper injections. Renal, pelvic, inguinal, and umbilical abscesses commonly arise from retroperitoneal infections, but are well-known for their intraperitoneal complications.

The bacteriology of abdominal abscesses can be approached in several ways. In the equine species, there appears to be a correlation with infections of the respiratory tract with pyogenic bacteria, notably *Streptococcus* equi, *S. zooepidemicus*, and *Corynebacterium spp*.[17,36] The significance of *E. coli* mentioned earlier[27] and a study of a series of 22 cases of peritonitis suggest the prevalence of enterobacteria in dogs.[37] A human study described intra-abdominal infections as polymicrobial, involving both aerobic and anaerobic bacteria, and ascribed pathogenicity to synergistic bacterial mechanisms. Anaerobes, the predominant organisms in the gastrointestinal tract, were isolated in 84% of the cases (multiple in 66%) and were the only organism in 39%. *E. coli* was the most commonly isolated of the gram-negative bacilli which accounted for 63% of the facultative anaerobes and strict aerobes isolated. By the use of specialized anaerobic laboratory techniques, the fastidious, obligate anaerobes, such as *Bacteroides fragilis*, have been identified as important causes of abdominal abscesses in humans. The study disputed the findings in cases of "sterile" pus, contending that to be due to inadequate testing methods.[21] Coliforms, such as *E. coli*, *Streptococcus fecalis* and Proteus spp. have been blamed for the majority of early deaths in acute bacterial peritonitis. In an experiment conducted on rats to evaluate the respective roles of coliforms and anaerobic bacteria, untreated controls exhibited a two-stage disease— an early acute stage claiming 37% mortality, attributed to coliforms principally, and a late stage charac-

terized by indolent intra-abdominal abscesses, due to anaerobic bacteria.[38] Another investigation done on the spontaneous bacterial peritonitis of cirrhotic ascites reflected the same relationship of early and late deaths, with obligate anaerobes being recovered from the indolent abscesses associated with the late deaths. However, this study emphasized that late abscess formation also required aerobic as well as anaerobic bacteria, returning to the earlier point of synergistic pathogenicity. An experiment with *E. coli*, enterococci, and *B. fragilis* proved nonvirulent in pure culture, but combinations of these organisms produced severe peritonitis.[23]

Other species of bacteria incriminated in intra-abdominal abscesses include *Clostridium perfringens*, the anaerobic gram-positive Peptococcus and Peptostreptococcus,[21] *Eubacterium tenue* and *aerofaciens*, *Fusobacterium varium*, Lactobacillus spp., alpha hemolytic streptococci,[38] Klebsiella spp.,[23] *Actinobacillus lignieresii*,[39] and *Actinomyces* spp.[40] The roles of other bacteria, protozoa, and fungi in peritonitis are discussed under subsequent headings.

Bile peritonitis has been listed as an aseptic peritonitis due to a noninfectious irritant;[1] however, more recent opinion holds that it is an inflammatory response to the presence of bile and bacteria.[41] Bile peritonitis results from extravasation of free bile into the peritoneal cavity from perforation of the gallbladder due to acute cholecystitis,[42] torsion and gangrene of the gallbladder, biliary tract surgery, penetrating and closed abdominal trauma,[3] percutaneous transhepatic cholangiography, choledochopancreatography,[43] carcinoma of the gallbladder[44] and rupture of choledochus cyst, subcapsular cholangitic abscess or amoebic abscess.[43,45] Impairment of bile flow has also been observed experimentally to result from the intrahepatic cholestasis caused by the action of *E. coli* endotoxins as are produced during bouts with such gram-negative bacterial infections.[46] Although not a true bile peritonitis, gangrene of the hepatic round ligament was credited as the cause of a diffuse, acute peritonitis in a 74-year-old-woman.[47]

In humans, perforation of the gallbladder due to cholecystitis is the most common cause and trauma the second most common.[41] Peritonitis is the commonest and most dangerous complication[45] and the cause of death is attributed to bacteria, fluid loss and toxic bile salts, all producing shock. Although gallbladder bile in dogs is often sterile, *Clostridium perfringens* and other bacteria are often isolated from peritoneal exudate. Experiments with gnotobiotic animals have established that bacteria are a major cause of death in bile peritonitis.[41] Bile-laden peritoneal fluid has been described as an excellent culture medium for growth of gram-negative organisms, including *Pseudomonas aeruginosa*.[43] Mortality rates are quite high when treatment is delayed or inadequate.[41,42]

Pancreatic peritonitis can result from acute pancreatitis, pancreatic surgery, trauma or perforations of the proximal duodenum with an outpouring of gastric juice, bile and pancreatic secretions, resulting in a chemical peritonitis. Much of the clinical course parallels the description of bile peritonitis, which is often coexistent. Differential diagnosis is based on testing peritoneal fluid sample for amylase content.[1,14,18,19,27]

Peritonitis has been the observed result of bacteremias, viremias and mycotic infections introduced through contaminated parenteral injections, peritoneal dialysis, and gastrointestinal leakage.

Spontaneous bacterial peritonitis has been reported as a frequent and silent infection in human patients with cirrhotic ascites.[48] As to the mode of transmission, two opinions prevail. One source states the most likely route to be direct inoculation of the peritoneum by transmural migration of enteric bacteria.[23] The second means is bacterial seeding during spontaneous, oftentimes occult, portal bacteremia. As expressed, "innocent bystander" effusions other than ascites, such as pleural,[49] pericardial and synovial fluids, might be similarly seeded. The contention is that any fluid in a closed space, in cirrhotic or non-cirrhotic patients, is at risk for infection during obscure bacteremias.[50]

In one series of 118 human cases of spontaneous bacterial peritonitis, all associated with hepatic cirrhosis, the following bacteriology results were obtained.[23]

Escherichia coli	46%
Streptococcus pneumoniae	17%
Other Streptococci	17%
Klebsiella pneumoniae	8%
Anaerobes or Microaerophiles	6%

Three bacteria that are common to animal species and that have been reported to cause spontaneous peritonitis in man are *Clostridium perfringens*,[51] *Pasteurella multocida*,[52] and *Campylobacter fetus*.[53] Pasteurella is a frequent animal pathogen, common to nose, mouth and throat, and in one human case the incriminated source of infections was the mouth of a pet cat.[52] Campylobacter is known as a cause of infectious abortion in cattle[53] and sheep. The organism has been isolated from placentas and gastric contents from aborted lamb fetuses, from feces of dogs with diarrhea, and from the intestinal tract of normal animals. It has recently been isolated from human patients with diarrhea.[54]

Candida peritonitis, due mostly to *Candida albicans* and *C. tropicalis*, is a complication of peritoneal dialysis, gastrointestinal surgery, or perforation of an abdominal viscus. Recent antibiotic therapy is regarded to be predisposing. It has been typified as localized in the abdominal cavity, with but rare cases of dissemination. The clinical course is that of bacterial peritonitis but with lower mortality in treated cases.[55] In one instance, Candida peritonitis occurred in the recipient of a kidney transplant due to a contaminated parenteral alimentation line. It was associated with acute pancreatitis and a pancreatic pseudocyst, regarded as complications in about 2% of kidney transplants. In addition, there was an *E. coli* septicemia.[56]

The principal example of viral peritonitis is to be found in feline infectious peritonitis, a viral-induced infectious disease of cats characterized by an effusive form, peritonitis and pleuritis, and a non-effusive or dry form affecting the liver, kidneys, eyes, brain, and spinal cord.[57] The peritonitis is described as fibrinous[58] and pyogranulomatous[59] with a characteristic viscid, yellow-colored fibrinous exudate which coagulates on standing.[58,60] The granulomatous plaques are found on all serous surfaces throughout the pleural as well as the peritoneal cavities,[59,61] and the abdominal lesions include focal necrosis in the liver, spleen, kidneys, and omentum.[58] Brain lesions include granulomatous meningitis, chorioependymitis, and acquired hydrocephalus.[57,62] This same pyogranulomatous reaction has been seen in the spinal cord along with cerebellar lesions.[63] Ocular signs have been described as an exudative choroiditis with multiple granulomatous lesions, perivascular infiltrates, retinal hemorrhages and detachment and a nonproductive conjunctivitis.[61] Virus particles have been identified in ascitic fluid and liver homogenates from natural and experimentally induced cases, and this virus has been characterized according to criteria which seem to justify its classification as a new member of the Coronaviridae family.[64,65] There is similarity to a human case of peritonitis due to *Diplococcus pneumoniae* that developed after an appendectomy in which there was a concomitant peritonitis and meningitis.[66]

Drug-Induced Peritonitis

A sclerosing peritonitis characterized by widespread peritoneal adhesions and thickening due to fibrosis with focal lymphocytic infiltration has been identified as being caused by prolonged treatment of human heart patients with practolol (Trasicor), a beta-blocking agent used with somewhat the same indications as propranolol (Inderal), for treatment of angina due to ischemic hypertensive heart disease due to myocardial infarction. Treatment periods have extended over periods ranging from months to years, with complications ensuing 7 to 18 months after treatment withdrawal. Clincal signs precipitating the discovery have usually been those of bowel obstruction, commonly small intestinal. Other untoward side-effects reported include psoriasis-like skin reactions, conjunctivitis, corneal involvement and reduction in tears. Identification of a positive anti-nuclear factor has prompted the question of drug-induced systemic lupus erythematosus.[28-31]

A somewhat related occurrence of spontaneous bacterial peritonitis was reported in two human patients that were being treated by selective infusions of vasopressin into the superior mesenteric or gastroduodenal arteries for upper gastrointestinal hemorrhage due to alcoholic cirrhosis. The presence of a polymicrobial population, including both aerobic and anaerobic organisms, suggested that the arteriolar vasocontriction had caused sufficient ischemia of the intestinal mucosal barrier to permit enterobacterial diapedesis into the ascitic pool within the peritoneal cavity.[67]

The preceding case study prompts a look at yet another bizarre instance of an enterocolitis with peritonitis in a child with pheochromocytoma. An 8-year-old boy presented with acute abdominal pain, rectal bleeding, peritonitis and shock. Clinical findings included inflammation and edema of the entire colon and terminal ileum, and two necrotic areas of the cecum, in addition to the tumor. Recovery followed removal of the tumor and a diverting loop ileostomy. Pheochromocytomas are catecholamine-producing tumors primarily of chromaffin tissue of adrenal medulla and paraspinal sympathetic ganglia. They have been incriminated as causing gastrointestinal bleeding, ileus, focal intestinal ischemia, or frank intestinal necrosis, plus hypertension attending the diarrhea.[68]

Thus, peritonitis may be drug-induced by both natural (endogenous) and artificial (exogenous) means with either infectious or noninfectious consequences. Considerable emphasis should be placed on the fact that exogenous induction is also iatrogenic. This discussion has served to introduce the next etiologic group of peritonitis-producing tumors.

Neoplasms and Cysts

In addition to the pheochromocytoma peritonitis described previously, and as further evidence of the vague demarcations that exist between causes of peritonitis, every example cited in this category has found appropriate location and discussion in previous categories. Other than confusing the diagnosis by resemblance to benign processes, carcinoma is often the cause of perforations of bowel and bile duct, resulting in either fecal or bile peritonitis.[18,44] Rupture of amebic abscesses of the liver and of choledochus cysts results in bacterial as well as biliary peritonitis.[69] Pancreatic pseudocyst associated with acute pancreatitis and Candida mycethemia has been involved with mycotic peritonitis.[56] Intraperitoneal rupture of ovarian cystic teratomas[16] and pseudomucinous cystadenomas of the ovary or appendix[1] have been the causes of irritant peritonitis. This ambiguity finds additional expression in the findings of one study that revealed 32.4% of the cases of feline infectious peritonitis were also positive for feline leukemia viral antigen as determined by indirect fluorescent antibody technique. This was almost half the incidence (73%) found in cases of lymphosarcoma and over four times the incidence (7.5%) found in 557 cats with various other lesions.[70] This suggests a relationship at least between some elements of feline infectious peritonitis and feline leukemia, both of which are of viral origin.

Peritonitis of Humans

A student of the subject cannot help but be struck by the great variety of etiologic types of peritonitis in the human. Nor is it an altogether safe assumption that peritonitis in animals does not possess the same diversity. But for the present, we must continue to review all the forms that are known to us, human and animal, with the expectation of recognizing the unusual and hitherto undescribed disease. Thus it is that this discussion of the etiology of peritonitis in animals concludes with mention of several types of the disease or elements of other diseases that have some bearing on the subject.

Periodic polyserositis is a familial disease occurring in the human populations indigenous to the Mediterranean. Its etiology is unknown but it is believed to be inherited as an autosomal recessive trait. It occurs in young people of both sexes and appears with a variable periodicity. Renal amyloidosis is the primary complication and the cause of death is usually renal failure. It does not respond to steroids and is not to be confused with lupus erythematosus.[2,71]

Eosinophilic peritonitis is a rare syndrome which produces edema, eosinophilic infiltration and a necrotizing angiitis of the serosa. Ascitic fluid has a high eosinophil count and peripheral blood may reflect the same picture. It may respond to corticosteroids and epinephrine and is thought to be allergic in nature.[2]

Lupus peritonitis is a complication of disseminated lupus erythematosus, which complication may result from vasculitis of the bowel wall, ulceration secondary to thrombosis of affected vessels, ulceration of the large bowel (resembling ulcerative colitis), an involvement of the appendix or gallbladder that mimics acute appendicitis or cholecystitis, and a similar association with acute pancreatitis or hepatitis. A generalized disease of unknown cause, it occurs most often in women in their thirties and forties. Treatment has included large doses of adrenocorticosteroids. In addition to gastrointestinal lesions, the nephrotic syndrome is listed as one of the major manifestations of systemic lupus erythematosus,[2] which offers some interesting connection with the spontaneous bacterial peritonitis seen in young patients with the nephrotic syndrome as described earlier in the chapter.[14,15] Acute phlegmonous gastritis, another poorly understood disease, is seen in old age, malnutrition, alcoholism, trauma, decreased gastric acid production, prior gastritis, and infectious foci elsewhere (e.g., pneumococcal endocarditis). Pathogens identified include Pneumococci, Klebsiella, alpha-hemolytic Streptococci, Clostridia, *E. coli*, and *Proteus vulgaris*. One case involved a patient with discoid lupus erythematosus. Pneumococcus was recovered on culture. The confusion on preoperative clinical diagnosis centered around the differentiation of acute phlegmonous gastritis from primary peritonitis and the peritonitis of collagen vascular disease. The contention was that primary peritonitis was usually associated with nephrosis (overlooking the patients with cirrhotic ascites) and an involvement of the general peritoneal viscera, rather than acute phlegmonous gastritis involving only the stomach (at least at the outset). On the other hand, lupus patients with diagnosis of intra-abdominal catastrophe had a sterile paracentesis (initially) and concomitant arthritis, positive lupus erythematosus (L.E.) preps and leukopenia. The question was whether a common denominator existed, such as an unidentified immunologic derangement, that might lead to peritonitis or acute phlegmonous gastritis in association with collagen disease.[72]

Scleroderma, another collagen disease (progressive systemic sclerosis), is characterized by diffuse sclerosis of connective tissue of the integument and other organs, including gastrointestinal involvement. Gastrointestinal scleroderma not uncommonly affects the small bowel, causing various clinical signs ascribed to pain and obstruction, malabsorption, and extension to the large bowel of edema, round cell infiltration of the mucosa and submucosa, and irregular replacement of muscle by collagen.[71] This led other investigators to suggest that the sclerosing peritonitis associated with prolonged practolol therapy might be a drug-induced systemic lupus erythematosus. They noted a positive antinuclear factor in their patients.[31] Bearing in mind the occurrence of rheumatoid arthritis and positive L.E. preps in animal patients, it would be interesting to know whether gastrointestinal complications and peritonitis had been observed and recorded in such cases.

Chyloperitoneum

Chylous ascites results from obstruction or perforation of abdominal lacteals or cisterna chyli by tumors, inflammation, or trauma. Paracentesis yields a fluid turbid with fat content (0.4 to 4 g/dl) and with a specific gravity > 1.012. Untreated cases have a high mortality rate. If sterile, the fluid can be citrated and returned to the patient by intravenous infusion for its nutritive value. The diagnosis may be confused with lymphosarcoma, which causes a milky (chyliform) ascites, but this fluid contains neoplastic cells, fibrin particles and blood cells, rather than fat globules.[2]

PATHOPHYSIOLOGY AND CLINICAL COURSE OF PERITONITIS

In health, the peritoneum is a smooth, moist dialyzing membrane capable of effecting rapid exchange of electrolytes rendered to ionic equilibrium with body fluids. Inflamed peritoneum becomes reddened and edematous with increased capillary permeability and subperitoneal vasodilation. Peritoneal effusion follows rapidly thereafter with accumulations of free fluid which gravitate in the peritoneal cavity. Chemotactic response to humoral elements causes intensified phagocytic activity and leads to suppuration in the presence of infection. Lymphatics are numerous and some have expressed the opinion that lymphatic activity is less in the pelvic end of the cavity.[14] In portal obstruction, either intra- or extrahepatic (as with some tumors) ascites may result. The horse appears to be much less predisposed to ascites due to intrahepatic portal obstruction than some of the other domestic animals or man, in whom it is quite common due to alcoholic cirrhosis.

Very soon after the initial insult, the peritoneum becomes covered with fibrin deposits, giving the smooth, moist, glistening surface a rough, dry appearance, shaggy with fibroplastic exudate and filmy adhesions. Visceral and parietal surfaces adhere to contiguous structures. The extent of this reaction is dependent upon: (1) the virulence of the pathogen, (2) the duration and extent of the contamination, (3) the source of the contamination, and (4) the efficacy of the treatment.[27] For example, monomicrobial infections may be regarded as less pathogenic than polymicrobial ones if the theory of synergistic potentiation between aerobic and anaerobic bacterial populations in closed space infections is accepted. However, no one would question the seriousness of a peritonitis caused by these species—*Clostridium perfringens* or *Mycobacterium tuberculosis.*

The natural defense mechanisms are comprised of the effective inflammatory reaction, the localizing adhesions and fibrin accumulations, sympathetic inhibition of peristalsis, gravitation of peritoneal fluid, heightened phagocytosis and antibody reaction, and inactivity imposed by pain. These are sufficient to protect the body against a single, transient contamination, or one that can be contained to a circumscribed location. However, when the insult is repetitive (e.g., a perforated ulcer), or so extensive at the outset as to overwhelm these natural defenses (e.g., rectal rupture), the peritonitis spreads, assisted by movements of bowel, urogenital tract, abdominal wall and diaphragm (respirations) as well as by shifting movements of the fluid effusion throughout the continuous spaces of the peritoneal cavity. The inflamed peritoneum becomes more permeable and provides an extensive surface for the absorption of toxins.[1,11,14,18,27]

As to the importance of the source of the contamination, it is recognized that the level at which the breach occurs in the bowel determines the type of peritonitis that is due to gastrointestinal origin. Breaks in the stomach and duodenum release gastric juice and pepsin (low pH) and bile and pancreatic enzymes (high pH), which cause an intensely irritating chemical peritonitis that spreads rapidly throughout the cavity.[18] Severe pain, pneumoperitoneum, and much effusion characterize this injury. It is quite common for the patient to succumb to massive shock peracutely and prior to any impressive degree of actual infection. Examples are numerous: the horse with gastric rupture due to acute dilatation, the giant breed of dog that overeats and suffers gastric volvulus with rupture, and the postparturient dairy cow that develops displacement and volvulus of the abomasum. Sudden onset, severe course, and acute death typify each of these.

Perforations occurring in the ileocecocolic regions produce a coliform peritonitis which may be rapid or deliberate in its course according to the extent of the contamination.[18] If the leakage stems from a small perforation that is walled-off by adhesions and does not itself cause bowel obstruction, the result may be a localized abscess. If the contamination is from a rent or rupture with gross soilage, diffuse peritonitis results. Although large effusions and chemical irritation may not characterize the early course, bacterial sepsis and endotoxemia may expectedly be even greater, with resultant high mortality, as exemplified by ruptures of the rectum and perforating diverticulitis of the colon.

Peritonitis exerts profound effects on circulatory homeostasis. In the acute, spreading infection characterized by great effusion, there is rapid and severe translocation of fluid, electrolyte and plasma protein into what has been called a third space,[1] in turn comprised of three "compartments"—the peritoneal cavity, the extraperitoneal tissues, and the lumen of the bowel. Pouring into the peritoneal cavity are such fluids as exudate (with a protein and electrolyte content approaching that of extracellular fluid), alimentary fluid, bile, pancreatic juice, urine, amniotic fluid, cystic fluid, chyle, and, of course, free blood. Fluid in the loose, extraperitoneal connective tissue consists mostly of edema, and this may accumulate around the walls of visceral organs and between the laminae of the mesenteries, as well as outside the parietal surfaces. The fluid accumulations in the static, atonic gut may account for the largest volume, either in the form of gastric and small intestinal secretions or as the entrapped component of the fluid flux in the colon when its prodigious water resorptive function is interrupted due to certain pathologic processes. Fluid loss into this "third space" has been compared to that of an extensive burn.[1]

Additional fluid deficit is due to diminished intake, vomition, and diarrhea. Where vomitus is the primary loss, the electrolyte derangement is likely to be a metabolic, hypokalemic alkalosis. With diarrhea, bicarbonate losses incline toward metabolic acidosis. Metabolic dysfunctions are also affected by respiratory insufficiency due to intense abdominal pain as well as intra-abdominal pressures exerted on the diaphragm by peritoneal effusions and bowel distention. The result is a respiratory acidosis superimposed on the metabolic defect. In both vomiting and diarrhea, severe hypovolemia and hemoconcentration is expected. In the protracted case, a severe anemia may supervene.

Death is due to a combination of factors, but shock is a common denominator, whether due to the gastroduodenal perforation and resultant chemical peritonitis, or to the more deliberate sepsis of fecal peritonitis. The intolerable derangements in the fluid-electrolyte balance, the loss of plasma protein into peritoneal effusions, the noxious effects of bacterial toxins and all of the end-products of anaerobic metabolism on vital organ systems, the debilitating effects of chronic empyema and abscess, and the progressive deterioration of body defenses are translated into a progression of failures: adrenocortical, hepatorenal, respiratory, and cardiovascular.

DIAGNOSIS

Heavy emphasis is placed on a careful history-taking and the physical examination. A knowledge of the type of injury or insult often leads to the diagnosis, whether complicated by infection or not. Exposure to certain respiratory infections, such as equine strangles, to feline colonies with a history of viral peritonitis, recent peritoneal dialysis, history of ingestion of ground hay from wire-bound bales, of barium enemas for contrast radiography, of bouts of venereal infections, all are good examples of the potential significance of a complete medical history.

Clinical signs include: pain, vomiting, adynamic ileus, tachycardia, fever, tachypnea, abdominal distention and tenderness, injected mucous membranes (later becoming cyanotic), dry fissured tongue, delayed capillary refill time, cold clammy skin and extremities, initial rise in blood pressure, followed by falling pressure later, and what has been described in the human as a Hippocratic facies, meaning an anxious expression and a reluctance to move. Abdominal splinting may vary somewhat with the species. Tactile percussion and palpation of the abdomen are easier in the small animal, and are easier in the cow than the horse. Palpation per rectum is understandably more valuable in the large animal.

Much of the demeanor of the patient can be attributed directly to pain, which has been classified as either visceral or parietal.[1,19] Visceral pain has been ascribed to that emanating from the sympathetic chain and splanchnic nerves and has been pictured as either steady or crampy, but vaguely defined, poorly localized, or referred pain. Parietal or somatic pain is that which originates from the parietal peritoneum supplied by sensory fibers from somatic nerves and is a sharp, well-defined symptom that signals the extension of the inflammatory process to the lining of the abdominal wall or pelvic cavity.

Interpreting pain in the animal case is fraught with miscues that may find parallel only in pediatric human medicine. In one series of 23 cases of emergency slaughter of cows, ostensibly for traumatic reticulitis, in all of which severe abdominal pain was observed, not any of the group exhibited

reticuloperitonitis on autopsy. However, all were affected with severe mastitis and a "septicaemia of the liver, gall bladder and spleen," which was attributed to the mastitis.[73]

A common sign of pain in herbivora is odontoprisis (bruxism) but it is not pathognomonic of peritonitis. Cattle with reticuloperitonitis will frequently exhibit an expiratory grunt, or audible groan. They may also elect to lie or stand uphill to relieve pressure and pain on the diaphragm, or to adopt a rigid stance with an arched back.

In other cases found in all species, pain may not be a conspicuous feature, but overshadowed by signs of depression and debilitation.[3,74]

Vomiting in peritonitis may be suspected as due to mechanical obstruction of the bowel or to functional interruption due to sympathetic inhibition. In either case, intestinal reflux causes secondary gastric filling and vomition. Adynamic ileus, indicated by the silent abdomen on auscultation, may be attended by either tympany or fluid distention of the bowel. Differentiation may be possible by palpation, percussion, auscultation and, in smaller individuals, abdominal radiography. The derangement of vital signs (fever, tachycardia, tachypnea, blood pressure changes, tissue perfusion) is an index of sepsis, fluid shift, electrolyte deficit, intoxication, ventilatory insufficiency, irritation of the diaphragm, intra-abdominal distention, and other related complications previously mentioned.

Special Diagnostic Procedures

Special procedures combine the efforts of the examination room, the clinical laboratory and the operating room. The procedures that are currently considered to be routine include: hematology and radiography, paracentesis, needle biopsy and microbial culture, laparoscopy, and minilaparotomy, as well as urinalysis and serology.[14,17,74-79]

Paracentesis (abdominocentesis) is done most often to aspirate a sample of the peritoneal fluid that has gravitated to the floor of the cavity; however, if necessary, a small catheter may be inserted to collect a peritoneal lavage sample. This is examined for bile, amylase, bacteria, vegetable fibers, and other foreign substances.[68] The protein content is expected to increase beyond 2.5 g/dl in the horse with peritonitis.[17] The leukocyte count and differential are considered to be highly significant even in the case of an occult bacterial ascites. One study set the arbitrary dividing line in humans with ascites due to alcoholic cirrhosis at < 300 WBC/mm^3 with 25% PMN. Less than this was acceptable, while more was suggestive of spontaneous bacterial peritonitis, even in the face of a negative culture.[76] Fortunately for the diagnostician, secondary bacterial peritonitis rarely requires such careful assessment, the leukocyte count usually being sufficient to alter the gross appearance of the specimen. It is the province of the clinical pathologist to decide whether the peritoneal fluid sample is exudative or transudative.

Needle biopsy in the context of this discussion is employed to explore for abscesses, such as ones found in the liver, or those that may have become walled off due to localized peritonitis. In addition, neoplasms, cysts, hematomas and masses due to aseptic sclerosing peritonitis must be differentiated. Although commonly performed as a percutaneous technique under local anesthesia, needle biopsy may also be done per laparotomy, culdoscopy, colpotomy or laparoscopy, according to need.

Laparoscopy was first done, interestingly enough, on a dog in 1901 by Kelling, using a standard Nitze cystoscope, and was not done on a human until 9 years later.[75] The technique has since been used in cattle, goats and horses, but remains to be accepted as a routinely employed method in the veterinary diagnostic clinic. It is widely used for both diagnostics and therapeutics in the human.[75]

The minilaparotomy[14] may be regarded as a procedure somewhat halfway between the laparoscopy and a conventional exploratory laparotomy. The concept has been used in veterinary surgery for years though not applying that particular phrase. It may be used for the dual purpose of installing drains and performing peritoneal lavage. In the large animal patient, the exploratory by manual palpation through a circumscribed opening in the paralumbar fossa may be rightly regarded as a minilaparotomy, when compared to the radical midline procedure done on the dorsal recumbent patient.

Radiographs of the abdomen in peritonitis often contain evidence of intestinal obstruction with widespread dilatation of gut loops.[1] The radiograph is of great value in the diagnosis of perforation with peritonitis, demonstrating pneumoperitoneum in the superior reaches of the peritoneal cavity owing to the escape of bowel gas through the perforation. In addition, consequential effusion, or escaped urine or other fluid accumulations present a visible fluid line in the dependent portions of the abdomen.[18] Contrast radiography, using intraperitoneal or retroperitoneal air or CO_2 and radiopaque media (e.g., Renografin or Hypaque), is employed to obtain further identification of the problem.[14] Gallium[67] scanning has been used to locate intra-abdominal inflammatory processes, such as peritoneal abscesses. The isotope is bound to leukocytes, which subsequently concentrate in abscesses and empyemas.[14]

Blood analysis for packed cell volume, blood gas and serum electrolyte concentrations is helpful as is the examination of peripheral blood, principally for total and differential leukocyte counts and plasma proteins. If the patient survives the initial insult for a sufficient number of hours, a leukocytosis occurs, but in protracted cases, this may be replaced by a degradative leukopenia. Total protein increases, consonant with rises in plasma fibrinogen ($>$ 400 mg/dl in horses)[17] and gamma globulin. However, abrupt increases in total protein are more likely a reflection of the dehydration and hemoconcentration. Albumin decreases, causing a lowered A:G ratio ($<$0.1 in horses with abdominal abscesses[17]). If peritonitis becomes chronic, with much effusion, the total protein may subsequently fall, reflecting a loss to the third space as well as the negative nitrogen balance and hepatic dysfunction. This hypoproteinemia lowers plasma osmotic pressure, further aggravating loss of fluids from the vascular compartment and increasing the edema and effusion. A study of plasma protein alterations in cattle suffering from acute peritonitis revealed a characteristic modification of the protein picture in both naturally occurring and experimentally induced cases. Considerable differences were noted in the postalbumin region of the electropherogram. One protein component increased in size, while another disappeared. Two weak components in normal sera were replaced by four discrete bands, specifically for peritonitis. In experimental cases, they were visible in 12 to 16 hours after induction.[77]

Urinalyses in peritonitis serve to assure that urine is being produced and to assess the status of renal function at a time when all vital organ systems are under threat of generalized sepsis as well as mounting intoxication from microbial sources and anaerobic metabolism. In a case study of a 3-year-old American Quarter Horse gelding with an acute, suppurative peritonitis of undisclosed origin, recovery was complicated by polyuria and polydypsia. Treatment consisted of high doses of chloramphenicol, initiated intravenously and maintained per os. Prednisolone sodium succinate 100 mg was administered intravenously at the outset. Other treatments were isonicotinic acid hydrazide per os for 8 weeks, and larvacidal doses of thiabendazole per os, 10 g/cwt on days 3 and 4. Urine specific gravity during hospitalization was 1.011. A sodium clearance, expressed as a percentage of creatinine clearance, was run to measure proximal tubular function.

Both sodium conservation and tubular function were judged to be normal, and true to prediction the horse made an uneventful recovery. The polyuria was interpreted as free water diuresis (borrowing the reasons given for the similar syndrome in the bitch with pyometra) due to a decreasing urine concentrating ability and presence of empyema. The diminished water reabsorption by the distal and collecting tubules has been attributed to ineffective ADH response presumably due to circulating endotoxins or absorption of antigen-antibody complexes from the large cavity of sepsis.[79]

Microbiologic examination should be a feature of every case workup where suppurative peritonitis is suspected. The lack of sophistication in sampling and culture techniques is only a part of the frequent failure to make an accurate accounting of the microbiologic characteristics of peritonitis. Much of the time paracentesis aspirates and abdominal biopsy samples are never submitted for culture, assuming the flora to be bacterial and of enteric origin. As has been amply stated in earlier discussion, this unwarranted assumption may lead to ineffectual treatment and unnecessary complications such as the late-occurring abdominal abscesses due to the difficult-to-culture microaerophilic *Bacteroides* spp., which may exist from the start with *Escherichia coli* and other facultative enterobacteria. It has been stated that a single type of coccal organism and pus cells justify the diagnosis of primary peritonitis, whereas if both gram-positive cocci and gram-negative rods are found, there is likely to be a gut perforation.[14]

There should be close working relationship between clinic and laboratory, including an understanding that pus is rarely sterile, and that microbial populations are often unpredictable. Finally, specific therapy is based upon a diagnosis which includes identification of the microbial agent and determination of the antibiotic sensitivity, which serves to introduce the subject of treatment.

TREATMENT

The broad approach to treatment of peritonitis is a reflection of the diverse causes and effects. Contraseptic therapy embraces the rational use of antibiotics. Support of homeostatic functions includes a repair of fluid, electrolyte and protein deficits as well as protection of the vital organ systems. Control of contamination is directed at the early removal or closure of the source, including management of external wounds. Peritoneal lavage is viewed as toilet of contaminated surfaces, a form of wet debridement. Decompression and drainage involve the gastrointestinal tract and peritoneal cavity primarily, the urogenital tract secondarily. Attention is called to complications such as clinical adhesions. Management of pain and discomfort fall under analgesia and nursing care.

Antibiotics

The rational use of antibiotics is dependent upon an understanding of the bacteriology of peritonitis and identifiable antibiotic sensitivities. From the recent literature it appears that these basic concerns are coming into a fuller appreciation, with certain impressions and misconceptions being challenged. The initiation of medication on the first encounter with peritonitis is oftentimes a presumptive choice, but it may be safe to say that there is less likelihood today that the contamination is assumed to be facultative gram-negative coliforms and nothing more of consequence. The role of anaerobic or micro-aerophilic bacteria is being questioned, and while improved laboratory methods are being used to identify these less conspicuous offenders, the clinician is learning to take such precautionary measures as to include these organisms in the spectrum of prescribed antibiotics. An interesting example of this evaluation of choices is found in the work of Hudspeth,[20] in which the progression went from penicillin and chloramphenicol to cephalothin and kanamycin, and, as most recently reported, to the combination of cephalothin, gentamicin and clindamycin, claimed to be the most efficacious treatment used by that investigator. Reasoning that synergistic bacterial mechanisms may be responsible for pathogenicity, and that if some of the organisms can be eliminated and this synergism removed, the natural host defenses may be able to overcome the remainder,[14,21] some have reported successful treatment of mixed aerobe-anaerobe infections by suppressing only the anaerobes.[21] In experimentally induced fecal peritonitis in rats, the respective roles of coliforms and anaerobic bacteria were studied with gentamicin and clindamycin.[38] Untreated controls had a two-stage disease characterized by an initial acute peritonitis (accounting for a 37% mortality rate) and a chronic peritonitis with indolent intra-abdominal abscesses in all survivors of the acute stage. Gentamicin treatment alone reduced the acute mortality rate to 4%, but 98% of the survivors had the indolent abscesses. Clindamycin treatment alone reduced the mortality rate only to 35%, but the abscess incidence dropped to 5%. The combination of gentamicin and clindamycin reduced the mortality rate to 7% and abscess rate to 6%. Coliforms were credited with the early mortalities versus the anaerobes as principal cause of the late abscesses. This experiment identified predominant species of facultative coliforms as *E. coli*, *Streptococcus fecalis*, *Proteus mirabilis* and *morgagni* and alpha hemolytic Streptococci. Dominant anaerobes were *Eubacterium tenue* and *aerofaciens*, *Bacteroides fragilis*, *Fusobacterium varium*, Clostridia spp., Peptococcus spp. and Lactobacillus spp.[38] A point of no small significance was the contention that Bacteroides, the most common obligate anaerobe isolated in a series of human cases of spontaneous bacterial peritonitis, was resistant to penicillin, cephalosporins and aminoglycosides, but was responsive to clindamycin. The demonstration of small, pleomorphic gram-negative bacilli suggestive of Bacteroides was considered to be an indication for clindamycin or chloramphenicol plus an aminoglycoside, to avert the acute early deaths and to reduce late abscess formation.[23] Another source calls attention to the fact that, while susceptibility of aerobic and facultative organisms like *E. coli* and Streptococcus spp. can be tested readily and reliably in the hospital laboratory with disc diffusion or tube dilution tests, these same methods are not applicable to test susceptibility of anaerobic bacteria. Ninety percent of *Bacteroides fragilis* strains are resistant to penicillin G and are "generally" resistant to cephalothin. Aminoglycosides such as kanamycin, gentamicin, neomycin, and streptomycin are almost totally ineffective against anaerobes. Tetracycline is now active against less than one half of the strains. On the other hand, clindamycin and chloramphenicol were cited as being active against nearly all anaerobes, including *B. fragilis*,[21] supporting the inclusion of one of these in medication of septic peritonitis of undetermined origin. Offered as an argument against the pharmacologic contraindication to simultaneous use of bactericidal and bacteriostatic antibiotics was the view that the advice held for monoclonal infections due to known species of bacteria, but was less applicable to enteric bacterial infections of multiple species with variable sensitivities.[14] Regardless of the validity of the argument, few would deny that the ultimate proving ground is in the wards. Clinical impressions, however, are no more reliable than careful documentation of the results and comparison with alternative methods. Veterinarians should be aware that clindamycin may be contraindicated in dogs. The untoward complication of pseudomembranous colitis has been repeatedly observed in association with its use in man.[79a]

Cases of amebic liver abscesses, strongyloides and ascarid parasitisms, and Candida peritonitis serve to warn against oversight of other important possibilities. In Candida infections, short-term, low-dosage systemic amphotericin B plus its use by intraperitoneal administration has reduced mortality rates.[55] Mannitol has been recommended as a nephroprotectant against both amphotericin and nephrotoxic antibiotics.[56]

It is generally acknowledged that the intravenous route is preferred for administration of antibiotics in the face of shock owing to the unreliable perfusion of tissues and the resultant delayed uptake and distribution from intramuscular injections or oral administration. This is also true in cases of peritonitis, since shock is an expected attendant. There is some controversy, however, over the advisability of intraperitoneal (IP) instillations. The methods include direct IP injections and periodic peritoneal lavage. Opponents of antibiotic delivery by peritoneal infusion maintain that the combination of ileus and fibroplastic adhesions prevent any beneficial circulation of antibiotic-laden fluids throughout the interstices of the peritoneal cavity.[20,80] In the instance of diffuse peritonitis with generalized adhesions, this is the probability. However, there are equally articulate spokesmen from the clinic floor who argue for the case based on their successful experiences.[27,37,81]

In a series of human patients with ascites and bacterial peritonitis, comparisons were made of parenterally administered antibiotic concentrations in the serum and the peritoneal fluid, using gentamicin, tobramycin, ampicillin, clindamycin, penicillin G, cephalothin, chloramphenicol, and cefazolin. All peritoneal concentrations achieved one-half or more of the serum values of the antibiotics and some, greater than 90% of the serum values. All antibiotics studied penetrated peritoneal fluid equally well and exceeded the minimal inhibitory concentration of the infecting organisms, suggesting little excuse for direct IP instillation except for the initial lag period between intravenous administration and appearance in the peritoneal fluid.[80]

In another study conducted in a rabbit peritonitis model, antibiotics were administered 3 hours after induction of peritonitis and serum peritoneal fluid concentrations were measured for 5 hours afterward. Amikacin, a new aminoglycoside, gentamicin and penicillin G were compared for penetration rates into exudate fluid. Peritoneal levels of each antibiotic exceeded the simultaneous serum levels by 1 hour after administration, and remained so thereafter. Amikacin reached 71.2% ± 12.7 of peak serum levels (immediately after dose), gentamicin reached

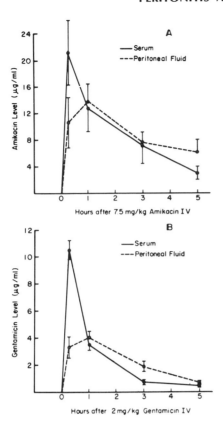

Figure 27–1. Serum and peritoneal fluid concentrations of amikacin and gentamicin after intravenous administration. Each antibiotic was given 3 hours after initiation of sterile peritonitis. The points represent mean concentrations in six animals, and the brackets indicate plus or minus standard errors of the means. (From MacGregor.[35])

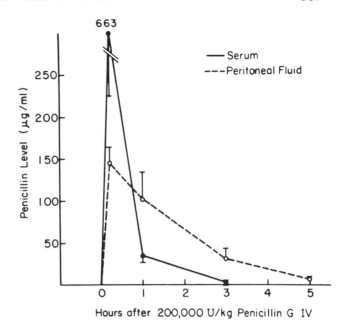

Figure 27–2. Serum and peritoneal fluid concentrations of penicillin G after intravenous administration. Conditions parallel those in Figure 27–1. (From MacGregor.[35])

37.1% ± 2.7, and penicillin G reached 23.2% ± 4.5, here again demonstrating the efficacy of parenteral administration (Figs. 27–1, 27–2, and 27–3).[35]

In peritonitis due to gram-negative rods (e.g., *E. coli*) aminoglycoside antibiotics offer the widest spectrum of efficacy. Amikacin, a relative of kanamycin A, is more active than kanamycin against most strains of Pseudomonas, including those that produce inactivating enzymes against gentamicin, tobramycin, and kanamycin.[35] However, some express preference for cephalothin because of its broad spectrum of activity and its minimal toxicity. Aminoglycosides are criticized for their otic and renal toxicity and may interact with anesthetics and muscle relaxants to cause muscle paralysis, respiratory depression, and reduction of cardiac output, systemic blood pressure, and myocardial contractile force.[81,82] Tetracyclines, colistin, lincomycin, and polymixin A and B are also incriminated.[82] Reportedly, cephalothin is free from these adverse effects.[81]

Other antibiotics advocated for treatment of peritonitis include ampicillin sodium, used both by IP administration and parenterally.[3,37] Despite what has been said in reference to clindamycin/chloramphenicol treatment of late-occurring abscesses caused by anaerobes, there are the notable examples of streptococcal abscesses in the horse that have

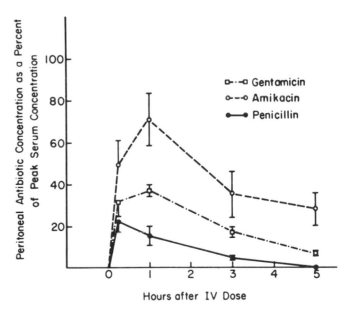

Figure 27–3. Concentration of the antibiotics in peritoneal exudate fluid after intravenous administration expressed as the percentage of peak serum concentration for each antibiotic. (From MacGregor.[35])

responded to long-term, high dosages of penicillin (40,000 to 100,000 U/kg for 10 days, followed by repositol penicillin alternate day therapy for 2 to 6 months).[17]

An interesting case was reported of a postoperative appendicitis, peritonitis and meningitis yielding *Diplococcus pneumoniae* that developed in the course of cephalothin therapy and responded to a combination of penicillin G and chloramphenicol sodium succinate IV for 10 days.[66] This seems to contradict the earlier statement that combinations of bactericidal and bacteriostatic antibiotics are indicated for polymicrobial infections as opposed to monoclonal ones,[14] but it must be appreciated that such remarks are at best only generalizations. Antibiotic sensitivity tests and patient response must be the final determinants in every individual case, and clinical judgment must be based on experience and careful observation.

Support of Homeostatic Functions

Repair of fluid-electrolyte deficits and protection of vital organ systems fall under the care of the total patient. As emphasized in earlier comments, cause of death is a combination of hypovolemia, sepsis, anaerobic metabolism and all of the aggravating factors including pain, bowel obstruction, ventilatory insufficiency, liver failure, renal shutdown, central nervous system depression and myocardial toxicity. Tissue perfusion and oxygenation are in jeopardy, and all efforts must be directed toward preservation of the life-support functions while treatment of the peritonitis is under way. Measures include replacement of the fluid-electrolyte-plasma protein deficit by prescription based on continuous monitoring of the peripheral blood values for packed cell volume, blood gases, serum electrolytes and plasma protein. Parenteral fluid therapy is discussed at greater length in Chapter 10.

Ventilation and, hence, oxygenation are assisted by reducing intra-abdominal distention. The peritoneal empyema should be evacuated, gastric suction or siphonage started, and intestinal decompression (fluids and gas) effected if and when possible. Control of abdominal pain by administration of analgesics (e.g., phenylbutazone) will also improve respiration by encouraging greater excursion of diaphragm and rib cage. Tracheal intubation by endotracheal or tracheotomy routes provides an easy avenue for direct oxygen infusion as well as mechanically assisted ventilation. Small animals can be placed in an oxygen chamber.

The inotropic effects on the myocardium of mega doses of adrenocorticoids (e.g., prednisolone sodium succinate, 30 mg/kg by intravenous injection) in the early stages of septic shock are a worthwhile consideration, by the same line of reasoning as the choice of antibiotics based upon potential cardiodepressant effects.

Assurance of urine output may be determined by monitored volume, with catheterization in some cases, in addition to regular assessment of blood urea nitrogen, serum creatinine, and urinalysis. The need for this is increased if the peritonitis is of urogenital origin, if bladder atony is a complication, or if aminoglycosides are used in treatment. Use of diuretics such as furosemide may be indicated in some cases, but should be followed carefully by serum electrolyte and hematocrit determinations.

Liver function may be assessed by measurements of serum bilirubin as well as the several enzyme tests (lactodehydrogenase, sorbitol dehydrogenase, ornithine carbamyl transferase, arginase, and, depending on the species, either SGOT in large animals or SGPT in small animals—dog, cat, and primate). As discussed earlier, needle biopsy may be employed in the case of chronic peritonitis. In the protracted case, it may be of value to correlate serum albumin, prothrombin time, and dye uptake-excretion tests (rose bengal, Bromsulphalein). Inasmuch as the liver is a primary target for the noxious effects of gram-negative bacterial endotoxins so oftentimes involved in secondary bacterial peritonitis, it may be assumed that a degree of hepatosis exists in all cases of septic peritonitis.

Surgical Management of Peritonitis

In the surgical management of peritonitis the decision must be made whether to operate or not. In cases of primary peritonitis (e.g., the spontaneous bacterial peritonitis of ascites) or deep-seated intra-abdominal abscesses remote to sites of surgical access, the more prudent alternative may well be the nonoperative course. Rumbaugh et al. make a strong case for the nonoperative management of internal abdominal abscesses due to Streptococcus spp. and Corynebacterium spp. in the horse. Twenty-five cases were treated successfully with high doses of penicillin over a long period of time.[17] Another example of nonoperative treatment is in the positioning of the patient, In the human, the semi-Fowler position is a 30° elevation of the upper body to induce gravitation of peritoneal exudate to the pelvis. This relieves pressure on the diaphragm and fosters localization of abscesses in the pelvis rather than under the diaphragm.[14] A remarkably similar maneuver has been advocated for years in the nonoperative management of traumatic reticuloperitonitis-pericarditis syndrome in the dairy cow. The cow is confined in a stanchion stall with a false floor elevated in the front to raise the forequarters of the cow, displacing the abdominal viscera toward the rear to relieve pressure on the diaphragm and possibly facilitate migration or gravitation of the foreign body backward into the reticulum. At least it results in symptomatic relief in some cases, and may either obviate immediate surgery or gain time to suppress the septicemia in order that the salvage value of the animal is protected.

On the other hand, where there is spreading peritonitis from an uncontrolled source of contamination (e.g., a perforated bowel) and where there is a mechanical ileus (e.g., a strangulation obstruction of the bowel), then operative surgery is mandatory if any lifesaving measures are undertaken. Procrastination in the face of these findings is not conservatism; it is criminal neglect. Delays are conscionable only for necessary stabilization of the patient's general physiologic state, such as administration of parenteral fluids and correction of major electrolyte deficits to reduce the anesthetic risk. As soon as this can be done, the abdomen should be opened.[14,18,20]

Operative Surgery

The operative management of peritonitis includes control of the source of the contamination, decompression of the bowel and other involved hollow organs, drainage of all abscesses, debridement of all detritus, pus and pseudomembranes, straightening of plications, separation of nonvascular planes, and vigorous lavage of all surfaces until the irrigant (sterile P.S.S. or Ringer's) is clear. The temperature of the irrigating solution can be adjusted to regulate body temperature.[20] Some advocate the addition of antibiotics to the irrigant such as 1% ampicillin,[3,37] kanamycin, cephalothin,[81] chloramphenicol,[37] neomycin and penicillin, mindful of the possible disadvantages of the aminoglycosides. Amphotericin B has been added to the lavage solution in cases of Candida peritonitis.[55] In renal failure, a peritoneal dialysing solution can be substituted for the Ringer's or saline solution.[27] The value of peritoneal lavage is dependent upon the containment or elimination of the source of the contamination. The distinction is made that lavage is not debridement in the full sense of the word.[20] It is useful to dilute contamination and flush away accumulations of feces, blood, urine, bile, pancreatic juice and pus; but lavage will not remove necrotic tissue, fibrinous adhesions, or pyogenic membranes.

If the source of the contamination is a perforating ulcer, it is advisable to excise the ulcer for biopsy. If this is not elected, the optional procedure is simple plication of the healthy adjacent gut wall. It may be an additional consideration to tack a piece of omentum over the repair. When more extensive injury has occurred to the bowel with gross contamination of the abdomen, or when the gut wall has been rendered friable by edema, ischemia, or prolonged distention so as to endanger the safety of an attempted anastomosis, the wiser course may be to do a temporary colostomy. This diverts accumulated intestinal contents and achieves decompression of the intestine without subjecting the patient to the additional hazard of a leaking anastomosis and all the ensuing complications.[11,18] If the patient survives the peritonitis, the colostomy can be closed and a reunion anastomosis effected with a second operation done as an elective rather than as an emergency procedure.

Unfortunately, colostomy technique in the animal patient has lagged behind other recent advances in abdominal surgery; and its obvious advantages, so commonly practiced in humans, are yet to be realized in veterinary surgery as a routine procedure.

If the source of contamination is in, or is contiguous to, surgically accessible abdominal wall, or if the infection has localized in such a site (e.g., the pelvic abscess that has extended forward to the inguinal region), the operation may entail either simple incision and drainage or a radical dissection and extirpation of the entire process. Thus, an umbilical abscess or omphalophlebitis, which is the common cause of neonatal peritonitis or septicemia, may require handling in either of two ways. If the process is localized to the cutaneous navel, incision and drainage may be all that is necessary. If a pervious urachus is refractory to conservative treatment and resection is elected, it must be treated as a septic process and completely isolated from contact with the peritoneal cavity during dissection.

If the location of the abscess is undetermined, an exploratory laparotomy may be performed through one incision and the infection drained through a secondary or counterincision chosen as a result of the exploratory.

In a classic series of 92 cases of spreading peritonitis where the source of contamination could be eliminated by surgical intervention, Hudspeth demonstrated that peritonitis could be treated successfully without external drainage. Of these 92 patients, all were critically ill and 90% had mechanical intestinal obstructions. The rationale of treatment started with preoperative supportive therapy and antibiotics. Through a vertical midline incision from xiphoid to pubis, the abdomen was explored throughout. All abscess cavities were entered and drained. The bowel was decompressed through long tube drainage either by nasogastric or jejunostomy routes. The patency of bowel and integrity of blood supply were reestablished by meticulous surgery. All pyogenic membranes were debrided and all surfaces cleansed, by both sharp dissection and irrigation with copious amount of PSS without antibiotics. Delayed primary closure was effected in one layer with large figure-8 stainless steel wire sutures. Postoperative, intensive care included fluid therapy, whole blood, combination of broad-spectrum antibiotics administered parenterally, and ventilatory support. External drainage was not used except following hysterectomy and then this was done per vaginum. All 92 patients recovered. The pertinent contention was that the general peritoneal cavity cannot be drained.[20] Another responsible source has stated that "most surgeons believe that it is impossible to adequately drain a peritoneal space involved with diffuse peritonitis" based on the fact that "a plastic reaction occurs very quickly around a drain so that drainage is effective only along the course of the drain itself."[18] However, there remain adequate justifications for the use of drains, namely, (1) near the site of the perforated viscus or an anastomosis at risk, (2) near the site of remaining necrotic tissue or where tissue is of questionable viability, (3) when hemostasis is insecure, (4) when there has been gross soilage of the peritoneal cavity (particularly in the large animal where complete peritoneal lavage is rarely possible), (5) where there has been disrupting injury to liver, pancreas, or kidney with leakage of secretions being a postoperative risk, (6) in the presence of exposed (and contaminated) retroperitoneal tissue, and (7) where dead space exists.[1,14,18,27,83]

Common types of drains include the Penrose tube, the double-lumen sump drain tube, and the fenestrated Silastic tube.[27,37] They may be simple, one-way exit drains or, for postoperative, intermittent peritoneal lavage, two-way, double lumen tubes that permit retrograde irrigation. The purpose of this is to clear the holes in the drain of accumulations of fibrin and tissue debris, and presumably to instill an antibiotic solution directly at the site of infection. That the latter is accomplished to any great advantage is subject to debate. Nevertheless, the practice has found its advocates. All agree as to the disadvantages, chief of which is the introduction of outside contamination, either by a passive, ascending (drain) infection or by the active process of retrograde irrigation. To avert this complication, aseptic management of drains and drainage wounds in the abdominal wall should be a requirement. The use of sterile, absorbent pads held in place by corset bandages and changed at frequent intervals is practicable in animal patients. The further use of self-contained suction packs may be advantageous in some cases. In the event drain catheters are left open to the outside, their ends should be covered with one-way rubber valves, such as a collapsible latex tube (Penrose, surgical glove finger, condom) that closes on itself when the lumen is wetted. This is the principle of the Heimlich valve used on thoracic drain catheters. The valve is no obstacle to drainage but prevents aspiration which will certainly occur otherwise with the movements of the abdomen during respiration, straining, and the like. Drainage of pelvic abscesses through the vagina and through the inguinal region is one example of indications for the open (uncovered) drain catheter.

Decompression of the gastrointestinal tract by long tube in the acute patient is usually a matter of gastric siphonage via nasogastric tube. This may be an indwelling tube, maintained in place by fixation at the external nares. If this is not well tolerated, the tube can be removed and reintroduced at intervals as dictated by enterogastric reflux. The important thing is to keep the stomach, and thus the small intestine, at least partially decompressed to relieve intra-abdominal pressure. In the chronic case, a relatively recent innovation is the pharyngostomy to bypass the nose and mouth. A point of major concern is iatrogenic alkalosis. Continued gastric siphonage results in a significant loss of H^+ and Cl^-, which, if not replaced in like amounts by parenteral infusion, results in a severe metabolic alkalosis. This is only aggravated by an unthinking parenteral administration of lactated Ringer's solution, or worse, Ringer's spiked with $NaHCO_3$; hence, iatrogenic alkalosis. It may provide the last straw.

Decompression of the large intestine distended with gas as well as fluid and ingesta, is a problem particularly in the large animal patient. Tympany can be relieved temporarily in the horse by cecal trocharization percutaneously through the right paralumbar fossa. The fact remains that decompression to any effective degree is accomplished only by evacuation per colotomy. This is done for the patient in acute abdominal crisis with colonic obstruction, but is rarely a definitive procedure for decompression due to the adynamic ileus of peritonitis.

It goes without saying that oral intake of fluids or feed is prohibited. If this advice seems pointless, it should be recalled that animals may exhibit intense thirst and either a true or an hysterical appetite during abdominal crisis. This may occur at intervals of relief from pain, or continuously as a result of anhydremia. It may occur immediately upon arrousal from general anesthesia following major abdominal surgery. The animal should be recovered and confined in quarters free of water or feedstuffs (including even inedible bedding), or else should be muzzled to prevent accidental ingestion until such time as bowel function returns, signaled by passage of flatus and feces and resumption of audible peristalsis. Only small amounts of water or normal electrolytes should be allowed at first; then, a gradual increase in easily digested feedstuffs given in small portions at frequent intervals.

Decompression of the urinary tract is easily accomplished by repeated catheterizations or the use of an indwelling catheter (e.g., Foley catheter). The primary indications are following surgical procedures on the bladder or urethra, in which bladder atony, dehiscence of freshly closed suture lines or possible secondary urethral obstruction must be anticipated. The same precautions apply for ascending tract infections as discussed in the use of abdominal drains.

Complications

In summary, complications of peritonitis include: (1) intraperitoneal or wound abscesses, (2) paralytic or mechanical ileus (supervening intestinal obstruction), (3) hypoventilation, atelectasis, pneumonitis and aspiration pneumonia, (4) thromboembolism, and (5) wound healing complications such as infection and disruption resulting in either herniation or evisceration.

The circumstances that produce *peritoneal adhesions* bear further discussion. Under optimum conditions the peritoneum heals defects in its mesothelial surface within 3 to 5 days. This results from implantation of free, desquamated mesothelial cells on the surface of the defect as well as from centripetal movement of uninjured cells around the margins of the defect. A metaplasia of stem cells in the base of the wounded surface also contributes to the remesothelialization. Fibroblasts and macrophages are important to the healing process. Contraction of the wound margins is not regarded as an essential feature of peritoneal healing. To the contrary, attempts to reconstruct peritoneal defects by placement of foreign bodies such as sutures may actually produce undesirable adhesions. Other examples include cotton fibers from surgical sponges, glove powder, and drain tubes. Sutures may be the primary stimulus for development of a fibrous band, raising the question of the advisability of suturing the peritoneum in abdominal wall reconstruction. The alternative recommended by proponents of this concept is the placement of abdominal wall sutures so that the peritoneum is not pierced.[84]

Studies were conducted on intraperitoneal oxygen and carbon dioxide tensions in experimental adhesion disease and peritonitis induced in rats by silica and by sigmoid perforation. Based on the biologic premise that repair processes require increased oxygen and nutrients, it was postulated that tissue ischemia provokes adhesion formation and, further, that reperitonealization of defects (by suture) caused tissue tension and ischemia, leading to adhesions. Venous stasis was regarded as even more deleterious than arterial ischemia (recalling the generalized splanchnic congestion in the acute abdominal crisis). During adhesion formation, the microclimate in the abdomen was one of hypoxia and hypercarbia. This was also true in fecal peritonitis. Arteriovenous shunting in the systemic vascular bed and in the area of peritonitis decreased PO_2 and increased PCO_2. There were also decreased erythrocyte levels of 2,3 diphosphoglycerate and increased affinity of O_2 to hemoglobin. In these rats with bacterial peritonitis, intermittent peritoneal lavage prevented ischemia by removing toxins and oxygen-consuming exudate from the abdomen. The deduction was that avoidance of surgical trauma and tissue ischemia was of great importance in the maintenance of a good supply of oxygen and nutrients and, thus, the reduction of incidence of unnecessary adhesion formation. It was advised that, whenever possible, serosal defects should be left open rather than pulled together under tension. When inevitable, sutures should be placed so that adhesions form to nonvital structures or so as not to interfere with normal function[85] (e.g., the Noble plication procedure).[12,84] Oxygen pneumoperitoneum is thought to have some possible use in adhesion prevention.[72]

The combination of promethazine HCl (Phenergan, Wyeth), a potent antihistamine, and cortisone has been reported to reduce or prevent adhesion formation in rats and dogs, possibly owing to the lathyrogenic qualities of promethazine. This needs further study. Fibrinolysis to prevent the formation of fibrous adhesions around deposits of fibrin is also a possibility for the future.[84] Mechanical displacement or dislodgment by manual manipulation per rectum has long been advocated to prevent fibrous adhesions to the uterus following cesarean section in the mare and cow. The recommended time has been around the fifth postoperative day. Clarifying a common misconception, fibrinous adhesions do not become fibrous adhesions in the sense of undergoing a transformation of one protein into another protein. However, fibrinous adhesions may provide a scaffold for the secondary formation of fibrous adhesions.[84] Agents used unsuccessfully to prevent adhesions include certain anticoagulants, proteolytic enzymes, dextran, polyvinyl-pyrrolidone, dimethylsulfoxide, corticosteroids, and mineral oil. The last mentioned did produce an oleogranulomatous peritonitis as an abortive result.[14] It should be remembered that the problem is not the formation of adhesions, but the development of intestinal obstruction as a result of the adhesions.[84] Thus, we speak of "clinical adhesions" in distinction from those that exist unknown and unseen. There are even reports of the mysterious disappearance of mature, fibrous adhesions that were known to have existed at a prior time.[83]

Nursing Care

In conclusion, the considerable benefits of good nursing should be emphasized. Making the patient as comfortable as a bad situation permits involves the diminution of pain by the regular administration of analgesics, stimulation of peristalsis by application of warm moist packs to the abdomen, correction of strained positions, shifting static recumbencies, control of environment by regulating air temperature, control of flies and other pests, regular attention to wounds, infusion tubes, drains, decompression tubes and surgical dressings, grooming the haircoat and regular removal of manure and wet or soiled bedding. The patient that is so fortunate as to receive this type of care stands a better chance of recovery for a multiplicity of reasons. The factors that aggravate shock are minimized. The homeostatic functions are monitored with greater care, so that essential adjustments are made in fluid-electrolyte therapy and ventilation while there is yet time for reparative measures. Patient response is more closely observed for assessment of the efficacy of the antibiotic regimen as well as other medications. Secondary or supervening infections are less likely to occur at drain sites because bandages are changed more frequently and wound toilet is more conscientious. Contamination from filthy bedding or soiled hair and skin surfaces is prevented. Aspiration pneumonia is avoided because the stomach is siphoned with regularity and the patient is not left for overlong periods of time in positions of lateral recumbency. The ruminant patient does not die of bloat because it is not left in the position of left lateral recumbency. Legs do not become functionless appendages because the patient is turned frequently and helped to stand and massaged to stimulate circulation.

Good nursing and good medicine are inseparable. Unfortunately, the doctor cannot prescribe compassion and concern to be translated into patient care. It cannot be ordered by specified quantity but the benefits are immeasurable. Patients with peritonitis are in dire distress and in great need of the best that nursing can provide. It is the doctor's responsibility to see that they receive it.

REFERENCES

1. Macbeth, R.A., and MacKenzie, W.C.: Chapter 21, The abdominal wall and peritoneum. *In* Christopher's Textbook of Surgery. Edited by Loyal Davis. Philadelphia, W. B. Saunders Co., 1968, p. 528.
2. Musgrove, J.E.: Chapter 20, Diseases of the peritoneum, mesentery and omentum. *In* Gastroenterology. Edited by Abraham Bogoch. New York, McGraw-Hill Book Co., 1973.
3. Obins, G.R.: Bile Peritonitis and Pleuritis. Veterinary Reference Service, Pet Practice Edition, Update 1977.
4. Vaughan, J.T.: Surgical Management of Rectal Ruptures in Mares. Proc. A. A. E. P., 23rd Annu. Conv., Vancouver, B.C., 1977.
5. Horwitz, M.A., and Bennett, J.V.: Nursery outbreak of peritonitis with pneumoperitoneum probably caused by thermometer-induced rectal perforation. J. Epidemiol. *104*:632, 1976.
6. Hofmeyr, C.F.B.: Chapter 11, The digestive system. *In* Textbook of Large Animal Surgery. Edited by F.W. Oehme and J.E. Prier. Baltimore, The Williams & Wilkins Co., 1974, p.178.
7. Rudel, J.A.: Traumatic peritonitis of the bovine. Southwest. Vet. *28*:63, 1975.
8. Reddy, C.R.R.M., Venkateswar Rao, D., Sarma, E.N.B., and Swamy, G.M.N.: Granulomatous peritonitis due to ascaris lumbricoides and its ova. J. Trop. Med. Hyg. *78*:146, 1975.
9. Limtermans, J.P.: Fatal peritonitis, an unusual complication of strongyloides stercoralis infestation. Clin. Pediatr. *14*:974, 1975.
10. Becker, R.L., Giles, R.C., and Hildebrandt, P.K.: Coitally induced peritonitis in a dog. J. A. A. H. A. *10*:53, 1974.
11. Welch, C.S., and Powers, S.R.: The Essence of Surgery. Philadelphia, W. B. Saunders Co., 1958, pp. 57 and 132.
12. Palmer, E.D.: Clinical Gastroenterology, 2nd ed., New York, Harper & Row Publishers, 1963, p. 109.
13. Monif, G.R.G., Welkos, S.L., Baer, H., and Thompson, R.J.: Cul-de-sac isolates from patients with endometritis-salpingitis-peritonitis and gonococcal endocervicitis. J. Obstet. Gynecol. *126*:158, 1976.
14. Rhoads, J.E. and Rhoads, J.E., Jr.: Chapter 27, The peritoneum. *In* Gastroenterology, Vol. 4. 3rd ed. Edited by Henry L. Bockus. Philadelphia, W. B. Saunders Co., 1976.
15. Rubin, H.M., Blau, E.B., and Michaels, R.H.: Hemophilus and pneumococcal peritonitis in children with the nephrotic syndrome. Pediatrics 56:598, 1975.
16. Waxman, M., and Boyce, J.G.: Intraperitoneal rupture of benign cystic ovarian teratoma. Obst. Gynecol. *48*:9s, 1976.
17. Rumbaugh, G.E., Smith, B.P., and Carlson, G.P.: Internal abdominal abscesses in the horse: a study of 25 cases. J. A. V. M. A. *172*:304, 1978.
18. Ballinger, W.F., and Zuidema, G.D.: Complications of Gastrointestinal Disease. Gastroenterologic Medicine. Edited by Moses Paulson. Philadelphia, Lea & Febiger, 1969, p. 1220.
19. Gius, J.A.: Fundamentals of General Surgery. Chicago, Year Book Medical Publishers, 1972, pp. 78, 127, 278, 302, 305, 306, 484.
20. Hudspeth, A.S.: Radical surgical debridement in the treatment of advanced generalized bacterial peritonitis. Arch. Surg. *110*:1233, 1975.
21. Lorber, B., and Swenson, R.M.: The bacteriology of intra-abdominal infections. Surg. Clin. North Am. 55:1349, 1975.
22. Walker, R., Wilder, M., and Valeri, C.R.: The effects of Staphylococcus aureus and Klebsiella pneumonial peritonitis in mice exposed to normal and hypoxic conditions on red cell oxygen transport function. J. Med. *6*:113, 1975.
23. Targan, S.R., Chow, A.W., and Guze, L.B.: Role of anaerobic bacteria in spontaneous peritonitis of cirrhosis. J. Med. *62*:397, 1977.
24. Hau, T., and Simmons, R.L./Browne, M.K.: Surgical Pros and Cons. Surgery Gynecol. Obstet. *144*:755, 1977.
25. Hau, T., Nelson, R.D., Fiegel, V. D., Levenson, R., and Simmons, R.L.: Mechanisms of the adjuvant action of hemoglobin in experimental peritonitis. II. Influence of hemoglobin on human leukocyte chemotaxis in vitro. J. Surg. Res. *22*:174, 1977.
26. Browne, M.K., and Leslie, G.B.: Animal models of peritonitis. Surg. Gynecol. Obstet. *143*:738, 1976.
27. Hoffer, R.E.: Chapter 15, The peritoneum. Current Techniques in Small Animal Surgery. Edited by M.J. Bojrab. Philadelphia, Lea & Febiger, 1975.

28. Allan, D., and Cade, D.: (Correspondence) Delayed fibrinous peritonitis after practolol treatment. J. Br. Med. *4*:40, 1975.
29. Baddeley, H.: (Correspondence) Sclerosing peritonitis due to practolol. J. Br. Med. *2*:193, 1977.
30. Kennedy, S.C., and Ducrow, M.: Fibrinous peritonitis. J. Br., Med. *1*:1598, 1977.
31. Panting, A.L., and Denham, H.E.H.: Drug-induced sclerosing peritonitis. J. N. Z. Med. *85*:10, 1977.
32. Reske, M., and Namiki, H.: Sclerosing mesenteritis. J. Clin. Pathol. *64*:661, 1975.
33. Sternlieb, J.J., McIlrath, D.C., van Heerden, J.A., and Harrison, E.G., Jr.: Starch peritonitis and its prevention. Arch. Surg. *112*:458, 1977.
34. Goodacre, R.L., Clancy, R.L., Davidson, R.A., and Mullens, J.E.: Cell-mediated immunity to corn starch in starch-induced granulomatous peritonitis. Gut *17*:202, 1976.
35. MacGregor, R.R.: Comparative penetration of amikacin, gentamicin, and penicillin G into exudate fluid in experimental sterile peritonitis. Antimicrob. Agents Chemother. *11*:110, 1977.
36. Page, E.H. and Amstutz, H.E.: Gastrointestinal disorders and peritonitis. *In* Equine Medicine and Surgery, 2nd ed. Wheaton, Il, American Veterinary Publications, 1972, p. 271.
37. Parks, J., Gahring, D., and Greene, R.W.: Peritoneal lavage for peritonitis and pancreatitis in twenty-two dogs. J. A. A. H. A. *9*:442, 1973.
38. Weinstein, W.M., Onderdonk, A.B., Bartlett, J.G., Louie, T.J., and Gorbach, S.L.: Antimicrobial therapy of experimental intra-abdominal sepsis. J. Infect. Dis. *132*:282, 1975.
39. Bisgaard, M.: Characterization of atypical actinobacillus lignieresii isolated from ducks with salpingitis and peritonitis. Nord. Vet. Med. *27*:378, 1975.
40. Chastain, D.B., Grier, R.L., Hogle, R.M., Glock, R.D., and Mitten, R.W.: Actinomycotic peritonitis in a dog. J. A. V. M. A. *168*:499, 1976.
41. Cohn, I., Jr.: Chapter 131, Bile peritonitis. *In* Gastroenterology, 3rd ed. Edited by Henry L. Bockus, Philadelphia, W. B. Saunders Co., 1976.
42. Dale, G., and Solheim, K.: Bile peritonitis in acute cholecystitis. Acta Chir. *141*:746, 1975.
43. Ramachandran, S., Induruwa, P.A.C., and Perera, M.V.F.: Bile peritonitis due to ruptured amoebic liver abscess. J. Trop. Med. Hyg. *78*:236, 1975.
44. Bakaleinik, M.: Biliary peritonitis due to double perforation of carcinoma of the gall bladder: case report. Milit. Med. *141*:551, 1976.
45. Adams, E.B., and MacLeod, I.N.: Invasive amebiasis. I. Amebic dysentery and its complications. II. Amebic liver abscess and its complications. Medicine *56*:315, 1977.
46. Utili, R. Abernathy, C.O., and Zimmerman, H.J.: Cholestatic effects of Escherichia coli endotoxin on the isolated perfused rat liver. Gastroenterology *70*:248, 1976.
47. Charuzi, I., and Freund, H.: Gangrene of the hepatic round ligament causing diffuse peritonitis. Am. Surg. *42*:926, 1976.
48. Conn, H.O.: Spontaneous bacterial peritonitis. Gastroenterology *70*:455, 1976.
49. Flaum, M.A.: Spontaneous bacterial empyema in cirrhosis. Gastroenterology *70*:416, 1976.
50. Murray, H.W., and Marks, S.J.: Spontaneous bacterial empyema, pericarditis, and peritonitis in cirrhosis. Gastroenterology *72*:772, 1977.
51. Brown, R.L., and Peter, G.: Clostridial spontaneous peritonitis. J. A. M. A. *236*:2095, 1976.
52. Gerding, D.N., Kahn, M.Y., Ewing, J.W., and Hall, W.H.: Pasteurella multocida peritonitis in hepatic cirrhosis with ascites. Gastroenterology *70*:413, 1976.
53. Targan, S.R., Chow, A.W., and Guze, L.B.: Spontaneous peritonitis of cirrhosis due to campylobacter fetus. Gastroenterology *71*:311, 1976.
54. Potter, M., and Blake, P.: Human campylobacteriosis, Bacterial Diseases Division, Bureau of Epidemiology, Center for Disease Control, Atlanta, GA, 1978.
55. Bayer, A.S., Blumenkrantz, M.J., Montgomerie, J.Z., Galpin, J.E., Coburn, J.W., and Guze, L.B.: Candida peritonitis—report of 22 cases and review of the English literature. J. Med. *61*:832, 1976.
56. Olivero, J.J., Lozano, J., and Suki, W.N.: Acute pancreatitis, pancreatic pseudocyst, and Candida peritonitis in recipient of a kidney transplant. South. Med. J. *69*:1619, 1976.
57. Krum, S., Johnson, K., and Wilson J.: Hydrocephalus associated with the noneffusive form of feline infectious peritonitis. J. A. V. M. A. *167*:746, 1975.
58. Jones, B.R.: Feline infectious peritonitis: a review. J. N. Z. Vet. Assoc. *23*:221, 1975.
59. August, J.R.: Feline infectious peritonitis—a case report. Auburn Vet. *33*:53, 1977.
60. Motensen, V.A., and Steensborg, K.: Infektis peritonitis hos katte (F.I.P.—Feline Infectious Peritonitis). Dansk Veterinaertidsskrift *18*:761, 1976.
61. Bullmore, C.C., and Twitchell, M.J.: A case of parenchymatous feline infectious peritonitis. Feline Practice *7*:46, 1977.
62. Fankhauser, R., Fatzer, R.: Meningitis und Chorioependymitis granulomatosa der Katze; mogliche Bezienhungen zur felinen infektiosen peritonitis (FIP). (Granulomatous meningitis and chorioependymitis in the cat: the possible relationship to feline infectious peritonitis (FIP)). Kleintierpraxis *22*:19, 1977.
63. Legendre, A.M., and Whitenack, D.L.: Feline infectious peritonitis with spinal cord involvement in two cats. J. A. V. M. A. *167*:931, 1975.
64. Horzinek, M.C., Osterhaus, A.D.M.E., and Ellens, D.J.: Feline infectious peritonitis virus. (I. Purification and electron microscopy.) Zentralbl. Veterinarmed. *5*:398, 1977.
65. Osterhaus, Von A.D.M.E., Horzinek, M.C., and Ellens, D.J.: Untersuchungenzur Ätiologie der Felinen Infektiosen Peritonitis. Berl. Munch. Tieraerztl. Wochenschr. *89*:135, 1976.
66. Dimond, M., and Proctor, H.J.: Concomitant pneumococcal appendicitis, peritonitis and meningitis. Arch. Surg. *111*:888, 1976.
67. Bar-Meir, S., and Conn, H.O.: Spontaneous bacterial peritonitis (SBP) induced by intraarterial vasopressin therapy. Gastroenterology *70*:418, 1976.
68. Fee, H.J., Fonkalsrud, E.W., Amment, M.E., and Bergstein, J.: Enterocolitis with peritonitis in a child with pheochromocytoma. Ann. Surg. *185*:448, 1977.
69. Nahrwold, D.L., and Demuth, W.E.: Diverticulitis with perforation into the peritoneal cavity. Ann. Surg. *185*:80, 1977.
70. Weijer, K.: The incidence of lymphosarcoma (leukemia) and feline leukemia virus (FeLV) in cats in the Netherlands. Tijdschr. Diergeneeskd. *100*:976, 1975.
71. MacDonald, W.C., and Fratkin, L.B.: Chapter 12, The small intestine. *In* Gastroenterology. Edited by Abraham Bogoch. New York, McGraw-Hill Book Co. 1973, p. 538.
72. Rakower, S.R., and Fazzini, E.: Acute phlegmonous gastritis: differentiation from primary peritonitis and the peritonitis of collagen vascular disease. Am. Surg. *41*:571, 1975.
73. Szazados, I., and Kadas, I.: Das Vorkommen und die Ursache des im Bereich der Vormagen lokalisierten Bauchschmerzes bei wegen Euterentzundung notgeschlachteten Kuhen. (Occurrence and Origin of Abdominal Pain in the Area of the Forestomachs in Cows Slaughtered Following Mastitis). D.T.W. *11*:471, 1976.
74. Coffman, J.R., and Tritschler, L.G.: Exudative peritonitis in two horses. J. A. V. M. A. *160*:871, 1972.
75. Boyce, H.W., and Palmer, E.D.: Techniques of Clinical Gastroenterology. Springfield, IL., Charles C Thomas Publisher, 1975, pp. 147, 463, 466.
76. Kline, M.M., McCallum, R.W., and Guth, P.H.: The clinical value of ascitic fluid culture and leukocyte count studies in alcoholic cirrhosis. Gastroenterology *70*:408, 1976.
77. Miclaus, I., and Brummerstedt, E.: Plasma protein alterations in cattle suffering from acute peritonitis. Nord. Vet. Med. *27*:203, 1975.
78. Swanwick, R.A., and Wilkinson, J.S.: A clinical evaluation of abdominal paracentesis in the horse. Aust. Vet. J. *3*:109, 1976.
79. Traver, D.S., Moore, J.N., Coffman, J.R., and Amend, J.F.: Peritonitis in a horse: a cause of acute abdominal distress and polyuria. J. Equine Med. Surg. *1*:36, 1977.
79a.Tedesco, F.J., Stanley, R.J. and Alpers, D.H.: Diagnostic features of clindamycin-associated pseudomembranous colitis. N. Engl. J. Med., *290*:841, 1974.
80. Gerding, D.N., Hall, W.H., and Schierl, E.A.: Antibiotic concentration in ascitic fluid of patients with ascites and bacterial peritonitis. Ann. Intern. Med. *86*:708, 1977.
81. Smith, E.B.: A rationale for intraperitoneally administered antibiotic. Surg. Gynecol. Obstet. *143*:561, 1976.
82. Steffy, E.P.: Effects of antibiotics on anesthesia. Vet. Anesth. *4*:49, 1977.
83. Frantz, V.K., and Harvey, H.D.: Introduction to Surgery, 4th ed. New York, Oxford University Press, 1959.
84. Peacock, E.E., and Van Winkle, W.: Surgery and Biology of Wound Repair, 2nd ed. Philadelphia, W.B. Saunders Co., 1976, p. 613.
85. Seppo, R., and Niinikoski, J.: Intraperitoneal oxygen and carbon dioxide tensions in experimental adhesion disease and peritonitis. J. Surg. *130*:286, 1975.

Chapter 28

METABOLIC AND ENDOCRINE DISEASE AND THE GASTROINTESTINAL SYSTEM

ROBERT H. WHITLOCK AND JOHN A. MULNIX

Many metabolic and endocrinologic diseases affect the gastrointestinal system and indirectly or directly produce clinical signs to suggest a primary gastrointestinal problem. The signs of gastrointestinal disease (anorexia, dysphagia, vomiting, diarrhea, and abdominal distention) discussed in Chapter 2 are outlined as they relate to endocrine and metabolic diseases. As most sick animals are anorectic, the diseases that are presented are only those in which anorexia or one of the other signs of digestive disease is a major or dominant sign.

ANOREXIA: EQUINE

Hypothyroidism

Anorexia is a nonspecific sign of many diseases and does occur with several endocrine and metabolic diseases. Partial anorexia or decreased feed intake, exercise intolerance, obesity, and laminitis have been suggested to be the major signs of equine hypothyroidism. However, in equine thyroid ablation experiments, obesity and laminitis were not observed. Thyroidectomized foals appeared dull and lethargic compared to controls. Thyroidectomized females consumed 46% less feed and gained 47% less weight than the controls. The decreased appetite in equine hypothyroidism is documented and seems to be a major sign of the disease. Mild anemia (PCV 24 to 30%), decreased bone growth, sensitivity to cold, failure to shed haircoats in the spring of the year, and dullness were additional clinical signs in athyroid horses.[1]

Documented cases of equine hypothyroidism where thyroid function was measured with the T4 test are few in number. Those reports suggesting obesity and chronic laminitis as the major signs have implicated hypothyroidism on the basis of response to thyroid hormone replacement. T4 values for horses decline with age, necessitating a critical evaluation of thyroid function with the thyroid stimulating hormone (TSH) response test. A fourfold increment is expected 24 hours after injection of 15 to 30 IU of thyrotropin.[2]

Diabetes Insipidus

Diabetes insipidus in horses is usually associated with adenomas of the pars intermedia of the pituitary and may result in decreased appetite or a ravenous appetite.[3] The appetite response depends on the extent of pathologic changes in the hypothalamus. Pituitary tumors are commonly encountered in aged horses and may present with a potpourri of clinical signs including anorexia, hirsutism, blindness, pendulous abdomen, polyuria, docility, and hyperhidrosis. An adenoma should be suspected[4] in any aged horse with one or more of these signs. Confirmation of the diagnosis may be obtained by hormone measurement and/or the dexamethasone suppression test. No effective treatment is available.

Hyperlipidemia

Hyperlipidemia occurs occasionally in ponies and less commonly in adult horses.[5] Partial to complete feed refusal may be the chief complaint in normal or obese pregnant ponies with hyperlipidemia. More than 90% of affected animals were in foal, had foaled, or had aborted. The hyperlipidemia is regarded as secondary to some other primary disease, such as a digestive disturbance or respiratory disease.

Hyperlipidemia is relatively easy to determine by noting visible milky turbidity (lactescence) in a blood sample. The plasma lipids can be quantitated and normally are less than 500 mg/dl,[6] but in hyperlipidemia they can increase to 7000 mg/dl.[7] During the period of negative energy balance, the lipid is mobilized from body fat depots and hyperlipidemia results. If left untreated and if the animal is not force-fed, the anorexia and hyperlipidemia become a self-perpetuating process. Death may result from the fatty liver, hypocalcemia, a ruptured liver, or the metabolic complications of a prolonged negative energy balance.

ANOREXIA: BOVINE

Parturient Paresis

Anorexia may be one of the early signs of parturient paresis, along with the signs of mild excitement and hypersensitivity. The cow often may shake her head, protrude the tongue, and grind her teeth (odontoprisis) in the initial stages of hypocalcemia. This stage is followed by dullness, recumbency, and death if not treated. The loss of appetite is often an important clinical sign to the owner, as this sign is associated with a decreased feed intake and subsequently rumino-intestinal stasis.[8] The alimentary tract stasis can occur either as a result of parturition or as a result of hypocalcemia; but, in any event, is an important contribution to the development of a more severe hypocalcemia.

The reduction in feed intake is greater in older cows approaching parturition than it is in younger cows.[9] If cows are on a high calcium diet, i.e., greater than 100 g calcium per day, anorexia may play an even more important role in the pathogenesis of milk fever. These cows are more dependent on continued intestinal calcium absorption to maintain normocalcemia than are cows on a lower calcium diet. Such cows will have a greater bone calcium turnover and are, therefore, better able to mobilize calcium from bone in order to correct the hypocalcemia caused by the temporary inappetence. Thus, anorexia can be both a prodromal sign and a factor responsible for the development of bovine parturient paresis.

Hypokalemia

Both naturally occurring and experimentally induced hypokalemia in cattle is associated with partial to complete inappetence, depending on the severity of the deficiency.[10] Since traditional ruminant diets are relatively rich in potassium, the continued anorexia further exacerbates the hypokalemia. Since hypokalemia commonly occurs with many bovine gastrointestinal obstructive diseases, the plasma or serum potassium concentration should be monitored.[11] If the concentration is below 2.5 mEq/L, supplementation with 30 to 60 g of potassium chloride should be given orally three to five times per day. Intravenous replacement is more time consuming, dangerous, and less effective than oral potassium.

Ketosis

In both ketosis and the fat-cow syndrome, anorexia is a predominate clinical feature of the disease. The owner first notes that the cow has failed to consume all her feed, and a reduction in milk production occurs promptly. In the absence of concurrent disease, the vital signs are normal. But often cows in this early postpartum period (10 to 60 days) will have concurrent diseases such as metritis, mastitis, and/or abomasal displacement.[12]

Dairy cows with primary ketosis usually have a strongly positive ketonuria and ketolactia, whereas cattle with the fatty liver syndrome have a moderate concentration of urinary or milk ketones. The diagnosis of the fat-cow syndrome is based on the history of excessive energy intake. Obesity and the presence of one or more periparturient diseases such as milk fever, ketosis, displaced abomasum, retained fetal membranes, and/or mastitis is diagnostic. Since a number of diseases may be present in this syndrome, it is very important to conduct a careful and complete physical examination to establish the diagnosis. The diagnosis is suggested by an unfavorable response to conventional effective therapy. A bromsulphalein (BSP) test is the best method to differentiate primary ketosis from the fat-cow syndrome. A BSP $T_{\frac{1}{2}}$ of greater than 10 minutes, in the absence of other disorders, is suggestive of a fatty liver—which can only be confirmed by a liver biopsy.[13]

Phosphorus Deficiency

Hypophosphatemia has been associated with infertility, pica, anemia, and anorexia.[14] Occasionally the hypophosphatemia may be so severe as to cause postparturient hemoglobinuria.[15] However, in these extreme life-threatening depletion syndromes, anemia and hemoglobinuria are the most obvious clinical signs and anorexia seems less important.

The diagnosis is based on a history of a phosphorus-deficient diet and a hypophosphatemia. The response to phosphorus supplementation is prompt.

Abdominal Fat Necrosis

Abdominal fat necrosis is a metabolic disease that may present with a chief complaint of anorexia or abdominal distention. The necrosis of abdominal fat usually causes few clinical signs, until it mechanically interferes with the passage of digesta. At that time cattle become anorectic, with concurrent signs of abdominal disease (diarrhea, constipation, or abdominal distention). With few exceptions, the disease occurs sporadically within a herd.[16]

A unique syndrome of fat necrosis occurs in the southeastern part of the United States where cattle grazing on highly fertilized (usually with poultry manure) fescue pastures may have a high incidence (up to 67%) of the disease.[16] When animals are removed from these pastures and fed a grass hay diet without concentrates, the lesions seem to regress slowly over a period of months. The association of herd problems with fat necrosis and ingestion of fescue grass is clear. The pathogenic factors of the grass are less obvious.

Hypervitaminosis D

Anorexia may be an important sign of diseases associated with hypercalcemia, i.e., hypervitaminosis D[17] and Manchester wasting disease.[18] Hypervitaminosis D usually occurs as an iatrogenic problem induced by overzealous therapy, especially in the prevention of postparturient paresis. Three plants, *Solanum malacoxylon*, *Cestrum diurnum*, and *Trisetum flavescens*, contain a vitamin D-like factor and give rise to a wasting disease characterized by stiffness and chronic anorexia.[19,20] These plants grow in several regions of the world and affect those animals that graze on the plants. Hypercalcemia (> 12 mg/dl) and hyperphosphatemia (> 6 mg/dl) are typical laboratory findings. The lesions at necropsy are essentially like those of hypervitaminosis D: widespread mineralization of soft tissue.

Cobalt Deficiency

One of the early clinical manifestations of cobalt deficiency in ruminants is decreased food intake.[21,22] Prolonged cobalt deficiency results in a wasting disease closely resembling and often confused with malnutrition or starvation. Anemia, characterized by pale mucous membranes and a lowered hematocrit, occurs late in the disease.[22] The cobalt deficiency syndrome in ruminants varies from an acute, often fatal disorder (rarely), to a mild, ill-defined, and often transient state of unthriftiness. As the disease is related to a deficiency, it occurs on a regional basis, especially in areas with sandy soils.

The documented response to cobalt supplementation or to vitamin B$_{12}$ is presumptive evidence of cobalt deficiency. Rumen cobalt values of < 0.5 ng/ml impede the synthesis of vitamin B$_{12}$ and blood values of B$_{12}$ fall, as they do in liver and other tissues. Liver cobalt concentration varies with dietary content, and a value less than 0.02 ppm dry matter is clearly deficient.[23] Liver vitamin B$_{12}$ values may be more sensitive than liver cobalt values in detecting a deficiency state, with less than 0.2 μg B$_{12}$ per gram wet weight being deficient. Ration concentrations of less than 0.08 ppm cobalt will result in B$_{12}$ deficiency.[22] Serum B$_{12}$ concentrations are of some value in the diagnosis of cobalt deficiency but are variable between animals on similar diets and often fluctuate from day to day.[24]

The clinical signs of wasting and cachexia are due to both the decreased appetite and the inefficient energy production. The weight loss can occur 30% faster in deficient animals compared to pair-fed controls.[21] Part of the biochemical defect is a failure of the transfer reactions responsible for the intermediate isomeric conversion of methyl malonyl coenzyme A to succinate with resultant increased concentration of methyl malonate.[23]

Diabetes Mellitus

Although diabetes mellitus is infrequently reported in cattle, anorexia is an important clinical sign.[25,26] Additional signs of polyuria, polydipsia, weight loss, and emaciation are present in most animals with diabetes mellitus, including cattle. Hyperglycemia with a diabetic-type glucose tolerance curve will help confirm the diagnosis. Ketonuria and ketolactia (if lactating) should be present in high concentrations in untreated cases. Insulin therapy is possible but not economically feasible in the ruminant.

ANOREXIA: CANINE

Anorexia can occur with several endocrine diseases in the dog. In a few diseases (i.e., hypoadrenocorticism, hyperparathyroidism), anorexia may be considered as a primary clinical sign. In other endocrine disorders of dogs (hypothyroidism, hyperthyroidism, diabetes mellitus, or diabetes insipidus) the sign of anorexia may be of only secondary or of minor significance.

Hypothyroidism

Hypothyroidism, either primary or secondary to TSH deficiency, may, on rare occasion, be present with a history of anorexia.[27] The history will more commonly indicate that the appetite is unaffected or there may be a poor appetite. The historic findings most frequently related by owners of hypothyroid dogs are an insidious development of slowing of physical and mental activities.[27] Other complaints may reflect the reduced metabolism such as intolerance to cold, reduced exercise tolerance, or, occasionally, skin and haircoat changes.

Signs of hypothyroidism also relate to the reduced metabolic activity.[27] Mental depression, lethargy, inactivity, a poor haircoat or alopecia, thickening of the skin, a "tragic expression" to the facial features,[27] and anestrus in intact bitches are frequently observed. In dogs, there is no particular combination of signs that constitutes the typical form of hypothyroidism.[28]

Laboratory findings that assist in the diagnosis of hypothyroidism are a mild or subclinical anemia and hypercholesterolemia. To prove the diagnosis it is necessary to measure circulating thyroxin (T4) levels by a method that is proven to be accurate in the dog. Radioimmunoassay (RIA) procedures for T4, before and after TSH stimulation, will provide an accurate diagnosis. If RIA procedures are not available, a thyroid biopsy can be utilized.

Hyperthyroidism

Anorexia may also be observed in dogs with hyperthyroidism.[27] However, this should be considered as an uncommon clinical sign. Dogs with hyperthyroidism may have a tremendous polydipsia and weight loss which could lead to an erroneous interpretation of anorexia. Cases have been reported in which anorexia alternated with polyphagia.[27] Hyperthyroidism in the dog is almost always secondary to a functional thyroid tumor; thus, an important clinical feature of this disease is a mass of variable size in the cervical region.[27,28] Other important clinical findings in decreasing order of significance are polyuria and polydipsia, weight loss, polyphagia, weakness and fatigue, heat intolerance and nervousness.[27] Other signs are occasionally observed.

Laboratory changes contribute little to confirmation of a diagnosis. The hemogram can be normal. The urine may be dilute (low specific gravity or low osmolality) secondary to the polyuria. Insufficient data is available on RIA studies for T4 hyperthyroid dogs to know whether abnormalities exist. Early surgical excision of the tumor with cessation of clinical signs would be very suggestive of the hyperthyroid state.

Adrenocortical Insufficiency

In primary adrenocortical insufficiency, the gastrointestinal sign of anorexia is common.[29,30,31] A history of recurrent, vague gastrointestinal signs (anorexia, vomiting, and diarrhea) in a young adult dog is very suggestive of hypoadrenocorticism, especially when parasitism and dietary factors have been eliminated.[28,31,32] Other significant clinical signs may include muscular weakness, depression, weak femoral pulse, occasionally bradycardia and complete collapse.[31] In the mild or chronic stages, gastrointestinal signs may predominate; however, complete collapse and a shock-like coma can occur.

The results of laboratory tests are usually necessary to confirm a diagnosis of adrenocortical insufficiency. A slight to moderate elevation of blood urea nitrogen concentration is a consistent finding.[31] Hyperkalemia and hyponatremia will also be observed.[30] Confirmation of the diagnosis can be made by measuring plasma cortisol values and thereby demonstrating that the adrenal glands are nonresponsive to an intravenous or intramuscular dose of corticotrophin (ACTH).[28,31]

Hyperparathyroidism

Anorexia in primary hyperparathyroidism is caused by the hypercalcemia that occurs in this disease.[28] Primary hyperparathyroidism is rare in the dog and is due to excessive secretion of parathormone by an adenoma of the parathyroid. Vomiting, constipation, generalized muscular weakness, and, occasionally, spontaneous fractures of long bones may be seen.[28]

Hypercalcemia is a consistent laboratory finding.[28] Elevation of serum alkaline phosphatase values may also be seen. Before a diagnosis of primary hyperparathyroidism can be made, other causes of hypercalcemia must be excluded. In the dog, pseudohyperparathyroidism can be caused by malignant neoplasms of non-endocrine origin,[28,33,34] vitamin D intoxication,[28] and malignant neoplasms with bone metastases.[28]

Diabetes Mellitus

Anorexia is not a common clinical sign in diabetes mellitus. The affected dog more commonly has an increased appetite, polyuria, polydipsia, and gradual weight loss.[28,32] As the diabetic state progresses, ketoacidosis and dehydration can develop. The animal will then become anorectic rather than polyphagic. Other complications such as vomiting and diarrhea may develop.[32]

Laboratory diagnosis of diabetes mellitus with ketoacidosis depends upon demonstrating glycosuria and acetonuria, and an absolute elevation of blood sugar concentration (generally above 200 mg/dl). Ketones can be detected in the plasma by using nitroprusside tablets (Acetest tablets, Ames Co.).[32]

DYSPHAGIA: EQUINE

Dysphagia is an uncommon clinical sign and when present usually engenders consideration of a neurologic deficit such as rabies, botulism, or cranial nerve injury, secondary to guttural pouch disease. However, dysphagia may be a prominent feature of equine eclampsia. Eclampsia or lactation tetany is an uncommon disease, but draft horses with a heavy milk flow are predisposed.[18] During these periods of hypocalcemia (4 to 6 mg/dl) the mare may make repeated attempts to eat and drink but appears unable to swallow, and passage of a stomach tube is difficult if not impossible. Profuse sweating, difficult moving due to muscular tetany, and rapid violent respirations with synchronous diaphragmatic flutter are commonly present. Affected animals respond rapidly and completely to intravenous calcium injections.

EMESIS: CANINE

The endocrine diseases that may cause vomiting are diabetes insipidus, hyperthyroidism, primary hyperparathyroidism, diabetes mellitus, and primary adrenocortical insufficiency.

Diabetes Insipidus

Diabetes insipidus is a disease state in which an inability to excrete a concentrated urine is usually associated with a deficiency of the antidiuretic hormone (ADH).[35,36,37,38] Varying degrees of polydipsia and polyuria are the chief clinical signs. Urine volume may approach 5 to 7 liters per day in some dogs. The only significant historic finding may be a sudden onset of polyuria and polydipsia.[36] In dogs that have severe polydipsia, vomiting may be seen secondary to severe gastric overload with water.

Routine laboratory findings, e.g., CBC, BUN, and other biochemical parameters, are usually within normal limits. Because of the constant state of dehydration in affected dogs, the plasma osmolality tends to be elevated. Urine analysis will usually reveal a very dilute urine (osmolality below 300 mOsm/l, or specific gravity below 1.005). Confirmation of a diagnosis of diabetes insipidus is based on demonstration of a lack of urine concentration with water deprivation, and increasing concentration following administration of exogenous ADH. These two procedures can be combined into one test procedure for convenience.[35,36] In dogs with severe diabetes insipidus, the deprivation procedure will seldom go beyond 4 hours, as most patients will lose 1 to 2% of their body weight per hour. An arbitrary 12-hour water deprivation test is contraindicated in a severely polyuric dog.

Hyperthyroidism and Hyperparathyroidism

Dogs with hyperthyroidism may also have severe polyuria and polydipsia and, like dogs with diabetes insipidus, will vomit secondary to gastric overloading with water. Vomiting in dogs with primary hyperparathyroidism occurs because of hypercalcemia.[28] Hypercalcemia may cause vomiting by at least two different mechanisms. The first is that the hypercalcemia may cause damage to the renal tubules,[39] which may in turn induce renal failure and signs of uremia, such as vomiting. In human beings, hypercalcemia may be a direct stimulus to increased gastric secretion,[40] causing ulceration and vomiting.

Diabetes Mellitus

Vomiting associated with diabetes mellitus may be caused by the pancreatitis that initially caused the diabetic state. Ketoacidosis may also cause vomiting in a diabetic dog. Ketoacidosis can be confirmed by demonstrating the presence of hyperglycemia and ketonemia.[32]

Adrenocortical Insufficiency

In chronic primary adrenocortical insufficiency vomiting may be only an occasional sign. However, it can occur as a severe clinical sign with complete collapse.[29,30,31] The exact mechanism of emesis is not known, but may relate to glucocorticoid deficiency and to metabolic changes of reduced renal perfusion.

DIARRHEA: BOVINE

Copper Deficiency

Intermittent chronic diarrhea is a major feature of severe chronic copper deficiency in cattle. In some parts of the world, this form of chronic copper deficiency is so prominent that it is called "scouring disease" or "peat scours."[22] Thus, from an epidemiologic viewpoint, this form of chronic diarrhea should affect several or many animals in a herd and distinct geographic regions should be predisposed. The diagnosis is easily confirmed by finding low concentrations of copper in the blood (< 0.6 μg/ml) and liver (< 30 ppm on a dry matter basis).[22]

Young steers with chronic diarrhea and confirmed copper deficiency have a marked depletion of cytochrome oxidase in the epithelium of the duodenum, jejunum, and ileum, with partial villous atrophy in the duodenum and jejunum. Enterocytes from these areas have mitochondrial abnormalities ranging from slight swelling to marked localized dilation. This type of lesion may be part of the explanation for the chronic diarrhea.

Magnesium Ingestion

Mild to moderate chronic diarrhea may result from excessive ingestion of magnesium ($> 1\%$ magnesium in the diet). The feces are usually soft to watery and contain excessive mucus. Tenesmus is not a feature. The high magnesium also depresses appetite and the animals show evidence of weight loss or may be stunted. High dietary magnesium levels are rarely the cause of mild chronic diarrhea. When it occurs, it is likely to result from feed mixing at the feed mill, rather then the ingestion of diets that are natually high in magnesium.

Salt Poisoning

Both diarrhea and vomiting may be associated with salt toxicosis in cattle. Additional signs of bovine salt poisoning include anorexia, polyuria, and mild abdominal pain. Subsequent nervous signs include blindness, paresis, and knuckling of the fetlock. Cattle with acute salt poisoning often die within 24 to 48 hours of the onset of signs; while in so-called chronic salt poisoning, the clinical signs are more gradual in onset, with mild anorexia, loss of body weight, dehydration, weakness, and intermittent diarrhea.[18]

The pathogenesis of the diarrhea in acute salt toxicosis is unclear, but may be related to the osmotic action of the salt in the intestinal lumen. High-producing milk cows in early lactation are more prone to salt toxicosis than are other cattle, because of their massive fluid and electrolyte fluxes. Salt toxicosis is best documented by measurement of serum sodium concentration, which should be more than 175 mEq/L. Although cattle may be on high salt diets (2 to 3% salt in the concentrate), they usually do not develop signs of salt toxicosis unless the salt-free water intake is restricted.

Amyloidosis

Mild chronic diarrhea resembling Johne's disease is often one of the early and most obvious clinical manifestations of amyloidosis in adult dairy cattle.[41,42] Other clinical signs consist of subcutaneous edema (bottle jaw) and renal enlargement as determined during rectal examination. Clinicopathologically, a heavy proteinuria (4+) and hypoproteinemia (< 4.0 g/dl) occur early in the disease, with azotemia occurring later. Histologically, amyloidosis is a multisystem disease with deposits in many organs including the liver, small intestine, colon, and especially the kidneys.[41] The pathogenesis of the chronic diarrhea has been attributed to the deposition of amyloid in the colon.[41] However, the lowered plasma oncotic pressure, due to the prominent hypoalbuminemia, may also be a major factor. In one cow with amyloidosis, the diarrhea diminished following plasma transfusion, relapsed as the plasma protein value decreased, responded to a second plasma transfusion, relapsed again, and at that time was debilitated. The cow was euthanatized for humane reasons.*

A tentative diagnosis of renal amyloidosis is justified by the determination of a persistent heavy proteinuria and a prominent hypoproteinemia. Confirmation is possible by histochemical staining of the kidney following renal biopsy. No effective treatment has been found.

DIARRHEA: CANINE

Adrenocortical Insufficiency

Diarrhea is an uncommon clinical sign with endocrine diseases in small animals except in the case of primary adrenocortical insufficiency. In this disease, diarrhea may be the chief complaint of the owner and, in more severe cases, it may even be bloody.[29,30,31]

ABDOMINAL DISTENTION: CANINE

Abdominal distention is an important clinical sign in dogs with hyperadrenocorticism.[28,43-47] It is related in part to loss of muscle tone as a result of excessive protein catabolism caused by the excessive production of glucocorticoids. Hepatomegaly may also contribute to the abdominal distention.

REFERENCES

1. Lowe, J.E., Baldwin, B.H., Foote, R.H., Hillman, R.B., and Kallfelz, F.A.: Equine hypothyroidism: the long term effects on metabolism and growth in mares and stallions. Cornell Vet. *64*:276, 1974.
2. Lowe, J.E., and Kallfelz, F.A.: Thyroidectomy and the T-4 test in the horse. Proc. Am. Assoc. Equine Pract. *16*:135, 1971.
3. Loeb, W.F., Capen, C.C., and Johnson, L.E.: Adenomas of the pars intermedia associated with hyperglycemia and glycosuria in two horses. Cornell Vet. *56*:623, 1966.
4. Gribble, D.H.: The endocrine system. *In* Equine Medicine and Surgery. Edited by E. J. Catcott and J. F. Smithcors. Wheaton, IL, American Veterinary Publications, 1972.
5. Schotman, A.J.H., and Wagenaar, G.: Hyperlipemia in ponies. Zentralbl. Veterinaermed. *16*:1, 1969.
6. Robie, S.M., Janson, G.G., Smith, S.C., and O'Connor, J.T., Jr.: Equine serum lipids: serum lipids and glucose in Morgan and Thoroughbred horses and Shetland ponies. Am. J. Vet. Res. *36*:1705, 1975.
7. Schotman, A.J.H., and Kroneman, J.: Hyperlipemia in ponies. Neth. J. Vet. Sci. *2*:60, 1969.

---

* Unpublished observation. R. H. Whitlock, University of Pennsylvania, New Bolton Center, Kennett Square, PA 19348

8. Payne, J.M.: Some recent work on the pathogenesis and prevention of milk fever. *In* Parturient Hypocalcemia. Edited by J. J. B. Anderson. New York, Academic Press, 1970.
9. Moodie, E.W., and Robertson, A.: Dietary intake of the parturient cow. Res. Vet. Sci. *2*:217, 1961.
10. Pradtron, K., and Hemken, R.W.: Potassium depletion in lactating dairy cows. J. Dairy Sci. *51*:1377, 1968.
11. Whitlock R.H., Tasker, J.B., and Tennant, B.C.: Hypochloremic metabolic alkalosis and hypokalemia in cattle with upper gastrointestinal tract obstruction. Am. J. Dig. Dis. *20*:595, 1975.
12. Whitlock, R.H.: Diseases of the abomasum associated with current feeding practices. J. A. V. M. A. *154*:1203, 1969.
13. Morrow, D.A.: Fat cow syndrome. J. Dairy Sci. *59*:1625, 1975.
14. Morrow, D.A.: Phosphorus deficiency and infertility in dairy heifers. J. A. V. M. A. *154*:761, 1969.
15. Parkinson, R., and Sutherland, A.K.: Postparturient hemoglobinuria of dairy cows. Aust. Vet. J. *30*:232, 1954.
16. Williams, D.J., Tyler, D.E., and Papp, E.: Abdominal fat necrosis as a herd problem in Georgia cattle. J. A. V. M. A. *154*:1017, 1969.
17. Capen, C.C., Cole, C.R., and Hibbs, J.W.: The pathology of hypervitamosis D in cattle. Pathol. Vet. *3*:350, 1966.
18. Blood, D.G., Henderson, J.A., and Radostits, A.M.: Veterinary Medicine. 5th Ed. Lea & Febiger, Philadelphia, 1978.
19. Wasserman, R.H., Krook, L., and Dirksen, G.: Evidence for antirachitic activity in the calcinogenic plant, *Trisetum flavescens*. Cornell Vet. *67*:333, 1977.
20. Collins, W.T., Capen, C.C., Dobereiner, J., and Tokarnia, C.H.: Ultrastructural evaluation of parathyroid glands and thyroid C cells of cattle fed *Solanum malacoxylon*. Am. J. Pathol. *87*:603, 1977.
21. Smith, R.M., and Marston, H.R.: Some metabolic aspects of vitamin B_{12} deficiency in sheep. Br. J. Nutr. *24*:879, 1970.
22. Underwood, E.J.: Trace Elements in Human and Animal Nutrition, 4th ed. New York, Academic Press, 1977.
23. Robertson, W.W.: Cobalt deficiency in ruminants. Vet. Rec. *89*:5, 1971.
24. Findlay, C.R.: Serum vitamin B_{12} levels and the diagnosis of cobalt deficiency in sheep. Vet. Rec. *90*:468, 1972.
25. Kaneko, J.J., and Rhode, E.A.: Diabetes mellitus in a cow. J. A. V. M. A. *144*:367, 1964.
26. Phillips, R.W., Knox, K.L., Pierson, R.E., and Tasker, J.B.: Bovine diabetes mellitus. Cornell Vet. *51*:114, 1971.
27. Rijnberk, A.: Iodine Metabolism and Thyroid Disease in the Dog. Thesis, Drukkenrij Elinkwijk, Utrecht, The Netherlands, 1971.
28. Capen, C.C., Belshaw, B.E., and Martin, S.L.: Endocrine disorders. *In* Textbook of Veterinary Internal Medicine. Edited by S. J. Ettinger, Philadelphia, W. B. Saunders Co., 1975, p. 1351.
29. Keeton, K.S., Schechter, R.D., and Schalm, O.W.: Adrenocortical insufficiency in dogs. Mod. Vet. Pract. *53*:25, 1972.
30. Mulnix, J.A.: Hypoadrenocorticism in the dog. J. A. A. H. A. *7*:220, 1971.
31. Mulnix, J.A.: Primary adrenocortical insufficiency. *In* Current Veterinary Therapy, Vol. VI. Edited by R. W. Kirk, Philadelphia, W. B. Saunders Co., 1977.
32. Siegel, E.T.: Endocrine Diseases of the Dog. Philadelphia, Lea & Febiger, 1977.
33. Osborne, C.A., and Stevens, J.B.: Pseudohyperparathyroidism in the dog. J. A. V. M. A. *162*:125, 1973.
34. Rijnberk, A.: Pseudohyperparathyroidism in the dog. Tijdschr. Diergeneeskd. *95*:515, 1970.
35. Joles, J.A., and Mulnix, J.A.: Primary adrenocortical insufficiency. *In* Current Veterinary Therapy, Vol. VI. Edited by R. W. Kirk. Philadelphia, W. B. Saunders Co., 1977.
36. Mulnix, J.A., Rijnberk, A., and Hendriks, H.J.: Evaluation of a modified water-deprivation test for diagnosis of polyuric disorders in dogs. J. A. V. M. A. *169*:1327, 1976.
37. Richards, M.A., and Sloper, J.C.: Diabetes insipidus. The complexity of the syndrome. Acta Endocrinol. *62*:627, 1969.
38. Richards, M.A.: Polydipsia in the dog. Symposium 1, 2, and 3. The differential diagnosis of polyuria syndromes in the dog. J. Small Anim. Pract. *10*:651, 1970.
39. Osborne, C.A., Low, D.G., and Finco, D.R.: Canine and Feline Urology. Philadelphia, W. B. Saunders Co., 1972.
40. Trudeau, W.L., and McGuigan, J.E.: Relations between serum gastrin levels and rates of gastric hydrochloric acid secretion. N. Engl. J. Med. *283*:408, 1971.
41. Murray, M., Rushton, A., and Selman, I.: Bovine renal amyloidosis: A clinico-pathological study. Vet. Rec. *90*:210, 1972.
42. Rooney, J.R.: Amyloidosis in a cow. Cornell Vet. *46*:369, 1956.
43. Lubberink, A.A.M.E., Rijnberk, A., der Kinderen, P.J., and Thijssen, J.H.H.: Hyperfunction of the adrenal cortex: a review. Aust. Vet. J. *47*:504, 1971.
44. Rijnberk, A., der Kinderen, P.J., and Thijssen, J.H.H.: Spontaneous hyperadrenocorticism in the dog. J. Endocrinol. *41*:397, 1968.
45. Rijnberk, A., der Kinderen, P.J., and Thijssen, J.H.H.: Canine Cushing's syndrome. Zentralbl. Veterinaermed. *16*:13, 1969.
46. Schechter, R.D., Stabenfeldt, G.H., Gribble, D.H., and Ling, G.V.: Treatment of Cushing's syndrome in the dog with an adrenocorticolytic agent (a, p'DDD). J. A. V. M. A. *162*:629, 1973.
47. Siegel, E.T., Kelly, D.F., and Berg, P.: Cushing's syndrome in the dog. J. A. V. M. A. *157*:2081, 1970.

Chapter 29

GASTROINTESTINAL MANIFESTATIONS OF URINARY DISEASES

CARL A. OSBORNE, JERRY B. STEVENS, AND DAVID J. POLZIN

Dysfunction of the alimentary system plays an important role in the syndrome of uremia. Unfortunately, differentiation of gastrointestinal signs associated with uremia from similar signs caused by primary non-urinary disorders is often difficult. The objective of this chapter is to provide an overview of current knowledge about the etiology and pathogenesis of gastrointestinal lesions and dysfunction caused by failure of one or more organs of the urinary tract. With this knowledge, clinical signs that mimic both gastrointestinal and urinary tract disorders may be rapidly localized to the appropriate system(s).

Overview of Normal Function provides a conceptual overview of normal function of the urinary system, knowledge of which is a prerequisite to localization and diagnosis of urinary tract disorders. *Renal Disease Versus Renal Failure* emphasizes important diagnostic and prognostic differences between renal diseases associated with adequate renal function, and renal diseases associated with renal failure. *The Polysystemic Nature of Uremia* provides a conceptual overview of uremia and its involvement of all systems of the body, including the gastrointestinal system. *Disorders Affecting Both the Gastrointestinal and Urinary Systems* emphasizes that both the urinary and gastrointestinal systems may be simultaneously affected by primary disorders of other body systems. *Etiopathogenesis of Gastrointestinal Manifestations of Urinary Diseases* has been organized to enhance understanding of recommendations made in *Localization of Signs Common to Urinary and Gastrointestinal Dysfunction*.

Unfortunately, evaluation of morphologic and functional changes in the alimentary system caused by renal failure in large domestic animals has been almost entirely neglected. Current understanding about gastroenteric disorders in veterinary medicine is therefore limited to in vitro and in vivo studies performed in humans, laboratory rodents,

dogs, and occasionally cats. Since there are significant species differences in gastroenteric anatomy, physiology, biochemistry, and pharmacology, there is great risk in formulating generalities concerning one species on the basis of observations made in another. Erroneous knowledge is often of greater detriment than lack of knowledge because it has a tendency to eliminate the search for correct information. A frightening outcome of such misconceptions is misdiagnosis, erroneous prognosis, and administration of ineffective or contraindicated therapy. Pending further studies, application of the following generalities to domestic animals must be accompanied with appropriate caution.

OVERVIEW OF NORMAL FUNCTION

The urinary system plays a major role in maintaining homeostasis by eliminating metabolic waste products from the body. In addition, the kidneys produce and degrade a variety of hormones. As is the situation to a greater or lesser degree with all body systems, effective function of the gastrointestinal system is dependent on adequate function of the urinary system, and vice versa.

A conceptual understanding of renal function is a prerequisite to detection of gastrointestinal diseases associated with primary and secondary renal disorders. Formation of urine by the kidneys results from three basic processes: glomerular filtration, tubular reabsorption, and tubular secretion. These mechanisms are modified by several hormones of nonrenal origin including antidiuretic hormone, aldosterone, parathormone, thyrocalcitonin, prohormone (vitamin) D, prostaglandins, calcitonin, and thyroxine.[1]

It is well established that formation of glomerular filtrate from plasma is a major function of glomeruli. Glomerular filtration is a passive process for the kidneys, deriving its energy from pressure generated by contraction of the left ventricle and the elasticity of vascular walls. Factors which influence the quantity and quality of glomerular filtrate in-

Table 29–1. Classification of azotemia

Cause	Classification
Decreased blood volume	Pre-renal
Decreased blood pressure	Pre-renal
Decreased colloidal osmotic pressure	Pre-renal
Decreased number of patent renal vessels	Primary renal
Decreased glomerular permeability	Primary renal
Increased renal interstitial pressure	Primary renal
Increased intratubular pressure	Primary renal (tubular obstruction)
	Post-renal (obstruction of ureters, bladder or urethra)

Table 29–2. Comparison of molecular weights of substances included in, and excluded from, glomerular filtrate

Substance	Molecular Weight	Presence in Glomerular Filtrate
Water	18	+
Urea	60	+
Creatinine	113	+
Glucose	180	+
Myoglobin	17,000	+
Amylase	50,000	+
Hemoglobin*	68,000	±
Albumin	69,000	±
Immunoglobulin-G	~150,000	–
Immunoglobulin-M	~1,000,000	–

* Probably excreted as a dimer with a monomeric molecular weight of approximately 32,000.

clude: (1) hydrostatic pressure; (2) volume of blood in glomerular capillaries; (3) colloidal osmotic pressure of blood in glomerular capillaries; (4) the number of patent renal vessels and glomerular capillaries; (5) the permeability of glomerular capillaries; (6) renal interstitial pressure; and (7) renal intratubular pressure (Table 29–1). Hydrostatic pressure is the major force that favors glomerular filtration. Forces that oppose glomerular filtration include colloidal osmotic pressure (which arises primarily from non-filtered protein molecules in glomerular capillary plasma), renal intratubular and interstitial pressure, and the selective permeability of glomerular capillary walls.

The glomerulus functions as a sieve which increasingly restricts passage of macromolecules of increasing diameter and molecular weight. Although the ability of substances to traverse glomerular capillary walls is primarily related to their molecular weight, the shape or configuration of molecules as well as their electrical charge also influence the degree to which they are filtered. Since cells, most proteins, and most lipoproteins are too large to pass through glomerular capillary walls, they are retained within the vascular compartment and are not present in glomerular filtrate in significant quantities. Most substances in glomerular filtrate of mammals have a molecular weight of less than 68,000[2,3] (Table 29–2). Thus glomerular filtrate is qualitatively similar to plasma with respect to the concentration of electrolytes and small molecular weight substances.

The common denominator of substances which appear in glomerular filtrate is not their potential value to the body, but rather their size, shape, and electrical charge. In order for the kidneys to regulate body fluid, electrolyte, and acid-base balance, it is essential that both beneficial and worthless metabolites of similar size be subjected to potential loss in urine. Some filtered substances (i.e., creatinine) cannot be reutilized by the body and are not reabsorbed by the tubules. Other filtered substances (i.e., amino acids, vitamins, glucose) are essential for body homeostasis, and are almost completely reabsorbed by the tubules. The body's requirement for water, electrolytes, and other filtered substances is variable, being dependent upon intake, metabolism and loss by nonrenal routes. Nephrons regulate conservation and excretion of these substances by selective partial tubular reabsorption and tubular secretion. Thus as glomerular filtrate passes through the tubules, it loses its original identity. The overall effect of these tubular functions is to balance the loss and gain of metabolites and water initially present in glomerular filtrate according to body need.

The kidneys are involved in regulation of erythropoiesis by production of erythrocyte stimulating factor, of calcium homeostasis by metabolizing vitamin (prohormone) D to its most metabolically active form, and of fluid and electrolyte balance by formation of renin and prostaglandins. The kidneys also degrade hormones including parathormone, insulin, and thyrotropic hormone.

The hydrodynamics associated with collection and unidirectional transport of urine from the renal pelvis to the bladder, and its subsequent elimination by the process of micturition are also essential for body homeostasis. Urine that accumulates in the renal pelvis initiates peristaltic movement of pelvic and then ureteral smooth muscle. As a result, elongated boluses of urine are propelled through the ureteral lumen to the urinary bladder. Anatomic ureterovesical sphincters are not present; however, the oblique course of the ureters through the bladder wall at the trigone form a flap valve that normally prevents retrograde flow of urine from the bladder. Ureterovesical valves protect the kidneys from abnormal retrograde pressure, and from contamination with infected bladder urine.

Micturition consists of the storage of urine in the urinary bladder, and its periodic complete elimination through the urethra. Discussion of the physiology of micturition is beyond the scope of this text, but has been reviewed elsewhere.[4,5] Micturition is fundamentally a reflex facilitated and inhibited by higher brain centers and, like defecation, is subject to voluntary initiation and inhibition.

RENAL DISEASE VERSUS RENAL FAILURE

Confusion caused by use of the terms renal disease and renal failure as synonyms may result in misdiagnosis and formulation of inappropriate, and even contraindicated, therapy.

Renal Disease

Renal disease indicates the presence of renal lesions of any size, distribution (focal or generalized), or cause (anomalies, infection, endogenous or exogenous toxins, obstruction to urine flow, neoplasms, ischemia, immune-mediated disorders, hypercalcemia, trauma) in one or both kidneys. The specific cause of renal disease(s) may or may not be known; however, quantitative information about renal function (or dysfunction) is not defined. Renal disease cannot be used synonymously with renal failure because of the tremendous functional reserve capacity of the kidneys. Depending on the quantity of renal parenchyma affected and the severity and duration of the lesions, renal diseases may or may not cause renal failure. Impairment of urine concentrating and diluting capacity of canine kidneys cannot be detected by evaluation of urine specific gravity or urine osmolality until approximately two thirds of the total renal parenchyma is surgically extirpated.[6] Although the serum concentrations of urea nitrogen and creatinine vary inversely with glomerular filtration rate, approximately three fourths of the nephrons of both kidneys must be nonfunctional before reduction in renal function is severe enough to be associated with significant elevations in either substance. It is obvious that renal disease can occur without renal failure. Unfortunately many renal diseases escape detection until they become so generalized that they induce clinical signs as a result of serious impairment of renal function.

Renal Failure

Renal failure implies that approximately three fourths or more of the functional capacity of the nephrons of both kidneys has been impaired. The term renal failure is analogous to liver failure or heart failure in that a level of organ dysfunction is described rather than a specific disease entity. Renal failure may be precipitated by acute or chronic, reversible or irreversible, pre-renal, renal or post-renal diseases. It may be associated with polyuria or oliguria. In some instances, uremic crises may suddenly be precipitated by pre-renal (i.e., pancreatitis, foreign body gastroenteritis, congestive heart failure) or less commonly post-renal (urethral obstruction, displacement of urinary bladder into perineal hernia) disorders which occur in patients with previously compensated primary renal failure.

Differentiation Between Renal Disease and Renal Failure

Differentiation between renal disease and renal failure must be based on knowledge of the fact that not all diagnostic procedures used to detect disorders of the urinary system provide information about renal functional capacity, nor is it always possible to differentiate inflammatory diseases of the lower urinary tract from the upper urinary tract (Table 29–3). For example, detection of significant numbers of casts in urine sediment provides reliable evidence of renal tubular involvement because it is known that casts form in the loops of Henle, distal tubules, and collecting ducts. One cannot infer that the presence of a large number of casts is indicative of renal failure, however, because their presence or absence cannot be correlated with the degree of renal dysfunction.

Differentiation between renal disease and renal failure is of great clinical significance when gastrointestinal, pancreatic, and hepatic diseases causing clinical signs similar to those associated with renal failure (vomiting, diarrhea, polydipsia, dehydration, depression, anorexia, and weight loss) secondarily induce pre-renal azotemia and ischemic tubular disease characterized by formation of variable numbers of epithelial cells and granular casts. Although extrarenal fluid loss and subsequent reduction in renal perfusion may be of sufficient magnitude to damage some nephrons, detection of concentrated urine (SG >1.025) indicates the presence of an adequate population of nephrons to prevent clinical signs associated with primary renal failure. Every effort should be made to restore renal perfu-

Table 29–3. Diagnostic procedures commonly used to detect disorders of the urinary system

Method	Renal Function	Localize to Kidney	Localize to Urinary System
Urea nitrogen (serum or plasma)	GFR	No*	—
Creatinine (serum or plasma)	GFR	No*	—
Specific gravity (urine)	Tubular reabsorption	No*	—
Osmolality (urine)	Tubular reabsorption	No*	—
Phenolsulphonphthalein (urine excretion)	RBF; tubular secretion	No*	—
Sodium sulfonilate (plasma retention)	GFR	No*	—
Intravenous urography	Crude index of RBF & GFR	Yes	Yes
Urinary casts	No	Yes	—
Renal biopsy	No	Yes	—
Significant bacteriuria	No	No	Yes†
Proteinuria	No	No‡	No
Pyuria	No	No§	Yes†
Hematuria	No	No§	Yes†

* Alterations in renal function are not always caused by diseases localized to the kidneys.
† Assuming urine not contaminated by genital tract.
‡ Large quantities of protein in absence of RBC and WBC suggest glomerular disease.
§ Unless present in urinary casts.
GFR = Glomerular Filtration Rate
RBF = Renal Blood Flow

sion, however, since progressive destruction of nephrons will ultimately result in primary ischemic renal failure.

THE POLYSYSTEMIC NATURE OF UREMIA

The pathophysiology and biologic behavior of the uremic syndrome have been primarily studied in humans, dogs, and laboratory rodents. Abnormalities that develop as a result of experimentally produced or naturally occurring primary renal failure in these species are similar. Although there is a paucity of information about the uremic syndrome in large domestic animals, enough observations have been made to support the view that the pathophysiology of uremia is similar in all species. Information in the following discussion is based primarily on experimental and clinical studies in humans, dogs, and cats.

When the structural and functional integrity of both kidneys has been compromised to such a degree that signs of renal failure become manifest clinically, a relatively predictable polysystemic symptom complex called uremia appears, regardless of underlying cause. Uremia is characterized by multiple metabolic and physiologic alterations that result from renal insufficiency. Renal insufficiency may be caused by any disease process that impairs the function of at least three fourths of the nephrons of both kidneys. Depending on the biologic behav-

ior of the disease in question, primary renal failure may be reversible or irreversible.

Primary renal failure may be associated with pathologic oliguria or pathologic polyuria (Table 29–4). Discussion of the pathophysiology of polyuric and oliguric primary renal failure is beyond the scope of this text, but has been described elsewhere.[7] Because there are significant differences in the type and magnitude of excesses and deficits of fluids, electrolytes, and acid-base metabolites that develop in oliguric and nonoliguric uremic patients, it is imperative to divide candidates for therapy into those with oliguria and those with polyuria (Table 29–5).

Table 29–4. Characteristic urine volume associated with different types of azotemia

Pre-renal Azotemia	Obstructive Post-renal Azotemia
Physiologic oliguria (U$_{SG}$ > 1.025)	Initial oliguria or anuria. Diuresis and polyuria following relief of obstruction.
Primary Acute Ischemic or Nephrotoxic Azotemia Initial oliguric phase (U$_{SG}$ = 1.007–1.024) Secondary polyuric phase (U$_{SG}$ = 1.007–1.024)	Primary Chronic Azotemia Polyuria (U$_{SG}$ = 1.007–1.024) Terminal oliguric phase (U$_{SG}$ = 1.008–1.012) Reversible oliguria may be caused by onset of nonrenal disorder that induces pre-renal azotemia. (U$_{SG}$ = 1.007–1.024)

Table 29–5. Similarities and differences of fluid, electrolyte, and acid-base balance in polyuric and oliguric primary renal failure

Factor	Polyuria	Oliguria
Urine specific gravity	1.007–1.024	1.007–1.024
BUN concentration	↑	↑
Serum creatinine concentration	↑	↑
Serum sodium concentration	Usually normal	Variable
Total body sodium concentration	Decreased	Variable
Serum potassium concentration	Usually normal	Increased
Blood pH	Normal to ↓	Marked ↓
Serum phosphorus concentration	Usually ↑	Usually ↑
Serum calcium concentration	Normal to ↓ *	Normal to ↓ †

* Unless renal failure caused by hypercalcemia.
† Anuric primary renal failure in the horse is associated with hypercalcemia.

Table 29–6. Interactions of multiple factors contributing to polysystemic manifestations of uremia

Abnormalities	Sequelae
Electrolyte Imbalances	
Sodium deficit	Dehydration
Sodium excess	Overhydration
Potassium deficit	Muscular weakness; decreased urine conc.
Potassium excess	Cardiotoxicity
Calcium deficit	Bone demineralization; tetany
Calcium excess	Calcium nephropathy, muscular atony
Acid-Base Imbalances	
Hydrogen ion retention	Metabolic acidosis
Increased bicarbonate utilization	Metabolic acidosis
Increased bicarbonate loss in urine	Metabolic acidosis
Decreased renal tubular production of ammonia	Metabolic acidosis
Fluid Imbalance	
Polyuria, vomiting, diarrhea	Dehydration
Oliguria, anuria	Overhydration
Endocrine Imbalance	
Decreased erythrocyte—stimulating factor production	Anemia
Decreased production of 1,25-dihydroxycholecalciferol	Hypocalcemia
Decreased degradation of parathormone	Bone demineralization
Decreased degradation and clearance of insulin	Increased sensitivity to exogenous insulin
Caloric Imbalance	
Anorexia, vomiting, diarrhea	Weight loss
Metabolic Waste Imbalance	
Decreased clearance of urea, creatinine, guanidines, phenols, and others	GI disorders; Neurologic disorders; Bleeding; Others

Clinical signs of uremia are not directly caused by renal lesions, but rather develop as a result of multiple metabolic deficits and excesses that develop as a result of decreased renal function caused by renal lesions. Clinical signs characteristic of uremia are manifestations of an interaction between: (a) autointoxication caused by reduction of renal function below that required to clear plasma of metabolic waste products, impaired ability to conserve vital metabolites in glomerular filtrate, and reduced production and degradation of several hormones (Table 29–6); and (b) the body's compensatory attempts to maintain homeostasis (Table 29–7). Signs caused by underlying renal lesions may also contribute to the spectrum of clinical findings.

In past years, a variety of toxins have been incriminated as underlying causes of polysystemic signs characteristic of uremia (Table 29–8).[8,9,10,11,12] Most so-called "uremic-toxins" are end-products of protein and nucleoprotein metabolism which accumulate in blood as a result of impaired renal clearance. Some are products of intestinal bacterial

Table 29–7. Compensatory reactions of the body to renal dysfunction

Disorder	Compensation
Polyuria	Polydipsia
Hypocalcemia	Hyperparathyroidism
Severe metabolic acidosis	Elimination of CO_2 by increased rate and depth of respiration
Retention of metabolic waste products	Vomiting = ?
Nephron destruction	Hypertrophy, hyperplasia, and increased function of viable nephrons

Table 29-8. Metabolites that have been incriminated as uremic toxins

Acetoin	Indole and its derivatives
Amines	Middle molecules
Aliphatic	Phenol and its derivatives
Aromatic	Pseudouridine
Creatine	Sulfates
Creatinine	Urea
Guanidine and its derivatives	
Guanidinoacetic acid	
Guanidinosuccinic acid	
Methylguanidine	

degradation and intestinal putrefaction. Some attain high extracellular concentrations, while others appear to attain high intracellular concentrations. It has been hypothesized that some of these toxic metabolites induce abnormalities by inhibiting intracellular enzymes.[8] Uremic toxins are not the sole cause for uremia, however, as evidenced by the inability to identify a substance that can induce a similar syndrome when administered to experimental animals. This observation, and the fact that the uremic syndrome has variable clinical manifestations, suggests that it is mediated by the summation of toxic metabolites in addition to fluid, acid-base, electrolyte, caloric, endocrine, and enzymatic imbalances.

Deficits due to loss of water and electrolytes in patients with renal failure are caused by one or a combination of the following: generalized nephron damage, polyuria, anorexia, vomiting, and diarrhea. These abnormalities have the potential to induce varying degrees of dehydration and negative body balance of sodium, chloride, calcium, and bicarbonate ions.

Excesses due to retention of water, electrolytes and non-electrolytes in patients with renal failure are caused by a reduction in renal clearance due to generalized nephron damage. This abnormality has the potential to induce varying degrees of edema (uncommon, and when present usually associated with generalized glomerular disease), hyperkalemia, hyperphosphatemia, retention of dietary nonvolatile acids, and retention of catabolic waste products (urea, creatinine, guanidines, phenols, indoles, and others).

Patients with oliguric or polyuric primary renal failure develop varying degrees of metabolic acidosis. This occurs because the tubules lose their ability to conserve buffer ions (especially bicarbonate) present in glomerular filtrate, because of reduction of glomerular clearance of dietary non-

volatile acids (sulfuric and phosphoric), and because the ability of the tubules to excrete hydrogen ion and ammonia is impaired.[13]

Because severe renal failure is associated with varying degrees of vomiting, diarrhea, and anorexia, a negative caloric balance develops. As a result the body must catabolize its own tissues for energy. Catabolism of proteins perpetuates abnormalities in acid-base and electrolyte balance because protein catabolism is associated with the release of intracellular potassium and phosphorus, and the production of protein waste products including nonprotein nitrogenous substances and nonvolatile acids. A negative caloric balance may also be aggravated by severe proteinuria.

Clinical evidence of disorders caused by abnormalities of water, electrolyte, acid-base, endocrine, and caloric balance are not invariably present in patients with generalized renal disease. This is related, at least in part, to the tremendous reserve capacity of the kidneys. Renal function adequate for homeostasis does not require that all nephrons be functional. In fact clinical signs of primary renal failure, including vomiting, diarrhea, depression, anorexia, dehydration, and weight loss, usually do not occur until 70 to 75% or more of the total nephron population have been functionally impaired. In addition, compensatory mechanisms of the body maintain a state of biochemical homeostasis despite significant renal dysfunction. A price is paid for loss of functional renal reserve capacity, however. Patients with presymptomatic primary renal failure have reduced capacity to respond to physiologic and pathologic stresses. A uremic crisis may be suddenly precipitated by decreased intake of water or nutrients, development of concomitant but unrelated diseases, and/or inappropriate administration of certain drugs.[14]

DISORDERS AFFECTING BOTH THE GASTROINTESTINAL AND URINARY SYSTEMS

Primary diseases of the gastrointestinal tract may secondarily affect the urinary system, and vice versa. Both the gastrointestinal and urinary systems may also be affected by disorders of other body systems, especially those associated with alterations in body fluid, electrolyte, and acid-base balance. Examples include hypercalcemia, heart failure, hypoadrenocorticism, metastatic neoplasia, and hypovolemic shock. Because of their clinical similarity to primary diseases of the gastrointestinal system, hypercalcemia and hypoadrenocorticism merit further discussion.

Hypercalcemia

Hypercalcemia, a disorder with many causes (Table 29–9), may induce dysfunction of many body systems, especially the gastrointestinal, urinary, and nervous systems.[15,16,17] Variations in functional and structural alterations of the kidneys and gastrointestinal tract are usually caused by variations in the severity and duration of hypercalcemia, rather than differences in the biologic behavior of the pathologic process that produced the hypercalcemia.

In man, dogs, and presumably other animals, increased serum calcium concentration depresses the excitability of nervous tissue, and the contraction of smooth, skeletal, and cardiac muscle. Generalized muscular weakness occurs as a result of decreased tonus of skeletal muscle. Loss of smooth muscle tonus of the gastrointestinal tract results in gastric atony associated with anorexia and vomiting, and intestinal atony associated with constipation.

Because hypercalcemia damages renal tubular epithelium, one of the earliest and most significant clinical manifestations of abnormal renal function is an impaired ability to concentrate urine which is unresponsive to endogenous or exogenous antidiuretic hormone. During early stages, the severity of impaired ability to concentrate urine is often much greater than would be predicted by evaluation of glomerular filtration rate. As the severity of renal damage progresses, however, GFR may decrease to a point where an increase in serum creatinine and urea nitrogen concentration may be detected. If the degree of calcium nephropathy is severe enough to cause primary renal failure, uremic signs may be observed.

Hypoadrenocorticism

Hypoadrenocorticism in dogs is associated with signs referable to the gastrointestinal system (vomiting, polydipsia, dark tarry feces), urinary system (pre-renal azotemia, variable specific gravity of urine), and cardiovascular system (cardiac conduction defects), in addition to nonlocalizing signs (anorexia, depression, dehydration, weight loss, collapse).[18,19]

Decreased production and release of mineralocorticoids caused by destruction of the adrenal glands is associated with impaired renal conservation of sodium and chloride, and subnormal renal tubular secretion of potassium. Loss of abnormal quantities of sodium in urine results in depletion of extracellular fluid volume, reduction in blood volume and pressure, and ultimately peripheral vascular collapse. In addition to hemoconcentration, reduction in vascular volume is associated with reduced renal perfusion and pre-renal azotemia.

Unlike most diseases associated with pre-renal azotemia, the urine specific gravity of dogs with hypoadrenocorticism is often below 1.025. Impaired release of antidiuretic hormone from the posterior pituitary gland as a result of hypo osmolality of plasma is not a tenable explanation of this observation since maxiumum output of ADH would be expected as a result of marked reduction in vascular volume. Impaired ability to concentrate urine may be caused by solute diuresis induced by natriuresis, and reduction in medullary hyperosmolality. The magnitude of diuresis is usually not sufficient to produce clinically evident polyuria. A high index of suspicion is required to prevent confusion of hypoadrenocorticism and pre-renal azotemia with primary oliguric renal failure.

Table 29–9. Causes of naturally occurring hypercalcemia in domestic animals and man

Cause	Species				
	Horse	Cow	Dog	Cat	Man
Primary hyperparathyroidism	NR	NR	Yes	NR	Yes
Paraneoplastic syndromes	Yes	NR	Yes	Yes	Yes
Hyperthyroidism	NR	NR	Yes (rare)	NR	Yes
Hypoadrenocorticism	NR	NR	Yes	NR	Yes
Disuse osteoporosis	NR	NR	NR	NR	Yes
Hypervitaminosis D	NR	NR	Yes	NR	Yes
Osteolytic neoplasia	NR	NR	Yes (uncommon)	NR	Yes
Toxic plants	Yes	Yes	NR	NR	NR
Primary renal failure*	Yes	NR	Yes	NR	Yes

* Primary renal failure is usually associated with normocalcemia or hypocalcemia, but on occasion is associated with hypercalcemia.
NR = Not Reported

Hyperkalemia caused by impaired renal secretion of potassium induces multiple cardiac arrhythmias and bradycardia, which further impair perfusion of organs and tissues.

Other than the obvious association with impaired production of mineralocorticoids and glucocorticoids, the specific cause(s) of gastrointestinal signs associated with hypoadrenocorticism have not been well documented.

ETIOPATHOGENESIS OF GASTROINTESTINAL MANIFESTATIONS OF URINARY DISEASES

The onset and spectrum of clinical signs of uremia may vary from patient to patient depending on the nature, severity, duration (acute or chronic), rate of progression of the underlying disease, presence or absence of coexistent but unrelated disease(s), and administration of therapeutic agents. In most instances, however, uremia is the clinical state toward which all progressive generalized renal diseases ultimately converge, and associated signs are more similar than dissimilar. In addition to manifestations of impaired renal function (azotemia, metabolic acidosis, oliguria or polyuria, hyponatremia, hypokalemia or hyperkalemia, hypocalcemia and hyperphosphatemia), signs indicative of variable involvement of the gastrointestinal, cardiovascular, pulmonary, neuromuscular, skeletal, hemopoietic, immune, genital, and endocrine systems, as well as of coagulation defects, may occur.[9,20,21]

Anorexia, Depression and Weight Loss

Anorexia, depression and weight loss are well-known signs of renal failure; however, the specific cause(s) of these nonspecific signs have not been carefully evaluated. Until recently, they have been regarded as sequelae to the polysystemic nature of uremia.

Chronic intoxication of normal dogs with methylguanidine, a suspected uremic toxin, induced many signs of uremia including anorexia, depression, and weight loss.[22] When conditions of uremia were produced by dialyzing anuric nephrectomized dogs against methylguanidine in the peritoneal dialysate solution, similar signs were observed.[23]

Studies in dogs indicate that anorexia is associated, at least in part, with stimulation of the medullary emetic chemoreceptor trigger zone (MECRTZ) by circulating toxins such as guanidines.[24] Ablation of the MECRTZ in nephrectomized dogs suppressed the onset of anorexia.

During recent years defects in intestinal absorption of calcium, proteins, and carbohydrates have been identified in uremic humans and animals. In addition to varying degrees of anorexia, vomiting, and diarrhea, it appears that these defects in intestinal function contribute to a low-grade malabsorption syndrome.

Impaired absorption of amino acids from the small intestine of uremic human beings has been reported.[25] Decreased activity of dipeptidases and disaccharidases was detected in biopsies of intestinal mucosa obtained from uremic human patients.[26] These enzymatic abnormalities were variably associated with elongation of villous crypts, invasion by plasma cells, increased fecal fat excretion, and a flat glucose tolerance curve after oral glucose administration.

On the basis of these findings it was postulated that disturbed function of the small intestine is common in human patients with chronic renal failure. It was also suggested that consumption of carbohydrate-rich diets commonly recommended for dietary management of renal failure may produce gastrointestinal disturbances because of inadequate digestion of disaccharidases.

Uremic Stomatitis

Dogs and cats with severe renal failure, especially if subacute or chronic, occasionally develop oral ulcers, brownish discoloration of the dorsal surface of the tongue, and fetor of breath. The mucous membranes may also become dry (xerostomia). These abnormalities, singly or collectively, are commonly called uremic stomatitis.

Experimental studies performed in dogs and clinical studies in humans incriminate the local caustic action of ammonia generated by bacterial decomposition of abnormally high concentrations of salivary urea as the cause of oral ulcers.[27,28] In one study, tartar scraped from the teeth of normal and nephrectomized dogs hydrolyzed urea to ammonia in a few minutes, suggesting that dental tartar contained urease.[27] It is probable that urease-producing bacteria were present in the tartar.[28] Ulcerations of the buccal mucosa and tongue of nephrectomized dogs occurred adjacent to teeth, and could be prevented by removal of dental tartar from nephrectomized azotemic dogs.[27] In man, poor oral hygiene and periodontal disease aggravate the severity of uremic stomatitis.[29] The fact that uremic stomatitis has been observed in completely edentulous humans indicates that urease does not solely originate from dental tartar, or that urease is not the only cause of uremic stomatitis.[28] Several species of bacteria produce urease, some of which are present in the normal oral flora in man. It is probable that a similar situation occurs in animals. Variations of the normal oral flora among different species, and individuals within species, may explain the sporadic occurrence of uremic stomatitis.

The observation that urea loading of azotemic humans by means of hemodialysis resulted in no consistent relationship between blood urea concentration and stomatitis suggests that other factors may be involved.[30] One hypothesis is that oral lesions represent only a local manifestation of a more generalized deterioration of gastrointestinal mucosa in the uremic syndrome.[29]

The cause of the brownish discoloration of the tongue of dogs and cats is unknown. Xerostomia may be caused by reduced production of saliva caused by dehydration, and compensatory hyperventilation associated with metabolic acidosis. Uremic fetor of breath may be caused by stomatitis and escape of volatile compounds such as ammonia and phenols which accumulate in the body as a result of renal failure.

Occasionally the first evidence of chronic progressive renal failure in dogs (especially when immature) owned by unobservant clients is demineralization of the skull associated with loosening of the teeth. This abnormality, sometimes called "rubber jaw," may be associated with distortion of facial bones by extensive proliferation of connective tissue (fibrous osteodystrophy), and is caused by progressive hypocalcemia and compensatory hyperparathyroidism.[13]

Vomiting

Vomiting is a well-known sign associated with renal failure in dogs, cats, and man. Contrary to popular opinion, however, it is not a consistent finding. Although it is often an early manifestation of acute onset uremia, it may not occur until late stages of chronic renal failure, especially if systemic disorders have been minimized by properly formulated symptomatic and supportive therapy.[21] The severity of vomiting does not always correlate with the severity of azotemia.

Vomiting associated with renal failure may be associated with any one or combination of the following causes: stimulation of the MECRTZ by circulating toxins, gastritis, attempts to force oral food or fluids, and intolerance to medications such as antibiotics and cardiac glycosides.

Injection of high doses of methylguanidine into normal dogs, and maintenance of high plasma concentrations of methylguanidine by selective peritoneal dialysis in anuric dogs was associated with a variety of signs typical of uremia including gastric and duodenal ulceration, hemorrhage of gastric and intestinal mucosa, and vomiting.[22,23] Recent studies suggest that methylguanidine arises from the metabolism of creatinine by intestinal bacteria.[10,31,32]

Studies involving ablation of the MECRTZ of nephrectomized dogs revealed that vomiting was induced by central stimulation of the MECRTZ prior to development of detectable lesions in the gastrointestinal tract.[24] Ablation of the MECRTZ essentially eliminated the emetic response to guanidine. In addition, denervation of the gastrointestinal tract by vagotomy and transection of the spinal cord did not delay the onset of vomiting associated with azotemia in nonablated nephrectomized dogs. The results of this study did not, however, exclude the probability that the severity of vomiting is intensified by local irritation following development of gastrointestinal lesions.

Hemorrhagic and occasionally ulcerative gastritis have been commonly observed in dogs and cats with severe primary renal failure.[33,34] Hemorrhagic gastritis is apparently uncommon in uremic cattle.[34] Gastric lesions in dogs are typically characterized by focal to generalized mucosal hemorrhage, focal ulcers, myoarteritis, and focal calcification of deep portions of the gastric mucosa. Even though gastric lesions are collectively described as gastritis, there is often a conspicuous absence of inflammatory cells.

The pathogenesis of hemorrhagic and ulcerative gastritis is unknown, nor has it been established that these lesions have a similar etiology. Popular hypotheses of their cause include local irritation by ammonia, alteration of the protective surface layer of mucus, uremic vasculitis, and/or coagulopathies.

The conclusion that local irritation by production of ammonia from urea results in gastric lesions appears to be based on the observation that the amount of urea entering the alimentary tract increases in proportion to elevations in plasma urea.[35] In addition, gastric mucosa of dogs, cats, and man has been reported to produce urease, and therefore is capable of hydrolyzing urea to ammonia.[36,37,38]

Support for the mucolytic effect of urea in the production of gastric lesions is based on the finding that urea dissolved the protective layer of mucus lining the stomach of dogs.[39,40] It was hypothesized that mucolysis may allow harmful back-diffusion of acid.[41] It is tempting to speculate that the high microbial urease content normally present in rumen ingesta may play some role in the low incidence of gastritis observed in cattle by degrading urea and minimizing mucolysis.

Vasculitis has been incriminated as a cause of

gastric ulceration in uremic dogs on the basis of detection of fibrinoid necrosis of arteries and arterioles adjacent to mucosal ulcers.[34,42,43] It is suggested that vascular occlusion results in focal ischemia of adjacent tissue which ultimately leads to necrosis and ulceration of the mucosa and submucosa.[41] Although vascular disease may result in the formation of gastric ulcers, studies in man and animals indicate that primary disorders of blood vessels do not play a significant role in the pathogenesis of gastrointestinal bleeding.[44]

Studies performed in uremic dogs and humans have revealed a major coagulation defect associated with an acquired, reversible qualitative defect in thrombocyte function.[30,44,45] Platelet numbers were not altered. This abnormality undoubtedly contributes to insidious but significant blood loss from the gastrointestinal tract. It may be associated with bloody diarrhea, less frequently gingival hemorrhage, and rarely hematemesis. The platelet dysfunction is characterized by diminished activation of platelet factor 3, decreased platelet adhesiveness and aggregation, and impaired prothrombin consumption. Studies in dogs with experimentally induced uremia revealed that the severity of abnormal coagulations was related to the severity of uremia.[46] Current evidence implicates circulating uremic toxins, especially guanidinosuccinic acid and hydroxyphenolacetic acid, in the etiopathogenesis of uremic platelet dysfunction.[44,47] Despite the potential for platelet dysfunction in uremic patients, bleeding has not been a significant problem in dogs and cats following needle punch biopsy of the kidney.[48]

Because the kidneys are the major route of excretion of active and metabolized drugs from the body, there is an increase in the frequency and severity of drug intolerance in patients with renal insufficiency. Some adverse effects of drugs which generally are of little significance in patients with normal renal function may become obvious in patients with renal insufficiency. Drugs are often administered to uremic patients without knowledge of the animals' normal metabolic pathways, and without knowledge of whether the drugs' pharmacologic actions will be affected by the uremic state. Because of lack of an adequate explanation, many atypical symptoms that appear are ignored or attributed to an unusual manifestation of the underlying disorder. In some patients with renal failure, clinical deterioration is often attributed to progession of the underlying disease, without considering that deterioration might be related, at least in part, to toxicity induced by the administration of drugs. Specific recommendations for use of drugs in azotemic dogs and cats have been reported.[14]

Although vomiting might by hypothesized as a compensatory response to aid in elimination of uremic toxins and minimize the severity of metabolic acidosis, it appears to aggravate the uremic syndrome. In addition to loss of gastric juices which augment imbalances in fluid and electrolytes, inhibition of compensatory polydipsia in patients with obligatory polyuria results in severe volume depletion and further reduction in glomerular filtration. Catabolism of body proteins for energy as a result of insufficient consumption of nutrients contributes further to retention of protein catabolic by-products in the body. Aspiration pneumonia may further complicate the patient's precarious balance between life and death.

Diarrhea

Diarrhea is not a constant finding associated with uremia. In fact dehydrated animals without a significant degree of enterocolitis may become constipated. The latter is thought to occur in response to conservation of intestinal fluids by the body in an attempt to restore fluid balance. In man, uremia may be associated with ileus.

Enterocolitis, manifested clinically as diarrhea, may occur in severely uremic dogs and cats, but is usually less severe than hemorrhagic gastritis. The lesions are similar to those observed in the stomach, except for lack of calcification of intestinal mucosa.[33,34] Intussusceptions have frequently been reported in dogs with experimentally produced uremia,[22,24,49,50,51] and we have observed them in dogs with naturally occurring uremia.

In contrast to dogs and cats, the most severe lesions in uremic cattle affect the large intestine.[34] Severe catarrhal or hemorrhagic inflammation may be present in the colon.[52]

Like gastric lesions, the etiology of hemorrhagic and ulcerative lesions in the large and small intestine is unknown. Several hypotheses have been proposed, including caustic action of ammonia, increased susceptibility of intestinal mucosa to pancreatic and bacterial enzymes, and abnormal coagulation.

Production of toxic substances capable of initiating local and systemic effects by action of intestinal bacteria on metabolites retained as a result of renal failure has been a popular hypothesis for many decades. For example, abnormal concentrations of methylguanidine may be produced by the action of enteric bacteria on creatinine.[10,31,32] High plasma concentrations of methylguanidine produce ulcerative lesions of the duodenum of dogs similar to those described in the stomach.[22,23]

The results of other studies also incriminate enteric bacteria in the genesis of uremic lesions. In one experiment, nephrectomized germ-free rats lived for a significantly longer period than nephrectomized rats with conventional enteric bacterial flora.[53] Uremic colitis of varying severity occurred in the majority of rats dying after bilateral nephrectomy, but was not detected in germ-free rats, or rats with limited bacterial flora.[54] Studies of uremic human patients were interpreted to indicate that a correlation existed between gastrointestinal lesions and areas of bacterial proliferation.[55] It is not unreasonable to assume that secondary invasion of damaged intestinal mucosa by resident enteric bacteria is associated with the etiopathogenesis of uremic lesions.

Caustic destruction of intestinal mucosa by ammonia formed from enteric bacterial degradation of abnormally high concentrations of urea has also been proposed. The observation that the concentration of urea in intestinal juices of uremic dogs parallels the serum concentration of urea, and that the number of strains of urease-producing bacteria increases as blood urea nitrogen increases, supports the hypothesis.[56,57] Arguments against the local caustic action of ammonia include studies indicating that the concentration of ammonia in feces of uremic humans is usually, but not invariably, normal.[35,58] The ammonia concentration in the feces of uremic animals has not been measured. In addition, administration of acetohydroxamic acid, a potent inhibitor of urease, to bilaterally nephrectomized rats reduced the mean colonic concentration of ammonia by 64%, but did not reduce the incidence of colitis.[59]

Experimental studies in dogs with acute uremia indicate that pancreatic secretions play a major role in the genesis of hemorrhagic intestinal lesions.[39] Prevention of exposure of intestinal mucosa to pancreatic exocrine secretions by ligation of pancreatic ducts resulted in fewer lesions in uremic dogs than occurred in nephrectomized dogs without pancreatic duct ligation. Intestinal lesions in control dogs were characterized by epithelial cell desquamation, hemorrhage, and loss of cellular components of the lamina propria, whereas intestinal lesions in dogs with ligated pancreatic ducts were limited to subtle epithelial changes. It was proposed that high concentrations of chyme in uremic dogs initiated dissolution of protective mucin and allowed proteolytic pancreatic enzymes to digest exposed intestinal mucosa.[39]

Reduction in the concentration of bicarbonate in pancreatic juice of humans with chronic renal failure has been incriminated as a cause of increased susceptibility of the intestinal mucosa to lesions.[60]

Reduction in the rate of villous epithelial cell renewal of uremic mice was hypothesized to increase their susceptibility to potentially toxic luminal factors.[61] Delayed physiologic regeneration of villous epithelium in mice with experimentally induced chronic uremia was associated with shortening of villi and crypts.[62] Impaired ability of the body to repair damaged tissue during uremia may also be involved in the pathogenesis of gastroenteric lesions.[63]

In addition to hemorrhagic and ulcerative lesions in the intestinal mucosa, diarrhea in uremic humans has been attributed to decreased production of disaccharidases and dipeptidases[26] and abnormal bile metabolism.[64]

Abdominal Distention

The most common causes of abdominal distention related to disorders of the urinary system are the nephrotic syndrome and rupture of the urinary bladder. Less common causes include chronic neurogenic dysfunction of the urinary bladder, profound chronic polyuria, hemoperitoneum caused by renal trauma, and enlargement of one or both kidneys.

Nephrotic Syndrome

Prolonged severe proteinuria and the resultant hypoproteinemia that occur secondary to damage of glomerular capillary walls initiate physiologic, metabolic and nutritional defects assocated with the nephrotic syndrome.[65] The nephrotic syndrome is characterized by proteinuria, hypoproteinemia, hypoalbuminemia, hypercholesterolemia, and frequently edema. In some respects it resembles the edematous syndrome caused by protein-losing enteropathies. It may or may not be associated with decreased glomerular filtration rate and azotemia.

Although the nephrotic syndrome is a documented complication of generalized glomerular disease in animals, it is not invariably present in all patients with generalized glomerular disease. Glomerular diseases with potential to cause the nephrotic syndrome in animals include amyloidosis and immune-complex glomerulonephritis.[66]

If the proteinuria that occurs secondary to damage to the filtration barriers of glomerular capillary walls is persistent and severe, urine protein (especially albumin) loss may exceed the capacity of the liver to maintain normal plasma protein concentration. In uremic patients, an increased rate of endogenous catabolism of albumin and decreased dietary intake of protein may also contribute to hypoalbuminemia. Since albumin molecules account for approximately 77% of plasma colloidal osmotic pressure, progressive hypoalbuminemia is associated with a proportionate decrease in plasma colloidal osmotic pressure. According to the Starling-Landis cycle of capillary-interstitial fluid exchange, a marked decrease in colloidal osmotic pressure will initiate an abnormal shift of fluid from the vascular compartment to the extravascular compartment, resulting in hypovolemia and edema. The edema is usually most severe in dependent portions of the body (ventral midline, limbs) because venous hydrostatic pressure is greatest in these locations. In severe cases, ascites and hydrothorax may develop.

In addition to the reduction in colloidal osmotic pressure that occurs as a result of glomerular loss of plasma protein, body compensatory mechanisms play a role in the development and maintenance of edema. As a result of loss of vascular fluid into the extravascular tissue spaces, vascular volume is reduced. Reduction of renal blood flow associated with decreased vascular volume initiates the compensatory release of aldosterone through the renin-angiotensin system. Reduction in vascular volume may also stimulate the release of antidiuretic hormone. These hormones promote the resorption of sodium and water from glomerular filtrate by the renal tubules. Because the resorbed sodium and water molecules are not large enough to be retained selectively in the vascular compartment by the capillary walls, they rapidly equilibrate with extravascular fluid compartments. The pharmacologic effects of these hormones tend to perpetuate and aggravate the edema in addition to expanding vascular volume.

Rupture of Urinary Bladder

Traumatic rupture of the urinary bladder is typically associated with a sudden increase in intravesical pressure in a bladder distended with urine. Traumatic rupture of the bladder in animals with no predisposing abnormalities of the urinary system has been most commonly encountered in male dogs and newborn foals. Traumatic rupture of the urinary bladder may occur in any species with partial or total obstruction of the urethra, especially if the integrity of the urinary bladder wall is altered by concomitant infection or neoplasia. Bladder rupture is a common sequela of the urethral obstruction

syndrome in male cats and steers, and occasionally occurs in female dogs with urethral calculi.

Because of the anatomic location of the urinary bladder in most domestic species of animals, rents in the bladder wall usually communicate with the peritoneal cavity.

Extravasation of urine from the excretory pathway of the urinary system into the peritoneal cavity is usually associated with severe ascites and peritonitis. Following accumulation of hyperosmolal urine in the peritoneal cavity, iso-osmolal fluid from the extravascular spaces moves into the peritoneal cavity in order to establish osmotic equilibrium. At the same time, high concentrations of solutes excreted in urine diffuse back into the body in order to establish solute equilibrium. The magnitude of these changes is dependent on urine osmolality and the rate of urine formation. If patients with ruptured urinary bladders are oliguric because of renal hypoperfusion associated with traumatic shock and/or loss of fluid into the peritoneal cavity, the onset of significant shifts in fluid balance may require more time to develop than would be the situation in patients with good renal function.

Because concentrated urine is irritating to tissues, peritonitis may develop. The severity of peritonitis may be aggravated by contamination with bacterial pathogens present in the urinary tract. Depending on the presence or absence of bacteria in urine at the time of rupture, cytologic evaluation of peritoneal fluid will reveal that it is an exudate (septic) or a modified transudate (nonseptic).

Enlargement of Urinary Bladder

Although uncommon, enlargement of the capacity of the urinary bladder of sufficient magnitude to cause visible distention of the abdomen may occur in dogs with neurogenic bladders or profound polyuria. Prolonged loss of ability of the detrusor muscle to contract as a result of impaired innervation may result in tremendous increase in the size of the urinary bladder. Neurogenic bladders with the capacity to hold up to 7 liters of urine have been observed in giant breeds of dogs.[13] We have also seen giant urinary bladders which are otherwise normal in dogs with profound polyuria caused by pituitary diabetes insipidus and portal vein anomalies.

Renal Trauma

Serious traumatic injuries to the kidneys are not a common clinical entity. This may be related to the fact that kidneys are not rigidly fixed in position, receive protection from vertebrae, ribs, and lumbar muscle mass, and are surrounded by a tough fibrous capsule.

Trauma of sufficient severity to cause large rents in the renal capsule and parenchyma may pose an immediate threat to life owing to exsanguination. Because of the tremendous blood supply to the kidneys, rupture of large renal arteries or veins, or avulsion of the renal artery and vein from the renal hilus may result in exsanguination and death in minutes. Traumatic rupture of the renal capsule and parenchyma may result in hemoperitoneum and eventually death if not corrected. Abdominal distention caused by hemoperitoneum may be associated with clinical signs characteristic of hypovolemic shock.

Renomegaly

Enlargement of one or both kidneys of sufficient magnitude to cause abdominal distention is uncommon, but may occur as a result of malignant neoplasms (renal cell carcinomas, nephroblastomas, leiomyosarcomas), unilateral hydronephrosis, and rarely polycystic disease.[13] Great enlargement of both kidneys will not occur in patients with bilateral hydronephrosis because death from uremia occurs before such extensive enlargement has time to develop.

Abdominal Pain

Abdominal pain may be caused by a wide variety of disorders including diseases of the urinary system. Unfortunately, little is known regarding its pathophysiology in animals.

The pattern of innervation of the parietal peritoneum is similar to the innervation of the skin and striated muscles in that it is characterized by numerous nerve endings without much overlapping.[67] Therefore lesions of the parietal peritoneum are typically associated with localized, severe, sharp pain. In contrast, the visceral peritoneum and abdominal viscera are supplied with fewer nerve endings per unit of tissue than the skin, and there is significant overlapping of areas supplied by different nerve fibers. Therefore inflammatory lesions that originate from abdominal viscera or visceral peritoneum are typically dull and poorly localized.[67]

Studies in man have revealed that renal pain is caused by stretching or compression of the peripelvic renal capsule and renal pelvis, by traction of the renal pedicle containing the renal artery and vein, and by intrarenal or extrarenal obstruction to urine outflow.[67,68,69] Portions of the renal capsule covering the greater curvature of the kidneys and the renal parenchyma itself apparently do not transmit sensations of pain. Presumably a similar situation occurs in animals.

It is known that renal pain is not associated with chronic generalized renal diseases, slowly growing neoplasms, chronic hydronephrosis or polycystic disease affecting dogs and cats. Although unproved, a similar situation would be expected to occur in other domestic animals. Since pain associated with renal disease occurs only when there is acute stretching or distention of the renal capsule, it would be expected to occur in association with acute obstruction to urine outflow at the level of the ureters or renal pelves, and with acute generalized nephritis or nephrosis.

Studies in man which may apply to animals indicate that so-called "ureteral colic" caused by ureteral calculi is not related to ureteral hyperperistalsis and spasm, but rather acute distention of the renal pelvis and upper ureter as a result of obstructed urine outflow.[68] The lower portion of the ureter of human beings is not sensitive to distention. The term ureteral colic is apparently a misnomer in that the pain originates from the kidneys rather than the ureters, and is constant rather than paroxysmal. The severity of the pain varies according to changes in the degree of ureteral obstruction.

Rupture of the urinary bladder associated with peritonitis may be associated with generalized severe abdominal pain if the parietal peritoneum is affected. If peritonitis is not severe and is localized to the caudal abdomen, abdominal pain may be less severe and more localized.

Overdistention of the urinary bladder caused by partial or complete obstruction of the urethra or herniation of the bladder into the perineum may be associated with discomfort and pain during digital palpation. Incorrect interpretation of client observations or superficial physical examinations may result in confusion of tenesmus caused by diseases of the lower intestinal tract with diseases of the lower urinary tract.

Azotemia

Azotemia is defined as the presence of abnormal concentrations of urea, creatinine, and other nonprotein nitrogenous substances in blood. Azotemia is a laboratory finding, and may or may not be caused by generalized lesions of renal parenchyma. Nonrenal causes of azotemia include decreased blood volume, decreased blood pressure, decreased colloidal osmotic pressure, and obstruction of both ureters, the bladder, or urethra (see Table 29–1).

Uremia is defined as the presence of abnormal quantities of urine constituents in blood caused by primary generalized renal disease and as the polysystemic toxic syndrome which occurs as a result of abnormal renal function. Although uremia is always accompanied by azotemia, azotemia may or may not be associated with uremia.

Serum concentrations of urea and creatinine are commonly used as a crude index of glomerular filtration rate. The basis for the statement that they are a crude index of glomerular filtration rate (GFR) is related to the fact that abnormal concentrations caused by damage to renal parenchyma cannot be detected until approximately three fourths of the functional capacity of the nephrons has been impaired. In addition the concentration of serum or plasma urea and creatinine may be affected by variables other than those associated with glomerular filtration rate.[13,70]

Despite the relative insensitivity of BUN and creatinine as indices of GFR, the ease with which they can be measured in plasma or serum, and the difficulty associated with more precise measurements of GFR, have resulted in their widespread clinical use. Meaningful interpretation of urea nitrogen and creatinine values, however, is dependent upon recognition of variables which influence glomerular filtration rate (see Table 29–1).

There is often significant variability between the serum concentration of urea nitrogen or creatinine and the severity of clinical signs of uremia. The latter may be related, at least in part, to the duration of the renal disease. Patients with acute renal failure often have severe polysystemic illness, even though their serum concentration of urea and creatinine is lower than that observed in asymptomatic patients with polyuric chronic renal failure. Progressive renal diseases that destroy renal parenchyma at a relatively slow rate allow the body to compensate for progressive but gradually developing alterations in fluid, acid-base, and electrolyte balance, and to minimize life-threatening imbalances. Because they survive for a longer period of time in a state of renal dysfunction, however, changes in other body systems are often much more severe in patients with chronic progressive primary renal failure.

Hyperamylasemia

Hyperamylasemia associated with naturally occurring primary renal failure has been observed in man[71,72] and dogs[73] without other clinical evidence of concomitant pancreatitis. Increased serum amylase activity has also been observed in dogs with experimentally induced renal failure.[74] Hyperamylasemia associated with primary renal failure is thought to occur, at least in part, as a result of impaired clearance of amylase by glomerular filtration. In one study of 28 dogs with spontaneously occurring primary renal failure, mean serum amylase activity was approximately 2.5 times normal as compared to amylase values of approximately seven times normal in dogs with histologically confirmed acute pancreatitis.[73] The mean serum amylase activity of dogs with probable acute pancreatitis was 2.5 times normal.

Although it is generally agreed that primary renal insufficiency may result in hyperamylasemia, the degree of elevation that may be attributed solely to renal malfunction is unclear. No obvious relationship existed between the degree of azotemia and the degree of hyperamylasemia in uremic dogs.[73] Detection of lesions in the pancreas of uremic humans and dogs has prompted speculation that uremia-induced pancreatitis may contribute to the magnitude of azotemic hyperamylasemia in some cases.[34,60,75] To date, however, the function of the exocrine pancreas has not been investigated in man or animals with renal failure, and involvement of pancreas in uremia is at best only a histologic entity.

Studies in dogs indicate that amylase may be eliminated from the circulation via the liver as well as by renal clearance.[76] In man, it has been estimated that only about 24% of the serum amylase is excreted in urine.[71] The fact that amylase may be removed from the circulation of extrarenal routes may explain why only modest increases in serum amylase activity occur in association with primary renal failure. This hypothesis is supported by the lack of correlation between serum and urine amylase activity in dogs with experimentally produced pancreatitis.[77]

Hyperlipasemia has been observed in uremic humans and rats but has not been carefully investigated in uremic domestic animals.[78,79]

Hypocalcemia

Abnormalities in serum calcium may be a cause (hypercalcemia) or a result (hypocalcemia) of renal failure in man, dogs, and laboratory rodents. Unlike the usual situation in man and other domestic animals, hypercalcemia has been reported in horses as a secondary manifestation of primary renal failure.[80] A few cases of hypercalcemia following onset of primary renal failure have been reported in man,[81,82] and we also have observed them in a few dogs with chronic primary renal failure. It is tempting to speculate that a possible cause of secondary hypercalcemia in uremic patients is impaired renal metabolism of parathormone or prostaglandins. Retention of calcium caused by reduced glomerular filtration and/or overproduction of parathormone by hyperplastic parathyroid glands may also be involved.

A variable degree of hypocalcemia and hyperphosphatemia typically develop in man and dogs as a result of renal failure, regardless of cause.[21] Although the precise mechanisms responsible for initiating and perpetuating hypocalcemia have not been established, they are thought to be related to one or more of the following abnormalities: (1) impairment of renal metabolism of vitamin D_3 to its metabolically active form, with resultant decreased intestinal absorption of calcium; (2) increased urinary excretion of calcium caused by impaired ability to reabsorb calcium; (3) decreased intake of calcium in protein-restricted diets; or (4) hyperphosphatemia which occurs as a result of decreased glomerular filtration. As a result of hyperphosphatemia, abnormal quantities of phosphorus enter the intestinal lumen and form nonabsorbable salts with dietary calcium. Hyperphosphatemia also alters the normal calcium-phosphorus ratio in plasma and results in precipitation of calcium salts in various body tissues.

Defective intestinal absorption of calcium is a significant cause of abnormal calcium balance in patients with severe uremia. Recent evidence suggests that impaired intestinal absorption of calcium is caused by an acquired defect in vitamin (prohormone) D metabolism.[18] Before acting on target cells in the intestine, vitamin D_3 must be converted to 25-hydroxycholecalciferol by liver mitochondrial enzymes, and then to 1,25-dihydroxycholecalciferol by mitochondrial enzymes in the kidney. 1,25-Dihydroxycholecalciferol is the most metabolically active known form of vitamin D, and available data indicate that it can be produced only by the kidneys.

Although it is not known when during the course of progressive chronic generalized renal disease that intestinal malabsorption occurs, it cannot be detected in human patients with mild renal failure.[83] Administration of small quantities of 1,25-dihydroxycholecalciferol to acutely uremic rats[84] and human beings with chronic renal failure[85] stimulated intestinal calcium transport and augmented calcium mobilization from bone. Vitamin D analogues have also been shown to improve intestinal calcium absorption from uremic human beings.[86]

Repeated administration of large doses of methyl-guanidine to normal dogs also decreased intestinal absorption of calcium.[87]

Hyperglycemia

Until recently, knowledge of the effect of chronic renal failure on glucose and insulin metabolism has been limited to two seemingly paradoxical clinical observations in man.[87] One is that hyperglycemia occasionally developed in patients with chronic renal failure, and the other was that insulin requirements of patients with diabetes mellitus decreased with the onset of renal insufficiency.

Glucose intolerance in patients with primary renal failure is sometimes called azotemic pseudodiabetes because patients have a diabetic-like glucose tolerance curve. In contrast to diabetes mellitus, however, azotemic pseudodiabetes is not associated with severe hyperglycemia, glucosuria, ketonuria, ketonemia, or severe metabolic acidosis.[9,88] Glucose intolerance in uremic patients is characterized by mild prolongation of hyperglycemia following oral or intravenous administration of glucose.[89] Fasting blood glucose concentrations in uremic dogs are usually normal, and when elevated do not exceed 150 mg/dl.[9] The degree of glucose intolerance is proportional to the degree of azotemia.

There is no evidence to suggest that glucose intolerance associated with azotemia is related to a primary defect in insulin secretion. In fact, an increase in plasma insulin concentration usually occurs.[90] It has been hypothesized that peripheral resistance to insulin-mediated uptake of glucose by tissues is the cause of azotemic glucose intolerance.[11,88] This hypothesis is supported by studies which indicate that the ability of exogenous insulin to lower plasma glucose concentration is impaired in uremic humans and dogs.[89] Although it appears that peripheral insulin resistance occurs in uremia, the underlying cause is obscure. Metabolic acidosis has been incriminated, but has been found to play only a minor role in dogs with experimentally induced renal failure.[9,89] Abnormal glucose tolerance curves have been induced in dogs with urea, but not methylguanidine.[87]

With the exception of the obvious need to differentiate azotemic pseudodiabetes from diabetes mellitus complicated by uremia, the clinical implications of abnormal glucose tolerance in uremia are not yet known. Peritoneal dialysate solutions with high concentrations of glucose should be used with caution.

Studies in dogs indicate that a profound effect of renal insufficiency on glucose and insulin metabolism is marked reduction in removal of insulin from plasma as a result of loss of functional renal parenchyma.[89] Dog kidneys remove approximately two thirds of the insulin that reaches the general circulation.[91] Since only a small amount of the insulin removed by the kidneys is excreted in urine, the kidneys appear to be an important site of insulin degradation.

The modest rise in serum creatinine concentration that occurs immediately following bilateral nephrectomy in dogs is associated with a considerable reduction in the rate of loss of insulin from plasma.[89] However, the onset of severe uremia several days following nephrectomy is not associated with further reduction in the half-life of insulin. These observations indicate that uremia per se has little effect on the rate of insulin removal from plasma, and that loss of renal parenchyma is primarily responsible for prolongation of the half-life of insulin in dogs with renal insufficiency. Impaired renal degradation of insulin is the best available explanation of the observation that uremic humans with diabetes mellitus require less insulin than nonuremic diabetics.

Studies in dogs also indicate that the net amount of insulin entering the general circulation decreases after nephrectomy.[89] It appears that the dog responds to impaired renal degradation of insulin by secreting less insulin.

LOCALIZATION OF SIGNS COMMON TO URINARY AND GASTROINTESTINAL DYSFUNCTION

In our opinion, the first step in the diagnostic process must be to define and verify the presence of clinical problems. These are essential beginning components since one must be able to define problems before they can be solved. Errors made in identification and verification of clinical problems may not only lead to the fruitless pursuit of nonexistent disorders; they may also result in a costly and time-consuming series of diagnostic and therapeutic plans before errors are identified.

Following accurate definition of problems from data collected from the history, physical examination, and (where appropriate) laboratory and radiographic procedures, a complete problem list should be constructed.[92,93] Problems should be stated at their highest level of refinement, and should be defined in such a way that their refinement can be defended with reasonable certainty on the basis of current knowledge about the patient. Listed from the lowest to the highest level of refinement, problems may be defined as: (1) a clinical sign (vomiting, polydipsia, diarrhea); (2) an abnormal laboratory finding (leukocytosis, hyperlipidemia, hyperamylasemia, bilirubinuria); (3) a pathophysiologic syndrome (nephrotic syndrome, renal failure); and (4) a diagnostic entity (pyelonephritis, renal carcinoma, renal amyloidosis).

When formulating a list of problems, it is useful to group signs (problems) according to the system or organ to which they are related. In other words, localization of problems should follow their definition and verification. For example, if a patient is examined because of vomiting, but no other abnormalities are initially identified, the problem should be listed as vomiting. Additional information is usually required to determine the location (esophagus, stomach, duodenum, kidneys, adrenal glands, liver, pancreas) and cause (anomalies, metabolic disturbances, neoplasia, infection, foreign body, exogenous or endogenous toxins) of the vomiting. On the other hand, if the vomitus contains exogenous foreign material, the problem might be defined as gastrointestinal foreign body accompanied by vomiting.

Disciplined thought is required to construct a meaningful problem list. When integrating problems to their highest level of refinement, it is important to consider that clinical manifestations of disease are usually a combination of: (1) signs induced by the disease (such as obligatory polyuria associated with primary renal failure); and (2) the compensatory reaction of the body to these signs (compensatory polydipsia that replaces fluid lost as a result of primary polyuric renal failure).

Anorexia, Depression, and Weight Loss

Anorexia, depression, and weight loss may occur as a result of such a variety of disorders that they usually are not of help in localizing their underlying cause to a body system or organ. Additional information must be obtained before these problems may be further refined. Anorexia, depression, and weight loss caused by renal dysfunction typically do not develop until approximately three fourths of the nephrons are damaged.

Uremic Stomatitis

Brownish discoloration of the dorsal aspect of the tongue, ulceration of the oral mucosa, and gingival hemorrhage are typically associated with other signs of severe renal failure including anorexia, depression, weight loss, vomiting, and dehydration. They are not pathognomonic of uremia, however.

Additional information must be obtained before these problems are further refined.

Vomiting

If clinical dehydration occurs in a vomiting patient with adequate renal function, the expected compensatory response by the kidneys is to conserve water in excess of solute by producing concentrated urine (physiologic oliguria). Therefore if clinical dehydration occurs in a vomiting patient with polyuria, it is evident that the kidneys are unable to conserve water in spite of the body's need for water. Under this circumstance, primary disorders of the esophagus, stomach and intestines, and acute pancreatitis would not be probable underlying causes of the vomiting.

In dogs and cats, vomiting, dehydration, and polyuria are frequently associated with primary polyuric renal failure, diabetic ketoacidosis, severe pyometra and, in some patients, with congenital or acquired generalized liver disease. Although polyuria, polydipsia and dehydration may be associated with pituitary diabetes insipidus, nephrogenic diabetes insipidus, hyperadrenocorticism and psychogenic polydipsia, these diseases are not typically associated with severe vomiting.

Disorders with the potential to cause impaired ability to concentrate urine, vomiting and dehydration are not always associated with polyuria. Acute oliguric primary renal failure and hypoadrenocorticism are notable examples of such diseases.

Diarrhea

Black tarry feces caused by renal failure is usually associated with other signs of uremia including vomiting, uremic stomatitis, anorexia, depression, and weight loss. It does not usually occur as an isolated uremic sign, and is not a constant finding associated with uremia.

Transudative Ascites

Since protein-losing glomerulopathies are not the only potential causes of transudative ascites and pitting edema of subcutaneous tissue, non-renal causes of abnormal fluid accumulation, including protein-losing enteropathies, hepatic cirrhosis, portal vein anomalies, and congestive heart failure, should be considered (Table 29–10).

The nephrotic syndrome is associated with proteinuria, hypoproteinemia, hypoalbuminemia, hypercholesterolemia, and usually edema. Pitting non-painful edema of the subcutaneous tissue of the ventral midline and rear limbs is common. Ascites, and less commonly hydrothorax, may occur in cases associated with severe hypoalbuminemia.

All types of glomerular disease have the potential to induce the nephrotic syndrome. A specific glomerular disease in its mildest form may result in mild proteinuria that is insufficient to cause hypoalbuminemia and other manifestations of the nephrotic syndrome. The same mild disease in another patient, or at a different stage in the same patient, may cause severe proteinuria and other signs of the nephrotic syndrome. Glomerulonephritic animals may develop all features of the nephrotic syndrome except edema. Even when present the edema varies greatly in severity from individual to individual and within the same individual. In fact clinical and biochemical manifestations may undergo complete remission without treatment.[65]

In addition to the biologic behavior of the underlying cause, the unpredictable variability of the natural clinical course of the nephrotic syndrome is related to fluctuations in the activity of aldosterone and antidiuretic hormone, and the concentration of electrolytes, colloids and water within the body compartments. Of these factors, the severity of the proteinuria and hypoalbuminemia is probably the

Table 29–10. Some distinguishing characteristics of common causes of transudative ascites

Factor	Nephrotic Syndrome	Protein-Losing Enteropathy	Cirrhotic Syndrome	Congestive Heart Failure
Subcutaneous edema	Variable	Variable	Usually absent	Absent
Ascites	Variable	Variable	Variable	Variable
Diarrhea	Usually absent	Present	Variable	Usually absent
Urine protein	Profound	Absent	Absent	Usually absent
Serum protein	Decreased	Decreased	Normal to decreased	Normal
Serum albumin	Decreased	Decreased	Normal to decreased	Normal
Serum globulins	Normal to increased	Normal to decreased	Variable	Normal
Serum cholesterol	Increased	Decreased	Variable	Normal
Intestinal fat absorption	Normal	Decreased	Normal	Normal
Intestinal D-xylose absorption	Normal	Normal to decreased	Normal	Normal
Hemoglobin	Normal to decreased	Normal to decreased	Normal	Normal to increased

most significant. As a generality, subcutaneous edema does not develop unless serum albumin concentration is less than 0.8 to 1.0 g per 100 ml. Because of variations in the capacity of the body to compensate for increased protein loss by increased hepatic protein synthesis, and because of fluctuations in the concentrations of the hormones and electrolytes, however, not all patients with serum albumin concentrations of this magnitude develop edema.

With the progression of glomerular lesions and the onset of primary renal failure, the severity of proteinuria, hypoproteinemia, and edema may decrease. This decrease occurs when reduction in glomerular perfusion with plasma is of such magnitude that it results in a significant reduction in the clearance of protein. In contrast to patients with remission of glomerular lesions, however, uremic nephrotic patients show a progressive increase in concentration of serum creatinine and urea nitrogen and a progressive loss of ability to concentrate or dilute urine.

Exudative Ascites

Rupture of the urinary bladder is the most common cause of exudative ascites that must be differentiated from other forms of peritonitis including rupture of the stomach, intestines, uterus, and gallbladder.

Clinical findings associated with rupture of the urinary bladder are variable, depending on the precipitating cause and duration of urine leakage. Significant findings in the history may include recent trauma, attempts to manually express a bladder distended with urine, and sudden onset of depression, vomiting, a stiff gait, and abdominal pain. Physical examination may reveal abdominal pain, spasm of abdominal musculature, ascites, inability to palpate the urinary bladder, and partial or total obstruction of the urethra.

Post-renal azotemia caused by rupture of the urinary bladder is characterized by azotemia, hyperphosphatemia, hemoconcentration, hyponatremia, and eventually hyperkalemia.[13,94] Microscopic evaluation of ascitic fluid removed by paracentesis typically reveals polymorphonuclear leukocytes, red cells, macrophages, degenerate mesothelial cells, and occasionally bacteria. The concentration of urea nitrogen in plasma and ascitic fluid is usually elevated to a similar degree. The concentration of creatinine in ascitic fluid is often higher than it is in serum or plasma. This may be related, at least in part, to the fact that creatinine has a larger molecular weight than urea (see Table 29-2).

Diagnosis of exudative ascites caused by rupture of the urinary bladder is best confirmed by positive contrast cystography.[13,94]

Abdominal Pain

When possible the presence or absence of renal pain should be evaluated by palpation of the kidneys rather than palpation of the lumbar muscles or vertebral column. Since pain localized to the area normally occupied by the kidneys can be caused by non-renal disorders (spinal cord disorders, bone diseases, intervertebral disc disease, gastrointestinal disorders), its significance should be evaluated by laboratory and/or radiographic techniques.

Azotemia

Dysfunction of the kidneys which is severe enough to cause reduction in glomerular filtration rate (GFR) and subsequent retention of metabolites (such as creatinine, urea and phosphorus) that are normally cleared from plasma by glomerular filtration is often associated with vomiting and anorexia. Serum and plasma concentrations of urea and creatinine are commonly used as crude indices of glomerular filtration rate. Abnormal concentrations of these nonprotein nitrogenous substances in blood, plasma, or serum is defined as azotemia.

Reduction in glomerular filtration may be caused by alterations in blood volume, blood pressure, colloidal osmotic pressure, the number of patent renal arteries and glomerular capillaries, the permeability of glomerular capillaries, renal interstitial pressure, and/or renal intratubular pressure. Thus glomerular filtration is dependent on pre-renal components (blood volume, blood pressure, colloidal osmotic pressure), renal components (patency of renal arteries and glomerular capillaries, permeability of glomerular capillaries, renal interstitial pressure, renal intratubular pressure), and post-renal components (influence of patency of ureters, bladder, and urethra on intratubular pressure). Therefore the cause(s) of reduction in glomerular filtration may be categorized as pre-renal, primary renal, and post-renal. Because of clinically significant differences in pathogenesis, prognosis, and treatment, it is recommended that causes of decreased glomerular filtration associated with azotemia always be localized according to this classification (see Table 29-1).

Pre-renal Azotemia

Nonurinary diseases, including gastroenteritis, pancreatitis, and hepatic disorders, may cause varying degrees of reduction in GFR as a result of decreased renal blood flow. Inadequate perfusion of normal glomeruli with blood, regardless of cause (dehydration, decreased cardiac output, hypovolemic shock, hypoadrenocorticism, decreased colloidal osmotic pressure), may cause pre-renal azotemia. Pre-renal azotemia is associated with structurally normal kidneys which are capable of quantitatively normal renal function, provided compromised renal perfusion is corrected prior to the onset of generalized ischemic nephron damage. Development of primary renal failure due to ischemia prolongs and reduces the likelihood of complete recovery. A diagnosis of pre-renal azotemia should be considered if abnormal elevation in the serum or plasma concentration of urea nitrogen or creatinine is associated with concentrated urine (specific gravity > 1.025) in patients with no specific evidence of generalized glomerular disease (Tables 29–4 and 29–11).[13] Such patients do not have a history of polyuria because they have compensatory physiologic oliguria. Detection of a urine specific gravity greater than approximately 1.025 in association with azotemia indicates that a sufficient quantity of functional nephrons are present to concentrate glomerular filtrate (i.e., at least one third of the total nephron population). Contrary to the once popular theory, acute renal diseases of sufficient severity to cause renal failure are not characteristically associated with elevated (> 1.025) specific gravities. Significant elevations in the serum or plasma concentration of urea nitrogen or creatinine due to primary renal failure cannot be detected until approximately 70 to 75% of the nephron population is nonfunctional. Concentration of urine (indicated by high specific gravity) associated with pre-renal

azotemia reflects a compensatory response by the body to combat low perfusion pressure and blood volume by secreting antidiuretic hormone (and possibly other substances) to conserve water filtered through glomeruli. Restoration of renal perfusion by appropriate volume replacement therapy is typically followed by a dramatic drop in the concentration of serum urea and creatinine to normal in approximately 1 to 3 days.

Another form of potentially reversible pre-renal azotemia may develop in patients with severe hypoalbuminemia caused by generalized glomerular disease, and perhaps by protein-losing enteropathies. Decreased renal blood flow and glomerular filtration which occur in association with marked reduction in vascular volume secondary to reduction in colloidal osmotic pressure may result in a proportionate degree of retention of substances normally cleared by the kidneys. Therefore the significance of an abnormal increase in the serum concentration of urea nitrogen or creatinine must be carefully defined in hypoproteinemic edematous patients. Azotemia cannot be accepted as indisputable evidence of severe renal lesions since it may be associated with a potentially reversible decrease in renal perfusion caused by hypoalbuminemia.

Glomerulotubular Imbalance

Abnormal elevation in the serum concentration of urea nitrogen or creatinine may also occur in association with an elevated urine specific gravity (~ 1.020) in some patients with primary renal failure caused by generalized glomerular disease.[66] A conceptual understanding of azotemia associated with primary renal failure and glomerulotubular imbalance is essential to differentiate this syndrome from pre-renal azotemia.

Caution should be used not to overinterpret the absolute value of urine specific gravity of proteinuric patients with glomerular disease, since it

Table 29–11. Common and distinguishing features of acute pancreatitis simulating primary renal failure

	Disorder	
Factor	Acute Pancreatitis and Pre-renal Azotemia	Primary Renal Failure
Serum amylase activity	Elevated	Elevated
Serum lipase activity	Elevated	Elevated
Serum urea concentration	Elevated	Elevated
Serum creatinine concentration	Elevated	Elevated
Urine volume	Physiologic oliguria	Pathologic oliguria or pathologic polyuria
Urine specific gravity	>1.025	1.007 to ±1.024

Table 29–12. Differentiation of pre-renal azotemia from glomerulotubular imbalance associated with primary azotemia

Factor	Pre-renal Azotemia	Glomerulotubular Imbalance
BUN	Increased	Increased
Creatinine	Increased	Increased
Urine specific gravity	>1.025	1.015–1.025
Proteinuria	Usually negative	Positive
Pre-renal cause	Present	Absent
Response to correction of renal perfusion	Within 1 to 3 days	Minimal

may be falsely elevated by the effect of protein. Addition of 400 mg of protein per 100 ml of urine will increase the urine specific gravity by approximately 0.001.[13]

The renal lesion in patients with primary azotemia and glomerulotubular imbalance must be characterized by glomerular damage which is sufficiently severe to impair renal clearance of urea and creatinine, but which has not yet induced a sufficient degree of ischemic atrophy and necrosis of renal tubular cells to prevent urine concentration. Thus glomerular filtrate that is formed can be concentrated, at least to some degree. The specific gravity rarely exceeds 1.025, however, possibly as a result of obligatory solute diuresis. This group of patients may be differentiated from patients with pre-renal azotemia by failure of a search for one of the non-renal causes of poor renal perfusion, by the presence of persistent proteinuria, and by lack of response to restoration of vascular volume and perfusion with appropriate therapy (Table 29–12).

Primary Renal Azotemia

The specific gravity of glomerular filtrate is approximately 1.008 to 1.012. Impaired ability to concentrate or dilute glomerular filtrate is a consistent finding in acute or chronic, oliguric or polyuric, reversible or irreversible, primary renal diseases (anomalies, infections, exogenous or endogenous toxins, ischemia, immune disorders, obstruction, neoplasia, trauma, hypercalcemia) that damage a sufficient population of nephrons. Because of the kidneys' tremendous reserve capacity, impairment of their ability to concentrate or dilute urine cannot be detected until at least two thirds of the total population of nephrons have been functionally incapacitated. Significant elevations in the serum or plasma concentration of urea nitrogen or creatinine that occur as a result of disorders localized to the kidney cannot be detected until 70 to 75% of the nephrons have been functionally incapacitated.

Total loss of ability to concentrate and dilute urine does not always occur as a sudden event, but often develops gradually. For this reason a urine specific gravity between approximately 1.007 and 1.024 associated with clinical dehydration or azotemia is indicative of primary renal azotemia (see Tables 29–4 and 29–5). Total inability of the nephrons to concentrate or dilute urine (so-called fixation of specific gravity) results in the formation of urine that is similar to that of glomerular filtrate (1.008 to 1.012).

If sufficient clinical evidence is present to warrant examination of the patient's renal function by determining the serum concentration of creatinine or urea nitrogen, the urine specific gravity should be evaluated at the same time. As emphasized in the section on pre-renal azotemia, a concentrated urine sample (SG >1.025) associated with azotemia suggests the probability of pre-renal disturbances (see Tables 29–4 and 29–11). If dehydrated and/or azotemic patients have impaired ability to concentrate or dilute urine (SG ≃ 1.007 to 1.024), it may be concluded that acute or chronic generalized renal disease is the probable underlying cause.

If the kidneys of a non-azotemic, dehydrated patient are unable to conserve water despite the stimulus for the release of antidiuretic hormone, either the kidneys are unable to respond to ADH because of generalized renal disease or renal diabetes insipidus, or the patient has pituitary diabetes insipidus. Azotemia in the absence of clinical dehydration, but associated with a urine specific gravity of approximately 1.007 to 1.024, also indicates the probability of primary renal failure. In this situation, impaired ability to concentrate and dilute urine is related, at least in part, to compensatory increase in glomerular filtration rate of viable glomeruli, decreased fractional tubular reabsorption of sodium and phosphorus by viable nephrons, loss of medullary hyperosmolality, and obligatory osmotic diuresis.[20]

If non-dehydrated, non-azotemic patients suspected of having pathologic polyuria do not have urine specific gravities that indicate the kidneys can definitely concentrate urine, further tests are required before meaningful conclusions can be established about the kidneys' capacity to concentrate urine. Following a water deprivation test, patients with adequate renal function will excrete urine with an elevated specific gravity (> 1.025), high osmolality, and relatively small volume.[21] Patients still unable to concentrate urine following water deprivation may be given an exogenous source of ADH to prove or disprove the presence of pituitary diabetes insipidus.

Post-Renal Azotemia

Post-renal azotemia is caused by diseases which prevent elimination of urine from the body. Causes include complete obstruction of the excretory pathway and communication of the excretory pathway with the peritoneal cavity. Unilateral ureteral occlusion is not associated with azotemia unless generalized disease of the nonobstructed kidney is also present.

Azotemia secondary to obstruction of urine outflow occurs as a result of abnormally high intratubular pressure which impairs or inhibits glomerular filtration. Like pre-renal azotemia, post-renal azotemia is initially associated with structurally normal kidneys that are capable of quantitatively normal renal function, providing the underlying cause is rapidly corrected. If the patient survives for a long enough period of time, however, renal lesions caused by increased renal pressure and decreased renal blood flow may develop. Untreated patients with complete obstruction to urine outflow usually die within 3 to 6 days, prior to development of significant structural lesions. Death is related to severe deficits and excesses in fluid and electrolyte, and to acid-base imbalance, and accumulation of metabolic waste products.

Azotemia which occurs as a sequela to rupture of the excretory pathway is primarily related to absorption of urine from the peritoneal cavity. Unless damaged as a result of hypovolemic shock secondary to the traumatic event that caused rupture of the excretory pathway or loss of fluid into the peritoneal cavity, the kidneys are structurally normal.

Because of its variability, the urine specific gravity of patients with post-renal azotemia is not relied on to the same degree as it is in patients with primary renal and pre-renal azotemia. Although a complete urinalysis should always be performed in such patients, the presence of azotemia in association with characteristic findings of obstruction or loss of continuity of the excretory pathway detected by history, physical examination, and radiography provide the best criteria with which to establish the presence of post-renal azotemia. Characteristic clinical findings include oliguria or anuria, dysuria, tenesmus, palpation of lesions obstructing the urethra, urinary bladder or both ureters, detection of urine in the peritoneal cavity by paracentesis, and radiographic evidence of lesions in the excretory pathway.

Primary Renal Azotemia with Concomitant Pre-renal or Post-renal Azotemia

Because kidneys with generalized disease have diminished ability to compensate for stresses imposed by concomitant diseases of other body systems, uremic crises may be abruptly precipitated by a variety of pre-renal, and less commonly post-renal, disorders which develop in patients with previously compensated chronic renal failure. For example, factors that accelerate endogenous protein catabolism (anorexia, infection and extensive tissue necrosis) may significantly increase the quantity of metabolic by-products in the body, since the kidneys have impaired capacity to excrete them. Stress states (fever, infection, and change in environment) are associated with release of glucocorticoids from the adrenal glands. Glucocorticoids stimulate conversion of proteins to carbohydrates (gluconeogenesis) and thus increase the quantity of protein metabolic by-products in the body. In these situations, uremic crises may be precipitated since protein by-products contribute significantly to the production of uremic signs in patients with renal failure. Any nonrenal abnormality that decreases renal perfusion (vomiting, diarrhea, decreased water consumption, shock, and cardiac decompensation) may also result in decomposition of primary renal failure.

Precipitation of uremic crises in patients with previously compensated primary renal failure by extrarenal diseases may be difficult to detect, especially if both disorders are associated with vomiting, polydipsia, dehydration, anorexia, depression, and weight loss. A high index of suspicion, and diagnosis by therapeutic trial is often necessary. Whereas patients with uremic crises precipitated by reversible extrarenal disorders (pancreatitis, hepatic disease, gastroenteritis) may rapidly respond to supportive and symptomatic therapy, patients with uremic crises caused by progressive irreversible destruction of nephrons will not respond rapidly.

Hyperamylasemia

Elevated serum amylase activity is not pathognomonic of acute pancreatitis since it may also be associated with primary renal failure. Knowledge of the serum concentration of urea or creatinine may not permit differentiation of pancreatitis from primary renal failure since vomiting induced by pancreatitis may result in fluid loss of sufficient magnitude to cause pre-renal azotemia. Evaluation of the ability of the kidneys to concentrate urine is of great value in distinguishing between acute pancreatitis and primary renal failure, however, provided both diseases are not present simultaneously (see Table 29–11). Acute pancreatitis in dogs is typically associated with severe hyperamylasemia (up to seven times normal values), occasionally azotemia, and ability of the kidneys to concentrate urine (SG > 1.025). Primary renal failure is typically associated with moderate azotemia, impaired ability to concentrate or dilute urine (SG = 1.007 to 1.024), and frequently, moderate hyperamylasemia (two to three times normal values).

Because of the potential value of urine specific gravity in evaluation of the cause of hyperamylasemia, it is essential that urine for analysis be collected prior to administration of fluids to correct dehydration. Once fluids have been administered, it is not possible to assess with certainty whether the formation of dilute urine occurred as a result of renal dysfunction or renal excretion of therapeutic fluids.

Since uremic hyperamylasemia in dogs is usually associated with serum amylase activity that is two to three times normal, larger elevations in serum amylase values in uremic patients suggest the concomitant presence of acute pancreatitis.

The value of serum lipase in providing information that will help to differentiate acute pancreatitis from primary renal failure in domestic animals is unknown. In a survey of 15 dogs with spontaneously-occurring primary renal failure at our practice, 10 had hyperamylasemia, hyperlipasemia, and azotemia. Five azotemic dogs had hyperamylasemia but did not have hyperlipasemia.

Hypocalcemia

Since serum calcium values vary with the analytic method employed, normal values should be determined for each laboratory. The significance of serum calcium concentration should be considered in association with the serum protein concentration, since approximately 50% of the serum calcium is bound to protein. It follows that hypoproteinemia (especially hypoalbuminemia) may be associated with a decrease in total serum calcium concentration, but a normal ionized calcium concentration. Hypoproteinemia associated with protein-losing enteropathies and protein-losing glomerulonephropathies are frequently associated with mild hypocalcemia (8.0 to 9.0 mg/dl).

Because of obvious differences in the spectrum and duration of associated clinical signs and laboratory abnormalities, hypocalcemia associated with chronic primary renal failure is not difficult to distinguish from the infrequently occurring hypocalcemia associated with acute pancreatitis.

Hyperglycemia

Most animals with primary renal failure have normal blood glucose concentrations. Blood glucose concentrations up to, but usually not greater than, 150 mg/dl have apparently been observed in dogs with primary renal failure.[9] Diabetic-like glucose tolerance curves have been observed in dogs with experimentally induced primary renal failure, and presumably occur in dogs with naturally occurring primary renal failure. In contrast to diabetes mellitus, however, azotemic pseudodiabetes is not associated with marked hyperglycemia, glucosuria, ketonuria, or ketonemia.

REFERENCES

1. Katz, A.I., and Lindheimer, M.D.: Actions of hormones on the kidney. Ann. Rev. Physiol. 39:97, 1977.
2. Monke, J.V., and Yuile, C.L.: The renal clearance of hemoglobin in the dog. J. Exp. Med. 72:149, 1940.
3. Bayliss, L.E., Tookey-Kerridge, M., and Russell, D.S.: The excretion of protein by the mammalian kidney. J. Physiol. 77:386, 1933.
4. Ganong, W.F.: Review of Medical Physiology, 7th ed. Los Altos, Lange Medical Publications, 1975.
5. Oliver, J.E., and Osborne, C.A.: Neurogenic urinary incontinence. In Current Veterinary Therapy, Vol. VI. Edited by R.W. Kirk. Philadelphia, W. B. Saunders Co., 1977.
6. Osborne, C.A., Low, D.G., and Finco, D.R.: Reversible versus irreversible renal disease in the dog. J. A. V. M. A. 155:2062, 1969.
7. Osborne, C.A., and Low, D.G.: The application of principles of fluid and electrolyte therapy to patients with renal failure. J. A. A. H. A. 8:181, 1972.
8. Bergstrom, J., and Biltar, E.E.: The basis of uremic toxicity. In The Biologic Basis of Medicine, Vol. VI. Edited by E.E. Biltar and N. Biltar. New York, Academic Press, 1969.
9. Bovee, K.C.: The uremic syndrome. J. A. A. H. A. 12:189–197, 1976.
10. Giovannetti, S., and Barsolti, G.: Uremic intoxication. Nephron 14:123, 1975.
11. Merrill, J.P., and Hampers, C.L.: Uremia. N. Engl. J. Med. 282:953 and 1014, 1970.
12. Schreiner, G.E., and Maher, J.F.: Uremia: Biochemistry, Pathogenesis, and Treatment. Springfield, IL, Charles C Thomas Publisher, 1961.
13. Osborne, C.A., Low, D.G., and Finco, D.R.: Canine and Feline Urology. Philadelphia, W. B. Saunders Co., 1972.
14. Osborne, C.A., and Klausner, J.S.: Adverse drug reactions in the uremic patient. In Current Veterinary Therapy, Vol. VI. Edited by R.W. Kirk. Philadelphia, W. B. Saunders Co., 1977.
15. Osborne, C.A., and Johnston, S.D.: Ectopic hormone production by nonendocrine neoplasms. In Current Veterinary Therapy, Vol. VI. Edited by R.W. Kirk. Philadelphia, W. B. Saunders Co., 1977.
16. Osborne, C.A., and Stevens, J.B.: Pseudohyperparathyroidism in the dog. J. A. V. M. A. 162:125, 1973.
17. Osborne, C.A., Stevens, J.B., and Yano, B.L.: Hypercalcemic nephropathy. In Spontaneous Animal Models of Human Disease. New York, Academic Press. In press.
18. Capen, C.C., Belshaw, B.E., and Martin, S.L.: Endocrine disorders. In Textbook of Veterinary Internal Medicine. Edited by S. J. Ettinger. Philadelphia, W. B. Saunders Co., 1975.
19. McDonald, L.E.: Veterinary Endocrinology and Reproduction, 2nd ed. Philadelphia, Lea & Febiger, 1975.
20. Finco, D.R., Osborne, C.A., and Low, D.G.: Physiology and pathophysiology of renal failure. In Textbook of Veterinary Internal Medicine. Edited by S. J. Ettinger. Philadelphia, W. B. Saunders Co., 1975.
21. Osborne, C.A., Finco, D.R., and Low, D.G.: Renal Failure: Diagnosis, treatment, and prognosis. In Textbook of Veterinary Internal Medicine. Edited by S. J. Ettinger. Philadelphia, W. B. Saunders Co., 1975.

22. Giovanetti, S., Biagini, M., Balestri, P.L., Navalesi, R., Giagnoni, P., deMatteis, A., Ferro-Milone, P., and Perfetti, C.: Uremia-like syndrome in dogs chronically intoxicated with methylguanidine and creatinine. Clin. Sci. 36:445, 1969.

23. Barsotti, G., Bevilacqua, G., Morelli, E., Cappelli, P., Balestri, P.L., and Giovanetti, S.: Toxicity arising from guanidine compounds: role of methylguanidine as a uremic toxin. Kidney Int. 7:S–299, 1975.

24. Borison, H.L., and Hebertson, L.M.: Role of medullary emetic chemoreceptor trigger zone in post-nephrectomy vomiting dogs. Am. J. Physiol. 197:850, 1959.

25. Gulyassay, P.F., Aviram, A., and Peters, J.H.: Evaluation of amino acid and protein requirements in chronic uremia. Arch. Intern. Med. 126:855, 1970.

26. Denneberg, T., Lindbein, T., Berg, N.O., and Dahlquist, A.: Morphology, dipeptidases, and disaccharidases of small intestinal mucosa in chronic renal failure. Acta Med. Scand. 195:465, 1974.

27. Bliss, S.: The cause of sore mouth in nephritis. J. Biol. Chem. 121:425, 1937.

28. Gruskin, S.E., Tolman, D.E., and Wagoner, R.D.: Oral manifestations of uremia. Minn. Med. 53:495, 1970.

29. Larato, D.C.: Uremic stomatitis: report of a case. J. Periodontol. 46:731, 1975.

30. Johnson, W.J., Hagge, W.W., Wagoner, R.D., Dinapoli, R.P., and Rosevear, J.W.: Effects of urea loading in patients with far-advanced renal failure. Mayo Clin. Proc. 47:21, 1972.

31. Giovanetti, S., Balestri, P.L., and Barsotti, G.: Methylguanidine in uremia. Arch. Intern. Med. 131:709, 1973.

32. Gonella, M., Barsotti, G., Lupetti, S., Giovanetti, S., Campa, V., and Falcone, G.: Role of Aerobic Gut Flora on Creatinine and Methylguanidine Metabolism. Proc. 6th Congr. Nephrol. Basel, S. Karger, 1976.

33. Bloom, F.: Pathology of the Dog and Cat. The Genitourinary System With Clinical Considerations. Evanston, IL, American Veterinary Publications, 1954.

34. Jubb, K.V.F., and Kennedy, P.C.: Pathology of Domestic Animals, Vol. 2, 2nd ed. New York, Academic Press, 1970.

35. Wilson, D.R., Ing, T.S., Metcalfe-Gibson, A., and Wrong, O.M.: The chemical composition of feces in uremia, as revealed by in-vivo fecal dialysis. Clin. Sci. 35:197, 1968.

36. Aoyagi, T., Engstrom, G.W., Evans, W.B., and Summerskill, W.H.J.: Gastrointestinal urease in man. Part I. Activity of mucosal urease. Gut 7:631, 1966.

37. Lieber, C.S., and Lefevre, A.: Ammonia as a source of gastric hypoacidity in patients with uremia. J. Clin. Invest. 38:1271, 1959.

38. VonKorff, R.W., Ferguson, D.J., and Glick, D.: Role of urease in the gastric mucosa. III. Plasma urea as source of ammonium ion in gastric juice of histamine-stimulated dogs. Am. J. Physiol. 165:695, 1951.

39. Bounous, G.: Role of pancreatic secretions in uremic gastroenterocolitis. Am. J. Surg. 119:264, 1970.

40. Davenport, H.W.: Destruction of the gastric mucosal barrier by detergents and urea. Gastroenterology 54:175, 1968.

41. Sleisenger, M.H., and Fordtran, J.S.: Gastrointestinal Disease: Pathophysiology, Diagnosis, Management. Philadelphia, W. B. Saunders Co., 1973.

42. McGill, H.C., Geer, J.C., Strong, J.P., and Holman, R.L.: Two forms of necrotizing arteritis in dogs related to diet and renal insufficiency. Arch. Pathol. 65:66, 1958.

43. Orbison, J.L., Christian, C.L., and Peters, E.: Studies on experimental hypertension and cardiovascular disease. Arch. Pathol. 54:185, 1952.

44. Rabiner, S.F.: Uremic bleeding. In Progress in Hemostasis and Thrombosis, Vol. I. Edited by T. Spact. New York, Grune and Stratton, 1971.

45. Eschback, J.W., Harker, L.A., and Dale, D.C.: The Hematological Consequences of Renal Failure. In The Kidney, Vol. II. Edited by B. M. Brenner and F. C. Rector. Philadelphia, W. B. Saunders Co., 1976.

46. Larrain, C., and Langdell, R.D.: The hemostatic defect of uremia. II. Investigation of dogs with experimentally produced acute urinary retention. Blood 11:1067, 1956.

47. Horowitz, H.I.: Uremic toxins and platelet function. Arch. Intern. Med. 126:823, 1970.

48. Osborne, C.A.: Clinical evaluation of needle biopsy of the kidney and its complications in the dog and cat. J. A. V. M. A. 158:1213, 1971.

49. Houck, C.R., Moore, M.W., Ellison, W.B., and Gilmer, R.: Intestinal intussusception in chronic nephrectomized dogs maintained by peritoneal dialysis. Science 119:845, 1954.

50. Kelly, G.E., Drummond, J.M., Rogers, J.H., and Sheil, A.G.R.: Intussusception in dogs following renal homograft transplantation. Aust. Vet. J. 47:597, 1971.

51. Low, D.G., Hiatt, C.W., Gleiser, C.A., and Bergman, E.H.: Experimental canine leptospirosis, I. Leptospira icterohemorrhagiae infections in immature dogs. J. Infect. Dis. 98:249, 1956.

52. Smith, H.A., Jones, T.C., and Hunt, R.D.: Veterinary Pathology, 4th ed. Philadelphia, Lea & Febiger, 1972.

53. Einheber, A., and Carter, D.: The role of the microbial flora in uremia: survival times of germfree, limited flora, and conventionalized rats after bilateral nephrectomy and fasting. J. Exp. Med. 123:239, 1966.

54. Carter, E., Einheber, A., Bauer, H., Rosen, H., and Burns, W.F.: The role of the microbial flora in uremia. II. Uremic colitis, cardiovascular lesions, and biochemical observations. J. Exp. Med. 123:251, 1966.

55. Jaffe, R.H., and Laing, D.R.: Changes of the digestive tract in uremia. A pathologic anatomic study. Arch. Intern. Med. 53:851, 1933.

56. Lee, Y.N.: Urea concentration in intestinal fluids in normal and uremic dogs. J. Surg. Oncol. 3:163, 1971.

57. Brown, C.L., Hill, M.J., and Richards, P.: Bacterial ureases in uremic men. Lancet 2:406, 1971.

58. Wrong, O., Wilson, D.R., Ing, T.S., and Metcalf-Gibson, A.: The metabolism of urea and ammonia in the normal and uremic colon. In Nutrition in Renal Disease. Edited by G. M. Berlyne. Baltimore, The Williams & Wilkins Co., 1969.

59. Swales, J.D., Tange, J.D., and Evans, D.J.: Intestinal ammonia in uremia: the effect of a urease inhibitor, acetohydroxamic acid. Clin. Sci. 42:105, 1972.

60. Bartos, V., Melichar, J., and Erben, J.: The function of the exocrine pancreas in chronic renal failure. Digestion 3:33, 1970.

61. McDermott, F.T., Dalton, M., and Galbraith, A.J.: Ileal epithelial cell migration in acute renal failure. Autoradiographic studies in the mouse. Dig. Dis. 19:1116, 1974.

62. Castrup, H.J., Lohrs, U., and Eder, M.: Zur entstehung der darmschleim haut veranderungen bei uramie. Klin. Wochenschr. 48:244, 1970.

63. Nayman, J.: Effect of wound healing on renal failure in dogs: response to hemodialysis following uremia induced by uranium nitrate. Ann. Surg. 164:227, 1966.

64. Gordon, S.J., Miller. L.J., Haeffner, L.J., Kinsey, M.D., and Kowlessar, O.D.: Abnormal intestinal bile acid distribution in azotemic man: a possible role in the pathogenesis of uremic diarrhea. Gut 17:58, 1976.

65. Osborne, C.A., Hammer, R.F., Resnick, J.S., Stevens, J.B., Yano, B.L., and Vernier, R.L.: Natural remission of nephrotic syndrome in a dog with immune complex glomerular disease. J. A. V. M. A. 168:129, 1976.

66. Osborne, C.A., Hammer, R.F., Stevens, J.B., Resnick, J.S., and Michael, A.F.: The glomerulus in health and disease: a comparative review in domestic animals and man. Adv. Vet. Sci. Comp. Med. 21:207, 1977.

67. Brooks, F.P.: Gastrointestinal Physiology. Edited by F. P. Brooks. New York, Oxford University Press, 1974.

68. De Wolf, W.C., and Fraley, E.E.: Renal pain. Urology 6:403, 1975.

69. Ray, B.S., and Neill, C.L.: Abdominal visceral sensation in man. Ann. Surg. 126:709, 1947.

70. Finco, D.R., and Duncan, J.R.: Evaluation of blood urea nitrogen and serum creatinine concentrations as indicators of renal dysfunction: a study of 111 cases and a review of related literature. J. A. V. M. A. 168:593, 1976.

71. Salt, W.B., and Schenker, S.: Amylase—its clinical significance. A review of the literature. Medicine 55:269, 1976.

72. Wolf, P.L., Williams, D., and Von der Muehll, E.: Practical Clinical Enzymology. New York, John Wiley & Sons, 1973.

73. Finco, D.R., and Stevens, J.B.: Clinical significance of serum amylase activity in the dog. J. A. V. M. A. 155:1686, 1969.

74. Meroney, W.H., Lawson, N.L., Rubini, M.E., and Carbone, J.V.: Some observations of the behavior of amylase in relation to acute renal insufficiency. N. Engl. J. Med. 255:315, 1956.

75. Baggenstoss, A.H.: The pancreas in uremia: a histopathologic study. Am. J. Pathol. 24:1003, 1948.

76. Hiatt, N., and Bonorris, G.: Removal of serum amylase in dogs and the influence of reticuloendothelial blockade. Am. J. Physiol. 210:133, 1966.

77. Brobst, D., Ferguson, A.B., and Carter, J.M.: Evaluation of serum amylase and lipase activity in experimentally induced pancreatitis in the dog. J. A. V. M. A. 157:1697, 1970.

78. Pasternack, A., Kuhlback, B., and Tallgren, L.G.: Serum lipase in acute and chronic nephropathies. Acta Med. Scand. (Suppl.) 412:87, 1964.

79. Sommer, H., Kasper, H., and Fosel, T.: Serum lipase activity in chronic renal failure. Acta Hepatogastroenterol. 22:248, 1975.

80. Tennant, B., Lowe, J.E., and Tasker, J.B.: Hypercalcemia and hypophosphatemia following bilateral nephrectomy in the horse. Fed. Proc. *3*:670, 1974.
81. Berghdahl, L., and Boquist, L.: Secondary hypercalcemic hyperparathyroidism. Virchows Arch. *358*:225, 1973.
82. deTorrente, A., Berl, T., Cohn, P.D., Kawamoto, E., Hertz, P., and Schrier, R.W.: Hypercalcemia of acute renal failure. Clinical significance and pathogenesis. Am. J. Med. *61*:119, 1976.
83. Coburn, J.W., Koppel, M.H., Brickman, A.S., and Massry, S.G.: Study of intestinal absorption of calcium in patients with renal failure. Kidney Int. *3*:264, 1973.
84. Wrong, R.G., Norman, A.W., and Reddy, C.R.: Biologic effects of 1,25-dihydroxycholecalciferol in acutely uremic rats. J. Clin. Invest. *51*:1287, 1972.
85. Brickman, A.S., Coburn, J.W., and Norman, A.W.: Action of 1,25-dihydroxycholecalciferol, a potent kidney-produced metabolite of vitamin D₃, in uremic man. N. Engl. J. Med. *287*:891, 1972.
86. Vergne-Marini, P., Parker, T.F., Pak, C.Y.C., Hull, A.R., DeLuca, H.F., and Fordtran, J.S.: Jejunal and ileal calcium absorption in patients with chronic renal disease: effect of 1∞-hydroxycholecalciferol. J. Clin. Invest. *57*:861, 1976.
87. Balestri, P.L.; Biagini, M., Rindi, P., and Giovanetti, S.: Uremic toxins. Arch. Intern. Med. *126*:843, 1970.
88. Hampers, C.L., Schupak, E., Lowrie, E.G., and Lazarus, J.M.: Long-term Hemodialysis. The Management of the Patient with Chronic Renal Failure. New York, Grune and Stratton, 1973.
89. Reaven, G.M., Weisinger, J.R., and Swenson, R.S.: Insulin and glucose metabolism in renal insufficiency. Kidney Int. (Suppl.) *6*:S–63, 1974.
90. Morton, E.S., Johnson, C., and Lebovitz, H.E.: Carbohydrate metabolism in uremia. Ann. Intern. Med. *68*:63, 1968.
91. Swenson, R.S., Silvers, A., Peterson, D.T., Kohatsu, S., and Reaven, G.M.: Effect of nephrectomy and acute uremia on plasma insulin 125-I removal rate. J. Lab. Clin. Med. *72*:829, 1971.
92. Osborne, C.A.: The transition of quality patient care from an art to a science: the problem oriented concept. J. A. A. H. A. *11*:250, 1975.
93. Osborne, C.A., and Low, D.G.: The Medical History Redefined: Idealism vs. Realism. Sci. Proc. 43rd Annu. Meet. Am. Anim. Hosp. Assoc. South Bend, 1976.
94. Burrows, C.F., and Bovee, K.C.: Metabolic changes due to experimentally induced rupture of the canine urinary bladder. Am. J. Vet. Res. *35*:1083, 1974.

Chapter 30

CONGESTIVE HEART FAILURE AND THE GASTROINTESTINAL SYSTEM

STANLEY G. HARRIS

The principal clinical instance in which spurious signs of gastrointestinal disease may actually arise from the cardiovascular system is when the patient is in congestive heart failure. When cardiovascular drugs are given to treat the failing heart, there may be anorexia, vomiting and/or diarrhea as signs of drug toxicity. These gastrointestinal problems are discussed in terms of how to distinguish the origin of the observed signs, in order that the problem may be correctly localized to the cardiovascular system and treated effectively. The discussion is phrased in terms of the dog but the principles have broad application across species lines.

GASTROINTESTINAL EFFECTS OF CONGESTIVE HEART FAILURE

Gastrointestinal function is dependent to a considerable extent on adequate cardiac function. Inadequate perfusion of the digestive tract first becomes evident in the liver and the intestine. Chronic passive congestion of the liver due to congestive heart failure not only results in hepatomegaly but is also reflected in a reduced rate of venous return through the portal vein, with an increasing tendency toward hypoxia of the intestinal mucosa as heart failure worsens.

Clinical Signs

The early stages of chronic passive congestion of the liver are clinically silent. The subsequent development of hepatomegaly, detectable in the dog at physical examination, may not be accompanied by other clinical evidence of liver disease. If the cardiac signs of heart failure are not detected, one may mistakenly persist in the attempt to diagnose and treat primary liver disease. Thus, one should always rule out primary cardiac disease, a very common cause of hepatomegaly in dogs, as an integral part of the initial workup of hepatomegaly.

The advancing sequence of events within the liver

results in ever-increasing engorgement with blood, distention of the central veins, and compression atrophy of liver cells with fatty degeneration. Affected dogs are not only less active at this point because of heart failure, but also tend to be somewhat depressed and may exhibit anorexia and vomiting. The triad of anorexia, vomiting, and hepatomegaly, being typical of primary or metastatic liver disease, may again mislead the unwary clinician toward liver disease and away from congestive heart failure. Granted that most failing hearts will have a murmur, an arrhythmia, or abnormal sounds at this stage, often with cough due to pulmonary congestion, but the fact remains that the cardiac findings are sometimes less obvious than is the big liver. Furthermore, some clients report the retching cough of the cardiac patient as "vomiting," further tending to mislead the unwary.

Hepatic pain may be present if there is rapid engorgement, leading to stretching of the pain fibers distributed along the vascular tree of the liver. Since there are no pain fibers in the capsule, stretching of the capsule does not produce pain.[1] Palpation of the anterior abdomen may elicit arching of the back, tensing of abdominal muscles, and whimpering.

Continuation of passive congestion leads to necrosis with focal regeneration and fibrous replacement of the hepatocytes. Hepatic function is then compromised to the extent that hepatic cellular destruction has occurred. Icterus may occur due to inability to excrete bile pigments, but is likely to be a very late complication of hepatopathy due to congestive heart failure.

Ascites, a common clinical sign of heart failure, probably results from an increase in postcaval pressure and an increase in the volume of extracellular fluid to accommodate retained sodium ions. These factors together with a limited capacity for lymph drainage cause transudation of the high-protein ascitic fluid in the form of droplets on the surface of the liver, which accumulates in the peritoneal cavity.[2] Protein content of the ascitic fluid formed in congestive heart failure is between 2.5 and 3.5 g/dl.[3]

Gradual weight loss is a common complication of congestive heart failure. Reduction in cardiac output results in decreased splanchnic blood flow which, with congestion of the portal system, leads to decreased intestinal absorption of nutrients and diarrhea.[4] The use of a low sodium diet as adjunct therapy for congestive heart failure may bring about weight loss because these diets, whether prepared commercially or in the client's home, tend to be lacking in palatability. The dog simply reduces its caloric intake. Therapeutic regimes of digitalis and aminophylline often further accelerate weight loss because of appetite suppression.

A decrease in splanchnic circulation due to congestive heart failure may result in edema of the gut and hypoxia, which increases capillary permeability. This is further complicated by declining plasma oncotic pressure as serum albumin values are decreased, thus worsening the edema.

Absorption of nutrients across the gut mucosa is inversely related to the severity of the edema. Patients with severe congestive heart failure may have pre-renal azotemia with signs of vomiting and anorexia.

Laboratory Tests

Blood biochemical tests indicating hepatic damage are qualitatively similar for congestive heart failure and for other hepatic diseases. However, hepatic enzyme values in heart failure (SGPT in the dog and SGOT in cattle) are not likely to be as high as those associated with severe hepatic necrosis due to infection or hepatotoxicosis. The physical examination must be relied upon to detect congestive heart failure, since laboratory tests must be interpreted in the light of physical findings.

Therapy

Conventional therapy for congestive heart failure is necessary when the diagnosis is made since symptomatic therapy for liver and bowel disease is likely to be unrewarding as long as congestive heart failure is unchanged. Dietary management with restricted sodium intake, digitalization, and diuresis are all indicated. Rest enforced by confinement may be beneficial. Hepatic function may be improved with the use of lipotropic factors (choline, methionine and inositol), if fatty change has occurred. Improvement in circulation by cardiac therapy will greatly improve

hepatic and intestinal function, with accompanying diminution of gastrointestinal signs.

GASTROINTESTINAL SIGNS ASSOCIATED WITH CARDIAC THERAPY

Both classes of drugs used in long-term therapy of congestive heart failure, digitalis glycosides and quinidine, may give rise to gastrointestinal signs when given in overdose.

Digitalis Glycosides

Widespread use of digitalis glycosides in cardiac disease often leads to digitalis intoxication, because of the narrow margin between therapeutic and toxic concentrations of the drug in blood. These toxic signs are largely of gastrointestinal origin. Anorexia ensues initially, often followed by nausea, ptyalism, and vomiting. Diarrhea is also often present when a dog or cat is being treated with a cardiac glycoside, and the therapy must be viewed as a possible cause of the gastrointestinal signs.

Formerly it was believed that the digitalis products, digoxin and digitoxin, produced direct irritation of the gastrointestinal tract, thereby leading to vomiting and diarrhea. However, parenteral administration of the drug will produce the same gastrointestinal signs; therefore factors other than direct irritation are operative. Reflex or direct central activation of the vomiting mechanism appears to explain the vomiting. Studies have shown that excitation of the chemoreceptor trigger zone by digitalis glycosides will induce vomiting.[5] Ptyalism or nausea should not be overlooked as signs of toxicity in dogs receiving digitalis.

The usual management of digitalis intoxication is temporary cessation of drug therapy. Severe long-term intoxication may require intestinal protectants to aid in control of diarrhea. Patients losing potassium may need supplementation with this electrolyte to treat or forestall hypokalemia. Antiarrhythmic therapy may be necessary if arrhythmias or numerous extrasystoles are present.

Antiarrhythmic Drugs

Quinidine and quinidine-like drugs produce gastrointestinal signs when toxic amounts are given. These include nausea, vomiting, abdominal pain, and diarrhea. Local irritation of the gastrointestinal tract by the drug is thought to produce the signs; however a central basis for the signs has also been shown.[6] Cessation of therapy will generally correct the signs within a day or two.

REFERENCES

1. Durant, T.M.: The interrelationship of cardiac and gastrointestinal disorders. *In* Gastroenterology, Vol. 4, 3rd ed. Edited by H. L. Bockus. Philadelphia, W. B. Saunders Co., 1976.
2. Brachfeld, N., and Ladue, J.S.: Congestive heart failure, coronary insufficiency, and myocardial infarction. *In* Pathologic Physiology, 4th ed. Edited by W. A. Sodeman and W. A. Sodeman, Jr. Philadelphia, W. B. Saunders Co., 1967.
3. Moore, W.E.: Personal communication, 1978.
4. Walters, M.B.: Relationships between the gastrointestinal and cardiovascular systems. *In* Gastroenterology. Edited by A. Bogoch. New York, McGraw-Hill Book Co., 1973.
5. Moe, S.K. and Farch, A.E.: Digitalis and allied cardiac glycosides. *In* The Pharmacological Basis of Therapeutics, 5th ed. Edited by L. E. Goodman and A. Gilman, New York, Macmillan Publishing Co., 1975.
6. Rollo, I.M.: Drugs used in the chemotherapy of malaria. *In* The Pharmacological Basis of Therapeutics, 5th ed. Edited by L. E. Goodman and A. Gilman, New York, Macmillan Publishing Co., 1975.

SOURCES OF ENDOSCOPY INSTRUMENTS

PHARYNGOSCOPY IN HORSES
1. American Cystoscope Makers, Inc.
   300 Stillwater Avenue
   Stamford, CT   06902
2. Olympus Corporation of America
   4 Nevada Drive
   New Hyde Park, NY   11042
3. American Optical
   Southbridge, MA   01550
   Distributed by:
   Western Serum Co., Inc.
   2318 S. Industrial Park Drive
   Tempe AZ   85282

ESOPHAGOSCOPY IN SMALL ANIMALS
1. American Cystoscope Makers, Inc.
   300 Stillwater Avenue
   Stamford, CT   06902
2. Olympus Corporation of America
   4 Nevada Drive
   New Hyde Park, NY   11042
3. George B. Pilling & Son Co.
   Delaware Drive
   Fort Washington, PA   19034
4. Electrosurgical Instrument Co.
   250 N. Goodman St.
   Rochester, NY   14607

GASTROSCOPY AND DUODENOSCOPY IN SMALL ANIMALS
1. Olympus Corporation of America
   4 Nevada Drive
   New Hyde Park, NY   11042
2. American Cystoscope Makers, Inc.
   300 Stillwater Avenue
   Stamford, CT   06902

LAPAROSCOPY IN SMALL ANIMALS
1. Dyonics
   Woburn, MA   01801

2. American Cystoscope Makers, Inc.
   300 Stillwater Avenue
   Stamford, CT   06902
3. Richard Wolf Medical Instrument Corp.
   7046 Lyndon Avenue
   Rosemont, IL   60018
4. Karl Storz Endoscopy—America Inc.
   658 South San Vicente Blvd
   Los Angeles, CA   90048
5. Olympus Corporation of America
   4 Nevada Drive
   New Hyde Park, NY   11042
6. Eder Instrument Co., Inc.
   5115 N. Ravenswood Avenue
   Chicago, IL   60640

COLONOSCOPY IN SMALL ANIMALS
1. Olympus Corporation of America
   4 Nevada Drive
   New Hyde Park, NY   11042
2. American Cystoscope Makers, Inc.
   300 Stillwater Avenue
   Stamford, CT   06902
3. Electrosurgical Instrument Co.
   250 N. Goodman St.
   Rochester, NY   14607
4. American Optical
   Southbridge, MA   01550
   Distributed by:
   Western Serum Co., Inc.
   2318 S. Industrial Park Drive
   Tempe AZ   85282

BIOPSY INSTRUMENTS
1. Tru-Cut needle—Abdominal Organs
2. Quinton Instruments—Esophagus, stomach, colon
   2121 Terry Avenue
   Seattle, WA   98121

INDEX